Orthopaedic Physical Therapy

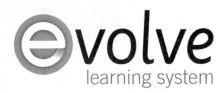
learning system

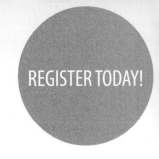

To access your Student Resources, visit:

http://evolve.elsevier.com/Donatelli/OrthopaedicPT/

Evolve Free Resources:

Instructor only

- **Electronic image collection**

Student and Instructor

- **Video clips showing exercises relevant to book content**
- **Reference lists with Medline links**

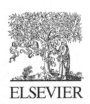
ELSEVIER

Orthopaedic Physical Therapy

FOURTH EDITION

Robert A. Donatelli
PhD, PT, OCS

Director of Sports Rehabilitation and
Outreach Programs
Physiotherapy Associates
Las Vegas, Nevada

Michael J. Wooden
MS, PT, OCS

Physiotherapy Associates
Decatur, Georgia
Continuing Education Coordinator
Physiotherapy Associates
Eaton, Pennsylvania
Instructor
Division of Physical Therapy
Department of Rehabilitation Medicine
Emory University
Atlanta, Georgia

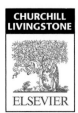

CHURCHILL
LIVINGSTONE

ELSEVIER

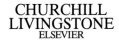

11830 Westline Industrial Drive
St. Louis, Missouri 63146

ORTHOPAEDIC PHYSICAL THERAPY, FOURTH EDITION   ISBN 978-0-443-06942-0

Library of Congress Control Number 2009930550

Vice President and Publisher: Linda Duncan
Executive Editor: Kathy Falk
Developmental Editor: Megan Fennell
Publishing Services Manager: Catherine A. Jackson
Senior Project Manager: Karen M. Rehwinkel
Design Direction: Amy Buxton

Printed in the United States of America

Last digit is the print number: 9 8 7 6 5 4 3 2 1

Contributors

Kenneth H. Akizuki, MD
Attending Physician
Sportsmed Orthopaedic Group, Inc.
San Francisco, California
Attending Physician
San Francisco Orthopaedic Residency Program
St. Mary's Medical Center
San Francisco, California

Carla Bader-Henderson, ORT/L, CHT
Hand Therapist
Stockbridge, Georgia

David S. Bailie, MD
Orthopaedic Surgeon
The Orthopaedic Clinic Association, PC (TOCA)
Scottsdale, Arizona

Charlie Baycroft, MD
Medical Director
Foot Science International
Christchurch, New Zealand

Turner A. Blackburn Jr., MEd, PT, ATC
Vice President Corporate Development
Clemson Sports Medicine and Rehabilitation
Manchester, Georgia
Adjunct Assistant Professor
University of St. Augustine for Health Sciences
St. Augustine, Florida

William G. Boissonnault, PT, DHSc, FAAOMPT
Assistant Professor
University of Wisconsin–Madison
Program in Physical Therapy
Madison, Wisconsin

Jean M. Bryan, PhD, MPT, OCS
Professor
U.S. Army–Baylor University Graduate Program in Physical
    Therapy
San Antonio, Texas

William Jay Bryan, MD
Professor
Department of Physical Therapy
Texas Woman's University
Surgeon
The Methodist Hospital
Houston, Texas

Kenji Carp, PT, OCS, ATC
Competency Certified Vestibular Therapist
Clinic Director
Physiotherapy Associates
Eugene, Oregon

Allen Carpenter, PT, Cert MDT
Clinic Director
Physiotherapy Associates
San Francisco, California

Chad Cook, PT, PhD, MBA, OCS, FAAOMPT
Associate Professor
Division of Physical Therapy
Department of Community and Family Medicine
Division of Experimental Surgery
Department of Surgery
Duke University
Durham, North Carolina

Lori DeMott, OTR/L,CHT
Hand ReHab
Program Coordinator
OhioHealth Physical Rehabilitation
Columbus, Ohio

Donn Dimond, PT, OCS
Physical Therapist
Physical Therapy Associates
Beaverton, Oregon

Sarah DoBroka, BS, PT, SCS
OrthoCarolina
Huntersville, North Carolina

Richard Ekstrom, PT, DSc, OCS
Associate Professor
Department of Physical Therapy
University of South Dakota
Vermillion, South Dakota

Todd S. Ellenbecker, DPT, MS, SCS, OCS, CSCS
Clinic Director
Physiotherapy Associates
Scottsdale Sports Clinic
National Director of Clinical Research
Physiotherapy Associates
Director of Sports Medicine—ATP Tour
Scottsdale, Arizona

Robert L. Elvey, BAppSc, Grad. Dip. Manip. Ther.
Senior Lecturer
Curkin University
Physiotherapy Consultant
Southcare Physiotherapy
Perth, Australia

Mary L. Engles, MS, PT, OCS, MTC
Private Practice
Sports Arena Physical Therapy
San Diego, California

William B. Farquhar, PhD
Associate Professor
Department of Health, Nutrition, and Exercise Sciences
University of Delaware
Newark, Delaware

Sharon Flinn, PhD, OTR/L, CHT, CVE
Assistant Professor
The Ohio State University
School of Allied Medical Professions
Division of Occupational Therapy
Columbus, Ohio

David Friedberg, MS, FACS
Austin, Texas

Linda Naomi Futamura, MS, PT
Physical Therapist
Physiotherapy Associates
Redwood City, California

Lisa M. Giannone, PT
Owner/Director
Active Care Physical Therapy and Sports Medicine Fitness Center
San Francisco, California

Joseph Godges, PT, DPT, MA, OCS
Assistant Professor
Department of Physical Therapy
Loma Linda University
Los Angeles, California

Bruce Greenfield, PT, PhD, OCS
Assistant Professor
Division of Physical Therapy
Department of Rehabilitation Medicine
Emory University School of Medicine
Atlanta, Georgia

Toby M. Hall, MSc, FACP
Specialist, Musculoskeletal Physiotherapist
Adjunct Senior Teaching Fellow
Curtin University
Perth, Australia
Visiting Lecturer
Trinity College
University of Dublin
Dublin, Ireland
Senior Teaching Fellow
University of Western Australia
Director Manual Concepts
Booragoon, Australia

Matt Holland, PT
Manager, Sports Rehabilitation
Methodist Sports Rehabilitation
The Methodist Hospital
Houston, Texas

Wendy J. Hurd, PT, PhD, SCS
Graduate Program in Biomechanics and Movement Science
University of Delaware
Newark, Delaware

†Scot Irwin, DPT, MA
Director
North Georgia Physical Therapy Practice
Dahlonega, Georgia

Frank W. Jobe, MD
Medical Director
Biomechanics Laboratory
Centinela Hospital Medical Center
Inglewood, California

---

†Deceased.

Marie A. Johanson, PT, PhD, OCS
Assistant Professor
Division of Physical Therapy
Department of Rehabilitation Medicine
Emory University School of Medicine
Atlanta, Georgia

Carrie Johnson, MPT
Physical Therapist
Seattle Sports
Seattle, Washington

Gregory S. Johnson, BS, PT
Associate Instructor
Physical Therapy Schools
University of St. Augustine
St. Augustine, Florida
Touro College
Long Island, New York
Codirector
Institute of Physical Art Continuing Education Institute
Steamboat Springs, Colorado

Victor Katch, MS, EdD
Professor of Movement Science
School of Kinesiology
Associate Professor of Pediatrics
Section of Pediatric Cardiology
School of Medicine
University of Michigan
Ann Arbor, Michigan

Steven L. Kraus, PT, OCS, MTC
Clinical Assistant Professor
Division of Physical Therapy
Department of Rehabilitation Medicine
Emory University School of Medicine
Atlanta, Georgia

Dianna Cole McNitt, PT
Facility Director
Physiotherapy Associates at the Littleton YMCA
Littleton, Colorado

Heather Moore, MPT, DPT
Director of Physical Therapy
Mishock Physical Therapy
Skippack, Pennsylvania

Scott Moorhead
Researcher
Department of Orthopedics
The Methodist Hospital
Houston, Texas

Caroline Nichols, PT, OCS, MTC, CSCS
Physical Therapist
Ladies Professional Golf Association
Daytona Beach, Florida

Lawrence M. Oloff, DPM
Surgeon
Foot and Ankle Surgery/Podiatry
Sports Orthopedic and Rehabilitation
Redwood City, California

Roy W. Osborn, PT, DPT, MS, OCS
Associate Professor
Department of Physical Therapy
The University of South Dakota

Grant D. Padley, DO
Orthopedic Surgeon
Valley Orthopedics
Goodyear, Arizona

Monique Ronayne Peterson, PT, OCT
Clinic Director
Physiotherapy Associates
Huntington Beach, California

Robert M. Poole, PT, MEd, ATC
Corporate Director
Human Performance and Rehabilitation Center
Atlanta, Georgia

Brian L. Shafer, MD
Sports Medicine
Arizona Bone and Joint Specialists
Scottsdale, Arizona

Lynn Snyder-Mackler, PT, ScD, FAPTA
Alumni Distinguished Professor
Department of Physical Therapy
Academic Director
Graduate Program in Biomechanics and Movement Science
University of Delaware
Newark, Delaware

†Robert B. Sprague, PT, PhD, GDAMT
Faculty
Maitland-Australian Physiotherapy Seminars
Cutchogue, New York

Thomas A. St. John, MD
Spine Surgeon
Orthopaedic Associates of Aspen & Glenwood
Aspen, Colorado

---

†Deceased.

Steven A. Stratton, PhD, PT, ATC
Clinical Associate Professor
University Health Science Center of San Antonio
School of Medicine
Physical Medicine and Rehabilitation Residency Program
San Antonio, Texas

Robert W. Sydenham, BSc, Dip. PT, MCPA, MAPTA, RPT, FCAMT
Fellow
The Canadian Academy of Orthopaedic Manipulative
   Therapists
Director
URSA Foundation
Edmonds, Washington
Clinical Director
Lifemark Health Facility
Edmonton, Canada

Megan M. Wenner, MS, ATC
Doctoral Candidate
University of Delaware
Newark, Delaware

Robbin Wickham-Bruno, PhD, PT
Physical Therapist
The Therapy Connection
Indianapolis, Indiana

Joseph S. Wilkes, MD
Clinical Associate Professor
Orthopaedics
Emory University
Active Staff Member
Piedmont Hospital
Specialty Consulting
Crawford Long Hospital
Atlanta, Georgia
Active Staff Member
Fayette Community Hospital
Fayetteville, Georgia

Steven B. Zelicof, MD, PhD
Associate Professor of Clinical Orthopaedic Surgery
New York Medical College
Valhalla, New York
Adjunct Clinical Assistant Professor of Orthopaedic Surgery
Weill Medical College of Cornell University
New York, New York
Assistant Professor of Medicine
New York Medical College
Valhalla, New York

My beautiful wife, Georgi, and my angels from God, Robby and Briana.
R.A.D.

To Bob Sprague: friend, mentor, colleague.
M.J.W.

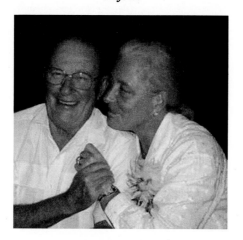

**Robert B. Sprague
PT, PhD, GDAMT**

June 30, 1929 – March 21, 2009

Preface

We are pleased and proud to present the fourth edition of *Orthopaedic Physical Therapy*. We have expanded and updated this volume to meet our goal as set forth in previous editions: to present the current state of orthopaedic physical therapy practice as it has been influenced by research, advanced education, and specialization. The book is written for the physical therapy student, the general physical therapy practitioner, and the physical therapist specializing in orthopaedics. It will also be a valuable reference for allopathic and osteopathic physicians, podiatrists, and non-medical practitioners who treat orthopaedic dysfunction. A new and exciting update to the fourth edition is the Evolve website that will allow the reader to download all of the figures in the book and have access to videos of exercises and special tests. Furthermore, the website will have all references from the book with links to Medline.

As before, this edition is divided into four main sections. The first section, Fundamental Principles, discusses the responses of the body tissues and systems to trauma, immobilization, and movement, and builds the foundation for safe and effective treatment.

The Upper Quarter and Lower Quarter sections emphasize treatment of the individual, not just the site of the dysfunction. Because dysfunction syndromes often develop as a result of abnormal posture or movement patterns, the entire region must be evaluated. Within each of these sections, the relationships and interdependence of anatomy, mechanics, and kinesiology are discussed. We are excited about the new chapters and authors we have added to the fourth edition. In the Upper Quarter section we have added a new chapter entitled "Strength Training Concepts in the Orthopaedic Patient". This chapter, written by Donn Dimond—an author new to the fourth edition—reviews the most up-to-date literature on the clinical concepts in strength training and the muscle physiological data on how muscle adapts to strength training.

In addition, Drs. William Boissonault and Joseph Godges have added a very valuable chapter on symptom investigation. This chapter has pertinent information regarding the assessment of pain and how to distinguish soft tissue dysfunction from disease. One of our most renowned authors, Dr. Frank Jobe, has contributed a chapter on surgery and rehabilitation of the elbow. Dr. Brian Shafer and Dr. Todd Ellenbecker, an experienced author and lecturer in our field, contributed to Dr. Jobe's chapter. Dr. Ellenbecker also co-authored with Dr. David S. Bailie a new chapter on arthroscopic surgery and rehabilitation of the shoulder. To complete the Upper Quarter we have two new authors, Sharon Flinn and Lori Demott, for the Dysfunction, Evaluation, and Treatment of the Wrist and Hand chapter.

The section on the Lower Quarter has a host of new authors and chapters. We have added Wendy Hurd and Dr. Lynn Snyder-Mackler, who produced an excellent chapter on neuromuscular rehabilitation. Another renowned author—Victor Katch—has added a new chapter called The Lumbopelvic System: Anatomy, Physiology, Motor Control, Instability, and Description of a Unique Treatment Modality. Another new author from Aspen Colorado, Dr. Thomas St. John, has added a chapter entitled Advances in Lumbar Spine Surgery. Dianna Cole-McNitt has written a very comprehensive chapter entitled Evaluation, Diagnosis, and Treatment of the Lumbar-Pelvic-Hip Complex. To complement Dianna's chapter, we were fortunate to get Dr. Steve Zelicof and Dr. David Friedburg to write a new chapter on the surgical treatment of the hip complex. Dr. Charlie Baycroft and Monique Peterson updated the chapter on the overview of foot orthotics and prescriptions.

In the Special Considerations section, Kenji Carp contributed a chapter on state-of-the-art somatosensory, vestibular, and visual sensory integration addressing implications for neuromuscular control and balance in orthopaedic practice. New author Allen Carpenter did an excellent job on Normal and Abnormal Mechanics of the Foot and Ankle, which includes information on running mechanics, the connection of the hip to the foot anatomically, and clinical applications.

The expertise of so many people behind the scenes has contributed to this book's production. We are grateful to Kathy

Falk for backing us all the way on this project, to Megan Fennell for keeping our shoulders to the wheel, and to Karen Rehwinkel for the finishing touches.

We have many people to thank. We are indebted, of course, to our contributors for their thorough, insightful, and timely chapters. Because of their efforts we are confident this book will greatly enhance patient care. And we are grateful to our co-workers, colleagues, mentors, and students who have taught us so much and inspired us through four editions.

Finally, we thank our wonderful families, whose love, patience, and encouragement are our greatest motivations.

Robert A. Donatelli
Michael J. Wooden

Contents

Orthopaedic Physical Therapy

CHAPTER

1

Heather Moore,
Caroline Nichols,
and Mary L. Engles

Tissue Response

For a rehabilitation specialist, it is important to know the responses of tissues found throughout the body. It is important to understand not only how they naturally exist, but also how they respond when mechanical loads are applied or trauma occurs, how they heal, and finally how they respond to interventions. Four main classes of tissues are present in the body: (1) muscle, (2) connective tissue (which has subclasses of connective tissue proper, bone, cartilage, and blood), (3) nerve, and (4) epithelium. Epithelium is not discussed in this chapter, as it is best left to other specialists.

Normal Tissue

MUSCLE

Macroscopic Muscle Structure

Muscles are attached to bone via tendons, which comprise densely packed connective tissue. Tendons, similar to muscles, are divided into fibrils, fibers, fiber bundles, and fascicles. However, the tendon functions as a whole to withstand high tensile forces.[1] A tendon consists of 55% to 70% water.[1] In all, 60 to 85% of the dry weight of the tendon is composed of collagen.[1]

Two layers of connective tissue cover the muscle: a thick outer layer called *fascia,* and a thin inner layer called the *epimysium.* Lying underneath the epimysium are bundles of tissue called the *fasciculi.* Each fasciculus is covered by a connective tissue layer call the *perimysium.* The fasciculi then are broken down into cells called *muscle fibers.* Again, a layer of connective tissue called the *endomysium* surrounds each of these muscle fibers. The three layers of connective tissue—epimysium, perimysium, and endomysium—play an important part in contraction of the muscle and provide access for blood vessels and nerves to reach the interior of the muscle.

Microscopic Muscle Structure

A microscopic look into a muscle begins with a view of the muscle fibers. Muscle fibers, which are the building blocks of muscle, have many different unique features. Muscle fibers are long, cylindrical cells that range from 10 to 100 μm in diameter and from 1 to 400 mm in length (Figure 1-1).[2] The diameter of muscle fibers is an important piece of information in that it will help one to determine muscle fiber strength. Type I fibers, the slow twitch fibers, have a smaller diameter and therefore have lower force output than Type II fibers.[3]

Sarcomeres, which are contained within the myofibril, make skeletal muscle contraction possible. Contained within the sarcomere are thick and thin myofilaments. The thick filaments are composed of myosin. The thin filaments are composed of actin, troponin, and tropomyosin. The sarcomere is divided into different bands: the dark A band and the light I band. The light and dark description comes from the appearance of the bands when viewed under a microscope. The A band, which consists mostly of myosin, is broad and contains both thick and thin filaments. The thin filaments are the anchors to the A band, and the thick filaments span the entire width. The I band, which contains just thin filaments, consists mostly of actin and anchors the A bands. The Z disc runs the entire length of a sarcomere and is a thick line seen in the middle of the I band. This is where the thin filaments are adjoined to the sarcomeres. Found in the middle of the A band is the H zone, which is visible only when the sarcomere is resting. It appears lighter than the A band because it is devoid of any actin filaments. When a contraction takes place, the actin filaments slide into this zone, causing it to look like the A band.

Surrounding each muscle fiber is a polarized plasma membrane, the sarcolemma, which fuses with the tendon and receives input from the nervous system. The sarcolemma contains sarcoplasm, which is a gel-like substance that consists of organelles, glycogen, fats, proteins, and minerals, and provides the medium for enzymatic reactions. It is comparable to the

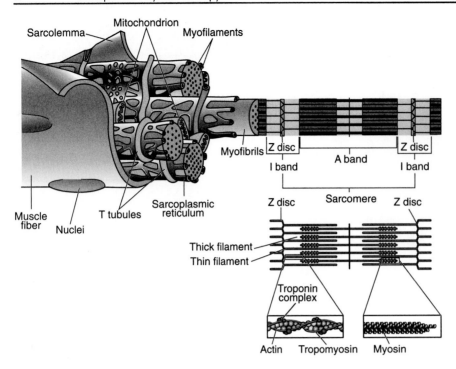

Figure 1-1 Organization of a muscle fiber. (From Donatelli R: Sports-specific rehabilitation. St. Louis, 2007, Churchill Livingstone.)

cytoplasm in cells but differs in the fact that it contains stored glycogen and myoglobin, an oxygen-binding compound.

Contained within the cytoplasm is a network of transverse tubules, T tubules, which pass through the muscle fiber. They are so named because of their perpendicular orientation to the cell. T tubules connect the sarcolemma to the sarcoplasmic reticulum; this junction is called a *triad*. T tubules are responsible for the spread of polarization on the inside of the cell, which triggers the sarcoplasmic reticulum to release calcium. The sarcoplasmic reticulum is a longitudinal network of tubules that run parallel to the myofibrils and are responsible for storing and releasing calcium.

The final microscopic structure to be discussed is the satellite cell. Although these cells play no important role in the contraction of skeletal muscle, they do have a significant role in remodeling and repair of skeletal muscle, which is discussed later in the chapter. The satellite cell is located between the basil lamina and the sarcolemma. The main purposes of satellite cells are to repair, revitalize, and mediate skeletal muscle tissue growth by differentiating into myocytes.[4] These cells become active only when injury to the skeletal muscle occurs. Upon injury, these cells multiply and are drawn to the injured site, where they fuse with the damaged area, donating their nuclei to the muscle fiber and helping in its regeneration. This process does not increase the number of muscle fibers but rather it increases the amounts of myosin and actin that are present. This proliferation of satellite cells can last up to 48 hours after the insult. Muscle fiber type determines the number of satellite cells present. In Type I fibers, satellite cell content is five to six times greater than in Type II fibers.[5] This can be attributed to increased quantities of blood and capillaries in the Type I fibers.[5]

It should be noted that most recent literature suggests that satellite cells do not all function in the same way.[6] Two populations of stem cells have been identified: those that are committed progenitor cells, which will become muscle cells and have a limited life span, and satellite stem cells, which are able to repopulate the satellite niche and self-renew.[6]

Muscle Architecture

Muscle architecture, or fiber orientation, plays a large part in determination of muscle function. An understanding of the direction and arrangement of fibers is imperative when one is designing a rehabilitation program. Muscle architecture functionality can be summarized in two statements: (1) muscle force is proportional to the physiologic cross-sectional area, and (2) muscle velocity is proportional to muscle fiber length.[7] Several types of muscle architecture are known: parallel, unipennate, and multipennate. Each arrangement is named for its direction in relation to the muscle's force-generating axis. Parallel fibers are arranged in a parallel fashion, for example, in the bicep muscle. Unipennate muscles are oriented in a single angle to force-axis, for example, the vastus lateralis muscle. The final category, multipennate muscles, is the one into which most muscles fall because of the fact that they are oriented at all different angles to the force production axis, similar to the gluteus medius. According to a study by Kawakami et al, increases in fiber angle may improve the force-generating capability of a muscle by allowing a greater number of attachment sites to attach to a given tendon.[8]

Muscle Fiber Type

A discussion of muscle structure without mention of muscle fiber type would be incomplete. However, only a short overview will be presented here, as this will be discussed in much greater depth in Chapter 3. Two main classifications of muscle fibers are known: type I and type II. Type I fibers are also termed slow oxidative, or slow twitch, fibers. These fibers are resistant to fatigue and have low peak forces. They exhibit high levels of oxidative enzyme activity and low levels of glycolytic enzyme activity. Muscles responsible for sustained posture activities are predominantly Type I. Type II fibers are broken into Type IIa and Type IIb. Type IIa are also called *fast oxidative glycolytic* fibers. These fibers have higher force production and are relatively fatigue resistant. Finally, Type IIb or fast glycolytic fibers can produce the maximum amount of force but only for a few contractions, as they fatigue quickly. Many factors determine the percentage of each fiber type that is present. In a study by Larsson, subjects in the 20- to 29-year-old age group had 39% Type I muscle fibers, and the 60- to 65-year-old age group had 66% Type I fibers.[9] However, this study was performed on sedentary men so is just an example of variant percentages within a given population. Again, the rehabilitation specialist's understanding of these different types of fibers is essential for the rehabilitation of patients.

Muscle Contraction

Proteins

Eleven proteins are contained within the myofibril complex and are necessary for the contraction of skeletal muscle. The first protein is myosin. It composes the thick filaments of the sarcomere. Each myosin strand contains several myosin heads. These heads are discussed further later in the chapter, when the sliding filament theory is discussed. Titin, which is a longitudinal filament, stabilizes myosin filaments on the longitudinal axis. Because of its elastic properties, titin, along with nebulin, another protein, may play a significant part in the contraction of muscle by maintaining the relationship between myosin, actin, and Z-lines throughout the contraction cycle. Wang has stated that titin and nebulin also aid in the sliding of actin and myosin during contraction of skeletal muscle.[10]

Two types of actin proteins are known: F-actin, or fibrous actin, and G-actin, or globular actin. Two F-actin strands coil together to form a single strand of actin. Along with the actin in the thin filaments, troponin and tropomyosin are present. Tropomyosin is an inhibitory protein that is found at intervals within the actin. Its action is to inhibit the active binding of actin, restricting actin and myosin activity during resting conditions. Three subunits of troponin have been identified: troponin C (Tn-C), troponin I (Tn-I), and troponin T (Tn-T). Tn-I is an inhibitory protein that blocks the actin-myosin binding site when at rest. Tn-C is a binding site for calcium. The binding of calcium to this site is necessary for muscle contraction. Finally, Tn-T binds troponin to tropomyosin.

The M-protein found on the M-line of the sarcomere is responsible for maintaining the structure and stability of the sarcomere. Another protein responsible for the structure and stability of the sarcomere is alpha-actinin. All of these proteins play an important part in muscle contraction and the sliding filament theory.

Excitation-Contraction Coupling

During the relaxed muscle state, myosin heads are vertical, and adenosine diphosphate and an inorganic phosphate molecule (ADP + Pi) are bound to the head. At this point, intracellular calcium is low. When an action potential (AP) is generated, it reaches the sarcolemma and spreads down the T tubules to the sarcoplasmic reticulum. This is termed *excitation-contraction coupling,* when depolarization reaches the muscle fiber. This depolarization spreads to the sarcoplasmic reticulum and causes the release of calcium from the lateral sacs of the sarcoplasmic reticulum, allowing for an increase in intracellular calcium. This increased intracellular calcium binds to troponin. The binding of calcium causes configuration changes to the calcium-troponin complex. This change also affects tropomyosin, which allows the opening of the actin-binding site. After these changes have occurred, the cross-bridge cycle begins.

The first step in the cross-bridge cycle occurs when the myosin heads bind to the actin site, which represents the formation of the cross-bridge. It is during the next step, the power stroke, that the actual contraction occurs. The myosin head swivels, which begins the sliding of the filaments. The thin filaments slide over the thick filaments toward the center of the sarcomere. The third step is the dissociation of actin and myosin. This happens when adenosine triphosphate (ATP) attaches to the myosin head. The final step is the breakdown of ATP. This breakdown allows the myosin heads to have energy to move the actin during the power stroke. This movement of the actin causes shortening of the sarcomeres, which results in muscle contraction. The cross-bridge cycle continues as long as intracellular calcium and ATP are present. Once AP is no longer being received, the extra calcium is pumped back into the sarcoplasmic reticulum, and the muscle rests. This process is discussed in greater detail in Chapter 3.

Types of Muscle Contraction

Three different types of muscle contraction have been observed: concentric, eccentric, and isometric. Understanding each of these contractions and their implications is imperative when one is designing a rehabilitation program.

An *eccentric contraction* is defined as lengthening of a contracting muscle by an external load (Figure 1-2). For example, during a bicep curl, the curl up would be a concentric contraction, and the lowering of weight would be the eccentric contraction. Throughout everyday life, periods that combine concentric and eccentric actions occur constantly; this phenomenon is referred to as the stretch-shorten cycle.[11]

Eccentric contractions produce the greatest force for skeletal muscle. They can produce two to three times the force that a concentric contraction can produce, and it is imperative to note this fact when one is designing a rehabilitation program. For example, following a rotator cuff repair, having the patient actively lower his arm could cause the tendon to rupture. That is why cuff repairs start with isometric strengthening. However, training eccentrics is an important part of the rehabilitation process when introduced at the appropriate stage. For example,

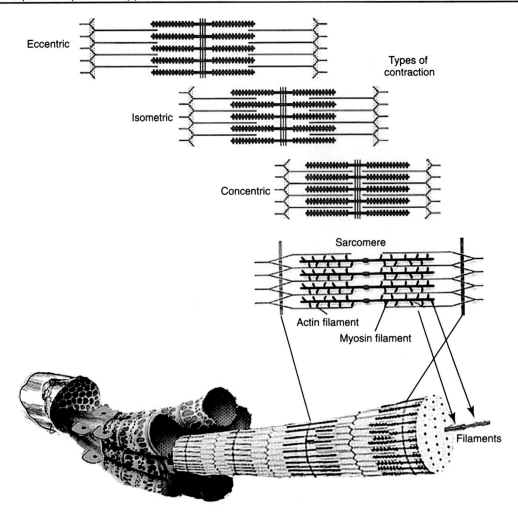

Figure 1-2 Types of muscle contraction. (From Huard J, Yong L, Fu F: Muscle injuries and repair: current trends in research, J Bone Joint Surg Am 84: 822-832, 2002.)

with training deceleration, eccentric training is a required part of the program.

Eccentric contractions cause muscle soreness 24 to 48 hours after exercise, which has been called *DOMS*, or *delayed-onset muscle soreness*. This occurs as the result of muscle swelling caused by damage to the muscle and a shift in the optimum length of the muscle to a longer length.[12] However, performing bouts of eccentric exercises through an adaptation called *the repeated bout effect* can prevent this damage.[13] Eccentric training can reduce injury and improve performance.[2]

With eccentric contraction, use of the word *contraction* can be a little confusing. *Contraction* by definition is the shortening of muscle, but when eccentric activity is discussed, this term actually refers to the lengthening of muscle. The American College of Sports Medicine still recommends use of the term *contraction* when eccentric activity is discussed because of its wide acceptance and nonspecific meaning.[14]

With a *concentric contraction,* the muscle produces a force that is greater than the external load, causing the muscle to shorten.[12] This second part of the stretch-shorten cycle occurs from day to day without specialized training.[12] When the stretch-shorten cycle occurs, it is almost impossible for only a concentric con-

traction to take place—a fact that is important to note when one is guiding rehabilitation of postsurgical patients.

Finally, an *isometric contraction* occurs when external force equals the force that the muscle is producing. These types of exercises are beneficial when one is treating the patient with low back pain. According to McGill, isometric contractions allow for continuous activation of the paraspinal muscles, but at a low load.[15] For example, in a study by Danneels et al, investigators found that static activation of the multifidus muscle produced greater hypertrophy and cross-sectional area then did general stabilization exercises and dynamic intensive lumbar resistance training.[16]

Sensory Feedback

Muscle has several components that provide sensory feedback. Sensory feedback from muscles forms the basis of proprioception, which is the detection of joint position. This joint position sense allows the body to maintain stability throughout static and dynamic positions, which is critical in the training and rehabilitation of all populations, especially athletes. Each of the different receptors discussed here provides different information. The muscle spindles provide information pertaining to position and velocity, whereas the Golgi tendon apparatus provides information regarding force.

Thus far, general reference has been made to muscle fibers. However, two types of muscle fibers are evident: intrafusal and extrafusal. Those discussed so far are the extrafusal muscle fibers, which are activated by alpha efferent motor neurons. Found deep within the muscles are the sensory specialization units of muscle tissue, called *muscle spindles.* Muscle spindles are noncontractile and are wrapped in two different afferent endings: Type I, or primary fibers, and Type II, secondary. Type I fibers are broken down further into Types Ia and Ib. Contained within these fluid-filled connective tissue capsules are the intrafusal muscle fibers, which are innervated by efferent nerves called *gamma motor neurons.* The muscle fibers react when muscle is stretched, allowing the number of action potentials to increase. This then causes the muscle to contract, which reduces tension on the muscle spindle, allowing the number of action potentials to decrease.

The Golgi tendon organ composed of type Ib fibers is another sensory feedback component. It consists of only afferent fibers but also responds to stretch. When too much force is placed on a muscle, the inverse myotatic reflex, which is mediated by the Golgi tendon organ, is initiated. This reflex causes the muscle to relax via an inhibitory neuron, which decreases the firing of motor neurons and allows constant force to be maintained. This phenomenon is often seen in bodybuilding; as a weightlifter lifts too much weight, he or she drops the weight when the Golgi tendon signals relaxation of the muscle.

Innervation

In general, muscles are innervated by efferent or motor neurons. These motor neurons leave the ventral root of the spinal cord and branch several times before synapsing with muscle fibers. Each motor neuron includes an axon that may attach to one or more muscle fibers. The collective group of muscle fibers innervated by an axon is called the *motor unit.* Motor units that contain a large number of fibers per unit, for example, the gluteus maximus, are used for gross motor skills, whereas fine motor skills are associated with many motor units.

Connective Tissue

Connective tissue is found nearly everywhere in the body and has many forms and functions. The major functions of connective tissue include (1) binding and support, (2) protection, (3) insulation, and (4) transportation of substances within the body.[17] Its main subclasses are connective tissue proper, cartilage, bone, and blood. Bone, blood, and cartilage usually are considered connective tissue, but because they differ so substantially from the other tissues in this class, the term *connective tissue proper* is commonly used to exclude those three. Connective tissue proper can be subdivided further into areolar (or loose) connective tissue and dense connective tissue (or, less commonly, fibrous connective tissue). Loose connective tissue consists of areolar, adipose, and reticular connective tissue. Dense connective tissue can be divided further into dense regular and dense irregular connective tissue. It forms ligaments and tendons. Three main types of cartilage have been identified: hyaline, elastin, and fibrocartilage. Connective tissues focused on here include connective tissue proper, bone, and cartilage.

Structural Elements of Connective Tissue

Connective tissue comprises three main elements. These include ground substance, fibers, and cells. Ground substance and fibers make up the extracellular matrix. Diversity in the arrangement of connective tissue enables it to perform its many different functions. It is the varying makeup of ground substance, cells, and fibers that determines connective tissue classes and subclasses. This variation is evident in the arrangement and composition of the extracellular matrix and in the properties of cells.[17]

Ground substance is an unstructured material that fills the space between cells and contains fibers. Ground substance provides a supporting framework for cells and acts as a lubricant to reduce friction between connective tissue fibers.[18] It contains glycosaminoglycans (GAGs), which are large, featherlike molecules with great affinity for water. This affinity for water greatly increases its space-occupying capability. Water and GAGs create a lubricating semi-fluid gel that maintains the distance between collagen fibers. This helps to prevent excessive collagen fiber cross-linkage, loss of collagen fiber gliding functions, and decreased connective tissue mobility.[19] Relative amounts and types of GAGs help to determine the mechanical and chemical properties of the matrix. As GAG content increases, ground substance becomes stiffer.[17]

Fibers also are found within the ground substance and help to provide support. They can be divided into collagen and elastin fibers. Elastin accounts for less than 1% of dry weight and helps the tissue to return to its prestretched length following physiologic loading.[2] Collagen is the most abundant fiber. It is extremely tough and provides high tensile strength to the matrix.[17] Alignment of collagen fiber bundles usually follows the lines of tension applied to the ligament or tendon. Collagen fibrils, when studied under polarized light microscopy, are seen to have a sinusoidal wave, or crimp pattern. This pattern allows them to elongate easily when a force is applied. When the force is removed, the fibers recoil and return to their original sinusoidal wave pattern.[2] Collagen Type I, the main component of ligaments and tendons, represents approximately 80% of the dry weight of connective tissue. Type I contributes largely to tensile stiffness.[2] The tensile strength of collagen has been estimated at 50 to 125 N/mm^2, depending on the specimen tested.[20] Some studies of human collagen report complete failure at 91 kilograms/force (kgf) for plantar fascia and at 40 kgf for anterior cruciate ligament.[21,22] Many other collagen types are present in lesser amounts. The roles of some types of collagen remain unclear, although the roles of other types have been explained by recent findings. Type III collagen is elevated during healing.[23] It lacks the strength and stability of Type I collagen. Type V collagen is believed to exist in association with Type I collagen and serves as a regulator of collagen fibril diameter.[24,25] Physiologically, collagen is a rather sluggish substance.[26] In most forms, it is inert and has a slow turnover rate. As collagen fibers mature, the cross-links increase in strength. Attempts to modify the structure or alignment of collagen therefore must be prolonged and must be made early after injury or immobilization. As collagen ages, a greater number of intermolecular cross-links form, and existing bonds become stronger.[27] The tissue thus becomes less extensible and more brittle.

The other component of connective tissue is the cell. Each class of connective tissue includes a fundamental cell type that exists in both immature and mature forms. If injury to the extracellular matrix occurs, the mature cells are able to revert back to a more active state to repair and regenerate the matrix.[17] The primary cell types in connective tissue (excluding bone) are mast cells, macrophages, plasma cells, and fibroblasts. Fibroblasts are responsible for the synthesis of collagen and other components of the extracellular tissue matrix during the repair process. Mast cells are immune cells whose function is to detect foreign substances in the tissue spaces and initiate local inflammatory responses against them. Macrophages are important in the immune response. Plasma cells produce and release antibodies. Both macrophages and plasma cells are important in the body's defense against specific pathogenic microorganisms.

Some studies indicate that not all connective tissue structures have identical ultrastructure or biochemistry.[28] Amiel et al[29] and Frank et al[30] identified histologic and biochemical differences between various ligaments and tendons. Lyon et al[28] reported differences in the cellular components of the medial collateral ligament (MCL) and the anterior cruciate ligament (ACL) of the knee. Using rabbits, they demonstrated that cell arrangement and quantity varied greatly between the two ligaments. This may contribute to the drastic disparity in healing capacity noted between the human ACL and MCL.

BONE

Functions of Bone

Bone performs several functions, including (1) support (it provides a framework for the body and an attachment for muscles), (2) protection (it helps to provide a framework for protection of internal organs such as brain, spinal cord, lungs, and heart), (3) movement (bones are the levers that move the body), (4) mineral storage (bones serve as storage centers for minerals, of which the two most important are calcium and phosphate), and (5) blood cell formation. The bulk of blood cell formation occurs within the marrow cavities of certain bones.[17]

Types of Bones

All bones have an outer shell of compact bone and an inner mass of spongy bone. It is the function and needs of bone that determine the percentages of the two. Compact, or dense, bone looks smooth and homogeneous. Spongy, or cancellous, bone is composed of small needlelike or flat pieces of bone called *trabeculae* and a lot of open space.[17] Compact and spongy bones differ in the amount of mineralized tissue present per total bone tissue volume. Compact bone is 5% to 30% porous, or nonmineralized, whereas spongy bone is 30% to 90% porous.[31,32]

Microscopic Structure of Bone

Compact Bone

The structural unit of compact bone is the osteon. An osteon is like a weight-bearing pillar and looks like rings in a tree. Each ring is called a *lamella*. Collagen fibers are aligned within lamellae in the same direction, and collagen fibers in adjacent lamellae run in opposite directions. This helps the bone to withstand torsion stresses. Within the core of each osteon is a canal that contains small blood vessels and nerve fibers. Nutrition to compact bone is provided through canaliculi, which tie together all the osteocytes within an osteon.

Spongy Bone

Spongy bone does not contain osteons. It consists of trabeculae, an irregular latticework of thin plates of bone.[33] This bone structure is designed to provide support along the shaft of a long bone, thus enhancing resistance of tension and bending. A dense portion of spongy bone appears as plates, such as those found in the pubis and the lateral angle of the scapula. The plate structure provides greater support near articular surfaces, which are subjected to compression and shear stresses. Nutrition in spongy bone is diffused through the canaliculi from the marrow spaces between trabeculae.

Chemical Composition of Bone

Bone is essentially a highly vascular, constantly changing, mineralized connective tissue. Bone is similar to other forms of connective tissue in terms of its main constituents, but it differs in terms of the quantities and exact types of various components. Bone includes a mineralized ground substance, whereas other connective tissues contain larger amounts of water and GAG. Bone receives a greater nutritional supply via its own blood vessels than do other connective tissues. Because of this greater vascularity and cellularity, bone is capable of more rapid change, including healing and remodeling, than are the other connective tissues. Bone contains inorganic components such as mineral salts, made up largely of calcium phosphates. These inorganic components account for its exceptional hardness, which allows it to resist compression. The combination of inorganic and organic components allows bone to be exceedingly durable and strong without becoming brittle. The strength of bone is correlated directly with its degree of mineralization and with the number and organization of its osteons.[32] Demineralized bone exhibits only 5% to 10% of the strength of mineralized bone. The strength and strain of bone decrease as the numbers of osteons increase because of the relative weakness of the cement lines between them.[29,31]

PERIPHERAL NERVE

Peripheral nerves are part of the somatic nervous system and contain nerves that connect the brain and spinal cord to muscles controlled voluntarily and to sensory receptors in the skin. These nerves exit the spinal cord via dorsal and ventral roots. Ventral roots contain motor or efferent neurons, and dorsal roots contain sensory or afferent neurons. After these nerves leave the spinal cord, some become a network of interwoven nerves called a *plexus*. Plexuses are known to innervate a specific part of the body, for example, the brachial plexus innervates the upper extremity.

The neuron is composed of a large cell body, which is connected to dendrites and an axon. Dendrites are considered receptive regions in that they have receptors for neurotransmitters. A neuron may have many dendrites but only one axon. Axons are nerve impulse generators and transmitters. Each axon ends in axonal terminals, which contain neurotransmitters. The release of these neurotransmitters and their attachment onto other dendrites is what causes neuron excitation. The axons then are covered in fatty tissue called *myelin*. This myelin sheath in the peripheral nervous system also contains Schwann cells. The Schwann cell nucleus and the bulk of the cytoplasm are covered by the myelin sheath. The peripheral parts of the Schwann cell that are not covered are referred to as the *neurilemma*. Schwann cells are similar to satellite cells in that they help peripheral nerves to function and regenerate.[34] Schwann cells are individual cells that are not continuous in nature; the spaces between the sheaths are called *nodes of Ranvier*. Damage to this myelin sheath can cause disruption or cessation of nerve impulses.

Much like muscle, each nerve fiber is wrapped in layers of connective tissue. The endoneurium is adjacent to the myelin sheath. The perineurium binds groups of fibers together into bundles called *fascicles*. Finally, the outer layer of connective tissue, the epineurium, binds all of the fascicles together.

MECHANICAL LOADING

Mechanical loading is the force per unit area that measures the intensity of internal forces acting within the body as a reaction to external applied force. Types of internal forces can be measured in different forms of stress such as shear, compressive, tensile, bending, and combined stress. Shear stress, which is seen parallel or tangential to the face of the material, measures the tendency of an object to slide on itself (Figure 1-3, *A*). Tensile stress is the stress that acts on either end of the object and leads to expansion or lengthening (Figure 1-3, *B*). Compressive stress is the stress that acts on either end of the material and causes compaction of the material (Figure 1-3, *C*). Torsion stress is a combination of compressive, shear, and

tensile stresses (Figure 1-3, *D*). Bending stress happens when a tensile stress is placed on one side and compression is placed on the other, creating a bend in the tissue (Figure 1-3, *E*). Finally, in a combined stress, two or more stresses, such as torsion and compression, are placed on the tissue (Figure 1-3, *F*). Although all figures here show the femur, these stresses can and do happen in all biological tissues of the body.

Most biological tissues, including tendons and ligaments, have viscoelastic properties, which means that they demonstrate solid- and fluid-like characteristics.[35] *Viscoelasticity* is the mechanical property of materials that describes the tendency of a substance to deform at a certain rate, regardless of the speed of the externally applied force. This is important to note because the viscoelasticity of an object determines how much mechanical loading the tissue can withstand. Viscoelastic properties are time and rate dependent, which can be plotted on a stress-strain curve, as is discussed in detail in the latter part of this chapter.

Mechanical loading is important for the body to endure, as it aids in metabolic responses and remodeling. Fibroblasts and muscle cells are highly responsive to mechanical loading.[1] These cells are involved in the adaptation of muscle and connective tissue. With respect to muscle, mechanical loading allows adaptations to be made that will make the tissue more resistant to future damage.[1] Tissue repair, flow dynamics, and the adaptability of connective tissue, muscle, nerve, and bone all are dependent on mechanical loading.

Tissue-Specific Response to Mechanical Loading

Muscle

The way that muscle responds to mechanical loading is seen best on a length-tension curve, with the length of muscle plotted on the *x*-axis and the tension plotted on the *y*-axis. Two muscle length-tension curves are plotted: the active tension curve and the passive tension curve.

The active tension curve is a theoretical curve that cannot be measured directly. It is determined by subtraction of the passive length tension curve from a curve that plots the muscle's isometric force at different lengths. The height of this graph represents the greatest number of actin-myosin binding sites seen when the muscle is at an intermediate length (Figure 1-4).[35,36]

The passive length tension curve demonstrates muscle length in relation to the tension provided. This passive tension, or stiffness, occurs whether the muscle is active or resting. Every muscle has its own degree of stiffness. This graph is also velocity dependent, meaning that the faster the muscle is elongated, the stiffer it will get. Three properties can affect muscle stiffness; these inherent properties of muscle consist of (1) connective tissue properties, as well as those of actin and myosin; (2) volitional contraction of the muscle; and (3) reflex stiffness (Figure 1-5).

Finally, if we combine the active and passive graphs, we see the length-tension curve for muscle. Each of these

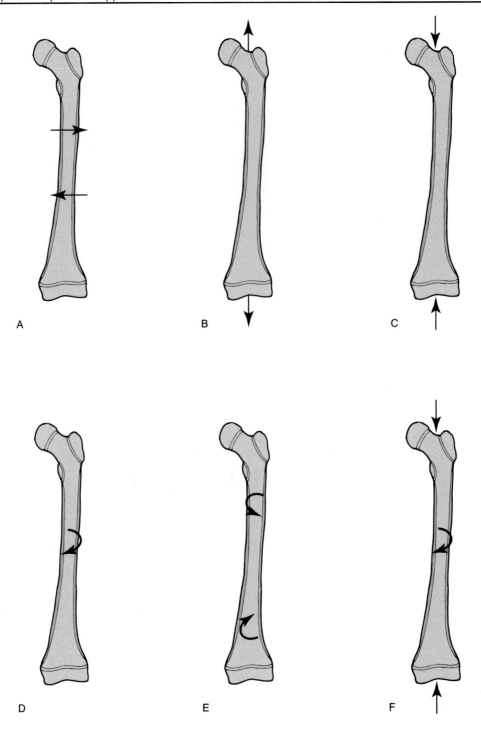

Figure 1-3 A, This picture represents shear stress on the femur. The force will cause the bone to slide on itself, thus creating a shear stress. **B,** This photo represents tensile stress, in which equal and opposite loads are applied to either end of the femur. **C,** This picture represents compressive forces on the bone, where equal loads are pushing both ends of the bone. **D,** This is an example of torsion stress, which is the point at which the bone twists around an internal axis. This represents a combination of compression, tension, and shear stresses. **E,** This is an example of bending stress, involving compression on the side of the femur where the arrows are located, which will result in tension stress on the opposite side. **F,** This is an example of the combined forces that can be applied to an object. Torsion is occurring while at either end the bone is being compressed.

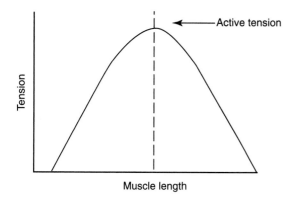

Figure 1-4 This figure represents the active length-tension curve of muscle.

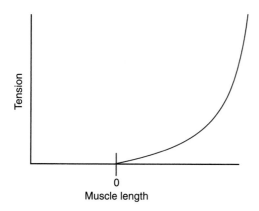

Figure 1-5 This graph shows the passive length-tension curve of muscle. It starts at zero because this is the resting length for muscle.

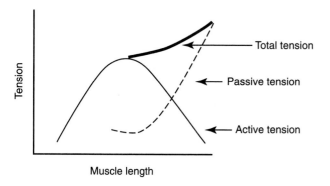

Figure 1-6 This graph depicts a length-tension curve for muscle. As shown, the two previous graphs are overlaid here.

characteristics is independent for each muscle; therefore, each muscle has its own length-tension curve. However, study of this curve reveals a few generalizations. First, at the beginning of the curve, excessive sarcomere overlap can be seen. Then, as actin-myosin binding occurs, optimal sarcomere overlap occurs around the intermediate length of the graph. Ultimately, at the end, sarcomere overlap is inadequate, leading to tissue failure (Figure 1-6).

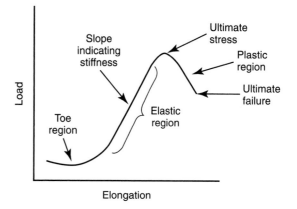

Figure 1-7 This graph is a representation of a nerve load-elongation graph. This also can be the stress-strain curve for connective tissue, with insertion of strain on the x-axis and stress on the y-axis. The toe region in the beginning is the place where the connective tissue is straightened. This is followed by a linear increase, which indicates stiffness up to the ultimate stress. After the ultimate stress point has been attained, the changes become permanent; thus begins the plastic region, which ultimately can lead to failure.

Connective Tissue

Mechanical forces are important regulators of connective tissue homeostasis. The force most often associated with connective tissue is tension stress. The effect of tension stress has been well documented via the stress-strain curve. Stress is a measure of force per area (y-axis), and strain is an expression of the percentage of elongation beyond resting length (x-axis) (Figure 1-7).

The stress-strain curve consists of three distinct regions: the toe region, the elastic region, and the plastic region. The toe region can also be called the *slack area,* hence the term "to take out the slack" in stretching. It indicates initial elongation of the tissue. What is occurring in the toe region is the straightening and flattening out of the wavy configuration of the tissues. Once the stretch has been removed, the tissue returns to it wavy configuration. Different connective tissues have different toe regions, depending on the waviness of the collagen pattern. Ligaments have longer toe regions compared with tendons.

In the elastic region, true elongation of the tissue occurs. The overall elasticity of a tissue is determined by the ratio of elastin to collagen. The length of the elastic region is determined by the amount of elasticity contained within a tissue. If the amount of deformation does not exceed the elastic range, the structure can return to its normal or original shape after the load has been removed. In connective tissue, most physiologic movements occur within the toe and early elastic regions.[37]

The plastic region is noted after the elastic region. In this region, progressive failure and microscopic tearing of collagen fibers are seen. Mechanical changes to tissue that occur in the plastic region are irreversible. If the load is removed, the tissue will not return to its original length. Continued stretching in the plastic region leads to a progressive increase in the number of fibers that fail. If the stretch is continued, complete rupture of the tissue occurs. For the tissue to return to normal length after plastic changes have occurred, it must exhibit inflammation and undergo repair.[38]

Connective tissue responds to mechanical stress in a time-dependent or viscoelastic manner.[39] Viscoelasticity, as related to connective tissue, involves a combination of stiff and elastic fibers embedded in a gel medium. Elasticity is the springlike element within the tissue, and viscous properties are the lubricating and dampening elements.[38]

Two primary behavioral responses have been reported when connective tissues are subjected to constant tension: creep and stress relaxation. *Creep* is an increase in deformation over time under a constant load or stress.[19] The greatest amount of creep occurs during the first 6 to 8 hours of tissue loading. *Stress relaxation* is a decline in stress over time under constant deformation or stress.[2] This is seen in repetitive loading sports such as running. Cyclic stress relaxation decreases tissue resistance to strain, and the result is a continuous decrease in peak stress for each cycle.[40,41] This may help to prevent fatigue failure in ligaments and tendons.[2]

With repeated loading, or cyclic loading, an increment of elongation occurs with each successive cycle. This increment of elongation decreases with every cycle until it plateaus, at which time the tissue will not elongate further. During the first four cycles of stretching, 80% of elongation takes place.[42] Changes reflect increased compliance (softening) of the tissue, increased early stiffness, and a decreased load to failure.[43,44] Softening of the tissue during the first cycle and subsequent cycles reflects a release of energy from the tissue, called *hysteresis*. It is thought that an increase in hysteresis could reduce risk of microinjuries due to fatigue at sites of local stress concentration within the tendon. It has been shown that unloaded tendon will lose hysteresis, thus becoming more susceptible to injury.[45] Application of cyclic loads usually leads to an enhanced matrix synthesis.[46]

Current findings suggest that human cartilage deforms very little in vivo during physiologic activities, and that it recovers from deformation within 90 minutes after loading.[47] Cartilage deformation becomes less notable with age. Gender and physical training do not seem to affect deformation.[47] If the rate of load application is increased, other mechanical responses change, to maintain a constant rate of deformation. Thus a rapidly applied load will produce less deformation before failure than a slowly applied load.

It has been shown through exercise that the extracellular matrix turnover of tendon is influenced by physical activity. Blood flow, oxygen demand, and levels of collagen synthesis and matrix metalloproteinase increase with mechanical loading. The mechanical loading of tendon enhances growth factors that are known to potentially stimulate synthesis of collagen and other intracellular matrix proteins.[48] These and other changes may contribute to training-induced adaptation of biomechanical properties.

Bone

Because of the rigidity and makeup of bone, it is unable to adapt quickly to stresses placed on it. It is able to functionally adapt to mechanical loading through bone remodeling. Three fundamental rules govern bone adaptation: (1) it is driven by dynamic, rather than static, loading; (2) only a short duration of mechanical loading is necessary to initiate an adaptive response; and (3) bone cells accommodate to a customary mechanical loading environment, making them less responsive to routine loading signals.[49]

Bones have the ability to alter their strength in response to mechanical stress. The mechanical stresses to which bone is subjected are those that result from the pull of skeletal muscle on bone when the weight of the body is supported against gravity. This is evidenced by a study showing that elite tennis players have greater bone density in the dominant extremity than in the nondominant extremity.[50] Bone adaptation can be stated by Wolff's law, which holds that adaptive changes in the structure and biomechanical properties of bone occur as the result of functional demands. In response to mechanical stress, bone produces very small currents of electricity, known as the *piezoelectric effect*.[33] Bone deposition occurs on the concave side as the result of a negative charge produced by pressure, or compression. The positive charge on the convex side, produced by tensile forces, favors bone resorption.[51]

As the result of an animal study, it has been suggested that short periods of exercise, with a 4- to 8-hour rest period between them, provide more effective stimulation of bone production than is provided by a single sustained session of exercise. The data also suggest that activities involving higher loading rates are more effective for increasing bone formation, even if the duration of the activity is short.[52] Another study looked at the long-term effects of mechanical loading and investigated whether "time off" improved the responsiveness of bone cells in increasing bone formation. Investigators concluded that mechanical loading of the rat ulna resulted in large improvements in bone formation during the first 5 weeks of loading, but that continual loading decreased the osteogenic response. Having time off facilitated bone formation.[53] Repetitive physiologic loading is widely believed to be beneficial in maintaining skeletal integrity but is associated with bone injury. One study looked at the effects of repetitive physiologic loading on bone turnover and mechanical properties in adult female and male rats. Researchers concluded that high cycles of low magnitude did not increase systemic bone resorption levels or substantially degrade the mechanical properties of long bone in adult rats. This lack of response is consistent with the idea that in addition to repetitive loading, a metabolic bone disturbance is needed for a stress fracture to develop.[54] Another study looked at whether cycle number directly affects bone response to loading, and whether cycle number for activation of formation varies with load magnitude at low frequency. Investigators concluded that as applied load or strain magnitude decreases, the number of cycles required to activate formation is dependent on strain, and as the number of cycles increases, so does bone response.[55]

As health care professionals, how can we have an impact on the overall health of patients' bones? Exercise should (1) be dynamic, not static; (2) exceed a threshold intensity; (3) exceed a threshold strain frequency; (4) be relatively brief but intermittent; (5) impose on bones an unusual loading pattern; (6) be supported by unlimited nutrient energy; and (7) be supported by adequate intake of calcium and cholecalciferol (vitamin D_3).[56]

Nerve

Nerves undergo exposure to various mechanical stresses on an everyday basis (e.g., posture habits place nerves under mechanical stress). These stressors are tensile stresses and may occur parallel or perpendicular to the nerve. Nerves also undergo compressive and shear forces on a daily basis. The amount and type of stress vary and are unique to each nerve. Nerves always follow the path of least resistance.[57] Therefore the location of connective tissue and muscle can greatly alter the amount of strain placed on a nerve. This is a critical point to consider in treatment, because factors such as poor posture or scar tissue can have a profound effect on the amount of mechanical stress placed on the nerve.

According to Millesi et al, joint motion causes elongation of the nerve bed, to which the nerve responds by elongating and gliding.[58] This nerve gliding in relation to the nerve bed is referred to as *excursion*.[57,59,60] The excursion of a nerve, to describe mechanical stresses, may be graphed on a load-elongation curve, or a stress-strain curve.[61]

During the "toe region" of the curve, minimal tension results structurally in straightening of connective tissue and axons.[62-64] Stiffness of the nerve is shown on this graph during the linear increase, with a steeper slope indicating increased stiffness and less elasticity in the nerve. A point of ultimate stress represents the transition between where the nerve is still elastic and recoverable and where it switches to permanent deformation or the plastic region.[61] It is after this plastic region that the nerve reaches ultimate failure and no longer can undergo additional mechanical stress.

Several factors may affect the ability of the nerve to elongate. These factors include nerve stiffness and velocity of movement. Nerve stiffness has been shown to be greater in nerves with long sections as opposed to multiple branches.[58] Also, velocity does affect its stiffness. The stiffness of nerve is greater when it is elongated quickly.[61]

Compression is another daily stress that nerves often encounter. This stress can be provided by adjacent tissue structures such as muscles and ligaments,[61] and it undergoes compressive forces as it elongates. As it elongates, the nerve is resisted by fluid and by the connective tissue in which it is contained.[58,65] Thus the nerve undergoes tensile stress, accompanied by compressive forces.

A few factors are affected when the nerve is placed under mechanical stress, whether compression or tension. With relief of the stressors (e.g., with improved posture), these factors can return to normal. The first is axoplasmic flow. When the axon plasma flow is interrupted, the static contraction weakens.[66] The blood supply to the nerve is also affected by mechanical stress, and the symptoms displayed will depend on whether deficiency is arterial or venous. With diminished arterial supply, weakness is seen with repeated effort, and with diminished venous supply, both weakness and pain occur.[66]

Trauma and Inflammation

TISSUE-SPECIFIC RESPONSES

Muscle

Muscle trauma and inflammation are very common, especially in the area of sports medicine. Following trauma, muscle undergoes distinct processes to repair itself, including inflammation, muscle regeneration, and development of fibrosis.[67]

Trauma to the muscle may be direct or indirect. An example of direct trauma is a contusion or laceration. Indirect trauma may be seen as a neurologic dysfunction or may be related to ischemia.[68,69] Most often, treatment is based on the severity of the injury, not necessarily on the type of injury. Both the type and the severity of injury determine the length of time that it takes to recover, but the healing process is the same regardless. In a recent study, a high-force concentric loading injury and a direct muscle injury were compared to determine whether utilizing knowledge of the type of injury would shorten recovery time.[70] Investigators concluded that the clinician who takes into account the type of injury knows the genes associated with that injury, allowing accelerated recovery time.[70]

The stages of healing start at approximately the same time for each injury. The inflammation stage begins almost immediately and lasts for approximately 1 week after the injury.[71] Muscle regeneration begins 7 to 10 days after the injury and peaks at around 14 days.[71] Finally, the fibrosis stage begins at approximately 14 days and increases over time until approximately 4 weeks post injury.[71] During the fibrosis stage, scar tissue is formed, signaling the end of the muscle repair process. According to Huard et al, because of the formation of scar tissue, complete regeneration of the muscle does not take place.[71]

The inflammatory period is characterized by an inflammatory cell response and necrosis of muscle tissue.[67] This stage is discussed in depth in Chapter 3; therefore only a brief overview is presented here. The immediate response is vascular changes, with immediate vasoconstriction to minimize blood loss. This is followed by the inflammatory cell response, whereby neutrophils arrive at the site within 1 to 6 hours after the initial insult. Neutrophils have been suggested to both help and hurt the muscle regeneration process. They aid the process through phagocytosis, or clearing the injured site of waste.[72] It has been suggested in the research, however, that neutrophils also hinder muscle regeneration by releasing free radicals and proteases, which injure the myotubes.[73] Neutrophils are followed by macrophages, which become predominant. Macrophages continue to facilitate phagocytosis[72,74] but also cause myoblast proliferation in vitro.[75-78]

The muscle regeneration phase is characterized by the activation of satellite cells. The release of satellite cells is triggered by lymphocytes, which have already arrived at the site of the injured muscle and have released growth factors and cytokines. The release of these causes satellite cells to self-renew, proliferate, and join with existing muscle cells to effect muscle regeneration.[79] Mononucleated satellite cells become multinucleated myotubes, which eventually combine with myofibers, thus promoting skeletal muscle regrowth.[80]

The final stage is fibrosis, or the formation of scar tissue. Scar tissue is formed from fibroblasts. It has been shown that transforming growth factor-β (TGF-β), which is active during this phase, stimulates fibroblast proliferation and collagen synthesis at low levels.[1] However, in high concentrations, TGF-β has been shown to inhibit fibroblast proliferation and therefore fibrosis.[1] Several antifibrotic agents, such as sumarin and decorin, have been shown to aid in the reduction of TGF-β and therefore have been effective in limiting scar tissue formation.[71]

Connective Tissue

Damaged tissues heal through a process of fibrous scar formation, not regeneration. The repair process is essentially the same in all connective tissue types. Connective tissue repair involves three primary stages: (1) inflammation, (2) fibroplasia, and (3) scar maturation.[19] Even though stages have been defined, it is important to note that healing stages overlap.

Inflammation

In response to damage, the body initiates a repair process called *inflammation.* The major roles of the process of inflammation include (1) protection of the body from infection and clearance of tissue debris from the site of injury, and (2) initiation of structural repair processes that take place at the site of damage.[38] Inflammation can be characterized as acute or chronic.

Acute Inflammation

Acute inflammation is the initial response to injury, lasting 3 to 4 days. The signs and symptoms of acute inflammation include increased tissue temperature, redness, and swelling. The function of acute inflammation is to localize and destroy pathogenic agents and foreign materials.[19] "It can be characterized by (1) vascular responses that result in excess fluid accumulation in the affected tissues, and (2) cellular responses that include proliferation of white blood cells and phagocytosis."[19] The vascular response that occurs during acute inflammation consists of (1) vasodilation, thus increasing blood flow, (2) increased vascular permeability, and (3) increased blood

viscosity, thus slowing blood flow.[19] This results in edema at the injury site. The cell responds during acute inflammation by localizing and destroying invading pathogenic microorganisms. This is accomplished primarily through the proliferation of white blood cells (leukocytes), whose role is to "clean up" the wound site. Successful cleanup of the wound site (phagocytosis) marks the end of the acute stage of inflammation.

Chronic Inflammation

Chronic inflammation occurs when persistent pathogenic microorganisms are still present after acute inflammation has occurred. In this case, chronic inflammation is an extension of the acute inflammatory response. This process can continue for months. Chronic inflammation also may have a gradual insidious onset that eventually becomes symptomatic.[19] Examples of these include bursitis and tenosynovitis. Macrophages continue their assault on pathogenic microorganisms and are joined in this stage by lymphocytes. The two types of lymphocytes seen in chronic inflammation are T cell and B cells. They function when previous levels of defense have failed.

Fibroplasia

With successful elimination of foreign material from the wound site, damaged tissue enters the second stage of repair: fibroplasia. This stage is marked by (1) the proliferation of fibroblasts, (2) collagen synthesis, (3) formation of granulation tissue, (4) wound contraction, and (5) dense fibrous scar formation.[38] When an injury occurs, the need for collagen deposition is increased. This is accomplished through the proliferation of fibroblasts within damaged tissues. As collagen synthesis occurs, temporary scaffolding, called *granulation tissue,* is laid down. It is formed from Type III collagen. This adhesion has little mechanical strength[38] because Type III collagen lacks the strength and stability of Type I collagen. This is important for physical therapists to know because this weak granulation tissue is very fragile and can be broken down easily by manual stretching. After wound contraction, scar formation occurs as the new tissue matrix slowly takes on the characteristics of dense fibrous connective tissue but does not duplicate the properties of normal connective tissue.[19] The transition from granulation tissue to dense fibrous tissue includes: "(1) a transition from Type III collagen to Type I collagen synthesis, (2) an increase in overall collagen deposition, and (3) resorption of small blood vessels in the vascular bed."[19] Increased Type I collagen formation and degradation of weaker Type III collagen contribute to greater tensile strength of the scar tissue matrix. In addition, a significant increase in collagen synthesis contributes to the increasing strength of the scar tissue matrix. In one study, investigators demonstrated that the ratios of collagen Types V to I and III to I in the healing MCL increased by 84% and 138%, respectively.[81] By week 52, the ratio of collagen Type III to Type I returned to normal levels, but that of collagen Type V to Type I remained elevated. This continued elevation of the ratio of V to I explains the uniform distribution of small collagen fibrils.[82] After 1 year, the number of collagen cross-links was reported only 45% of normal.[83]

Scar Maturation

During this stage, biomechanical properties and strength of the scar tissue matrix are determined. Scar maturation is a slow process that evolves over several months to longer than a year. "The primary factors that contribute to scar maturation are (1) the rate of collagen turnover, (2) an increased number of stronger collagen cross-links, and (3) linear alignment of collagen fibers."[19] As scar maturation occurs, the rate of collagen synthesis versus lysis gradually approaches normal levels. During scar maturation, collagen cross-linkage is seen in the scar matrix. This contributes to increased density but less pliability than is seen with an immature scar.[19] The linear alignment of collagen fibers has been shown to correlate directly with improvement in the bone-ligament complex.[40,84]

Bone

As was noted in the previous section, soft connective tissue heals by scar formation. Bone heals by regeneration. This restores the normal structural and biomechanical properties of the bone. The repair process can be described in four phases: (1) hematoma formation, (2) fibrocartilaginous callous formation, (3) bony callous formation, and (4) remodeling.

When a fracture occurs, bleeding is seen and a hematoma develops around the bone ends at the fracture site. This hematoma, along with the inflammatory response, represents the normal initial stage of bone healing. The inflammatory response is described in the previous connective tissue section. The fracture hematoma also is the place at which the osteogenic cells necessary for collagen synthesis and new bone formation proliferate.[19] Shortly after the hematoma is formed, bone cells deprived of nutrition begin to die, and tissue at the fracture site becomes swollen, painful, and inflamed.[17]

A fibrocartilaginous callus is formed. Fibroblasts and osteoblasts (bone-forming cells) enter the fracture site to begin to reconstruct the bone. Fibroblasts make chondrocytes. As a result, cartilage develops in the outer part of the callus. Phagocytic cells invade the area to clean the debris. Capillaries grow into the hematoma. As osteoblasts and osteoclasts continue to work, the fibrocartilaginous callus is converted gradually to a hard callus that is made of spongy bone. Formation of callus generally begins 3 to 4 weeks after injury.[17]

Remodeling begins as stability of the fracture site is restored. This is the process by which bones resume their normal structure, size, and shape.[19] Cartilage is replaced with bone as the intercellular substance deposited between chondrocytes becomes calcified and cells die. The matrix of dead bone is removed gradually by osteoclasts. Osteoblasts move into the spaces opened by removal of dead bone, and new living bone is deposited. The callus is removed gradually by replacement of cartilage with bone and by conversion of spongy bone to compact bone.

Nerve

Peripheral nerve trauma and inflammation may have many causes and may result in a myriad of orthopaedic problems. Again, similar to muscle and connective tissue, nerve goes through its own inflammation and healing process. However, because of the complex nature of nerves and their healing process, complete return to function is not always possible.

One of the most common ailments is peripheral neuropathy. It must be noted that this is a general term encompassing hundreds of different types of disorders that can vary in severity from intermittent numbness and tingling to paralysis. It is important to remember that nerves may be motor, sensory, or autonomic. Therefore the branch that is impaired will determine the magnitude and exactness of the signs and symptoms.

Peripheral neuropathies may be inherited or acquired. Inherited peripheral neuropathy can result from genetic mutations. Acquired peripheral neuropathy may be seen as trauma to a nerve (e.g., constriction from connective tissue), infection, autoimmune deficiency, or systemic disease. Again, whether acquired or inherited, these neuropathies manifest in different forms from mild to extremely severe.

Although clinically, peripheral nerve injury presents with a myriad of signs and symptoms, the nerve itself exhibits only a few specific responses: neuropraxia, axonotmesis, and neurotmesis. In neuropraxia, axonal conduction is disrupted segmentally. The myelin sheath may be somewhat gone, but nerve transmission although slower will continue. Depending on the extent of injury that occurs to the myelin sheath, transmission may be interrupted altogether. Patients may exhibit pain, weakness, or loss of sensation.[85]

Axonotmesis is the loss of axon continuity with continuation of connective tissue. On the distal axon, Wallerian degeneration occurs, along with changes in the cell body that take place over 5 to 12 days.[86] Finally, neurotmesis occurs as the complete separation of the axon; it is the most severe of all nerve injuries.

Three different modes of nerve recovery are known: remyelination, collateral sprouting from surviving axons, and axonal regeneration.[87] Recovery from neuropraxia generally requires remyelination and takes 6 to 8 weeks.[88] Axonotmesis requires two processes for recovery, depending on the percentage of axons involved. If only 20 to 30% of axons are involved, then the nerve will heal via collateral axon sprouting, which occurs over 2 to 6 months.[87] When more than 90% of the axons are damaged, regeneration must occur.[89,90] This rate of recovery differs between proximal regeneration, which involves 6 to 8 mm per day, and distal regeneration, which occurs at a rate of 1 to 2 mm per day.[91] However, regeneration must take place within an 18- to 24-month time frame, because this is when Schwann cells are viable; after this period has ended, regeneration is not possible.[90]

As was stated previously, these injuries manifest differently, and patients can show up in the clinic with a variety of different symptoms. Signs and symptoms may be motor, sensory, or autonomic. Motor symptoms may present as weakness or muscle wasting. Generally, nerve injuries involve a hypotonic state. Sensory loss can be seen in a single digit or in the whole hand. It also may occur as loss of pressure-touch, loss of position sense, or loss of temperature. Sensory impairment in the hands or feet may be evident as constant tingling. However, one must be sure to rule out ischemic pain of peripheral vascular disease before automatically attributing tingling and sensation impairment to nerve damage. Unlike the motor component, the sensory nerve may produce hyperesthesia, or exaggerated sensation. The autonomic response to nerve injury is usually orthostatic hypotension without a change in the pulse rate. Others such as excessive sweating may occur, but the clinician must do a thorough evaluation to determine whether autonomic factors truly are the result of peripheral nerve injury. Finally, in the presence of demyelinating nerve injury, the stretch reflex may be decreased. This reflex may be diminished or may not be present at all.

Immobilization

MUSCLE

Many adverse effects may occur with immobilization of muscle. Although immobilization sometimes is necessary for proper recovery, it is imperative that the clinician understand that these adverse effects begin almost immediately and, depending on the duration of immobilization, can become significant, with longer periods being more detrimental.

The most obvious effect that immobilization has on muscle is loss of muscle mass. The most significant atrophy happens in the early stages of immobilization and may occur as early as 48 hours after immobilization.[92,93] In a study by Max, it was demonstrated that only 3 days of immobilization resulted in a 30% loss of the gastrocnemius in rats, and at 15 days of immobilization, a 50% loss of muscle mass was noted.[94] In a study done on humans, specifically young soccer players, an 11% to 17% loss of muscle mass was evident in the thigh after 31 days of immobilization.[95] The maximum cross-sectional area of the triceps surae muscle was found to be reduced by 20% to 32% after 8 weeks of cast immobilization, with the greatest loss reported within the first 2 weeks of immobilization.[96] In addition, a 21% decrease in cross-sectional area of the quadriceps femoris was seen after 4 weeks of cast immobilization.[97] Therefore it is imperative for clinicians to be aware that when a patient is immobilized, muscle atrophy can begin to happen almost immediately.

Coinciding with the loss of muscle mass is the loss of muscle force, which also has a direct correlation to the amount of time spent immobilized. However, it should be noted that loss of muscle mass alone does not cause a decrease in muscle force; metabolic and neurologic factors also play a part.[98] In a study by Shaffer et al, a 45% decrease in plantar flexion peak torque was observed after cast immobilization 8 weeks after surgery for open reduction–internal fixation (ORIF) of an ankle fracture.[98] The most significant loss has been shown to occur within the first week, at 1% to 6% per day.[98,99] Although the rate of decrease slowed as time went on, by 6 to 8 weeks, force production had decreased by 50%.[97,98,100-102]

It is important to note that physical exercise of surrounding joints and muscles, as much as is allowed, helps to prevent this atrophy. It has been shown that a 30% maximum isometric contraction for 5 seconds once a day has been enough to prevent disuse atrophy.[103] Recent studies have gone on to prove that the use of electrical stimulation of the muscle will limit the amount of atrophy caused by immobilization.[104-106]

A significant effect on neural activation was reported in a study by Hortobágyi et al.[107] This study demonstrated strength loss and muscle fiber atrophy after 3 weeks of immobilization.[107] However, the amount of strength loss, 47%, did not correlate with the amount of muscle fiber loss, 11%.[107] A study by Deschenes et al showed that after 14 days of immobilization, cortisol levels significantly increased; this was a precursor to atrophy, and no change to muscle fiber size or type was seen,[108] suggesting that neural changes, not contractile changes, affected the muscle.[108]

One thing that seems to increase after immobilization is muscle fatigue. Many studies show that immediately after immobilization, the affected leg seems to exhibit increased resistance to muscle fatigue.[98,108] Shaffer et al postulated that this had more to do with metabolic reasons but went on to point out that an increase in fatigue resistance did not correlate to lower extremity fatiguing less rapidly than it did in the non-immobilized limb.[98]

The effect that immobilization has on muscle fiber type is inconsistent throughout the literature. However, fast twitch fibers are most susceptible to disuse atrophy. One study that demonstrated support of slow twitch muscle atrophy was done by Lieber et al on the immobilization of a dog's quadriceps for 10 weeks; researchers found that the postural muscles in fact were most susceptible to disuse atrophy.[109] However, support for fast twitch muscle atrophy is found more commonly. Edgerton et al conducted a study on astronauts and reported a loss of cross-sectional area in the vastus lateralis muscle, along with a decrease in the number of fiber types, with Type IIb showing the greatest loss, followed by IIa and finally I.[110,111] Additional support was offered by Widrick et al, who measured cross-sectional area and muscle fiber types in the soleus muscle of astronauts 45 days before they were in space and again 17 days after they were in space.[112] Researchers found that Type IIa cross-sectional area had decreased by 26%, and Type I had decreased by only 15%.[112] Some studies have gone on to state that fiber type loss presents itself more specifically to the extensor muscle groups, as opposed to the flexor muscle groups.[113,114]

Significant changes to the muscle were seen at the cellular level. A study by Oki et al showed sarcomere dissolution, accumulation of connective tissue, and endothelial degradation.[111,115] Many studies have reported a decrease in the number of mitochondria.[116,117] However, one of the most significant findings has been the disappearance of the myonuclear number.[118] An understanding of the myonuclear domain theory is needed before this last statement can be appreciated fully.

The myonuclear domain theory proposes that each nucleus of a muscle cell is responsible for controlling a finite volume of cytoplasm or muscle tissue. Therefore, for a muscle to hypertrophy, it must increase its number of nuclei to control muscle tissue. These nuclei are derived from satellite cells that fuse with the muscle and donate their nuclei.[119] The disappearance of myonuclear number was shown by Smith et al after immobilization of a rabbit's hind limb.[118] Outcomes, however, differ greatly on whether the number of myonuclei or the myonuclear domain is decreased. Additional research is needed in this area, so that researchers can learn the exact effect that immobilization has on myonuclear domain and number.

It is of significant importance to note that positioning of a muscle, even if it is not being used, will greatly affect results immediately following the period of disuse. Most research in this area has been performed on unloaded limbs as opposed to immobilized limbs. Limb immobilization studies always reported significantly greater deficits immediately following the period of disuse. Although certainly detrimental effects did occur during unloading, differences among them must be noted. One author hypothesized that differences may be due to the shortened position that the muscle must maintain constantly during immobilization.[107] His study found a 47% loss in quadriceps muscle strength,[107] as opposed to another study, which conducted limb unloading for the same time period and showed only a 20% reduction in quadriceps strength.[120]

Ultimately, what immobilization leads to is lack of functional ability. All of the changes to muscle described previously will correlate with a loss in functional ability. Clinicians need to focus on restoring these functional deficits. Functional loss is relative, and understanding the patient and his or her lifestyle will allow the rehabilitation specialist to focus treatment on the deficits that need to be treated. For example, a retired 70-year-old who lives a sedentary lifestyle may need to gain ambulation for only short periods to be functional, but a 70-year-old school janitor must regain the ability to perform steps, ambulate long distances, and stand for long periods of time. It is important to document all of this information when taking a complete history.

CONNECTIVE TISSUE

Akeson and associates have done several classic studies on the effects of immobilization on connective tissue.[121,122] After immobilization of rabbit knee joints, they reported the following findings: (1) loss of ground substance and water, (2) no net collagen loss until 9 to 13 weeks, (3) formation of collagen interfiber cross-links at microscopic and macroscopic levels, and (4) a haphazard lying down of newly synthesized collagen and fibro fatty infiltrates visible at the macroscopic level. The authors theorized that loss of water and GAGs, although total collagen remained the same, would decrease the space between collagen fibers in the connective tissue, thus altering free movement between fibers. This lack of free movement tended to make the tissue less elastic, less plastic, and more brittle. Also,

the increase in fibro fatty infiltrates and the random pattern of the new collagen inhibited normal gliding movement and increased the likelihood of adhesions.[121,122]

In immobilized joints, cartilage surface irregularities appeared after 2 weeks and progressed rapidly to plateau after 8 weeks.[123] The overall thickness of cartilage is affected by immobilization. It is decreased up to 9%, and the deformation rate under test load is increased up to 42% (after 11 weeks of immobilization).[124] One study performed on human spinal cord patients at 6, 12, and 24 months post trauma showed progressive thinning (atrophy) of human cartilage in the absence of normal joint loading and movement.[125] Detrimental changes to cartilage are also seen with partial weight bearing. Findings revealed changes in the partial weight-bearing limb, whereas no change was observed in the contralateral knee.[126]

With immobilization, ligaments lose strength and stiffness, and their insertion points are weakened.[127,128] Ligaments immobilized for 8 weeks showed a decrease in maximum load to failure, a decrease in energy absorbed at failure, and an increase in extensibility.[129] A study done by Woo on ligaments showed that ultimate loads and energy absorbed at failure of the femur-MCL-tibia complex were only 31% and 18%, respectively, of contralateral nonimmobilized controls.[130] A study on the effects of physical activity on ligament insertions in the knees of dogs showed that failure occurred at the tibial insertion rather than at the midsubstance because of increasing orthoclastic activities at the insertion site.[131] It also has been shown that different ligaments demonstrate different changes in tensile properties after immobilization.[132]

Effects on immobilized tendons are similar to those on ligaments. Immobilized tendons atrophy, with degradation of their mechanical properties.[133] The space between the tendon and its sheath is decreased significantly or is eliminated completely as a result of adhesions. This restricts the gliding action of the tendon within its sheath.[134] The vascular supply also is affected by immobilization. Poor, random growth of blood vessels is the result of immobilization.[38]

Increased joint stiffness is commonly seen after immobilization. It has been shown that after 9 weeks of immobilization, the amount of torque required to initially extend a rabbit knee is increased significantly.[135,136] The joint capsule also failed at lower loads than in control joints. Changes in the force required for motion and in the load at failure were evident after 16 days of immobilization.

BONE

Bones are immobilized for various reasons and in different ways. It is important during fracture repair/healing that fracture fragment position is maintained and protected to permit solid bony union.[19] Although immobilization may be necessary for fracture healing, as well as healing of other injuries, it has detrimental effects on bone. Bone accretion and absorption are maintained in equilibrium by weight bearing and muscular contraction.[137-140] Immobilization changes the equilibrium and induces a very rapid increase in osteoclast activity. This significant rise in osteoclastic activity can be seen within 24 hours of immobilization.[141] The mineral content of the bone also is diminished during immobilization, as can be seen by increased secretion of urinary calcium. The mechanical properties of bone also change with the loss of its organic and inorganic components.

The hardness of bone steadily decreases with the duration of immobilization. After 12 weeks of immobilization, hardness is reduced from normal bone by 55% to 60%.[137] Elastic resistance also is decreased, making the bone brittle and more susceptible to fracture. The extent of bone mineral loss and the potential for restoration appear to be related to the duration of immobilization. The longer the immobilization period, the greater are the detrimental effects.[142] Immobilization should be continued long enough for a solid bony union to occur but should be discontinued as soon as mechanical loading can begin safely.[19]

NERVE

A nerve can be immobilized through various media such as casting or splinting. Many changes to a nerve's biological structure can be implemented during the period of immobilization. The length of time that a limb is immobilized will have a significant bearing on the number of changes that occur. Unfortunately, research in this area is very sparse, and most of the findings discussed in this section were derived from the Topp and Boyd article,[61] which is an excellent article on peripheral nerves.

During periods of immobilization, various changes occur to the axon, axon terminals, myelin, and connective tissues. These changes are not positive and most likely cause the nerve to be unable to tolerate physical stress.[61] In a study by Pachter and Eberstein, the effect of immobilization for 3 weeks on the hind limb of rats was examined, and decreases in myelin were found, along with myelin debris, at the neuromuscular junction.[61,143]

Additional studies went on to look at collagen deposition in the endoneurium and found that with immobilization in rats for 6 weeks, collagen deposits were increased, and large-diameter myelinated fibers were altered.[61,144] This alteration in large-diameter fibers was shown in other studies that documented an increase in the ratio of small- to large-diameter fibers, which resulted in an overall reduction in mean fiber diameter.[61,144-146] As immobilization progressed to 16 weeks, fiber diameter grew smaller and myelinated fibers were lost.[61,145,147]

Remobilization

MUSCLE

Muscles very rarely undergo complete functional recovery because of slow healing times and the formation of fibrotic tissue, which actually can set the muscle up for recurring injury.[71] Formation of scar tissue usually begins at the second to third week after injury, and scar tissue increases in size as time goes by.[71] A study that examined whether immobilization or suturing was better for fibrotic tissue concluded that suturing allowed the prevention of fibrous tissue deep in the muscle but still allowed some scar tissue to form superficially, whereas immobilization allowed scar tissue to form both deep within the muscle and superficially.[148] Garrett et al reported that when lacerations in rabbits were repaired, the muscle was able to return to being useful, but because of fibrosis formation, full functional recovery did not occur.[149]

Therefore one of the goals of remobilization is the prevention of scar tissue buildup. Although the formation of scar tissue is part of the natural healing process of muscle, scar tissue can and does prevent motion. Scar tissue buildup can be prevented through motion, and the amount of motion is relative.[150] Studies have shown that this fibrotic tissue actually may be a contributing factor in recurring strains.[71,151-156]

Despite the fact that full functional recovery is not always possible after muscle injury, most often the factors affected by immobilization are completely reversible with proper physical training. In a study conducted by Shaffer and colleagues, in which plantar flexion torque was measured, investigators demonstrated that in the first 5 weeks post immobilization, the casted lower limb had regained 70% of the muscle force found in the plantar flexors.[98] Hortobágyi et al found that 2 weeks post immobilization for 3 weeks of the lower limb, 90% recovery of strength deficits occurred, along with 95% recovery of fiber type.[107] Yue et al reported that strength in the upper extremity, the elbow extensors to be precise, returned at 100% 2 weeks after a 4-week immobilization period.[157] This recovery seemed to be independent of whether the muscle was a postural muscle[107,120] or a nonpostural muscle.[102,107,157] In the case of vascular density at the myotendinous junction of rats, after 8 weeks of remobilization, density returned to the level of controls.[158]

Berg and Tesch conducted a study of 10-day unilateral limb unloading in healthy males followed by a 4-day recovery period.[159] They examined knee extensor torque, angular velocity, and quadriceps electromyography (EMG) and observed that torque and angular velocity were decreased immediately after unloading. However, when subjects were retested after 4 days of weight bearing, all values had returned to normal, indicating that in this case recovery took less time than with actual immobilization.[159] However, it should be noted that investigators in the previous study used healthy subjects and performed limb unloading, not casting. Therefore, subjects were able to contract inadvertently and use their unloaded limb.

Studies performed on animals with remobilization have taken a look at younger compared with older skeletal muscle. Overall findings of these studies on rats show that younger skeletal muscle returned to its pre-atrophy state, but older skeletal muscle did not.[160-165]

Although muscle can regenerate to almost as it was before, care must be taken not to reinjure the muscle while rehabilitating it. For example, eccentric activities can cause muscle damage.[166] Therefore when the skeletal muscle has been damaged, isometric exercises and concentric exercises should be started before any eccentric training is provided. However, proper use of eccentric activity can cause the muscle to recover faster. Hortobágyi found that return to normal strength occurred 2 weeks faster when eccentrics were used as opposed to only concentric training.[107] Eccentric exercises have been shown to greatly increase isometric strength, further proving their importance in recovery training at appropriate times.[167]

Clinicians must have a good understanding of tissue response with regard to healing. Using a sound rationale, the clinician can provide a fast, functional recovery with minimum scar tissue buildup and minimum risk of reinjury.

CONNECTIVE TISSUE

Strong evidence indicates that periodic moderate stress is essential for connective tissue nutrition, homeostasis, and repair.[168-170] In many studies, remobilization was initiated with passive movement,[171-175] but moderate active movement also has been shown to be beneficial in assisting tissue recovery after injury and immobilization.[133,169,176]

Movement encourages normal collagen turnover and helps align collagen along the lines of mechanical stress. This provides the tissue with better tensile properties. Movement also helps to improve the balance of GAGs and water content within the tissue. This aids in lubrication, helps to maintain interfibril distance, and decreases the risk of formation of abnormal cross-links and adhesions.[38]

Passive movement has been shown to stimulate various aspects of repair in ligaments. If a knee is mobilized shortly after injury, the ligaments show greater strength and stiffness compared with immobilized ligaments. This holds true as long as movements are not excessive and scar formation is not disturbed.[177] Repaired ligaments have been shown to have greater strength in animals that were allowed to exercise.[178] Remobilization of the knee joint after immobilization reveals that the mechanical properties of the MCL substance in the functional range return to normal values relatively quickly.[130] Although mechanical properties may return to a functional range, the histologic and morphologic appearance of healed ligaments does not return to its preinjury state.[2] As is seen with transmission electron microscopy, the number of collagen fibrils is increased over the number in an uninjured ligament, but the diameters of the healed ligaments are uniformly small. This remains evident 2 years post injury.[82,83] The collagen fiber alignment of the healing ligament remains abnormal for up to 1 year.[83,84]

After surgery, tendons that undergo mobilization have greater tensile strength and rupture less often than immobilized tendons.[179,180] Early tendon mobilization reduces the proliferation of fibrous tissue and decreases the formation of adhesions between the tendon and its sheath.[179,181] Animal experiments have shown that tendons undergoing early mobilization are stronger than immobilized tendons.[38] In tendons,

early mobilization has been shown to stimulate the reorientation and revascularization of blood vessels at the site of repair in a more normal pattern. This better enables the blood vessels to withstand the mechanical forces imposed on the tissue.[38] Tendons and ligaments that have been injured have displayed abnormal viscoelastic properties. Under static and cyclic loading, healing MCLs of animals exhibited significantly more stress relaxation when compared with normal controls.[182]

One study suggests that cartilage is never fully restored after prolonged immobilization. A study was done on the hind limbs of beagle dogs that were immobilized for 11 weeks and then remobilized for 50 weeks. After 50 weeks of remobilization, full restoration of articular cartilage glycosaminoglycan concentration was not attained. This may have an effect on the well-being of articular cartilage.[176]

BONE

It has been well documented that acute bone loss may occur after injury. The long-term effects of remobilization have been less well documented. After immobilization, the processes of bone deterioration do not cease immediately upon resumption of normal mechanical loading.[183] It has been seen with as little as 2 weeks of immobilization, and bone density had not returned to normal after 4 weeks of normal activity.[184] Another study had a similar conclusion. One forelimb of a horse was immobilized for 7 weeks; this was followed by 8 weeks of increasing exercise. After 8 weeks, bone mineral density had not returned to normal.[185]

As was stated previously, bone adapts to the stresses placed on it, as stated by Wolff's law. Bone remodeling at a fracture site, as well as restoration of normal bone density and bone mass lost during immobilization, is enhanced by mechanical loading. A step approach to mechanical loading can start the restoration process earlier, bringing a quicker return to full function. Static muscle contraction within a cast or splint (as deemed appropriate with injury healing) initiates controlled mechanical loading. Progression to active range of motion and passive range of motion as safe healing allows continues to slowly increase the stress placed on bone. With lower extremity involvement, progression of weight bearing adds to mechanical stress. It has been shown that when limb-loading frequency is matched, swimming may equal if not provide better benefits than treadmill running.[186] This graduated level of functional loading stimulates bone deposition and increases osteoblast activity but reduces the risk of excessive mechanical forces that could lead weakened bone to refracture.[187] The amount of bone mass increase that can be achieved through physical activity appears to depend on the initial bone mass.[187] This study supported a reversal of bone atrophy after immobilization and the fact that bone mass restoration can potentially return to pre-immobilization levels. Another study indicated the need for greater than normal activity to restore bone mineral content and bone mineral density to normal levels after immobilization. It also found that the benefits of intensified remobilization are lost if activity is terminated. Bone-loading activities should be continued so that bone density and bone mineral gains can be maintained.[188]

NERVE

The effects of remobilization of nerve have not been widely investigated. No studies to date have measured how much compression, tension, or excursion a nerve is able to incur after remobilization. However, specific techniques must be followed after remobilization of the limb.

Topp and Boyd hypothesized that a reduction in axon girth and loss of myelin cause tissue to be less tolerant of absolute stresses placed upon it.[61] During the rehabilitation and remobilization process, care must be taken to monitor pain, paresthesia, and reflexes that may indicate stress to the nerve.[61]

During the remobilization process, specific sensation training is performed because axon regeneration to new locations may occur. This type of training has three phases: desensitization, early-phase discrimination, and tactile gnosis.[189] It is important to follow these phases so as not to cause undue stress on the nerve. Desensitization is a gradual process that begins with the introduction of graded stimuli. When the patient is able to tolerate a 30-cps tuning fork, the localization phase, which consists of distinguishing between static and dynamic touch, begins.[189] Finally, in the last stage, emphasis is placed on the ability to discern differences between intricate parts of objects.[189]

During the remobilization process, it is important for the clinician to be aware of lengthening stresses placed on the nerve. According to Topp and Boyd, a nerve can handle 6% to 8% for short duration, but acute strains greater than 11% may cause long-term damage.[61] This lengthening of the nerve is affected greatly by limb positioning, a matter about which the clinician must be constantly aware.

The therapist must be aware of more than just length and positioning stresses imposed by the clinician. Nerve injuries due to cumulative trauma, such as postural stresses and repetitive motions, have risen over the past 15 years and are especially prevalent with high-force and high-repetition activities.[190,191] For example, a job that requires an excessive amount of deviation at the wrist predisposes the patient to median nerve trauma.[191,192]

Comorbidities also predispose nerves to stress, which may hinder or exacerbate issues during the remobilization process. For example, lumbar stenosis places excessive pressure on the nerves.[193] This pressure is evident while the patient is in extension postures, so care must be taken to place the patient in a lumbar flexion posture to help reduce stress on the tissues.[194]

The clinician must be aware that immobilization of other tissues in the body, such as muscle, causes the nerve to undergo immobilization stresses. With the formation of fibrosis, this can influence the amount of stress that is put on the nerve, and the patient may develop sensory impairments that were not present before the muscle or connective tissue injury occurred. A focus on making sure that the nerve is able to glide unimpeded must be included in rehabilitation for any injury.

Impedance of a nerve's path may occur through improper everyday postures that happen at work and home. Posture education for daily activities must be a matter of focus in any rehabilitation program. Postures that the patient needs to be taught can be decided after a thorough history is taken. Postures can and will change through the mobilization and remobilization process; therefore, maintenance of minimum stress on the nerve must be a focus of treatment. Injury to a tissue that leads to mobilization affects not just that specific tissue but all of the tissues involved in immobilization and remobilization.

TISSUE RESPONSE TO REMOBILIZATION

Various methods have been employed by physical therapists as part of the remobilization process. Some of these include manual joint mobilization, low-load prolonged stretch (LLPS) modalities, and passive range of motion (PROM). Devices such as Dynasplint (Dynasplint Systems, Inc., Severna Park, MD) and Joint Active Systems (JAS; Joint Active Systems, Inc., Effingham, IL) may facilitate the remobilization process. All of these treatments focus on restoring the range of motion to a joint, and many share the same school of thought; however, the literature is unclear as to which is the preferred method. That is why it is imperative for physical therapists to understand the rationale behind performing each of these treatment techniques. No matter which intervention is chosen, the goal always should be to provide plastic deformation to the tissues.

LLPS and Dynasplint follow similar theories. They are based on a similar biomechanical rationale, but they differ in terms of their approach to static vs. dynamic. The basic principle is that when tissues are exposed to a low load over a particular period of time, deformation will occur based on their viscoelastic properties. This property is called *creep,* and the principle is called *creep-based loading.* The Dynasplint applies a constant low-load prolonged force for several hours, that is, for 6 to 8 hours daily. Low-force long-duration stretching causes plastic deformation, whereas high-force short-duration stretching allows only for elastic deformation.[195] This high-force stretch, which often is used in the clinic setting, causes pain and possible rupture of tissue.[196]

The low-load principle has been found to be more beneficial than a higher-load, briefer stretch. In a study by Light et al, knee flexion contractures were treated with the use of LLPS for 1 hour, twice a day, five times a week for 4 weeks, or with high-load brief stretches. High-load stretches consisted of three 1-minute bouts, twice a day, five times a week for 4 weeks. The study concluded that the LLPS group had more beneficial outcomes than did the high-load group.[197]

In addition, this low load must be provided over a prolonged period of time. Zito et al investigated short-duration stretching by using two 15-second bouts of stretches for the ankle dorsiflexors.[198,199] No significant changes occurred during the 24-hour retesting period. Bohannon increased the time to 8-minute hamstring stretches over 3 days, which again showed no significant change in straight leg raise range of motion.[199,200]

However, despite multiple studies that proved ineffectiveness with short duration, the exact length of time that the stretch should be held is controversial.[198,199]

LLPS has been utilized heavily in the physical therapy industry, and many devices have been used to perform this process mechanically. However, the benefits of these devices remain unclear. A study by Steffan et al examined bilateral knee flexion contractures in the elderly nursing home patient using the Dynasplint on one lower extremity and PROM and manual stretching on the other contracture.[201] The Dynasplint was used for 3 hours per day, 5 days per week, and PROM and manual stretching were done two times per week subsequent to a standard protocol. The entire study lasted 5 months. Investigators concluded that use of the Dynasplint over this period did not improve the contracture or the function of the patient versus PROM and manual stretching.[201]

However, some studies point to the effectiveness of the use of an intermediary, such as Dynasplint. In a study by Willis et al that examined shoulder external rotation in patients with stage II adhesive capsulitis, a significant increase in range of motion was seen in both groups of patients, one of which used only the Dynasplint and the other, physical therapy and the Dynasplint.[202] In a study that examined elbow flexion contractures in neurologic patients, it was found that Dynasplint did in fact aid in the restoration of range of motion.[203]

The JAS system (Figure 1-8) works under a principle called *static progressive stretch,* which employs the stress-relaxation concept. Stress-relaxation loading involves holding the tissue at a constant length and gradually reducing the force over time.[204,205] Bonutti et al found that with only 30 minutes twice a day, the tissues would become permanently elongated.[206] With reduction in stress to the tissues, plastic deformation occurs as the result of realignment of fibers and elongation of tissue.[204] The amount of force required for application of the stress-relaxation theory is beyond the "toe" region of the curve, just beyond where the slack is taken out of the tissues.[204] This length must be maintained for a plastic deformation to occur; otherwise, if the load is removed, tissue will be in the elastic phase and will return to normal length. Donatelli et al used a JAS device in treating adhesive capsulitis and found that use of the JAS combined with manual therapy had a significant effect on improving passive glenohumeral external rotation and active glenohumeral abduction.[204]

One of the major differences between the two devices—JAS and Dynasplint—is the duration of time that a patient must wear them before the desired result is achieved. Dynasplint must be worn 6 to 8 hours per day to achieve plastic deformation. JAS, however, must be worn three times per day for 30 minutes for the principles of stretch relaxation to apply. These factors must be considered when one is choosing the best device for the patient, because patient compliance is mandatory for positive outcomes to occur.

Some studies have shown the effectiveness of applying two interventions, such as modalities and low-load prolonged duration stretch. Peres et al found that LLPS used in conjunction with pulsed short-wave diathermy yielded an increased dorsiflexion range of motion compared with LLPS alone.[207] In a

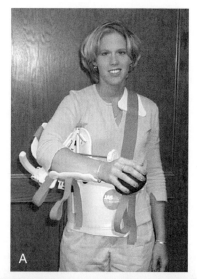

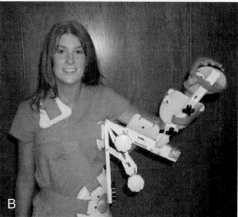

Figure 1-8 Joint active systems (JAS) shoulder arthrosis as a useful adjunct for treatment of frozen shoulder. (From Donatelli R: Physical therapy of the shoulder, 4th edition, 2005, Churchill Livingstone.)

study on rat tail tendons, the greatest increase in range of motion was seen when the LLPS was applied while the tendon was being heated vigorously.[208]

Passive Range of Motion

Passive motion has a positive effect on the quality of repair of different structures and is used postoperatively to facilitate joint repair.[209-211] Early PROM has multiple benefits. Early passive movement will help to decrease joint swelling by activating the trans-synovial pump. It also helps to increase the rate of improvement in range of motion after surgery or injury.[210,212,213] Passive range of motion helps to stimulate production of small amounts of cartilage.[171] In animals, it has been shown to promote repair of minor cartilage damage.[214] As stated in the remobilization section on connective tissue, PROM improves the quality of repair of ligaments, tendons, and synovial tissue. Passive range of motion also has been shown to reduce pain. In one study, a 12-minute daily session of PROM of the low back into flexion and extension cycles produced significant relief of low back pain.[215]

Passive range of motion for acute or chronically inflamed joints should be within the pain-free range and should not involve stretching. For connective tissue, movement should occur in the toe or the early elastic region of the joint on the stress-strain curve. For muscle, change occurs in the plastic region. Beyond this, damage may occur.[19] It can be concluded that patients who receive early PROM for joint surgery tend to have reduced hospital stay times and are able to return to normal daily activities earlier.[216]

Massage

Massage has been shown to increase muscle flexibility. Dynamic soft tissue mobilization (which consists of standard soft tissue mobilization techniques followed by distal to proximal longitudinal strokes performed during passive, active, and eccentric loading of the hamstring) was performed.[217] Dynamic soft tissue mobilization has been shown to increase hamstring flexibility.[217]

Massage to the muscle belly for a short time has been shown to reduce motor neuron excitability.[218] One study compared two intensities of massage. Higher-intensity massage produced greater motor neuron inhibition.[219] Similar results of reduced motor neuron excitability were found in patients with spinal cord injury.[219]

Massage also can be effective for gating pain. Gating is a form of competition involving sensory information.[38] During a massage, stimulation of proprioceptors competes with nociceptive information. This is a form of sensory gating. Another example of sensory gating can be seen right after an injury, when a person is stroking or rubbing the skin over an area of injury.[220]

Traditional massage techniques were found to be ineffective in increasing blood flow through the muscle. Mild exercise was found to be more effective in increasing blood flow.

Mobilization

No studies in the literature have explored the direct effect that mobilization has on joint structures, and although mobilization is a large part of physical therapy practice, little evidence reveals the effectiveness of mobilization. "Mobilization is the skilled passive movement to a joint and or related soft tissue at varying speeds and amplitudes, including a small amplitude high velocity therapeutic movement."[66] In this paper, mobilization and manipulation are synonymous. Research has concluded that end-range mobilization is effective in increasing range of motion,[221,222] and high-grade mobilization is more effective than low-grade mobilization for adhesive capsulitis of the shoulder.[223] Another study concluded that dorsal and ventral translational mobilization caused improvements in range of motion in abduction on the glenohumeral joint.[224] Although no direct evidence is available to support what is occurring at microscopic and macroscopic levels in the joint and in surrounding tissue, the inference can be made that mobilization aids in the alignment of collagen, improves the balance of GAGs and water content within the tissue, decreases the formation of adhesions, improves tensile properties, and encourages collagen turnover. These changes help to promote healing to ultimately increase range of motion and restore function.

REFERENCES

1. Kjaer M: Role of extracellular matrix in adaptation of tendon and skeletal muscle to mechanical loading, Physiol Rev 84:649-698, 2004.
2. Donatelli R: Sports-specific rehabilitation, St. Louis, 2007, Churchill Livingstone.
3. Billeter R, Hoppeler H: Muscular basis of strength. In Komi P: Strength and power in sport, Oxford, 1992, Blackwell Scientific Publications.
4. Zammit P, Beauchamp J. Differentiation: the skeletal muscle satellite cell: stem cell or son of the stem cell? London, 2001, Blackwell Wissenschafts-Verlag.
5. Hawke T, Garry D: Myogenic satellite cells: physiology to molecular biology, J Appl Physiol 91:534-551, 2001.
6. Kuang S, et al: Asymmetric self-renewal and commitment of satellite stem cells in muscle, Cell 129(5):999-1010, 2007.
7. Sacks R, Roy R: Architecture of the hindlimb muscles of cats: functional significance, J Morphol 173:185-195, 1982.
8. Kawakami Y, Abe T, Fukunaga T: Muscle-fiber pennation angles are greater in hypertrophied than in normal muscles, J Appl Physiol 74:2740-2744, 1993.
9. Larsson L, Sjödin B, Karlsson J: Histochemical and biomechanical changes in human skeletal muscle with age in sedentary males ate 22-65 years, Acta Physiol Scand 103:31-39, 1978.
10. Wang K: Sarcomere-associate cytoskeletal lattices in striated muscle. In Shay J, editor: Cell muscle motility, vol 6, New York, 1985, Plenum Publishing.
11. Enorka R: Eccentric contractions require unique activation strategies by the nervous system, J Physiol 123:2339-2346, 1996.
12. Proske U, Morgan D: Muscle damage from eccentric exercise: mechanism, mechanical signs, adaptation and clinical application, J Physiol 537:333-345, 2001.
13. McHugh M: Recent advances in the understanding of the repeated bout effect: the protective effect against muscle damage from a single bout of eccentric exercise, Scand J Med Sci Sports 13(2):88-97, 2003.
14. Raven P: Contraction: a definition of muscle action, Med Sci Sports Exer 23(7):777-778, 1991.
15. McGill S: Ultimate back fitness and performance, Ontario, 2004, Wabuno.
16. Danneels L, Vanderstraeten G, Cambier D, et al: Effects of three different training modalities on the cross sectional area of the lumbar multifidus muscle in patients with chronic low back pain, Br J Sports Med 35:186-191, 2001.
17. Marieb E: Human anatomy and physiology, ed 3, Redwood City, Calif, 1995, The Benjamin/Cummings Publishing Company, Inc.

18. Juanqueira LC, Carneiro J, Kelly RO: Basic histology, ed 8, Norwalk, Conn, 1995, Appleton and Lange.

19. Delforge G: Musculoskeletal trauma implications for sports injury management, Champaign, Ill, 2002, Human Kinetics.

20. Soderberg GL: Kinesiology: application to pathological motion, Baltimore, 1986, Williams and Wilkins.

21. Lieber RL, Brown CG, Trestik CL: Model of muscle-tendon interaction during frog semitendinosis fixed-end contractions, J Biomech 25:421, 1999.

22. Lieber RL, et al: Frog semitendinosus tendon load-strain and stress-strain properties during passive loading, Am J Physiol 261:C86-C92, 1991.

23. Liu SH, et al: Collagen in tendon, ligament, and bone healing: a current review, Clin Orthop Rel Res 318:265-278, 1995.

24. Birk DE, Mayne R: Localization of collagen types I, III, and IV during tendon development: changes in collagen types I and III are correlated with changes in fibril diameter, Eur J Cell Biol 72(4):352-361, 1997.

25. Linsenmayer TF, et al: Type V collagen: molecular structure and fibrillar organization of the chicken al(V) Nh2-terminal domain, a putative regulator of corneal fibrillogenesis, J Cell Biol 121(5):1181-1189, 1993.

26. Donatelli R, Owens-Burkhardt H: Effects of immobilization on the extensibility of periarticular connective tissue, J Orthop Sports Phys Ther 3:67, 1981.

27. Akeson WH, Ameil D, Woo SL-Y: Immobility effects of synovial joints: the pathomechanics of joint contracture, Biorheology 17:95, 1980.

28. Lyon RM, et al: Ultrastructural difference between the cells of the medial collateral ligament and the anterior cruciate ligament, Clin Orthop 272:279, 1991.

29. Amiel D, et al: Tendons and ligaments: a morphological and biomechanical comparison, J Orthop Res 1:257, 1984.

30. Frank C, et al: Normal ligament properties and ligament healing, Clin Orthop 196:15, 1985.

31. Reigger CL: Mechanical properties of bone. In Davies GJ, Gould JA, editors: Orthopedic and sports physical therapy. ed 2, St. Louis, 1985, Mosby, and Reigger-Krugh CL: Bone. In Malone TR, McPoil TG, Nitz AJ, editors: Orthopaedic and sports physical therapy, ed 3, St Louis, 1997, Mosby.

32. Frankel VH, Nordin M: Basic biomechanics of the skeletal system, Philadelphia, 1980, Lea & Febiger.

33. Tortora G, Anagnostakos N: Principles of anatomy and physiology, ed 6, New York, 1990, Harper Collins Publishers.

34. Syroid D, et al: Cell death in the Schwann cell lineage and its regulation by neuregulin, Proc Natl Acad Sci USA 93:9229-9234, 1996.

35. Zhang G: Evaluating the viscoelastic properties of biological tissues in a new way, J Musculoskelet Neuronal Interact 5(1):85-90, 2005.

36. Lieber L, Bodine-Fowler S: Skeletal muscle mechanics: implications for rehabilitation, Phys Ther 73:844-856, 1993.

37. Smith L, Weiss E, Lehmkuhl D: Brunnstrom's clinical kinesiology, ed 5, Philadelphia, 1996, F.A. Davis.

38. Lederman E: The science and practice of manual therapy, ed 2, 2005, Churchill Livingstone.

39. Butler DL et al: Biomechanics of ligaments and tendons, Exerc Sport Sci Rev 6:126, 1979.

40. Woo SL-Y et al: Anatomy, biology and biomechanics of tendon and ligaments: orthopaedic basic science, 2nd edition, 581-616, Rosemont, Ill, 2000, American Academy of Orthopaedic Surgeons.

41. Woo SL-Y, Gomez MA, Akeson WH: The time and history-dependent viscoelastic properties of the canine medial collateral ligament, J Biomech Eng 103(4):293-298, 1981.

42. Taylor DC, et al: Viscoelastic properties of muscle-tendon units: the biomechanical effects of stretching, Am J Sports Med 18(3):300-309, 1990.

43. Poo MM: Rapid lateral diffusion of functional ACh receptors in embryonic muscle cell membrane, Nature 295:332-334, 1982.

44. Fukuda E: Mechanical deformation and electrical polarization in biological substances, Biorheology 5:199, 1968.

45. Eliasson P, et al: Unloaded rat achilles tendons continue to grow, but lose viscoelasticity, J Appl Physiol Aug;103(2):459-463, 2007, Epub 2007 Apr. 5.

46. Rannou F, Poiraudeau S, Revel M: Cartilage: from biomechanics to physical therapy, Ann Readapt Med Phys 44(5):259-267, 2001.

47. Eckstein F, Hudelmaier M, Putz R: The effects of exercise on human articular cartilage, J Anat 208(4):491-512, 2006.

48. Kjaer M, et al: Metabolic activity and collagen turnover in human tendon in response to physical activity, J Musculoskelet Neuronal Interact Mar;5(1):41-42, 2005.

49. Turner CH: Three rules for bone adaptation to mechanical stimuli, Bone Nov;23(5):399-407, 1998.

50. Krahl H, et al: Stimulation of bone growth through sports, Am J Sports Med 22:751-757, 1994.

51. Salter RB: Textbook of disorders and injuries of the musculoskeletal system, ed 3, Baltimore, 1999, Williams and Wilkins.

52. Burr DB, Robling AG, Turner CH: Effects of biomechanical stress on bones in animals, Bone 30(5):781-786, 2002.

53. Saxon LK et al: Mechanosensitivity of the rat skeleton decreases after a long period of loading, but is improved with time off, Bone 36(3):454-464, 2005.

54. Yingling VR, Davies S, Silva MJ: The effects of repetitive physiologic loading on bone turnover and mechanical properties in adult female and male rats, Calcif Tissue Int 68(4):235-239, 2001, Epub 2001 Apr 11.

55. Cullen DM, Smith RT, Akhter MP: Bone-loading response varies with strain magnitude and cycle number, J Appl Physiol 91(5):1971-1976, 2001.

56. Borer KT: Physical activity in the prevention and amelioration of osteoporosis in women: interaction of mechanical, hormonal and dietary factors, Sports Med 35(9):779-830, 2005.

57. Dilley A, et al: Quantitative in vivo studies of median nerve sliding in response to wrist, elbow, shoulder, and neck movements, Clin Biomech 18: 899-907, 2003.

58. Millesi H, Zoch G, Reihsner R: Mechanical properties of peripheral nerves, Clin Orthop Relat Res 314:76-83, 1995.

59. McLellan D, Swash M: Longitudinal sliding of the median nerve during movements of the upper limb, J Neurol Neurosurg Psychiatry 39:566-570, 1976.

60. Erel E, Dilley A, Greening J, et al: Longitudinal sliding of the median nerve in patients with carpal tunnel syndrome, J Hand Surg Br 28:439-443, 2003.

61. Topp K, Boyd B: Structure and biomechanics of peripheral nerves: nerve reponses to physical stresses and implications for physical therapist practice, Phys Ther 86:92-109, 2006.

62. Sunderland S: The anatomy and physiology of nerve injury, Muscle Nerve 13:771-784, 1990.

63. Kwan M, et al: Strain, stress, and stretch of peripheral nerve: rabbit experiments in vitro and in vivo, Acta Orthop Scand 63 :267-272, 1992.

64. Pourmand R, Ochs S, Jersild R Jr: The relation of the beading of myelinated fibers to the bands of Fontana, Neuroscience 61:373-380, 1994.

65. Walbeehm E, et al: Mechanical functioning of peripheral nerves: linkage with the "mushrooming" effect, Cell Tissue Res 316:115-121, 2004.

66. Paris S, Loubert P: Foundations of clinical orthopedics. ed 3, St. Augustine, Fla, 1999, Institute Press.

67. Yong L, Fu F, Huard J: Cutting edge muscle recovery: using antifibrosis agents to improve healing, The Physician and Sports Medicine 33(5), 2005.

68. Trojanowska M, et al: Pathogenesis of fibrosis: type 1 collagen and the skin, J Mol Med 76(3-4):266-274, 1998.

69. Schmid P, et al: Enhanced expression of transforming growth factor-beta type I and type II receptors in wound granulation tissue and hypertrophic scar, Am J Pathol 152(2):485-493, 1998.

70. Warren G, et al: Mechanisms of skeletal muscle injury and repair revealed by gene expression studies in mouse models, J Physiol May 3, 2007.

71. Huard J, Yong L, Fu F: Muscle injuries and repair: current trends in research, J Bone Joint Surg Am 84 :822-832, 2002.

72. Papadimitriou JM, et al: The process of new plasmalemma formation in focally injured skeletal muscle fibers, J Struct Biol 103:124-134, 1990.

73. Pizza FX, et al: Neutrophils injure cultured skeletal myotubes, Am J Physiol Cell Physiol 281:C335-C341, 2001.

74. Mitchell CA, McGeachie JK, Grounds MD: Cellular differences in the regeneration of murine skeletal muscle: a quantitative histological study in SJL/J and BALB/c mice, Cell Tissue Res 269:159-166, 1992.

75. Cantini M, Carraro U: Macrophage-released factor stimulates selectively myogenic cells in primary muscle culture, J Neuropathol Exp Neurol 54:121-128, 1995.

76. Massimino ML, et al: ED2+ macrophages increase selectively myoblast proliferation in muscle cultures, Biochem Biophys Res Commun 235:754-759, 1997.

77. Merly F, et al: Macrophage enhance muscle satellite cell proliferation and delay their differentiation, Muscle Nerve 22:724-732, 1999.

78. Robertson TA, et al: The role of macrophages in skeletal muscle regeneration with particular reference to chemotaxis, Exp Cell Res 207:321-331, 1993.

79. Grounds M: Towards understanding skeletal muscle regeneration, Pathol ResPract 187(1):1-22, 1991.

80. Hurme T, et al: Healing of skeletal muscle injury: an ultrastructural and immunohistochemical study, Med Sci Sports Exerc 23(7):801-810, 1991.

81. Niyibizi C, et al: Type V collagen is increased during rabbit medial collateral ligament healing, Knee Surg Sports Traumatol Arthrosc 8(5):281-285, 2005.

82. Hart RA, Woo SL-Y, Newton PO: Ultrastructural morphometry of anterior cruciate and medial collateral ligaments: an experimental study in rabbits, J Orthop Res 10(1):96-103, 1992.

83. Frank C, McDonald D, Shrive N: Collagen fibril diameters in the rabbit medial collateral ligament scar: a longer term assessment, Connect Tissue Res 36(3):261-269, 1997.

84. Frank C, Schachar N, Dittrich D: Natural history of healing in the repaired medial collateral ligament, J Orthop Res 1(2):179-188, 1983.

85. Miller RG: Acute versus chronic compressive neuropathy, Muscle Nerve 7:427, 1984.

86. Schlaepfer WW, Bunge RP: The effects of calcium ion concentration on the degradation of amputated axons in tissue culture, J Cell Biol 59:456, 1973.

87. Quan D, Bird S: Nerve conduction studies and electromyography in the evaluation of peripheral nerve injuries, U of Penn Ortho J 12:45-51, 1999.

88. Chaudry V, Cornblath DR: Wallerian degeneration in human nerves: a serial electrophysiologic study, Muscle Nerve 15:687, 1992.

89. Trojaborg W: Rate of recovery in motor and sensory fibers of the radial nerve: clinical and electrophysiologic aspects, J Neurol Neurosurg Psychiatry 33:625, 1970.

90. Miller RG: Injury to peripheral motor nerves, Muscle Nerve 10:689, 1987.

91. Bird SJ, Brown MJ: Peripheral nerve. In Dee R, et al, editors: Principles of orthopaedic practice, New York: 1997, McGraw-Hill, p 129.

92. Goldspink DF: The influence of activity on muscle size and protein turnover, J Physiol (Lond) 264:283-296, 1977.

93. Goldspink DF: The influence of immobilization and stretch on protein turnover of rat skeletal muscle, J Physiol (Lond) 264:267-282, 1977.

94. Max SR, Maier RF, Vogelsang L: Lysosomes and disuse atrophy of skeletal muscle, Arch Biochem Biophys 146:227-232, 1971.

95. Halkjaer-Kristensen J, Ingemann-Hansen T: Wasting of the human quadriceps after knee ligament injuries, Scand J Rehabil Med Suppl 13:5-11, 1985.

96. Vandenborne K, et al: Longitudinal study of skeletal muscle adaptations during immobilization and rehabilitation, Muscle Nerve 21:1006-1012, 1998.

97. Veldhuizen JW, et al: Functional and morphological adaptations following four weeks of knee immobilization, Int J Sports Med 14:283-287, 1993.

98. Shaffer M, et al: Effects of immobilization on plantar-flexion torque, fatigue resistance, and functional ability following an ankle fracture, Phys Ther 80(8):769-780, 2000.

99. Stillwell DM, McLarren GL, Gersten JW: Atrophy of quadriceps muscle due to immobilization of the lower extremity, Arch Phys Med Rehabil 48:289-295, 1967.

100. Duchateau J, Hainaut K: Effects of immobilization on contractile properties, recruitment, and firing of human motor units, J Physiol (Lond) 422:55-65, 1990.

101. Appell HJ: Muscular atrophy following immobilization: a review, Sports Med 10:42-58, 1990.

102. MacDougall JD, et al: Effects of strength training and immobilization on human muscle fibres, Eur J Appl Physiol 43 :25-34, 1980.

103. Muller EA: Influence of training and of inactivity on muscle strength, Arch Phys Med Rehabil 51(8):449-462, 1970.

104. Buckely DC, et al: Transcutaneous muscle stimulation promotes muscle growth in immobilized patients, J Parenteral Enteral Nutr 11(6):547-551, 1987.

105. Gould N, et al: Transcutaneous muscle stimulation as a method to retard disuse atrophy, Clin Orthop 164:215-220, 1982.

106. Gould N, et al: Transcutaneous muscle stimulation to retard disuse atrophy after open meniscectomy, Clin Orthop 178:190-197, 1983.

107. Hortobágyi T, et al: Changes in muscle strength, muscle fibre size, and myofibrillar gene expression after immobilization and retraining in humans, J Physiol 524.1:293-304, 2000.

108. Deschenes M, et al: Neural factors account for strength decrements after short-term muscle unloading, Am J Physiol Regul Integr Comp Physiol 282(2):R578-R583, 2002.

109. Lieber RL, et al: Differential response of the dog quadriceps muscle to external skeletal fixation of the knee, Muscle Nerve 11(3):193-201, 1988.

110. Edgerton V, et al: Human fiber size and enzymatic properties after 5 and 11 days of space flight, J Appl Physiol 78:1733-1739, 1995.

111. Boonyarom I: Atrophy and hypertrophy of skeletal muscles: structural and functional aspects, Acta Physiologica 188(2):77-89, 2006.

112. Widrick J, et al: Effect of a 17-day space flight on contractile properties of human soleus muscle fibres, J Physiol 516:915-930, 1999.

113. Fitts R, Riley D, Widrick J: Physiology of a microgravity environment. Invited review: microgravity and skeletal muscle, J Appl Physiol 89:823-839, 2000.

114. Tischler M, et al: Spaceflight on STS-48 and earth-based unweighting produce similar effects of skeletal muscle of young rats, J Appl Physiol 74:2161-2165, 1993.

115. Oki D, et al: Capillaries with fenestrae in the rat soleus muscle after experimental limb immobilization, J Electron Microsc 44:307-310, 1995.

116. Rifenberick D, Gamble J, Max S: Response of mitochondrial enzymes to decreased muscular activity, Am J Physiol 225:1295-1299, 1973.

117. Mujika I, Padilla S: Muscular characteristics of detraining in humans, Med Sci Sports Exerc 33:1297-1303, 2001.

118. Smith H, et al: Nuclear DNA fragmentation and morphological alterations in adult rabbit skeletal muscle after short-term immobilization, Cell Tissue Res 302:235-241, 2000.

119. Hawke T: Muscle stem cells and exercise training, Exercise and Sport Science Reviews 33:63-68, 2005.

120. Berg H, et al: Effects of lower limb unloading on skeletal muscle mass and function in humans, J App Physiol 70:1882-1885, 1991.

121. Akeson WH, Woo SL, et al: The connective tissue response to immobility: biochemical changes in periarticular connective tissue of the immobilized rabbit knee, Clin Orthop Rel Res 93:356-362, 1973.

122. Akeson WH, et al: The collective tissue response to immobility: an accelerated aging response, Exp Gerontol 3:289-301, 1968.

123. Trudel G, et al: Measurement of articular cartilage surface irregularity in rate knee contracture, J Rheumatol Oct;30(10):2218-2225, 2003.

124. Vanwanseele B, Lucchinetti E, Stussi E: The effects of immobilization on the characteristics of articular cartilage: current concepts and future directions, Osteoarthritis Cartilage 10(5):408-419, 2002.

125. Vanwanseele B, et al: Knee cartilage of spinal cord-injured patients displays progressive thinning in the absence of normal joint loading and movement, Arthritis Rheum 46(8):2073-2078, 2002.

126. Hinterwimmer S, et al: Cartilage atrophy in the knees of patients after seven weeks of partial load bearing, Arthritis Rheum 50(8):2516-2520, 2004.

127. Frank C, et al: Physiology and therapeutic value of passive range of motion, Clin Orthop Rel Res 185:113-125, 1984.

128. Amiel D, et al: The effect of immobilization on collagen turnover in connective tissue: a biochemical-

biomechanical correlation, Acta Orthopaedica Scandinavica 53:325-332, 1982.

129. Dehne E, Torp RP: Treatment of joint injuries by immediate mobilization: based on the spinal adaptation concept, Clin Orthop 77:218, 1971.

130. Woo SL, et al: The biomechanical and morphological changes in the medial collateral ligament of the rabbit after immobilization and remobilization, J Bone Joint Surg Am 69(8):1200-1211, 1987.

131. Laros GS, Tipton CM, Cooper RR: Influence of physical activity on ligament insertions in the knees of dogs, J Bone Joint Surg Am 53(2):275-286, 1971.

132. Newton PO, et al: Immobilization of the knee joint alters the mechanical and ultrastructural properties of the rabbit anterior cruciate ligament, J Orthop Res 13(2):191-200, 1995.

133. Montgomery RD: Healing of muscle, ligaments, and tendons, Semin Vet Med Surg (Small Animal) 4(4):304-311, 1989.

134. Gelberman RH, et al: Flexor tendon repair, J Orthop Res 4:119-128, 1985.

135. Woo SL-Y, et al: Connective tissue response to immobility: correlative study of biomechanical and biochemical measurements of normal and immobilized rabbit knees, Arthritis Rheum 18(3):257-264, 1975.

136. LaVigne AB, Watkins RP: Preliminary results on immobilization-induced stiffness of monkey knee joints and posterior capsule. In Perspectives in biomedical engineering. Proceedings of a symposium, Biological Engineering Society, University of Strathclyde, Glasgow, June 1972. Baltimore: 1973, University Park Press.

137. Steinberg FU: The immobilized patient: functional pathology and management, New York, 1980, Plenum.

138. Little K, De Valderama JF: Some mechanisms involved in the osteoporotic process, Gerontologia 14:109, 1968.

139. Hardt AB: Early metabolic responses of bone to immobilization, J Bone Joint Surg 54(a):119, 1972.

140. Geiser M, Trueta J: Muscle action, bone rarification and bone formation, J Bone Joint Surg 40(b):282, 1958.

141. Heer M, et al: Immobilization induces a very rapid increase in osteoclastic activity, Acta Astronautica 57(1):31-36, 2005

142. Raney RB, Brashear HR: Shand's handbook of orthopaedic surgery, ed 8, St. Louis, 1971, Mosby.

143. Pachter B, Eberstein A: The effect of limb immobilization and stretch on the fine structure of the neuromuscular junction in rat muscle, Exp Neurol 92:13-19, 1986.

144. Malathi S, Batmanabane M: Effects of varying periods of immobilization of a limb on the morphology of a peripheral nerve, Acta Morphol Neerl Scand 21:185-198, 1983.

145. Malathi S, Batmanabane M: Effects of immobilization of a limb on the maturation of a peripheral nerve in kittens, Acta Anat 132:191-196, 1988.

146. Eisen A, et al: The effects of muscle hyper- and hypoactivity upon fiber diameters of intact and regenerating nerves, J Neurol Sci 20:457-469, 1973.

147. Appenzeller O, Ogin G, Palmer G: Fiber size spectra and cyclic AMP content of sciatic nerves: effect of muscle hypoactivity and hyperactivity, Exp Neurol 50:595-604, 1976.

148. Menetrey J, et al: Suturing versus immobilization of a muscle laceration: a morphological and functional study in a mouse model, Am J Sports Med 27:222-229, 1999.

149. Garrett W, et al: Recovery of skeletal muscle after laceration and repair, Am J Hand Surg 9(5):683-692, 1984.

150. Beredjiklian P: Biologic aspects of flexor tendon laceration and repair, Am J Bone Jt Surg 85:539-550, 2003.

151. Kasemkijwattana C, et al: Use of growth factors to improve muscle healing after strain injury, Clin Orthop 370:272-285, 1999.

152. Lehto M, Jarvinen M, Nelimarkka O: Scar formation after skeletal muscle injury: a histological and autoradiographical study in rats, Arch Orthop Trauma Surg 104:366-370, 1986.

153. Li Y, Cummins J, Huard J: Muscle injury and repair, Curr Opin Orthop 12:409-415, 2001.

154. Chan Y, et al: Antifibrotic effects of suramin in injured skeletal muscle after laceration, J Appl Physiol 95:771-780, 2003.

155. Taylor D, et al: Experimental muscle strain injury: early functional and structural deficits, and the increased risk for reinjury, Am J Sports Med 21:190-194, 1993.

156. Menetrey J, et al: Growth factors improve muscle healing in vivo, J Bone Joint Surg Br 82:131-137, 2000.

157. Yue G, et al: Task-dependent effect of limb immobilization on the fatigability of the elbow flexor muscles in humans, Exp Physiol 82:567-592, 1997.

158. Kvist M, et al: Vascular density at the myotendinous junction of the rat gastrocnemius muscle after immobilization and remobilization, Am J Sports Med 23:359-364, 1995.

159. Berg H, Tesch P: Changes in muscle function in response to 10 days of lower limb unloading in humans, Acta Physiologica Scandinavica 157(1):63-70, 1996.

160. Booth F: Regrowth of atrophied skeletal muscle in adult rats after ending immobilization, J Appl Physiol 44:225-230, 1978.

161. Iway S, et al: Potential role for Id myogenic repressors in apoptosis and attenuation of hypertrophy in muscles of aged rats, Am J Physiol Cell Physiol 283:C66-C76, 2002.

162. Childs T, et al: Temporal alterations in protein signaling cascades during recovery from muscle atrophy, Am J Physiol Cell Physiol 285:C391-C398, 2003.

163. Degens H, Alway S: Skeletal muscle function and hypertrophy are diminished in old age, Muscle Nerve 27:339-347, 2003.

164. Pattison S, Folk L, Madsen R, Booth F: Selected contribution: identification of differentially expressed genes between young and old rat soleus muscle during recovery from immobilization-induced atrophy, J Appl Physiol 95:2171-2179, 2003.

165. Blough E, Linderman J: Lack of skeletal muscle hypertrophy in very aged male Fischer 344 x Brown Norway rats, J Appl Physiol 88:1265-1270, 2000.

166. Chargé S, Rudnicki M: Cellular and molecular regulation of muscle regeneration, Physiol Rev 84:209-238, 2004.

167. Lastayo P, et al: Chronic eccentric exercise: improvements in muscle strength can occur with little demand for oxygen, Am J Physiol 276:R611-R615, 1999.

168. Hargens AR, Akeson WH: Stress effects pm tissue nutrition and viability. In Hargens AR, editor: Tissue nutrition and viability, New York, 1986, Springer-Verlag.

169. Buckwalter JA, Grodzinsky AJ: Loading of healing bone, fibrous tissue, and muscle: implications for orthopaedic practice, J Am Acad Orthop Surg 7(5):291-299, 1999.

170. Eckstein F, et al: Functional adaptation of human joints to mechanical stimuli, Osteoarthritis and Cartilage 10(1):44-50, 2002.

171. Viidik A: Functional properties of collagenous tissue, Review of Connective Tissue Research 6:144-149, 1970.

172. Arnoczky SP, et al: Activation of stress-activated protein kinases (SAPK) in tendon cells following cyclic strain: the effects of strain frequency, strain magnitude, and cytosolic calcium, J Orthop Res 20(5):947-952, 2002.

173. Bosch U, et al: Effect of cyclical stretch on matrix synthesis of human patellar tendon cells, Unfallchirurg 105(5):437-442, 2002.

174. Graf R, et al: Mechanosensitive induction of apoptosis in fibroblasts is regulated by thrombospondin-1 and integrin associated protein (CD47), Apoptosis 7(6):493-498, 2002.

175. Zeichen J, van Griensven M, Bosch U: The proliferative response of isolated human tendon fibroblasts to cyclic biaxial mechanical strain, Am J Sports Med 28(6):888-892, 2000.

176. Haapala J, et al: Incomplete restoration of immobilization induced softening of young beagle knee articular cartilage after 50-week remobilization, Int J Sports Med 21(1):76-81, 2000.

177. Fronek J, et al: The effect of intermittent passive motion in the healing of medial collateral ligament, Proceedings of the Orthopaedic Research Society 8:31, 1983 (abstract).

178. Vailas AC, et al: Physical activity and its influence on the repair process of medial collateral ligament, Connective Tissue Research 9:25-31, 1981.

179. Gelberman RH, et al: Effects of early intermittent passive mobilization on healing canine flexor tendons, J Hand Surg 7(2):170-175, 1982.

180. Pneumaticos SG, et al: The effects of early mobilization in the healing of Achilles tendon repair, Foot and Ankle International 21(7):551-557, 2000.

181. Savio SL-Y, et al: The importance of controlled passive mobilization on flexor tendon healing, Acta Orthop Scand 52:615-622, 1981.

182. Chimich D, et al: Water content alters viscoelastic behavior of the normal adolescent rabbit medial collateral ligament, J Biomech 25(8):831-837, 1992.

183. Trebacz H: Disuse-induced deterioration of bone strength is not stopped after free remobilization in young adult rats, J Biomechanics 34(12):1631-1636, 2001.

184. Trebacz H, Dmowska M, Baj J: Age-dependent effect of limb immobilization and remobilization on rat bone, Folia Biol (Krakow) 50(3-4):121-127, 2002.

185. van Harreveld P, et al: Effects of immobilization followed by remobilization on mineral density, histomorphometric features, and formation of the bones of the metacarpophalangeal joint in horses, Am J Vet Res 63(2):276-281, 2002.

186. Warner SE, Shea JE, Miller SC, Shaw JM: Adaptations in cortical and trabecular bone in response to mechanical loading with and without weight bearing, Calcif Tissue Int 79(6):395-403, 2006, Epub 2006 Dec 8.

187. Whiting WC, Zernicke RF: Biomechanics of musculoskeletal injury. Champaign, Ill, 1998, Human Kinetics.

188. Kannus P, Jarvinen TL, Sievanen H, et al: Effects of immobilization, three forms of remobilization, and subsequent deconditioning on bone mineral content and density in rat femora, J Bone Miner Res 11(9):1339-1346, 1996.

189. Payne H: Nerve repair and grafting in the upper extremity, J South Orthop Assoc 10(2):173-181, 2001.

190. Putz-Anerson V, editor: Cumulative trauma disorders: a manual for musculoskeletal diseases of the upper limbs, New York, 1988, Taylor and Francis.

191. Mueller M, Maluf K: Tissue adaptation to physical stress: a proposed "physical stress theory" to guide physical therapist practice, education and research, Phys Ther 82(4):383-403, 2002.

192. Novak C, Mackinnon S: Repetitive use and static postures; a source of nerve compression and pain, J Hand Ther 10:151-159, 1997.

193. Nowakowski P, Delitto A, Erhard R: Lumbar spinal stenosis, Phys Ther 76:187-190, 1996.

194. Penning L, Wilmink J: Posture-dependent bilateral compression of L4 or L5 nerve roots in facet hypertrophy: a dynamic CT-myelographic study, Spine 12:488-500, 1987.

195. Hepburn G, et al: Multi-center clinical investigation of the effect of incorporating Dynasplint® treatment into standard physical therapy practice for restoring range of motion of elbows and knees, presented at the New York APTA State Chapter Meeting, New York, April 26, 1985.

196. Sapega A, et al: Biophysical factors in range-of-motion exercise, Physician Sportsmed 9(12):57-65, 1981.

197. Light KE, et al: Low-load prolonged stretch versus high-load brief stretch in treating knee contractures, Phys Ther 64:330-333, 1984.

198. Zito M, et al: Lasting effects of one bout of two 15-second passive stretches on ankle dorsiflexion range of motion, J Orthop Sports Phys Ther 24:214-221, 1997.

199. Blanton S, Grissom S, Riolo L: Use of a static adjustable ankle-foot orthosis following tibial nerve block to reduce plantar-flexion contracture in an individual with brain injury, Phys Ther 82(11):1087-1097, 2002.

200. Bohannon RW: Effect of repeated eight-minute muscle loading on the angle of straight-leg raising, Phys Ther 64:491-497, 1984.

201. Steffan T, Mollinger L: Low-load, prolonged stretch in the treatment of knee flexion contractures in nursing home residents, Phys Ther 73:886-895, 1995.

202. Willis B, Neffendorf C, Gaspar P: Device and physical therapy unfreeze shoulder motion, Biomech, January 2007.

203. MacKay-Lyons M: Low-lad, prolonged stretch in treatment of elbow flexion contractures secondary to head trauma: a case report, Phys Ther 69(4):292-296, 1989.

204. Donatelli R, et al: Frozen shoulder encapsulates therapy challenges, Biomech Feb 2006.

205. Nordin M, Frankel VH: Basic biomechanics of the musculoskeletal system, ed 3, Philadelphia, 2001, Lippincott, Williams & Wilkins.

206. Bonutti PM, et al: Static progressive stretch to reestablish elbow range of motion, Clin Orthop Relat Res 303:128-134, 1994.

207. Peres S, et al: Pulsed shortwave diathermy and prolonged long-duration stretching increase dorsiflexion range of motion more than identical stretching without diathermy, J Athletic Training 37(1):43-50, 2002.

208. Warren CG, Lehmann JF, Koblanski JN: Heat and stretch procedures: an evaluation using rat tail tendon, Arch Phys Med Rehabil 57(3):122-126, 1976.

209. McCarthy MR, et al: The effects of immediate continuous passive motion on pain during the inflammatory phase of soft tissue healing following anterior cruciate ligament reconstruction, J Orthop Sports Phys Ther 17(2):96-101, 1993.

210. Raab MG, et al: Early results of continuous passive motion after rotator cuff repair: a prospective, randomized, blinded, controlled study, Am J Orthop 25(3):214-220, 1996.

211. Korcock M: Motion, not immobility, advocated for healing synovial joints, JAMA 246(18):2005-2006, 1981.

212. Simkin PA, et al: Continuous passive motion for osteoarthritis of the hip: a pilot study, Rheumatology 26(9):1987-1991, 1999.

213. O'Driscoll SW, Giori NJ: Continuous passive motion (CPM): theory and principles of clinical application, J Rehab Res Dev 37(2):179-188, 2000.

214. Williams JM, et al: Continuous passive motion stimulates repair of rabbit knee articular cartilage after matrix proteoglycan loss, Clinical Orthopedics 304:252-262, 1994.

215. Oron A, et al: Continuous passive mobilization to the lower vertebral column—a controlled randomized study, Department of Orthopaedics, Assaf Harofeh Medical Center, Zerifin, Israel (unpublished), 2003.

216. Johnson DP: The effect of continuous passive motion on wound-healing and joint mobility after knee arthroplasty, J Bone Joint Surg (American) 72(3):421-426, 2000.

217. Hopper D, et al: Dynamic soft tissue mobilization increases hamstring flexibility in healthy male subjects, Br J Sports Med Sep;39(9):594-598, 2005.

218. Sullivan SJ, et al: Effects of massage on alpha neuron excitability, Physical Therapy 71(8):555-560, 1991.

219. Goldberg J, et al: The effect of therapeutic massage on H-reflex amplitude in persons with spinal cord injury, Physical Therapy 74(8):728-737, 1991.

220. Hannington-Kiff JG: 1981 Pain, London, 1981, Yodate Publications.

221. Yang J-I, et al: Mobilization techniques in subjects with frozen shoulder syndrome: randomized multiple-treatment trial, Phys Ther 87(10):1307-1315, 2007.

222. Vermeulen H, et al: End-range mobilization techniques in adhesive capsulitis of the shoulder joint: a multiple-subject case report, Phys Ther 80(12):1204-1213, 2000.

223. Vermeulen H, et al: Comparison of high-grade and low-grade mobilization techniques in the management of adhesive capsulitis of the shoulder: randomized controlled trial, Phys Ther 86(3):355-368, 2006.

224. Hsu A-T, et al: Changes in abduction and rotation range of motion in response to simulated dorsal and ventral translational mobilization of the glenohumeral joint, Phys Ther 82(6):544-556, 2002.

Exercise Treatment of the Rehabilitation Patient
Cardiopulmonary and Peripheral Responses

Rehabilitation services provided after injury or surgery often fail to include a fitness training program. In view of statistics suggesting that physical activity participation is generally low in the United States,[1] and coupled with statistics suggesting that the prevalence of obesity is rising,[2,3] a therapist's recommendation to increase habitual physical activity and encourage participation in a regular exercise program is important. Once the injured extremity or spine has achieved an acceptable level of function, program goals should be adjusted to achieve an overall state of cardiovascular fitness that is at least equal to that of the preinjured state.

This chapter discusses the completion of rehabilitation through endurance exercise training, with the goal of increasing cardiorespiratory fitness level. First, the cardiovascular responses to acute exercise and the physiologic benefits of endurance exercise training are discussed. Second, data on the physiologic consequences of physical inactivity are reviewed. Changes that occur within the cardiovascular system as a result of extreme physical inactivity, such as bed rest, are striking. Although the effects are more subtle, even partial bed rest, immobilization, or simply reduced habitual physical activity can set in motion the same physiologic changes. Third, individual patient risk stratification is presented, to allow the therapist to determine whether it is appropriate for a patient to begin exercise immediately, or if further medical workup is warranted. Fourth, basic exercise prescription is reviewed. This chapter is not intended to replace the many excellent sources on this topic,[4] but rather to provide the therapist with a brief overview of the exercise prescription process. The guidelines presented in this chapter are consistent with the goals of the new initiative of the American College of Sports Medicine (ACSM) entitled "Exercise Is Medicine." The vision of this recent initiative is "to make physical activity and exercise a standard part of a disease prevention and treatment medical paradigm in the United States"[4] and "for physical activity to be considered by all healthcare providers as a vital sign in every patient visit …"[4] Additional information on this initiative can be found at http://www.exerciseismedicine.org.

CARDIOVASCULAR RESPONSES TO EXERCISE

During dynamic exercise, heart rate, stroke volume, and systolic blood pressure are increased. Cardiac output (the product of heart rate and stroke volume) thus increases, allowing more blood to circulate to the working muscles. The initial increase in cardiac output during acute exercise is the result of increases in both heart rate and stroke volume (to approximately 40% of oxygen consumption [$\dot{V}O_2$] maximum), whereas with more vigorous exercise, additional elevations in cardiac output are caused by increases in heart rate. As the intensity or workload becomes greater, $\dot{V}O_2$ rises.

Oxygen demand of the working tissues also rises during exercise of working tissues. To supply the working muscles with more oxygen, blood flow is redistributed in the periphery. Specifically, vasodilation to exercising skeletal muscles (to allow for greater blood flow) occurs, while blood vessels to non-exercising tissues such as the splanchnic region (i.e., the GI tract and liver) are constricted. Vasoconstriction to non-exercising tissues allows more blood to move to working skeletal and heart muscle. Also, an increase in the arteriovenous oxygen (a-vO_2) difference during an exercise bout shows that more oxygen is being extracted by the working tissues: at $\dot{V}O_2$ max, 80% to 85% of the oxygen is extracted from the blood.[5]

Maximum oxygen uptake—or $\dot{V}O_2$ max—is the gold standard of cardiorespiratory fitness. $\dot{V}O_2$ max is calculated by using the Fick equation as follows:

$$\dot{V}O_2 \max = (HR \ max) \times (SV \ max) \times (a\text{-}vO_2 \ diff \ max)^5$$

Both central and peripheral adaptations contribute to an increase in $\dot{V}O_2$ max (or whole-body oxygen consumption) with endurance training. During endurance training, resting heart rate is reduced, allowing more time in diastole for the heart to fill with blood. Stroke volume and contractility are also greater; thus, the heart pumps more efficiently. Resting blood pressure is modestly reduced as a result of regular endurance training.[6] Physical activity also results in an increase in blood volume. As depicted in Figure 2-1, the initial increase

---

†Deceased.

in blood volume with exercise training is due primarily to increases in plasma volume, whereas sustained elevations in blood volume are due to an increase in both plasma volume and RBC volume; the result is an 8% to 10% increase in blood volume.[7]

Physically active individuals have 20% to 25% more blood volume compared with sedentary individuals,[8] and Convertino demonstrated a positive linear correlation between blood volume and $\dot{V}O_2$ max.[8] Increases in both plasma and blood volume in response to endurance training allow for greater

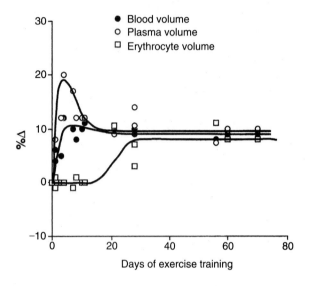

Figure 2-1 Initial and long-term changes to blood, plasma, and red blood cell volume attained through exercise training. (From Sawka MN, Convertino VA, Eichner ER, Schnieder SM, Young AJ: Blood volume: importance and adaptations to exercise training, environmental stresses, and trauma/sickness. Med Sci Sports Exerc 32(2):332-348, 2000.)

venous return to the heart. This increased venous return increases stroke volume. Thus cardiac output—and ultimately $\dot{V}O_2$ max—increases as a result of endurance training. This increase in $\dot{V}O_2$ max with training is illustrated in Figure 2-2.[5] As an individual moves from sedentary to normally active to conditioned, not only workload but also $\dot{V}O_2$ max is increased. The maximum oxygen consumption is determined when the individual reaches a plateau in terms of oxygen uptake.[5]

Increased blood volume causes structural changes to the heart, particularly to the left ventricle. Endurance training can cause an increase in left ventricular mass and chamber size (i.e., left ventricular hypertrophy or volume hypertrophy). This is commonly seen in runners and in rowing athletes and sometimes is referred to as "the athlete's heart."[9] In addition to these central adaptations, exercise training causes peripheral changes. The number and density of capillaries per muscle fiber, for example, increase in active skeletal muscle, allowing for better gas exchange.

Age-related declines in cardiovascular function during exercise do occur and include increases in resting and exercising blood pressure and decreases in exercising heart rate max, cardiac output, and $\dot{V}O_2$ max.[10,11] Therefore, aging may be viewed as a model of deconditioning. Although differences in cardiovascular response to acute exercise have been noted between young and old individuals,[10,11] the cardiovascular adaptations that occur as a result of endurance training are similar.[11,12] However, the increase that occurs in $\dot{V}O_2$ max in older adults may be due to increases in the a-vO_2 difference max (peripheral effects).[12]

Regular physical activity improves cardiovascular function. Any progress along the physical activity spectrum[13] (i.e., increasing regular physical activity per guidelines stated later in this chapter) can reduce the risk of mortality (Figure 2-3).[14] However, certain injuries or diseases may impair daily living

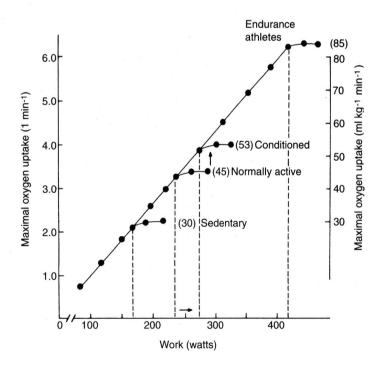

Figure 2-2 Increase in maximum oxygen consumption ($\dot{V}O_2$ max) attained through endurance training. (From Rowell LB: Human circulation: regulation during physical stress. New York, 1986, Oxford University Press.)

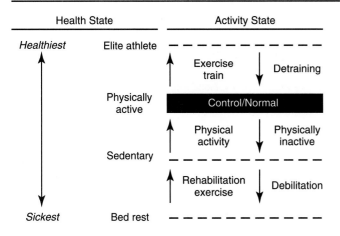

Figure 2-3 The health-activity spectrum. (From Booth FW, Lees SJ: Physically active subjects should be the control group. Med Sci Sports Exerc 38(30):405-406, 2006.)

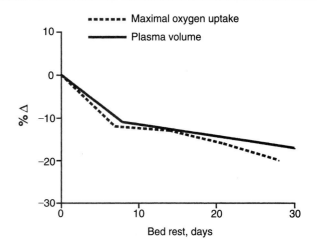

Figure 2-4 Plasma volume lost in bed rest. (From Convertino VA: Cardiovascular consequences of bed rest: effect on maximal oxygen uptake. Med Sci Sports Exerc 29(2):191-196, 1997.)

and the individual's ability to be physically active or to exercise. The most severe case of physical inactivity is bed rest. Several studies have used bed rest as a model to examine the cardiovascular response to physical inactivity.

PHYSIOLOGIC CONSEQUENCES OF PHYSICAL INACTIVITY

As depicted on the health-activity spectrum (see Figure 2-3), bed rest is viewed as the "sickest state."[13,15] Certain populations, such as patients with stroke and spinal cord injury, are at increased risk for suffering the physiologic effects of immobilization or bed rest, as seen in declines in cardiovascular function, bone mineral density, and muscle atrophy due to drastically reduced activity. Even patients with simply decreased activity, such as those with lower extremity injuries, can suffer physiologic consequences. Patients with severe injury (fracture or torn ligament) and those with chronic disease are frequently subjected to periods of immobilization, inactivity, and possibly bed rest. Several research models, including patients on bed rest, patients with spinal cord injuries, and stroke patients, as well as immobilization studies, are used to examine the physiologic consequences of physical inactivity.

Cardiovascular health should be an important consideration in rehabilitation. Within the first 24 to 72 hours of bed rest, 10% to 30% decrease is seen in plasma and blood volume, primarily because of reduced water and electrolyte retention by the kidney.[8,16] A reduction in blood volume (i.e., hypovolemia)[17,18] causes a decrease in venous return to the heart, less cardiac filling, and therefore a lower stroke volume during exercise.[16,18] This decrease in maximum stroke volume from bed rest or inactivity is the major causal factor in decreased cardiac output despite an increased heart rate response during exercise.[16] Increased sympathetic activity and beta-receptor sensitivity of the heart may be the mechanism by which heart rate max increases during bed rest.[16] The factors mentioned above (decrease in blood volume, stroke volume, and cardiac

output) then contribute to the large decline in $\dot{V}O_2$ max that occurs with bed rest.

Numerous studies have documented this reduction in $\dot{V}O_2$ max with bed rest.[16,18-21] As was mentioned previously, a relationship between plasma volume and $\dot{V}O_2$ max has been noted.[8] The decline in aerobic capacity during bed rest and deconditioning is related directly to the loss in plasma volume, as depicted in Figure 2-4.[16,21] It is important to note that this loss of plasma and blood volume during bed rest is also associated with orthostatic intolerance,[22,23] because loss of hydrostatic pressure occurs during bed rest.

Along with deficits in central cardiac function are peripheral effects from bed rest and deconditioning. Oxygen delivery to the tissues is reduced during exercise as a result of decreased cardiac output and red blood cell volume, as was discussed previously.[16] However, aerobic capacity also is dependent on oxygen utilization by the tissues; the a-vO$_2$ difference does not change during bed rest.[16] Prolonged bed rest not only demonstrated a decrease in capillary length, but mitochondrial volume, muscle oxidative capacity, and enzyme activity also were reduced.[20] Thus bed rest induced a decrease in peripheral oxygen diffusion and utilization.[20]

With bed rest or immobilization, decrements in muscle mass (particularly in the lower extremity) occur. Physical inactivity results in a decrease in muscle cross-sectional area, along with a decline in both slow and fast twitch muscle fiber area.[20,24,25] Muscle strength also is reduced, most likely as the result of a decrease in motor unit activation[24]; however, it is important to note that exercise training can reverse these neuromuscular deficits.[24]

Because of the decrease in gravitational forces that occurs when a person is bedridden, bone mineral density also can decline (Figure 2-5) as the result of an imbalance between bone formation and reabsorption.[24,26] The lumbar spine and the lower limbs are primarily affected.[24,26] Stroke patients may suffer from periods of immobilization as a result of hemiplegia, and the duration of paralysis is significantly correlated to bone

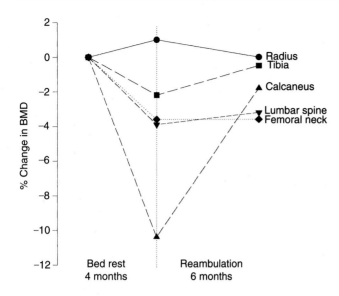

Figure 2-5 Changes in bone mineral density after bed rest. (From Bloomfield SA: Changes in musculoskeletal structure and function with prolonged bed rest. Med Sci Sports Exerc 29(2):197-206, 1997. Leblanc AD, Schneider VS, Evans HJ, Engelbretson DA, Krebs JM: Bone mineral loss and recovery after 17 weeks of bed rest. J Bone Miner Res 5(80):843-850, 1990.)

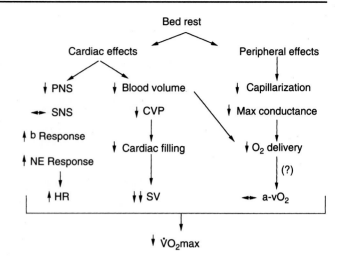

Figure 2-6 Effect of bed rest on maximum oxygen consumption ($\dot{V}O_2$ max). (From Convertino VA: Cardiovascular consequences of bed rest: effect on maximal oxygen uptake. Med Sci Sports Exerc 29(2):191-196, 1997.)

mineral density loss in the trochanter and the femoral neck.[27] Patients who are able to walk during the first 2 months after stroke incur less bone loss in the femoral neck compared with those who are wheelchair bound.[28] Thus, assuming an upright position and the ability to walk are important in reducing bone loss in stroke patients. When elderly patients or those with osteopenia are rehabilitated, care should be taken in performing strengthening exercises because of the increased risk of fracture after prolonged bed rest, and because bone recovers at a slower rate compared with muscle mass.[24]

Bed rest also changes venous and arterial properties. As was stated previously, hydrostatic forces are reduced during bed rest, thus altering bone mineral density and causing fluid shifts.[24] Changes in plasma and blood volume that occur during bed rest (as discussed earlier) may cause patients to be more likely to experience orthostatic intolerance after prolonged bed rest. One potential mechanism for this may be related to properties of the venous system. For example, prolonged bed rest was associated with a decrease in muscle blood flow[29] and a decrease in leg (but not arm) venous compliance.[22] Although this reduction in venous compliance was not related to orthostatic intolerance,[22] the lack of hydrostatic pressure in the supine position and the resultant decrease in venous pooling of the lower extremity may contribute to a decrease in VO_2 max.[30] Similar to bed rest, unilateral lower limb suspension caused a decrease in calf blood flow, along with a reduction in diameter of the femoral artery in the affected limb.[31] Within the first 4 weeks of bed rest, a 12% to 13% decline in femoral artery diameter was noted[31,32]; however, functional electrical stimulation has been shown to increase femoral artery diameter and to enhance leg blood flow in 2 weeks in patients with spinal cord injury.[33]

Exercise can attenuate the physiologic consequences of immobilization and bed rest. Isotonic exercise on a cycle ergometer during bed rest, for example, maintained plasma and red cell volumes and peak $\dot{V}O_2$.[17] The exercise was performed for 30 minutes twice a day, and consisted of short-duration (2 min) high-intensity cycling. The reduction in red cell volume and $\dot{V}O_2$ peak was less in subjects who performed isokinetic exercise (high intensity) compared with controls, despite a similar decline in plasma volume.[17] Muscle strength and endurance also tend to be greater if isokinetic exercise is performed during bed rest than in controls.[21] Therefore, exercise (either isotonic or isokinetic) performed during bed rest can maintain or minimize the decline in $\dot{V}O_2$ that occurs as the result of inactivity. Exercise can also attenuate the loss in bone mineral density that occurs with bed rest. Specifically, resistance exercise training attenuated the loss in bone mineral density and muscle mass that occurs during bed rest.[34]

In summary, inactivity or bed rest results in a decrease in $\dot{V}O_2$ max caused by both central and peripheral changes (Figure 2-6). Certain populations such as stroke and spinal cord–injured patients are at increased risk of suffering the physiologic effects of immobilization or bed rest, such as declines in cardiovascular function and bone mineral density, as well as muscle atrophy. However, exercise (even during bed rest) can minimize these deficits.

EVALUATION

As reviewed above, orthopaedic injuries that limit physical activity often result in a reduction in cardiorespiratory fitness level. The degree to which cardiorespiratory fitness declines is determined by the type, extent, and length of time of the injury. Therefore each patient should be given an individualized exercise prescription to restore and/or improve his or her cardiorespiratory fitness level. The first step in formulating an individualized exercise prescription is risk stratification. Risk stratification should allow the therapist to answer the following questions: Is it safe for a particular patient to begin an endurance training program? Is further medical workup warranted before he or she begins?

The best single source of information for risk stratification as related to formulating an exercise prescription is the Seventh Edition of ACSM's *Guidelines for Exercise Testing and Prescription.*[4] The information is summarized briefly here, but the reader is encouraged to consult the ACSM text for additional details. To stratify an individual patient, the therapist must obtain the following information: (1) age, (2) major signs or symptoms suggestive of cardiovascular, pulmonary, or metabolic disease, and (3) risk factors for coronary artery disease (CAD). This information then can be used to determine whether an individual is at low, moderate, or high risk. In this context, "risk" refers to the probability that a particular patient will experience a cardiac event during an exercise bout. The higher the risk, the more screening should take place before the patient can begin an exercise program.

Low risk is defined as men younger than 45 and women younger than 55 years of age with no symptoms (e.g., chest discomfort, dyspnea) and no more than one CAD risk factor (e.g., hypertension, dyslipidemia, cigarette smoking). Moderate risk is defined as men older than 45 and women older than 55 years of age, and those with two or more CAD risk factors. High risk is defined as those with symptoms or diagnosed cardiovascular, pulmonary, or metabolic disease. Standardized questionnaires[4] and medical history forms can be used to obtain this information. The individual classification will allow the therapist to determine whether a formal medical evaluation and/or diagnostic exercise test is needed before the patient can begin an endurance exercise training program. The exercise intensity of the planned exercise program will factor into this decision. However, to simplify in this brief chapter, we will assume that the exercise program to be prescribed will be of a moderate nature (40% to 59% of heart rate or oxygen consumption reserve) and not vigorous (more on this later). This is a reasonable assumption, in that moderate-intensity exercise should be the long-term goal of the vast majority of patients who come through orthopaedic rehabilitation.

Individual patients deemed to be at low risk do not need to undergo a specific medical evaluation or diagnostic exercise test before beginning a moderate-intensity exercise program. Clearly, information obtained from a medical evaluation and exercise test can be useful in formulating an exercise prescription; however, for a "low-risk" individual, this added step should not become a barrier to exercise participation. On the other end of the spectrum, those deemed to be at high risk do need to be given a medical examination and a diagnostic exercise test before beginning a moderate-intensity exercise program. Even if (for example) coronary artery disease is already "diagnosed," the diagnostic exercise test in this context can be used to ensure that the patient can exercise up to a given intensity level without symptoms, ECG changes suggesting

ischemia, or arrhythmias. Generally speaking, those deemed to be at moderate risk do not need a medical evaluation or a diagnostic exercise test before beginning a moderate-intensity exercise program. However, some caution is warranted here, and clinical judgment may result in some of these individuals being referred on for a medical evaluation and a diagnostic exercise test. These recommendations should not be viewed as absolutes, rather they should be viewed as a guide or an aid to decision making.

Once the patient has been stratified appropriately, and—if needed—the additional medical screening has been performed, the next step for the therapist is to formulate the individual exercise prescription.

EXERCISE PRESCRIPTION: THE BASICS

The basis of most individualized exercise prescriptions is a fitness (exercise) test. If the patient completed a graded, symptom-limited diagnostic exercise test as part of the evaluation process (detailed earlier), then this information can be used to help formulate the exercise prescription. If not, the therapist may decide to perform a submaximum or maximum fitness test using a cycle ergometer or a treadmill. Details on conducting fitness tests are beyond the scope of this chapter but may be found elsewhere.[4]

Although many similarities in fitness testing and diagnostic testing are known, the goals of these tests are different. In addition, clinical and/or diagnostic exercise tests are performed in laboratories associated with cardiologists, whereas fitness tests are performed more commonly in health and fitness facilities, or perhaps in the physical therapy (PT) clinic. Figure 2-7[4] provides the oxygen cost at different stages of the Bruce treadmill protocol and different workloads on a cycle ergometer (i.e., metabolic equivalents [METs]; 1 MET = 3.5 ml $\cdot$ kg^{-1} $\cdot$ min^{-1}, which is normal resting oxygen consumption; METs express oxygen uptake relative to resting values: 10 METs is 10× the resting value of oxygen consumption, or 35 ml $\cdot$ kg^{-1} $\cdot$ min^{-1}).

In some instances, the exercise prescription is formulated without information obtained from a fitness test. This is probably the norm, although exercise/fitness testing before an endurance exercise program is begun should be encouraged. Not only does it allow the therapist to more precisely prescribe exercise, it also allows progress to be tracked. Tracking progress can inform the therapist about the effectiveness of the program and can serve as a source of motivation for the patient.

An individualized exercise prescription is made up of five components: frequency, intensity, time, type, and rate of progression. The first four of these components often are abbreviated "FITT." Each of these factors can be varied to achieve specific goals and to accommodate specific patients. Based on the most recent (2007) guidelines from the American College of Sports Medicine (ACSM) and the American Heart Association (AHA),[1] generalized guidelines for those aged 18 to 65 years old are as follows:

FUNCTIONAL CLASS	CLINICAL STATUS	O_2 COST ml/kg/min	METS	BICYCLE ERGOMETER (FOR 70 KG BODY WEIGHT Kpm/min (WATTS))	BRUCE 3 MIN STAGES MPH/%AGR
NORMAL AND I	HEALTHY, DEPENDENT ON AGE, ACTIVITY	73.5	21		
NORMAL AND I	HEALTHY, DEPENDENT ON AGE, ACTIVITY	70	20		5.5 / 20
NORMAL AND I	HEALTHY, DEPENDENT ON AGE, ACTIVITY	66.6	19		
NORMAL AND I	HEALTHY, DEPENDENT ON AGE, ACTIVITY	63	18		
NORMAL AND I	HEALTHY, DEPENDENT ON AGE, ACTIVITY	59.5	17		5.0 / 18
NORMAL AND I	HEALTHY, DEPENDENT ON AGE, ACTIVITY	58.0	16		
NORMAL AND I	HEALTHY, DEPENDENT ON AGE, ACTIVITY	52.5	15		
NORMAL AND I	HEALTHY, DEPENDENT ON AGE, ACTIVITY	49.0	14	1500 (245)	
NORMAL AND I	HEALTHY, DEPENDENT ON AGE, ACTIVITY	45.5	13		4.2 / 16
NORMAL AND I	HEALTHY, DEPENDENT ON AGE, ACTIVITY	42.0	12	1350 (221)	
NORMAL AND I	HEALTHY, DEPENDENT ON AGE, ACTIVITY	38.5	11	1200 (197)	
NORMAL AND I	SEDENTARY HEALTHY	34.0	10	1050 (172)	3.4 / 14
NORMAL AND I	SEDENTARY HEALTHY	31.5	9		
NORMAL AND I	SEDENTARY HEALTHY	28.0	8	900 (148)	
NORMAL AND I	SEDENTARY HEALTHY / LIMITED	24.5	7	750 (123)	2.5 / 12
II	SEDENTARY HEALTHY / LIMITED / SYMPTOMATIC	21.0	6	600 (98)	
II	SEDENTARY HEALTHY / LIMITED / SYMPTOMATIC	17.5	5	459 (74)	
III	SEDENTARY HEALTHY / LIMITED / SYMPTOMATIC	14.0	4	300 (49)	1.7 / 10
III	LIMITED / SYMPTOMATIC	10.5	3	150 (24)	
III	LIMITED / SYMPTOMATIC	7.0	2		
IV	SYMPTOMATIC	3.5	1		

RAMP — PER 30 SEC MPH/%GR

MPH	%GR
3.0	25.0
3.0	24.0
3.0	23.0
3.0	22.0
3.0	21.0
3.0	20.0
3.0	19.0
3.0	18.0
3.0	17.0
3.0	16.0
3.0	15.0
3.0	14.0
3.0	13.0
3.0	12.0
3.0	11.0
3.0	10.0
3.0	9.0
3.0	8.0
3.0	7.0
3.0	6.0
3.0	5.0
3.0	4.0
3.0	3.0
3.0	2.0
3.0	1.0
3.0	0
2.5	0
2.0	0
1.5	0
1.0	0
0.5	0

Figure 2-7 Oxygen cost of different stages of the Bruce treadmill protocol. (From Whaley MH, editor: ACSM's guidelines for exercise testing and prescription. Seventh ed, Philadelphia: 2006, Lippincott Williams & Wilkins.)

Frequency	5 days per week
Intensity	Moderate (40% to 59% of HRR)
Time	30 minutes (continuous or multiple bouts)
Type	Aerobic (endurance)
Rate of progression	Gradual

HRR, Heart rate reserve.

The ACSM/AHA position paper provides examples of combining moderate and vigorous activities throughout the week, but—as was stated earlier—to simplify this presentation, the focus here is only on moderate-intensity physical activity, which is appropriate for most physical therapy patients. Moderate-intensity exercise, as defined specifically by ACSM, is 40 to 59% of heart rate or oxygen consumption reserve (Table 2-1).[4,35]

This is where it is helpful to obtain data from a fitness test; a more precise and customized intensity can be given, including a training heart rate range and MET range. As an example, a 40-year-old male with no risk factors or symptoms (risk stratification: low) has a resting heart rate of 78 beats per

Table 2-1	Classification of Physical Activity Intensity					
	Relative Intensity		Absolute Intensity Ranges (METs) Across Fitness Levels			
Intensity	$\dot{V}O_2R$, % HRR, %	Maximum HR, %	12 MET $\dot{V}O_2$ max	10 MET $\dot{V}O_2$ max	8 MET $\dot{V}O_2$ max	6 MET $\dot{V}O_2$ max
Very light	<20	<50	<3.2	<2.8	<2.4	<2.0
Light	20-39	50-63	3.2-5.3	2.8-4.5	2.4-3.7	2.0-3.0
Moderate	40-59	64-76	5.4-7.5	4.6-6.3	3.8-5.1	3.1-4.0
Hard (vigorous)	60-84	77-93	7.6-10.2	6.4-8.6	5.2-6.9	4.1-5.2
Very hard	≥85	≥94	≥10.3	≥8.7	≥7.0	≥5.3
Maximal	100	100	21	10	8	6

Data from U.S. Department of Health and Human Services. Physical activity and health: A report of the Surgeon General, 1996; American College of Sports Medicine, Position Stand: The recommended quantity and quality of exercise for developing and maintaining cardiorespiratory and muscular fitness, and flexibility in healthy adults. Med Sci Sports Exerc 30:975-991, 1998. Howley ET: Type of activity: Resistance, aerobic and leisure versus occupational physical activity. Med Sci Sports Exerc 33:5364-5369, 2001. In Whaley MH, editor. ACSM's Guidelines for Exercise Testing and Prescription. Seventh ed: Lippincott Williams & Wilkins; 2006.

HR, Heart rate; HRR, heart rate reserve; MET, metabolic equivalent; $\dot{V}O_2$ max, maximum oxygen uptake.

Table 2-2	50th Percentile Values (in METs) for $\dot{V}O_2$ max				
Age, yr	29-29	30-39	40-49	50-59	60-69
Male	12.3	12.3	10.9	9.7	8.0
Female	10.0	9.0	8.0	7.4	6.3

Data from Howley ET. Type of activity: resistance, aerobic and leisure versus occupational physical activity. Med Sci Sports Exerc 33(6 Suppl):S364-S369, 2001, discussion S419-S420; Canada Fitness Survey. Fitness and Lifestyle in Canada. Ottawa, ON: Fitness and Amateur Sport; 1983.

METs, Metabolic equivalents; VO2 max, maximum oxygen uptake.

minute. He completes 9 minutes of a Bruce protocol, with an ending speed of 3.4 mph and an ending grade of 14%. He reaches a peak heart rate of 178 beats per minute and a peak blood pressure of 190/86. No symptoms or arrhythmias are noted. Estimated METs for this speed and grade are 10 (see Figure 2-7). This particular patient, with a MET value of 10, is just below the 50th percentile value of 10.9 for 40- to 49-year-old men (as depicted in Table 2-2).[35,36]

In this example, we will take 40% to 59% of the heart rate reserve to come up with a training heart rate. Heart rate reserve (HRR) is calculated as follows: (Peak exercise heart rate − Resting heart rate) (Desired intensity) + Resting heart rate. In our example, to calculate 40% of HRR, do the following: (178 − 78) (0.4) + 78 = 118 bpm. To calculate 59% of HRR, do the following: (178 − 78) (0.59) + 78 = 137 bpm. Therefore, for this hypothetical patient the heart rate training range is 118 to 137 bpm. We also can provide this patient with an MET training range. To calculate the appropriate MET training range, a similar procedure is followed. Oxygen consumption reserve (using METs) is calculated as follows: (Peak METs − Resting METs) (Desired intensity) + Resting METs. To calculate 40% of oxygen consumption reserve, do the follow-

ing: (10 − 1) (0.4) + 1 = 4.6 METs. To calculate 59% of oxygen consumption reserve: (10 − 1) (0.59) + 1 = 6.3 METs. Thus the appropriate MET range for our hypothetical patient is 4.6 to 6.3. This can be very useful in helping the patient select appropriate activities. Table 2-1[4] links subjective intensities (i.e., moderate-intensity exercise) with the appropriate objective heart rate reserve and oxygen consumption reserve ranges. As was noted earlier, moderate-intensity exercise is 40% to 59% of heart rate and oxygen consumption reserve; for an individual with a cardiorespiratory fitness level of 10 METs, the appropriate MET range would be 4.6 to 6.3; calculations are demonstrated above. MET charts can be consulted for examples of activities.[37] Walking at a brisk pace (4.0 mph) on a flat surface would put this patient just below the low end of the desired MET range (4.6 to 6.3 METs); heart rate during this activity can be used to modify the intensity (below 118, speed up; above 137, slow down).

Without exercise or fitness testing data, a training heart rate still can be determined by using 220 − Age to estimate peak exercise heart rate, and then going through the same calculations as illustrated above (as above, resting heart rate needs to be assessed). Also, without data from a fitness test, a reasonable assumption is that brisk walking at a pace of 3 to 4 mph represents moderate-intensity exercise for most adults. To further guide exercise intensity, a rating of perceived exertion (0 to 10 scale) of 5 to 6 can be viewed as "moderate-intensity" exercise.[1,38] If using the 6 to 20 Borg Rating of Perceived Scale, moderate-intensity exercise would be 12 to 13.[35,36,39] It is also important to incorporate a brief warm-up and cool-down into the exercise session (5 to 10 minutes each should suffice). To encourage lifelong participation, care should be taken to ensure that the person enjoys doing the activity that is being prescribed. Resistance training is also very important but is discussed elsewhere in this text.

Several other approaches can be used to provide a patient with an appropriate heart rate and intensity training range.

Discussion of these other methods is beyond the scope of this chapter.

SUMMARY

The goal of this chapter was to provide a straightforward approach to prescribing exercise for the vast majority of patients who come through rehab. This is especially important in view of data suggesting that less than half of U.S. adults meet the minimum physical activity recommendations.[1] This chapter has reviewed (1) the physiologic benefits of endurance exercise, (2) the physiologic consequences of extreme physical inactivity, (3) a simple method for stratifying the individual patient based on risk, and (4) a straightforward approach to prescribing endurance exercise. Clinically, physical therapists should strive to incorporate some form of endurance exercise training into their patient care programs, or should provide a referral so every patient has the opportunity to increase his or her cardiorespiratory fitness level. As reviewed earlier, the new ACSM Exercise Is Medicine™ initiative specifically calls on "physicians to assess and review every patient's physical activity program at every visit." We similarly call on physical therapists to assess and review every patient's physical activity program at every visit.

REFERENCES

1. Haskell WL, Lee IM, Pate RR, et al: Physical activity and public health: updated recommendation for adults from the American College of Sports Medicine and the American Heart Association, Med Sci Sports Exerc 39(8):1423-1434, 2007.
2. Ogden CL, Carroll MD, Curtin LR, et al: Prevalence of overweight and obesity in the United States, 1999-2004. JAMA 295(13):1549-1555, 2006.
3. Wang YC, Colditz GA, Kuntz KM: Forecasting the obesity epidemic in the aging U.S. population, Obesity (Silver Spring) 15(11):2855-2865, 2007.
4. Whaley MH, editor. ACSM's guidelines for exercise testing and prescription, ed 7, Philadelphia, 2006, Lippincott Williams & Wilkins.
5. Rowell L: Human cardiovascular control, New York: Oxford University Press; 1993.
6. Pescatello LS, Franklin BA, Fagard R, et al: American College of Sports Medicine position stand: exercise and hypertension, Med Sci Sports Exerc 36(3):533-553, 2004.
7. Sawka MN, Convertino VA, Eichner ER, et al: Blood volume: importance and adaptations to exercise training, environmental stresses, and trauma/sickness. Med Sci Sports Exerc 32(2):332-348, 2000.
8. Convertino VA: Blood volume response to physical activity and inactivity, Am J Med Sci 334(1):72-79, 2007.
9. Pluim BM, Zwinderman AH, van der Laarse A, van der Wall EE: The athlete's heart: a meta-analysis of cardiac structure and function, Circulation 101(3):336-344, 2000.
10. Booth FW, Lees SJ: Physically active subjects should be the control group, Med Sci Sports Exerc 38(3):405-406, 2006.
11. Booth FW, Laye MJ, Lees SJ, et al: Reduced physical activity and risk of chronic disease: the biology behind the consequences. Eur J Appl Physiol 2007.
12. Julius S, Amery A, Whitlock LS, Conway J: Influence of age on the hemodynamic response to exercise, Circulation 36(2):222-230, 1967.
13. Stratton JR, Levy WC, Cerqueira MD, et al: Cardiovascular responses to exercise: effects of aging and exercise training in healthy men, Circulation 89(4):1648-1655, 1994.
14. McGuire DK, Levine BD, Williamson JW, et al: A 30-year follow-up of the Dallas Bedrest and Training Study: II. Effect of age on cardiovascular adaptation to exercise training, Circulation 104(12):1358-1366, 2001.
15. Erikssen G, Liestol K, Bjornholt J, et al: Changes in physical fitness and changes in mortality, Lancet 352(9130):759-762, 1998.
16. Convertino VA: Cardiovascular consequences of bed rest: effect on maximal oxygen uptake, Med Sci Sports Exerc 29(2):191-196, 1997.
17. Greenleaf JE: Intensive exercise training during bed rest attenuates deconditioning, Med Sci Sports Exerc 29(2):207-215, 1997.
18. Saltin B, Blomqvist G, Mitchell JH, et al: Response to exercise after bed rest and after training, Circulation 38(5 Suppl):VII1-78, 1968.
19. DeBusk RF, Convertino VA, Hung J, Goldwater D: Exercise conditioning in middle-aged men after 10 days of bed rest, Circulation 68(2):245-250, 1983.
20. Ferretti G, Antonutto G, Denis C, et al: The interplay of central and peripheral factors in limiting maximal O_2 consumption in man after prolonged bed rest, J Physiol 501(Pt 3):677-686, 1997.
21. Greenleaf JE, Bernauer EM, Ertl AC, et al: Work capacity during 30 days of bed rest with isotonic and isokinetic exercise training, J Appl Physiol 67(5):1820-1826, 1989.
22. Bleeker MW, De Groot PC, Pawelczyk JA, et al: Effects of 18 days of bed rest on leg and arm venous properties, J Appl Physiol 96(3):840-847, 2004.
23. Melchior FM, Fortney SM: Orthostatic intolerance during a 13-day bed rest does not result from increased leg compliance, J Appl Physiol 74(1):286-292, 1993.
24. Bloomfield SA: Changes in musculoskeletal structure and function with prolonged bed rest, Med Sci Sports Exerc 29(2):197-206, 1997.
25. Hather BM, Adams GR, Tesch PA, Dudley GA: Skeletal muscle responses to lower limb suspension in humans, J Appl Physiol 72(4):1493-1498, 1992.
26. Leblanc AD, Schneider VS, Evans HJ, et al: Bone mineral loss and recovery after 17 weeks of bed rest, J Bone Miner Res 5(8):843-850, 1990.
27. Demirbag D, Ozdemir F, Kokino S, Berkarda S: The relationship between bone mineral density and immobilization duration in hemiplegic limbs, Ann Nucl Med 19(8):695-700, 2005.
28. Jorgensen L, Jacobsen BK, Wilsgaard T, et al: Walking after stroke: does it matter? Changes in bone mineral

density within the first 12 months after stroke: a longitudinal study, Osteoporos Int 11(5):381-387, 2000.

29. Pawelczyk JA, Zuckerman JH, Blomqvist CG, et al: Regulation of muscle sympathetic nerve activity after bed rest deconditioning, Am J Physiol Heart Circ Physiol 280(5):H2230-H2239, 2001.

30. Convertino VA, Sandler H, Webb P, Annis JF: Induced venous pooling and cardiorespiratory responses to exercise after bed rest, J Appl Physiol 52(5):1343-1348, 1982.

31. Bleeker MW, De Groot PC, Poelkens F, et al: Vascular adaptation to 4 weeks of deconditioning by unilateral lower limb suspension, Am J Physiol Heart Circ Physiol 288(4):H1747-H1755, 2005.

32. Bleeker MW, De Groot PC, Rongen GA, et al: Vascular adaptation to deconditioning and the effect of an exercise countermeasure: results of the Berlin Bed Rest study, J Appl Physiol 99(4):1293-1300, 2005.

33. Thijssen DH, Ellenkamp R, Smits P, Hopman MT: Rapid vascular adaptations to training and detraining in persons with spinal cord injury, Arch Phys Med Rehabil 87(4):474-481, 2006.

34. Shackelford LC, LeBlanc AD, Driscoll TB, et al: Resistance exercise as a countermeasure to disuse-induced bone loss, J Appl Physiol 97(1):119-129, 2004.

35. Howley ET: Type of activity: resistance, aerobic and leisure versus occupational physical activity, Med Sci Sports Exerc 33(6 Suppl):S364-S369, 2001, discussion S419-S420.

36. Canada Fitness Survey. Fitness and Lifestyle in Canada. Ottawa, Fitness and Amateur Sport, 1983.

37. Ainsworth BE, Haskell WL, Leon AS, et al: Compendium of physical activities: classification of energy costs of human physical activities, Med Sci Sports Exerc 25(1):71-80, 1993.

38. Nelson ME, Rejeski WJ, Blair SN, et al: Physical activity and public health in older adults: recommendation from the American College of Sports Medicine and the American Heart Association, Med Sci Sports Exerc 39(8):1435-1445, 2007.

39. Borg GA: Psychophysical bases of perceived exertion, Med Sci Sports Exerc 14(5):377-381, 1982.

Sarah DoBroka,
Robbin Wickham-Bruno,
and Lynn Snyder-Mackler

Theory and Practice of Muscle Strengthening in Orthopaedic Physical Therapy

Muscle strengthening is a core focus of orthopaedic physical therapy practice. This chapter addresses issues of muscle physiology, skeletal muscle force generation, muscle fatigue, tissue healing, immobilization, and physiologic changes in training to provide a theoretical basis for muscle strengthening in training and rehabilitation. Case presentations are used to illustrate how the science can inform practice.

MUSCLE PHYSIOLOGY

Contraction of a skeletal muscle cell is the result of a five-step process: (1) An action potential arrives at the sarcolemma, and the intracellular calcium (Ca^{2+}) concentration rises; (2) Ca^{2+} ions bind to troponin, a regulatory protein associated with tropomyosin, causing a change in orientation of the troponin/tropomyosin complex (Figure 3-1); (3) cross-bridges form between the actin and myosin filaments; (4) Ca^{2+} dissociates from troponin once the stimulus is removed; and (5) actin returns to its resting state, and further cross-bridge formation is disallowed. This five-step process is called the *contraction-relaxation cycle.*[1] We now will take a closer look at the specific mechanisms involved in this process.

Contraction of a muscle under voluntary control begins with an impulse generated in the motor cortex of the brain. The impulse is carried from the central nervous system to the muscle via a peripheral nerve that synapses at the sarcolemma of an individual muscle cell. Generation of an action potential changes the permeability of the cell membrane, and sodium and calcium ions from the extracellular fluid flow into the cell. The influx of extracellular Ca^{2+} by itself is insufficient to cause a conformational change in the troponin/tropomyosin complex. However, the increased intracellular Ca^{2+} concentration stimulates the sarcoplasmic reticulum (SR) to release its stored Ca^{2+}. Calcium ions from the SR increase the cytosolic concentration of Ca^{2+} to more than 1 μM. At cytosolic Ca^{2+} concentrations greater than 1 μM, Ca^{2+} binding sites on troponin are fully occupied, thus increasing the space occupied by this complex.[2] Steric hindrance causes rotation of the tropomyosin and actin filaments, leading to exposure of the cross-bridge binding site, and the cross-bridge on the myosin filament binds to the actin filament. Rotation of the cross-bridge head from a 90-degree angle to a 45-degree angle shortens the sarcomere (Figure 3 2). Cross-bridge cycling continues until no additional action potentials are received. Throughout the action potential, the SR is actively resequestering Ca^{2+}. In the absence of a new action potential, the rate of Ca^{2+} uptake exceeds the rate of release, returning the cytosolic Ca^{2+} concentration to the resting level.[2] Actin resumes its resting conformation, with the cross-bridge binding site blocked, and the skeletal muscle cell returns to the relaxed state.

Different types of muscle contraction have different adenosine triphosphate (ATP) requirements. During a concentric contraction, many cross-bridges are formed, dissociated, and re-formed at the next available cross-bridge site on the actin filament. Each cycle, cross-bridge binding and dissociation, requires energy input of one ATP. At low loads, the rate of fiber shortening is high and cross-bridge cycling is rapid. ATP expenditure is consequently high. As the load is increased, the rate of muscle shortening decreases with a subsequent decrease noted in ATP hydrolysis, because the rate of cross-bridge cycling is decreased. If the load is further increased to the point where the muscle is unable to generate a force sufficient to overcome the load, no shortening occurs and the muscle contracts isometrically. ATP still is needed because the cross-bridges cycle but return to the same binding site during each cycle. An eccentric contraction requires no ATP expenditure because the cross-bridge remains in a high-energy state during dissociation and therefore can bind to the actin filament again without further energy input.[2]

Muscle requires a constant supply of ATP for contraction. ATP promotes dissociation of the actin-myosin cross-bridge (actomyosin complex). Energy resulting from hydrolysis often activates the dissociated cross-bridge, and another actomyosin complex can be formed. ATP also provides the energy for active resequestering of Ca^{2+} from cytosol by the SR via the Ca^{2+}-ATPase pump. In the absence of ATP, rigor mortis ensues because the intracellular Ca^{2+} concentration remains elevated and the cross-bridge is held in a fixed position on the actin filament.[1,2]

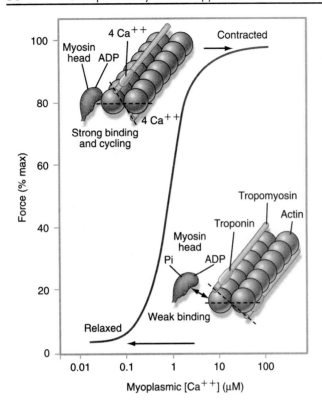

Figure 3-1 Calcium (Ca^{2+}) ions bind to troponin, a regulatory protein associated with tropomyosin, causing a change in the orientation of the actin filament. (From Koeppen B, Stanton B, Levy M, et al: Physiology, ed 4. St. Louis, 1998, Mosby.)

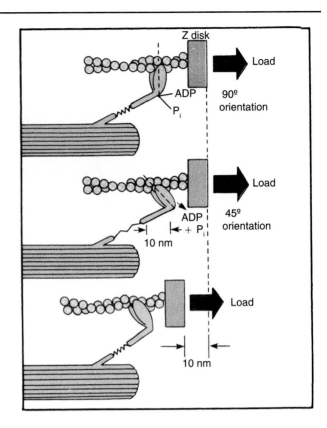

Figure 3-2 Sarcomere shortening as a conformation of cross-bridge changes. (From Levy M, Berne R: Principles of Physiology, ed 3. St. Louis, 2000, Mosby.)

Although ATP is the energy currency for all mammalian cells, other compounds, including reduced nicotinamide adenine dinucleotide (NADH) and flavin adenine dinucleotide (FADH$_2$), serve as energy vouchers that can be converted to ATP under aerobic conditions. At rest, mammalian cells have minimum energy requirements and intracellular ATP concentrations are high. A high ATP concentration inactivates the enzyme pathways of energy production to conserve resources for times of need. At the onset of exercise, the muscles use intracellular ATP stores as the initial energy source, but the cell can store only enough ATP for the first 2 to 3 seconds of exercise. The cells need a way to replenish ATP if additional work is to be performed. A small amount of ATP is formed from the phosphorylation of adenosine diphosphate (ADP) via the phosphocreatine (PCr) system. PCr donates a high-energy phosphate group to ADP under enzymatic control to regenerate ATP. However, direct phosphorylation from PCr provides energy for only 10 to 20 seconds.[3,4]

Energy released in macronutrient (carbohydrate, fat, and protein) degradation serves the crucial purpose of ATP resynthesis. The specific pathways of breakdown differ depending on the nutrients metabolized. Carbohydrates are the only macronutrients whose stored energy generates ATP anaerobically. Glucose degradation occurs in two stages. In glycolysis, the first stage, a series of 10 enzymatically controlled chemical reactions rapidly create two molecules of pyruvate from the anaerobic breakdown of glucose. Two ATPs are also formed from substrate level phosphorylation during glycolysis. During strenuous exercise, the circulatory system sometimes is unable to supply sufficient oxygen to meet cellular needs, and the respiratory chain cannot process all of the hydrogen joined to NADH. Under these conditions, nonoxidized hydrogens temporarily combine with pyruvate to form lactic acid. Skeletal muscle is unable to use lactic acid for further energy production. Therefore, it is removed from the muscle by the Cori cycle and is transported to the liver, where it is converted back to pyruvate and muscle glycogen (gluconeogenesis).

When the pyruvate formed in anaerobic glycolysis irreversibly converts to acetyl-coenzyme A (CoA), it enters the second stage of carbohydrate breakdown, known as the citric acid cycle (also called the Krebs cycle). During the citric acid cycle, each molecule of pyruvate yields four NADH, one FADH$_2$, and one guanosine triphosphate (GTP) (an energy equivalent of ATP). Thus, one molecule of glucose gives two GTP, eight NADH, and two FADH$_2$ from the citric acid cycle.[5] NADH and FADH$_2$ must undergo further processing to be converted to the energy-rich compound ATP.

During oxidative phosphorylation, NADH and FADH$_2$ transfer two electrons to a series of cytochromes within the mitochondrial inner membrane, which are alternately oxidized and reduced. Oxygen serves as the final electron acceptor in the electron transport or respiratory chain. Electron transfer is accompanied by the release of hydrogen ions (H^+). The hydrogen ion concentration increases in the mitochondrial matrix, creating a proton gradient. ATP is produced by pumping the protons across the inner membrane when oxygen is present. This process yields 2.5 ATP for every NADH molecule and 1.5 ATP for every $FADH_2$. Overall, under aerobic conditions, one molecule of glucose will generate 2 ATP, 2 GTP, 22.5 ATP from NADH, and 3 ATP from $FADH_2$, for a total of approximately 30 ATPs that actually will enter the cytoplasm of the cell.[6] Aerobic breakdown of a carbohydrate is more efficient for generating rapid energy compared with fatty acid breakdown for energy production.

Fats, or triglycerides, consist of a glycerol backbone and three fatty acid side chains. Relative to carbohydrates and protein, stored fat provides almost unlimited energy. Accumulation of triglycerides in adipose cells functions as energy storage during times of plenty (postprandial). Cells cannot use fats directly to form ATP. The fats first must be hydrolyzed to constituent parts, and some carbohydrate catabolism is required to process fat into energy. After a series of chemical reactions, glycerol is converted to pyruvate to form ATP during substrate level phosphorylation (glycolysis). Fatty acids undergo further degradation via the consecutive removal of two carbon fragments with subsequent conversion into acetyl-CoA through a process called beta oxidation. Each round of beta oxidation also yields one NADH and one $FADH_2$. Acetyl-CoA has direct entry into the citric acid cycle, and NADH and $FADH_2$ are oxidized in the electron transport chain. Fats can be oxidized only in the mitochondria, and under anaerobic conditions, fat breakdown is brought to a halt.[4]

Naturally occurring fatty acids have an even number of carbons. The 16- and 18-carbon chains are most common in biological systems. For example, palmitic acid, a 16-carbon fatty acid, goes through seven cycles of beta oxidation, yielding eight acetyl-CoA, seven NADH, and seven $FADH_2$. Each acetyl-CoA yields the equivalent of 10 ATP in the citric acid cycle. Thus, the total ATP produced by the complete oxidation of one molecule of palmitic acid is 108 ATP. Because 2 ATP is used to activate the breakdown process, the net ATP is 106 (compared with 30 ATP per glucose molecule).[7]

Carbohydrates and fats ideally serve as the primary energy substrates, but dietary intake determines which fuels will be utilized most by the body. Ingested protein is used to maintain muscle, blood plasma, and visceral tissue protein. However, protein can be used as a major source of energy production during extreme endurance-type activities and arduous training, or during starvation conditions.[4] The conversion of protein to ATP is beyond the scope of this book, and the reader is referred to physiology, nutrition, or molecular biology books for additional details.

The relative amount of carbohydrate usage compared with fat utilization depends on the intensity and duration of exercise. As the activity level increases, the percentage of usage of each substrate changes. At rest, the body uses almost double the quantity of fatty acids to fuel metabolic processes compared with carbohydrates. During light to moderate activity, fats and carbohydrates each generate almost half of the energy needed by the body. Carbohydrate utilization rises precipitously during exercise about the ventilatory threshold where the Krebs cycle is saturated, and glycolysis again plays a primary role in energy generation for exercise. It is important to note that carbohydrate is the only substrate that can be used in glycolysis. This explains why high-intensity sprint and endurance activities require a very high percentage of carbohydrates compared with a very low percentage of fats.[4]

SKELETAL MUSCLE FORCE GENERATION

The force that an individual muscle can generate is modulated over a wide range. (Think of holding an egg versus gripping a baseball bat.) Grading of force can be accomplished by rate coding or recruiting motor units. Rate coding refers to increasing or decreasing the frequency of motor neuron discharge, thus changing the firing rate of muscle fibers within the motor unit. The components of a motor unit are the alpha motor neuron and the muscle fibers it innervates. A muscle consists of thousands of motor units. Within a single motor unit, the fiber type is constant. Different motor units within a single muscle include different types of fibers, and the proportion of the three fiber types within the muscle depends on the function of the muscle. Individual fibers in a motor unit cannot function independently. Therefore, an action potential that causes one fiber to fire results in firing of all fibers within that motor unit. This is known as the *all-or-none phenomenon.*

Skeletal muscle fibers are classified into three groups based on the energy production system, contents of the cytoplasm, structural characteristics, and the ability to generate tension. Type I fibers (slow oxidative [SO]) rely on aerobic pathways for energy production. Consequently, oxidative enzyme concentrations, mitochondrial content, capillary density, and myoglobin concentrations are high. These cells generate extra ATP per oxidized glucose molecule. Therefore, the amount of intracellular glycogen (the storage form of glucose) is typically low.[8] As can be seen in Figure 3-3, Type I fibers take longer to reach peak force, and the twitch lasts longer. However, despite a longer twitch, peak force output is low.[9] Neural impulses to slow oxidative fibers are delivered in long trains of low-frequency pulses.[10] This combination of high oxidative capacity, low force output, and low-frequency neural input bestows fatigue resistance on Type I fibers.

Type IIb fibers (fast glycolytic or fast fatigue [FF]) have a large cross-sectional area (CSA) composed primarily of contractile proteins. These fibers rely predominantly on anaerobic glycolysis for energy production. Because oxygen utilization is minimal, the number of mitochondria, the capillary density, and the myoglobin concentration are low. Glycolytic enzyme levels are high, as are glycogen stores.[8] These fibers are capable of generating large forces quickly (time to peak force is fast, and twitch duration is short), but they fatigue rapidly.[9] Nerves that supply Type IIb fibers generate short bursts of high-frequency impulses.[10]

Type IIa fibers use both aerobic and anaerobic energy production systems and are identified as fast oxidative-glycolytic,

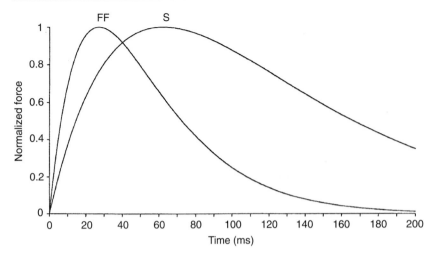

Figure 3-3 Model twitches of fast fatigable (FF) and slow (S) motor units. (From Clamann HP: Motor unit recruitment and the gradation of muscle force. Phys Ther 73:830, 1993.)

or fast fatigue-resistant (FR), fibers. Type IIa fibers represent an intermediate fiber type, where oxidative and glycolytic enzymes are present in moderate amounts. Myoglobin, mitochondria, and capillary density also are found in moderate amounts. Glycogen stores are high to provide substrate for the less efficient glycolytic system. These FR fibers are capable of generating large forces.[8] The action potential that follows short, high-frequency bursts of stimulation resembles that of Type IIb fibers.[9,10] Generally speaking, the FF motor units in a particular muscle generate more force than the FR fibers, and the FR motor units produce greater force than the SO fibers. However, this single muscle generalization does not apply when force output is compared across different muscles within the same organism.[9]

The proportion of different fiber types in a muscle is determined in part by genetic predisposition, the type of activity performed, and neural input. Buller et al[11] demonstrated the influence of neural input on muscle by switching the nerves supplying an SO muscle (soleus) and those supplying an FF muscle (medial gastrocnemius). Upon reinnervation, the FF muscle took on properties of its new innervation and became slower, while the SO muscle became faster. Recent studies have established that fast-to-slow fiber type conversion involves morphologic and biochemical changes that result in altered contractile properties and endurance capacities. Functional adaptations of skeletal muscle cell electrophysiologic properties also occur. Motor neuron firing patterns control the expression of isoforms of contractile proteins and metabolic enzymes on muscle fibers. Continuous electrical stimulation has mimicked these firing patterns, promoting the conversion of FF fibers to SO fibers.[12] The exact cellular signaling mechanisms involved in fiber type conversion still are poorly understood, but changes in intracellular free Ca^{2+} concentration seem to be essentially involved.[13] This conversion phenomenon has been utilized as a treatment for heart failure. In dynamic cardiomyoplasty, the latissimus dorsi is conditioned via electrical stimulation to assume characteristics of cardiac muscle to augment left ventricular ejection.[14,15] It is important to note that stimulation programs that promote the reverse—conversion of SO to FF—have yet to be elucidated.

Training techniques also influence the proportion of muscle fibers in a muscle. Training may develop the fibers best suited to perform a certain task while minimizing the development of other fibers. This has the effect of making the percentage of the developed fiber type greater on cross-sectional area while not changing the absolute number of each fiber type.

The strength of a motor unit depends on the fiber type, the number of fibers, and the force per unit area (specific tension). Contraction strength is variable, with a twitch contraction being on average only one-fifth as strong as a tetanic contraction. Rate coding, or increasing the frequency of stimulation of a motor unit, accounts for a fivefold increase in force production (average range = 2 to 15).[9] The muscle responds to the need for greater force by recruiting additional motor units. Recruitment order is a function of motor unit size, activation threshold, and maximum force capability. Small, low-threshold motor units with low strength capacity are recruited first.[97,98] This pattern of recruitment provides incremental increases in force production by the muscle (proportional control). For maximum force output, the largest motor units with high thresholds must be recruited and activated at a high rate.

MUSCLE FATIGUE

Muscle fatigue can be defined as any acute impairment in the ability to exert force or power, regardless of whether the task itself still can be performed successfully. Fatigue subsequently can result in feelings of tiredness, exhaustion, and lack of energy. It is a symptom, not a disease. Certain health problems can result in muscle fatigue, but their discussion is beyond the scope of this chapter. Often, the fatigability of a muscle is characterized by endurance time (sustaining force or power) or the extent of reduction of force or power.[16] How quickly the muscle fatigues is dependent upon how efficient the body is in utilizing anaerobic and aerobic metabolism (i.e., how quickly the body can keep generating ATP for energy). Aging also plays a role in the fatigability of a muscle, in that a shift toward a greater proportion of SO (Type I) muscle fibers in the body should result in improved muscle endurance capacity.[17-19]

Fatigue can occur at central or peripheral sites. Central fatigue is a progressive exercise-induced reduction in the level of voluntary activation of a muscle that appears to be task dependent. Studies have shown that people who were unfamiliar with a fatigue task showed greater predisposition for central fatigue.[16] Another study revealed that voluntary fatigue may occur as a result of conscious or unconscious mechanisms. A person may decide that a sensation is unacceptable and may deliberately reduce the level of activity. Alternatively, afferent information from working muscles, joints, or tendons may inhibit motor activity at spinal or supraspinal levels.[20] Despite numerous studies, controversy still surrounds the exact role that central activation plays in healthy individuals.[21]

Peripheral factors responsible for muscle fatigue include decreased muscle membrane excitability and failure in the excitation-contraction (EC) mechanism. EC failure typically occurs during action potential propagation and/or during calcium regulation at the level of the contractile elements. In conjunction with neuromuscular contributions, muscle blood flow has an important role in the development of muscle fatigue. Blood flow alters the depletion of energy substrates and the accumulation of metabolic byproducts, which ultimately affects the contractile properties of the exercising muscle.[16] Blood flow occlusion during a muscle contraction also can occur in those with larger muscle mass, resulting in premature fatigue.[19] All of these factors must be taken into consideration when one is designing a scientifically based training or rehabilitation program.

TISSUE HEALING

After injury occurs, regardless of origin (e.g., trauma, bacterial infection, surgery), the damaged tissue undergoes a typical physiologic response.[22] The first 24 to 72 hours, the inflammatory stage, is characterized by redness, swelling, warmth, pain, and loss of function. The goal of the inflammatory phase is to "put out the fire," thus preventing injury to surrounding tissues. The immediate response is arteriolar vasoconstriction to minimize blood loss. Injury to the tissue stimulates release of chemical messengers, including prostaglandins, histamine, thromboxanes, and bradykinin. These chemical messengers cause local vasodilation and increase vascular permeability. Vasodilation decreases the rate of blood flow through the vessel (think of the effect of opening and closing a nozzle on a water hose), allowing blood cells, especially leukocytes, to move toward the vessel wall (margination). Increased permeability results from contraction of the capillary endothelial cells, creating space between adjacent cells. Blood cells and large plasma proteins can leave the vessel through these spaces and collect in the interstitial space, creating an osmotic gradient. Water is attracted to the hyperosmotic area, and edema results. Although edema formation is an undesirable outcome, increased capillary permeability brings leukocytes (neutrophils, monocytes, and lymphocytes) and platelets to the area. Neutrophils are the first subpopulation of white blood cells (WBCs) to enter a traumatized or stressed tissue, but macrophages (converted monocytes) soon follow. Neutrophils are drawn to the injury site by chemotaxis, and they pass from circulation into the tissue through a process called *diapedesis*. The mechanisms responsible for recruiting macrophages remain unknown, but speculations suggest that injured tissue releases a signal. The interactions between neutrophils and macrophages remain poorly understood, but early removal of bacteria and cellular debris by phagocytosis has been shown to have a direct effect on tissue repair and regeneration.[23] Lymphocytes tag invading bacteria for destruction by the immune system, and platelets prevent further bleeding by depositing a fibrin mesh that forms blood clots.

The acute inflammatory responses seen after an injury are important to the healing process. Debate is ongoing regarding which form of analgesia is most conducive to promoting early healing while simultaneously providing pain relief. Recent animal studies have examined the effects that nonsteroidal anti-inflammatory drugs (NSAIDs) have on tendon healing. Findings suggest detrimental biomechanical effects, including decreased failure loads and increased rates of failure, when the medicine was initiated immediately postoperatively.[24,25] Ibuprofen appeared to be the one exception as it showed no effect on healing strength. Based on these conclusions, it is recommended that acetaminophen and opiates be prescribed more often, and that NSAIDs be used more judiciously in the acute hours following an injury.[24]

Goals of rehabilitation during the inflammatory phase are to decrease pain caused by irritating chemical agents (histamine, bradykinin, and prostaglandins), decrease swelling, and promote range of motion. Effective medications were discussed previously, but other physical agents can be used in conjunction to provide additional relief. Cold modalities are used not only for their analgesic effects, but also to decrease the metabolic rate of surrounding healthy tissue to minimize hypoxic injury from reduced blood supply to these tissues.

Repair and regeneration of injured tissue characterize the second phase of tissue healing. Tissue repair depends on resolution of inflammation, elimination of dead tissue, restoration of the blood supply, and formation of scar tissue. Certain tissues (epidermis, bone, and ciliated epithelial) can heal with native tissue in a process called *tissue regeneration*. Scar tissue is formed by fibroblasts that deposit a collagen and ground substance connective matrix. Decreased oxygen and elevated metabolic activity in the injured area stimulate the formation of capillary buds from healthy vessels in nearby tissues. The new capillaries interconnect to form a capillary bed that supplies nutrients and removes waste from the healing tissue.

Anti-inflammatory medications are useful during this phase, as a prolonged inflammatory response delays healing. Rehabilitation during the repair phase is focused on restoring range of motion and applying controlled stress to newly formed tissue to promote alignment of collagen fibers and minimize adhesions. Because the collagen fibers are weak, it is important not to overstress the tissue and disrupt the fragile collagen scar.

Tissue healing is completed when the scar matures and remodels to its final form. Mature scar tissue is fibrous and inelastic and has no vascular supply. The scar is integrated into the injured tissue and the collagen fibers become thicker, increasing tensile strength, although never to the strength of the original tissue. Goals of rehabilitation during the maturation phase are to increase strength and neuromuscular control, with return to everyday activities and recreational pursuits.

IMMOBILIZATION

Muscle

Immobilization has a profound and devastating effect on skeletal muscle, with atrophy noted after 1 to 2 weeks. Numerous experiments have demonstrated decreases in muscle weight[26] and CSA[27-29] after immobilization. Heslinga et al[30] reported an increased rate of atrophy in fast twitch fibers compared with slow twitch fibers. Immobilization in a shortened position has the further consequence of decreasing the number of series sarcomeres, with subsequent loss of muscle length.[31-33] Other structural changes observed following immobilization include a 50% decrease in muscle/tendon contact area, with degenerative changes noted at the myotendinous junction,[99] formation of capillary fenestrae,[34] mitochondrial swelling with myofibrillar damage,[35] and deposition of connective tissue within the muscle.[34] Metabolic changes also occur during periods of immobilization. Protein synthesis is reduced as the result of decreased protein translation.[100] Immobilization promotes insulin resistance in muscle, leading to decreased glycogen stores when glucose is not transported into the cell and glycogen synthase enzyme activity is reduced.[101] The number of sodium (Na^+,K^+-ATPase) pumps in the sarcolemma is decreased,[29] serum creatine kinase levels are elevated,[35] the inorganic phosphate/phosphocreatine ratio (Pi/PCr) is elevated,[28] succinate dehydrogenase activity is decreased,[102] and cytoplasm antioxidant enzyme activity is increased in response to the formation of peroxide radicals and superoxides during muscle degeneration.[103] These structural and metabolic changes lead to strength deficits of 50%.[28,29] After immobilization, human subjects were unable to achieve maximum contraction during a burst superimposition test (a short burst of high-intensity electrical stimulation superimposed on a volitional contraction), indicating a central activating deficit.[28]

Bone

Immobilization is associated with reduced bone mass, osteopenia, and osteoporosis, with a subsequent increased risk of fracture when normal mechanical stress is applied to the weakened bone. Absence of stress on the bone leads to decreased osteoblast activity,[36] while osteoclast activity remains constant. Bone mineral loss does not resolve immediately upon return of normal stresses.

Houde et al[37] reported decreased bone mineralization 5 weeks after remobilization of the hand and wrist following cast immobilization. Bone growth is regulated locally by many factors, including insulin-like growth factor I (IFG-I). Decreased expression of IGF-I or membrane receptor resistance

may play a role in the reduction of bone growth. Bikle and colleagues[104] found increased IGF-I expression during immobilization, implicating a membrane receptor defect as the causative factor in cessation of bone growth.

Connective Tissues

Immobilization adversely affects musculoskeletal tissues other than muscle and bone. Tissues that experience reduced stress undergo physiologic and structural changes, resulting in decreased load-bearing capacity. Immobilized ligaments that have less fibronectin,[38] fewer menisci,[39] and less articular cartilage[40] show reduced aggregating proteoglycans (aggrecans), and their water content is increased. Evidence of reduced collagen content in ligaments,[38,41] tendons,[41] and menisci[42] has been found because these tissues become catabolic with disuse. The newly forming collagen is deposited in a haphazard pattern, with resultant low tensile strength.[43] Changes in composition of the connective tissue matrix also are observed. Alterations in the matrix reduce tensile stiffness and limit the capacity to resist deforming forces. Articular cartilage becomes thinner in the absence of normal joint stresses.[44] Joint capsule adhesions formed during immobilization result in decreased range of motion (ROM) and joint volume with increased intracapsular pressure.[45]

PHYSIOLOGIC CHANGES OF TRAINING

Endurance Training

When exposed to different functional demands, muscle fibers display considerable plasticity that extends to all aspects of their biomechanical and morphologic properties.[46] Low-load, high-repetition exercise promotes endurance gains by increasing mitochondrial density in the muscle.[47] The advantages of increased mitochondrial density include greater efficiency of energy production, increased use of fatty acids as an energy substrate, and decreased use of muscle glycogen. Concomitant with the increase in mitochondria per unit area is an increase in the activity of enzymes associated with aerobic energy production.[48,49] Prolonged low-intensity exercise also stimulates capillary growth, so that the oxygen diffusion distance remains low as the muscle enlarges.

In response to endurance training regimens, changes in fiber type expression and fiber CSA may be observed. If the intensity of repeated muscle contractions is low, the transition from fast to slow fiber type is slowed. On the contrary, high-intensity endurance training appears to induce a greater proportion of fast-to-slow fiber type conversions, as well as an increase in the proportion of SO fibers. The CSA of fibers remains unchanged or even decreases after endurance training.[46]

Strength Training

Skeletal muscle changes are more pronounced with heavy resistance exercise. Within a few weeks of the start of a resistance training program, changes in the myosin heavy chain (MHC) isoform (one of three polypeptide chains in the myosin filament) are observed.[50] The MHC isoform has a high degree of correlation with muscle fiber type. The total quantity of contractile proteins increases, leading to muscle hypertrophy and an increase in the CSA of the muscle fiber. Increased amino acid uptake is stimulated by tension on the myofilaments.[51] A study by Staron et al[52] showed that high-intensity resistance training of the thigh musculature led to increases in maximum force output. A significant decrease in Type IIb fibers was observed in as little as 2 weeks (four training sessions), whereas a simultaneous increase was noted in Type IIa MHC proteins.[52] The shift to a greater percentage of Type IIa muscle fibers denoted an increase in oxidative capacity. Concomitant increases in capillary density and citrate synthase activity further supported an increase in oxidative capabilities.[53] The fate of Type I fibers remains unclear because some studies show increases in Type I fibers,[46,54-57] and others demonstrate no change in their relative percentage.[58-60]

Heavy resistance training activates the high- and low-threshold motor units. Without question, high-resistance strength training leads to increased muscle CSA, where gains of 4.5% to 19.3% are observed in the first few months of training.[60-62] Whether this improved CSA is attributed to muscle hypertrophy (increase in the radial diameter of fibers within the muscle) or to muscle hyperplasia (increase in the number of fibers) is not fully known. Proponents of the hyperplasia theory point to increased numbers of muscle fibers in body-builders[63,64] and to the small fiber diameter in the hypertrophied deltoid muscle of wheelchair athletes.[65] A proposed explanation favoring hyperplasia states that a muscle fiber has a predetermined maximum volume, and that cell growth exceeding that volume causes the fiber to split into two daughter cells.[66] Most scientific studies do not support the role of hyperplasia in muscle enlargement, rather they support hypertrophy during high-resistance strength training. Muscle hypertrophy occurs via an increase in the size and number of myofibrils.[67] Actin and myosin content within the cell increases, along with the number of series sarcomeres. The accumulation of contractile proteins is accomplished by an increase in protein synthesis, a decrease in protein degradation, or both.[63,67]

Another area of controversy revolves around the "interference effect" seen in strength development and muscle hypertrophy, when strength training is performed concurrently with endurance training. As was mentioned previously, strength and endurance training regimens may yield differences with regard to the degree of fast-to-slow fiber type conversions and changes in fiber CSA. Recent studies have shown that concurrent strength and endurance training paradigms are antagonistic and limit the development of muscle strength,[46] while others show no difference.[57] Variances in training frequency and intensity between studies account for the differences in results.

Many other physiologic changes also occur as the result of resistance training. Converted Type IIa fibers show increased oxidative enzymatic activity,[68] while the enzymes of anaerobic glycolysis, phosphofructokinase, and lactate dehydrogenase remain unchanged.[69-71] Glycogen, phosphocreatine, and ATP stores are not increased as muscle fibers are able to generate sufficient ATP via oxidative phosphorylation.[70] The capacity to supply the cell with nutrients and oxygen is enhanced by increased capillarity[58] and increased myoglobin concentration. Reports of decreased capillary and myoglobin density[63] can be explained by the dilution effect of greater hypertrophy compared with capillary ingrowth or mitochondrial expression.

Strength Training in the Elderly

A remarkable decrease in both muscle mass and bone mineral density (BMD) is related to aging. Loss of muscle mass is attributed primarily to loss of alpha motoneurons and incomplete reinnervation of muscle cells by remaining intact motor units. The result is muscle atrophy, or sarcopenia, and loss of individual muscle fibers, predominantly Type II fibers.[72,73] Muscle strength declines by 15% per decade at between 50 and 70 years of age, and by 30% per decade thereafter.[74,75] More recent data demonstrate significant gender-related differences in the regulation of human skeletal muscle function at the muscle and single-fiber levels. In general, older men exhibit a decline in voluntary muscle force production, and older women experience a greater decrease in muscle contraction regulation, which contributes to greater frailty of overall muscle function.[73]

In the early 1980s, a study by Aniansson et al[72] revealed that low-intensity training led to very modest strength gains. These results misled the community into thinking that elderly persons could not combat sarcopenia with strength training. Recently, high-intensity resistance programs with elderly subjects have been implemented, and strength gains of 200% have been reported with increases in Type I and Type II fibers.[76] Decreases in musculotendinous and musculoarticular stiffness also were correlated with strength training.[77] Regimens typically consisted of three sets of eight to ten repetitions at 80% of one repetition maximum in two to three sessions per week. Strength gains are even observed in those older than 87 years at intensities of 1 RM. More important is the functional carryover of increased walking speeds, improved stair climbing, better balance, and overall increased movement throughout the day.[78]

In conjunction with strength gains, resistance training has the added benefit of reducing the loss of bone density, or osteoporosis, that accompanies aging. Both osteoporosis and a handicap at the skeletal muscle level are highly associated with a decreased ability to perform activities of daily living such as stair climbing and transfers, and they impair balance reactions, which increases the risk for falls. Hip fractures resulting from a fall can lead to significant morbidity and are the number one predictor of an inability to return to independent living. Elderly persons who train at 80% of 1 RM can increase BMD,[79] or can significantly retard the loss of BMD through a process called *osteogenesis,* or new bone growth, resulting from application of stress to the bone.[80] The ACSM and the AHA recently developed physical activity guidelines for older adults.[81] Parameters for both strength and endurance exercises for a variety of diagnoses can be found at www.acsm-msse.org.

Strengthening

Strength refers to the ability of a muscle to generate force and depends on muscle CSA, length, fiber type distribution, and velocity of movement.[105] As was described earlier, muscle CSA reflects the myofibril content of the muscle. Larger muscles have a greater number of myofibrils and therefore are able to generate increased force. The length of the muscle fiber also influences force development according to Starling's law. Simply stated, muscle has an optimum length at which it is capable of generating the greatest force (length-tension curve). When the muscle is shortened (active insufficiency), myosin filaments collide with the Z discs, and actin filaments overlap, preventing further shortening. If the muscle is stretched beyond its optimum length, the myosin-actin overlap is reduced, and some of the cross-bridges are unable to bind during cross-bridge cycling. Lengthening beyond the optimum length leads to passive insufficiency. Muscles with a higher percentage of Type II fibers generally are able to generate greater force than muscles with high Type I content. Finally, during concentric contraction, the muscle is able to generate greater force at lower speeds compared with higher speeds. Previously, isokinetic testing within the first 12 weeks after anterior cruciate ligament (ACL) reconstruction with a patellar tendon graft was conducted at a rate of 180 to 300 degrees per second to decrease the tensile forces on the patellar tendon and patella. During eccentric contractions, the opposite holds true, and the muscle is able to generate greater force at high speeds.

DeLorme[82] introduced strength training with weights in the early 1940s. He demonstrated that strength gains could be maximized with low-repetition, high-resistance programs. Further work showed that maximum strength gains occur when a load with resistance greater than 66% of 1 RM is lifted 10 times.[106] For continued strength gains, the load must be increased progressively. Failure to increase resistance progressively results in less muscle activation, as fewer motor units are recruited to lift the unchanging load. Presently, weight lifting is a component of the training program for all athletes. Sports-specific resistance training increases strength, power, and endurance, enhancing the athlete's performance.

Strength training programs change throughout the year, reflecting the different training seasons (preseason, in-season, off-season). Strength and conditioning specialists are experts in developing periodized strength training programs to accomplish the goals of each season. Although a complete discourse on the methods of periodized program design is beyond the scope of this book, it is helpful for the rehabilitation specialist to understand the basic tenants of periodization. A periodized program cycles volume and intensity over specific time periods. It consists of three cycles: macrocycle, mesocycle, and microcycle. The macrocycle describes an entire training period (usually a year for a competitive athlete) and typically is composed of several mesocycles. Mesocycles usually begin with a high-volume phase and end with a high-intensity peaking phase that corresponds to the different training seasons. Microcycles deal with daily and weekly variations in volume, intensity, loading, and exercise selection.[83] Exercises typically are chosen to mimic the movement patterns of the sport. The order of performance progresses from lifts or drills involving large muscle groups or multiple joints to lifts or drills specific for smaller muscle groups. Volume and intensity can be manipulated to create heavy and light lifting days. Rest between sets and exercise days can be changed to vary the intensity of the total workout. To increase strength, the weight chosen is usually less than 6 RM; 20 RM may be used to improve endurance.[84]

Periodization applies equally to the rehabilitation process of an injured patient. Table 3-1 depicts a periodized program for ACL reconstruction. A close resemblance to the criterion-based rehabilitation program previously described by Manal and Snyder-Mackler can be seen.[85] The macrocycle encompasses the time from injury until return to play. Mesocycles may include the preoperative phase, the early postoperative phase (days 1 to 7), the mid-postoperative phase (weeks 2 to 4), the late postoperative phase (weeks 5 to 12), and the return to activity phase (weeks 13 to 26). Microcycles are the specific exercises and treatment parameters that are used within each daily session. Consideration for protecting healing structures is imperative when a strengthening program is developed for the injured patient population.

Electrical Stimulation for Strengthening

Neuromuscular electrical stimulation (NMES) also can be used to increase muscular strength.[86] Electrically elicited muscular contraction, when used properly, can be more effective than volitional exercise during periods of decreased volitional control or reduced willingness to recruit the desired musculature. Evidence for effectiveness is strong.[86,87] A clear dose-response relationship has been noted between electrically elicited force and strengthening. Guidelines suggest a current intensity sufficient to elicit 50% of the volitional isometric force of the targeted musculature, which is the minimum dose for strength gains to be realized.[88] The intensity of stimulation needed to produce the necessary force of contraction can be uncomfortable for the patient, and the therapist must be willing and able to carry out the treatment at therapeutic intensities. The therapist also must have a method of measuring the force output (dose) so as to determine whether therapeutic levels are being reached.

Neural Adaptation

Early strength gains observed during resistance training programs cannot be explained by muscle changes, as contractile protein content and muscle CSA are unchanged. Increased strength in the absence of muscle hypertrophy is attributed to neural adaptation with training. As was noted previously, force output is increased by recruiting additional motor units or by increasing the rate of firing of active motor units. Strength gains also can be achieved by coordinating firing of the synergists to the prime mover, or by inhibiting antagonist contraction.

Motor learning, or the integration of movement patterns within the motor cortex, plays a role in the strength gains

Table 3-1	Periodized ACL Program	
Mesocycle	**Goals**	**Microcycle (Sample Treatment)**
Preoperative	Full knee extension	Quad sets, straight leg raise (3) ×3 (10 min)
Early postoperative (days 1 to 7)	Quadriceps activation	NMES ×3 (10 min)
	Decrease effusion	Ice, elevation, compression ×3 (10 min)
	ROM 0 to 90 degrees	Wall slides ×3 (5 min)
Mid-postoperative (weeks 2 to 4)	Quadriceps contraction	Patellar mobilizations superior, inferior, and diagonals ×3 (5 min)
	Ambulating without crutches	Gait training knee extension at heel strike
	Flexion within 10 degrees*	Cycling ×3 (10 min)
		Tibiofemoral mobilization with rotation (grade III/IV)
	Full knee extension*	Prone hangs (with weights) ×3 (10 min)
		Superior patella glide ×3 (5 min)
	Quadriceps strength >50%	Isokinetic intervals at 180 degrees per second, 360 degrees per second (2) × 3 (10 min)
		NMES ×3 (10 min)
		Wall squats (3) ×3 (10 min)
	Stairs, foot over foot	Step-ups and step-downs with a 6- to 8-inch block (3) ×3 (10 min)
Late postoperative (weeks 5 to 12)	Full ROM*	Prone quad stretch (5) × 3 (45 sec)
	Quadriceps strength >80%	Standing terminal knee extensions (3) ×3 (10 min)
		Leg press (3) ×3 (10 min)
		Single leg cycling ×3 (10 min)
		Squats (3) ×3 (10 min)
	Coordinate muscle firing	Perturbation training (3) ×3 (1 min each exercise)
	Normal gait	Treadmill ×3 (10 min)
Return to activity (weeks 13 to 26)	Quadriceps strength >95%	Increase intensity of exercises (3) ×3 (20 min)
	Hop test >85%	Agility drills ×3 (10 min)
		Treadmill running ×3 (10 min)
		Sport-specific perturbation training ×3 (15 min)

*Comparable with that of the uninvolved limb.

observed early in training. Practice is an integral part of this learning process. Research has shown that strength gains achieved through one type of muscle contraction have little carryover to other ranges. Multi-angle isometrics therefore are used to strengthen muscles surrounding a painful joint. Dynamic muscle contractions exhibit a similar specificity for training. Higbie et al[89] found that subjects trained with eccentric isokinetic exercise were stronger with eccentric testing, and those trained concentrically exhibited greater strength on concentric testing.

Co-contraction of antagonist muscles is apparent during the initial performance of any task. (Remember the first time you tried to ice skate.) Antagonist contraction limits motor unit activation in agonist muscles. Furthermore, antagonist inhibition as a result of training would be represented as increased prime mover strength.

Electromyography (EMG) is used to study the rate of action potentials and force output. The area under the curve, the integrated EMG (I-EMG), indicates the total force output during a contraction. Prime mover activation can be studied easily by surface EMG. These studies demonstrate a correlation between increases in strength and increases in I-EMG,[90] indicating that strength training improves activation of the prime mover by recruiting additional motor units and by increasing

the firing rate. It has been found that training one limb leads to increased strength in the contralateral limb, signifying a crossover effect in central processing.[91]

Measuring changes in firing rate or motor unit recruitment in synergistic muscles is more difficult, but strength gains certainly suggest greater activation of synergist muscles. Increased synergistic activation with training implies an inability to maximally activate the prime mover. However, Sale[92] reviewed studies of motor unit activation and concluded that untrained subjects were able to maximally activate tested muscles. He postulated that the complex multi-joint movements involved in weightlifting may result in central activation inhibition not observed in simple, single-joint test motions.

Synchronicity of muscle firing also can be evaluated with EMG. Strength training promotes synchronized firing of motor units during short, maximum contractions.[93] The exact role that synchronized firing plays in strength gains is unclear because asynchronous motor unit firing leads to greater force output during submaximum contraction.[92]

Central and peripheral neural adaptation does not technically strengthen the muscle, but it is inextricably linked to strengthening paradigms and programs. The therapist needs to exploit neural adaptation principles for therapeutic benefit.

CASE STUDY 3-1

A 19-year-old collegiate athlete originally dislocated her shoulder playing lacrosse in May. She underwent arthroscopic Bankart repair and rehabilitation. She was deemed adequately rehabilitated to return to playing field hockey in September because her shoulder would not be put in a compromised position by the demands of the sport. At the completion of her field hockey season in November, she asked to participate in two weekend lacrosse tournaments. Her surgeon was concerned about whether her shoulder was strong enough to withstand the rigors of lacrosse and referred her to a physical therapist for consultation.

Physical examination revealed excellent active and passive ROM, with no pain on any active or resisted motions. Strength and proprioceptive testing also revealed no abnormalities in any testing below 90 degrees of flexion or abduction. Above 90 degrees, however, strength and control deficits were significant. Based on this evaluation, the athlete was not cleared to participate in lacrosse tournaments. Instead, rehabilitation was reinstituted to prepare her for the upcoming lacrosse season in February.

Diagnostic classification: Musculoskeletal 4D: Late effects of dislocation (05.6)

This case illustrates the principles of motor learning, neural adaptation, and specificity of exercise. Rehabilitation focused on exercises that were progressively more challenging in elevated ROM. Abduction and posterior rotator cuff strengthening exercises were instituted above 90 degrees, with the shoulder moving into external rotation. A manually resisted D2 flexion (proprioceptive neuromuscular facilitation [PNF]) pattern was used, beginning at 90 degrees of flexion and moving to full flexion. Rhythmic stabilization exercise was begun in the supine position and progressed to the sitting position, again in elevated ROM. Plyometric external rotation was begun in the supine position and progressed to the sitting position, and finally to standing. A weight training program modified for her stabilization surgery was instituted,[94] and within 1 month, functional progression of lacrosse activities (throwing, catching, and cradling) was instituted. Return to play in February was uneventful.

CASE STUDY 3-2

A 24-year-old professional football running back who tore his left ACL in training camp was referred to physical therapy 10 days post injury and 2 days after ACL reconstruction using an Achilles tendon allograft. Upon initial evaluation, the patient was wearing a postoperative knee immobilizer and was weight bearing as tolerated using axillary crutches. Both the immobilizer and the surgical dressing were removed, which revealed the tibial incision along with several arthroscopic portals covered with Steri-Strips. His knee was swollen and a bit warm, but he had no real pain. Initially, he was a bit tentative about moving his knee, but he responded well to encouragement.

An early goal was to restore full extension equal to the opposite side within the first week.[95] Range of motion was 1 degree hyperextension to 95 degrees flexion as measured goniometrically in the supine position. He was instructed in active wall slide and quadriceps setting exercises for ROM. He also was able to pedal on a raised-seat stationary bike and maintained 60 RPMs for several minutes.

The athlete demonstrated good quadriceps contraction with a small lag during leg elevation. This lack of control was attributed to his knee effusion and resulting quad inhibition.[96] He began the NMES protocol with his knee flexed to 60 degrees.[85] Two 3 × 5-inch self-adhesive electrodes were placed over the medial quadriceps distally and the lateral quadriceps proximally. A 2500-Hz alternating current with a 50% duty cycle at 75 bursts per second was delivered for 10 seconds, with a 50-second rest period. His maximum voluntary isometric contraction torque was approximately 75 ft/lb, but electrically elicited forces of nearly 100 ft/lb were measured by the end of 10 contractions.

Diagnostic classification: Musculoskeletal 4I: ACL tear (717.8)

Subsequent initial therapy interventions included effusion control, patellar mobilizations, gait training without crutches, and scar mobility once the stitches were removed. He had a history of previous surgeries but did not appear to develop keloid scarring. Left leg strengthening was performed in the clinic with the use of both open and closed kinetic chain exercises, and the athlete was responsible for upper body and right leg weight training on non-therapy days.

The athlete was seen for 12 visits over 4 weeks before his care was transferred back to the athletic training staff. After 4 weeks, he exhibited equal extension bilaterally and nearly full flexion ROM. His quadriceps weakness was minimal as he demonstrated only a 20% strength deficit left versus right. Therefore it was recommended that NMES be discontinued. His incisions were well healed, and he had a normalized gait pattern. With continued strengthening and functional progression training, he returned to play the following spring.

SUMMARY

Strength training is essential for countering the muscle weakness that occurs with injury, disuse, and aging. Morphologic and physiologic characteristics of muscle can provide information that can be used to design more effective training regimens, especially for patients with muscle weakness. This chapter has endeavored to provide a systematic assessment of the physiologic response of muscle to repetitive contraction under conditions that occur during exercise (rest, fatigue, and recovery) in vivo, and to examine its relationship to existing and proposed strength training programs for rehabilitation and training.

REFERENCES

1. Murphy RA: Contractile mechanisms of muscle cells. In Berne RM, Levy MN, editors: Physiology, ed 4, St. Louis, 1998, Mosby, p 269.

2. Murphy RA: Skeletal muscle physiology. In Berne RM, Levy MN, editors: Physiology, ed 4, St. Louis, 1998, Mosby, p 282.

3. Whitney EN, Rolfes SR: Fitness: physical activity, nutrients, and body adaptations. In Understanding nutrition, ed 7, West Minneapolis, Minn, 1995, p 509.

4. McArdle WD, Katch F, Katch V: Sports and exercise nutrition, ed 2, Philadelphia, 2005, Lippincott Williams and Wilkins.

5. Stryer L: Citric acid cycle. In Biochemistry, ed 4, New York, 1995, WH Freeman, p 509.

6. Stryer L: Oxidative phosphorylation. In Biochemistry, ed 4, New York, 1995, WH Freeman, p 529.

7. Stryer L: Fatty acid metabolism. In Biochemistry, ed 4, New York, 1995, WH Freeman, p 603.

8. Rose SJ, Rothstein JM: Muscle mutability. Part 1: general concepts and adaptation to altered patterns of use. Phys Ther 62:1773, 1982.

9. Clamann HP: Motor unit recruitment and the gradation of muscle force, Phys Ther 73:830, 1993.

10. Hennig R, Lomo T: Firing patterns of motor units in normal rats, Nature 314:164, 1985.

11. Buller AJ, Eccles JC, Eccles RM: Differentiation of fast and slow muscles in the cat hind limb, J Physiol 150:399, 1960.

12. Salmons S, Vrbova G: The influence of activity on some contractile characteristics of mammalian fast and slow muscles, J Physiol (Lond) 201:535, 1969.

13. Zebedin E, Sandtner W, Galler S, et al: Fiber type conversion alters inactivation of voltage-dependent sodium currents in murine C2C12 skeletal muscle cells, Am J Physiol Cell Physiol 287:C270-C280, 2004.

14. Dimengo JM: Surgical alternatives in the treatment of heart failure, AACN Clin Issues 9:192, 1998.

15. Lucas CMHB, Debelaar ML, Vanderveen FH, et al: A new stimulation protocol for cardiac assist using the latissimus dorsi muscle, PACE 16:2012, 1993.

16. Allman B, Rice C: Neuromuscular fatigue and aging: central and peripheral factors, Muscle Nerve 25:785-796, 2002.

17. Kent Braun JA, le Blanc R: Quantitation of central activation failure during maximal voluntary contractions in humans, Muscle Nerve 19:861-869, 1996.

18. Stevens JE, Binder Macleod SA, Snyder Mackler L: Characterization of the human quadriceps muscle in active elders, Arch Phys Med Rehabil (in press).

19. Baudry S, Klass M, Pasquet B, Duchateau J: Age-related fatigability of the ankle dorsiflexor muscles during concentric and eccentric contractions, Eur J Appl Physiol 100:515-525, 2007.

20. Maffiuletti N, Jubeau M, Munzinger U, et al: Differences in quadriceps muscle strength and fatigue between lean and obese people, Eur J Appl Physiol 101:51-59, 2007.

21. Snyder-Mackler L, De Luca PF, Williams PR, et al: Reflex inhibition of the quadriceps femoris muscle after injury or reconstruction of the anterior cruciate ligament, J Bone Joint Surg 76A(4):555-560, 1994.

22. Reed BV: Wound healing and the use of thermal agents. In Michlovitz SL, editor: Thermal agents in rehabilitation, ed 3, Philadelphia, 1996, FA Davis.

23. Butterfield T, Best T, Merrick MA: The dual roles of neutrophils and macrophages in inflammation: a critical balance between tissue damage and repair, J Ath Train 41(4):457-465, 2007.

24. Ferry S, Dahners L, et al: The effects of common anti-inflammatory drugs on the healing rat patellar tendon, Am J Sports Med 35:8, 2007.

25. Cohen DB, Kawamura S, Ehteshami JR, Rodeo SA: Indomethacin and celecoxib impair rotator cuff tendon to bone healing, Am J Sports Med 34:1-8, 2006.

26. Nicks DK, Beneke WM, Key RM, et al: Muscle fiber size and number following immobilization atrophy, J Anat 163:1, 1989.

27. Veldhuizen JW, Verstappen FT, Vroemen JP, et al: Functional and morphological adaptations following four weeks of knee immobilization, Int J Sports Med 14:283, 1993.

28. Vandenborne K, Elliott MA, Walter GA, et al: Longitudinal study of skeletal muscle adaptations during immobilization and rehabilitation, Muscle Nerve 21:1006, 1998.

29. Leivseth G, Clausen T, Everts ME: Effects of reduced joint mobility and training on Na,K ATPase and Ca ATPase in skeletal muscle, Muscle Nerve 15:843, 1992.

30. Heslinga JW, te Kronnie G, Huijing PA: Growth and immobilization effects on sarcomeres: a comparison between gastrocnemius and soleus muscles of the adult rat, Fur J Appl Physiol 70:49, 1995.

31. Appell HJ: Skeletal muscle atrophy during immobilization, Int J Sports Med 7:1, 1986.

32. Heslinga JW, Huijing PA: Effects of short length immobilization of medial gastrocnemius muscle of growing young adult rats, Fur J Morphol 30:257, 1992.

33. Williams PE: Use of intermittent stretch in the prevention of serial sarcomere loss in immobilized muscle, Ann Rheum Dis 49:316, 1990.

34. Oki S, Desaki J, Matsuda J, et al: Capillaries with fenestrae in the rat soleus muscle after experimental limb immobilization, J Electron Microsc Tokyo 44:307, 1995.

35. Kauhanen S, Leivo I, Michelsson JE: Early muscle changes after immobilization: an experimental study on muscle damage, Clin Orthop 297:44, 1993.

36. Kannus P, Jozsa L, Kvist M, et al: Expression of osteocalcin in the patella of experimentally immobilized and remobilized rats, J Bone Miner Res 11:79, 1996.

37. Houde JP, Schulz LA, Morgan WJ, et al: Bone mineral density changes in the forearm after immobilization, Clin Orthop 317:199, 1995.

38. AbiEzzi SS, Foulk RA, Harwood FL, et al: Decrease in fibronectin occurs coincident with the increased expression of its integrin receptor alpha5beta1 in stress deprived ligaments, Iowa Orthop J 17:102, 1997.

39. Djurasovic M, Aldridge JW, Grumbles R, et al: Knee joint immobilization decreases aggrecan gene expression in the meniscus, Am J Sports Med 26:460, 1998.

40. Palmoski MJ, Perrione E, Brandt KD: Development and reversal of proteoglycan aggregation defect in normal canine knee cartilage after immobilization, Arthritis Rheum 22:508, 1979.

41. Harwood FL, Amiel D: Differential metabolic responses of periarticular ligaments and tendon to joint immobilization, J Appl Physiol 72:1687, 1992.

42. Dowdy PA, Miniaci A, Arnoczky SP, et al: The effect of cast immobilization on meniscal healing: an experimental study in the dog, Am J Sports Med 23:721, 1995.

43. Padgett LR, Dahners LE: Rigid immobilization alters matrix organization in the injured rat medial collateral ligament, J Orthop Res 10:895, 1992.

44. Jurvelin J, Diviranta I, Tammi M, et al: Softening of canine articular cartilage after immobilization of the knee joint, Clin Orthop 207:246, 1986.

45. Schollmeier G, Uhthoff HK, Sarkar K, et al: Effects of immobilization on the capsule of the canine glenohumeral joint: a structural functional study, Clin Orthop 304:37, 1994.

46. Putman C, Xu X, Gillies E, et al: Effects of strength, endurance and combined training in myosin heavy chain content and fibre-type distribution in humans, Eur J Appl Physiol 92:376-384, 2004.

47. Holloszy JO, Coyle EF: Adaptations of skeletal muscle to endurance exercise and their metabolic consequences, J Appl Physiol 56:831, 1984.

48. Holloszy JO: Biochemical adaptations in muscle: effects of exercise on mitochondrial oxygen uptake and respiratory enzyme activity in skeletal muscle, J Biol Chem 242:2278, 1967.

49. Morgan TE, Cobb LA, Short FA, et al: Effects of long term exercise on human muscle mitochondria. In Pernow B, Saltin B, editors: Muscle metabolism during exercise, New York, 1971, Plenum, p 87.

50. Staron RS, Johnson P: Myosin polymorphism and differential expression in adult human skeletal muscle, Comp Biochem Physiol 106B:463, 1993.

51. Goldberg A, Ettinger JD, Goldspink DF, et al: Mechanisms of work induced hypertrophy of skeletal muscle, Med Sci Sports 7:248, 1975.

52. Staron RS, Karapondo DL, Kraemer WJ, et al: Skeletal muscle adaptations during the early phase of heavy resistance training in men and women, J Appl Physiol 76:1247, 1994.

53. Frontera WR, Meredith CN, O'Reilly KP, et al: Strength training and determinants of $\dot{V}O_2$ max in older men, J Appl Physiol 68:329, 1990.

54. Pyka G, Lindenberger E, Charette S, et al: Muscle strength and fiber adaptation to a year long resistance training program in elderly men and women, J Gerontol 49:M22, 1994.

55. Sipila S, Elorinne M, Alen M, et al: Effects of strength and endurance training on muscle fiber characteristics in elderly women, Clin Physiol 17:459, 1997.

56. Taaffe DR, Pruitt L, Phka G, et al: Comparative effects of high and low intensity resistance training on thigh muscle strength, fiber area, and tissue composition in elderly women, Clin Physiol 16:381, 1996.

57. Häkkinen K, Alen M, Kraemer WJ, et al: Neuromuscular adaptations during concurrent strength and endurance training versus strength training, Eur J Appl Physiol 89:42-52, 2003.

58. Hather BM, Tesch PA, Buchanan P, et al: Influence of eccentric actions on skeletal muscle adaptations to resistance training, Acta Physiol Scand 143:177, 1991.

59. Adams GR, Hather BM, Baldwin KM, et al: Skeletal muscle myosin heavy chain composition and resistance training, J Appl Physiol 72:911, 1993.

60. Hakkinen D, Newton RU, Gordon SC, et al: Changes in muscle morphology, electromyographic activity and force production characteristics during progressive strength training in young and older men, J Gerontol Biol Sci 53:8415, 1998.

61. Narici MV, Hoppeler H, Kayser B, et al: Human quadriceps cross sectional area, torque and neural activation during 6 months strength training, Acta Physiol Scand 157:175, 1996.

62. Sipila S, Sirominen H: Effects of strength and endurance training on thigh and leg muscle mass and composition in elderly women, J Appl Physiol 78:334, 1995.

63. MacDougall JD, Sale DG, Moroz JR, et al: Mitochondrial volume density in human skeletal muscle following heavy resistance training, Med Sci Sports 11:164, 1979.

64. Tesch PA, Larsson L: Muscle hypertrophy in body builders. Eur J Appl Physiol 49:301, 1982.

65. Tesch PA, Karlsson J: Muscle fiber type characteristics of m. deltoideus in wheelchair athletes: comparison with other trained athletes. Am J Phys Med 62:239, 1983.

66. Gonyea WJ: Muscle fiber splitting in trained and untrained animals, Exp Sports Sci 8:19, 1980.

67. Gordon EE, Kowalski K, Fritts W: Changes in rat muscle fiber with forceful exercise, Arch Phys Med Rehabil 48:577, 1967.

68. Ploutz LL, Tesch PA, Biro RL, et al: Effects of resistance training on muscle use during exercise, J Appl Physiol 76:1675, 1994.

69. Tesch PA, Komi PV, Hakkinen K: Enzymatic adaptations consequent to long term strength training, Int J Sports Med 8(suppl):66, 1987.

70. Tesch PA, Thorsson A, Colliander EB: Effects of eccentric and concentric resistance training on skeletal muscle substrates, enzyme activities and capillary supply, Acta Physiol Scand 140:575, 1990.

71. Houston ME, Froese EA, Valeriote SP, et al: Muscle performance, morphology and metabolic capacity during strength training and detraining: a one leg model, Fur J Appl Physiol 51:25, 1983.

72. Aniansson A, Grimby G, Hedberg M, et al: Muscle morphology, enzyme activity and muscle strength in elderly men and women, Clin Physiol 1:87, 1981.

73. Yu F, Hedström M, Cristea A, et al: Effects of ageing and gender on contractile properties in human skeletal muscle and single fibres, Acta Physio 190:229-241, 2007.

74. Danneskoild Damsoe B, Kofod V, Munter J, et al: Muscle strength and functional capacity in 77 81 year old men and women, Fur J Appl Physiol 52:123, 1984.

75. Larsson L: Histochemical characteristics of human skeletal muscle during aging, Acta Physiol Scand 117:469, 1983.

76. Frontera WR, Meredith CN, O'Reilly KP, et al: Strength conditioning in older men: skeletal muscle hypertrophy and improved function, J Appl Physiol 64:1038, 1988.

77. Ochala J, Lambertz D, Van Hoecke J, Pousson M: Changes in muscle and joint elasticity following long-term strength in old age, Eur J Appl Physiol 100:491-498, 2007.

78. Fiatarone MA, O'Neill EF, Ryan ND, et al: Exercise training and nutritional supplementation for physical frailty in very elderly people, N Engl J Med 330:1769, 1994.

79. Nelson ME, Fiatarone MA, Morganti CM, et al: Effects of high intensity strength training on multiple risk factors for osteoporotic fractures, JAMA 272:1909, 1994.

80. Ryan AS, Treuth MS, Hunter GR, et al: Resistive training maintains bone mineral density in postmenopausal women, Calcif Tissue Int 62:295, 1998.

81. Nelson M, Rejeski WJ, Blair SN, et al: Physical activity and public health in older adults: recommendation from the American college of sports medicine and the American Heart Association, Med Sci Sports Exerc 39(8):1435-1445, 2007.

82. DeLorme TL: Restoration of muscle power by heavy-resistance exercises, J Bone Joint Surg 27:645, 1945.

83. Stone MH: Muscle conditioning and muscle injuries, Med Sci Sports Exerc 22(4):457-462, 1990.

84. Kraemer WJ, Duncan ND, Volek JS: Resistance training and elite athlete's adaptations and program considerations, J Orthop Sports Phys Ther 28:110, 1998.

85. Manal TJ, Snyder-Mackler L: Practice guidelines for anterior cruciate ligament rehabilitation: a criterion based rehabilitation progression, Oper Tech Orthop 6:190, 1996.

86. Snyder Macker L, Delitto A, Bailey S, et al: Quadriceps femoris muscle strength and functional recovery after anterior cruciate ligament reconstruction: a prospective randomized clinical trial of electrical stimulation, J Bone Joint Surg 77A:1166-1173, 1995.

87. Snyder Mackler L, Ladin Z, Schepsis AA, et al: Electrical stimulation of thigh muscles after reconstruction of the anterior cruciate ligament, J Bone Joint Surg 73 A:1025-1036, 1991.

88. Snyder-Macker L, Delitto A, Stralka SW, et al: Use of electrical stimulation to enhance recovery of quadriceps femoris muscle force production in patients following anterior cruciate ligament reconstruction, Phys Ther 74:901-907, 1994.

89. Higbie EJ, Cureton KJ, Warren GL, et al: Effects of concentric and eccentric training on muscle strength, cross sectional area, and neural activation, J Appl Physiol 81:2173, 1996.

90. Hakkinen D, Komi PV: Training induced changes in neuromuscular performance under voluntary and reflex conditions, Eur J Appl Physiol 55:147, 1986.

91. Moritani T, deVries HA: Neural factors vs. hypertrophy in time course of muscle strength gains, Am J Phys Med Rehabil 58:115, 1979.

92. Sale DG: Neural adaptation to resistance training, Med Sci Sports Exerc 20(suppl):S135, 1988.

93. Milner Brown HS, Stein RB, Lee RG: Synchronization of human motor units: possible roles of exercise and supraspinal reflexes, Electroencephalogr Clin Neurophysiol 38:245, 1975.

94. Fees M, Decker T, Snyder-Mackler L, et al: Upper extremity weight training modifications for the injured athlete, Am J Sports Med 26:732-742, 1998.

95. Axe MJ, Linsay K, Snyder-Mackler L: The relationship between knee hyperextension and articular pathology in the anterior cruciate ligament deficient knee, J Sports Rehabil 5:120-126, 1996.

96. Palmieri-Smith RM, Kreinbrink J, et al: Quadriceps inhibition induced by an experimental knee joint effusion affects knee joint mechanics during a single-legged drop landing, Am J Sports Med 35:8, 2007.

97. Zajac Fe, Faden JS: Relationship among recruitment order, axonal conduction velocity, and muscle unit properties of type identified motor units in cat plantaris muscle, J Neurophysiol 53:1303, 1985.

98. Fleshman JW, Munson JB, Sypert GW, et al: Rheobase, input resistance, and motor unit type in medial gastrocnemius motoneurons in the cat, J Neurophys 46:1326, 1981.

99. Kannus P, Jozoa L, Kvist M, et al: The effect of immobilization on myotendinous junction: an ultrastructural, histochemical and immunohistochemical study, Acta Physiol Scand 144:387, 1992.

100. Booth FW, Criswell DS: Molecular events underlying skeletal muscle atrophy and the development of effective countermeasures, Int J Sports Med 18:S265, 1997.

101. Nicholson WF, Watson PA, Booth FW: Glucose uptake and glycogen synthesis in muscles from immobilized limbs, J Appl Physiol 56:431, 1984.

102. Haggmark T, Jansson E, Eriksson E: Fiber type area and metabolic potential of the thigh muscle in man after knee surgery and immobilization, Int J Sports Med 2:12, 1981.

103. Kondo H, Miura M, Itokawa Y: Antioxidant enzyme systems in skeletal muscle atrophied by immobilization, Pflugers Arch 422:404, 1993.

104. Bikle DD, Harris J, Halloran BP, et al: Skeletal unloading induces resistance to insulin like growth factor I, J Bone Miner Res 9:1789, 1994.

105. Jones DA: Strength of skeletal muscle and the effects of training, Br Med Bull 48:592, 1992.

106. Costill DL, Coyle EF, Fink WF, et al: Adaptations in skeletal muscle following strength training, J Appl Physiol 46:96, 1979.

107. Moritani T, deVries HA: Potential for gross muscle hypertrophy in older men, J Gerontol 35:672, 1980.

Strength Training Concepts in the Orthopaedic Patient

This chapter will cover the physiological adaptations within the muscle following strength exercises by providing examples of the changes that occur with neural adaptations within muscle. The major contributors to improving muscle strength will be discussed, and the differences between strength, power, and endurance will be explained. The reader will be able to distinguish between how to train Type I, Type IIA, and Type X (IIB) muscle fiber types and will be able to describe the changes that take place in tendons secondary to strengthening. The reader will also be able to identify the number of repetitions, sets, and the amount of resistance needed to increase muscle strength and hypertrophy, describe the effects of aging on muscle, and describe the differences between eccentric, concentric, and isometric exercises. To illustrate the strength training concepts there is a 7-page series of general strengthening exercise images, including exercises of the shoulders, arms, chest, back, hips, and core.

Strengthening is an important part of any patient's rehabilitation. If a patient is to attain optimal strengthening and progress, numerous variables must be considered. The therapist should consider the type of exercise, the frequency, the intensity, and the duration. All of these variables will determine the success of any strengthening program. The therapist also must understand the physiologic and neural adaptations that occur within the muscle, and how long it takes to make these changes. Can we convert muscle fiber types through strength training? Should eccentric, concentric, and/or isometric exercises, or a combination of all three, be used? Is it necessary to periodize the patient's strength training program, and would this result in significant changes in muscle strength? How does the therapist incorporate neuromuscular exercises into a strengthening program? Answers to these questions are essential to professionals who are responsible for prescribing resistance exercise to improve a patient's way of life, be it on the field of play or in terms of everyday function.

Simply stated, *strength* is the ability of the muscle to exert a maximum force at a specified velocity.[1] *Power* is defined as the force exerted multiplied by the velocity of movement.[1] *Muscular power* is a function of both strength and speed of movement. *Endurance* is the ability to sustain an activity for extended periods of time.[1] Local muscle endurance is best described as the ability to resist muscular fatigue.[1] It is the opinion of the authors of this chapter that a good strength base, a foundation of muscular power, and muscular endurance are important for reestablishing function and/or improving performance.

In today's therapy environment, much emphasis is placed on functional exercise. Unfortunately, most of the exercises regarded as functional seem to be performed in a weight-bearing position with significant muscular co-contraction. In fact, strengthening exercises have been labeled as nonfunctional because they are performed in the open kinetic chain (OKC). For the purposes of this chapter, a *functional exercise* is defined as an exercise specific to the muscle groups that are important to the activity the patient wishes to return to; sufficient resistance, repetitions, and sets are used to stimulate the muscle to adapt by increasing strength. Several studies have demonstrated that when OKC exercises were used to strengthen the glenohumeral rotators, significant gains were made both in the velocity of a baseball during a pitch and in the velocity of a tennis ball in a tennis serve.[2,3] Therefore, strength training for the rotators of the glenohumeral joint performed by moving the shoulder into internal and external rotation in an OKC position is a functional exercise. Another study found that by strength training with weight machines, subjects between 60 and 83 years of age were able to decrease the amount of time it took them to climb a flight of stairs.[4] Finally, another study found that combining OKC exercise with functional exercise yielded better outcomes than did functional exercise by itself in patients who had undergone anterior cruciate ligament (ACL) reconstruction.[5]

This chapter begins by describing different types of muscle action. Neural adaptations both at the local level and within the central nervous system that result from strength training are discussed. Muscle cellular adaptations, including fiber conversion, changes in sarcomeres, and hypertrophy versus hyperplasia, are discussed. Mechanical muscles changes produced by strength training, as well as connective tissue changes, are explained. Discussion of hormonal and metabolic changes is followed by discussion of the effects of aging on muscle and exercise adaptations in the elderly. Gender differences and muscles changes are described. Finally, time frames for developing strength gains, in addition to the amount of resistance and the numbers of sets and repetitions needed to make these changes, are put forth. An understanding of the cellular and molecular adaptations of skeletal muscle in response to strength training is important for the clinician who seeks to provide a framework for improving performance in the athlete and for enhancing health and quality of life in the general population, with or without chronic disease.

TYPES OF MUSCLE ACTIONS

Three main muscle-strengthening actions have been identified: eccentric, concentric, and isometric. Simply stated, an eccentric action occurs whenever opposing forces acting on a muscle exceed the force produced by that muscle.[6] This causes the muscle to lengthen while it is being activated. Eccentric actions are characterized by their ability to achieve high muscle forces—an enhancement of the tissue damage associated with muscle soreness—and perhaps require unique control strategies.[7] Eccentric actions are used frequently throughout everyday life, and especially in athletic competition. A common human movement strategy is to combine concentric and eccentric actions into a sequence called the *stretch-shorten cycle*.[7] This cycle typically involves a small-amplitude eccentric contraction of moderate to high velocity that is followed by a concentric contraction.[7] Eccentric contractions are mechanically efficient, can attenuate impact forces, and serve to maximize performance.[7]

The second type of action is a concentric contraction. A concentric contraction occurs when the force produced by the muscle exceeds the external force or load.[6] This contraction causes the muscle to shorten and is the latter action of the stretch-shorten cycle. This cycle, as pointed out earlier, happens during most day-to-day activities and occurs without specialized training.[6] Enorka[6] considered that only when a concentric contraction is performed without an eccentric action would muscle performance be decreased.[5,6]

The last type of muscle action is called an *isometric action*. Isometric strengthening occurs when the force generated by muscle and the external force are the same, and no lengthening or shortening of the muscle occurs. Isometric strengthening has been shown to be very joint angle specific with minimum carryover to other joint angles. Only a 20-degree carryover is seen either way, from where the muscle was trained, although one study showed that carryover throughout the entire range is greater when the muscle has been trained isometrically in the lengthened position.[8]

NEURAL ADAPTATIONS

The first signs of muscle adaptation to strengthening exercises are neural adaptations. Several studies have demonstrated that early strength gains induced by resistance training are primarily due to modifications of the nervous system. These modifications can occur both at the local level and at the central nervous system level. Moritani and DeVries[9] in a landmark study found that "neural factors" accounted for significant improvements observed during the first 4 weeks of an 8-week resistance-training program. Staron et al[10] demonstrated that only after 6 weeks of training was significant muscle fiber hypertrophy detected. The neural adaptations elicited by resistance training include decreased co-contraction of antagonists and expansion in dimensions of the neuromuscular junction, indicating increased content of presynaptic neurotransmitter and postsynaptic receptors.[11-13] Greater synchronicity of the discharge of motor units after strength training also has been reported.[14] Aagaard et al[15] suggest that increases in motoneuronal output induced by strength training can cause increased central motor drive, elevated motoneuron excitability, and reduced presynaptic inhibition. Laqerquist et al[16] described similar increases in strength in the trained and the untrained soleus of subjects who were trained for 5 weeks. Based on their results, investigators concluded that the increase in strength of the untrained limb may be due to supraspinal mechanisms. They go on to suggest that increased force production of the trained limb versus the untrained limb may be due to a synergistic effect of increased somatosensory stimuli and descending supraspinal commands. Another study found that the cross-education effect may be controlled in part by adaptations in the sensorimotor cortex and the temporal lobe.[17] In fact, one paper recommends that motor learning theory and imagined contractions should be incorporated with strength training.[18] It is important to note that eccentric contractions have been found to induce greater cross-education effects than concentric and isometric muscle actions. Zhou[19] found increases of 5% to 35% in force production for the untrained limb during both isometric and concentric muscle actions, although Hortobagyi et al[20] reported increases as high as 104% during eccentric muscle action in the untrained limb.

Conflicting views present the relative contributions of neural versus muscle adaptation, with strength training lasting longer than 2 to 3 months. Deschenes et al[1] indicate that with prolonged resistance training, the degree of muscle hypertrophy is limited, and significant hypertrophic responses can occur within a finite period of time, lasting no longer than 12 months. A secondary neural adaptation explains the continued strength gains with prolonged resistance training. The secondary phase of neural adaptations takes place between the sixth and twelfth month. In contrast, Shoepe et al[21] demonstrated substantial muscle hypertrophy as a result of several years of resistance training, when compared with a group of sedentary individuals.

CELLULAR ADAPTATIONS

To review, muscles are made up of hundreds of thousands of muscle cells, which also are referred to as *muscle fibers*. These muscle fibers are made up in part by hundreds of myofibrils, which extend along the length of the muscle fibers. The myofibrils are made up of two types of protein filaments, called thick filaments and thin filaments. A *sarcomere* is the small structural unit that makes up the myofibril and contains both thick and thin filaments. When a muscle contracts, the sarcomeres shorten. Thick filaments are made up of a contractile protein called *myosin.* Thin filaments are made up of three different contractile proteins called *actin, tropomyosin,* and *troponin.* The turnover rate of these muscle proteins is one of the slowest in the body. Within skeletal muscle synthesis, growth of contractile proteins lags behind that of other proteins such as mitochondria and sarcoplasmic reticulum.[22,23] It is the synthesis and accretion of contractile proteins that account for the hypertrophy that occurs with resistance training. This hypertrophy, in addition to hypertrophy within the whole muscle (5% to 8%), occurs mostly within the intracellular myofibrils (25% to 35%).[1,24]

It is important to note that different types of muscle fibers are found in the human body: Type I, Type IIa, and Type IIx (used to be referred as Type IIb). Also within any muscle, hybrids of these fiber types can be found, including Type I/IIa, Type IIa/IIx, and Type I/IIa/IIx.[25] Type I fibers tend to have a slower contraction time, high resistance to fatigue, and low force production. Type IIa fibers have a fast contraction time, intermediate resistance to fatigue, and high force production. Type IIx fibers have a very fast contraction time, low resistance to fatigue, and very high force production.

MUSCLE FIBER TYPE–SPECIFIC ADAPTATIONS

Malisoux et al[25] found that 8 weeks of training involving stretch-shortening cycle exercises increased single fiber diameter, peak force, and shortening velocity, leading to enhanced fiber power. All of these changes were seen in Type I, IIa, and IIa/IIx fibers. In addition, peak power was improved in Type IIa fibers.

It is well documented that a prolonged program of resistance training brings about fiber type conversion within the muscle. The most common finding is an increase in the percentage of Type IIA fibers, along with a decrease in percentage of Type IIB (Type IIx) fibers.[26-28] It appears that as soon as a Type IIB (IIx) muscle fiber is stimulated, it starts a process of transformation toward Type IIA by changing the quality of proteins and expressing different types and amounts of myosin adenosine triphosphatase (mATPase).[29] At the end of a resistance-training program, very few Type IIB (IIx) fibers remain; this situation is reversed during detraining. However, when resistance training is started again, the conversion from Type IIB (IIx) to Type IIA is quicker. Although resistance training promotes hypertrophy in all three major muscle fiber types in humans—I, IIA, IIB (IIx)—the amount of hypertrophy differs in each fiber type. Based on examination of pretraining to posttraining muscle samples, it has been established that muscle hypertrophy is greatest in Type IIA fibers, followed by Type IIB (IIx), with Type I fibers demonstrating the least amount of hypertrophy.[10,26-28,30]

CHANGES IN SARCOMERES

Besides fiber type adaptations at the cellular level, other structural signs may indicate muscle damage. Under electron microscope, it has been shown that sarcomeres may become out of register, Z-line streaming is evident, regions of overextended sarcomeres are found, and regional disorganization of myofilaments and T-tubule damage may occur.[31] Evidence suggests that an increase in sarcomeres occurs after bouts of eccentric exercise.[32] In fact, one study found an 11% increase in sarcomere number after eccentric loading.[31]

HYPERTROPHY VERSUS HYPERPLASIA

Resistance exercise is a potent stimulus for increasing the size of muscle. For a muscle to become larger, it must increase in cross-sectional area (hypertrophy), or the number of muscle fibers (hyperplasia) must be increased. It generally is believed that the number of muscle fibers is innate and does not change during life.[33] In contrast, several researchers have reported that muscle is capable of increasing in size as the result of an increase in fiber number.[34,35] The exact mechanism responsible for muscle hypertrophy is uncertain, although several theories have been expressed in the literature. Skeletal muscles are capable of remodeling under various conditions. The activation of myogenic stem cells within the muscle is one of the most important events that occur during skeletal muscle remodeling.[35] Muscle (myogenic) stem cells remain dormant under the basement of the myofibers; upon stimulation, they differentiate into satellite cells to form myofibers.[35] Muscle, or myogenic, stem cells start to generate, and through a series of cell divisions, daughter cells become satellite cells. Evidence suggests that strength training induces a significant increase in satellite cell content in skeletal muscle, and that strength training downregulates the expression of myostatin, which is responsible for inhibiting satellite cell activation.[36] Because the myonuclei in mature muscle fibers are not able to divide, it is suggested that the incorporation of satellite cell nuclei into muscle fibers results in the maintenance of a constant nuclear/cytoplasmic ratio. Therefore, new muscle fibers are formed following strength training. When resistance or endurance exercises promote satellite cell proliferation, and differentiation can be detected in injured fibers and those with no discernible damage, muscle hyperplasia occurs in human skeletal muscle.[34,35,37,38]

Force developed by the myofilaments (actin and myosin) may stimulate the uptake of amino acids, thus resulting in muscle tissue growth.[39] Heavy forces encountered during resistance training lead to disruption in the Z-lines. Disorganization after disruption of the Z discs may cause the myofibril to split and grow back at full size.[40] Furthermore, disruption and rebuilding of the muscle result in an increase in connective tissue surrounding the muscle fibers.

In summary, as a result of strength training exercises, physiologic adaptations of muscle result in an increase in strength.

These adaptations include hypertrophy (within the first 6 to 8 weeks), hyperplasia, hormonal changes, increased connective tissue surrounding muscle fibers, disruption of the myofilaments, and neuromuscular changes (within the first 2 weeks of training). In addition, metabolic adaptations within the muscle fiber enhance the ability of the muscle to generate adenosine triphosphate (ATP) for anaerobic metabolism. Anaerobic metabolism requires that the muscle increase phosphocreatine (PC) and glycogen stores, leading to an increase in the enzyme creatine phosphokinase that breaks down PC, as well as an increase in the rate-limiting enzyme phosphofructokinase (PFK) of glycolysis.

MECHANICAL CHANGES IN PASSIVE AND DYNAMIC MUSCLE STIFFNESS

At the mechanical level, evidence of increased dynamic and passive muscle stiffness can be found.[41] Whitehead et al[32] states that the rise in passive muscle tension is dependent on the range of length over which the muscle is worked. With bicep brachii eccentric loading, the sense organs of the muscle and the body's ability to sense joint position have shown both an increase and a decrease in the flexed position. This seems to be dependent on whether a muscle spindle injury actually occurs (which increases the flexed position), or whether sarcomere disruption is present (which decreases the flexed position), the former happening with high intensity strengthening.[7] Mechanically, signs of a shift in the muscle's optimum length can be seen, toward longer muscle length, decreased active tension, increased passive tension, and muscle swelling and soreness.[31] Muscle swelling and soreness lead to delayed-onset muscle soreness (DOMS), which is thought to be purely mechanical and is not an inflammatory response.[41]

Connective Tissue Changes

Not only are changes in the muscles and their respective cells evident, but changes also take place in the tendons. As you will see, tendons in trained individuals are different from those in untrained individuals. Data from humans show that a larger cross-sectional area (CSA) of the trained tendon results in less stress on the tendon during maximal isometric contractions in trained compared with untrained individuals, and it provides a more injury-resistant tendon.[42] Ying et al[43] found that the Achilles tendons of individuals with a history of physical activity had a larger CSA than those of their sedentary counterparts. An adaptive response that results in the increased net synthesis of Type I collagen in the peritendinous tissue around the Achilles tendon has been found to take place after 4 weeks of training.[44] Type I collagen is the thicker fiber among all collagen fibers. Although an initial increase in Type I collagen occurs, this does not lead to an immediate increase in the CSA of a nonpathologic tendon. It seems that a prolonged training effect in nonpathologic tendons is needed for an increase in CSA to occur. One study found that CSA was increased by 20% to 30% in long distance runners versus untrained subjects.[45] Yet another study reported no increase in CSA after just 6 months

of recreational running.[46] When an injury process is in place though, a tendency toward a quicker response to resistance training is seen within the tendon in its normal state. Kadi[47] showed that with eccentric training in patients with Achilles tendinosus, both pathologic Achilles tendon width and pain were decreased over a 12-week period. Because most of the studies discussed earlier used isotonic or concentric resistance training as their mode of exercise, it would be interesting to see what types of changes would take place when eccentric resistance training is used in healthy subjects, and whether Achilles tendon CSA and maximal strain would increase more quickly with eccentric loading versus concentric or isotonic contractions.

It is important to note that with a chronic overload injury to a tendon, upregulation of Type I and Type III collagen occurs, with a preference for Type III.[42] Type III collagen is thinner than Type I and has been shown to be more prevalent at rupture sites in the Achilles tendon than at other areas in the same tendon.[42] It is interesting to note that training can increase Type I collagen production and can improve patients' overall symptoms involving tendinopathy; training also may decrease their chances for acute rupture.[42]

In summary, resistance training not only changes muscles, it has an effect on connective tissue as well. Connective tissue can increase in size and strength, which may help to decrease the incidence of injury. Although the length of this training in healthy subjects remains uncertain, through eccentric loading of a pathologic tendon, one can improve a patient's symptoms and can normalize tendon size within 12 weeks.

Hormonal Responses

Resistance training has been shown to elicit a significant acute hormonal response, which is more critical for tissue growth and remodeling than are chronic changes in resting hormonal concentrations. Anabolic steroids such as testosterone and the growth hormones (GH) have been shown to become elevated over 15 to 30 minutes of high-volume exercise that is moderate to high in intensity, with short rest periods and stressing a large muscle mass, when compared with low-volume, high-intensity protocols in which long rest intervals are provided.[47]

Although single bouts of exercise can cause a significant acute rise in serum total and free testosterone concentrations in males, no significant rise is seen in females, regardless of age.[48] Other anabolic hormones such as insulin and insulin-like growth factor-I (IGF-I) are critical for skeletal muscle growth. Blood glucose and amino acid levels regulate insulin. However, following resistance exercise, elevations in circulating IGF-I have been reported, presumably in response to GH-stimulated secretion.[47] A significant rise in growth hormone occurs regardless of gender, but not in elderly women.[48]

Aging and Muscle Changes

Professional athletes are performing longer and longer over the past decade. Demographic data clearly illustrate that, overall, the U.S. population is growing older. Aging causes loss of functional capacity, resulting from a decrease in muscle mass (sarcopenia).[49] Approximately one-third of total muscle mass is lost between 30 and 80 years of age.[50] This muscle loss is primarily the result of selective loss and remodeling of motor units. By the seventh decade of life, some muscles may include only half the number of motor units, and 75% of the total number of fibers, present in the muscles of young adults.[51] Type II fibers appear to be the most seriously affected; they gradually decrease in both size and number with advancing age. Loss of fiber begins at approximately 25 years of age and accelerates thereafter.[52] However, it appears that training can reverse aging atrophy and can maintain fiber type distribution in elderly individuals similar to that found in the young. Several studies have determined that strength improvements in the elderly are coupled with cellular and whole muscle hypertrophy.[11,53-55] Also, muscle hypertrophy responses to resistance training have been found to be indistinguishable between young and elderly people.[11,56]

Recently research has suggested that power (high velocity) training may be more effective than strength training in improving physical function in community-dwelling adults.[57] Another study found that using 80% of 1 rep max for resistance was the most effective way to achieve simultaneous improvements in muscle strength, power, and endurance in older adults.[58] It is interesting to note that another study reported that power training increases balance over that seen in a nontraining group, especially when a load of 20% 1 rep max is used.[59]

Although in general, two to three sets of strength training is most beneficial, some studies have found that in elderly individuals who do one set, exercise is sufficient to significantly enhance muscle function and physical performance (chair rise, 6-meter backward walk, 400-meter walk, and stair climbing test), although gains in muscle strength and endurance are greater in the three-set group.[60] Another study found that regardless of intensity (high = 80% 1 RM, and low = 50% 1 RM), significant improvements in strength, endurance, and stair climbing time were attained by doing a single set of 12 reps.[61] Another interesting note is that elderly individuals who supplemented their exercise regimen with creatine exhibited a greater increase in fat free mass and total body mass as compared with the placebo group with strength training.[62] The recommendations for the strength training variables noted below are beneficial for use with the elderly or with the young athlete and/or patient:

- Strength training reps, 6 to 12
- Multiple sets, 2 to 3
- At least 2 days per week and a maximum of 3 days per week of strength training
- 90 seconds to 2 minutes rest between sets
- Train the large muscle groups before the smaller muscle groups
- Choice of exercise should be based on an evaluation of muscle strength and of muscles that are important to the type of activity the patient wishes to return to. The greater the intensity of the activity the patient wishes to return to, the greater is the intensity of the recommended rehabilitation and/or training.

Gender Differences and Muscle Changes

Gender differences are apparent in muscle cross-sectional examination both before and after training; Type IIA fibers are the largest among men, whereas Type I fibers are of greatest size among women.[63] Furthermore, Staron et al[26] demonstrated that with heavy resistance training, the conversion of Type IIB (IIx) fibers to Type IIA fibers occurred at 2 weeks in females and at 4 weeks in males.

One study found that when muscle quality (maximal force production per unit of muscle mass) was measured, young women (20 to 30 years) were seen to have significantly greater gains than young men, old men, and old women after 9 weeks of strength training.[64] In fact, after 30 weeks of detraining, young women still had greater muscle quality than did members of the other three groups. In another study that looked at muscle volume in response to strength training in both old and young men and women, young men made up the only group that was able to maintain gains in muscle volume after 31 weeks of detraining.[65]

Apparent differences also can be seen in relation to eccentric strength across genders and the life span. In both men and women, concentric peak torque was seen to decrease farther than eccentric peak torque with age.[66] Investigators in another study found that women tended to better preserve muscle quality with age for eccentric peak torque.[67] In addition, older women seemed to have an enhanced capacity, about a decade longer, to store elastic energy better than similarly aged men and younger men and women.[67]

TYPES OF MUSCLE ACTION ADAPTATIONS

Eccentric Strengthening

After a bout of eccentric exercise, an adaptation takes place. This adaptation can be called the *repeated bout effect*. When one performs an eccentric bout of exercise, a repeated bout effect adaptation will protect the muscle against further damage from subsequent eccentric bouts.[41] This can help to improve performance and prevent injury. With eccentric strengthening and the above adaptations, strength, CSA, and neural activation are increased.[68] Along with muscle adaptation, possible tendon adaptations have been discussed. With bicep brachii eccentric loading, muscle sense organs and the body's ability to sense joint position have shown both an increase and a decrease in the flexed position. This seems to be dependent on whether a muscle spindle injury has actually occurred (increase flexed position), or only sarcomere disruption (decreased flexed position), the former happening with high-intensity strengthening.[7] Increased signal from a muscle spindle has been shown with heavy eccentric strength, although no studies have shown more evidence of significant neural adaptation than those involving concentric strengthening.

Typically, eccentric contractions can generate two to three times more force than concentric contractions.[69] This has led some authors to believe that eccentric training rather than concentric strengthening leads to a greater capability of overloading the muscle to a greater extent, thereby enhancing muscle mass, strength, and power.[69] This generalization may seem fair but may be too simple.

Many studies have shown an increase, a decrease, or no change in functional performance, concentric strength, and eccentric strength after eccentric training.[70-81] Outcomes noted in the previous section can be attributed to different training protocols and methods of assessment.[70] Current research has shown that eccentric training is more effective than concentric training in developing eccentric strength, and that concentric strengthening is more effective in developing concentric strength.[71] The specificity of training noted here represents another application of the specific adaptations to imposed demands (SAID) principle.

The degree of strength gain is relative to the volume/intensity and velocity of eccentric exercise. In most studies, the load used was appropriate to induce failure in the muscle. The actual volume does vary, but the findings of one study support the use of low-volume eccentric exercise.[81] Another study found that when compared with high-intensity eccentric training, low-intensity eccentric training is seen to cause the same amount of muscle damage, but without the large drop in muscle performance.[82] Based on these two studies, it can be seen that a high-intensity/volume model may not be needed to attain eccentric strength gains. Other research has shown that to obtain the greatest hypertrophy and strength gains, one must work eccentrically 180 degrees per second over the range.[83] Keep in mind though that this study was performed with isokinetic equipment, and the carryover to isotonic equipment is unknown.

Concentric Strengthening

As was discussed earlier, neural, contractile, and muscle fiber–type adaptations are made in strength training. Most athletes will use a combination of eccentric, concentric, and isometric contractions. To address the need to control a load when returning it to the starting position, most strengthening studies have used a combination of eccentric and concentric actions. As was noted previously, the stretch-shorten cycle is initiated by an eccentric action followed by a concentric contraction, but an eccentric contraction can happen by itself. Because of this fact, whenever anyone works isotonically, he or she is working eccentrically, even if concentrating on the shortening contraction. In the real world, it is almost impossible to work only concentrically. That is what makes it so difficult to discuss the adaptations of concentric only contractions. What follows is an attempt to discuss concentric strengthening adaptations. The changes associated with concentric strength training are poorly understood.[84]

Concentric only strengthening does not produce as much exercise-induced muscle injury as is produced by eccentric strengthening.[85] In fact, more muscle damage is produced when a muscle is loaded eccentrically than when it is loaded eccentrically and concentrically, regardless of whether this is done alternately or at separate times.[86] Whereas eccentric strengthening carry-over seems to be very specific to intensity,

mode, and velocity of training, concentric strengthening may be more general in terms of its carryover. In one study, investigators found that velocity-specific concentric only strengthening resulted in increased peak torques above and below the training velocity,[87] although another study found that concentric training was less mode and speed specific versus corresponding eccentric training.[88,88a]

Isometric Strengthening

The question remains regarding what types of adaptations the muscle undergoes during isometric strengthening. One study has reported that this is dependent on the type or rate of contraction. Progressive contractions produce modification of the nervous system at the peripheral level, whereas ballistic contractions affect the muscle's contractile properties.[89] Another study found that increased isometric strength might be due to factors associated with hypertrophy, independent of neural adaptations.[90]

Clinical Application

How does one apply this information to a clinical situation? First, we as clinicians need to integrate eccentric strengthening into our practice. This involves more than just lowering the weight after a concentric contraction. Because of current research findings, we know that to rehabilitate a patient for functional tasks or to train an athlete, we must have them perform eccentric movements. Remember, in the definition of a stretch-shorten cycle, an eccentric contraction is a low-amplitude, moderate- to high-velocity contraction. Therefore, eccentric movements must be faster than concentric contractions. Eccentric isotonic training must produce force that is two to three times greater than that of its concentric counterpart to achieve the proper intensity. This does not necessarily mean that the isotonic load should be doubled or tripled. Force that is generated during exercise is dependent on the amount of resistance used; the greater the resistance, the slower is the speed. (Force equals mass times acceleration.) Because an eccentric action should be happening at greater speed, one may have to increase the load by only 20% to 30% if the limb is moved twice as fast as the concentric contraction. We then need to allow a rest period greater than 48 hours. We have to work with patients in a specific eccentric manner to obtain maximum gain through their rehabilitation and performance training. How to do this isotonically and safely and effectively in a controlled clinical setting is the first question that must be answered.

What injuries or muscle groups would benefit the most from eccentric strengthening? Numerous studies have discussed the use of eccentric strengthening in the treatment of patients with Achilles tendinosus, patellar tendinopathy, iliotibial band syndrome (runners), and chronic isolated posterior cruciate ligament (PCL)-injured knees.[91-95] MacLean et al[94] showed that in knees with a PCL deficit, a significantly decreased eccentric/concentric ratio was noted compared with the contralateral hamstring. In the study by Mafi et al,[91] investigators found that a greater number of patients with chronic Achilles tendinosus experienced better overall satisfaction and decreased pain with eccentric strengthening training than with concentric strengthening training. Another study by Young et al[95] showed that eccentric training with a decline squat protocol was superior to a traditional eccentric protocol, with decreased pain and improved sporting function noted over 12 months in elite volleyball players who had suffered patellar tendinopathy. Kadi[47] showed that with eccentric training in patients with Achilles tendinosus, an actual decrease in Achilles tendon width occurred, along with decreased pain. These studies tell us that eccentric strengthening should definitely be included as part of any tendinopathy treatment.

Other applications may include use of eccentric actions and loading on muscle groups that primarily work concentrically but that have been immobilized. Take, for example, a patient who is status post anterior cruciate ligament repair. If the knee has been braced and the quadriceps group has been maintained in a shortened position, we know that muscular atrophy will occur, along with a decrease in the number of sarcomeres. This remolding can occur within the first 5 days of immobilization.[7] If we eccentrically load the quadriceps group properly in the open chain, we will produce sarcomere lengthening, along with an increase in the actual number of sarcomeres. This adaptation will help to speed up the return of a good quadriceps eccentric action and possibly the concentric contraction as well. Also note that with eccentric loading of the tibia in the open chain position, the tibia will be gliding posteriorly, and this will eliminate any anterior shear force on the ACL. With a concentric open chain quadriceps contraction, the force generated will be an anterior shear.

When working with patients and athletes, we must consider what the specific function of a muscle is in relation to that athlete's sport. Consider a track sprinter who is going through rehabilitation from a hamstring group strain. If the athlete's hamstring were properly loaded eccentrically, this may help to prevent further injury due to the repeated bout effect. The same is true with a baseball pitcher, who by eccentrically training the rotator cuff muscles may be able to adapt to higher eccentric forces, thereby decreasing his chances of suffering from a deceleration injury. To gain these benefits from eccentric training, the athlete most likely would need to be trained very specifically through training of the same muscle groups with the same intensity as needed by the particular sport. One study showed a decrease in the occurrence of hamstring strain injuries in elite soccer players who underwent eccentric overload training.[96]

Examples of when not to use an eccentric loading action would include the time during initial rehabilitation after a tendon repair, or during the initial stages of muscle healing. Because the force generated by an eccentric action can be two to three times greater than that of a concentric contraction, failure may be generated at the repair site, or at the site of tissue injury. For example, if a patient has just gone through a supraspinatus tendon repair and is status post 2 weeks, eccentric loading obviously should be avoided. However, if the same patient is working on active assistive range of motion with wall walks, and at the top of the exercise starts to lower his arm without assistance from the wall, he will eccentrically load that tendon and may re-rupture the tendon repair. Because concentric loading generates less force, it may be more beneficial when working with a repaired tendon to initially use concentric only strengthening when the tissue has healed enough to withstand an external load.

Isometric contractions seem to be most beneficial when used to increase the endurance of those muscles that function as spinal stabilizers.[97] This will help to maintain low but continuous activation of the paraspinal and abdominal wall muscles that function as stabilizers.[98] According to recent research findings, isometric contractions lend themselves more to a neural than to a contractile adaptation.[98]

Exercise Variables

If one is to achieve the physiologic adaptations described earlier, several variables must be considered. The variables that must be planned for carefully in the development of an exercise program include choice of exercise, order of exercises, number of sets, number of repetitions, intensity of exercise, duration of rest between sets and exercises, and frequency of training.

The type of exercise chosen should be specific to the specific muscle deficits revealed in the initial evaluation. Furthermore, the type of exercise used should be specific to the muscle groups that are important in improving the performance of the athlete. For example, in the overhead throwing athlete, the external rotators—infraspinatus and teres minor—provide a breaking action in deceleration of the shoulder. Eccentric loading to the external rotators is a specific exercise for strengthening the external rotators, and eccentric activity of the external rotators is specific to the movement pattern and to exercise performed by the athlete in competition. Furthermore, high-speed eccentric loading is very damaging to the muscle. When the eccentric strength of the external rotators is increased, greater protection from damage is provided to the muscle. This concept is discussed in greater detail later in this chapter.

The order of exercises performed by the athlete typically involves performance of large muscle group exercises before smaller muscle group exercises. Because metabolic demand is greater for large muscle group exercises, exercises that recruit more than one muscle group, such as closed kinetic chain exercises, should be performed before isolation exercises are performed.[29]

Once again, debate is evident in the literature regarding the numbers of sets and the frequency of strength training. For the athlete, the numbers of sets within a workout are directly related to the individual training goals. Multiple-set programs optimize the development of strength and local muscular endurance.[99] Gains in strength occur more rapidly with multiple-set programs than with single-set protocols.[100] Single-set exercise programs may be effective for individuals who are untrained, or for those who are just beginning a resistance training program. Single-set workouts are also useful in maintenance programs. Furthermore, strength changes over a short-term training period, and nonperiodized multiple-set programs may not be different between one, two, and three sets of 10 to 12 RM.[101] However, when a single-set protocol is compared with multiple-set periodized programs, significantly superior results are observed with multiple-set periodized programs that last longer than 1 month.[102] Gotshalk et al[102] demonstrated that higher volumes of total work produced significantly greater increases in circulating anabolic hormones during the recovery phase after multiple-set heavy resistance exercise protocols.

McLester et al[103] showed that training 1 day per week was an effective way to increase strength, even in experienced recreational weightlifters. However, this study reported superior results with training 3 days per week when compared with 2 days per week when the total volume of exercise was held constant.

Advanced training frequency varies considerably. Hoffman et al[104] demonstrated that football players who trained 4 to 5 days per week achieved better results than those who trained 3 or 6 days per week. Frequencies as high as 18 sessions per week have been reported in Olympic weightlifters.[105]

The intensity of the exercise or the amount of resistance used for a specific exercise is the most important variable in resistance training. The most common method of determining the amount of resistance that should be used in a strength-training program is to identify the maximal load that can be lifted in a given number of repetitions within one set. The greatest effects on strength measures, or maximal power outputs, are achieved when strength-training repetitions range between 6 and 12.[29] In other words, the maximum weight that can be lifted 6 times and 6 times only is the amount of resistance to start with. Sets and repetitions are added at subsequent workouts until 3 sets of 12 repetitions (reps) is reached. After the above reps and sets goal is reached, reps are reduced down to 8, and weight is added, allowing only 8 repetitions. It has been demonstrated that once 15 repetitions are achieved with a specific weight, the muscle no longer continues to improve in strength. However, lighter loads that allow 15 to 20 repetitions are very effective in increasing absolute local muscle endurance.[106,107]

Maximizing power requires a good strength base. Given that both force and time components are relevant for maximizing power, training to increase muscle power requires two general loading strategies. First, heavy resistance training must recruit high-threshold fast twitch muscle fibers needed for strength. The second strategy is to incorporate lighter loads; depending on the exercise, this may encompass 30% to 60% of 1 RM.[108,109] Weight training for power has been referred to as *explosive strength training*. Paavolainen et al[110] demonstrated that explosive strength training was able to improve a running time for 5 kilometers by improving running economy and muscle power, although a large volume of endurance training was performed concomitantly. The maximum amount of resistance used in the explosive strength training exercises was 40% of 1 RM. When performing explosive weight training exercises, the athlete moves as fast as possible throughout the range of motion, resulting in loss of contact with the ground in an explosive squat, or loss of contact with the bar in a bench press. During traditional bench press and squat weight training exercises performed at an explosive velocity, a recent study has shown that 40% to 60% 1 RM and 50% to 70% 1 RM, respectively, may be most beneficial in the development of power.[111]

The final variable that is important for muscle adaptation from strength training is the time interval between sets. The rest interval is dependent upon the intensity of the training. For example, it has been shown that acute force and power production may be compromised by short rest periods of 60 seconds or less.[112] Longitudinal studies have shown that greater strength increases are seen with long rest periods between sets, that is, 2 to 3 minutes versus 30 to 40 seconds.[113,114,115]

In conclusion, the authors of this chapter believe that if one is to make progressive, efficient, major strength gains in the athlete, one must apply numerous concepts. The patient must be worked specifically toward his goals, whether they consist of strength, hypertrophy, power, or endurance in the context of life and/or sport. At the same time, the patient must vary his strengthening program with periodization if he will be training for extended periods. The basic concept of periodization involves changing the intensity, velocity, and volume of exercise as needed. Consideration also must be given to the type of muscle action needed (eccentric, concentric, and isometric) and the amount of focus that that action will require if one is to help the athlete in his sport. The authors recommend the exercise variables listed below for rehabilitating and/or training a patient:

- Strength training of 8 to 12 repetitions for strength and hypertrophy, 4 to 6 repetitions for power, and 12 to 15 repetitions for endurance
- Multiple sets for all types of strengthening
- At least 2 days of strength training per week
- 1- to 2-minute rest for smaller muscle groups, and 2- to 3-minute rest for larger muscle groups
- Starting with multiple-joint exercise, and finishing with single-joint exercise
- Intensity starting at 8 repetition (rep) max for strength and 10 rep max for hypertrophy, 6 rep max for power at high or moderate velocity, and 15 rep max for muscular endurance
- Velocity that is slow, moderate, or fast depending on specific goals
- Focus on eccentric strengthening for deceleration muscles and on eccentric and concentric training for acceleration muscles
- Need for periodization any time an athlete requires strength training for longer than 4 weeks
- Choice of exercises based on evaluation of muscle strength and of muscles that are important to the type of activity in which the patient participates (As was noted previously, the greater the intensity of the activity, the greater the intensity of the strength training should be.)

General Strengthening Exercises

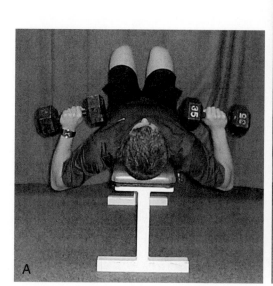
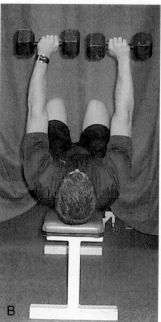

Figure 4-1 Bench and reach. (From Donatelli RA: Sports-specific rehabilitation, St. Louis, 2008, Churchill Livingstone.)

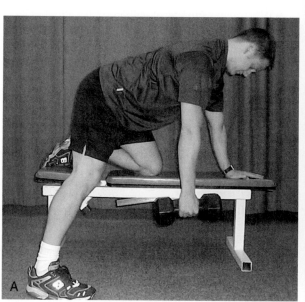
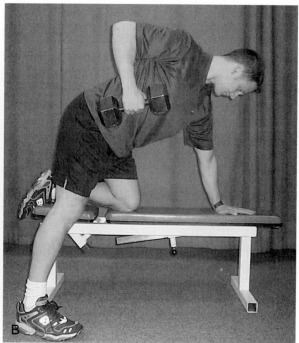

Figure 4-2 Arm row. (From Donatelli RA: Sports-specific rehabilitation, St. Louis, 2008, Churchill Livingstone.)

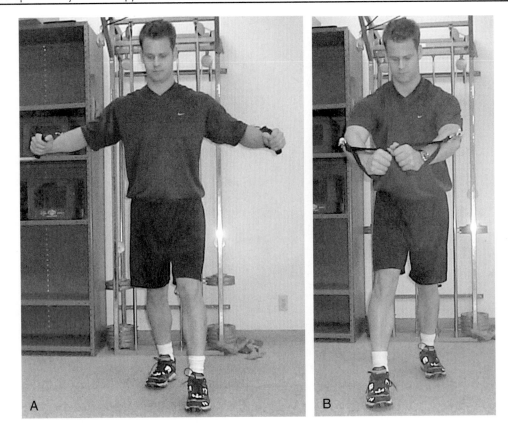

Figure 4-3 Dynamic hug. (From Donatelli RA: Sports-specific rehabilitation, St. Louis, 2008, Churchill Livingstone.)

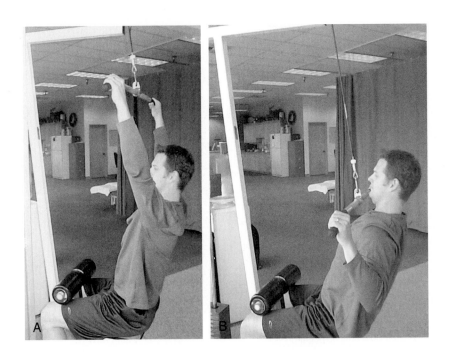

Figure 4-4 Lateral pulldown. (From Donatelli RA: Sports-specific rehabilitation, St. Louis, 2008, Churchill Livingstone.)

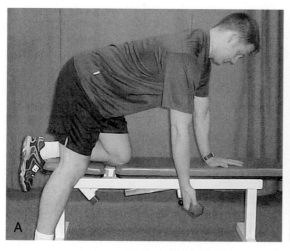
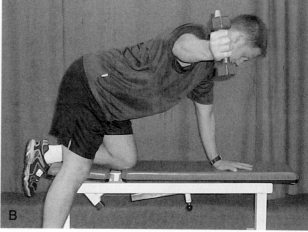

Figure 4-5 Mid trap lift. **A,** Infraspinatus. **B,** Supraspinatus. (From Donatelli RA: Sports-specific rehabilitation, St. Louis, 2008, Churchill Livingstone.)

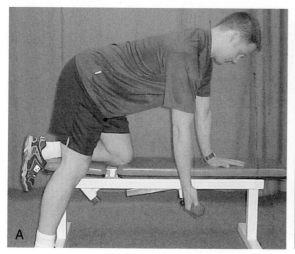
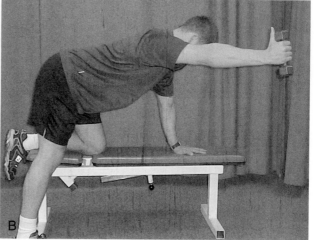

Figure 4-6 Lower trap lift. (From Donatelli RA: Sports-specific rehabilitation, St. Louis, 2008, Churchill Livingstone.)

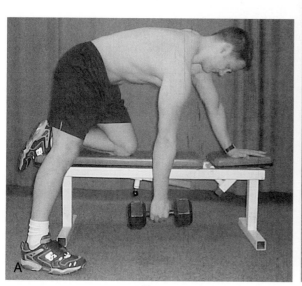
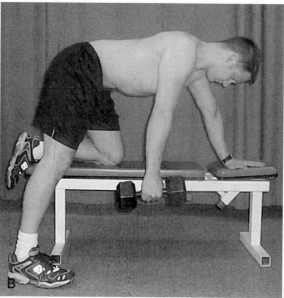

Figure 4-7 Scapular retraction. (From Donatelli RA: Sports-specific rehabilitation, St. Louis, 2008, Churchill Livingstone.)

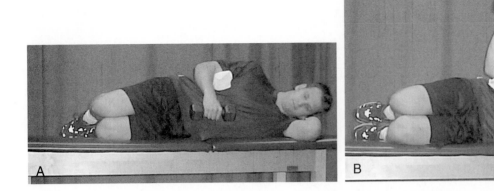

Figure 4-8 Side-lying external rotation. (From Donatelli RA: Sports-specific rehabilitation, St. Louis, 2008, Churchill Livingstone.)

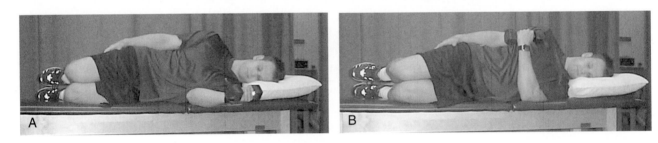

Figure 4-9 Side-lying internal rotation. (From Donatelli RA: Sports-specific rehabilitation, St. Louis, 2008, Churchill Livingstone.)

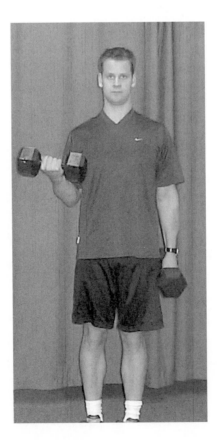

Figure 4-10 Bicep curl. (From Donatelli RA: Sports-specific rehabilitation, St. Louis, 2008, Churchill Livingstone.)

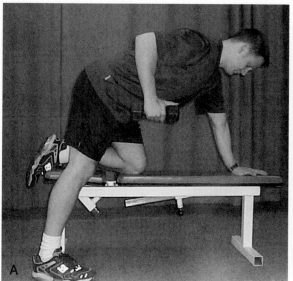 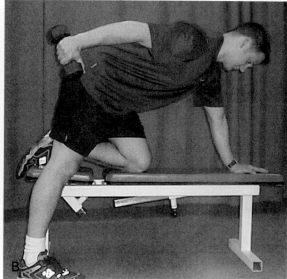

Figure 4-11 Tricep kickback. (From Donatelli RA: Sports-specific rehabilitation, St. Louis, 2008, Churchill Livingstone.)

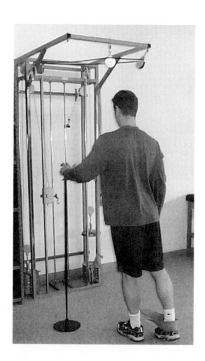

Figure 4-12 Standing pulley hip extension. (From Donatelli RA: Sports-specific rehabilitation, St. Louis, 2008, Churchill Livingstone.)

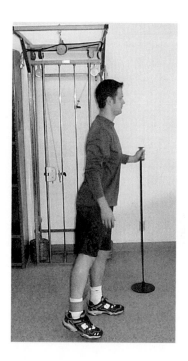

Figure 4-13 Standing pulley hip abduction. (From Donatelli RA: Sports-specific rehabilitation, St. Louis, 2008, Churchill Livingstone.)

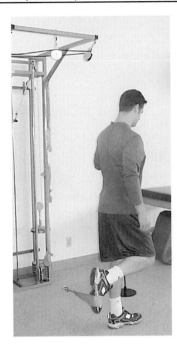

Figure 4-14 Standing pulley hip external rotation. (From Donatelli RA: Sports-specific rehabilitation, St. Louis, 2008, Churchill Livingstone.)

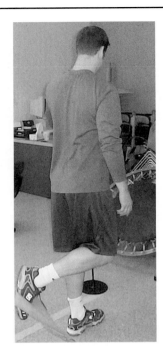

Figure 4-15 Standing pulley hip internal rotation. (From Donatelli RA: Sports-specific rehabilitation, St. Louis, 2008, Churchill Livingstone.)

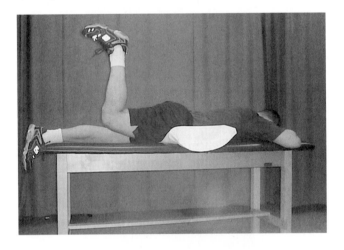

Figure 4-16 Prone hip extension. (From Donatelli RA: Sports-specific rehabilitation, St. Louis, 2008, Churchill Livingstone.)

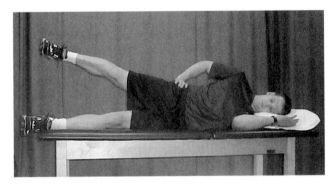

Figure 4-17 Side-lying hip abduction. (From Donatelli RA: Sports-specific rehabilitation, St. Louis, 2008, Churchill Livingstone.)

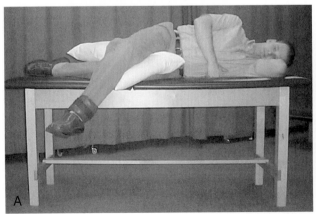
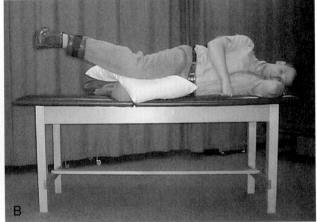

Figure 4-18 Side-lying hip internal rotation. (From Donatelli RA: Sports-specific rehabilitation, St. Louis, 2008, Churchill Livingstone.)

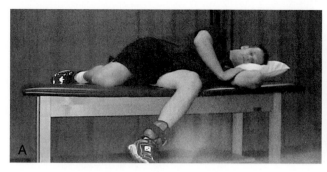
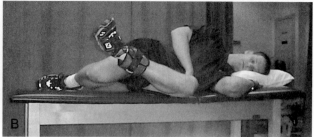

Figure 4-19 Side-lying hip external rotation. (From Donatelli RA: Sports-specific rehabilitation, St. Louis, 2008, Churchill Livingstone.)

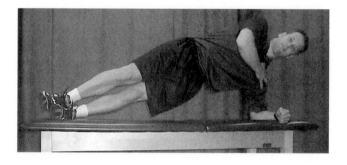

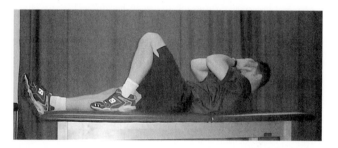

Figure 4-20 Sidebridge. (From Donatelli RA: Sports-specific rehabilitation, St. Louis, 2008, Churchill Livingstone.)

Figure 4-21 Curl up. (From Donatelli RA: Sports-specific rehabilitation, St. Louis, 2008, Churchill Livingstone.)

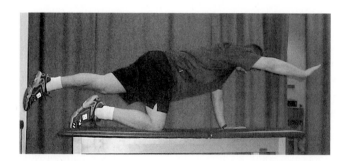

Figure 4-22 Advanced back extensor. (From Donatelli RA: Sports-specific rehabilitation, St. Louis, 2008, Churchill Livingstone.)

REFERENCES

1. Deschenes M, Kraemer W: Performance and physiologic adaptations to resistance training, Am J Phys Med Rehab 81(11):3-16, 2002.
2. Monte M, Cohen D, Campbell K, et al: Isokinetic concentric versus eccentric training of shoulder rotators with functional evaluation of performance enhancement in elite tennis players, Am J Sports Med 22(4):513-517, 1994.
3. Wooden M, Greenfield B, Johanson M, et al: Effects of strength training on throwing velocity and shoulder muscle performance in teenage baseball players, J Ortho Sports Phys Ther 15(5):223-227, 1992.
4. Vincent KR, Braith RW, Feldman RA, et al: Resistance exercise and physical performance in adults aged 60 to 83, J Am Geriatr Soc Jun;50(6):1100-1107, 2002.
5. Mikkelsen C, Werner S, Eriksson E: Closed kinetic chain alone compared to combined open and closed kinetic chain exercises for quadriceps strengthening after anterior cruciate ligament reconstruction with respect to return to sports: a prospective matched follow-up study, Knee Surg Sports Traumatol Arthrosc 8(6):337-342, 2000.
6. Enorka RM: Eccentric contractions require unique activation strategies by the nervous system, J Physio 123:2339-2346, 1996.
7. Proske U, Morgan DL: Muscle damage from eccentric exercise: mechanism, mechanical signs, adaptation and clinical applications, J Physio 537(2):333-345, 2001.
8. Bandy WD, Hanten WP: Changes in torque and electromyography activity of the quadriceps femoris muscles following isometric training, Phys Ther 73(7):455-465, 1993.
9. Moritani T, DeVries H: Neural factors versus hypertrophy in the time course of muscle strength gain, Am J Phys Med 58:115-130, 1979.
10. Staron RS, Leonardi MJ, Karapondo DL: Strength and skeletal muscle adaptations in heavy-resistance-trained women after detraining and retraining, J Appl Physiol 70:631-640, 1991.
11. Hakkinen K, Alen M, Kallimen M: Neuromuscular adaptation during prolonged strength training, detraining, and re-strength-training in middle-aged and elderly people, Eur J Appl Physiol 83:51-62, 2000.
12. Hakkinen K, Kallimen M, Izquierdo M: Changes in agonist-antagonist EMG, muscle CSA, and force during strength training in middle aged and older people, J Appl Physiol 84:1341-1349, 1998.
13. Dechenes MR, Judelson DA, Kraemer WJ: Effects of resistance training on neuromuscular junction morphology, Muscle Nerve 23:1576-1581, 2000.
14. Milner-Brown H, Stein R, Lee R: Synchronization of human motor units: Possible roles of exercise and supraspinal reflexes, Electroencephalogr Clin Neurophysiol 38:245-254, 1975.
15. Aagaard P, Simonsen E, Andersen J, et al: Neural adaptations to resistance training: changes evoked in V-wave and H-reflex responses, J Appl Physiol 92:2309-2318, 2002.
16. Laqerquist O, Zehr E, Docherty D: Increased spinal reflex excitability is not associated with neural plasticity underlying the cross education effect, J Appl Physiol 100:83-90, 2006.
17. Farthing J, Borowsky R, Chilibeck P, et al: Neurophysiological adaptations associated with cross-education of strength, J Sci Med Sport 8:255-263, 2005.
18. Gabriel D, Kamen G, Frost G: Neural adaptations to resistive exercises: mechanisms and recommendations for training practices, Sports Med 37:1-14, 2007.
19. Zhou S: Chronic neural adaptations to unilateral exercise: mechanisms of cross education, Exerc Sports Sci Rev 28:177-184, 2000.
20. Hortobagyi TK: Cross education and the human central nervous system, Eng Med Biol Mag 24:22-28, 2005.
21. Shoepe T, Stelzer J, Garner D, Widrick J: Functional adaptability of muscle fibers to long-term resistance exercise, Med Sci Sports Ex 35(6):944-951, 2003.
22. Balogopal P, Rooyacker O, Adey D: Effects of aging on in vivo synthesis of skeletal muscle myosin heavy-chain and sarcoplasmic protein in humans, Am J Physiol 273:E790-800, 1997.
23. Rooyackers O, Adey D, Ades P: Effect of age on in vivo rates of mitochondrial protein synthesis in human skeletal muscle, Proc Natl Acad Sci 93:15364-15369, 1996.
24. McCall G, Byrnes W, Fleck S: Acute and chronic hormonal responses to resistance training designed to promote muscle hypertrophy, Can J Appl Physiol 24:96-107, 1999.
25. Malisoux L, Francaux M, Nielens H, Theisen D: Stretch-shortening cycle exercises: an effective training paradigm to enhance power output of human single muscle fibers, J Appl Physiol 100:771-779, 2006.
26. Staron RS, Karapondo DL, Kraemer WJ: Skeletal muscle adaptations in heavy resistance training in men and women, J Appl Physiol 76:1247-1255, 1994.
27. Kraemer W, Patton J, Gordon S: Compatibility of high intensity strength and endurance training on hormonal and skeletal muscle adaptations, J Appl Physiol 78:976-989, 1995.
28. Volek J, Duncan N, Mazzetti S: Performance and muscle fiber adaptations to creatine supplementation and heavy resistance training, Med Sci Sports Exerc 31:1147-1156, 1999.
29. Kraemer W, Duncan N, Volek J: Resistance training and elite athletes: adaptations and program considerations, J Orth Sports Phy Ther 28(2):110-119, 1998.
30. Johnson T, Klueber K: Skeletal muscle following tonic overload: functional and structural analysis, Med Sci Sports Exerc 23:49-55, 1991.
31. Yu JG, Malm C, Thornell: Eccentric contractions leading to DOMS do not cause loss of desmin nor fibre necrosis in human muscle, Histochem Cell Biol 118(1):29-34, 2002.

32. Whitehead NP, Morgan DL, Gregory JE, Proske U: Rises in whole muscle passive tension of mammalian muscle after eccentric contractions at different lengths, J Appl Physiol 95:1224-1234, 2003.

33. Malina R: Growth of muscle tissue and muscle mass. In Faulkner F, Tanner J (editors): Human growth: a comprehensive treatise, Vol 2, New York, 1986, Plenum Press, pp 77-99.

34. Larsson L, Tesch P: Motor unit fiber density in extremely hypertrophied skeletal muscle in men: muscle electrophysiological signs of fiber hyperplasia, Eur J Appl Physiol 55:130-136, 1986.

35. Yan Z: Skeletal muscle adaptation and cell cycle regulation, Ex Sport Sci Reviews 2801:24-26, 2000.

36. Kim J, Cross J, Bamman M: impact of resistance loading on myostatin expression and cell cycle regulation in young and older men and women, J Appl Physiol 101:53-59, 2006.

37. Irintchev A, Wernig A: Muscle damage and repair in voluntarily running mice: strain and muscle differences. Cell Tissue Res 249:509-521, 1987.

38. Rosenblatt JD, Parry DJ: Adaptation of rat extensor digitorum longus muscle to gamma irradiation and overlaid, Pflugers Arch 423:255-264, 1993.

39. Goldberg A, Etlinger J, Goldspink D, Jablecki, C: Mechanisms of work-induced hypertrophy of skeletal muscle, Med Sci Sports 7:248-261, 1975.

40. Goldspink G: Changes in striated muscle fibers during contraction and growth with particular reference to myofibril splinting, J Cell Sci 9:123-127, 1971.

41. McHugh MP: Recent advances in the understanding of the repeated bout effect: the protective effect against muscle damage from a single bout of eccentric exercise, Scand J Med Sci Sports 13(2):88-97, 2003.

42. Kjaer M: Role of extracellular matrix in adaptation of tendon and skeletal muscle to mechanical loading, Physiol Rev 84:649-698, 2004.

43. Ying M, Yeung E, Li B, et al: Sonographic evaluation of the size of achilles tendon: the effect of exercise and dominance of the ankle, Ultrasound Med Biol 29:637-642, 2003.

44. Langberg H, Rosendal L, Kjaer M: Training-induced changes in peritendinous type I collagen turnover determined by microdialysis in humans, J Physiol 534:397-402, 2001.

45. Rosager S, Aagaard P, Dyhre-Poulsen P, et al: Load displacement properties of the human triceps surae aponeurosis and tendon in runners and non-runners, Scand J Med Sci Sports 12:90-98, 2002.

46. Magnusson SP, Hansen P, Kjaer M: Tendon properties in relation to muscular activity and physical training, Scand J Med Sci Sports 13:211-233, 2003.

47. Kadi F: Adaptation of human skeletal muscle to training and anabolic steroids, Acta Physiologica Scandinavica Supplementum 168:4-53, 2000.

48. Hakkinen K, Pakarinen A, Kraemer W, et al: Basal concentrations and acute response of serum hormones and strength development during heavy resistance training in middle aged and elderly men and women, Scand J Rheumatol 34:309-314, 2005.

49. Tzanoff S, Norris A: Effects of muscle mass decrease on age related BMR changes, J Appl Physiol 43:1001-1006, 1977.

50. Doherty T, Vandrervoot A, Taylor A, Brown W: Effects of motor unit losses on strength in older men and women, J Appl Physiol 74:868-874, 1993.

51. Larrson L, Sjodin B, Karlsson J: Histochemical and biochemical changes in human skeletal muscle with age in sedentary males, age 22-65 years, Acta Physiol Scand. 103:31-39, 1978.

52. Fromtera W, Meredith C, O'Reilly K, et al: Strength conditioning in older men: skeletal muscle hypertrophy and improved function, J Appl Physiol 64:1038-1044, 1988.

53. Taafe D, Marcus R: Dynamic muscle strength alterations to detraining and retraining in elderly men, Clin Physiol 17:311-324, 1997.

54. Esmarck B, Anderson J, Olsen S, et al: Timing of post-exercise protein intake is important for muscle hypertrophy with resistance training in elderly humans, J Physiol 535:301-311, 2001.

55. Newton R, Hakkinen K, Hakkinen A, et al: Mixed-methods of resistance training increases power and strength of young and older men, Med Sci Sports Ex 34:1367-1375, 2002.

56. Lindstedt SL, Reich TE, Keim P, LaStayo PC: Do muscles function as adaptable locomotor springs? J Exper Biol 205:2211-2216, 2002.

57. Miszko T, Cress M, Slade J, et al: Effect of strength and power training in physical function in community dwelling older adults, J Gerontol A Biol Sci Med 57:168-172, 2002.

58. de Vos N, Singh N, Ross D, et al: Optimal load for increasing muscle power during explosive resistance training in older adults, J Gerontol A Biol Sci Med Sci 61:78-85, 2006.

59. Orr R, de Vos N, Singh N, et al: Power training improves balance in healthy older adults, Clin Physiol Funct Imaging 26:305-313, 2006.

60. Galvao D, Taaffe D: Resistance exercise dosage in older adults: single versus multiset effects on physical performance and body composition, J Am Geriatr Soc 50:1100-1107, 2002.

61. Vincent K, Braith R, Feldman R, et al: Resistance exercise and physical performance in adults aged 60 to 83, J Am Geriatr Soc 55:B95-105, 2000.

62. Brose A, Parise G, Tarnopolsky M: Creatine supplementation enhances isometric strength and body composition improvements following strength exercise training in older adults, J Am Geriatr Soc 53:2090-2097, 2005.

63. Staron R, Hagerman F, Hikida R: Fiber type composition of the vastus lateralis muscle of young men and women, J Histochem Cytochem 48:623-629, 2000.

64. Atha J: Strengthening muscle, Exerc Sports Sci Rev 9:1-73, 1981.

65. Ivey F, Tracy B, Lemmer J, et al: Effects of strength training and detraining on muscle quality: age and gender comparisons, Scand J Med Sci Sports 14:16-23, 2004.

66. Ivey F, Roth S, Ferrell R, et al: Effects of age, gender, and myostatin genotype on the hypertropic response to heavy resistance strength training, J Appl Physiol 86:195-201, 1999.

67. Porter MM, Myint A, Kramer JF, Vandervoort AA: Concentric and eccentric knee extension strength in older and younger men and women, Can J Appl Physiol 20(4):429-439, 1995.

68. Lindle RS, Metter EJ, Lynch NA, et al: Age and gender comparisons of muscle strength in 654 women and men aged 20-93 yr, J Appl Physiol 83(5):1581-1587, 1997.

69. Higbie EJ, Cureton KJ, Warren III GL, Prior BM: Effects of concentric and eccentric training on muscle strength, cross-sectional, and neural activation, J Physiol 19:2173-2181, 1996.

70. LeStayo PC, Woolf JM, Lewek MD, et al: Eccentric muscle contractions: their contribution to injury, prevention, rehabilitation, and sport, J Ortho Sports Phys Ther 33:557-571, 2003.

71. Tomberlin JP, Basford JR, Schwen EE, et al: Comparative study of is kinetic eccentric and concentric quadriceps training, J Orthop Sports Phys. Ther 14:31-36, 1991.

72. Colliander EB, Tesch PA: Effects of eccentric and concentric muscle actions in resistance training, Acta Physiol Scand 140:31-39, 1990.

73. Komi P, Buskirk ER: Effect of eccentric and concentric muscle conditioning on tension and electrical activity of human muscle, Ergonomics 15:417-434, 1972.

74. Colliander EB, Tesch PA: Responses to eccentric and concentric resistance training in females and males, Acta Physiol Scand 141:149-156, 1990.

75. Jones DA, Rutherford OM: Human muscle strength training: the effects of three different regimes and the nature of the resultant changes, J Physiol Lond 391:1-11, 1987.

76. Dudley GA, Tesch PA, Miller BJ, Buchanan P: Importance of eccentric actions in performance adaptations to resistance training, Aviat Space Environ Med 62:543-550, 1991.

77. Johnson BL, Adamczyk JW, Tennoe KO, Stromme SB: A comparison of concentric and eccentric muscle training, Med Sci Sports Exercise 8:35-38, 1976.

78. Duncan PW, Chandler JM, Cavanaugh DK, et al: Mode and speed specificity of eccentric and concentric exercise training, J Orthop Sports Phys Ther 11:70-75, 1989.

79. Johnson BL: Eccentric vs concentric muscle training for strength development, Med Sci Sports Exercise 4:111-115, 1972.

80. Ellenbecker TS, Davies GJ, Rowinski MJ: Concentric versus eccentric isokinetic strengthening of the rotator cuff: objective data versus functional test, Am J Sports Med 16:64-69, 1988.

81. Hortobagyi T, Katch FI: Role of concentric force in limiting improvement in muscular strength, J Appl Physiol 68:650-658, 1990.

82. Paddon-Jones D, Abernethy PJ: Acute adaptation to low volume eccentric exercise, A Med Sci Sports Exerc 33(7):1213-1219, 2001.

83. Paschalis V, Koutedakis Y, Jamurtas AZ, Mougios V, Baltzopoulos: Equal volumes of high and low intensity of eccentric exercise in relation to muscle damage and performance, J Strength Cond Res 19(1):184-188, 2005.

84. Farthing JP, Chilibeck PD: The effects of eccentric and concentric training at different velocities on muscle hypertrophy, Eur J Appl Physiol 89(6):578-586, 2003.

85. Weir JP, Housch DJ, Housch TJ, Weir LL: The effect of unilateral concentric weight training and detraining on joint angle specificity, cross training, and the bilateral deficit, J Orthop Sports Phys Ther 25(4):264-270, 1997.

86. Clarkson PM, Hubal MJ: Exercise-induced muscle damage in humans, Am J Phys Med Rehabil 81:S52-S69, 2002.

87. Nosaka K, Lavender AP, Newton MJ: Effect of alternating eccentric and concentric versus separated eccentric and concentric actions on muscle damage, American College of Sports Medicine 2004 Annual Meeting, June 2-5, 2004; Indianapolis. Annual Meeting Abstracts: A-25: Athlete Care: Treatment and Prevention.

88. Housch DJ, Housch TJ: The effects of unilateral velocity-specific concentric strength training, J Orthop Sports Phy Ther 17(5):252-256, 1993.

88a. Seger JY Thorsteensson A: Effects of eccentric versus concentric training in thigh muscle strength and EMG, Int J Sports Med 26(1):45-52, 2005.

89. Maffiuletti NA, Martin A: Progressive versus rapid rate of contraction during 7 wk of isometric resistance training, Med Sci Sports Exerc 33(7):1120-1127, 2001.

90. Ebersole KT, Housch TJ, Johnson GO, et al: Mechano-myographic and electromyographic responses to unilateral isometric training, J Strength Cond Res 16(2):192-201, 2001.

91. Mafi N, Lorentzon R, Alfredson H: Superior short term results with eccentric calf muscle training compared to concentric training in a randomized prospective multicenter study on patients with chronic achilles tendinosis, Knee Surgery, Sports Traumatology, Arthroscopy 9(1):42-47, 2001.

92. Peers KH, Lysens RJ: Patellar tendinopathy in athletes: current diagnostic and therapeutic recommendations, Sports Med 35(1):71-87, 2005.

93. Fredericson M, Wolf C: Iliotibial band syndrome in runners: innovations in treatment, Sports Med 35(5):451-459, 2005.

94. MacLean CL, Taunton JE, Clement DB, Regan W: Eccentric and concentric isokinetic moment characteristics in the quadriceps and hamstrings of the chronic isolated posterior cruciate ligament injured knee, Br J Sports Med 33:405-408, 1999.

95. Young MA, Cook JL, Purdam CR, et al: Eccentric decline squat protocol offers superior results at 12 months compared with traditional eccentric protocol for patellar tendinopathy in volleyball players, Br J Sports Med 39(2):102-105, 2005.

96. Askling C, Karlsson J, Thorstensson A: Hamstring injury occurrence in elite soccer players after preseason strength training with eccentric overload, Scand J Med Sci Sports 13(4):244-250, 2003.

97. Biering-Sorensen F: Physical measurements as risk indicators for low back trouble over a one year period, Spine 9:106-119, 1984.

98. McGill S: Low back disorders: evidence-based prevention and rehabilitation, Champaign, Ill, 2000, Human Kinetics.

99. McDonagh M, Davies C: Adaptive response of mammalian skeletal muscle to exercise with high loads, Eur J Appl Physiol 52:139-155, 1984.

100. Baker J, Cooper S: Strength and body composition: single versus triple set resistance training programmes, Med Sci Sports Exerc 36(5):S53, 2004.

101. Fleck S, Kraemer W: Designing resistance training programs, ed 2, Champaign, Ill, 1997, Human Kinetics.

102. Gotshalk L, Loebel C, Nindl B, et al: Hormonal responses of multiset versus single set heavy resistance exercise protocols, Can J Appl Physiol 22(3):244-255, 1997.

103. McLester J, Bishop P, Guilliams M: Comparison of 1 day and 3 day per week of equal-volume resistance training in experienced subjects, J Strength Conditioning Res 14(3):273-281, 2000.

104. Hoffman J, Kraemer W, Fry A, et al: The effects of self-selection for frequency of training in a winter conditioning program for football, J Appl Sport Sci Res 3:76-82, 1990.

105. Kraemer W, Ratamess N: Fundamentals of resistance training: progression and exercise prescription, Med Sci Sports Ex 36:674-688, 2004.

106. Campos G, Luecke H, Wendeln, et al: Muscular adaptations in response to three different resistance-training regimes: specificity of repetition maximum training zones, Eur J Appl Physiol 88:50-60, 2002.

107. Stone W, Coulter S: Strength/endurance effects from three resistance-training protocols with women, J Strength Cond Res 8:231-234, 1994.

108. Wilson G, Newton R, Murphy A, Humphries B: The optimal training load for the development of dynamic athletic performance, Med Sci Sports Exerc 25:1279-1286, 1993.

109. Baker D, Nance S, Moore M: The load that maximizes the average mechanical power output during jump squats in power-trained athletes, J Strength Cond Res 15:92-97, 2001.

110. Paavolainen L, Hakkinen K, Hamalainen I, et al: Explosive-strength training improves 5km running time by improving running economy and muscle power, J Appl Physio 86:1527-1533, 1999.

111. Siegel J, Gilders R, Staron R, Hagerman F: Human muscle power output during upper and lower body exercises, J Strength Cond Res 16:173-178, 2002.

112. Kraemer W: A series of studies-the physiological basis for strength training in American football: fact over philosophy, J Strength Cond Res 11:131-142, 1997.

113. Pincivero D, Lephart S, Karunakara R: Effects of rest interval on isokinetic strength and functional performance after short-term high-intensity training, Br J Sports Med 31:229-234, 1997.

114. Robinson J, Stone M, Johnson C, et al: Effects of different weight-training exercise/rest intervals on strength, power, and high-intensity exercise endurance, J Strength Cond Res 9:216-221, 1995.

115. Evans W, Campbell W: Sarcopenia and age-related changes in body composition and functional capacity, J Nutr 123:465-468, 1993.

5

Joseph Godges
and William G. Boissonnault

Symptom Investigation*

This chapter will describe the types of patient data that fall under the category of symptom investigation, including the information that constitutes a red flag requiring physician contact. It will also summarize symptoms/signs associated with medical disorders that may result in patient pain syndromes common to the practice of physical therapy. Finally, it will present medical-screening questionnaires and allow the reader to incorporate them into an examination scheme for patients with common pain syndromes. To accomplish these tasks the chapter will also cover the questions necessary in a clinician's evaluation of a patient, potential red flags when dealing with various types of pain, and possible causes of referred pain.

Investigating a patient's presenting disorder usually reveals the reason why the patient has consulted the physical therapist (PT). Symptoms such as lower back, shoulder, or knee pain that interferes with daily activities motivate many people to seek physical therapy services.[1-3] Many of these patients assume that their symptoms are related to a sprain, a strain, poor posture, or an arthritic condition. For a percentage of these patients, however, the symptoms are related to a more serious medical condition. For example, low back pain, an extremely common reason that patients seek care in ambulatory clinics, can be mechanical in nature or may be related to cancer, infection, visceral disease, or fracture. Jarvik and Deyo[4] estimate that of patients with low back pain who present to ambulatory primary care clinics, 4% will have symptoms associated with an osteoporosis-related fracture, 2% with a spondylolisthesis/spondylolysis, 2% with visceral disease, 0.7% with cancer, and 0.5% with infection. The clinician must promptly recognize the patient at risk for such conditions and must make the appropriate referral.

A primary objective of the examination process is for the practitioner to decide whether (1) PT intervention is appropriate, (2) consultation with another health care provider is required along with PT intervention, or (3) PT intervention is not indicated and the patient should be managed by another provider.[5] The patient's description of symptoms is the initial focus of the patient interview process and often is the point in the examination process at which the PT's suspicion of a potentially serious cause of symptoms is first raised. This suspicion is based on an atypical description of symptoms provided by the patient—a description that does not make sense based on the PT's understanding of basic and clinical sciences, and the PT's clinical experiences.

Symptom investigation involves subcategories of symptom location, onset (history) of symptoms, and behavior of symptoms. The patient's description of the symptoms will cause the PT to ask about when and how the symptoms began, and how the symptoms fluctuate over a defined period of time (e.g., 24 hours). Just as important, the location of symptoms should alert the PT to other possible "pain generators" (disease entities) that would warrant a referral if present. The PT must know what diseases could produce local pain or referred pain in a particular region, so he or she can screen for other symptoms or signs associated with these conditions.

This chapter discusses the medical screening principles used in the investigation of patients' chief presenting symptoms. Follow-up questions associated with red flags also will be discussed. For example, night pain (pain that wakes a patient from sleep) is considered a red flag and is possibly associated with serious pathology. Yet some authors have associated night pain with degenerative joint disease, especially of the lumbar spine, hip, and knee joints, and others have noted that night pain occurs in a large proportion of patients who apparently do not have a serious disease. So, when is night pain a red flag, suggestive of a potentially life-threatening disorder? Can the clinician determine the seriousness of this symptom through further questioning after the patient has revealed the night pain?

In addition, this chapter lists and describes diseases that are possible "pain generators" in the low back, pelvis/hip/thigh, knee/leg/ankle/foot, thorax, cervical spine/shoulder, head/face, and elbow/wrist/hand regions. Many of these diseases, if suspected, would prompt communication with a physician. Initiating a plan of care for an apparent musculoskeletal disorder

*From Boissonnault WG: Primary care for the physical therapist. St. Louis, 2005, Saunders.

that is actually produced by a more serious underlying medical condition can lead to grave consequences for the patient.

For example, delaying referral of a patient who complains of lower leg pain and swelling resulting from an acute anterior compartment syndrome while a trial of physical agents is undertaken to relieve the leg pain and inflammation could result in unnecessarily serious disability (e.g., paresis, paralysis) for the patient. In another example, a patient might seek physical therapy services for the management of calf pain. Implementing a treatment of soft tissue mobilization/manipulation, ultrasound, and therapeutic exercise could result in medical complications for the patient if the actual cause of the symptoms is a deep vein thrombosis. This chapter describes other potential symptoms and signs besides pain that are associated with each of the disorders. Finally, a summary table and a self-report medical screening questionnaire for each of the seven body regions are offered as "quick clinical reference guides."

LOCATION OF SYMPTOMS

To help document symptoms, the authors recommend the use of a body diagram for noting the exact locations of symptoms, including pain, paresthesia, numbness, and weakness. Questioning should start with the patient's chief symptom, that is, the symptom(s) that is (are) interfering most with function, assuming this is the reason why physical therapy services have been initiated.

After the PT has heard the description of the chief symptom (e.g., ache, stiffness, pressure), the PT asks, "Do you have symptoms anywhere else?" For example, Figure 5-1 shows that

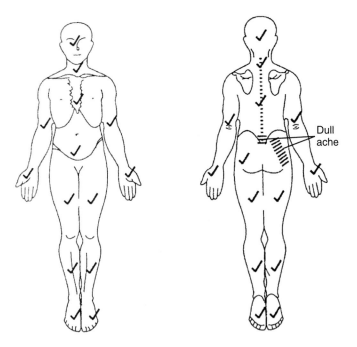

Figure 5-1 Example of a body diagram used to illustrate symptomatic and asymptomatic body regions. (From Boissonnault WG: Examination in physical therapy practice: screening for medical disease, ed 2, New York, 1995, Churchill Livingstone.)

this patient presented with low lumbar and right buttock pain (dull ache). After reporting these symptoms, the patient stated, "That is all of the symptoms I have."

The next follow-up question is, "So you don't experience any pain, pins and needles, weakness, or numbness down the backs of your legs, on the bottoms of your feet, up the front of your body, including the pelvis, stomach, chest, neck, or face, or between your shoulder blades, and you don't experience any headaches?" Noting where the patient does not have symptoms is just as important as documenting where the patient does have symptoms. Patients may not volunteer that they have belly pain or facial pain. Their rationale may be, "Why does the PT need to know if my stomach hurts? I am here for my low back pain," or "My physician takes care of my stomach problem, not my PT."

In addition, one of the ways in which disease-related symptoms may be missed is that the patient has such severe or intense symptoms in one area that he or she pays little attention to a mild ache that was present before the injury. This aching may not be limiting function at all, and if the patient has seen a physician, the patient might not have mentioned the ache. Asymptomatic areas should be noted on the body diagram with a check mark or some other notation, as shown in Figure 5-1.

Investigation of symptoms also includes the patient's description of the symptoms. Sometimes the patient may use more than one descriptor for a symptom. For example, the patient may state that he or she has pain and stiffness, aching, and sharp soreness over the right iliac crest region. The PT must assess each descriptor independently of the others, including the onset and pattern of symptoms. Hearing a similar pattern (aggravating and alleviating factors) for each of the descriptors would lead the PT to believe that all three symptoms are related to the same lesion, but hearing different patterns for these symptoms should lead the PT to consider that iliac crest symptoms might have more than one source.

Pain from visceral structures typically would be thought to be located in the anterior chest wall or abdominal region, but several viscera are located in the retroperitoneal region of the trunk. These structures include portions of the duodenum, ascending and descending colon, abdominal aorta, pancreas, and kidneys, and if diseased, back pain rather than belly pain may manifest. This leads to considerable "overlap" between pain location patterns associated with visceral disorders and common musculoskeletal disorders (Figure 5-2 and Table 5-1). In addition, many pain-generating diseases simply present as a dull ache, stiffness, or mild to moderate soreness in their early or middle stages; these are very common conditions for many patient populations. The location of symptoms by itself rarely is significant in helping the clinician decide whether a referral is in order. Exceptions to this rule are the patient with a symptom of chest pain or pressure with pain extending into the left upper extremity. PTs (and many patients) rightly would suspect possible involvement of the heart in this scenario. Descriptors such as throbbing, pulsating, and pounding also suggest involvement of the vascular system rather than pain of musculoskeletal origin.

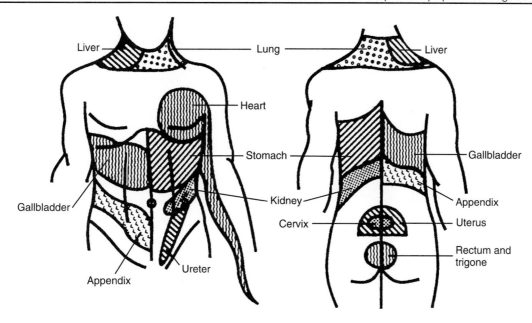

Figure 5-2 Possible local and referred pain patterns of visceral structures. (From Boissonnault WG: Examination in physical therapy practice: screening for medical disease, ed 2, New York, 1995, Churchill Livingstone.)

Although symptom location only occasionally helps to differentiate diseases from impairments, these patient data do play an important role in the medical screening process. Knowledge of potential pain patterns associated with viscera can guide the PT in selecting the organ systems to screen with review-of-systems questioning. Finally, knowing the pain patterns associated with various diseases will help the PT to know which disorders should be suspected as he or she carries out the examination.

SYMPTOM HISTORY

For many patients, the current episode of symptoms is not the first episode, but the most relevant information in the initial visit is a description of the most recent injury or flare-up. If the patient is asked, "When did your symptoms begin?" the reply may be, "20 years ago," and after a 5-minute discussion of the incident of 20 years ago, the PT might conclude that he or she has learned nothing that influences today's clinical decision making. To promote practice efficiency, start with the current or most recent episode, then work backward chronologically to the initial event.

Impairment-related symptoms typically are associated with a traumatic incident, an accident, repetitive overuse, or sustained postural strain. These events may include lifting an object, falling, or taking an extended car ride or plane trip, or the patient may report shoulder or back pain after a day of heavy yard work. However, many patients cannot relate the onset of their symptoms to any particular incident or accident. Careful questioning by the PT will reveal a likely cause, such as the patient's beginning to run after not running for 3 months, being promoted to an administrative position that requires sitting for 8 hours per day, or beginning gardening or

yard work after a winter of inactivity. If the onset of symptoms is truly insidious, if new symptoms occur insidiously during the course of treatment, or if resolved symptoms return for no apparent mechanical reason, the PT should be concerned about the underlying nature of the condition.[6]

Investigation of previous episodes of the chief presenting complaint also may produce relevant examination information. One way that pain-generating diseases may "slip through" the health care system occurs when a patient with chronic neck pain has a new episode. In the patient's mind, this is his or her "usual" neck pain, and if a PT already has seen this patient a few times for these symptoms, the PT may make the same assumption. These assumptions may lead the patient to fail to report a unique finding about his or her current episode and may cause the PT to skip steps in the examination process. In the past, flare-ups might have been associated with prolonged travel or time at a computer, but neither might be the case for this episode. The current episode in fact could be related to the previous condition, but any change in symptom descriptors, onset of symptoms, or 24-hour report of symptoms compared with previous episodes should alert the PT that this condition may have a different source.

BEHAVIOR OF SYMPTOMS

The patient report of changes in symptom site and intensity over a defined period of time provides information vital to the medical screening process. The PT should ask questions about (1) the relationship that symptoms have to rest, activities, time of day (morning, midday, evening, or night), and positions/postures, and (2) the constancy, frequency, and duration of symptoms, including fluctuations in intensity.[7]

Table 5-1	Visceral Local and Referred Pain Patterns	
Structure	**Segmental Innervation**	**Possible Areas of Pain Location**
Pelvic Organs		
Uterus, including uterine ligaments	T1-L1, S2-S4	Lumbosacral junction
		Sacral
		Thoracolumbar
Ovaries		Lower abdominal
		Sacral
Testes	T10-T11	Lower abdominal
		Sacral
Retroperitoneal Region		
Kidney	T10-L1	Lumbar spine (ipsilateral)
		Lower abdominal
		Upper abdominal
Ureter	T11-L2, S2-S4	Groin
		Upper abdominal
		Suprapubic
		Medial, proximal thigh
		Thoracolumbar
Urinary bladder	T11-L2, S2-S4	Sacral apex
		Suprapubic
		Thoracolumbar
Prostate gland	T11-L1, S2-S4	Sacral
		Testes
		Thoracolumbar
Digestive System Organs		
Esophagus	T4-T6	Substernal and upper abdominal
Stomach	T6-T10	Upper abdominal
		Middle and lower thoracic spine
Small intestine	T7-T10	Middle thoracic spine
Pancreas	T10	Upper abdominal
		Lower thoracic spine
		Upper lumbar spine
Gallbladder	T7-T9	Right upper abdominal
		Right middle and lower thoracic spine, aspect scapula
Liver	T7-T9	Right middle and lower thoracic spine
		Right cervical spine
Common bile duct	T8-T10	Upper abdominal
		Middle thoracic spine
Large intestine	T11-L1	Lower abdominal
		Middle lumbar spine
Sigmoid colon	T11-T12	Upper sacral
		Suprapubic
		Left lower quadrant of abdomen
Cardiopulmonary System		
Heart	T1-T5	Cervical anterior
		Upper thorax
		Left upper extremity
Lungs and bronchi	T5-T6	Ipsilateral thoracic spine
		Cervical (diaphragm involved)
Diaphragm (central portion)	C3-C5	Cervical spine

From Boissonnault W, Bass C: Pathological origins of trunk and neck pain: parts I, II, III, J Orthop Sports Phys Ther 12(5):191-221, 1990.

For many patients with neuromusculoskeletal disorders, a description of how symptoms do or do not change over a 24-hour period is adequate. For patients with disorders such as multiple sclerosis, stroke, or head injury, the time frame may be 3 to 6 months.

Besides insidious onset of symptoms, a report of an unexpected or atypical behavior of symptoms may be the initial clue that raises the suspicion of a serious underlying condition. Symptoms associated with impairments or movement disorders typically fluctuate accordingly as the mechanical loads on the body increase or decrease with time of day, onset or cessation of specific activities, and the assumption or avoidance of certain postures. This expected behavior of symptom pattern fits many patients who seek physical therapy services, with or without a pathoanatomic cause of symptoms. In a study of pain profiles for patients with low back pain, Boissonnault and DiFabio[8] found no difference in the time of day that pain was most intense, in movements and postures that altered symptoms, or in frequency of night pain in patients with disc pathology (degeneration, internal disruption, herniation, or bulging) versus those with no pathoanatomic findings on magnetic resonance imaging (MRI) or computed tomography (CT) scans. If the symptom pattern reveals no pattern, the PT should begin to question whether physical therapy intervention is warranted. This inconsistent symptom pattern should alert the PT that specific body systems should be screened later in the examination.

Symptoms associated with visceral disease vary in their behavior depending on the severity of the disorder and the function of the structure. Therefore, a patient report of intermittent pain does not rule out the possibility of disease. If the patient's thoracic spine pain is the result of a duodenal ulcer, gastrointestinal system activity may alter the symptoms. For example, the pain associated with the ulcer probably will be reduced shortly after the patient eats, because the food acts as a buffer, and a few hours after eating, the pain will return or intensify. The patient probably will not make the connection between eating and pain level; in fact, the patient may attribute the symptoms to certain activities, or to working at a computer for a number of hours. Careful questioning about changes in symptoms over a 24-hour period may reveal inconsistencies that catch the clinician's attention.

Another example of visceral pain that may mimic mechanical pain patterns is colicky pain. Spasm of the smooth muscle wall of a hollow visceral structure will result in a deep cramping, gnawing, achy sensation that is intermittent. Pain intensity will vary depending on the intensity of the spasm of the smooth muscle wall; the spasms often are mild initially but build to a crescendo over a period of minutes. Although spasms may occur at a variety of times (e.g., while the patient is sitting, standing, lying down, or walking), the patient may be pain free much of the time. Gastroenteritis, constipation, menstruation, gallbladder disease, and ureteral obstruction all have been implicated as causes of colicky pain in the belly or back area.[9]

Finally, an inconsistent pattern of change in symptom intensity is not the only warning sign that may be discovered during behavior-of-symptom questioning. Symptoms that move from one body location to another for no apparent mechanical reason are also an atypical report for many patients who seek physical therapy services. For example, a patient may note right shoulder and wrist pain during the initial visit, and at the second visit may report right and left shoulder and left elbow and wrist pain. This patient cannot describe any reason why the apparently new pains have started. Primary neurologic, endocrine, or rheumatic disorders or adverse drug reactions may account for a symptom pattern such as this.

The investigation of symptom behavior over a defined period of time (often 24 hours) includes questions about night pain. Night pain (pain that wakes someone from sleep) has been associated with serious diseases such as cancer and infection.[10-13] Many studies have described night pain as being associated with degenerative joint disease, especially of the lumbar, hip, and knee regions.[14-19] In addition, a significant percentage of patients with low back pain have reported night pain with no evidence of serious disease. So, when is night pain a red flag? When night pain is reported, follow-up questions should include the following:

- How many nights per week do you have night pain?
- Do you wake up at a consistent time?
- How does the intensity of the night pain compare with pain experienced at other times of the day?
- What do you have to do to fall back to sleep?

Boissonnault and DeFabio[8] noted that 53% of patients with a complaint of back pain reported night pain. Only one member of this group stated that night pain was more intense than pain in the morning, midday, or evening, and almost 80% stated that they simply had to change position in bed to fall back to sleep. This pattern would be expected for the patient with nonacute low back pain. The practitioner would assume that the low back area would be mechanically loaded to a greater degree, and therefore would be more painful, when the patient was physically active. In addition, many patients with low back pain start the night sleeping supine with a pillow under the knees, or sidelying with a pillow between the legs, to support the lumbar region, but wake up with pillows on the floor and lying halfway onto their stomach. Low back discomfort wakes them up, but they fall back to sleep with minimal effort after the pillows are back in place. Greater concern would be warranted if the night pain was the patient's most intense pain, and if it took more than minimal effort for the patient to fall back to sleep (nonacute conditions).

Finally, another patient report that would cause concern is a report that night pain episodes were becoming more frequent and severe with no "mechanical" explanation for the worsening. Based on current evidence, one must conclude that the presence of night pain as the sole red flag has little diagnostic value but must be considered in the context of other examination findings.

In summary, symptom investigation often is the step that first alerts the PT to the possible need for a patient referral. Careful questioning will reveal a pattern of symptoms that is unusual for patients with impairment-driven conditions. Using a body diagram to document the locations of symptoms and a description of the symptoms can save documentation time for the PT. A well-organized sequence of questions will allow a patient to give an accurate history of his or her reasons for seeking medical care:

- In which area do symptoms interfere most with functions or daily activities?
- Describe the symptom(s) to me (e.g., ache, pins, needles).
- Do these symptoms spread to any other body regions or parts?
- Was there a recent injury or flare-up? If so, when?
- If not, can you explain why these symptoms may have begun?
- Are the symptoms constant, or do they come and go?
- What makes the symptoms worse or better?
- Can you rate the intensity of the symptoms on a 0 to 10 scale?
- Do the symptoms wake you up at night?
- Have you had any previous episodes like this?
- Do you have symptoms anywhere else? (If so, repeat the above line of questioning.)

REGIONAL PAIN PATTERNS AND ASSOCIATED DISEASES AND DISORDERS

Low Back Pain

Consider a 55-year-old patient with a recent history of low back pain who is being examined by a PT. Four serious conditions that may present as low back pain are tumor, spinal infection, vertebral fracture, and cauda equina syndrome.[10] As this patient is describing the pain and activity limitations, he reports that his pain has not resolved with rest or anti-inflammatory medications over the past 6 weeks. The PT recalls that lack of improvement in a patient over the age of 50 years with acute low back pain is a red flag, increasing the index of suspicion that the patient's low back pain is caused by a tumor, rather than by a relatively less serious musculoskeletal disorder such as a lumbar or sacroiliac ligament sprain.[20]

This patient's reported lack of improvement leads the PT to verify the patient's age and to ask whether the patient has a history of cancer or has experienced recent, unexplained weight loss. Evidence supporting the value of these inquiries is found in a study by Deyo and Diehl on patients with low back pain who had cancer. Deyo and Diehl[21] reported that, of 13 patients whose low back pain was caused by cancer (out of a total subject pool of 1975 patients with low back pain), all 13 were older than 50 years of age, had a history of cancer, had experienced unexplained weight loss, or had failed to improve with conservative therapy.

The PT thus asks our 55-year-old patient the following questions to increase or decrease the index of suspicion that this patient's low back pain is caused by cancer:

- Do you have a history of cancer? If so, what type of cancer did you have (e.g., lung, breast, prostate)?

- Have you lost weight recently, even though you have not been attempting to eat less or to exercise more? If so, how much?

In our example, the patient responds "no" to each question. Next, the PT considers three other serious pathologies that may cause low back pain. One of these conditions is a back-related infection, such as spinal osteomyelitis.[22] All red flags that raise the suspicion of osteomyelitis as a cause of low back pain are factors that put the patient at risk for spinal infection. These factors include current recent bacterial infection (e.g., urinary tract or skin infection), intravenous drug use and/or abuse, and concurrent suppression of the patient's immune system. The PT thus asks the following questions to increase or decrease the index of suspicion that this patient's low back pain is caused by a back-related infection:

- Have you recently had a fever?
- Have you recently taken antibiotics or other medicines for an infection?
- Have you been diagnosed with an immunosuppressive disorder?
- Does your pain ease when you rest in a comfortable position?

Again, the patient responds "no" to the all of the above questions. Negative responses to the first three questions reduce the suspicion that this patient has a back-related infection. A negative response to the fourth question, however, suggests that the patient's low back pain is not due to a musculoskeletal disorder, because pain related to musculoskeletal disorders typically is eased when the patient rests in a comfortable position.

To rule out the likelihood of spinal fracture as a cause of this patient's low back pain, the patient is asked whether any trauma to the spine triggered the onset of pain. In addition, the PT asks whether the patient has any history of osteoporosis, because minor strains or falls may produce an unsuspected spinal fracture in an individual with osteoporosis. The PT also asks whether the patient has a history of other disorders that may increase the risk for decreased bone density, including hyperparathyroidism, renal failure, chronic gastrointestinal disorders, and long-term use of corticosteroids:

- Have you recently had a major trauma, such as a vehicle accident or a fall from a height?
- Have you ever had a medical practitioner tell you that you have osteoporosis or other disorders that could cause "weak bones"?

The PT asks our 55-year-old patient these questions and receives negative responses; this greatly reduces the suspicion of fracture as a cause of this patient's low back pain.

Finally, to rule out cauda equina syndrome associated with this patient's low back pain, the PT relies on both historical and physical examination data. The PT asks the following questions:

- Have you noticed a recent onset of difficulty with retaining your urine?
- Have you noticed a recent need to urinate more frequently?

Table 5-2	Red Flags for the Low Back Region
Condition	**Red Flags**
Back-related tumor[21]	• Age >50 years • History of cancer • Unexplained weight loss • Failure of conservative therapy
Back-related infection (spinal osteomyelitis)[12]	• Recent infection (e.g., urinary tract or skin infection) • Intravenous drug user/abuser • Concurrent immunosuppressive disorder
Cauda equina syndrome[10]	• Urine retention or incontinence • Fecal incontinence • Saddle anesthesia • Global or progressive weakness in the lower extremities • Sensory deficits in the feet (i.e., L4, L5, S1 areas) • Ankle dorsiflexion, toe extension, and ankle plantar flexion weakness
Spinal fracture[10,20]	• History of trauma (including minor falls or heavy lifts for osteoporotic or elderly individuals) • Prolonged use of steroids • Age >70 years

Table 5-3	Medical Screening Questionnaire for the Low Back Region

	Yes	No
Have you recently had a major trauma, such as a vehicle accident or a fall from a height?		
Have you ever had a medical practitioner tell you that you have osteoporosis?		
Do you have a history of cancer?		
Does your pain ease when you rest in a comfortable position?		
Have you recently had a fever?		
Have you recently lost weight even though you have not been attempting to eat less or exercise more?		
Have you recently taken antibiotics or other medicines for an infection?		
Have you been diagnosed as having an immunosuppressive disorder?		
Have you noticed a recent onset of difficulty with retaining your urine?		
Have you noticed a recent need to urinate more frequently?		
Have you noticed a recent onset of numbness in the area of your bottom where you would sit on a bicycle seat?		
Have you recently noticed your legs becoming weak while you are walking or climbing stairs?		

Adapted from Bigos S, Bowyer O, Braen G, et al: Acute lower back problems in adults. Clinical practice guideline no 14. AHCPR publication no 95-0642, Rockville, MD, December 1994, Agency for Health Care Policy and Research, Public Health Service, US Department of Health and Human Services.

• Have you noticed a recent onset of numbness in the area of your bottom where you would sit on a bicycle seat?
• Have you recently noticed that your legs become weak while walking or climbing stairs?

A positive response to any of these questions increases the suspicion that the patient has a cauda equina syndrome. The PT follows these inquiries with a physical examination, assessing the sensory integrity of the perianal and perineal areas, as well as the L4, L5, and S1 dermatomes. The PT also assesses the motor integrity of the L4 (quadriceps and tibialis anterior), L5 (extensor hallucis longus and foot everters), and S1 (ankle plantar flexors) musculature. In our example, all of the history and physical examination findings that suggest a cauda equina lesion were negative. Table 5-2[3,12,13,43] summarizes red flags for the low back region, and a low back medical screening questionnaire is shown in Table 5-3.

In summary, our patient's response that his pain does not ease when he rests in a comfortable position suggests a non-spinal pathology mimicking a back problem. This justifies examination for a possibly serious condition in an adjacent region (see the discussion below on colon cancer). However, the PT found no other red flags that suggest a back-related tumor or infection, spinal fracture, or cauda equina syndrome. A review of the function of the gastrointestinal, urogenital, and vascular systems may be especially helpful in patients with low back pain whose presentation and symptoms suggest a non-musculoskeletal disorder.

Pelvis, Hip, and Thigh Disorders

Serious medical conditions that may mimic common musculoskeletal disorders of the pelvis, hip, and thigh include colon cancer, pathologic fracture of the femoral neck, osteonecrosis of the femoral head, Legg-Calvé-Perthes disease, and slipped capital femoral epiphysis. Colon cancer, the third most common cancer among both women and men,[23] is a result of malignant neoplasms that develop in the large intestine, from the cecum to the rectum. Colon cancer is most common in people 50 years and older and who have a family history of colon cancer. Initial symptoms usually include a change in bowel habits, such as blood in the stools (if the lesion is near the rectum) or black stools (if the lesion producing the bleeding is located in the more proximal portion of the colon).

Colon cancer is an especially deadly disease because malignant neoplasms can develop undetected for many years before the onset of bowel symptoms. Thus PTs, along with other health care professionals, must stress the importance of routine screening examinations for colon cancer (e.g., sigmoidoscopy, colonoscopy) for individuals with a family history of this disorder. Polyps, which are the precursor to cancerous lesions in the colon, often can be excised if they are discovered during a colonoscopy examination. In the later stages of colon cancer, a palpable mass may be felt in the abdominal cavity.

Because PTs often see patients with midback and thoracic cage pain, they should remember that the most common metastatic presentation of colon cancer includes the thoracic spine and the rib cage. The following details, collected by a PT during a history or physical examination, could serve as red flags for colon cancer[24]:

• Age greater than 50 years
• History of colon cancer in an immediate family member (first-degree relative)
• Bowel disturbances (e.g., rectal bleeding, black stools)
• Unexplained weight loss
• Back or pelvic pain that is unchanged by position or movement

Disorders of the proximal femur represent another type of serious condition that the PT may encounter. As the elderly population increases, PTs will be more likely to detect and manage patients with pathologic fracture of the femoral neck. Pathologic fracture of the femoral neck occurs as the result of disease and often in the absence of trauma. These fractures are most common in people older than 50 years (women more often than men) who have a history of metabolic bone disease, such as osteoporosis or Paget's disease. A history of a fall from a standing position often is reported, along with a feeling of a sudden, painful snap in the hip region and a giving way. Acute groin pain usually is reported, but pain also may be felt in the anteromedial thigh or in the trochanteric region. Physical examination usually reveals that the involved extremity appears shortened when compared with the contralateral side and typically is held in an externally rotated position.[25]

Another serious disorder of the proximal femur is osteonecrosis (also known as *avascular necrosis*) of the femoral head. Osteonecrosis of the femoral head is the result of an insufficient arterial supply to this region. This ischemic process eventually results in death of the bony tissue of the femoral head and can be associated with hip trauma, such as fracture or dislocation. It also can be associated with nontraumatic conditions, such as sickle cell disease, and with long-term corticosteroid administration, as in patients receiving corticosteroid therapy for the management of rheumatoid arthritis, systemic lupus erythematosus, or asthma. Nontraumatic osteonecrosis of the femoral head may be bilateral in up to 60% of cases.[26]

A similar condition that occurs in children (most common in 5- to 8-year-old boys) is Legg-Calvé-Perthes disease. This disorder results from an idiopathic loss of blood supply from the lateral ascending cervical artery to the femoral head. Patients with osteonecrosis and Legg-Calvé-Perthes disease often report pain in the groin, thigh, and knee that worsens with weight-bearing activities, resulting in an antalgic gait. Common clinical findings in children with Legg-Calvé-Perthes disease also include shortening of the involved extremity and limited internal rotation and abduction of the involved hip.[27] Internal rotation typically is tested in these cases with the patient prone, with both extremities simultaneously internally rotated, and with the angles of the tibial shaft compared relative to the table. Abduction is tested with the patient supine in the hook-lying position (with the knees flexed to approximately 90 degrees and both feet positioned on the table adjacent to the midline). The patient then is instructed to relax his or her adductor muscles and to allow the knees to fall out to the "frog-leg" position (i.e., horizontally abducted toward the table). This test allows easy comparison of involved and uninvolved hips; abduction is measured by using the angles of the tibial shaft relative to the table, with the femora at approximately 45 degrees of hip flexion.[28]

A hip disorder that occurs in adolescence is slipped capital femoral epiphysis, which involves progressive displacement of the femoral head relative to the neck through the open growth plate. It is more common in males (male-to-female ratio, 2.5:1), who are typically, but not always, overweight. Patients with slipped capital femoral epiphysis usually experience groin, thigh, or knee pain that is described as diffuse and vague (i.e., difficult to pinpoint). Common findings on physical examination include antalgic gait, position of the involved extremity in external rotation, and hip internal rotation range-of-motion limitations.[29] Red flags for slipped capital femoral epiphysis, as well as for other serious conditions of the pelvis, hip, and thigh region, are listed in Table 5-4. Table 5-5 offers a self-report questionnaire that can help the clinician in screening for these conditions.

Knee, Lower Leg, and Ankle/Foot Pain

Remaining regions of the lower quarter that should be considered are the knee, leg, ankle, and foot regions. Two important conditions—compartment syndrome and deep vein thrombosis (DVT)—are described here in detail, as are three other potentially serious conditions of the knee, leg, ankle, and foot that a PT is likely to encounter: peripheral arterial occlusive disease, septic arthritis, and cellulitis.

Peripheral arterial occlusive disease, also known as *peripheral vascular disease*, is the manifestation of atherosclerosis below the bifurcation of the abdominal aorta. This disease is common, which is not surprising when we consider that the risk factors for heart disease that are so widespread in our society (i.e., history of type 2 diabetes, smoking, and sedentary lifestyle) are also the risk factors for peripheral arterial occlusive disease. In fact, people who have a history of ischemic heart disease should be assumed to have peripheral arterial occlusive disease until proven otherwise. A primary clinical feature of this disease is intermittent claudication. A patient with intermittent claudication often complains of aching in the buttock and of thigh and calf pain that is precipitated by walking, intensifies with walking, and disappears with rest. In addition, the patient may complain that the distal extremities feel cold. Physical examination findings that suggest peripheral occlusive arterial disease include decreased pedal pulses (i.e., posterior tibialis and dorsalis pedis arteries), a unilateral cool extremity, and wounds and sores on the toes or feet.

Two special tests that the PT can perform that aid in confirming the presence of peripheral vascular disease are the reactive hyperemia test and the ankle-to-arm systolic pressure (ankle/brachial index; ABI) index. The reactive hyperemia test assesses the integrity of the vascular system in redistributing blood with postural changes. One performs this test by elevating the leg of a patient who is lying supine to 45 degrees of hip flexion (i.e., a unilateral straight leg test to 45 degrees).

Table 5-4	Red Flags for the Pelvis, Hip, and Thigh Region

Condition	Red Flags
Colon cancer[24]	• Age >50 years • Bowel disturbances (e.g., rectal bleeding, black stools) • Unexplained weight loss • History of colon cancer in immediate family • Pain unchanged by position or movement
Pathologic fracture of the femoral neck[25]	• Older females (>70 years) with hip, groin, or thigh pain • History of a fall from a standing position • Severe, constant pain, worse with movement • A shortened and externally rotated lower extremity
Osteonecrosis of the femoral head[26] (also known as avascular necrosis)	• History of long-term corticosteroid use (e.g., in patients with RA, SLE, asthma) • History of AVN of the contralateral hip • Trauma
Legg-Calvé-Perthes disease[13]	• 5- to 8-year-old boys with groin/thigh pain • Antalgic gait • Pain symptoms aggravated by hip movement, especially hip abduction and internal rotation
Slipped capital femoral epiphysis[29]	• Overweight adolescent • History of a recent growth spurt or trauma • Groin aching exacerbated by weight-bearing • Involved leg held in external rotation • ROM limitations of hip IR and abduction

AVN, Avascular necrosis; IR, internal rotation; RA, rheumatoid arthritis; ROM, range of motion; SLE, systemic lupus erythematosus.

Table 5-5	Medical Screening Questionnaire for the Pelvis, Hip, and Thigh Region

	Yes	No
Have you recently had a trauma, such as a fall?		
Have you ever had a medical practitioner tell you that you have osteoporosis?		
Have you ever had a medical practitioner tell you that you have a problem with the blood circulation in your hips?		
Are you currently taking steroids or have you been on prolonged steroid therapy?		
Does your pain ease when you rest in a comfortable position?		
Do you have a history of cancer?		
Has a member of your immediate family (i.e., parents or siblings) been diagnosed with cancer?		
Have you recently lost weight even though you have not been attempting to eat less or exercise more?		
Have you had a recent change in your bowel functioning, such as black stools or blood in your rectum?		
Have you had diarrhea or constipation that has lasted for more than a few days?		
Do you have groin, hip, or thigh aching or pain that increases with physical activity, such as walking or running?		

The lower extremity is maintained in this position for 1 to 3 minutes, or until the color of the foot, ankle, and lower leg is blanched. The examiner then lowers the limb and measures the number of seconds required for the limb to turn pink. Normal time is 1 or 2 seconds. A venous filling time greater than 20 seconds indicates peripheral occlusive arterial disease.

The PT obtains the ankle-to-arm systolic pressure index by measuring the highest systolic blood pressure at the ankle (using the dorsalis pedis and posterior tibial arteries) with a hand-held Doppler flowmeter, and dividing it by the blood pressure in the brachial artery. An ankle-to-arm systolic pressure index that is less than 0.97 indicates the presence of peripheral occlusive arterial disease.[30,31]

One of the major therapies for patients with peripheral vascular disease is aerobic exercise, such as progressive walking.

Thus PTs often may help to design and monitor exercise programs for patients with this disorder. However, the PT must remember that when a screening examination of a lower extremity musculoskeletal disorder suggests peripheral occlusive vascular disease, the PT must assume the presence of ischemic heart disease until it is proven otherwise. Therefore, physician evaluation (often including an exercise tolerance test) and medical management (often including medications) of the underlying cardiovascular disorder are essential, so the PT can proceed with the plan of care, confident about the patient's safety.

Another serious condition of the lower extremity that may appear initially as a musculoskeletal strain is DVT. A DVT is a spontaneous obstruction of the popliteal vein of the calf; it may present as a gradual or sudden onset of calf pain, and typically is intensified with standing or walking and reduced with rest and elevation. Up to 50% of patients with DVT will not experience calf pain. Risk factors that predispose an individual to DVT include recent surgery, malignancy, trauma, prolonged immobilization of the extremities (including placement of the limb in a cast or immobilizer and a long car ride or plane trip, especially for those already at risk for DVT), and pregnancy. Physical examination findings that increase suspicion of a DVT are localized calf tenderness, calf swelling and edema, and skin warmth. The diagnosis of DVT is confirmed by contrast venography or other imaging procedures. The possibility that the blood clot may travel proximally toward or into the pulmonary vessels is the risk that makes DVT a serious condition that requires referral to a physician for a medical examination and for possible intervention, including anticoagulant medication. Red flags that suggest the presence of a DVT are listed in Table 5-6.[6,31,47]

PTs often help in the management of patients who have experienced trauma or overuse (i.e., repetitive trauma) strain to the legs. The inflammatory phase of healing that accompanies these traumas can lead to an abnormal rise in pressure in one of the fascial compartments of the leg. This abnormal rise in pressure that results from acute swelling inside a fascial

Table 5-6	Red Flags for the Knee, Leg, Ankle, or Foot Region
Condition	**Red Flags**
Peripheral arterial occlusive disease[30,31]	• Age >60 years • History of type 2 diabetes • History of ischemic heart disease • Smoking history • Sedentary lifestyle • Concurrent intermittent claudication • Unilaterally cool extremity • Decreased pedal pulses: posterior tibial artery, dorsalis pedis artery • Prolonged venous filling time • Abnormal ankle-to-arm systolic pressure
Deep vein thrombosis[32]	• Calf pain, edema, tenderness, warmth • Calf pain that is intensified with standing or walking and is relieved by rest and elevation • Recent surgery, malignancy, pregnancy, trauma, or leg immobilization
Compartment syndrome	• History of blunt trauma, crush injury, or unaccustomed exercise • Severe, persistent leg pain that is intensified by stretch applied to involved muscles • Swelling, exquisite tenderness, and palpable tension (hardness) of involved compartment • Paresthesia, paresis, and pulselessness
Septic arthritis[32]	• Constant aching and/or throbbing pain, joint swelling, tenderness, warmth • History of recent infection, surgery, or injection • Coexisting immunosuppressive disorder
Cellulitis[32]	• Pain, skin swelling, warmth, and an advancing, irregular margin of erythema/reddish streaks • Fever, chills, malaise, and weakness • History of recent skin ulceration or abrasion, venous insufficiency, CHF, or cirrhosis

CHF, Congestive heart failure.

connective tissue compartment is called a *compartment syndrome.* The vascular occlusion and nerve entrapments that are possible sequelae of a compartment syndrome make this condition a medical emergency. Thus the PT must know the red flags that signify the presence of a compartment syndrome when examining musculoskeletal disorders of the lower extremity.

Patients with compartment syndromes have a history of a blunt trauma or crush injury, or of participating in an unfamiliar physical activity involving the lower extremities, such as rapidly increasing the amount of running distance (e.g., while training for a marathon) or walking distance (e.g., while participating in a long hike). The patient often reports severe, persistent leg pain that is intensified when stretch is applied to the involved muscles. Physical examination reveals swelling, exquisite tenderness, and palpable tension (i.e., hardness) of the involved compartment. The nerve entrapment or compression noted in this condition results in paresthesias and possibly in paresis or paralysis. The vascular compromise that accompanies this condition results in diminished peripheral pulses (i.e., dorsalis pedis or posterior tibial). A mnemonic that clinicians use to remember the signs of a compartment syndrome are the five "P's": *p*ain, *p*alpable tenderness, *p*aresthesias, *p*aresis, and *p*ulselessness.

Two remaining potentially serious conditions that may mimic lower extremity musculoskeletal disorders are related to infection. One is septic arthritis, which is inflammation in a joint that is caused by bacterial infection, and the other is cellulitis, which is an infection in the skin and underlying tissues that follows bacterial contamination of a wound. Patients who have septic arthritis complain of a constant aching and or throbbing pain and swelling in a joint. The involved joint usually is tender and warm when palpated. Patients who develop septic arthritis often are immunosuppressed or have preexisting joint disease. This immunosuppression may be the result of corticosteroid administration, alcohol abuse, renal failure, malignancy, diabetes mellitus, intravenous drug abuse, collagen vascular disease, organ transplantation, or acquired immunodeficiency syndrome.

Examples of preexisting joint diseases that predispose individuals to septic arthritis are rheumatoid arthritis, osteoarthritis, and psoriatic arthritis. The cause of septic arthritis usually is associated with a local or distant site of infection, or a history of recent joint surgery or intra-articular injection. An example of a distant infection site is a gonococcal infection. Thus individuals who are sexually active and are exposed to gonorrhea may develop gonococcal septic monoarthritis or gonococcal septic polyarthritis.[33]

Infection in the tissues—cellulitis—exhibits the classic signs of pain, skin swelling, warmth, and an advancing, irregular margin of erythema or reddish streaks. Upon further inquiry, patients with these findings may report other classic signs of infection such as fever, chills, malaise, and weakness. Individuals predisposed to developing cellulitis are those with congestive heart failure, lower extremity venous insufficiency, diabetes mellitus, renal failure, liver cirrhosis, and advancing age. The precipitating factor to the development of cellulitis is typically a recent skin ulceration or abrasion.[33]

Table 5-7	Medical Screening Questionnaire for the Knee, Leg, Ankle, or Foot Region		
		Yes	No
Have you recently had a fever?			
Have you recently taken antibiotics or other medicines for an infection?			
Have you recently had surgery?			
Have you recently had an injection into one or more of your joints?			
Have you recently had a cut, scrape, or open wound?			
Have you been diagnosed as having an immunosuppressive disorder?			
Do you have a history of heart trouble?			
Do you have a history of cancer?			
Have you recently taken a long car ride, bus trip, or plane flight?			
Have you recently been bedridden for any reason?			
Have you recently begun a vigorous physical training program?			
Do you have groin, hip, thigh, or calf aching or pain that increases with physical activity, such as walking or running?			
Have you recently sustained a blow to your shin or any other trauma to either of your legs?			

The management of septic arthritis and cellulitis includes (of course) monitored administration of antibiotic therapy; thus referral of the patient to a physician should be expedited. Red flags and medical screening questionnaires for peripheral arterial occlusive disease, DVT, compartment syndrome, septic arthritis, and cellulitis are found in Tables 5-6 and 5-7.

Thoracic Pain: Cardiac/Pulmonary Disorders

The thoracic spine and the rib cage lie close to many organ systems; when these are diseased, local or referred pain to the thoracic cage usually results. In addition, both metastatic disease and bone disease usually manifest as pathologic fractures of the thoracic vertebrae and ribs.[13] Thus the PT should remember that the patient who reports "back pain" may have an underlying serious medical condition when the reported back pain is in the thoracic region. This section briefly discusses the clinical presentation and red flags of cardiac (myocardial infarction, unstable and stable angina), pulmonary (lung cancer, pneumothorax, pneumonia, pleurisy, and pulmonary embolus), gastrointestinal (peptic ulcer and cholecystitis), and urogenital (pyelonephritis) conditions.

Myocardial infarction (MI; an acute blockage of a coronary artery resulting in death of a portion of the myocardium) has the highest mortality rate of any of the disorders discussed in this chapter. A cardinal clinical feature of MI is angina, that is, chest symptoms described as discomfort, pressure, tightness, or squeezing with potential referral into the arm, neck, or jaw regions. The classic presentation of pain in the left chest and

the left upper extremity is not necessarily the norm for women or the elderly. Pain experienced in the epigastric, midthoracic spinal, and right shoulder/neck regions may be the presentation for these patients. PTs should realize that one of every three patients diagnosed with MI does not have chest pain on initial presentation to a hospital emergency room.[34] Instead of pain as the primary manifestation, MI may appear with the clinical features of dyspnea, nausea or vomiting, palpitations, syncope, or cardiac arrest. Risk factors for this atypical presentation of MI include a history of diabetes, older age, female sex, nonwhite racial or ethnic group, and a history of congestive heart failure and stroke.[34]

Two related terms that PTs should understand are *stable* and *unstable angina pectoris*. Stable angina, as the name implies, is substernal chest pain or pressure with possible pain referral to the left upper extremity that occurs with predictable exertion or known precipitating events, such as exercise or exertion at an intensity level higher than usual. The chest pain that occurs with stable angina is predictably alleviated by a change in the precipitating event (e.g., rest) or by self-administration of sublingual nitroglycerin. Chest pain that occurs with stable angina is relatively benign, especially if relief is attained with rest and administration of nitroglycerin.

Unstable angina, also as the name implies, is chest pain that occurs outside of a predictable pattern and that does not respond to nitroglycerin. Individuals who are experiencing unstable angina must be monitored closely. Signs suggesting MI, such as substernal squeezing or crushing pressure, pain radiation to both arms, shortness of breath, pallor, diaphoresis, or angina that lasts longer than 30 minutes, should alert the PT that this is an emergency condition, and that immediate transportation to an appropriate emergency room or coronary care facility is indicated. The survival rate of those who experience an MI is improved greatly if therapy known to improve survival is available and is used appropriately. These therapies include thrombolysis of primary angioplasty, aspirin, beta-blocker therapy, and heparin.[35]

Chest pain that extends to the left shoulder and possibly down the left arm also may reveal pericarditis. This chest pain usually is accompanied by fever; it increases with lying down, inhalation, or coughing, and is alleviated by forward lean while sitting. Pericarditis is an inflammation of the pericardium, a sac that surrounds the heart to keep it in place, to prevent overfilling with blood, and to protect the heart from chest infection. The pericardium becomes inflamed by bacterial, viral, or systemic disease, such as kidney failure, systemic lupus, rheumatoid disease, heart failure, or increased fluid around the heart with leakage from an aortic aneurysm. This inflammation around the heart prevents complete expansion, because the additional pressure caused by resulting inflammation results in less blood leaving the heart. To make up for the reduced stroke volume, and to get enough oxygen to the tissues, the heart beats faster. If increased heart rate cannot compensate enough, the person may start to breathe heavily, the veins in the neck may become distended, and blood pressure may drop drastically during inhalation. This condition is termed *cardiac tamponade* and is often a medical emergency.

Emergency medical care is needed to remove pressure on the heart and to restore proper cardiac output.

Pulmonary embolus is a pulmonary condition that may produce angina-like pain. An acute massive pulmonary embolism can even produce crushing chest pain that mimics MT, especially if the blood clot, usually traveling from the calf, thigh, or pelvic veins, reaches a major pulmonary artery. The location of the chest pain usually is substernal, but it can be located anywhere in the thorax depending on the location of the embolus. This may include shoulder pain or upper abdominal pain. In addition to chest pain, patients with a pulmonary embolus may develop dyspnea, wheezing, and a marked drop in blood pressure. Factors that increase the risk for blood clots in the lower extremities or pelvis and subsequent embolus include immobilization and recent surgery; these are two patient types that PTs frequently treat. Pulmonary embolism also has a high mortality rate, so if the PT suspects this condition, he or she should immediately refer the patient to emergency care, so that a definitive diagnosis can be made and appropriate anticoagulant therapy (e.g., intravenous streptokinase, heparin) can be administered.

Two other pulmonary conditions that can cause chest pain are pleurisy and pneumothorax. *Pleurisy* is an irritation of the pleural membranes that make up the lining between the lungs and the inner surface of the rib cage. The pain that pleurisy produces is characteristically described as sharp and stabbing and is worsened by deep inspiration and by other rib cage movements, such as a cough. Passive movement testing of the rib cage and the thoracic spine also may produce pleuritic pain. Pleurisy may have multiple causes, such as viral infection or tumor, and is associated with disorders such as rheumatoid arthritis. Each of these conditions requires a definitive diagnosis and intervention by a physician. Suspicion of this disorder should lead the PT to auscultate over the thorax, while listening for a "pleural rub" sound.

A pneumothorax—air in the thoracic cage—produces chest pain that is intensified upon deep inspiration. A pneumothorax can be a spontaneous, usually pathologic event that is associated with rupture of the wall of the lung lining. Such a rupture prevents the lung from maintaining negative pressure during diaphragmatic and rib cage motions. A simple pneumothorax may begin without any precipitating event, or it may follow a bout of extreme coughing or strenuous physical activity. Physical examination findings associated with a pneumothorax include a limited ability of the affected side of the chest to expand, hyperresonance of the affected area upon percussion, and markedly reduced breath sounds. A small pneumothorax may resolve within a few days without therapy. A large pneumothorax, however, will require aspiration of air from the lung. Factors predisposing individuals to pneumothorax are menstruation (in young women), asthma, chronic obstructive lung disease, cystic fibrosis, and lung cancer. A tension pneumothorax usually is a consequence of a trauma, such as a penetrating wound to the rib cage or a severe blow to the rib cage that may occur in contact sports or during an automobile injury (with the patient hitting the steering wheel). Signs of a tension pneumothorax include severe pleuritic-type chest wall pain, extreme shortness of breath, tracheal deviation, distended neck veins, tachycardia, hypotension, and hyperresonance to percussion of the involved (painful) side of the chest. Tension pneumothorax can be an extreme emergency requiring insertion of a chest tube with a seal or a Heimlich valve.[33]

Finally, another cause of pleuritic-type chest pain is pneumonia, which is a bacterial or viral infection of the lungs. Signs of systemic infection, such as chills, fever, malaise, nausea, and vomiting, typically accompany the pleuritic pain. The fever may be absent in the elderly, with onset or worsening of confusion being the primary manifestation. A distinguishing characteristic of pneumonia is a cough that produces sputum of varying coloration, from light green to dark brown.

Gastrointestinal Disorders

Gastrointestinal disorders are common in the general population and may present as comorbidities during the examination process. The PT should routinely ask patients about bowel movement characteristics, vomiting, unexplained weight loss, or extended use of nonsteroidal anti-inflammatory drugs (NSAIDs). Common gastrointestinal disorders include gastric or peptic ulcer disease and cholecystitis. Ulcers occur when the lining of the digestive tract is exposed to digestive acids and are named according to their anatomic location. An ulcer in the duodenum is called a *duodenal ulcer* and is associated with the presence of *Helicobacter pylori* bacteria in the stomach. Duodenal ulcers present as dull, gnawing, or burning pain in the epigastric region, in the midthoracic (T6-T10) region, or in the supraclavicular region. These symptoms occur when the stomach is empty and are relieved with eating or taking of antacids. Relief is temporary, however, and symptoms return within 2 to 3 hours. If the ulcer is located in the stomach (a gastric ulcer), eating may increase, rather than relieve, the symptoms. These ulcers are more common in the elderly because of increased use of NSAIDs.

Unlike duodenal ulcers, gastric ulcers can be malignant and require the attention of a doctor even if symptoms spontaneously resolve when the drugs are stopped. With esophageal ulcers, the person experiences pain upon swallowing or when lying down. Symptoms of these ulcers include black, tarry-colored stools; bright red or reddish-brown clumps (coffee ground emesis) in the vomit; relief or intensification of pain with eating; and pain in the chest, back, or supraclavicular area.

The other common gastrointestinal disorder is cholecystitis, an inflammation of the gallbladder. The initial symptom often is pain in the right upper abdominal quadrant or in the interscapular or right scapular region,[36] which can be constant and intense. Pain usually is severe enough to cause nausea and vomiting. Murphy's sign is positive (inspiration inhibited by pain on local palpation in the right upper abdominal quadrant) in more than 50% of patients with cholecystitis.[37] Patients initially may seek pain control from a PT but should be referred to their physician or local emergency room. Inflammation of the gallbladder usually is caused by a gallstone lodged in the cystic duct; medical help is needed to remove the gallstone.

Kidney Disorders

Disorders of the kidney such as pyelonephritis and renal stones result in pain in the posterior lateral aspect of the thoracic cage and the upper lumbar area. PTs may see the term *costovertebral angle (CVA)* or *flank* in physician notes referring to this region. Both conditions present with chills, fever, nausea, vomiting, and renal colic. Renal colic is excruciating intermittent pain from the CVA or flank that spreads across the lower abdomen into the labia in women and into the testicles and penis in men. The pain is associated with spasms in a ureter and may extend as far down as the inner thighs.

Pyelonephritis is an infection in the kidney, usually caused by an infection in the ascending urinary tract. Thus those at risk for pyelonephritis are individuals with recent or coexisting urinary tract infection. Blood-borne pathogens or conditions that cause obstruction of urine flow (benign prostatic hyperplasia or kidney stones) also may cause renal infection.

Kidney stones (nephrolithiasis if in the kidney, urolithiasis if anywhere else in the urinary tract) are hard masses of salts that precipitate from the urine when it becomes supersaturated with a particular substance. Most stones are composed of calcium; less common are stones composed of uric acid, cystine, or struvite (a combination of magnesium, ammonium, and phosphate). Risk factors for developing kidney stones are warm, humid atmospheric temperatures and diseases (such as leukemia) that involve high cell turnover. The incidence of kidney stones in men is four times greater than in women.[32] Caucasian men have three times as many stone episodes as black men. About 5% to 15% of the population is expected to have kidney stones during their lifetime.[32] Still, the best predictor of kidney stones is a past episode, as about 50% of patients experience at least one recurrence.[38] A PT who suspects these conditions should refer the patient for medical attention. Tables 5-8 and 5-9 offer a summary of red flags for thoracic symptoms and a questionnaire for screening.

Shoulder and Cervical Pain

Patients with shoulder and cervical symptoms make up a large portion of the caseload of an orthopaedic PT.[1-3] Fewer serious disorders involve the shoulder and neck regions compared with the thorax. For example, metastasis does not occur in the cervical region nearly as often as in other regions of the axial skeleton.[13] PTs should be familiar with a few conditions, however, including central cord syndromes, ligamentous instability, brachial plexus neuropathies, and Pancoast's tumor.

The PT should rule out a ligamentous injury after trauma such as a motor vehicle accident or a fall, but trauma is not the only condition that should alert the PT to the possibility of ligamentous instability. People with rheumatoid arthritis, Down syndrome, or ankylosing spondylitis, and even those who merely use oral contraceptives, should be screened for ligamentous instability of the neck. The alar and transverse ligaments maintain the proper relationship of C1 on C2, while the ligamentum flavum, anterior and posterior longitudinal ligaments, and interspinous and intertransverse ligaments help maintain proper alignment through the entire cervical region. Resultant instability can lead to significant neurologic and cardiovascular consequences, and PTs should routinely screen for such symptoms.

Neurologic symptoms associated with ligamentous instability can include the typical presentation of tingling, numbness, weakness, or burning pain. The PT should be concerned about possible compromise of the spinal cord if the patient has these symptoms in more than one extremity. In addition, dizziness, vertigo, or nystagmus associated with head or neck movements should alert the PT. Symptoms such as these in a patient who has been involved in a traumatic event or has a positive history of the disorders mentioned previously that can lead to instability should prompt the PT to conduct special stability tests such as the Sharp-Purser test and alar and transverse ligament stress tests. Other potential signs to note during the physical examination include clonus and a positive Babinski sign.[39]

Brachial plexus neuropathies can occur as the result of repetitive overuse, postural syndromes, and trauma. Nerves affected by such neuropathies fall into three categories: sensory, motor, and mixed. Emphasis is placed on motor nerves, but the therapist should remember that there is no such thing as a pure motor nerve. A motor nerve carries efferent commands to the muscles but returns with information from muscles, joints, and associated ligamentous structures. A nerve that innervates a muscle also augments sensation from the joint upon which that muscle acts. Pain produced by a motor nerve entrapment neuropathy is not well localized, is present at rest, and has a retrograde distribution. Innervated muscles can be tender to palpation, and if the neuropathy has been present for an extended time, muscle atrophy may occur, although the patient may not be aware of the weakness. The greatest challenge with entrapment neuropathies is not treatment but diagnosis. These neuropathies often are the cumulative result of many small traumas or longstanding compression, or they may be of mechanical origin.

With evaluation of any new patient, the PT should conduct a thorough examination of motor and sensory function and reflexes in the area of interest. The PT should observe the area carefully, preferably with the area disrobed to allow for bilateral comparison of muscle bulk and visualization of possible atrophy. If the PT suspects a specific nerve, he or she should consider the muscles and sensory distribution that would be affected. The PT should palpate bilaterally along the path of the suspected nerve, looking for bone, joint, or soft tissue abnormalities. Local tenderness or a positive Tinel sign will help reveal the site of nerve entrapment. Suspicion can be resolved by the use of electromyography (EMG) and/or nerve conduction studies (NCS).[40]

If a patient presents with weakness of shoulder abduction and cannot shrug a shoulder, the PT should suspect a nerve entrapment of the spinal accessory nerve. The patient typically will have dull pain, weakness, drooping of the shoulder, and paralysis of the trapezius muscle, and winging of the scapula usually is present. The spinal accessory nerve can be injured by blunt trauma to the posterior triangle of the neck or a traction

Table 5-8	Red Flags for the Thoracic Spine and Rib Cage Region
Condition	**Red Flags**
Myocardial infarction	Chest pain
	Pallor, sweating, dyspnea, nausea, palpitations
	Presence of risk factors: previous history of coronary artery disease, hypertension, smoking, diabetes, elevated blood serum cholesterol (>240 mg/dL)
	Men over age 40, women over age 50
	Symptoms lasting longer than 30 minutes and not relieved with sublingual nitroglycerin
Unstable angina pectoris	Chest pain that occurs outside of a predictable pattern
	Not responsive to nitroglycerin
Stable angina pectoris	Chest pain/pressure that occurs with predictable levels of exertion
	Symptoms predictably alleviated with rest or sublingual nitroglycerin
Pericarditis	Sharp/stabbing chest pain that may be referred to the lateral neck or either shoulder
	Increased pain with left-side lying
	Relieved with forward lean while sitting (supporting arms on knees or a table)
Pulmonary embolus	Chest, shoulder, or upper abdominal pain
	Dyspnea
	History of, or risk factors for developing, a deep vein thrombosis
Pleurisy	Severe, sharp, "knife-like" pain with inspiration
	Dyspnea, decreased chest wall excursion
	History of a recent or concurrent respiratory disorder (e.g., infection, pneumonia, tumor, tuberculosis)
Pneumothorax	Chest pain, intensified with inspiration
	Difficulty ventilating or expanding rib cage
	Recent bout of coughing or strenuous exercise or trauma
	Hyperresonance on percussion
	Decreased breath sounds
Pneumonia	Pleuritic pain, may be referred to shoulder
	Fever, chills, headache, malaise, nausea
	Productive cough
Cholecystitis	Colicky pain in right upper abdominal quadrant with accompanying right scapular pain
	Symptom worsening with ingestion of fatty foods
	Symptoms not increased by activity nor relieved by rest
Peptic ulcer	Dull or gnawing pain or "burning" sensation in the epigastrium, midback, or supraclavicular region
	Symptoms relieved with food
	Localized tenderness at the right epigastrium
	Constipation, bleeding, vomiting, tarry-colored stools, coffee ground emesis
Pyelonephritis	Recent or coexisting urinary tract infection
	Enlarged prostate
	Kidney stone or past episode of kidney stone
Nephrolithiasis (kidney stones)	Sudden, severe back or flank pain
	Chills, fever, nausea, or vomiting
	Renal colic
	Symptoms of urinary tract infection
	Residence in hot and humid environment
	Past episodes of kidney stone, with 50% of patients experiencing a recurrence

injury, or injury can result from cervical surgery, such as for head and neck cancers.[41] The spinal accessory nerve is susceptible to trauma at the posterior triangle because of its superficial location, but the SCM would be spared because the injury would be distal to its innervation. A traction force that depresses the shoulder while laterally flexing the head in the opposite direction stretches and can damage the nerve. The patient will become aware of damage to the spinal accessory nerve when he or she notices a reduced ability to use his or her shoulder because of lack of scapular stabilization or a reduced ability to shrug the shoulder.

Weakness of shoulder abduction and flexion should raise the suspicion of a possible axillary nerve entrapment or injury. The axillary nerve arises from the posterior cord of the brachial plexus and contains fibers from C5 and C6 nerve roots. After branching from the brachial plexus, the nerve travels laterally and downward, passing just below the shoulder joint and into the quadrilateral space.[41] The nerve then curves around the posterior and lateral portion of the proximal humerus to innervate the deltoid and teres minor muscles, while supplying sensation to the lateral aspect of the upper arm.[41] A typical axillary nerve injury is caused by trauma such as a direct blow

Table 5-9	Medical Screening Questionnaire for the Thoracic Spine and Rib Cage Region		
		Yes	**No**
Do you have a history of heart problems?			
Have you recently taken a nitroglycerin tablet?			
Do you have diabetes?			
Do you take medication for hypertension?			
Have you been or are you now a smoker?			
Does your pain ease when you rest in a comfortable position?			
Have you had recent surgery?			
Have you recently been bedridden?			
Have you recently noticed that it is difficult for you to breathe, laugh, sneeze, or cough?			
Have you recently had a fever, infection, or other illness?			
Have you recently received a blow to the chest, such as during a fall or motor vehicle accident?			
In the past few weeks, have you noticed that when you cough, you easily cough up sputum?			
Are your symptoms relieved after eating?			
Does eating fatty foods increase your symptoms?			
Do you currently have a urinary tract infection, or have you had one in the past 2 months?			
Do you currently have a kidney stone, or have you had one in the past?			
Do you experience severe back or flank pain that comes on suddenly?			

to the shoulder or a dislocation that stretches the nerve where it curves around the humerus. Patients will be aware of weakness with shoulder flexion and abduction, but numbness will not necessarily be present. The PT should refer such a patient to his or her doctor for surgical intervention.

Scapular winging may be due to trapezius involvement or may be related to serratus anterior paralysis. The serratus anterior is innervated by the long thoracic nerve after it branches from cervical roots 5, 6, and 7. The nerve passes down the posterolateral aspect of the chest wall, and its superficial course makes it susceptible to injury. The nerve can be damaged by excessive use of the shoulder, prolonged traction to the nerve, or trauma to the lateral chest wall. A patient with entrapment or injury of the long thoracic nerve will experience pain in the shoulder girdle, a reduction in active shoulder motion caused by loss of scapulohumeral rhythm, and scapular winging that becomes especially evident when doing a wall push-up.

Poorly localized shoulder pain may be related to a rotator cuff tear or to suprascapular nerve entrapment. Suprascapular nerve entrapment often is confused with a rotator cuff tear, because both exhibit wasting of the supraspinatus or infraspinatus with loss of strength in abduction and external rotation of the shoulder. The suprascapular nerve, like the long thoracic nerve, is a motor nerve, and pain resulting from its irritation is deep and poorly localized. The suprascapular nerve derives

from the upper trunk of the brachial plexus, formed from the roots of C5 and C6. The nerve runs in the posterior triangle of the neck, sometimes passing through the body of the middle scalene, and past the anterior border of the trapezius on its way to the upper border of the scapula. After arriving at the scapula, the suprascapular nerve passes through the suprascapular notch. The notch is roofed by the transverse scapular ligament, making the U-shaped notch into a foramen. Here the nerve gives off innervation for the supraspinatus muscle; it then continues around the lateral border of the spine of the scapula. The nerve passes through the spinoglenoid notch to reach its destination in the infraspinatus muscle.[41]

Entrapment of the suprascapular nerve most often occurs at the suprascapular foramen, resulting in weakness and atrophy of the supraspinatus and infraspinatus muscles. Entrapment also has occurred, however, at the spinoglenoid notch, resulting in isolated involvement of the infraspinatus muscle. Trauma, whether in the form of repetitive microtrauma or distal trauma, causes a traction injury to the suprascapular nerve. A person with poor scapular stability will exhibit additional motion at the suprascapular foramen against the suprascapular nerve, causing pain and inflammation through repetitive microtrauma.

A distal trauma can result from a fall onto an outstretched arm that is fully supinated, extended, and somewhat adducted. With this type of fall, the scapula remains fixed at the end of the upper extremity, while the inertia of the trunk keeps the body moving down, and the nerve is injured directly, before protective crumpling or a Colles' fracture occurs. Conservative treatment consisting of rest, NSAIDs, and physical therapy is often unsuccessful, and surgical decompression may be necessary.[41]

As stated earlier, shoulder and cervical pathologies make up a large portion of the caseload of an orthopaedic PT. Thoracic outlet syndrome, cervical disc disease, and intrinsic shoulder disorders (e.g., bursitis, tendonitis, frozen shoulder) are very common disorders. Most PTs think that they fully understand these diagnoses and can confidently guide a patient through rehabilitation, but do they understand the relationship of these diagnoses to Pancoast's tumor? All of these diagnoses are common misdiagnoses of Pancoast's tumor.

Pancoast's tumor is a malignant tumor in the upper apices of a lung; it may be referred to as a superior pulmonary sulcus tumor. Pancoast's tumor has the highest occurrence in men over 50 with a history of cigarette smoking. In more than 90% of patients, shoulder pain, rather than pulmonary symptoms, appears first.[42] Pulmonary symptoms are rare, and shoulder or disc problems are suspected because the tumor grows into the thoracic inlet, affecting the eighth cervical and first thoracic nerve roots, the subclavian artery and vein, and the sympathetic chain ganglions.

The patient with Pancoast's tumor initially suffers only "nagging" pain in the shoulder and along the vertebral border of the scapula as the tumor irritates the parietal pleura. As the tumor continues to invade the thoracic inlet, the pain becomes more burning, extending down the arm and into the ulnar nerve distribution. Over time, the intrinsic hand muscles atrophy, and the tumor occludes the subclavian vein. Occlusion causes venous distention of the ipsilateral arm. It is during this progressive decline that the patient seeks medical attention, and the disorder is misdiagnosed for an average of 6.8 months (ranging from 1 to 24 months).[42] Misdiagnosis by doctors and mistreatment by PTs and chiropractors reduce the odds of survival, as with any malignant cancer.

The goal is to prevent metastasis to the mediastinal lymph nodes or other peripheral sites. If a PT is treating a patient (especially one with the above profile: male older than 50 years and a smoker) for neck or shoulder diagnoses mentioned previously and does not notice any change in pain after three to four treatments, a referral back to the doctor may be warranted. Table 5-10[38] summarizes the red flags for patients with cervical and shoulder pain, and Table 5-11 offers a medical screening questionnaire for these patients.

Craniofacial Pain

PTs have become increasingly involved in the treatment of conditions of the head, face, and temporomandibular joint (TMJ). When seeing a patient for TMJ dysfunction, Bell's palsy, stroke, or even conditions of the back or neck, PTs should consider the possibility of meningitis, a primary brain tumor, or a subarachnoid hemorrhage. Quick detection of all of the aforementioned conditions by an alert PT can greatly increase the chance of survival and can possibly minimize morbidity.

Meningitis is a relatively rare infection that affects the meninges, causing brain swelling, bleeding, and death in 10% of cases.[43] The most common and most serious type of meningitis is bacterial meningitis. Bacteria that are responsible for bacterial meningitis are present in the external environment and even in our own respiratory system. The bacteria somehow cross the blood-brain barrier after a head injury, because of a depressed immune system, or for some unidentifiable reason. Bacterial meningitis can cause death within hours, and a child younger than 2 years old with an unexplained fever should be seen by a doctor immediately.

Viral meningitis, caused by a viral intestinal infection, mumps, or a herpes infection, is generally the least serious, clearing on its own within 1 to 2 weeks. Antiviral medications may be used in more serious cases of infection, depending on the type of viral infection. Acyclovir is effective against herpes simplex, which can cause herpes encephalitis and severe brain damage if not treated. Acyclovir, although effective against the herpes virus, does little to most other viruses and must be given before the person lapses into a coma.

Fungal meningitis affects 10% of patients with acquired immunodeficiency syndrome (AIDS) and should be considered when one is seeing these patients.[43] Fungal meningitis is spread from pigeon droppings and is treated with antifungal medications after it is detected.

Meningitis is more common in people with compromised immune systems, such as patients with AIDS and those who have suffered a facial trauma leading to infection that spreads to the cerebrospinal fluid (CSF). Meningitis is most common

Table 5-10	Red Flags for the Cervical Spine and Shoulder Region
Condition	**Red Flags**
Myocardial infarction	• Chest pain • Pallor, sweating, dyspnea, nausea, palpitations • Presence of risk factors: previous history of coronary artery disease, hypertension, smoking, diabetes, elevated blood serum cholesterol (>240 mg/dL) • Men over age 40, women over age 50 • Symptoms lasting longer than 30 minutes and not relieved by sublingual nitroglycerin
Cervical ligamentous instabilities with possible cord compromise	• Major trauma such as a motor vehicle accident or a fall from a height • Rheumatoid arthritis or ankylosing spondylitis • Oral contraceptive use • Long track neurologic signs, especially those present in more than one extremity, dizziness, nystagmus, vertigo with head/neck movements/positions, clonus, positive Babinski sign
Cervical and shoulder girdle peripheral entrapment neuropathies	• Paresthesias • Pain present at rest, possibly with a retrograde distribution • Innervated muscles tender to palpation • Muscles and sensory distribution that follows a specific nerve pattern
Spinal accessory nerve	• Weakness of shoulder abduction • Inability to shrug the shoulders • Dull pain, weakness, and drooping of the shoulder • Lack of scapular stabilization
Axillary nerve	• Weakness of shoulder abduction and flexion • Lack of sensation in the lateral aspect of the upper arm
Long thoracic nerve	• Serratus anterior weakness with scapular winging • Loss of scapulohumeral rhythm
Suprascapular nerve	• Presentation similar to rotator cuff tear because of wasting of the supraspinatus and/or infraspinatus muscle • Loss of strength in abduction and external rotation of the shoulder • Pain that is deep and poorly localized
Pancoast's tumor[42] (superior sulcus lung tumor)	• Men older than 50 years with a history of cigarette smoking • "Nagging"-type pain in the shoulder and along the vertebral border of the scapula • Pain that has progressed from nagging to burning in nature, often extending down the arm and into the ulnar nerve distribution

Table 5-11	Medical Screening Questionnaire for the Cervical Spine and Shoulder Regions

	Yes	No
Have you had a direct blow to your shoulder or a shoulder dislocation?		
Have you recently used your shoulder excessively?		
Have you had a traction injury to your arm?		
Have you had a direct blow to the lateral chest wall?		
Have you recently fallen onto an outstretched arm?		
Have you noticed difficulty lifting your arm or any other muscle weakness?		
Have you been experiencing pins and needles anywhere in your body?		
Do you experience pain that does not improve with rest?		
If you do have pain, where is your pain?		
Does your pain move into the arm?		
Do you currently smoke?		
Do you have a history of smoking?		

in children younger than 2 years old and people living in close quarters, such as college dormitories or military training camps.

If meningitis is suspected, a slump test is performed. In this test, the neck and trunk are fully flexed, causing pain that is relieved when neck flexion ceases. Different variants of the test are used with the trunk flexed and the leg straightened, but all forms stress the meninges.[7] If meningeal inflammation is present, a positive test should result, as pain in the back, neck, or head is relieved when the meninges are no longer stressed. Other signs include headache, high fever, stiff neck, nausea and vomiting, photophobia, confusion, sleepiness, and seizures. A patient with this type of presentation should be referred immediately to an emergency room or back to his or her primary care physician for proper testing. A physician must perform a lumbar puncture to obtain a sample of CSF for analysis, to make the diagnosis, and to determine appropriate treatment.

Another possible intracranial disorder that requires vigilance is brain cancer. A primary brain tumor occurs relatively infrequently, in six to nine people per 100,000,[44] but the central nervous system (CNS) is a common site for metastasis. Lung cancer accounts for about one-half of all metastatic brain lesions, and breast cancer and melanomas often metastasize to the brain. Therefore, PTs treating patients with a history of these primary cancers should be vigilant for symptoms that suggest CNS metastases. Although headache is a symptom associated with a brain tumor, neurologic deficits are a more common symptom in the early and middle stages of this disorder.[45] Change in mentation, vomiting with or without nausea, visual changes, seizures, ataxia, and speech impairment all are possible presentations, with or without the headache. Symptoms of this type would warrant a detailed neurologic screening.

Table 5-12	Red Flags for the Head, Face, and Temporomandibular Joint Regions

Condition	Red Flags
Meningitis	• Positive slump sign • Headache • Fever • Gastrointestinal signs of vomiting and symptoms of nausea • Photophobia • Confusion • Seizures • Sleepiness
Primary brain tumor	• Ataxia • Speech deficits • Sensory abnormalities • Headache • Gastrointestinal signs of vomiting and symptoms of nausea • Visual changes • Altered mental status • Seizures
Subarachnoid hemorrhage	• Headache of sudden onset (the worst headache of his or her life) • Brief loss of consciousness • Brain tumor signs (neurologic dysfunction, nausea and vomiting) • Meningeal irritation signs (nuchal rigidity, fever, photophobia, nausea and vomiting)

The third condition affecting the head, face, and TMJ region is subarachnoid hemorrhage. Hemorrhage is caused most often by rupture of a saccular intracranial aneurysm or rupture of an arteriovenous malformation. Signs and symptoms can be very similar to those of a brain tumor and of meningitis. The patient will describe a headache of sudden onset that is the worst headache of his or her life, and the patient even may experience a brief loss of consciousness. Meningeal irritation symptoms and signs (nuchal rigidity, fever, photophobia, nausea, and vomiting) and brain tumor symptoms and signs (neurologic dysfunction, nausea, and vomiting) also are possible. If a PT suspects a subarachnoid hemorrhage, emergency medical care should be instituted. Early diagnosis is critical and can prevent devastating neurologic effects. See Table 5-12 for a summary of the red flags for patients with craniofacial pain and Table 5-13 for a medical screening questionnaire for these patients.

Elbow, Wrist, and Hand Pain

Injuries involving the elbow, wrist, and hand are common, and pain in specific locations should alert the PT to the possibility of a more serious disorder. For example, a patient with osteoporosis or other conditions that can compromise bone density who suffers a fall is more likely to sustain a fracture. A patient

Table 5-13	Medical Screening Questionnaire for the Head, Face, and Temporomandibular Joint Regions		

	Yes	No
Do you have a depressed immune system?		
Have you recently had an intestinal infection, mumps, or herpes?		
Have you had recent contact with pigeons or pigeon droppings?		
Have you recently been living in close quarters, such as in a dormitory or military training camp?		
Have you recently had a head trauma?		
Do you currently have a high fever, or have you had a fever recently?		
Have you been experiencing nausea or vomiting?		
Have you had difficulty with light sensitivity?		
Have you noticed a recent inability to concentrate?		
Have you recently had a seizure?		
Do you experience abnormal sensations in the skin?		
Have you recently had difficulty with speaking?		
Have you noticed increased clumsiness or lack of coordination?		
Have you recently experienced a loss of consciousness?		

who takes corticosteroids for chronic respiratory problems will be more likely to suffer a tendon rupture or ligamentous injury during the same fall. Finally, a patient who is immunosuppressed for any number of reasons is more susceptible to a space infection in the hand. This section discusses the red flags associated with specific fractures, tendon ruptures, space infections of the hand, Raynaud's disease, and complex regional pain syndrome (reflex sympathetic dystrophy).

Fractures

A fracture at the elbow most likely will have been caused by a fall onto an outstretched arm or by direct trauma to the elbow itself. An olecranon fracture will cause posterior pain, swelling, and tenderness. Elbow extension is the function most often impaired, and a gap may be palpable between the olecranon and the trochlear notch of the humerus. A fall also may cause anterolateral pain and tenderness or an inability to supinate and pronate the forearm, or it may cause the arm to be held against the side with the elbow flexed. This would be typical of a radial head fracture, and flexing the elbow would produce the least pressure within the elbow capsule. This loosely packed position of 70 degrees of ulnohumeral flexion and 10 degrees of supination also will compensate for the effusion of the elbow joint that is usually present.[46]

The radius may be fractured distally during a fall onto an outstretched arm. A fracture of the distal radius, Colles' fracture, typically presents with local pain, tenderness, swelling, and ecchymoses, and wrist extension in particular is painful.[46] The same fall onto an outstretched arm and extended wrist can cause a scaphoid fracture. The patient will have similar signs

and symptoms, but these will be localized to the anatomical snuffbox. The wrist will be very stiff as the result of swelling. Radiographs, if performed with all four views plus a navicular view, have a 100% diagnostic sensitivity.[33] If films are negative, however, the patient is put into a spica cast, and radiographs are repeated after 2 weeks. The main concern with scaphoid fractures is the possibility of avascular necrosis related to disruption of the blood supply.

The final types of fracture discussed here are a lunate fracture or dislocation and a capitate fracture. Lunate fractures are rare and often are related to osteonecrosis. Lunate fractures can cause diffuse synovitis with generalized wrist swelling, pain, and decreased motion, and even reduced grip strength. The best way to identify a lunate fracture is through radiographic imaging, especially a T1-weighted magnetic resonance image to detect loss of bone marrow. A capitate fracture is more common and will present with similar symptoms of wrist pain, swelling, and tenderness at the mid-dorsal wrist area. Capitate fractures are the result of trauma involving maximal wrist flexion or extension, rather than of osteonecrosis.

Soft Tissue Injuries

Falls, traumas, and sports-related injuries cause problems not only with bones but also with local soft tissue structures. The flexor forearm muscle mass, including the pronator teres, flexor carpi radialis, palmaris longus, and flexor carpi ulnaris, can be strained or even ruptured. A grade I muscle strain is defined as stretching of the muscle fibers without disruption. A grade II tear occurs as a partial tearing of the muscles with maintenance of the overlying fascia. This injury will involve local tenderness, swelling, muscle spasms, a hematoma, and pain with motion and with passive elongation of the tissue. Strains of grades I and II can be treated conservatively with the RICE (rest, ice, compression, elevation) technique. Grade III tears signify complete tearing of the muscle and its investing fascia. This injury results in a total loss of motion, and surgical repair is needed. Swelling, tenderness, ecchymoses of the overlying skin, and a palpable defect in the muscle are characteristic of a grade III rupture of the flexor forearm muscle mass and would warrant referral of the patient to a physician as soon as possible.

Infection

The hand often is traumatized as the result of puncture wounds, abrasions, cuts, or other injuries, and a break in the skin brings the increased possibility of an infection. Hands have several spaces (e.g., midpalmar space, web space, thenar space) that can serve as prime areas for development and spread of infection. Fingers also have such spaces on the volar surface, such as the pulp space of the proximal, middle, and distal phalanx. Any of these spaces can become infected after a direct puncture, formation of an abscess, or purulent tenosynovitis of tendons that pass through the space. These spaces also can become infected as the result of trauma or poor nail care. A patient will present with typical signs of local inflammation, and swelling will cause the finger pads to be tense and painful with resultant loss of motion. Infection must be treated quickly, or it may spread to the adjacent web space of the hand and beyond.

If the web space becomes infected, swelling, pain, tenderness, warmth, and erythema will be present in the palm and over the dorsum of the hand proximal to the involved area of the involved space. Edema can cause the metacarpal bones to become splayed, resulting in loss of normal hand shape. Causes are similar to those listed above, and, as mentioned, can be caused by progression of a pulp space infection.

Midpalmar space infections appear very similar to web space infections in their presentation, with inflammation of the palm and dorsum of the hand and loss of concavity of the palm caused by swelling. Even the midpalmar space can become infected by the second, third, and fourth web spaces through the lumbrical canals.[33] Direct puncture also can infect the midpalmar space or can produce tenosynovitis of the flexor tendons of the second or fourth finger.

The thenar space is the equivalent of the midpalmar space, but for the thumb. Direct puncture tenosynovitis of the second flexor tendon or from an adjacent space, such as the midpalmar space, can infect this area. This space is treated in the same way as the spaces mentioned previously, that is, by drainage with a course of antibiotics specific to the organism causing the infection. If the patient is not seen by a doctor quickly, the infection could drain through a necrotic area of the skin, increasing the possibility of osteomyelitis or septic arthritis. The infection also can spread, causing high fever, chills, weakness, and malaise. Ultimately, the infection may lead to sepsis and amputation of fingers or parts of the hand.[47] As with any infection, people who are immunocompromised are at greatest risk. Space infections also have been seen in recipients of cardiac transplants, because of the need for long-term immunosuppression to prevent rejection of the donor heart.[47]

Raynaud's Disease

Another disorder that may affect patients who see PTs is Raynaud's disease, or Raynaud's phenomenon. This disorder affects one or both hands and the feet. One or more digits may be involved, and progression of the disease involves additional digits. When a person is exposed to cold or to emotional upset, the hands blanch, become cyanotic, and then turn red. During the rubor stage, the patient has pain and paresthesias as the blood returns to the hands or feet. This entire phase lasts only 15 to 20 minutes, and the patient can alleviate it by running the hands under warm water. As mentioned, exposure to cold or stress usually precipitates episodes, but Raynaud's phenomenon is more common in patients with rheumatoid arthritis or occlusive vascular disease, those who smoke, and people taking beta-adrenergic blocking drugs to treat migraine, angina, or hypertension.

Reflex sympathetic dystrophy (RSD; also known as *complex regional pain syndrome*) is a disorder that varies in severity and often follows trauma to the elbow, wrist, or hand. The trauma may involve a fracture, sprain, dislocation, or crush injury, or surgery such as a carpal tunnel procedure. A lag period often

Table 5-14	Red Flags for the Elbow, Wrist, and Hand Regions
Condition	**Red Flags**
Fracture	• Recent fall or trauma • Pain, tenderness, swelling, and ecchymosis • History of osteoporosis • Extended use of steroids (e.g., respiratory problems) • Pathology with improper bone remodeling
Radial head fracture	• Fall onto an outstretched arm that is supinated • Anterolateral pain and tenderness at the elbow • Inability to supinate and pronate the forearm • Elbow held against the side with 70 degrees of flexion and slightly supinated
Distal radius (Colles') fracture	• Fall onto outstretched arm with forceful wrist extension • Wrist held in neutral resting position • Wrist swelling • Painful movements into wrist extension
Scaphoid fracture	• Fall onto outstretched arm • Wrist swelling • Wrist held in neutral position • Pain in the "anatomical snuff box"
Lunate fracture or dislocation	• Diffuse synovitis • Generalized wrist swelling and pain • Decreased motion • Decreased grip strength (rule out capitate fracture)
Long flexor tendon rupture	• Grade I and II muscle tear: local tenderness, swelling, muscle spasms, hematoma, pain with motion and with passive stretch • Grade III muscle rupture: total loss of motion and palpable defect in the muscle, swelling, tenderness, ecchymosis of overlying skin
Space infection of the hand	• Recent puncture of skin • Presence of an abscess • Purulent tenosynovitis of tendons that go through a space • Typical signs of inflammation: swelling in palm, dorsum of hand, or fingertips • Pain, tenderness, warmth, and erythema • Signs of long-standing infection: high fever, chills, weakness, and malaise
Raynaud's phenomenon or Raynaud's disease	• Hands or feet that blanch, go cyanotic, and then turn red when exposed to cold or emotional stress • Pain and tingling in hands or feet when they turn red • Past medical history significant for rheumatoid arthritis, occlusive vascular disease, smoking, or use of beta-blockers
Complex regional pain syndrome (reflex sympathetic dystrophy)	• Trauma, including fracture, dislocation, or surgery • Severe aching, stinging, cutting, or boring pain that is not typical of injury; hypersensitivity • Area swollen (pitting edema), warm, and erythematous • Pain not responsive to typical analgesics

Table 5-15	Medical Screening Questionnaire for the Elbow, Wrist, and Hand Regions		
		Yes	No
Have you recently had a trauma, such as a fall?			
Has a medical practitioner ever told you that you have osteoporosis?			
Are you currently taking steroids or have you been on prolonged steroid therapy?			
Do you have pathology with improper bone remodeling?			
Have you noticed an inability to move your elbow normally?			
Have you noticed an inability to move your wrist normally?			
Do you have difficulty turning your hand upward or downward (e.g., turning a doorknob)?			
Have you recently had an infection?			
Do you have any open wounds, cuts, swelling, or redness on your hands or arms?			
Have you noticed weakness in your hands or frequent dropping of objects?			
Have you recently experienced a high fever, chills, weakness, or malaise?			
Do your hands or feet blanch, go blue, and then turn red when exposed to cold or emotional stress?			
Do you have a medical history of rheumatoid arthritis, occlusive vascular disease, or use of beta-blockers?			
Do you currently smoke or have a history of smoking?			
If you have pain, does it respond to typical pain medications?			

occurs between the injury and the onset of symptoms of complex regional pain syndrome. Symptoms include severe aching, stinging, cutting, or boring pain that is out of proportion to the injury, corrective surgery, or normal tissue healing.[12,48] The pain does not respond to typical analgesics, and regional nerve blocks usually produce only temporary relief. The hand often becomes swollen, warm, and erythematous.

Hyperhidrosis is often present. The other hand may support the involved limb, and the patient is often resistant to letting a practitioner handle the hand because of hypersensitivity. Nerve blocks are a common treatment and are performed in conjunction with physical therapy to maintain function and assist the patient with strategies for pain management.

See Table 5-14 for a summary of red flags for patients with distal upper extremity pain and Table 5-15 for a medical screening questionnaire for these patients.

SUMMARY

The investigation of symptoms produces information vital in determining why the patient has sought physical therapy services. While the patient describes the location, onset, and behavior of symptoms, the PT must decide whether the patient's narrative makes sense based upon our understanding of basic and clinical sciences and our experiences. This information helps the PT make a diagnosis and decide whether to refer the patient to a physician. Information gathered during the initial patient visit also helps guide the PT (1) in choosing body systems to screen later during the history, (2) in determining whether a lower quarter or an upper quarter screening examination is warranted, and (3) in identifying the components of these examinations that are most relevant.

Finally, the location of symptoms should alert the PT to the possibility of certain disorders that may be responsible for the patient's symptoms. Knowledge of such disorders will enable the PT to recognize specific symptoms and warning signs for these disorders. The clinician also is encouraged to use the accompanying tables and figures to collect this patient information in an effective and efficient manner.

REFERENCES

1. Boissonnault W: Prevalence of comorbid conditions, surgeries, and medication use in a physical outpatient population: a multicentered study, J Orthop Sports Phys Ther 29:506-519, 1999.
2. DiFabio R, Boissonnault W: Physical therapy and health-related outcomes for patients with common orthopaedic diagnoses, J Orthop Sports Phys Ther 27:219-230, 1998.
3. Jette AM, Davis KD: A comparison of hospital-based and private outpatient physical therapy practices, Phys Ther 71:366-375, 1991.
4. Jarvik JG, Deyo RA: Diagnostic evaluation of low back pain with emphasis on imaging, Ann Intern Med, 137:586-597, 2002.
5. Delitto A, Erhard RE, Bowling RW: A treatment-based classification approach to lower back syndrome: identifying and staging patients for conservative treatment, Phys Ther 75:470-489, 1995.
6. Zohn DA, Mennell JM: Diagnosis and physical treatment, musculoskeletal pain, Boston, 1976, Little, Brown, pp 20, 36, 49.
7. Maitland GD, Hengeveld E, Banks K, et al, editors: Maitland's vertebral manipulation, ed 6, Oxford, 2001, Butterworth-Heinemann, pp 41-43.
8. Boissonnault W, DiFabio R: Pain profile of patients with low back pain referred to physical therapy, J Orthop Sports Phys Ther 24:180-191, 1996.
9. Raj PP: Prognostic and therapeutic local anesthetic block. In Cousins MJ, Bridenbaugh PO, editors: Neural blockade in clinical anesthesia and management of pain, ed 2, Philadelphia, 1988, JB Lippincott, p 908.
10. Bigos S, Bow yer O, Braen G, et al: Acute lower back problems in adults: clinical practice guideline no 14. AHCPR publication no 95-0642, Agency for Health Care Policy and Research, Public Health Service, US Department of Health and Human Services, Rockville, Md, December, 1994.
11. Schofferman L, Schofferman J, Zucheman J, et al: Occult infection causing persistent low back pain, Spine 14:417-419, 1989.

12. Vanharanta H, Sachs BI, Spivey M, et al: A comparison of CT/discography, pain response and radiographic disc height, Spine 13:321-324, 1988.

13. Weinstein JN, McLain RF: Primary tumors of the spine, Spine 12:843-851, 1987.

14. Acheson RM, Chan YK, Payne M: New Haven survey of joint diseases: the interrelationships between morning stiffness, nocturnal pain and swelling of the joints, J Chron Dis 21:533-542, 1969.

15. Farrell JP, Twomey LT: Acute low back pain: comparison of two conservative approaches, Med J Aust 1:160-164, 1982.

16. Foldes K, Balint P, Gaal M, et al: Nocturnal pain correlates with effusions in diseased hips, J Rheumatol 19:1756-1758, 1992.

17. Jayson MI, Sims-Williams H, Young S, et al: Mobilization and manipulation for low back pain, Spine 6:409-416, 1981.

18. Jonsson B, Stromquist B: Symptoms and signs in degeneration of the lumbar spine: a prospective, consecutive study of 300 operated patients, J Bone Joint Surg 75B:381-385, 1993.

19. Siegmeth W, Noyelle RM: Night pain and morning stiffness in osteoarthritis: a crossover study of flurbiprofen and diclofenac sodium, J Intern Med Res 16:182-188, 1988.

20. Deyo RA, Rainville J, Kent DL: What can the history and physical examination tell us about lower back pain? JAMA 268:760-765, 1992.

21. Deyo RA, Diehl AK: Cancer as a cause of back pain: frequency, clinical presentation, and diagnostic strategies, J Gen Intern Med 3:230-238, 1988.

22. Waldvogel FA, Vasey H: Osteomyelitis: the past decade, N Engl J Med 14:360-370, 1980.

23. Jemal A, Murray T, Samuels A, et al: Cancer statistics, 2003, CA Cancer J Clin 53:5-26, 2003.

24. Suadicani P, Hein HO, Gyntelberg F: Height, weight, and risk of colorectal cancer, an 18-year follow-up in a cohort of 5249 men, Scand J Gastroenterol 28:285-288, 1993.

25. Tronzo RG: Femoral neck fractures. In Steinburg ME, editor: The hip and its disorders, Philadelphia, 1991, Saunders, pp 247-279.

26. Stulberg BN, Bauer TW, Belhobek GH, et al: A diagnostic algorithm for osteonecrosis of the femoral head, Clin Orthop 249:176-182, 1989.

27. Wenger DR, Ward WT, Herring JA: Current concepts review: Legg-Calve-Perthes disease, J Bone Joint Surg 73:778-788, 1991.

28. DeRosa GP. The child. In D'Ambrosia RD, editor: Musculoskeletal disorders: regional examination and differential diagnosis, ed 2, Philadelphia, 1986, JB Lippincott, pp 595-598.

29. Busch MT, Morrissey RT: Slipped capital femoral epiphysis, Orthop Clin North Am 18:637-647, 1987.

30. Boyko EJ, Ahroni JH, Davignon D, et al: Diagnostic utility of the history and physical examination for peripheral vascular disease among patients with diabetes mellitus, J Clin Epidemiol 50:659-668, 1997.

31. McGee SR, Boyko EJ: Physical examination and chronic lower-extremity ischemia: a critical review, Arch Intern Med 158:1357-1364, 1998.

32. Wiener SL: Differential diagnosis of acute pain by body region, New York, 1993, McGraw-Hill, pp 532, 542, 616, 645, 678, 680.

33. Canto JG, Shlipak MG, Rogers WJ, et al: Prevalence, clinical characteristics, and mortality among patients with myocardial infarction presenting without chest pain, JAMA 283:3223-3229, 2000.

34. Henderson JM: Ruling out danger: differential diagnosis of thoracic spine, Phys Sports Med 20:124-131, 1992.

35. Doran FSA: The sites to which pain is referred from the common bile duct in man and its implication for the theory of referred pain, Br J Surg 54:599-606, 1967.

36. Liu, K, Atten M: Coping with kidney stones, Am Surg 63:519-525, 1997.

37. Wells K: Nephrolithiasis with unusual initial symptoms, J Manipulative Physiol Ther 23:196-205, 2000.

38. Saklayen M: Medical management of nephrolithiasis, Med Clin North Am 81:785-799, 1997.

39. Meadows JTS: Orthopedic differential diagnosis in physical therapy, New York, 1999, McGraw-Hill.

40. Kopell H, Thompson W: Peripheral entrapment neuropathies, Malabar, Fla, 1976, Robert I Krieger Publishing, pp 146-153,156,167.

41. Lorei M, Hershman E: Peripheral nerve injuries in athletes, Sports Med 16:130-147, 1993.

42. Spengler D, Kirsh M, Kaufer H: Orthopaedic aspects and early diagnosis of superior sulcus lung tumor, J Bone Joint Surg 55:1645-1650, 1973.

43. Bruce M, Rosenstein N, Capparella J, et al: Risk factors for meningococcal disease in college students, JAMA 286:688-693, 2001.

44. Snyder H, Robinson K, Shah D, et al: Signs and symptoms of patients with brain tumors presenting in the emergency department, J Emerg Med 11:253-258, 1993.

45. Isaacs ER, Bookhout MR: Screening for pathologic origins of head and facial pain. In Boissonnault WG, editor: Examination in physical therapy practice: screening for medical disease, ed 2, New York, 1995, Churchill Livingstone, pp 181-182.

46. Magee DJ: Orthopedic clinical assessment, Philadelphia, 1997, Saunders, p 38.

47. Klein M, Chang J: Management of hand and upper-extremity infections in heart transplant recipients, Plast Reconstr Surg 106:598-601, 2000.

48. Van de Vusse AC, Stomp-van den Berg SGM, de Vet HWC, et al: Interobserver reliability of diagnosis in patients with complex regional pain syndrom, Eur J Pain 7:259-265, 2003.

C H A P T E R

6

Bruce Greenfield

Upper Quarter Evaluation
Structural Relationships and Interdependence

As physical therapists, we are concerned about the process of disablement, or the consequences of disease on the musculoskeletal system that can lead to impairments in body function and structure.[1] Impairments in body function and structure often result in secondary joint and soft tissue injuries.[2] The main areas of impairment affecting the upper quarter of the body—the cervical spine, the shoulder complex, the thoracic outlet, and the craniomandibular complex—may be involved simultaneously, especially in chronic conditions, often resulting in numerous and overlapping signs and symptoms. As a result, referred symptoms of pain due to musculoskeletal injury are a common problem facing many clinicians. Consequently, physical therapists should be trained to rule out secondary and tertiary impairments as sources of pain and dysfunction in the musculoskeletal system as part of their routine clinical evaluation.

The discussion in this chapter of the interrelationships of structure and function in the upper quarter is designed to help clinicians screen and identify multiple impairments in the upper quarter of the body that may be contributing to their patients' signs and symptoms. One purpose of this chapter is to review the structural interrelationships in the upper quarter of the body, with a focus on posture and postural impairment as a sequel of movement impairment and tissue injury. Elements of an upper quarter screening evaluation are reviewed as a systematic method of evaluating all structures that could contribute to or be the sole cause of the patient's chief complaint. A case study illustrates the use of the upper quarter screening evaluation in a patient who presents with shoulder pain.

STRUCTURAL INTERRELATIONSHIPS IN THE UPPER QUARTER

The upper quarter includes the occiput, the cervical and upper thoracic spine, the shoulder girdle, the upper extremities, asso-

ciated soft tissues, and related nerves and blood vessels.[3] The relationships among these structures are such that changes in the position and function of one structure may influence the position and function of another. Additionally, many of these structures that share similar spinal innervations have overlapping patterns of referred pain. A cursory review of functional anatomy will help to clarify these relationships.

Functional Anatomy

The shoulder girdle, which consists of the clavicle, humerus, and scapula, is largely suspended by muscles to allow mobility.[3,4] The clavicle provides the only direct connection of the shoulder girdle to the axial skeleton. The clavicle articulates at its medial and more movable end with the sternum, and at its lateral end, through a slightly movable sliding joint, with the scapula.

The clavicle is important as a brace that keeps the shoulder joint positioned far enough laterally to allow movement of the humerus. Limited excursion of the upper extremity at the glenohumeral joint under normal circumstances is dependent on movements of the scapula. Forward, upward, and downward movements of the humerus typically are accompanied by a turning of the glenoid cavity in the corresponding direction. The mobility of the scapula, in turn, depends in part on the mobility of its one bony brace, the clavicle.

The occiput, mandible, cervical spine, and shoulder girdle are joined by numerous soft tissue and muscular attachments. Superficial and deep fibers of the cervical fascia join the superior nuchal line of the occipital bone, the mastoid process, and the base of the mandible above to the acromion, clavicle, and manubrium sterni below. Muscles that in part are responsible for scapular movement, namely, the upper fibers of the trapezius and the levator scapulae, connect the occiput and the cervical spine to the superior lateral and superior medial borders of the scapula, respectively. Anteriorly, the sternocleidomastoid muscle attaches from the mastoid process of the cranium to the sternum and clavicle.[4]

The deep muscles in the cervical and thoracic spine can be divided anatomically and functionally into a longer and a shorter group. Muscles of the longer group, which includes the iliocostalis, longissimus, and spinalis muscles, originate and insert across several segments. These muscles function as prime movers for spinal extension and counteract the forces of gravity in the spinal column during upright posture.

The shorter group, which includes the multifidus, rotatores, interspinales, and intertransversarii, arise from and insert more closely into the intervertebral joints. These muscles function during spinal movement by stabilizing and steadying bony segments. According to Basmajian,[5] during movement and standing, the shorter or intrinsic muscles in the back act as dynamic ligaments by adjusting small movements between individual vertebrae. Conversely, movements of the vertebral column are performed by the larger muscles with better leverage and with a mechanical advantage.

The deep suboccipital muscles connecting the axis, atlas, and occipital bones are the rectus capitis posterior minor and major and the obliquus capitis superior and inferior. These muscles have a high innervation ratio, with approximately three to five fibers innervated by one neuron. These muscles, therefore, rapidly alternate tension within milliseconds, allowing for subtle postural adjustments in the head and neck during standing.[6] Joint stiffness or degenerative joint disease that alters suboccipital joint mobility influences suboccipital muscle function. Impairments in muscle structure and performance commonly accompany degenerative joint disease. Jowett and Fiddler[7] demonstrated, in the presence of degenerative spinal disease, histochemical changes in the multifidus muscle, resulting in an increase in slow twitch muscle fibers. They concluded that the multifidus, in the presence of spinal segmental instabilities and joint disease, functions less as a dynamic spinal stabilizer than as a postural muscle. One may speculate that degeneration in the craniovertebral joints may alter the phasic or fast twitch capabilities of the suboccipital muscles toward a more postural mode. The result may be a loss of the quick muscle reaction necessary for normal upper quarter equilibrium and control.

An important area of soft tissue connections is that between the cranium, mandible, hyoid bone, cervical spine, and shoulder girdle. The cranium and the mandible are joined by the temporalis and masseter muscles. The mandible is joined to the hyoid bone by the suprahyoid muscles, including the digastric, stylohyoid, mylohyoid, and geniohyoid. The infrahyoid muscles connect the hyoid bone to the shoulder girdle and indirectly, through soft tissue connections, to the cervical spine. These muscles include the sternohyoid, sternothyroid, thyrohyoid, and omohyoid. Specifically, the hyoid bone is joined to the scapula by the omohyoid muscle and to the sternum and clavicle by the sternohyoid muscle.

Using a model and substituting pieces of elastic for muscles, Brodie demonstrated how tension in one group of muscles may result in tension in another group.[8] The mandible, during normal standing posture, remains balanced with the cranium through tensile forces produced by normal function of the suprahyoid and infrahyoid muscles.[9] The activity of these muscles is related to those of the neck and trunk, as well as to the direction of the gravitational forces acting on the system. Changes in head position in a relaxed subject will alter the position of the mandible at rest. When the head is inclined backward, the mandible moves away from the maxilla into a retruded position.[10] The influence of the cervical spine on the position and function of the mandible is well documented.[11-14] Further discussion of this relationship is presented later in this chapter and in Chapter 7.

Like all synovial joints, the cervical facet joint capsule contains mechanoreceptors. Afferent impulses for the static and dynamic regulation of body posture arise from receptor systems in the connective tissue structures and muscles around these joints. Muscle tone is regulated by these and other afferent impulses in the joint capsules, the synovial membrane, the ligaments, and the tendons. Activation of these specialized receptors and pain receptors in the presence of impairment or injury to musculoskeletal tissues may alter motor activity in the neck and limb musculature. Subsequent changes in muscle tone about the head, neck, and shoulder girdle result in distortions in posture, movement patterns, and joint mobility.

Summary

The upper quarter functions as a mechanical unit that is interconnected by numerous soft tissue links. These links, or articulations, are functionally and reflexly interdependent on one another. The simple act of picking up a pencil involves movement at the head, neck, shoulder, elbow, hand, and fingers. Performance of a precision task requires adequate freedom of motion in various joints (arthrokinematics), proper muscle control and length, and proper neurophysiologic responses. The relative alignment of body segments influences motor function. Alignment of body segments is a function of postural control. Normal posture is the state of muscular and skeletal balance that protects supporting structures of the body against injury and deformity and occurs in the presence of normal joint and soft tissue mobility.[15] Postural alignment provides the muscular and skeletal base of support during movement to influence normal neuromuscular control. Maintaining good alignment in the upper quarter, therefore, is necessary for normal function. Good alignment allows for normal joint integrity and muscle balance and promotes normal arthrokinematic movements. Long-term changes in normal postural alignment resulting in muscle imbalance and compromising joint arthrokinematics may result in motor impairments and tissue pathology.

POSTURE

In referring to posture, an important distinction should be made between dynamic and static posture. Although all posture to some degree is dynamic, for our purposes *dynamic posture* refers to positional changes that occur during function, and *static posture* is the position of a subject while relaxed, standing, sitting, or lying down.

Relaxed, standing posture is defined by Kendall and her colleagues[15] in terms of the relationships of the parts of the body to the line and center of gravity. For example, in the sagittal plane, the ideal erect posture is one in which the line of gravity corresponds with the following points: (1) midpoint of the mastoid process, (2) a point just in front of the shoulder joints, (3) the greater trochanter (or a point just behind it), (4) a point just in front of the center of the knee joint, and (5) a point just in front of the ankle joint (Figure 6-1). Conversely, in the frontal plane, the ideal erect posture is one in which the line of gravity bisects the skull, midway between the scapulae, in line with the spine, in line with the gluteal fold, and midway between the lower extremities and feet. The right and left halves of the skeletal structures are essentially symmetrical. In the upper quarter of the body, the scapulae should be positioned symmetrically approximately 3 inches from the mid spinal line situated between the spinal levels of T2 and T8. Keep in mind that ideal posture does not mean normal posture; very few of us actually exhibit ideal postural alignment but get along quite well within a range of ideal.

The scapulae sit in the plane of the scapula (scaption) approximately 30 degrees anterior to the frontal plane. In this position, the glenoid fossae face anterior lateral and superior. Changes in scapular positions and alignment have been closely associated with muscle imbalances and movement impairments that result in shoulder impingement problems.[16,17]

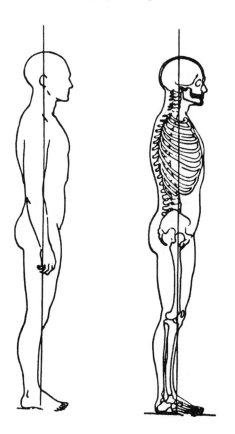

Figure 6-1 Erect posture relative to the line of gravity. (From Bamajian JU: Muscles alive, ed 4, Baltimore, 1979, Williams & Wilkins.)

Maintenance of normal posture is influenced by the forces of weight bearing (e.g., leg length difference, uneven terrain) and by several physiologic processes, including respiration, deglutition, sight, vestibular balance, and hearing. Solow and Tallgren[18] found, during cephalometric postural recording, that subjects looking straight into a mirror held their head and neck approximately 3 degrees higher than did subjects who used their own feeling of natural head balance. Vig et al[19] demonstrated that experimental nasal obstruction in humans resulted in progressive extension of the head, and that removal of this obstruction led to a return to the normal baseline head position. Cleall et al[20] showed that a consistent pattern of head extension and flexion during normal swallowing is altered in subjects with a grade II malocclusion and tongue thrust.

Relaxed, standing posture, therefore, is dynamic, requiring constant neurophysiologic and accommodative adjustments. These normal adjustments maintain a balance of equal weight in front of and behind the central gravity line. In more accurate, mechanical terms, the moment of the forces anterior to the central gravity line must equal the moment of the forces posterior to that line.[21] Therefore, if more weight of a body part is displaced forward of the central gravity line, an equal shift of another body part backward must occur. Thus, if the pelvis shifts anteriorly, lumbar lordosis and thoracic kyphosis are increased. The cervical spine shifts forward, resulting in decreased midcervical lordosis. Backward bending occurs in the occipitoatlantal joint, leaving one in a position to look straight ahead.

Similarly, body weight in the frontal plane must be divided equally between the two legs, and in normal posture, equal weight is supported by each foot. A considerable margin of lateral shift of the central gravity line is possible, however, because each leg can support all of the body's weight at any time. A lateral shift, in the presence of uneven terrain or a leg length difference, of parts of the body away from the central gravity line results in compensatory shifts somewhere else. For example, if one side of the pelvis drops, a lateral curve is created in the lumbar spine to the opposite side, along with a compensating convexity toward the same side higher up in the spine. These accommodative shifts maintain the upper quarter within the central gravity line, allowing for normal balance and function.

Neurophysiology and Normal Posture

Vestibular sensation results in part from the orientation of the semicircular canals in the head. The head is held so that the horizontal semicircular canals are actually in a horizontal plane. Proprioceptive impulses from nerve endings in ligaments, joint capsules, tendons, and muscles form a very large part of the input pattern and are related most closely to postural tone. Muscle spindles are the specialized receptors involved in tendon reflexes. Postural or antigravity muscles are richly supplied with muscle spindles. When muscles are lengthened—for example, the posterior cervical muscles when the central gravity line in the cervical spine shifts forward—the parallel muscle spindles also are lengthened. This lengthening stimulates the muscle spindles to send afferent impulses to the homonymous alpha motor neurons, which carry excitatory impulses to related muscles. Afferent impulses also may send inhibitory impulses through interneurons to alpha motor neurons of antagonistic muscles, causing reflex inhibition of the anterior cervical or prevertebral muscles. Other afferent fibers from the muscle spindles carry impulse patterns of approximate muscle length to the central nervous system, where these patterns are integrated in higher centers with patterns of changing tension and position that have originated in other proprioceptors.[22]

Summary

Posture during weight bearing consists of subtle accommodative movements to maintain body segments along the central gravity line. Normal posture, therefore, depends on a variety of factors, including normal joint arthrokinematics, muscle balance, and normal neurophysiologic responses. Muscular contractions, required to maintain normal balance, are controlled and coordinated by the nervous system. Changes in joint range of motion (ROM) or muscle function may interfere with the normal accommodative responses necessary to maintain normal posture. Poor accommodative responses may result, in turn, in long-term postural deviations, pain, muscle imbalances, and pathologic conditions.

INTERDEPENDENCE OF FUNCTION AND STRUCTURE DURING NORMAL POSTURE

An excellent example of the interdependence of function and structure in the upper quarter is illustrated during shoulder elevation.

Shoulder elevation, or elevation of the humerus, is commonly described with reference to several different body planes: the coronal or frontal plane, the sagittal plane, and the plane of the scapula. The plane of the scapula is approximately 30 to 45 degrees anterior to the frontal plane. Movement of the humerus in this plane allows the muscles surrounding the glenohumeral joint to function in an optimal length-tension relationship.

Elevation of the humerus in the plane of the scapula depends on smooth, synchronous motion involving every component of the shoulder girdle complex. Normal scapulohumeral rhythm requires full ROM at each joint and well-coordinated muscle balance. The ratio of humeral to scapular motion is a matter of controversy, but many authors agree that the humerus and scapula move in rhythm, so that for every 15 degrees of elevation of the arm, 10 degrees is provided by elevation at the glenohumeral joint and a corresponding 5 degrees by rotation of the scapula. Thus full overhead elevation of the arm (180 degrees) requires 60 degrees of scapular rotation and 120 degrees of glenohumeral elevation.

Movement of the scapula is accompanied by movement of the acromioclavicular (AC) and sternoclavicular (SC) joints. Movement of the SC joint is most evident from 0 to 90 degrees of elevation, and that of the AC joint primarily before 30 degrees and beyond 135 degrees. Half of the scapular rotation (30 degrees) is reached by clavicular elevation. The remaining 30 degrees occurs by rotation of the crank-shaped clavicle as it exerts pull on the coracoid process through the coracoclavicular ligaments.

Elevation of the humerus results from a series of muscular force couples acting at the glenohumeral and scapulothoracic joints. A force couple is formed when two parallel forces of equal magnitude but opposite direction act on a structure, producing rotation.[23]

Rotation at the glenohumeral joint is produced by the upward pull of the deltoid and by the combined inward and downward pull of the rotator cuff muscles. Similarly, scapular rotation results from the upward pull of the upper fibers of the trapezius and the downward pull of the lower fibers of the trapezius. The serratus anterior also helps to rotate and glide the scapula along the thoracic wall.

Elevation of the upper extremities results in motion in the cervical and upper thoracic spine, as well as in the atlantoaxial joint. Unilateral elevation of an upper extremity in the plane of the scapula results in rotation of the midcervical spine to the ipsilateral side.[24] Pure rotation does not occur within the midcervical spine but is accompanied by side flexion to the ipsilateral side. Contralateral side flexion with ipsilateral rotation occurs at the occipitoatlantal joint and upper thoracic spine to enable the head to remain in the sagittal plane. This counterrotation occurs only in the axially extended or neutral position. In the presence of a forward head posture, these compensatory motions are lost and excessive forces are placed on the midcervical spine.

Overhead work requiring bilateral elevation of the upper extremities results in extension of the head and thorax. This "habitual extension" induces flexion of the upper thoracic spine, extension of the midcervical spine, and extension of the atlanto-occipital joint, thus restoring the weight of the skull in the line of gravity.[24] Specifically, during midcervical extension, the superior articular facets slide posteriorly and inferiorly on the inferior facets, as well as tilting posteriorly, thus increasing the anterior interspace of the facet joint. The posterior tilting of the related spinal segment is restrained by the intervertebral disc and its associated longitudinal ligaments, and by the osseous impact of the posterior neural arches, as well as the capsule of the facet joints.

Forces generated during limb, trunk, and neck movements are also responsible for the repeated piston-like movement of the nerve complex within the intervertebral foramen of the cervical and upper thoracic spine. Overstretching of the nerve roots, according to Sunderland,[25] is prevented by the nerves' elastic properties, as well as by their attachment by fibrous slips to gutters in the corresponding transverse processes. Overstretching or friction on the nerve roots often occurs in the presence of postural deviations, such as forward head posture.

Postural Impairments and Tissue Changes

A musculoskeletal impairment produces a chain of reflexes that involve the whole motor system. The reflex changes and impairment not only may result in clinical manifestations of pain arising from impaired function but also may influence the results of the whole process of motor reeducation.

Changes in muscle function play an important role in the pathogenesis of many painful conditions of the motor system and are an integral part of postural defects. One theory holds that certain muscles usually respond to dysfunction by tightening or shortening, whereas others react by inhibition, atrophy, and weakness.[26] Muscles that have become tight tend to pull the body segments to which they attach, causing deviations in alignment. The antagonistic muscles may become weak, allowing deviation of body parts through their lack of support. These muscle responses follow typical patterns and have been described by Janda.[26]

Investigators have demonstrated that muscles are sensitive to long-term changes in length.[27,28] Sahrmann[2] observed that in the presence of long-term postural impairments, certain muscles are maintained in a chronically shortened position, and other muscles are maintained in a chronically lengthened position. For example, individuals with rounded shoulders often have excessively abducted scapular positions (greater than 3 inches from the mid spine). In this situation, the middle trapezius and rhomboid muscles are chronically lengthened, while the serratus anterior muscle is chronically shortened. Williams and Goldspink[27] demonstrated that muscles that are chronically shortened or lengthened lose and gain sarcomeres in series, respectively. The result is the length-tension curve of muscle changes; the shortened muscle length-tension curve shifts to the left (it is able to generate maximum tension in its shortened position). Conversely, the lengthened muscle length-tension curve shifts to the right (it is able to generate maximum tension in its lengthened position)[29] (Figure 6-2).

The structures of connective tissue, bone, and muscle also adapt to alterations in function.[23] Known as *Wolff's law*, when

stresses are applied to a bone, the trabeculae within that bone develop and align themselves to adapt to these lines of stress. Pressure within the physiologic limits of force exerted by the musculature stimulates or enhances osteogenesis. Excessive pressure causes necrosis with delayed osteogenesis. Pressure exerted perpendicular to the axis of a long bone is more likely to cause resorption of bone, whereas pressure acting in the line of the bone axis is more likely to cause osteogenesis. Therefore, postural deviations that cause malalignment and asymmetrical stresses on bone and cartilage can result in reabsorption and degeneration.[30]

Continued asymmetrical stresses on soft tissues can result in degeneration. Salter and Field[31] found in animal models that continuous compression of opposing joint surfaces causes pressure necrosis of articular cartilage. The connective tissue response to immobility is well documented.[32,33] Changes in the joint capsule include loss of glycosaminoglycan and water, random deposition of newly synthesized collagen with abnormal cross-linking, and infiltration of joints by fibrofatty material. Results include increased joint stiffness (resistance to passive stretch) and altered arthrokinematics. Similar changes may occur in joint capsules shortened as a result of long-term postural deviations.

Postural Impairment and Shoulder Dysfunction

Guide to Physical Therapist Practice,[34] published by the American Physical Therapy Association (APTA), describes preferred practice patterns containing generally accepted elements of patient management that physical therapists provide for patient diagnostic groups. Diagnostic groups are classified by clustering primary impairments together with a patient's functional loss. *Guide to Physical Therapist Practice* identifies 11 diagnostic groups for musculoskeletal rehabilitation. Included among these diagnostic groups is impaired posture. Impaired posture includes appendicular postural deficits, cumulative effects of poor habitual posture in addition to poor work-related posture, pregnancy-related postural changes, and scoliosis or other excessive spinal curvatures. Patients with functional limitations related to impaired posture present with associated muscle weakness or imbalance, associated pain, structural or functional deviation from normal posture, and suboptimal join mobility. The forward head posture typifies a postural impairment reflective of muscle imbalance that may result in pain and suboptimal mobility.[35-37] For example, the relationship between forward head posture and pain was examined in 88 otherwise healthy subjects by Griegel-Morris et al.[37] Subjects with increased thoracic kyphoses and rounded shoulders had an increased incidence of interscapular pain, and those with a forward head posture had an increased incidence of cervical interscapular and headache pain. Forward head posture is characterized by protracted and medially rotated scapulae, internal rotation at the glenohumeral joints, increased kyphoses of the upper thoracic spine, increased cervical spine lordosis, and craniomandibular backward bending. A second variation of forward head posture is characterized by reversal of the cervical

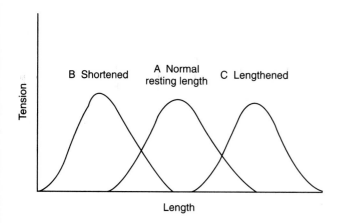

Figure 6-2 Effect of muscle length-tension capabilities. **A,** Normal resting muscle length. **B,** Shift of the length-tension curve to the left in a muscle that has shortened as the result of loss of sarcomeres. **C,** Shift of the length-tension curve to the right in a muscle that has lengthened because of a gain in sarcomeres.

lordoses, or flattening out of the midcervical spine, without craniomandibular backward bending. This type of forward head posture occurs commonly after a cervical injury.

The muscles and other soft tissues of the upper quarter change in response to changes in forward head posture. Excessive compression of the facet joints and posterior surfaces of the vertebral bodies occurs, as well as excessive lengthening, with associated weakness of the anterior vertebral neck flexors and tightness of the neck extensors. Additional changes include shortening of the suboccipital and suprahyoid musculature and lengthening of the infrahyoid muscles with elevation of the hyoid bone. Increased tension in the suprahyoid muscles pulls the mandible posteriorly and inferiorly, increasing the distance between the maxilla and the mandible. The temporalis, masseter, and medial pterygoid muscles must contract against the shortened antagonistic muscles to close the jaw. Excessive tension in the muscles of mastication can result in myofascial strain and painful trigger points.[35,38] Stomatognathic problems are discussed further in Chapter 7.

Elevation of the hyoid bone increases tension on the omohyoid muscle and its attachment to the upper portion of the scapula. With the head moving anteriorly and the posterior aspect of the occiput moving posteriorly and inferiorly, shortening of the upper trapezius muscle and of the levator scapulae occurs. Shortening of these muscles results in scapular elevation.[11]

The increased thoracic kyphosis tends to abduct or protract the scapulae and lengthen the rhomboid middle and lower trapezius muscles while shortening the serratus anterior, latissimus dorsi, subscapularis, and teres major muscles. Also, the increased scapular abduction shortens the pectoralis major and minor muscles, which, by their attachment to the coracoid process of the scapula, tend to pull the scapula over the head of the humerus. The humerus rotates internally, shortening the glenohumeral ligaments and the anterior shoulder capsule.[39]

Muscle tone changes in response to afferent impulses from the joint capsule, resulting in inhibition or facilitation of selected muscles. Several muscle imbalances result because a tight muscle inhibits its antagonist.[26] Weakness of the lower trapezius muscle may result from shortening of the upper trapezius and levator scapulae muscles, whereas inhibition of the rhomboid muscles may occur in response to shortening of the teres major muscle. Increased glenohumeral internal rotation shortens the glenohumeral medial rotators, with lengthening and inhibition of the lateral rotators. These changes in normal muscle length may result in alteration of the normal scapulohumeral rhythm.

Weakness of the supraspinatus, infraspinatus, and teres minor alters the force couple at the glenohumeral joint during elevation of the humerus. The function of these muscles in maintaining the humeral head at the glenoid fossa and resisting the upward pull of the deltoid is lost. The repetitive upward pull of the deltoid during glenohumeral elevation results in abutment of the humeral head and associated soft tissues against an unyielding coracoacromial ligament. Impingement of the rotator cuff tendons may result in inflammation, with subsequent pain and loss of function.[16]

Reduction in the normal amount of scapular rotation during elevation of the humerus results from muscle imbalance at the scapulohumeral articulation.[2] Increased strain is placed on the rotator cuff muscles to elevate the arm overhead. The result may be inflammation of the rotator cuff tendons. Investigators have observed that inadequate scapular outward rotation and posterior tipping during overhead elevation is strongly associated with shoulder impingement. Overactivity of the rotator cuff muscles to compensate for reduced scapular rotation results in painful trigger points.

Abnormal Posture and the Cervical Spine

Forward head posture produces compensatory motions in the cervical and upper thoracic spine, as well as in the atlantoaxial joint. Unilateral elevation of an upper extremity, as mentioned previously, results in rotation with ipsilateral side bending in the midcervical spine.[24] Compensatory, contralateral side flexion with ipsilateral rotation occurs in the upper thoracic spine and in the occipitoatlantal joint to maintain the head and neck in the central gravity line. However, these compensatory motions occur only in the axially extended or neutral position. The forward head posture results in increased flexion in the upper thoracic spine and extension in the upper cervical spine. Compensatory motions, therefore, are lost, and excessive forces are placed on the midcervical spine during unilateral elevation of the upper extremity. Traumatic changes in the intervertebral disc and neural arches may result in transverse intradiscal tears, most commonly seen at the C5-C6 and C6-C7 segments. Degeneration of the intervertebral disc leads to reabsorption and approximation of related segments.[30] Osteophytic spurs may develop in the uncovertebral joints and in the posterior facet joints. The result during repetitive extension and rotation of the degenerated midcervical spine is friction of the nerve roots by osseofibrous irregularities in the intervertebral foramen or traction on nerve roots fixed in the gutters of related transverse processes.[24,25]

Pressure or traction on a nerve can result in mechanical irritation of that nerve, producing pain and dysfunction.[28] The initial response of a nerve to mechanical irritation, according to Sunderland,[25] is an increase in intrafunicular pressure in the nerve, obstructing venous drainage and slowing capillary drainage. Capillary circulation slows and intrafunicular pressure rises. The incarcerated nerve fibers are compressed, and their nutrition is impaired by hypoxia to the point where they become hyperexcitable and begin to discharge spontaneously. Spontaneous firing of selective large, myelinated fibers occurs, resulting in hyperesthesia in the related dermatome. A steady increase in intrafunicular pressure can result in spontaneous firing of gamma-efferents fibers, leading to hypertonicity of segmentally related muscles.

Chronic anoxia damages the capillary endothelium, with leakage of protein through the capillary walls, fibroplasia, and intraneural scarring.[25] In patients with a long history of recurrent sciatica, Lindahl and Rexed[40] observed histologic changes at the L5 and S1 nerve roots, including hyperplasia of the perineurium with infiltration of lymphocytes and degeneration of nerve fibers. Resultant demyelination of selected nerve fibers may increase the sensitivity of segmentally related structures. According to Gunn,[41] deep muscle tenderness may be caused by denervation sensitivity of nociceptors at the neurovascular hilus. Long-term denervation can result in decreased total collagen in segmentally related soft tissues and muscles. Muscle atrophy occurs, with progressive destruction of the fiber's contractile element, resulting in decreased fiber diameter and decreased speed of muscle contraction. Changes in collagen content and degenerated muscle fibers can increase the susceptibility of related tissues to microtears or macrotears, resulting in inflammation and dysfunction. Lee[24] has suggested denervation of the C6 nerve root in the cervical spine as a possible extrinsic cause of lateral epicondylitis. Examination of a musculoskeletal lesion therefore should include local contractile and noncontractile tissues, as well as the integrity of the related spinal and/or peripheral nerve.

ABNORMAL POSTURE AND ENTRAPMENT NEUROPATHIES

Thoracic Outlet

Compression of the nerves of the brachial plexus and of the great vessels in the region of the thoracic outlet may occur in a variety of ways, some caused in part by poor posture.[42]

The clavicle holds the shoulder up, out, and back, thus producing a short, broad outlet canal. The angle between the anterior and middle scaleni muscles is broad enough to allow passage of the nerve roots of the brachial plexus. The loss of muscle tone and drooping shoulders seen in persons with forward head posture can result in depression of the anterior chest wall. The depression of the sternum pulls the anterior thoracic cage down. This, in turn, pulls the shoulder girdle down, forward and closer to the chest wall. As a result, the angle between the scaleni muscles is decreased, and the outer

end of the clavicle and the shoulder girdle are pulled closer to the lateral chest wall, as well as down and forward. These changes decrease the width and increase the length of the outlet canal, which makes the nerve trunks of the brachial plexus and the subclavian artery more vulnerable to compression or kinking as they pass through the scaleni triangle[43] (Figure 6-3). Thoracic outlet problems are discussed further in Chapter 8.

Dorsal Scapular Nerve

The dorsal scapular nerve arises from the upper trunk of the brachial plexus and pierces the body of the scalene medius muscle. The scaleni muscles are prime movers of the cervical spine. When the myoligamentous system (i.e., the stabilization mechanism for vertebral function) is inadequate, the prime movers go into compensatory hyperactivity.

Myoligamentous laxity may result from increased tension in the anterior cervical spine with forward head posture. Hyperactivity and hypertrophy of the scalene muscle may result in entrapment of the dorsal scapular nerve. When the dorsal scapular nerve is compressed at the entrapment point in the scalene medius muscle, the slack necessary to compensate for head and arm motion is prevented.[39] A tense nerve moving against taut muscles can set up the initial mechanical irritation in the nerve.[25] The resultant nerve ischemia, as outlined previously, can produce scapular pain, as well as diffuse pain that radiates down the lateral surface of the arm and forearm. Soft tissue changes in response to denervation neuropathy may result along the segmental distribution of the nerve.

Suprascapular Nerve

The suprascapular nerve is derived from the upper trunk of the brachial plexus, which is formed from the roots of C5 and C6. The nerve passes through the suprascapular notch at the upper border of the scapula. The notch is roofed over by the transverse

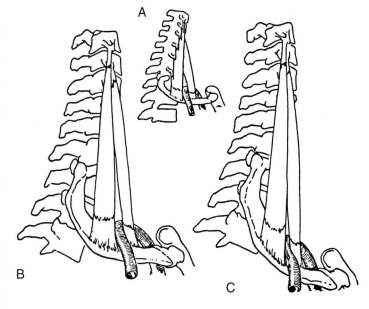

Figure 6-3 Descent of the sternum with maturation and aging. **A,** Position at birth. **B,** Position in an adult man. **C,** Position in an adult woman. (From Overton: The causes of pain in the upper extremities: a differential diagnosis study, Clin Orthop 51:27, 1967.)

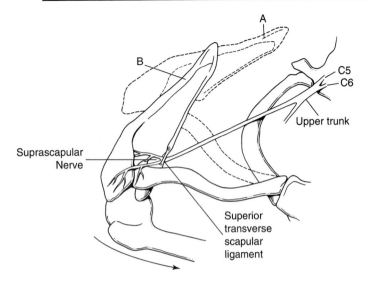

Figure 6-4 The effect of shoulder abduction on the course of the suprascapular nerve. **A,** Position of the scapula when the arm is in the anatomical position. **B,** Position of the scapula when it is abducted across the thoracic wall. (From Thompson WAL, Kopell HP: The effect of shoulder abduction on the course of suprascapular nerve, N Engl J Med 260:1269, 1959.)

scapular ligament. This nerve supplies the supraspinatus muscle, the glenohumeral and acromioclavicular joints, and the infraspinatus muscle.

Forward head posture, resulting in increased scapular abduction and medial rotation, may cause traction in the brachial plexus at the origin of the suprascapular nerve[39] (Figure 6-4). The abducted position increases the total distance from the origin of the nerve to the suprascapular notch, placing tension on the suprascapular nerve.

Changes in normal scapulohumeral rhythm in such conditions as frozen shoulder may result in suprascapular nerve neuropathy. Limited glenohumeral motion in the frozen shoulder forces a greater range of scapular motion for a desired degree of shoulder motion. This abnormal excursion of the scapula may induce a neuropathy at the entrapment point of the suprascapular nerve. Pain may be felt in the lateral and posterior aspects of the shoulder, with secondary radiation down the radial nerve axis to the region of the common extensor group.

Summary

Impairment of upper quarter function may result in, and from, postural deviations. The interdependence of the motor system suggests that a functional disturbance produces a chain of reflexes that may involve the whole upper quarter. Therefore, although upper quarter dysfunctions may appear locally, the subsequent success of treatment may necessitate evaluation of the motor system as a whole.

UPPER QUARTER EVALUATION

Several experts in the practice of musculoskeletal rehabilitation have emphasized the importance of including a musculoskel-

etal screening examination as part of the overall patient evaluation.[44-46] The skillful performance of a screening evaluation has become increasingly important with increasing emphasis on prevention and wellness in contemporary practice physical therapy. Typically, the screening evaluation can occur after the patient history and can help the clinician organize and prioritize the performance of subsequent tests and measures. Proper performance of the elements of an upper quarter screening evaluation offers a systematic method of evaluating all structures that could contribute to or be the sole cause of the patient's chief complaint. Proper interpretation of each test designed to differentiate tissues and structures is based on our knowledge of anatomy, mechanics, and typical causative and pathologic processes.

History

A detailed history will help the clinician to identify potential secondary and tertiary areas of impairment and sites of referred pain. A patient referred to physical therapy with shoulder impingement who reports stiffness and pain in his neck due to osteoarthritis may have referred pain to his shoulder from the cervical spine. Routine questions are asked to determine the onset of the problem, the area and nature of the pain, the behavior of pain (what activities increase or decrease the intensity or alter the type of pain), previous treatment, functional losses, and associated health problems. A patient with a previous history of cervical spondylosis who presents with intermittent numbness and tingling in his upper extremity should be screened for cervical radiculopathy, thoracic outlet syndrome, and signs of neural tension. A patient who presents with chronic temporal and orbital headaches with clicking and pain in his craniomandibular joints should be screened for forward head posture, cervical ROM, and increased tone and active trigger points in the upper trapezius and sternocleidomastoid muscles. Because the different lesions that produce pain and impairment about the shoulder and upper extremities may have their origin in the cervical spine, the thoracic outlet, the craniomandibular area, or the arm itself, the clinician must have knowledge of the patterns of pain referral.

Embryology

Many structures are innervated by nerve fibers from more than one spinal segment. Limb buds in the developing embryo comprise a mass of undifferentiated mesenchymal cells. The anterior primary divisions of the spinal nerves invade the developing limb buds to innervate the muscle masses. Because of the intertwining of segmental nerves throughout the regional plexus, and because the muscle masses tend to divide or fuse with one another, a muscle typically receives innervation from more than one segment, and a segmental nerve tends to innervate more than one muscle.

Overlapping of myotomes, dermatomes, and sclerotomes results from a change in the orientation of developing limb buds from a position in the frontal plane at approximately 90 degrees of abduction, with the palms facing forward, to the fetal position. Growth of the arm bud draws the lower cervical and uppermost thoracic segments out into itself. The scapula and surrounding muscles are derived from the middle and lower cervical segments, whereas the overlying skin and ribs are formed from the thoracic segments. Therefore, pain felt in the upper posterior part of the thorax into the shoulder and upper limb has a cervical or scapular origin, and pain felt in the upper posterior thorax radiating into the upper chest has an upper thoracic origin.

Patterns of Pain Referral

Several authors have investigated the patterns of pain referral. Robinson found that similar patterns of referred pain in the upper extremity area were reproduced by stimulating different structures in the cervical spine. Robinson exposed the anterior portions of the cervical vertebrae and adjacent muscles of patients under local anesthesia. The same referred pain was reproduced by plucking with a needle the anulus fibrosus of more than one intervertebral disc. Similarly, identical pain was reproduced by plucking the edge of the longus colli muscle. Feinstein et al[47] studied patterns of deep somatic pain referral after paravertebral injections of a 6% saline solution from the occiput to the sacrum. Pain distributions were found to approximate a segmental plan, although the pain patterns overlapped considerably and differed in location from conventional dermatomes.

Studies by Kellgren[48] identified specific reproducible patterns of pain activated when selective connective tissues and muscle structures were irritated (Figures 6-5 and 6-6). Inman and Saunders demonstrated that pain resulting from the stimulation of joints and other structures deep to the skin had no superficial component. These authors used needles with or without hypertonic saline to produce pains that commonly arise from the deeper structures. Such a pain, Inman and Saunders[49] concluded, unlike that of a cut in the skin, cannot be localized with any precision. The best distance for radiation, they found, varied proportionately with the intensity of the stimulus.[49] Activation of trigger points in muscles about the shoulder and neck was shown by Simons to refer pain consistently to the hand, wrist, and elbow, and to produce pain at the site of the lesion.[51]

To summarize, pain arising from the muscles, deep ligaments, and joints of the cervical spine and shoulder girdle area tends to be referred segmentally. Because of the similarity of the type and distribution of pain referred to the upper extremities from different structures, the clinician should consider every case with careful attention to all potential pain-producing structures and tissues.

Upper Quarter Screening Examination

The goal of the upper quarter examination is to scan quickly the entire upper quarter to rule out sources of impairment and to note areas that need more specific testing. The entire examination should require approximately 5 to 10 minutes. The physical therapist can sequence the order of the examination in several ways, depending in part on information obtained in the

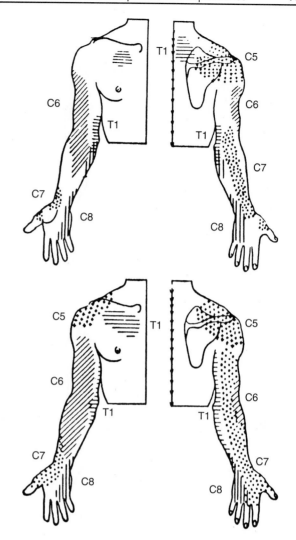

Figure 6-5 Mappings of referred pain from local irritation of the rhomboids (crosses), the flexor carpi radialis (oblique hatching), the abductor pollicis longus (stippling), the third dorsal interosseus (vertical hatching), and the first intercostal space (horizontal hatching). (From Kellgren J: Observations of referred pain arising from muscle, Clin Sci 3:175, 1938.)

history. This author's preference is to perform the most global and least invasive components of the screen first (i.e., posture), then the more invasive and specific tests and measures (palpation/provocation tests).

Postural screen requires observation for postural impairments such as forward head posture or changes in the normal rest position of the scapulae. From behind, the therapist should observe the positions of the scapulae for protraction, retraction, elevation, or winging of the medial border, as well as the relative positions of the cervical spine on the thorax and the cranium on the cervical spine. Deviations from the midsagittal spine (scoliosis, rotation, or tilting of the head and neck) should be recorded.

Laterally, the alignment of the upper quarter segments should be compared with the hypothetical plumb mentioned previously. Increased cervical inclination or increased cervical lordosis with backward bending of the cranium on the cervical

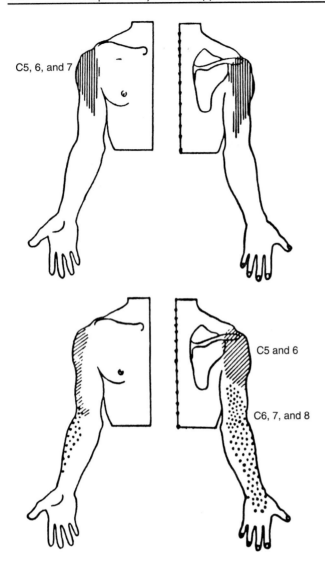

C5, 6, and 7

C5 and 6

C6, 7, and 8

Figure 6-6 Mappings of referred pain from local irritation of the serratus anterior (oblique hatching) and the latissimus dorsi (stippling). (From Kellgren J: Observations of referred pain arising from muscle, Clin Sci 3:175, 1938.)

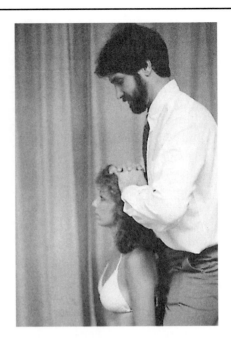

Figure 6-7 Axial compression as part of the screening evaluation.

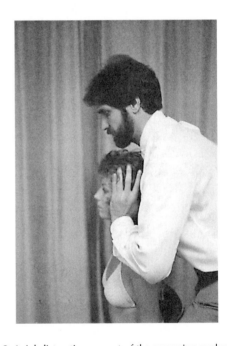

Figure 6-8 Axial distraction as part of the screening evaluation.

spine indicates postural impairment and potential dysfunction. Anteriorly, the position of the cervical spine and cranium relative to the midsagittal plane again should be noted. Positional changes at the shoulder (internal or external rotation, elevation, or depression) together or relative to each other are recorded.

In the next step, the function of the cervical spine is examined with respect to mechanics (degree and quality of motion) and pain (location and severity). After each active motion, overpressure is applied while the pain is located and its severity assessed. Janda[50] has suggested that rotation should be tested in ventroflexion and dorsiflexion, as well as in the vertical position. If the cervical spine is flexed maximally, the segments below C2 and C3 are blocked, and therefore the movement restriction is a sign of impaired mobility of the upper cervical segments. Conversely, during maximum dorsiflexion, the upper segments are blocked. Limited rotation is then a

symptom of impaired mobility of the segments distal to C2 and C3. Cervical spine tests are performed to identify or exclude pathology originating in the cervical region.

Axial compression (Figure 6-7) and axial distraction (Figure 6-8) are applied manually by the clinician to provoke or change the patient's symptoms. Additional cervical tests include the cervical quadrant tests to the left and right. The quadrant test also known as Spurling's test is used to determine the presence of a spinal nerve impingement as it exits the neural foramen.

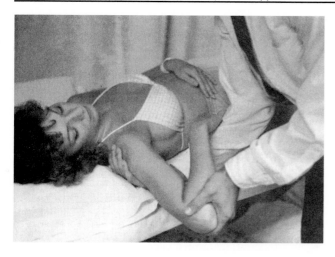

Figure 6-9 Locking maneuver: Internal rotation and abduction of the shoulder.

The patient's cervical spine is moved passively into extension, rotation, and side bending to the left or right (depending on history), to reproduce signs and symptoms of nerve root compression. Although these tests have been widely reported in the orthopaedic literature, their validity and reliability are unknown. The vascular examination, which is described elsewhere in this text, includes Adson's, costoclavicular, and hyperabduction testing to rule out vascular entrapment in the area of the thoracic outlet.

Each peripheral joint is tested for mechanics and pain during overpressure. For example, active shoulder movement with passive overpressure can be performed for shoulder flexion, abduction, hand to opposite shoulder, hand to the back of the neck, and hand behind and up the back. The locking position (Figure 6-9) and the quadrant position can be performed on the shoulder to test for impingement and anterior capsule inflammation and/or laxity, respectively. Reproduction of the patient's symptoms is recorded.

The clinician should quickly screen myotomes for areas of weakness. Examples include resisted shoulder abduction (C5), internal and external rotation, as well as resisted elbow flexion (C6), elbow extension (C7), forearm pronation and supination (C7), finger abduction (C8), and finger adduction (T1). Sensory testing is performed for the C4-T1 dermatomes with the use of light touch or sharp-dull discrimination. Reflex testing includes jaw jerk (cranial nerve V), as well as testing of the biceps (C5, C6), triceps (C7, C8), and brachioradialis (C5, C6).

Palpation should be added to the screening evaluation to differentiate and recognize changes in skin, subcutaneous tissue, ligaments, and muscles. Patterns of pain referral should be recorded. Special attention should be paid to the muscles. Spasm, tenderness, hyperirritability, tightness, or hypotonia should be noted. A characteristic and specific chain of muscle changes and imbalances should be assessed. A proposed sequence of palpation in the head and neck is as follows: trapezius and levator scapulae, followed by the scaleni, sternocleidomastoid, and suprahyoid muscles, followed in turn by the lateral and medial pterygoid, masseter, and temporalis muscles.

The steps required for upper quarter screening evaluation are listed below:

- Posture examination
- Cervical testing
- Active ROM with overpressure
- Cervical distraction/compression/quadrant testing
- Peripheral joint testing
- Active ROM with overpressure to the shoulder, elbow, forearm, and wrist and hand
- Provocation testing: locking/quadrant tests
- Myotomes
- Resisted tests
- Reflex tests
- Dermatomes
- Sensory tests
- Palpation

In conclusion, the screening examination affords the clinician a quick, precise scan of upper quarter structure and function. A specific test that provokes the patient's symptoms alerts the clinician to the potential site of the musculoskeletal lesion; this should be followed by a thorough evaluation of that area.

The following case provides an example of the manner in which an upper quarter screening examination is integrated into an overall clinical evaluation. It is the author's belief that an upper quarter evaluation often yields additional information on the impairments contributing to or perpetating a patient's functional loss, to be included in the overall treatment program.[1]

This case illustrates the use of components of upper quarter screening in a patient with shoulder pain and dysfunction. An initial history is followed by a physical therapy evaluation. Upper quarter screening is incorporated into the physical therapy evaluation. An assessment outlines the physical therapy problem list, impairments or treatment goals, and plan. Actual treatments are beyond the purview of this chapter and are not reviewed. The reader is encouraged to review subsequent chapters in this text that examine specific treatment techniques.

CASE STUDY 6-1

History

The patient is a 36-year-old woman who developed gradual right shoulder pain and stiffness. She is right hand dominant and works as a secretary in a law firm. She reports that her pain started approximately 6 months earlier, after she painted a room in her house. Since that time, her shoulder has become progressively more painful and stiff. Her pain is located along the lateral and anterior aspects of her shoulder and radiates along the right cervical spine and the right interscapular area. She describes her pain as a diffuse dull ache, which becomes sharp during elevation of her right extremity. Her pain and stiffness are worse in the morning and tend to decrease when she begins to move her arm. However, at the end of her workday, she reports that the pain, particularly along the cervical and interscapular areas, is worse. She has difficulty sleeping on that shoulder at night. She is taking anti-inflammatory medicine. Significant past and current medical histories were unremarkable. She enjoys tennis but is unable to play because of her shoulder problem.

Upper Quarter Screening

- Posture: forward head posture with rounded shoulders (protracted and medially rotated scapulae). The right scapula was slightly elevated relative to the left.
- Cervical testing: cervical right rotation slightly limited and painful, with overpressure at the end of the range. However, this test, as well as the cervical compression or distraction test, did not reproduce the patient's pain. As a result of cervical testing, the therapist decided to examine cervical and thoracic passive segmental mobility.
- Passive mobility testing: restricted segmental mobility in the mid and upper thoracic spine and midcervical spine.
- Myotome dermatome and reflex tests: negative.
- Vascular tests (i.e., thoracic outlet tests): negative.
- Shoulder tests: bypassed until later in the evaluation.
- Peripheral joints: ROM and overpressure in related peripheral joints did not reproduce the patient's pain.
- Palpation: elevated tone and muscle trigger points were palpated in the muscle bellies of the right upper trapezius, rhomboids, and subscapularis muscles. Palpation of the trigger point in the upper trapezius muscle reproduced the patient's right cervical pain. Palpation of the trigger point in the rhomboid muscles reproduced the interscapular pain. Palpation of the subscapularis trigger point reproduced most of the anterior and lateral shoulder pain.
- Active/passive ROM in right shoulder: limited in capsular pattern, with external rotation most limited, followed by abduction in the plane of the scapula, followed

by internal rotation. In this case, internal rotation was tested by having the patient reach behind her back and by assessing the spinal level she could touch with her thumb. All movements were painful and stiff concomitantly at the end of the range. Her passive external rotation was most limited with the extremity positioned at neutral abduction, with greater external rotation available from 60 to 90 degrees of abduction.

- Scapulohumeral rhythm: lateral rotation of the scapula initiated within the first 30 degrees of humeral elevation.
- Accessory testing: limited inferior and anterior glenohumeral joint glides.
- Resisted tests: moderately weak but painless for shoulder abduction and external rotation.
- Special tests: impingement test negative; quadrant test difficult to perform because of anterior glenohumeral joint tightness.
- Palpation: tender anterior glenohumeral capsule.

Assessment:

1. Medical diagnosis: adhesive capsulitis.
2. Stage of reactivity: moderate.
3. Physical therapy diagnosis (problem list of impairments):
   a. Restricted passive/active ROM in right shoulder, both physiologic and accessory movements.
   b. Decreased strength in shoulder abduction and external rotation.
   c. Postural impairments (i.e., forward head posture with rounder shoulders perpetuating muscle imbalances about the shoulder) (spinal segmental restrictions perpetuating forward head posture).
   d. Myofascial pain with active trigger points as secondary sources of shoulder pain. The trigger point in the subscapularis reflected chronic tightness and resulted in limited external rotation of the humerus in the neutral position. The elevated tone and trigger point in the right upper trapezius also reflected muscle tightness, resulting in an elevated scapula and an increased in right cervical spine pain and motion restriction. The trigger point in the rhomboid muscles resulted from stretch weakness caused by the protracted scapula.

Diagnostic classification: Musculoskeletal 4D: Adhesive capsulitis (726.0)

Goals of Treatment

1. Restore active/passive ROM to right shoulder. Treatments:
   a. Stretch subscapularis.
   b. Mobilize glenohumeral anterior and inferior capsules.

CASE STUDY 6-1—cont'd

c. Strengthen rotators and force the couple mechanism in both the glenohumeral joint and the scapulothoracic junction.
2. Decrease myofascial pain. Treatment: Eliminate trigger points in upper trapezius, rhomboid, and subscapularis muscles.
3. Improve upper quarter posture. Treatment: Promote axial extension.
   a. Mobilize segmental restrictions in mid and upper thoracic spine and midcervical spine.
   b. Correct muscle imbalances (i.e., stretch tight muscles and strengthen weak antagonists).

Summary

This case represents a typical shoulder dysfunction that is complicated by upper quarter changes. Failure to evaluate the structure and function of the upper quarter thoroughly and systematically in this patient would result in failure to resolve a large component of her pain and dysfunction and would perpetuate her shoulder problem. The upper quarter screening was incorporated into the total physical therapy evaluation, and certain steps in the upper quarter evaluation were omitted or implemented later in the overall evaluation.

CASE STUDY 6-2

John is a 34-year-old carpenter with a diagnosis of lateral epicondylitis in the right elbow. The problem began 2 weeks ago after the patient began work on a job of renovating a house. The patient is right hand dominant. His pain is described as a dull ache located along the lateral aspect of the elbow. The patient describes the pain as radiating along the lateral aspect, posterior surface of the forearm, and proximal to the middle one-third of the upper arm. The patient reports occasional tingling and numbness in the same area of the pain in his arm and forearm. Symptoms are worsened with repetitive gripping and with reaching activities.

Upper Quarter Screening

- Posture: lateral or sagittal plane alignment of the cervical spine and upper thoracic spine is unremarkable. In the frontal plane (anterior view), the cervical spine is in slight right-side bending and left rotation.
- Function tests: cervical spine right rotation and side bending with overpressure reproduces paresthesia in the right upper extremity. The cervical compression test reproduces paresthesia in the right upper extremity. Cervical distraction eliminates right upper extremity paresthesia.
- Neurologic examination: manual muscle testing indicates the following:

	Right	Left
Lateral shoulder rotation	5/5	5/5
Abduction of shoulder	5/5	5/5
Elbow flexion	4/5	5/5
Elbow extension	4/5	5/5
Wrist extension	3+/5	5/5
Wrist flexion	4/5	4/5
Forearm supination	4/5	5/5
Forearm pronation	5/5	5/5
Finger abduction	4/5	5/5
Finger adduction	4/5	5/5

Manual muscle testing produces right lateral elbow pain for wrist extension and forearm supination on the right.

	Deep Tendon Reflexes	
	Right	Left
Biceps C5	Normal	Normal
Triceps C6	Decreased	Normal
Brachioradialis C7	Decreased	Normal

- Sensation: decreased to light touch and pinprick along the posterior aspect of the right proximal arm and forearm to the wrist.
- Thoracic outlet tests: positive for right upper extremity pain and paresthesia with the Adson's and costoclavicular tests. However, no signs and symptoms of vascular compromise were present, including diminished radial pulse.
- Palpation: elevated tone and muscle spasms in the right scalene and sternocleidomastoid muscles. Palpation along the cervical spine elicited tenderness along the lower cervical posterolateral facet joints at the C6-C7 and C7-T1 levels.
- Peripheral joints: shoulder has full ROM and no pain; the elbow has full motion; passive wrist and finger flexion with forearm pronation reproduces right lateral elbow pain.
- Accessory testing: side glide of C6 on C7 and C7 on T1 to the left is painful and limited.
- Resisted tests: painful, with resisted wrist extension and forearm supination.
- Palpation: tender along the right lateral epicondyle and proximal muscle–tendinous junction of the wrist and finger extensor muscles.

Assessment

1. Medical diagnosis: lateral epicondylitis of the right elbow. The screening evaluation indicates a secondary problem characterized by a C7 nerve root radiculopathy.

Continued

CASE STUDY 6-2—cont'd

Findings that indicate this problem include positive spine provocation tests that reproduce paresthesia along the C7 dermatome, tenderness at the C6-C7 interspace, and sensory motor and reflex changes consistent primarily with C7 spinal innervation.

2. Stage of reactivity: moderate for both the lateral epicondyle and cervical radiculopathy.

3. Physical therapy problem list:
   a. Tender lateral epicondyle.
   b. Pain with passive wrist extension, forearm supination, and finger flexion.
   c. Pain and mild weakness with wrist extension and forearm supination.
   d. Limited and painful cervical spine side bending and rotation to the right.
   e. Tender lower cervical facet joints.
   f. Spasms, scalenes, and sternocleidomastoid muscles.
   Diagnostic classification: Musculoskeletal 4D: Lateral epicondylitis (726.32)

Goals of Treatment

1. Eliminate tenderness of the right lateral epicondyle. Treatments: anti-inflammatory modalities, including iontophoresis, ice massage, pulsed or low-intensity, continuous ultrasound, and rest from harmful activities, including repetitive gripping activities.

2. Increase passive wrist flexion, forearm supination, and finger flexion. Treatment: gradual low load stretch into the ranges identified in Assessment (2) above.

3. Increase pain-free wrist extension and forearm supination strength. Treatments: Begin with submaximal isometrics to the forearm supinators and wrist extensors, and progress to partial range concentrics and finally full-range eccentrics.

4. Reduce signs and symptoms of C7 radiculopathy. Treatment: cervical traction.

5. Increase passive and active cervical side bending and rotation. Treatment: cervical mobilization using an initial grade of I and II for the left-side glide at C6 through T1. As reactivity decreases, progress to grades III and IV.

6. Eliminate muscle spasms in right scalenes and sternocleidomastoid muscles. Treatments: heat; continuous ultrasound, soft tissue massage, and stretching.

Summary

This case illustrates a secondary problem that resulted in a considerable number of impairments, in addition to those resulting from lateral epicondylitis. Although a tentative medical diagnosis is given on the basis of the physical therapy evaluation, this was done for continuity to present case findings, not to illustrate this author's general approach to patient care. If this were an actual situation, the author would contact the referring physician to discuss additional clinical findings of the screening evaluation, so the physician can make the decision regarding an additional medical workup.

SUMMARY

The information presented in this chapter underscores the importance of a screening evaluation as part of the overall physical therapy evaluation for musculoskeletal rehabilitation. The interdependent nature of the upper quarter indicates that impairments often occur in clusters, and several tissues and structures may be involved in producing pain and functional loss. The presenting signs and symptoms often are confusing, particularly to the novice practitioner. A systematic approach that briefly but concisely examines all relevant pain-producing tissues will help to clarify potential confusing presentations for effective treatment planning.

REFERENCES

1. Jette A: Toward a common language for function, disability, and health. Phys The 86(5):726-734, 2006.
2. Sahrmann S: Diagnosis and treatment of movement impairments, St. Louis, 2002, Mosby.
3. Hollinshead WH: The back and the limbs: anatomy for surgeons, vol 3, New York, 1969, Harper and Row.
4. Warwick R, Williams P: Gray's anatomy, Philadelphia, 1973, Saunders.
5. Bamajian JU: Muscles alive, ed 4, Baltimore, 1979, Williams & Wilkins.
6. Grieve GP: Vertebral joint problems, New York, 1981, Churchill Livingstone.
7. Jowett RI, Fiddler MW: Histochemical changes in the multifidus in mechanical derangements of the spine, Orthop Clin North Am 6:145, 1975.
8. Brodie AG: Anatomy and physiology of head and neck musculature, Am J Orthod 36(831), 1950.
9. Rocabado M: Biomechanical relationship of the cranial, cervical and hyoid regions, J Craniomandib Pract 11:3, 1983.
10. Mohl NO: Head posture and its role in occlusion, NY State Dent J 42:17, 1976.
11. Ayub E, Glasheen-Wary M, Kraus S: Head posture: a study of the effects on the rest position of the mandible, J Orthop Sports Phys Ther 5:179, 1984.

12. Gresham HSPA: Cervical and mandibular posture, Dent Rec 74:261, 1954.

13. Darling PW, Kraus S, Glasheen-Wary MB: Relationship of head posture and the rest position of the mandible, J Prosthet Dent 16:848, 1984.

14. Goldstein DF, Kraus SL, Williams WB, et al: Influence of cervical posture on mandibular movement, J Prosthet Dent 52:421, 1984.

15. Kendall FP, McCreary EK, Provance PG, et al: Muscles: testing and function with posture and pain, ed 5, Baltimore, 2005, Lippincott Williams & Wilkins.

16. Ludewig PM, Cook TM: Alterations in shoulder kinematics and associated muscle activity in people with symptoms of shoulder impingement, J Orthop Sports Phys Ther 80:276, 2000.

17. McClure PW, Bialker J, Neff N, et al: Shoulder function and 3-dimensional kinematics in people with shoulder impingement syndrome before and after a 6-week exercise program, J Orthop Sports Phys Ther 84:832, 2004.

18. Solow B, Tallgren A: Natural head position in standing subjects, Acta Odontol Scand 29:591, 1971.

19. Vig PS, Showfety KJ, Philips C: Experimental manipulation of head position, Am J Orthod 77(3), 1980.

20. Cleall JR, Alexander WJ, McIntyre HM: Head posture and its relationship to deglutition, Angle Orthod 36:335, 1966.

21. Bailey H: Theoretical significance of postural imbalance, especially the "short leg", J Am Osteopath Assoc 77:452, 1978.

22. Guyton AC: Organ physiology: structure and function of the nervous system, ed 2, Philadelphia, 1976, Saunders.

23. Nordin M, Frankel VH: Basic biomechanics of the musculoskeletal system, ed 3, Philadelphia, 2001, Lippincott Williams & Wilkins.

24. Lee D: Tennis elbow, J Orthop Sports Phys Ther 8(3), 1986.

25. Sunderland S: Traumatized nerves, roots and ganglia: musculoskeletal factors and neuropathologic consequences. In Korr IM, ed. The neurobiologic mechanisms in manipulative therapy, New York, 1978, Plenum.

26. Janda V: Muscles, central nervous motor regulation and back problems. In Korr IM, editor: The neurobiologic mechanisms in manipulative therapy, New York, 1978, Plenum.

27. Williams P, Goldspink G: Changes in sarcomere length and physiologic properties in immobilized muscle, J Anat 116:45, 1978.

28. Tabary JC, Tardieu C, Tardieu G, et al: Experimental rapid sarcomere loss with concomitant hypoextensibility, Muscle Nerve 4:198, 1981.

29. Lieber RL: Skeletal muscle, structure, function, and plasticity, ed 2, Philadelphia, 2002, Lippincott Williams & Wilkins.

30. Eggers GWN, Shindler TO, Pomeral CM: Osteogenesis: influence of the contact-compression factor on osteogenesis in surgical fractures, J Bone Joint Surg Am 31:693, 1949.

31. Salter RB, Field P: The effects of continuous compression on living articular cartilage: an experimental investigation, J Bone Joint Surg Am 42(31), 1960.

32. Akeson WH, Amiel D, Mechanis GL, et al: Collagen cross-linking alterations in joint contractures: changes in the reducible cross-links in periarticular connective tissue collagen after nine weeks of immobilization, Connect Tissue Res 5(15), 1977.

33. Woo S, Mathews JU, Akeson WH, et al: Connective tissue response to immobility: correlative study of biomechanical and biochemical measurements of normal and immobilized rabbit knees, Arthritis Rheum 18(3), 1975.

34. APTA: Guide to physical therapist practice, ed 2, Phys Ther 81(1), 2003.

35. Cimbiz A, Beydemir F, Manisaligil U: Evaluation of trigger points in young subjects, J Musculoskeletal Pain 14(4):27-35, 2006.

36. Fernandez-de-las-Penas C, Alonso-Blanco C, Cuadrado ML et al: Trigger points in the suboccipital muscles and forward head posture in tension-type headache, Headache 46(3):454-460, 2006.

37. Griegel-Morris P, Larson K, Mueller- Klaus K, et al: Incidence of common postural abnormalities in the cervical, shoulder, and thoracic regions and their associations with pain in two age groups of healthy subjects, Phys Ther 72(6):425-430, 1992.

38. Mannheimer JS, Anttansio R, Cinotti WR, et al: Cervical strain and mandibular whiplash: effects upon the craniomandibular apparatus, Clin Prev Dent 11:29-32, 1989.

39. Kopell HP, Thompson WAL: Peripheral entrapment neuropathies, ed 2, New York, 1976, Robert E. Krieger.

40. Lindahl O, Rexed B: Histologic changes in spinal nerve roots of operated cases of sciatica, Acta Orthop Scand 20:215, 1951.

41. Gunn CC: Prespondylosis and some pain syndromes following denervation supersensitivity, Spine 5(2), 1980.

42. Edgelow PI: Neurovascular consequences of cumulative tissue disorders affecting the thoracic outlet: a patient-centered treatment approach. In Donatelli R, editor: Physical therapy of the shoulder, ed 4, St. Louis, 2004, Churchill Livingstone.

43. Overton. The causes of pain in the upper extremities: a differential diagnosis study, Clin Orthop 51:27, 1967.

44. Boissonnault WG: Primary care for the physical therapist: examination and triage, St. Louis, 2005, Elsevier Saunders.

45. Dutton M: Orthopaedic examination, evaluation, and intervention, New York, 2004, McGraw-Hill.

46. Hertling D, Kessler RM: Management of common musculoskeletal disorders: physical therapy principles and methods, ed 4, Philadelphia, 2006, Lippincott Williams & Wilkins.

47. Feinstein B, Langton JNK, Jameson RM, et al: Experiments of pain referred from deep somatic tissues, J Bone Joint Surg Am 36(5), 1954.

48. Kellgren J: Observations of referred pain arising from muscle, Clin Sci 3:175, 1938.

49. Inman VT, Saunders JB: Referred pain from skeletal structures, J Nerv Ment Dis 99:660, 1944.

50. Janda V: Some aspects of extracranial causes of facial pain, J Prosthet Dent 56(4), 1986.

51. Trauell JG, Simon DG: Myofascial pain and dysfunction: the trigger point manual, Baltimore, 1984, Lippincott Williams & Wilkins.

7

Steven L. Kraus

Temporomandibular Disorders, Head and Orofacial Pain*
Cervical Spine Considerations

Head and orofacial pain originates from dental, neurologic, musculoskeletal, otolaryngologic, vascular, metaplastic, or infectious disease and is treated by many health care practitioners, such as dentists, oral surgeons, and physicians who specialize in this pathology. This article focuses on the nonpathologic involvement of the musculoskeletal system as a source of head and orofacial pain. Areas of the musculoskeletal system that are reviewed include the temporomandibular joint (TMJ) and muscles of mastication, which are collectively referred to as temporomandibular disorders (TMDs), and cervical spine disorders.[1]

Conservative treatment is recommended for most patients who experience TMDs and cervical spine disorders.[1,2] Physical therapists offer conservative treatment in rehabilitation of TMDs and cervical spine disorders. The American Physical Therapy Association (APTA) defines physical therapy as "...the care and services provided by or under the direction and supervision of a physical therapist."[3] The position of the APTA is "... only physical therapists provide or direct the provision of physical therapy."[4] The most valuable contribution that physical therapists make regarding the management of TMDs and cervical spine disorders involves the proper identification of components in the musculoskeletal system that contribute to a patient's symptoms and functional limitations. This is done by collecting a detailed history from the patient and conducting an appropriate physical assessment based on the history.[4] An evaluation that is properly performed by a physical therapist determines the type of treatment to be offered, and results in optimal and meaningful functional outcomes.

Consequently, the validity of research that investigates physical therapy intervention for TMDs and head and orofacial pain should be questioned when it is unclear whether a physical therapist participated in evaluation of the patient or provided physical therapy treatment. Referring to physical therapy only as a modality is misleading, and conclusions made about the therapeutic value of physical therapy may be inaccurate.[5,6] The objective of this article is to demonstrate the extent to which

a physical therapist who is trained in the specialty of TMDs and cervical spine disorders contributes to the successful management of this condition.

The first part of this article highlights the role of physical therapy in the treatment of TMDs. The second part discusses cervical spine considerations in the management of TMDs and head and orofacial symptoms. This article concludes with an overview of evaluation and treatment of the cervical spine.

Physical Therapy Management of Temporomandibular Disorders

TMDs can be divided into arthrogenous disorders, which involve the TMJ, and myogenous disorders, which involve the muscles of mastication.[1] An extensive subclassification has been developed for arthrogenous and myogenous disorders.[1] The common arthrogenous and myogenous disorders that are seen clinically by physical therapists, dentists, oral surgeons, and physicians are addressed in this chapter (Box 7-1). Diagnostic criteria for each of the common TMD conditions that follows are referenced in the literature and are not covered in this article.[1,7-9] The objective of this portion of the chapter is to highlight physical therapy treatment for common TMDs.

TEMPOROMANDIBULAR DISORDERS: ARTHROGENOUS

Inflammation

Inflammation can originate from TMJ tissues, such as the capsule, medial and lateral collateral ligaments, the TMJ ligament, or the posterior attachment. TMJ tissue inflammation can result from blunt trauma and microtrauma caused by parafunctional activity. Parafunctional activity is nonfunctional activity, which, when it occurs in the orofacial region, includes nail biting, lip or cheek chewing, abnormal posturing of the jaw, and bruxism.[1] Bruxism is diurnal or nocturnal clenching,

*From Kraus S: Temporomandibular disorders, head and orofacial pain: cervical spine considerations. Dent Clin North Am 51(1):161-93, vii. Jan 2007.

BOX 7-1	Common Temporomandibular Disorders (TMDs) With Corresponding International Classification of Diseases, Ninth Revision (ICD-9) Codes

TMD Arthrogenous	TMD Myogenous
Inflammation 524.62	Masticatory muscle pain
Hypermobility 830.1	728.85
Fibrous adhesions 524.61	
Disc displacements 524.63	
Disc displacement with reduction	
Disc displacement without reduction	
Chronic disc displacement without reduction	

bracing, gnashing, and grinding of the teeth.[1] Inflammation also can result from arthritic conditions.

Physical therapy treatment for TMJ inflammation involves patient education regarding dietary and oral habits.[9] Iontophoresis, phonophoresis, and interferential electrical stimulation are therapeutic modalities that are used to decrease TMJ inflammation.[10-12] Patients who are diagnosed with TMJ inflammation may have altered mandibular dynamics due to intracapsular swelling and resultant joint pain. Physical therapists teach patients range of motion exercises that maintain functional mandibular dynamics during the rehabilitation phase without increasing inflammation.

Hypermobility

Hypermobility is excessive translation of the mandibular condyle during opening of the mouth.[13] With condylar hypermobility, the condyle translates anteriorly during opening while following the slope of the articular eminence past the articular crest onto the articular tubercle.[13] Hypermobility that occurs unilaterally may be associated with deviation of the mandible, which is observed during mouth opening. Deviation is the mandible moving away from midline, but returning to midline at the completion of opening.[9] Although hypermobility may cause disc displacement of the TMJ, the cause and effect relationship has not been established.[14,15] Hypermobility is a common, frequently benign, condition.

Patients who exhibit hypermobility without pain do not require treatment.[14] Controlling hypermobility is necessary only when other TMJ conditions exist. If the patient has TMJ inflammation, hypermobility may perpetuate the inflammation when the patient opens his/her mouth wide during yawning. In the presence of TMJ inflammation, full mouth opening, regardless of whether hypermobility exists, needs to be avoided.

Dislocation of the condyle can result from uncontrolled hypermobility. Diagnosis of condylar dislocation is made if a patient complains that his or her jaw catches on closing from a full, open mouth position. Hypermobility also may be accompanied by palpable joint noises. Palpable joint noises are noises that are heard by the patient and felt by the clinician while palpating over the TMJ during opening and closing movements of the mandible. Joint noises that are associated with hypermobility must be differentiated from joint noises that are associated with a disc displacement. Although the patient may not have pain with jaw movement, the experience of joint noise, the feeling of a condyle catching on closing, and awareness of deviation of the mandible on opening are events that are disconcerting to the patient.

The most important aspect regarding treatment for hypermobility is patient education. Physical therapists should inform their patients that noises and deviations of the jaw are not necessarily signs of significant pathology, and that they can be controlled with proper muscular reeducation strategies. When mouth closing is associated with catching, the amount of mouth opening needs to be controlled through neuromuscular coordination exercises that are taught by a physical therapist who is knowledgeable in exercise interventions for TMJ hypermobility.[9]

Disc Displacement

Disc displacement can be classified into three stages: disc displacement with reduction, disc displacement without reduction, and chronic disc displacement without reduction.[16] Not all disc displacements are painful or interfere with functional movements of the mandible. Treatment is necessary when a patient experiences pain with or without functional limitations of the jaw.[17] Treatment choices for disc displacements that are painful or interfere with function consist of repositioning the disc to the condyle or allowing the disc to remain displaced while improving function and decreasing pain in intra-articular and associated periarticular/myofascial tissues about the TMJ.

When the choice is made to reposition the disc to the condyle, the options are arthrotomy and an anterior repositioning appliance. Because of the progressive nature of disc displacement, which is accompanied by increasing pathologic changes in the disc itself and in its peripheral attachments, restoring a satisfactory functional disc–condyle relationship may be difficult.[17] Consequently, arthrotomy and anterior repositioning appliances have led to mixed results in maintaining a normal long-term disc-condyle relationship.[18-22]

Arthrotomy is a treatment choice for patients who do not respond to conservative care. Conservative care consists of physical therapy, medication, and a full-coverage acrylic appliance that does not reposition the mandible.[23]

An anterior repositioning appliance, which repositions the mandible, is the most controversial treatment option for repositioning the disc to the condyle.[24] The controversy relates to whether the anterior-repositioning appliance actually recaptures the disc.[24] During the use of an anterior-repositioning appliance, the absence of joint noises and pain with functional mouth opening does not necessarily indicate that the disc has been recaptured.[20,24] Studies in which preoperative and postoperative computed tomography (CT) and magnetic resonance imaging (MRI) was used showed that permanent long-term disc recapture using an anterior-repositioning appliance was noted in only 10% to 30% of patients.[20] When an anterior-repositioning appliance is discontinued, some patients may require orthodontics and possible orthognathic surgery. For the most part, an anterior-repositioning appliance should be considered on a case-by-case basis, and should be used only as an infrequent treatment option for repositioning disc displacements.[24]

If the choice is not to reposition the disc to the condyle, the treatment options include arthroscopy (in its simplest format involving lavage/lysis), arthrocentesis, and physical therapy. The therapeutic value common to arthroscopy, arthrocentesis, and physical therapy interventions relates to the facilitation of adaptive responses of articular tissues to the disc displacement. The human TMJ can adapt or remodel in response to articular disc displacement, regardless of the type of intervention, and often best when no intervention is provided. For example, the posterior attachment of the disc (superior and inferior strata and retrodiscal pad) becomes a pseudo disc that can withstand loading of the condyle during function.[17,25] Restoring a normal disc position is not a necessary component for treating pain and functional resolution.[17] Nonpainful disc displacements are so prevalent in patient and nonpatient populations that they may be considered a normal anatomical variant.[26-28] Because adaptive responses of the articular tissues within the TMJ are common in relation to disc displacement—and in most cases lead to pain-free and functional outcomes—perhaps the most therapeutic intervention should be the least invasive (i.e., physical therapy).

Disc Displacement Without Reduction

An article that has reviewed the literature comparing arthrocentesis, arthroscopic surgery, and physical therapy for the treatment of disc displacement without reduction has demonstrated no significant difference in the effects of maximum mandibular opening, pain intensity, or mandibular function.[29] The decision to perform arthroscopy or arthrocentesis instead of physical therapy should be based upon an evidence-based evaluation and on the needs of the informed patient. When noninvasive treatment is recommended, physical therapy that is performed by a licensed physical therapist with an orthopaedic specialty—and preferably, a subspecialty in TMDs—should be the first choice in the treatment of disc displacements without reduction.

Physical therapy procedures may be successful in the treatment of pain and limited mouth opening associated with disc displacement without reduction.[30-33] Using various active and passive jaw exercises, as well as intraoral mobilization techniques, physical therapists may restore functional mandibular dynamics without pain when the disc is displaced. Inflammation that results from disc displacement or that coexists with disc displacement may be treated as identified previously. An oral appliance that is fabricated by a dentist also may facilitate the reduction of inflammation, especially if the patient bruxes. If physical therapy and the use of an oral appli-

ance have not reduced pain to a satisfactory level, or have not restored functional movements of the jaw after 4 to 12 weeks, the patient should consult with an oral surgeon to discuss surgical options.

Disc Displacement With Reduction and Chronic Disc Displacement Without Reduction

Patients who experience a disc displacement with reduction or a chronic disc displacement without reduction may be capable of functional movements of the mandible without pain.[17] The first goal of physical therapy consists of educating the patient on the cause of his or her joint noises (i.e., reciprocal click or crepitus), so that he or she is aware of the aggravating factors of the condition. If the patient has TMJ pain that is due to inflammation, the goal of physical therapy is to reduce pain and improve mandibular function through manual therapy and exercise interventions, despite the disc displacement. An oral appliance that is fabricated by a dentist also may facilitate the reduction of inflammation, especially if the patient bruxes. A patient who has joint inflammation that does not respond to an oral appliance or to 4 to 12 weeks of physical therapy may be referred to an oral surgeon for discussion of surgical options.

A physical therapist may attempt to eliminate or decrease joint noises associated with a disc displacement with reduction. Clinically, the goal of physical therapy is to have functional mandibular dynamics without pain and without noises, despite the fact that the disc is being displaced permanently. The following criteria are used for patient selection:
- Joint noises are disturbing to the patient.
- Patient experiences intermittent catching/locking with or without pain during mouth opening.
- Patient understands that the treatment may (a) cause joint pain, or (b) cause limited mouth opening, or (c) result in TMJ surgery because (a) or (b) could not be resolved.
- Patient consulted previously with a dentist or oral surgeon.

Exercises and intraoral manual procedures for treating a reducing disc are not the same as exercises and intraoral manual procedures for increasing limited mouth opening associated with a nonreducing disc and fibrous adhesions. Progressing a reducing disc to a nonreducing disc involves the application of exercises and intraoral manual procedures that prevent the disc from reducing on opening. Preventing the disc from reducing on opening elongates the posterior attachment. Once sufficient elongation of the posterior attachment occurs, the patient can achieve functional opening without popping, with the disc remaining displaced.[9,34,35] The patient may go through a short period with limited opening and possible pain. In the author's experience, 4 to 12 weeks is a sufficient time to achieve functional mandibular dynamics without pain and with in the absence of joint noises even with the disc displaced permanently.

Fibrous Adhesions

Fibrous adhesions may appear in the capsular-ligament tissues and in the upper joint space of the TMJ.[36] Fibrous adhesions can result from chronic inflammation, blunt trauma, postoperative healing of a capsular incision, or immobility that occurs with intermaxillary fixation or from limited opening that is associated with a disc displacement without reduction. The physiologic changes that are associated with fibrous adhesions are documented in the literature.[37-40] Physical therapy procedures and modalities for the treatment of fibrous adhesions are similar, but not identical, to those that are used for treating a disc displacement without reduction. Treating fibrous adhesions involves applying an intraoral mobilization technique that is referred to as "lateral glide." A lateral glide passive intraoral mobilization procedure may be performed at the same time that the patient opens his or her mouth actively. Clinically, this passive/active mobilization force targets restrictions in the lateral aspect of the capsular-ligament complex of the TMJ. Clinical decisions that are necessary to determine the duration, intensity, frequency, and progression of exercise intervention strategies require skill and experience. The effectiveness of a mobilization technique is related to proper patient selection, appropriate choice of technique, effective execution of the procedure, and adjustments based on tissue response and patient feedback. Inappropriate management of a mechanical dysfunction of the TMJ by untrained personnel may lead to exacerbation of symptoms and worsening of the condition.

TEMPOROMANDIBULAR DISORDERS: MYOGENOUS

Masticatory Muscle Pain

Masticatory muscle pain is a common clinical finding in patients who experience head and orofacial pain.[41] The relationship between bruxism and masticatory pain is unclear[42]; however, parafunctional activity, such as bruxism, may be a predisposing, precipitating, or perpetuating factor in masticatory muscle pain.[43,44] The common treatment for managing bruxism/masticatory pain is an oral appliance.[1] Oral appliances have been shown to be effective in the treatment of masticatory pain.[45,46]

Physical therapists may provide modalities and therapeutic procedures that offer symptomatic relief in masticatory muscle pain. Modalities, such as iontophoresis, ultrasound, and electrical muscle stimulation, may help to reduce muscle pain.[9] Intraoral and extraoral soft tissue mobilization to the muscles of mastication also may provide symptomatic relief.[9] Therapeutic exercises to the mandible that consist of isometric, isotonic, and eccentric contractions have been observed clinically to reduce masticatory muscle pain.[30] Patient education strategies that are related to oral modifications and enhanced self-awareness about aggravating factors have been shown to provide relief of masticatory muscle pain.[47] Oral modifications consist of dietary changes and elimination or limitation of oral habits, such as gum chewing and nail, lip, or cheek biting. Self-awareness strategies include instructing the patient on the proper rest position of the tongue and mandible. Patients who take an active role in making oral modifications and performing neuromuscular exercises may achieve satisfactory daytime relief from masticatory muscle pain. Decreasing cumulative loading during the day also may provide relief of nighttime pain associated with bruxism. Nocturnal bruxism is more difficult to treat, even when the patient wears an oral appliance. Physical therapists can assist in reducing nocturnal bruxism by addressing head and neck positioning while sleeping. Instructing the patient on proper selection and usage of pillow support that is appropriate for his or her cervical spine alignment and motion function may help to lessen the tendency for bruxism at night by enabling a more restful mandibular position. Cervical spine disorders that may contribute to bruxism are discussed in a later section.

Cervical Spine Considerations in the Management of Temporomandibular Disorders and Head and Orofacial Pain

The coexistence of neck pain and TMD is common.[48-61] One study found that neck pain is associated with TMD 70% of the time.[55] A high occurrence of neck pain also has been found in patients who have facial pain. A study was conducted on 200 consecutive female patients who were referred to a university facial pain clinic. Patients were asked to mark all painful sites on sketches that showed contours of a human body in frontal and rear views.[62] Analysis of the pain distribution according to the arrangements of dermatomes revealed three distinct clusters of patients: (1) those with pain restricted to the region innervated by the trigeminal nerve (N = 37); (2) those with pain in the trigeminal dermatomes and any combination involving the spinal dermatomes C2, C3, and C4, but no other dermatomes (N = 32); and (3) those with pain sites involving dermatomes in addition to those listed in (1) and (2) (N = 131).

In summary, the pain distribution of the 200 patients who had facial pain is more widespread than is commonly assumed.[62] Of 200 patients, 163 had pain that extended outside of the head and face to areas that included the C2, C3, and C4 dermatomes.[62] Other studies also have concluded that patients who have head and orofacial pain often experience widespread pain in the neck and shoulder areas.[63,64]

A systematic review of the association between cervical posture and TMDs has been conducted.[65] This review examined 12 studies that satisfied the same inclusion criteria for participants. It concluded that an association between TMDs and cervical posture is unclear. The uncertainty of the association between TMDs and cervical posture was related to the poor methodologic quality of the 12 studies.[65] Determining the typical resting posture of the head and neck for a study that evaluates upper body positional relationships is difficult, because all individuals assume many different head and neck postures during the course of a day's activities. Perhaps future studies that investigate cervical spine and TMD relationships should account for the dynamics of the cervical spine, instead of focusing on rest positions. The relationship of mandibular dynamics to the cervical spine needs to be analyzed in future studies through the use of reliable clinical instrumentation that compares active movements of the cervical spine vs. mandibular opening and closing or masticatory muscle pain. The following section highlights cervical spine considerations in the management of TMD; it is followed by a discussion on cervical spine considerations for head and orofacial pain.

Cervical Spine Considerations With Temporomandibular Disorders— Arthrogenous Involvement

The TMJ is a load-bearing joint.[1] TMJ inflammation may be perpetuated by bruxism that loads the joint excessively.[66,67] An oral appliance helps to control bruxism[24]; however, not all patients respond favorably to an oral appliance that is designed to control bruxism. Many variables can contribute to bruxism, which is why an oral appliance may not always be therapeutic in controlling bruxism. One variable is cervical spine involvement. Decreasing the intensity and duration of bruxism by managing cervical spine disorders may reduce the pain that originates from arthrogenous involvement. Cervical spine involvement as a cause of masticatory muscle pain or bruxism is discussed later in this article.

Typically, full mouth opening is accompanied by extension of the head, whereas mouth closing typically is accompanied by flexion of the head.[68] A frequently observed abnormal posture involves an extended head-neck position, which is a component of "forward head posture." Forward head posture may facilitate wider mouth opening during functional activities, such as yawning and eating a large sandwich. Increasing patient awareness of forward head posture and providing instruction in correcting forward head posture during sitting, standing, and walking may control excessive mouth opening associated with hypermobility; this approach should be incorporated into the conservative management program for every patient with a diagnosis of TMD.

On the other hand, if the objective is to facilitate mouth opening, physical therapists may position the patient's head and neck in slight extension during procedures (e.g., intraoral mobilization, static-dynamic jaw exercises) that increase mouth opening. When the patient stands for mouth-opening exercises, he or she is instructed to allow the head to extend slightly while opening the mouth.

Patients often believe that their head and orofacial pain is due entirely to their disc displacement. Many patients believe that the only way to feel better is to have the disc "put back into place." This may be true, however, in only a small percentage of patients who have a disc displacement. Often, the source of the patient's pain is independent of the disc displacement. Instead, it originates from TMJ inflammation, overactive masticatory muscles, and irritation of the pain-sensitive structures of the cervical spine. Cervical spine involvement as a source of head and orofacial pain is discussed later.

Cervical Spine Considerations With Temporomandibular Disorders: Myogenous Involvement

Bruxism is more common in patients who have myofascial pain in the masticatory and cervical spine muscles.[51] Patients who have TMDs report neck symptoms more frequently than do patients who do not have TMDs; patients who have neck pain report more signs and symptoms of TMDs than do healthy controls.[58] Neck and shoulder pain is more prevalent in patients who have a TMD with a myogenous component than in patients who have a TMD with an arthrogenous component.[56] Therefore, the prevalence of neck pain coexisting with masticatory pain may be more than a coincidence. Cervical spine involvement as a predisposing, precipitating, or perpetuating variable to masticatory muscle pain or bruxism is highlighted in the following three theories.

Theory One

The first theory is that afferent input that is associated with neck pain converges onto trigeminal motor neurons in the trigeminocervical nucleus, which results in an increase in masticatory muscle hyperactivity and pain. Motor activity of trigeminal innervated muscles of mastication increases when tissues that are innervated by upper cervical spine segments are irritated experimentally.[69-73] Little information on human subjects is available regarding the influence of experimental pain in the neck and shoulder muscles on motor activity in the orofacial region. One study was done to clarify the effects of experimental trapezius muscle pain on pain spread and on jaw motor function.[74] Experimental pain was induced in the superior border of the trapezius muscle of 12 subjects, aged 25 to 35 years of age, by injection of 0.5 ml of hypertonic (6%) saline. Results showed pain spread over a wide area to include the temporomandibular region, with pain referral accompanied by a reduction in mouth opening.[74] Afferent nociceptive input from the neck muscles may excite efferent (motor) neurons of cranial nerve V, which results in contraction of masticatory muscles.[75,76] Similar convergences and central excitation phenomena as seen with cervical and trigeminal sensory neurons also may exist for trigeminal motor neurons.[77,78]

Theory Two

The second theory is that masticatory muscles contract in response to the contraction of cervical spine muscles. Neurophysiologic interplay involves a synergistic relationship between the cervical spine and the muscles of mastication under normal circumstances.[79-85] Synergistic co-contraction can be observed with jaw and neck muscles during activities involving chew, talk, and yawn. Reciprocal innervation of opposing muscles has been demonstrated.[82] The cervical spine muscles and the muscles of mastication can be viewed as agonistic and antagonistic to one another.[83] In overt motor patterns, such as walking, augmentation and diminution of antagonistic muscles that contract concurrently (co-contraction) with agonist muscles has been demonstrated.[84,85]

Sometimes common daily events may cause the muscles of mastication to contract disproportionately in response to contraction of cervical muscles. Head, neck, shoulder girdle, and upper extremity posture must be positioned precisely during eye-hand coordination activities, such as writing, painting, computer work, and driving. A task that involves a specific head and neck posture requires a constant low-level contraction of muscles of the cervical spine. The longer a subject spends maintaining a specific head-neck posture, the more likely it is that an exaggerated contraction of the muscles of mastication will occur in response to contraction of cervical spine muscles.

Isometric, isotonic, or eccentric contractions of cervical spine muscles occur during lifting, carrying, pushing, pulling, and reaching activities. When cervical spine muscles perform repetitive activity, under load, and over a long duration, the more likely it is that the muscles of mastication will contract disproportionately.

Theory Three

The third theory is that the patient bruxes in response to neck pain. Patients start to brux, or the intensity and frequency of their bruxing may be exacerbated by their response to acute or chronic neck pain.

Thus, a neurophysiologic interplay exists between the muscles of mastication and the cervical spine; this must be addressed by thorough management of the patient with a TMD. Although these three theories should be further examined by clinical research, physical therapists observe that treating cervical spine pain often decreases masticatory muscle pain. Consequently, neck pain should be added to the list of factors that contribute to bruxism and masticatory muscle pain.

Cervical Spine Considerations With Oral Appliances

Common treatments for masticatory muscle pain include medication and application of an oral appliance, both of which can be offered by a dentist or oral surgeon.[24] Physical therapists should be familiar with the different structural designs of splints and must be able to explain the rationale and therapeutic benefits of oral appliance use.[46,86,87]

One common feature of the use of oral appliances and postural reeducation/manual therapy intervention for cervical spine dysfunction is that both treatment strategies influence the rest position of the mandible. The rest position of the mandible determines the initial path of closure into tooth-to-tooth contact or contact of teeth with an appliance.[88] The design of an oral appliance influences the vertical and horizontal positions of the mandibular rest position; this changes the path of mandibular closure and affects how the teeth and the oral appliance make contact.[89]

Conversely, head and neck posture also influences the vertical and horizontal positions of the mandibular rest position, which subsequently alters the path of closure into teeth-to-

teeth contact.[90-98] Mohl[90] stated, "if the rest position is altered by a change in head position, the habitual path of closure of the mandible must also be altered by such a change." Clinically, physical therapists have recognized that cervical spine motion restrictions and forward head posture affect mandibular closure, which, in turn, alters how the teeth and the oral appliance make contact.

Patients may complain that they do not "hit," "bite," or "make contact" evenly on their appliance. If the patient's complaint cannot be explained by interferences that are caused by the appliance design, the dentist should consider a mechanical disorder within the cervical spine that affects the path of closure of the mandible onto the appliance. Patients who do not to respond to an oral appliance within a 4-week period may not need to spend more time wearing the appliance, and they may not need a change in the design of the appliance.[1] Another alternative is to have a physical therapist evaluate the cervical spine to assess for possible dysfunctions that might be interfering with the effectiveness of the oral appliance. Clinically, cervical spine dysfunction with respect to abnormal posture or motion impairment can be treated before, during, or after the use of an oral appliance. Favorable outcomes are more likely to be achieved when cervical spine treatment is rendered concurrently with the use of an oral appliance, according to physical therapists who are experienced in managing masticatory muscle pain.

Cervical Spine Considerations With Head and Orofacial Pain

Symptoms that originate from the cervical spine and require immediate medical attention for spinal pathology include gross mechanical instability that may affect spinal cord function, primary bone tumor, metastatic disease, infection, fracture, and dislocation.[99] Symptoms also may be referred to the cervical spine as the result of visceral pathology.[100] "Red flags" that suggest a visceral pathology should alert the clinician to a nonmusculoskeletal origin of the patient's pain (Box 7-2). Imaging studies and erythrocyte sedimentation rates can help the clinician in detecting whether underlying pathology is present.[101]

Most cervical spine–related symptoms are not caused by spinal or visceral pathology.[102] Nonpathologic symptoms may originate from disc disorders, nerve root irritation, spinal cord compromise related to spinal stenosis, facet joint dysfunction, and myofascial pain. Common medical diagnoses for each cervical spine tissue are listed in Box 7-3. Patients frequently have more than one cervical spine–related tissue that is the source of their cervical spine–related symptoms. Multiple cervical spine tissue involvement can be referred to collectively as *cervical spine disorders*. Cervical spine disorders can cause pain or functional limitations of the cervical spine in which symptoms vary with physical activity or static positioning and may develop gradually or follow trauma.

The prevalence of nonpathologic neck pain is high. Approximately 70% of the general population is affected by neck pain at some time in their lives[103] and 54% of the general

---

BOX 7-2 Pathologic Conditions Suspected With the Following "Red Flags"

- Fever
- Unexplained loss of weight
- History of inflammatory arthritis
- History of malignancy
- Osteoporosis
- Vascular insufficiency
- Blackouts
- History of drug abuse, AIDS, or other infection
- Immunosuppression
- Lymphadenopathy
- Severe trauma
- Minor trauma or strenuous lifting in an older patient
- Increasing or unremitting pain

Data from Jarvik J, Deyo R: Diagnostic evaluation of low back pain with emphasis on imaging, Ann Intern Med 137:586-597, 2002.

BOX 7-3 Common Sources of Neck Symptoms With Corresponding International Classification of Diseases, Ninth Revision (ICD-9) Codes

Disc: 722.6, degeneration; 722.2, herniation
Nerve root: 723.4, cervical radiculopathy
Spinal cord: 721.1, cervical myelopathy
Facet joint: 719.5, hypomobility
Muscle: 728.5, muscle spasm; 729.1, myalgia

BOX 7-4 Classification and Diagnostic Criteria for Headache Disorder, Cranial Neuralgia, and Facial Pain

1. Migraine headache
2. Tension-type headache
3. Cluster headache and chronic paroxysmal hemicrania
4. Miscellaneous headache, unassociated with structural lesion
5. Headache associated with head trauma
6. Headache associated with vascular disorder
7. Headache associated with nonvascular intracranial disorder
8. Headache associated with substances or withdrawal
9. Headache associated with noncephalic infection
10. Headache associated with metabolic disorder
11. Headache or facial pain associated with disorder of cranium, neck, eyes, ears, nose, sinuses, teeth, mouth, or other facial or cranial structures
    11.1 Cranial bones, including the mandible
    11.2 Neck
    11.3 Eyes
    11.4 Ears
    11.5 Nose and sinuses
    11.6 Teeth and related oral structures
    11.7 Temporomandibular joint
    11.8 Masticatory muscles
12. Cranial neuralgias, nerve trunk pain, and deafferentation pain
13. Headache not classified

Adapted from International Headache Society, Classification Committee: Classification and diagnostic criteria for headache disorders, cranial neuralgias and facial pain, Cephalalgia 8(Suppl 7):9-96, 1998.

---

population has experienced neck pain in the past 6 months.[104] The general population has a point prevalence of neck pain that varies between 9.5% and 22%.[105]

Head and Orofacial Pain of Cervical Spine Origin

The International Headache Society has created a list of 144 different headache types that fall into one of 13 categories (Box 7-4).[106] The cervical spine is listed as a possible source of headaches and is reported as "neck" in classification 11, subclassification 11.2.

The literature is clear that cervical spine tissues refer pain to the head and orofacial areas.[77,107] The neuroanatomical mechanism that explains referred pain is the convergence between trigeminal afferents and afferents of the upper three cervical nerves.[108] This convergence occurs in an area that is referred to as the *trigeminocervical nucleus.*[109] The trigeminocervical nucleus is located in the upper cervical spinal cord within the pars caudalis portion of the spinal nucleus of the trigeminal nerve (Figure 7-1).[110,111]

Primary sources of head and orofacial pain that originates from the cervical spine are the structures that are innervated by C1 to C3 spinal nerves.[111] The lower segmental levels, C4 through C7, also may contribute to head and orofacial pain through the trigeminocervical nucleus.[112] Box 7-5 lists the tissues with sensory innervation from the upper three cervical nerves that contribute to symptoms referred to the head and orofacial areas.[111]

The greater occipital nerve (GON) branches off from the C2 nerve root.[113] GON cutaneous branches and their innervations are as follows:

- Medial branch: innervates the occipital skin
- Lateral branch: innervates the region above the mastoid process and behind the pinna (the projecting part of the ear lying outside of the head)
- Intermediate branches: run rostrally and ventrally across the top of the skull as far as the coronal suture. Anastomosis of the GON to the supraorbital nerve, which is a trigeminal branch, occurs at the coronal suture.

Trauma or suboccipital muscle tightness may involve the GON; this is referred to as *occipital neuralgia.*[114] Symptoms that are associated with occipital neuralgia refer to the occipital area, the top of the skull, the TMJ area, and the area in or around the ear.[115,116]

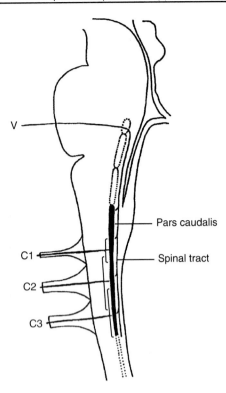

Figure 7-1 A sketch of the "trigeminocervical nucleus." Afferent fibers from the trigeminal nerve (V) enter the pons and descend within the spinal tract to upper cervical levels, sending collateral branches into the pars caudalis of the spinal nucleus of the trigeminal nerve and the gray matter of the C1 to C3 spinal cord segments. Afferent fibers from the C1, C2, and C3 spinal nerves ramify in the spinal gray matter at their segment of entry and at adjacent segments. The column of gray matter that receives trigeminal and cervical afferents constitutes the trigeminal nucleus *(black)*. (From Bogduk N: Cervical causes of headache and dizziness. In Grieve G, editor: Modern manual therapy, ed 2, Edinburgh, 1986, Churchill Livingstone, p 317.)

Cervicogenic Headache

The term *cervicogenic headache* was used first in 1983 by Sjaastad and colleagues.[117] Cervicogenic headache refers to head and orofacial pain that originates from the cervical spine tissues. Cervicogenic headache can be a perplexing pain disorder.[118] The following is a clinical presentation of cervicogenic headache as described by Sjaastad et al[117]: "The pain is usually unilateral but when severe can be felt on the opposite side. It is a head pain and not just a neck pain. The main manifestation of the headache is in the temporal, frontal, and ocular areas. It has a fluctuating long-term course with remissions and exacerbations; some patients have a continuous basal headache, others do not. During the headache attack, there may be the following accompanying phenomena; ipsilateral blurring and reduced vision, a "migrainous" phenomena[on] like nausea and loss of appetite; there may even be vomiting. Phonophobia and photophobia occur frequently. Some patients complain of dizziness and of difficulty swallowing during symptomatic periods. Even between attacks, patients may feel stiffness and reduced mobility of the neck."

BOX 7-5   Sensory Innervations From the Upper Three Cervical Nerves

- C1 sensory innervation
  - Suboccipital tissues and muscles
  - Atlanto-occipital and atlantoaxial facet joints
  - Paramedian dura of the posterior cranial fossa and dura adjacent to the condylar canal
  - Upper prevertebral muscles (longus capitis and cervicis and rectus capitis anterioris and lateralis)
- C2 sensory innervation
  - Skin of the occiput
  - Upper posterior neck muscles; semispinalis capitis, longissimus capitis and splenius capitis, sternocleidomastoid, trapezius, and prevertebral muscles
  - Atlantoaxial facet joint
  - Paramedian dura of the posterior cranial fossa
  - Lateral walls of the posterior cranial fossa
- C3 sensory innervation
  - Multifidus, semispinalis capitis, sternocleidomastoid, trapezius, and prevertebral muscles
  - Suboccipital skin
- C2/3 facet joint
  - Cervical portion and intracranial branches of the vertebral artery

---

Prevalence of Cervicogenic Headache

Cervicogenic headache is one of the three large headache groups; the other two are tension-type headache and common migraine without aura.[119] Cervicogenic headache accounts for 15% to 35% of all chronic and recurrent headaches.[119-121]

Although cervicogenic headache has been diagnosed frequently over recent years, it also has been misdiagnosed because of the considerable overlap in symptoms with more popular causes of headache (tension-type and migraine).[117,122,123] Cervical pain and muscle tension are common symptoms of a migraine.[124,125] In a study of 50 patients who had migraine, 64% reported neck pain or stiffness associated with their migraine, with 31% experiencing neck symptoms during the prodrome, 93% experiencing neck symptoms during the headache phase, and 31% experiencing neck symptoms during the recovery phase.[124] Other studies show that neck pain often coexists with migraine headache.[126,127] In addition, cervical muscles may play a role in the pathogenesis of migraine headache.[128] Patients often suffer several headache types concurrently.[129] Patients may require medications for migraine, application of an oral appliance for tension headache, and physical therapy for cervicogenic headache. In summary, many patients are misdiagnosed to have migraine or tension-type headache, when in fact these patients actually have headache of cervical origin. Therefore, the appropriate treatment should be targeted to mechanical dysfunction or to muscle tension in the cervical spine.

Dizziness

Dizziness and vertigo refer to a false sensation of motion of the body, which patients describe as a spinning or swaying feeling.[130,131] These are synonymous terms that are used to describe spinning, swaying, the subjective accompaniments of ataxia, and a variety of other colloquially described sensations. Dizziness may result from involvement of the eyes, the parietal and temporal lobes, and the cerebellum—most commonly as a result of disease affecting the labyrinth or the vestibular nuclei.[132,133] In the absence of disease, the vestibular nuclei can be affected by disorders of the neck in two ways: through ischemic processes or by disturbances of neck proprioceptors.[133] Disturbance of the vestibular nuclei associated with dysfunctional neck proprioceptors is addressed in this discussion.

Afferent input from neck proprioceptors (i.e., facet joints and muscles) is believed to affect vestibular nuclei activity, which results in a variety of motor and subjective abnormalities.[133] Cervical facet joints and muscles may produce a generalized ataxia, with symptoms of imbalance, disorientation, and motor incoordination.[134-139] Vertigo, ataxia, and nystagmus were induced in animals and in man by injection of local anesthetic into the neck.[140] These injections presumably interrupted the flow of afferent information from joint receptors and neck muscles to the vestibular nuclei. Vertigo following a whiplash injury (an extension/flexion movement of the head and neck) may be due to afferent excitation that originates from cervical muscles, ligaments, facet joints, and sensory nerves.[141] Patients who do not respond to treatment for dizziness that is believed to be originating from the eye, inner ear, or sinus should be suspected of having cervicogenic vertigo. Patients who experience cervicogenic vertigo may complain of pain, stiffness, and tightness in the neck; they are good candidates for physical therapy intervention that focuses on the cervical spine.[142,143]

Subjective Tinnitus and Secondary Otalgia

Objective tinnitus is characterized by physiologic sounds and represents only 1% of cases of tinnitus. Subjective tinnitus is an otologic phenomenon of phantom sounds. Although 10% of the population suffers from subjective tinnitus, its cause remains unknown.[144]

Subjective tinnitus has been related to cervical spine involvement. The sensory upper cervical dorsal roots and the sensory components of four cranial nerves (V, VII, IX, X) converge on a region of the brain stem that is known as the *medullary somatosensory nucleus*.[145] Subjective tinnitus is a neural threshold phenomenon, and cervical muscle contraction alters the neural activity that is responsible for tinnitus.[146] One hundred fifty patients were tested through a series of head and neck maneuvers to assess whether any of these maneuvers changed their subjective tinnitus. Eighty percent of patients had increased tinnitus during the test.[146] A similar study tested 120 patients who had subjective tinnitus and 60 subjects who did not have tinnitus.[147] Findings showed that forceful head and neck contractions, as well as loud sound exposure, were significantly more likely to modulate ongoing auditory perception in individuals who had tinnitus than in those who did not have tinnitus.[147] This study supports the concept that subjective tinnitus has a neural threshold.[147]

Secondary otalgia (i.e., earache not caused by primary ear pathology) is common in patients who are suffering from earache.[148] In a standardized examination and interview of 100 subjects, 91 subjects were found to have secondary otalgia, and 9 were found to have primary otalgia.[149] An epidemiologic study examined subjects who had secondary otalgia during a 2-year follow-up period.[150] Subjects who had secondary otalgia experienced pain with palpation over the masticatory muscles and TMJ, and they reported neck and shoulder pain more frequently than did individuals who did not have secondary otalgia.[150] Kuttila and colleagues[149] investigated whether secondary otalgia is associated with cervical spine disorder, TMDs, or both.[149] Most of the subjects who reported secondary otalgia also had signs and symptoms of cervical spine and TMD involvement. An examination of the cervical spine and the TMD is recommended as a routine diagnostic process for patients who have secondary otalgia.

Cervical Spine Examination

History

Orthopaedically related cervical spine problems are suspected first during the history. Primary symptoms of cervical spine disorders include neck, shoulder, and upper extremity pain and headache (cervicogenic). Cervicogenic headache is described by patients as pain that projects from the neck to the forehead, orbital region, temples, vertex, or ears. Symptoms for cervicogenic headache as identified by the International Headache Society criteria for cervicogenic headache are listed in Box 7-6.[151] Symptoms such as dizziness, ear pain (secondary), and subjective tinnitus also may have a cervicogenic origin. A complete list of cervical spine–related symptoms in given in Box 7-7.[152]

BOX 7-6   International Headache Society Criteria for Cervicogenic Headache

A. Pain localized in the neck and occipital region. May project to the forehead, orbital region, temples, vertex, or ears.

B. Pain is precipitated or aggravated by special neck movements or sustained neck posture.

C. At least one of the following occurs:
 1. Resistance to or limitation of passive neck movements
 2. Changes in neck muscle contour, texture, tone, or response to active and passive stretching and contraction
 3. Abnormal tenderness in neck muscles

D. Radiologic examination reveals at least one of the following:
 1. Movement abnormalities in flexion/extension
 2. Abnormal posture
 3. Fractures, congenital abnormalities, bone tumors, rheumatoid arthritis, or other distinct pathology (not spondylosis or osteochondrosis)

Adapted from International Headache Society: Classification and diagnostic criteria for headache disorders, cranial neuralgias and facial pain, Cephalalgia 8(Suppl 7):9-96, 1998.

BOX 7-7	Symptoms That May Originate From Cervical Spine Disorders

- Neck/shoulder pain
- Reduced/painful neck movements
- Numbness, tingling, or pain in arm or hand
- Reduced/painful jaw movement
- Headache
- Dizziness/unsteadiness
- Nausea/vomiting
- Difficulty swallowing
- Ringing in the ears
- Vision problems
- Numbness, tingling, or pain in leg or foot
- Lower back pain
- Memory problems
- Problems concentrating

Data from Spitzer WO, Skovron ML, Salmi LR, et al: Scientific monograph of the Quebec Task Force on Whiplash-Associated Disorders: redefining "whiplash" and its management, Spine 20(8 Suppl):1S-73S, 1995.

BOX 7-8	Procedures Used to Diagnose Cervical Spine Disorders (Disc, Nerve Root, Spinal Cord, Facet Joint, and Muscle)

- Neurologic testing for nerve function
  - Deep tendon reflex
  - Sensation
  - Strength
  - Spurling's test
  - Hoffman's reflex
  - Lhermitte's test
  - Nerve tension tests
  - Active range of motion
  - Passive range of motion
  - Cardinal plane movement
  - Intersegmental movement
- Muscle contraction (isometric/isotonic/eccentric)
- Palpation
  - Muscles
  - Facet joints
  - Greater occipital nerve
- Manual traction
- Posture

The patient's symptoms can be quantified by documenting their frequency, intensity (visual analog scale), and duration. This information can be used to monitor the patient's response to treatment. The Copenhagen Neck Functional Disability Scale or the Functional Rating Index can be used to document improvement.[153,154] Duration of sleeping and sitting and the patient's ability to reach, pull, and lift are documented in a measurable manner. Change in medication intake also can be used to monitor the patient's response to treatment.

Physical Examination

A physical examination of the cervical spine involves tests that incriminate nerve involvement. Often, neurologic signs are the result of nerve root compromise and are referred to as *cervical radiculopathy*, whereas spinal cord compromise is referred to as *cervical myelopathy*. Aside from physical tests that evaluate nerve function (manual muscle tests, sensory tests, reflex responses, and nerve tension tests), the physical therapy examination assesses for motion impairment of the cervical spine that influences gross range of motion or results in abnormal segmental vertebral motion that corresponds to the patient's symptoms and functional limitations. Palpatory tests are used to evaluate myofascial pain and dysfunction with respect to tenderness and tightness. Pain also can be accessed upon contraction of the muscle. Manual muscle and neuromotor tests are used to assess strength and coordination. A postural analysis is included to evaluate for possible areas of stress concentration. Physical therapists often determine the patient's response to manual traction during the initial examination, so they can evaluate the need for mechanical cervical traction treatment. Physical examination procedures are listed in Box 7-8. Imaging studies may be needed if findings of the history and physical examination are questionable or vague.

Treatment Strategies for Cervical Spine and Related Symptoms

Invasive Procedures

Treatment guidelines, such as the Scientific Monograph of the Quebec Task Force on Whiplash-Associated Disorders and Evidence-based Practice Guidelines for Interventional Techniques in the Management of Chronic Spinal Pain, recommend a noninvasive approach in the treatment of cervical spine symptoms with or without neurologic signs.[152,155] Only after unsuccessful conservative treatment has occurred should invasive procedures be considered.[156] Invasive procedures include epidural injections, nerve root injections, facet joint denervation, myofascial trigger point injections, and surgery (i.e., cervical fusion).

Unless neurologic signs suggest otherwise, patients who have symptoms of radiculopathy or myelopathy should be considered for surgery after conservative care has failed. Three studies examined the effects of surgery and conservative care on pain for sensory loss and weakness in patients who had minimal to moderate cervical radiculopathy or myelopathy. Two studies were prospective, randomized studies that evaluated a total of 130 patients; the other study was a randomized study that involved 68 participants.[157-159] No differences were found in sensation or motor strength between patients who were treated surgically and those who were managed conservatively in follow-up examinations at 24 and 36 months. Therefore, patients should be informed that long-term outcomes for conservative treatment of minimal to moderate cervical radiculopathy or myelopathy may be the same as those reported for surgical intervention, and in some cases, the only reason for selecting a surgical approach may be to achieve faster pain relief.

Conservative Care

Patients who have neck pain can choose from several complementary/alternative treatments that may be part of a physical therapist's knowledge and skill base. Complementary and alternative medicine (CAM) involves a diverse group of health-related professionals who have not documented the therapeutic value of their alternative treatments (e.g., magnet therapy, crystal application) through randomized clinic trials.[160] Physical therapy, however, is not CAM. Physical therapists offer evidence-based treatments for TMDs and cervical spine disorders based on data that are well documented in peer-reviewed journals.[161-167] Physical therapists follow evidence-based guidelines when using a multimodal conservative treatment approach for cervical spine symptoms that consists of manual therapy, exercise, patient education, and mechanical cervical traction.

A multicenter, randomized, controlled trial with unblinded treatment and blinded outcome measures was conducted to investigate the efficacy of physical therapy management of cervicogenic headache.[168] A group of 200 participants who met the diagnostic criteria for cervicogenic headache were randomized into four treatment groups: manipulative therapy, exercise therapy, combined therapy, and no treatment. The primary outcome measured was a change in headache frequency. Other outcomes evaluated included changes in headache intensity and duration, improvement in the Northwick Park Neck Pain Index, reduction in medication intake, and patient satisfaction. The physical outcomes evaluated included pain on neck movement, upper cervical joint tenderness, a craniocervical flexion muscle test, and a photographic measure of posture. The treatment period was 6 weeks, with follow-up assessment after treatment, then at 3, 6, and 12 months. At the 12-month follow-up assessment, manipulative therapy and specific exercise had reduced headache frequency and intensity and neck pain significantly, and effects were maintained ($P < .05$ for all). In summary, manipulative therapy and specific therapeutic exercise reduce the symptoms of cervicogenic headache over the short and the long term.[168]

Manual Therapy

Manual therapy techniques consist of a continuum of skilled passive movements to joints or related soft tissues that are applied at varying speeds and amplitudes, including a small-amplitude/high-velocity therapeutic movement.[169] Mobilization (nonthrust) or manipulation (thrust), when used with exercise, is effective for alleviating persistent pain and improving function when compared with no treatment. When compared with each other, neither mobilization nor manipulation is superior.[161] The psychological, neurophysiologic, and mechanical benefits of manual therapy have been discussed adequately in the literature.[170,171]

Exercise

Exercise may be effective in treating and preventing neck pain.[172] Specific exercises combined with manual therapy may be effective in the treatment of subacute and chronic neck pain, with or without headache, over the short and the long term.[155,173] Physical therapists can identify muscles of the cervical, shoulder, and thoracic areas that are tight and weak, and for which regulation of tension levels may be difficult. Physical therapists instruct patients in exercise programs that consist of stretching, strengthening, conditioning, and coordinating that are specific to the patient's needs. Modification of the exercise program frequently is necessary after reevaluation of the patient; this is dependent upon changes in the patient's signs and symptoms. A successful home exercise program is a function of proper patient performance and diligence. The skill of the physical therapist in teaching correct exercise form, making modifications in the exercises based on patient response, and motivating the patient to perform his or her home program is critical for obtaining an optimal outcome.

Patient Education

Patient education focuses on many elements of patient care and often involves instructing the patient on proper sitting and sleep postures. Support for and encouragement of patients also are important in helping them to overcome fear, anxiety, and misconceptions about their condition. Frequently, well meaning advice from friends or family members may interfere with recovery because of misbeliefs or incorrect information. In some cases, incorrect information is received from online computer resources that the patient has read. Frequently, physical therapists must dispel myths that the patient may have obtained from different sources, to alleviate anxiety and fear and to manage pain.[174,175]

Patients are educated by physical therapists about the meaning of their diagnosis because physical therapists typically spend more time with the patient than do medical professionals. Patients often perceive that "something is wrong" (i.e., irreversible) from a medical diagnosis such as degenerative joint disease, when degenerative joint disease in itself is neither predictive of, nor strongly correlated with, the patient's symptoms. In this way, a medical diagnosis may enhance the feelings of fear and anxiety, which can intensify symptoms and lead the patient to believe that a cure is not available.[176] Patients can become preoccupied with their diagnosis and often seek invasive treatment in an attempt to "fix" the condition. The health practitioner must understand that a patient's fear, misunderstanding, and beliefs about the meaning of pain may determine whether he or she progresses from acute to chronic neck pain.[177] A patient is less likely to develop a chronic pain mentality when he or she is educated about the condition after information is obtained regarding the medical diagnosis and symptoms. The physical therapist plays a major role in reducing patient anxiety and fear by keeping the patient focused on functional goals.

Mechanical Cervical Traction

Traction is a treatment that is based on application of a longitudinal force to the axis of the spinal column. Medically accepted uses for spinal traction include soft tissue tightness, joint stiffness, cervical radiculopathy, and cervical myelopathy, which are caused by disc degeneration or disc herniation.[178] The therapeutic value of traction was demonstrated in a trial of 30 patients who had unilateral C7 radiculopathy.[179] Patients were assigned randomly to a control group or an experimental group. The application of cervical traction, combined with electrotherapy and exercise, produced an immediate improvement in hand-grip function in patients who had cervical radiculopathy compared with the control group, which received electrotherapy/exercise treatment.[179] Although this is only one study that provides support for the use of mechanical traction, it does demonstrate its potential for radicular signs and symptoms.

The benefits of neck traction are optimal when it is performed with the patient in a supine position. The traction unit should not pull through the mandible, but only through the base of the skull/mastoid process area. Guidelines are available that recommend angle of pull, poundage, and duration of pull.[178] A physical therapist considers the patient's signs and symptoms to adjust the force and duration of stretch, to get the desired results.

SUMMARY

Physicians, dentists, oral surgeons, and physical therapists must work together to achieve the best outcomes for patients who experience TMDs and head and orofacial pain. Physical therapists play an important role in the conservative care of TMDs and cervical spine disorders that cause head and orofacial pain. Physicians and dentists should keep in mind that not all physical therapists have specialty practices that focus on TMDs and cervical spine disorders. Therefore, referral to an orthopaedic physical therapist who specializes in TMDs and cervical spine disorders is important for appropriate management of the patient.

Physical therapists treat patients with TMDs that are caused by inflammation, hypermobility, disc displacement, fibrous adhesions, and masticatory muscle pain and bruxism. Studies have shown that masticatory muscle pain and bruxism may be perpetuated by cervical spine involvement. Research evidence suggests a neurophysiologic interplay between the muscles of mastication and the cervical spine muscles. The cervical spine should be evaluated and treated when patients' TMD symptoms do not respond to medication and an oral appliance.

Often, cervical spine involvement is a misdiagnosed or unrecognized source of head and orofacial pain (i.e., headache), dizziness, subjective tinnitus, and secondary ear pain. Head and orofacial pain that originates from the cervical spine is referred to as cervicogenic headache. Cervicogenic headache symptoms can be similar to those of other common headache disorders, such as migraine or tension-type headache.

Cervical spine disorders that are treated by physical therapists who use evidence-based interventions, such as manipulation/mobilization and therapeutic exercise, can decrease the protracted course of costly treatment and can reduce the patient's pain. Physical therapists, therefore, have an important role in the management of head-neck and orofacial pain. Patients who present with TMD and cervical spine disorder many times can be treated effectively by a physical therapist who has specialized skills and experiences. Consequently, physical therapists should be an important member of the group of health practitioners who work with patients who have head, neck, and orofacial pain.

REFERENCES

1. Differential diagnosis and management considerations of temporomandibular disorders. In Okeson JP, editor. Orofacial pain: guidelines for assessment, diagnosis, and management, Carol Stream, Ill, 1996, Quintessence Publisher Co., Inc, p 45-52.
2. Hoving JL, Gross AR, Gasner D, et al: A critical appraisal of review articles on the effectiveness of conservative treatment for neck pain, Spine 26(2):196-205, 2001.
3. A guide to physical therapist practice, volume I, A description of patient management, Phys Ther 75:70756, 1995.
4. APTA House of Delegates Policies HOD#06–93–22–43. Alexandria, Va, 1996, American Physical Therapy Association.
5. Clark G, Seligman D, Solberg W, et al: Guidelines for the treatment of temporomandibular disorders, J Craniomandib Disord 4:80-88, 1990.
6. Feine J, Widmer C, Lund J: Physical therapy: a critique. Presented at the National Institutes of Health Technology Assessment Conference on Management of Temporomandibular Disorders, Bethesda, Md, April 29-May 1, 1996.
7. McNeill C, editor. Temporomandibular disorders: guidelines for classification, assessment and management, ed 2, Carol Stream, Ill, 1993, Quintessence Publishing Co., Inc.
8. Dworkin S, LeResche L: Research diagnostic criteria for temporomandibular disorders: review, criteria, examination and specifications critique, J Craniomandib Disord 6:301-355, 1992.
9. Kraus SL: Temporomandibular disorders. In Saunders HD, Saunders Ryan R, editors. Evaluation, treatment and prevention of musculoskeletal disorders, vol 1, Spine, ed 4, Chaska, Minn, 2004, The Saunders Group, Inc, p 173-210.
10. Schiffman E, Braun B, Lindgren J, et al: Temporomandibular joint iontophoresis: a double blind randomized clinical trial, J Orofac Pain 10:157-165, 1996.
11. Shin S-M, Choi J-K: Effect of indomethacin phonophoresis on relief of TMJ pain, J Craniomandibular Pract 15(4):345-348, 1997.
12. Watson T: The role of electrotherapy in contemporary physiotherapy practice, Man Ther 5(3):132-141, 2000.

13. Dijkstra PU, de Bont LGM, Leeuw R, et al: Temporomandibular joint osteoarthrosis and temporomandibular joint hypermobility, J Craniomandibular Pract 11:268-275, 1993.

14. Westling L, Mattiasson A: General joint hypermobility and temporomandibular joint derangement in adolescents, Ann Rheum Dis 51:87-90, 1992.

15. Dijkstra PU, de Bont LGM, Stegenga B, et al: Temporomandibular joint osteoarthrosis and generalized joint hypermobility, J Craniomandibular Pract 10:221-227, 1992.

16. Moffett BC: Definitions of temporomandibular joint derangements. In Moffett BC, Westesson P-L, editors: Diagnosis of internal derangements of the temporomandibular joint, vol 1, Double-contrast arthrography and clinical considerations. Proceedings of a Continuing Dental Education Symposium, Seattle, 1984.

17. Milam S: Pathophysiology of articular disk displacements of the temporomandibular joint. In Fonseca RJ, editor: Oral and maxillofacial surgery: temporomandibular disorders, vol 4, Philadelphia, 2000, Saunders, p 46-72.

18. Montgomery MT, Gordon SM, Van Sickels JE, et al: Changes in signs and symptoms following temporomandibular joint disc repositioning surgery, J Oral Maxillofac Surg 50(4):320-328, 1992.

19. Assael LA: Arthrotomy for internal derangements. In Kaplan AS, Assael LA, editors: Temporomandibular disorders: diagnosis and treatment, Philadelphia, 1991, Saunders, p 663-679.

20. Orenstein ES: Anterior repositioning appliances when used for anterior disk displacement with reduction: a critical review, J Craniomandib Pract 11(2):141-145, 1993.

21. Chen CW, Boulton J, Gage JP: Splint therapy in temporomandibular joint dysfunction: a study using magnetic resonance imaging, Aust Dent J 40(2):71-78, 1995.

22. de Leeuw R: Clinical signs of TMJ osteoarthrosis and internal derangement 30 years after nonsurgical treatment, J Orofac Pain 8:18-24, 1994.

23. Bays R: Surgery for internal derangement. In Fonseca RJ, editor: Oral and maxillofacial surgery: temporomandibular disorders, vol 4, Philadelphia, 2000, Saunders, p 275-300.

24. Sollecito T: Role of splint therapy in treatment of temporomandibular disorders. In Fonseca RJ, editor: Oral and maxillofacial surgery: temporomandibular disorders, vol 4, Philadelphia, 2000, Saunders, p 145-160.

25. Blaustein DI, Scapino RP: Remolding of the temporomandibular joint disc and posterior attachment in disc displacement specimens in relation to glycosaminoglycan content, Plast Reconstr Surg 79:756-764, 1986.

26. Turell J, Ruiz HG: Normal and abnormal findings in temporomandibular joints in autopsy specimens, J Craniomandib Disord 1:257-275, 1987.

27. Kircos LT, Ortendahl DA, Mark AS, et al: Magnetic resonance imaging of the TMJ disc in asymptomatic volunteers, J Oral Maxillofac Surg 45:852-854, 1987.

28. Westesson PL, Eriksson L, Kurita K: Reliability of a negative clinical temporomandibular joint examination: prevalence of disk displacement in asymptomatic temporomandibular joints, Oral Surg Oral Med Oral Pathol 68:551-554, 1989.

29. Kropmans TJ, Dijkstra PU, Stegenga B, et al: Therapeutic outcome assessment in permanent temporomandibular joint disc displacement, J Oral Rehabil 26:357-363, 1999.

30. Kraus SL: Physical therapy management of temporomandibular disorders. In Fonseca RJ, editor: Oral and maxillofacial surgery: temporomandibular disorders, vol 4, Philadelphia, 2000, Saunders, p 161-193.

31. Segami N, Murakami K-I, Iizuka T: Arthrographic evaluation of disk position following mandibular manipulation technique for internal derangement with closed lock of the temporomandibular joint, J Craniomandib Disord 4:99-108, 1990.

32. Van Dyke AR, Goldman SM: Manual reduction of displaced disk, J Craniomandib Pract 8:350-352, 1990.

33. Minagi S, Nozaki S, Sato T, et al: A manipulation technique for treatment of anterior disk displacement without reduction, J Prosthet Dent 65:686-691, 1991.

34. Scapino RP: The posterior attachments: its structure, function, and appearance in TMJ imaging studies, part 1, J Craniomandib Disord 5(2):83-94, 1991.

35. Scapino RP: The posterior attachments: its structure, function, and appearance in TMJ imaging studies, part 2, J Craniomandib Disord 5(3):155-166, 1991.

36. Holmlund AB: Arthroscopy. In Fonseca RJ, editor: Oral and maxillofacial surgery: temporomandibular disorders, vol 4, Philadelphia, 2000, Saunders, p 255-274.

37. Hardy MA: The biology of scar formation, Phys Ther 69(12):22-32, 1989.

38. Akeson WH, Amiel D, Woo S: Immobility effects of synovial joints the pathomechanics of joint contracture, Biorheology 17:17-95, 1980.

39. Salter RB: The biologic concept of continuous passive motion of synovial joints: the first 18 years of basic research and its clinical application, Clin Orthop Relat Res 242:12-25, 1989.

40. Frank C, Akeson WH, Woo SL, et al: Physiology and therapeutic value of passive joint motion, Clin Orthop Relat Res 185:113-125, 1984.

41. Moss R, Rum M, Sturgis E: Oral behavioral patterns in facial pain, headache, and nonheadache populations, Behav Res Ther 6:683-697, 1984.

42. Dao TTT, Lund JP, Lavigne GJ: Comparison of pain and quality of life in bruxers and patients with myofascial pain of the masticatory muscles, J Orofac Pain 8:350-356, 1994.

43. Faulkner KDB: Bruxism: a review of the literature, part I, Aust Dent J 35:266-276, 1990.

44. Faulkner KDB: Bruxism: a review of the literature, part II, Aust Dent J 35:355-361, 1990.

45. Boero RP: The physiology of splint therapy: a literature review, Angle Orthod 59(3): 165-180, 1989.

46. Al-Ani MZ, Davies SJ, Gray RJM, et al: Stabilisation splint therapy for temporomandibular pain dysfunction syndrome, Cochrane Database Syst Rev (1):CD002778, 2004.

47. Molina OF, Santos JD, Mazzetto M, et al: Oral jaw behavior in TMD and bruxism: a comparison study by severity of bruxism, J Craniomandib Pract 19:114-122, 2001.

48. Clark GT: Examining temporomandibular disorder patients for craniocervical dysfunction, J Craniomandib Pract 2:56-63, 1984.

49. Clark GT, Green EM, Doman MR, et al: Craniocervical dysfunction levels in a patient sample from a temporomandibular joint clinic, J Am Dent Assoc 115:251-256, 1987.

50. Kirveskari P, Alanen P, Karskela V, et al: Association of functional state of stomatognathic system with mobility of cervical spine and neck muscle tenderness, Acta Odont Scand 46:281-286, 1988.

51. Isaacsson G, Linde C, Isberg A: Subjective symptoms in patients with temporomandibular joint disc displacement versus patients with myogenic craniomandibular disorders, J Prosthet Dent 61:70-71, 1989.

52. Cacchiotti DA, Plesh O, Bianchi P, et al: Signs and symptoms in samples with and without temporomandibular disorders, J Craniomandib Disord 5:167-172, 1991.

53. Braun BL, DiGiovanna A, Schiffman E, et al: A cross-sectional study of temporomandibular joint dysfunction in post-cervical trauma patients, J Craniomandib Disord 6:24-31, 1992.

54. De Laat A, Meuleman H, Stevens A: Relation between functional limitations of the cervical spine and temporomandibular disorders [abstract], J Orofac Pain 1:109-110, 1993.

55. Padamsee M, Mehta N, Forgione A, et al: Incidence of cervical disorders in a TMD population [abstract], J Dent Res 186, 1994.

56. Lobbezoo-Scholte AM, De Leeuw JRJ, Steenks MH, et al: Diagnostic subgroups of craniomandibular disorders, part 1: self-report data and clinical findings, J Orofac Pain 9:24-36, 1995.

57. de Wijer A, Steenks A, de Leeuw MH, et al: Symptoms of the cervical spine in temporomandibular and cervical spine disorders, J Oral Rehabil 23(11):742-750, 1996.

58. de Wijer A, de Leeuw JRJ, Steenks MH, et al: Temporomandibular and cervical spine disorders: self-reported signs and symptoms, Spine 21:1638-1646, 1996.

59. De Laat A, Meuleman H, Stevens A, et al: Correlation between cervical spine and temporomandibular disorders, Clin Oral Investig 2:54-57, 1998.

60. Ciancaglini R, Testa M, Radaelli G: Association of neck pain with symptoms of temporomandibular dysfunction in the general adult population, Scand J Rehab Med 31:17-22, 1999.

61. Visscher CM, Lobbezzo F, de Boer W, et al: Clinical tests in distinguishing between persons with or without craniomandibular or cervical spinal pain complaints, Eur J Oral Sci 108:475-483, 2000.

62. Turp JC, Kowalski CJ, O'Leary N, et al: Pain maps from facial pain patients indicate a broad pain geography, J Dent Res 77(6):1465-1472, 1998.

63. Hagberg C, Hagberg M, Koop S: Musculoskeletal symptoms and psychological factors among patients with craniomandibular disorders, Acta Odontol Scand 52:170-177, 1994.

64. Sipila K, Ylostalo P, Joukamaa M, et al: Comorbidity between facial pain, widespread pain, and depressive symptoms in young adults, J Orofac Pain 20:24-30, 2006.

65. Olivo SA, Bravo J, Magee DJ, et al: The association between head and cervical posture and temporomandibular disorders: a systematic review, J Orofac Pain 20(1):9-23, 2006.

66. Molina OF, dos Santos J, Nelson SJ, et al: Prevalence of modalities of headache and bruxism among patients with craniomandibular disorders, J Craniomandib Pract 15: 314-325, 1997.

67. Trenouth MJ: The relationship between bruxism and temporomandibular joint dysfunction as shown by computer analysis of nocturnal tooth contact patterns, J Oral Rehabil 6:81-87, 1979.

68. Eriksson PO, Zafar H, Nordh E: Concomitant mandibular and head-neck movements during jaw opening-closing in man, J Oral Rehab 25:859-870, 1998.

69. Hu JW, Yu XM, Vernon H, et al: Excitatory effect on neck and jaw muscle activity of inflammatory irritant applied to cervical paraspinal muscles, Pain 55:243-250, 1993.

70. McCouch G, Deering I, Ling T: Location of receptors for tonic neck reflexes, J Neurophysiol 14:191-196, 1951.

71. Sumino R, Nozaki S, Katoh M: Trigemino-neck reflex. In Kawamura Y, Dubner R, editors: Oral-facial sensory and motor functions, Tokyo, 1981, Quintessence Books Publishing Co Inc, p 81-88.

72. Wyke BD: Neurology of the cervical spinal joints, Physiotherapy 65:72-76, 1979.

73. Funakoshi M, Amano N: Effects of the tonic neck reflex on the jaw muscles of the rat, J Dent Res 52:668-673, 1973.

74. Komiyama O, Arai M, Kawara M, et al: Pain patterns and mandibular dysfunction following experimental trapezius muscle pain, J Orofac Pain 19:119-126, 2005.

75. Svensson P, Arendt-Nielsen L: Muscle pain modulates mastication: an experimental study in humans, J Orofac Pain 12:7-16, 1998.

76. Komiyama O, Arai M, Kawara M, et al: Effects of experimental pain induced in trapezius muscle on mouth opening, J Jpn Soc TMJ 15:173-177, 2003 [in Japanese].

77. Sessle BJ, Hu JW, Amano M, et al: Convergence of cutaneous, tooth pulp, visceral, neck and muscle afferents onto nociceptive and nonnociceptive neurons in trigeminal subnucleus caudalis and its implications for referred pain, Pain 27:219-235, 1986.

78. Carlson CR, Okeson JP, Falace DA, et al: Reduction of pain and EMG activity in the masseter region by trapezius trigger point injection, Pain 55:397-400, 1993.

79. Clark GT, Browne PA, Nakano M, et al: Co-activation of sternocleidomastoid muscles during maximum clenching, J Dent Res 72:1499-1502, 1993.

80. Ehrlich R, Garlick D, Ninio M: The effect of jaw clenching on the electromyographic activities of 2 neck and 2 trunk muscles, J Orofac Pain 13:115-120, 1999.

81. Eriksson PO, Haggman-Henrikson B, Nordh E, et al: Coordinated mandibular and head-neck movements during rhythmic jaw activities in man, J Dent Res 79:1378-1384, 2000.

82. Sherrington CS: The integrative action of the nervous system, ed 2, New Haven, Conn, 1906, Yale Press.

83. Kapandji IA: The physiology of the joint, The Trunk and Vertebral Column 3:170-251, 1974.

84. Ralston HJ, Libet B: The question of tonus in skeletal muscle, Am J Phys Med 32:85-92, 1953.

85. Smith AM: The coactivation of antagonist muscles, Can J Physiol Pharmacol 59:733-747, 1981.

86. Major PW, Nebbe B: Use and effectiveness of splint appliance therapy: review of literature, J Craniomandibular Pract 15:159-166, 1997.

87. Clark GT: A critical evaluation of orthopedic interocclusal appliance therapy: design, theory and overall effectiveness, J Am Dent Assoc 108:359-364, 1984.

88. Posselt U: Studies on the mobility of the human mandible, Acta Odontol Scan 10:1-50, 1952.

89. Lawrence ES, Razook SJ: Nonsurgical management of mandibular disorders. In Kraus SL, editor: Temporomandibular disorders, ed 2, New York, 1994, Churchill Livingstone, p 125-160.

90. Mohl N: Head posture and its role in occlusion, New York State Dent J 42:17-23, 1976.

91. McLean LF: Gravitational influences on the afferent and efferent components of mandibular reflexes [doctoral dissertation]. Philadelphia, 1973, Thomas Jefferson University of Philadelphia.

92. Lund P, Nishiyama T, Moller E: Postural activity in the muscles of mastication with the subject upright, inclined, and supine, Scand J Dent Res 78:417-424, 1970.

93. Eberle WR: A study of centric relation as recorded in a supine position, J Am Dent Assoc 42:15-26, 1951.

94. Mclean LF, Brenman HS, Friedman MGF: Effects of changing body position on dental occlusion, J Dent Res 52:1041-1045, 1973.

95. Goldstein DF, Kraus SL, Williams WB, et al: Influence of cervical posture on mandibular movement, J Prosthet Dent 52:421-426, 1984.

96. Darling DW, Kraus SL, Glasheen-Wray MB: Relationship of head posture and the rest position of the mandible, J Prosthet Dent 52:111-115, 1984.

97. Root GR, Kraus SL, Razook SJ, et al: Effect of an intraoral appliance on head and neck posture, J Prosthet Dent 58:90-95, 1987.

98. Mohl ND: The role of head posture in mandibular function. In Solberg WK, Clark GT, editors: Abnormal jaw mechanics diagnosis and treatment, Chicago, 1984, Quintessence Publishing, p 97-111.

99. Mausner JS, Kramer S: Screening in the detection of disease. In Mausner, Baum, editors. Epidemiology: an introductory text, Philadelphia, 1985, Saunders, p 214-237.

100. Ness TJ, Gebhart GF: Visceral pain: a review of experimental studies, Pain 41:167-234, 1990.

101. Jarvik J, Deyo R: Diagnostic evaluation of low back pain with emphasis on imaging, Ann Intern Med 137:586-597, 2002.

102. Spitzer WO, LeBlanc FE, Dupuis M, et al: Scientific approach to the assessment and management of activity-related spinal disorders: a monograph for Clinicians Report of the Quebec Task Force on Spinal Disorders, Spine 12:S4-59, 1987.

103. Cote P, Cassidy JD, Carroll L: The Saskatchewan Health and Back Pain Survey: the prevalence of neck pain and related disability in Saskatchewan adults, Spine 23:1689-1698, 1998.

104. Andersson HI, Ejlertsson G, Leden I, et al: Chronic pain in a geographically defined general population: studies of differences in age, gender, social class, and pain localization, Clin J Pain 9:174-182, 1993.

105. Bovim G, Schrader H, Sand T: Neck pain in the general population, Spine 19:1307-1309, 1994.

106. International Headache Society Classification Committee: classification and diagnostic criteria for headache disorders, cranial neuralgias and facial pain, Cephalalgia 8(Suppl 7):9-96, 1998.

107. Bogduk N: The neck and headaches, Neurol Clin 22:151-171, 2004.

108. Kerr FWL: Structural relation of the trigeminal spinal tract to upper cervical roots and the solitary nucleus in cat, Exp Neurol 4:134-148, 1961.

109. Bogduk N: The anatomical basis for cervicogenic headache, J Manipulative Physiol Ther 15:67-70, 1992.

110. Bogduk N: Anatomy and physiology of headache, Biomed Pharmacother 49:435-445, 1995.

111. Bogduk N: Cervical causes of headache and dizziness. In Grieve G, editor: Modern manual therapy, ed 2, Edinburgh, 1994, Churchill Livingstone, p 317-331.

112. Michler RP, Bovim G, Sjaastad O: Disorders in the lower cervical spine: a cause of unilateral headache? A case report, Headache 31:550-551, 1991.

113. Bogduk N: The clinical anatomy of the cervical dorsal rami, Spine 7(4):319-329, 1982.

114. Bogduk N: The anatomy of occipital neuralgia, Clin Exp Neural 17:167-184, 1980.

115. Hildebrandt J, Jansen J: Vascular compression of the C2 and C3 roots—yet another cause of chronic intermittent hemicrania? Cephalalgia 4:168-170, 1984.

116. Rosenberg W, Swearingen B, Poletti C: Contralateral trigeminal dysaesthesias associated with second cervical nerve compression: a case report, Cephalalgia 10:259-262, 1990.

117. Sjaastad O, Saunte C, Hovdahl H, et al: "Cervicogenic" headache: an hypothesis, Cephalalgia 3:249-256, 1983.

118. Biondi DM: Cervicogenic headache: a review of diagnostic and treatment strategies, J Am Osteopath Assoc 105(4):16S-22S, 2005.

119. Nilson AN: The prevalence of cervicogenic headache in a random population sample of 20-59 year olds, Spine 20:1884-1888, 1995.

120. Pfaffenrath V, Kuabe H: Diagnostics of cervical spine headache, Funct Neurol 5:157-164, 1990.

121. Balla J, Lansek R: Headache arising from disorders of the cervical spine. In Hopkins A, editor: Headache: problems in diagnosis and management, London, 1988, Saunders, p 241-267.

122. Vernon H, Steiman I, Hagino C: Cervicogenic dysfunction in muscle contraction headache and migraine: a descriptive study, J Manipulative Physiol Ther 15:418-429, 1992.

123. Yi X, Cook AJ, Hamill-Ruth RJ, et al: Cervicogenic headache in patients with presumed migraine: missed diagnosis or misdiagnosis? J Pain 6(10):700-703, 2005.

124. Blau JN, MacGregor EA: Migraine and the neck, Headache 34:88-90, 1994.

125. Bartch T, Goadsby PJ: The trigeminocervical complex migraine: current concepts and synthesis, Curr Pain Headache Rep 7:371-376, 2003.

126. DeNarinis M, Accornero N: Recurrent neck pain as a variant of migraine: description of four cases, J Neurol Neurosurg Psychiatry 62:669-670, 1997.

127. Marcus D, Scharff L, Mercer MA, et al: Musculoskeletal abnormalities in chronic headache; a controlled comparison of headache diagnostic groups, Headache 39:21-27, 1999.

128. Shevel E, Spierings E: Cervical muscles in the pathogenesis of migraine headache, J Headache Pain 5(1):12-14, 2004.

129. Lance J: Mechanism and management of headache, ed 5, Oxford, UK, 1993, Butterworth-Heinemann.

130. Brown J: A systemic approach to the dizzy patient, Neurol Clin 8:209-224, 1990.

131. Fisher CM: Vertigo in cerebrovascular disease, Arch Otolaryngol 85:529-534, 1967.

132. Hoffman RM, Einstadter D, Kroenke K: Evaluating dizziness, Am J Med 107:468-478, 1999.

133. Reker V: Cervical nystagmus caused by proprioceptors of the neck, Laryngol Rhinol Otol Stuttgart 62:312-314, 1983.

134. Cohen L: Role of eye and neck proprioceptive mechanisms in body orientation and motor coordination, J Neurophysiol 24:1-11, 1961.

135. Abrahams VC: The physiology of neck muscles; their role in head movement and maintenance of posture, Can J Physiol Pharmacol 55(3):332-338, 1977.

136. Manzoni D, Pompeiano O, Stampacchia G: Tonic cervical influences on posture and reflex movements, Arch Ital Biol 117(2):81-110, 1979.

137. Cope S, Ryan GMS: Cervical and otolith vertigo, J Laryngol Otol 73:113-120, 1959.

138. Gray LP: Extra labyrinthine vertigo due to cervical muscle lesions, J Laryngol Otol 70(6):352-361, 1956.

139. Weeks VD, Travell J: Postural vertigo due to trigger areas in the sternocleidomastoid muscle, J Pediatr 47(3):315-327, 1955.

140. De Jong PTVM, De Jong JMBV, Cohen B, et al: Ataxia and nystagmus induced by injection of local anesthetics in the neck, Ann Neurol 1:240-246, 1977.

141. Hinoki M: Vertigo due to whiplash injury: a neurotological approach, Acto Otolaryngol (Stockh) 419(Suppl): 9-29, 1985.

142. Norre ME: Neurophysiology of vertigo with special reference to cervical vertigo: a review, Acta Belg Med Phys 9:183-194, 1986.

143. Phillipszoon A: Neck torsion nystagmus, Pract Otorhinolaryngol (Basel) 25:339-344, 1963.

144. Rubinstein B: Tinnitus and craniomandibular disorders: is there a link? Swed Dent J Suppl 95:1-46, 1993.

145. Young ED, Nelken I, Conley RA: Somatosensory effects on neurons in dorsal cochlear nucleus, J Neurophysiol 73:743-765, 1995.

146. Levine RA: Somatic (craniocervical) tinnitus and the dorsal cochlear nucleus hypothesis, Am J Otolaryngol 20:351-362, 1999.

147. Abel MD, Levine RA: Muscle contractions and auditory perception in tinnitus patients and nonclinical patients, J Craniomandibular Pract 22(3):181-191, 2004.

148. Paparella MM, Jung TTK: Odontalgia. In Paparella MM, Shumrik DA, Gluckman JL, editors: Otolaryngology, Philadelphia, 1991, Saunders, p 1237-1242.

149. Kuttila S, Kuttila M, Le Bell Y, et al: Characteristics of subjects with secondary otalgia, J Orofac Pain 18(3):226-234, 2004.

150. Kuttila S, Kuttila M, Le Bell Y, et al: Aural symptoms and signs of temporomandibular disorder in association with treatment need and visits to a physician, Laryngoscope 109:1669-1673, 1999.

151. Olsen J, editor: Classification and diagnostic criteria for headache disorders, cranial neuralgias and facial pain, Copenhagen, 1990, The International Headache Society.

152. Spitzer WO, Skovron ML, Salmi LR, et al: Scientific monograph of the Quebec Task Force on Whiplash-Associated Disorders: redefining "whiplash" and its management, Spine 20(8 Suppl):1S-73S, 1995.

153. Jordan A, Manniche C, Mosdal C: The Copenhagen Neck Functional Disability Scale: a study of reliability and validity, J Manipulative Physiol Ther 21(8):520-527, 1998.

154. Feise RJ, Micheal MJ: Functional rating index: a new valid and reliable instrument to measure the magnitude of clinical change in spinal conditions, Spine 26(1):78-87, 2001.

155. Manchikanti LS, Peter SS, Vijay S, et al: Evidence-based practice guidelines for interventional techniques in the management of chronic spinal pain, Pain Phys 6:3-81, 2003.

156. Abenhaim L, Rossignol M, Valat J-P, et al: International Paris Task Force on Back Pain, Spine 25(4 Suppl):1S-31S, 2000.

157. Persson LCG, Carlsson C-A, Carlsson JY: Long-lasting cervical radicular pain managed with surgery, physiotherapy, or a cervical collar, Spine 22:751-758, 1997.

158. Bednarik J, et al: The value of somatosensory- and motor-evoked potentials in predicting and monitoring the effect of therapy in spondylotic cervical myelopathy: prospective randomized study, Spine 24(15):1593-1598, 1999.

159. Kadanka Z: Approaches to spondylotic cervical myelopathy: conservative versus surgical results in a 3-year follow-up study, Spine 27(20):2205-2210, 2002.

160. Raphael KG, Klausner JJ, Nayak S, et al: Complementary and alternative therapy use by patients with myofascial temporomandibular disorders, J Orofac Pain 17:36-41, 2003.

161. Gross AR, Hoving JL, Haines TA, et al: Cervical overview group manipulation and mobilisation for mechanical neck disorders, Cochrane Database Syst Rev (1):CD004249, 2004.

162. Aker PD, Gross AR, Goldsmith CH, et al: Conservative management of mechanical neck pain: systematic overview and meta-analysis, Br Med J 313(7068):1291-1296, 1996.

163. Hurwitz EL, Aker PD, Adams AH, et al: Manipulation and mobilization of the cervical spine: a systematic review of literature, Spine 21:1746-1760, 1996.

164. Jordan A, Bendix T, Nielsen H, et al: Intensive training, physiotherapy, or manipulation for patients with chronic neck pain: a prospective single-blinded randomized clinical trial, Spine 23:311-319, 1998.

165. Nelson BW, Carpenter DM, Dreisinger TE, et al: Can spinal surgery be prevented by aggressive strengthening exercises? A prospective study of cervical and lumbar patients, Arch Phys Med Rehabil 80:20-25, 1999.

166. Rodriquez AA, Bilkey WJ, Agre JC: Therapeutic exercise in chronic neck and back pain, Arch Phys Med Rehabil 73:870-875, 1992.

167. Swezey RL, Swezey AM, Warner K: Efficacy of home cervical traction therapy, Am J Phys Med Rehabil 78(1):30-32, 1999.

168. Jull GA, Trott P, Potter H, et al: A randomized, controlled trial of exercise and manipulative therapy for cervicogenic headache, Spine 27(17):1835-1843, 2002.

169. Farrell JP, Jensen GM: Manual therapy: a critical assessment of role in the profession of physical therapy, Phys Ther 12(2):11-20, 1992.

170. Goldstein M: The research status of spinal manipulative therapy 1975. US Department of Health, Education, and Welfare, Rockville, Md, Publication No. (NIH) 76-998, NINCDS Monograph No.15.

171. Korr IM: The neurobiologic mechanisms in manipulative therapy, New York, 1978, Plenum Press.

172. O'Leary S, Falla D, Jull G: Recent advances in therapeutic exercise for the neck: implications for patients with head and neck pain, Aust Endod J 29(3):138-142, 2003.

173. Kay TM, Gross A, Santaguida PL, et al: Cervical Overview Group. Exercises for mechanical neck disorders, Cochrane Database Syst Rev (3):CD004250, 2005.

174. Al-Obaidi S, et al: The role of anticipation and fear of pain in the persistence of avoidance behavior in patients with chronic low back pain, Spine 25(9):1126-1131, 2000.

175. Wrubel J, et al: Social competence from the perspective of stress and coping. In Wine J, Smye M, editors: Social competence, New York, 1981, Guilford Press, p 61-99.

176. Pincus T: A systematic review of psychological factors as predictors of chronicity/disability in prospective cohorts of low back pain, Spine 27(5):E109-E120, 2002.

177. Waddell G, Newton M, Henderson I, et al: A fear-avoidance beliefs questionnaire (FABQ): the role of fear-avoidance belief in chronic low back pain and disability, Pain 52:157-168, 1993.

178. Wong A, et al: The traction angle and cervical intervertebral separation, Spine 17(2): 136-138, 1992.

179. Joghataei MT, Arab AM, Khaksar H: The effect of cervical traction combined with conventional therapy on grip strength on patients with cervical radiculopathy, Clin Rehabil 18(8):879-887, 2004.

8

Steven A. Stratton
and Jean M. Bryan

Dysfunction, Evaluation, and Treatment of the Cervical Spine and Thoracic Inlet

Many patients present to physical therapy with complaints of pain caused by cervical dysfunction. The cervicothoracic region is complex and requires a thorough evaluation if the disorder is to be treated appropriately. The clinician must understand the applied anatomy and biomechanics of this region to recognize pathology. This chapter covers the pertinent anatomy and kinesiology of the cervical and upper thoracic spine, the evaluation procedure, and the correlation of findings required for initiation of treatment.

Functional Anatomy

UPPER CERVICAL SPINE

The joints of the upper cervical spine region, also known as the craniovertebral joints, include the occipitoatlantal (OA) joint, the atlantoaxial (AA) joint, and the articulations between the second and third cervical vertebrae (C2-C3), including facet joints, intervertebral disc, and joints of von Luschka. Clinically, the upper cervical spine is considered a functional region because of the interdependency of these joints associated with movement.

The Atlas

The first and second cervical vertebrae have characteristics that make them different from the more typical cervical vertebrae, C3 to C7. The atlas (C1) is best thought of as a "washer" between the occiput and the axis (C2).[1] Two distinguishing features of the atlas are its long transverse processes and its lack of a spinous process. The superior articulating surfaces, which articulate with paired, convex occipital condyles, are concave

both anteroposteriorly and mediolaterally. The articulating surfaces are oval (Figure 8-1).[2]

The Axis

Besides being the largest cervical vertebra of the upper cervical region, the axis (C2) has several other distinguishing features (see Figure 8-1). Its most striking landmark is the odontoid process (the dens), which passes up through the middle of the atlas, articulates with the anterior arch, and acts as a pivot for the OA joint. The axis also has a large vertebral body. The superior articular facets are oriented superiorly and laterally, are convex anteroposteriorly, and are flat transversely. The spinous process of the axis is bifid, like that of other cervical vertebrae, but is larger in mass. The inferior articular processes of C2 are attached below the pedicle, face inferiorly and anteriorly, and correspond to the superior articular processes of C3. Both the C1 and C2 transverse processes have a vertical foramen for the vertebral artery.[2]

OCCIPITOATLANTAL AND ATLANTOAXIAL LIGAMENTS

Alar Ligaments

The alar ligaments are irregular, quadrilateral, pyramid-like trunks that attach from the medial occipital condyle to the lateral surface of the dens (Figure 8-2). The function of the alar ligament is to assist in controlling movements of extension and rotation.[1,3] During extension of the head, the alar ligament is stretched; during flexion, it is relaxed. During rotation of the OA joint, the ligament of the opposite side is stretched and drawn against the dens of the axis. For example, with rotation to the right, the left alar ligament is stretched and the right alar ligament is relaxed. During sidebending, the alar ligament on the same side relaxes and the opposite alar ligament causes a forced rotation of the axis to the sidebending side. The forced rotation is due to the attachment of the alar ligament to the dens (Figure 8-3).[1,2]

The opinions expressed herein are solely those of the authors and are not to be construed as reflecting official doctrine of the U.S. Army Medical Department.

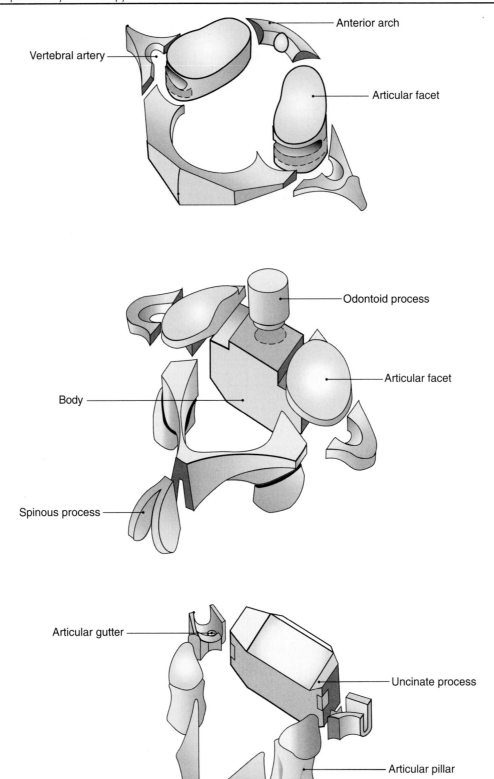

Figure 8-1 The upper cervical vertebrae. (From Kapandji I: Physiology of the joints, ed 2, vol III, The trunk and vertebral column, Edinburgh, 1974, Churchill Livingstone.)

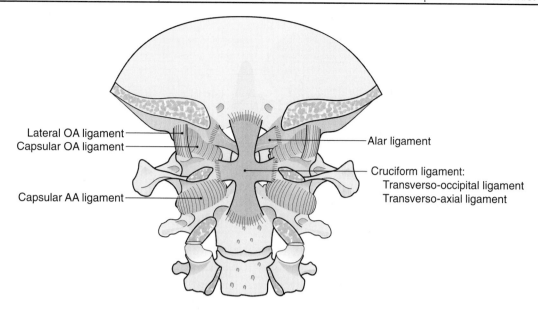

Figure 8-2 Ligaments of the upper cervical spine complex. AA, Atlantoaxial; OA, occipitoatlantal. (From Kapandji I: Physiology of the joints, ed 2, vol III, The trunk and vertebral column, Edinburgh, 1974, Churchill Livingstone.)

Table 8-1	**Structures That Restrict Occipitoatlantal and Atlantoaxial Joint Range of Motion About the Transverse Axis**
Flexion	**Extension**
Bony limitation	Bony limitation
Posterior muscles of the neck	Anterior muscles of the neck
Longitudinal fibers of the cruciform ligament	Sternocleidomastoid and scalene muscles
Tectorial membrane	Tectorial membrane
Nuchal ligament	Alar ligaments
Posterior longitudinal ligament	Anterior longitudinal ligament

Cruciform Ligament

The cruciform ligament consists of a horizontal transverse ligament of the atlas and the vertical attachments to the occiput and axis, respectively called the transverso-occipital and transversoaxial ligaments. The transverse ligament arises from the medial surfaces of the lateral mass of the atlas and guarantees physiologic rotation of C1-C2 while protecting the spinal cord from the dens.[2] The other ligaments of the craniovertebral complex—tectorial membrane, anterior longitudinal ligament, OA ligament, facet capsules, and ligamentum nuchae—all help to provide support; however, only certain ligaments restrict flexion and extension (see Figure 2-2; Table 8-1).[1]

Occipitoatlantal Motion

The upper surface of the occipital condyles is concave; thus, arthrokinematically, movement of the occiput on the atlas requires opposite joint glide in relation to physiologic move-

ment.[4] The articulations are divergent at approximately 30 degrees, so the joint surfaces are not in the true sagittal plane. The sagittal axial angle of the joints is 50 to 60 degrees in the adult. The sagittal angle of the joint axes from the occipital condyles, as described by Ingelmark,[5] reveals a 28 degree divergence of the articular surfaces anteriorly (Figure 8-4). Werne[3] described the OA joint as condyloid, with free flexion and extension (nodding) and limited sidebending. Flexion and extension take place around a transverse axis, and sidebending around a sagittal axis. Flexion and extension range from 16 to 20 degrees and are limited by bony structures. Sidebending measures approximately 4 to 5 degrees. Maximum sidebending is possible with the head in a slightly flexed position; when the head is extended, sidebending is prohibited by the alar ligaments.[6]

Different findings have been reported in the literature regarding the possibility of rotation at the OA joint. Fielding et al,[6,7] Werne,[3] White and Panjabi,[8] and Penning[9] found no rotation. Recent investigations reveal one-side axial rotation between C0 and C1 in the range of 3 to 8 degrees. Clark and colleagues[10] reported an average of 4.8 degrees. Dvorak and colleagues,[11] using computed axial tomography in vivo, noted an averaged one-side axial rotation of 4.3 degrees. Panjabi and associates[12] reported 8 degrees with the use of three-dimensional analysis. Dupreux and Mestdagh[13] contend that up to 5 degrees of rotation exists, with an average of 3.2 degrees. Attempts to explain this rotation often describe the atlas as a washer, interposed between the occiput and the atlas like a meniscus, which would imply a gliding or linear movement (Table 8-2).[1]

Atlantoaxial Motion

The AA joint has four articulations for movement: the bursa atlantodentalis together with the middle and two lateral articu-

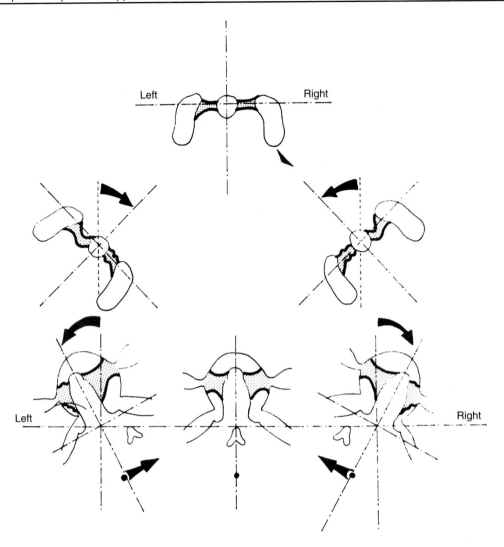

Figure 8-3 Role of the alar ligament in upper cervical spine motion.

Table 8-2	Active Range of Motion of the Upper Cervical Spine			
	Active Range of Motion			
Vertebral Unit	Flexion	Extension	Sidebending*	Axial Rotation*
C0-C1 (occipitoatlantal joint)	0-15 degrees	0-20 degrees	5-0-5 degrees	8-0-8 degrees
C1-C2 (atlantoaxial joint)	0-10 degrees	0-10 degrees	3-0-3 degrees	40-0-40 degrees

*Range available on either side of neutral.

lations. The bursa atlantodentalis is a space between the transverse ligament of the atlas and the dens of the axis. The middle AA articulation is located between the dens of the axis and the posterior surface of the anterior arch of the atlas. Most movement at the AA joint occurs at the lateral AA articulations, which are the superior articular surfaces between the atlas and the axis.[2] The articular surfaces of the atlas are convex, and those of the axis are relatively flat.[1] The range of motion to each side is 40 to 50 degrees, which constitutes half of the total rotation of the cervical spine.[6] Werne[3] reported 47 degrees of

rotation to one side, whereas Panjabi and colleagues[12] measured 38.9 degrees. As in the OA joint, rotation is limited primarily by the alar ligaments. Only minimal (10 to 15 degrees) flexion-extension occurs because of the bony geometry and the securing ligamentous structures. Sidebending between C1 and C2 is possible only with simultaneous rotation about the axis.[1] Lewit[14] and Jirout[15] described this movement as forced rotation that is mainly a result of the physiologic function of the alar ligaments. When forced rotation is produced, lateral displacement of the articular margin of the lateral joint of the atlas as

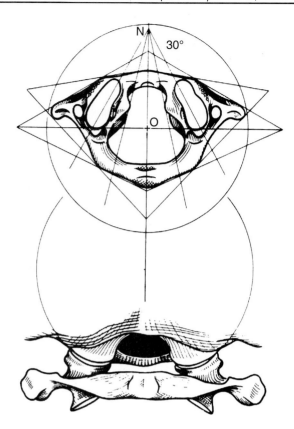

Figure 8-4 Occipitoatlantal joint sagittal axis from the occipital condyles. (From Kapandji I: Physiology of the joints, ed 2, vol III, The trunk and vertebral column, Edinburgh, 1974, Churchill Livingstone.)

compared with the lateral margin of the axis is seen.[2] Sixty percent of axial rotation of the entire cervical spine and occiput is found in the upper cervical spine (C0-C2).[16]

THIRD CERVICAL VERTEBRA

The third cervical vertebra is typical of the remaining cervical vertebrae, C3 to C7 (see Figure 8-1). The vertebral body is wider than it is high, and its superior surface is raised laterally to form the uncinate processes (uncovertebral joints or joints of von Luschka). The inferior vertebral surface resembles the superior surface of the inferior vertebra, and the anterior border shows a beaklike projection facing downward. These articular processes, which are part of the posterior arch, have both superior and inferior articulating facets. The superior facet is oriented superiorly and posteriorly and corresponds to the inferior facet of the overlying vertebra; the inferior facet faces inferiorly and anteriorly and corresponds to the superior facet of the underlying vertebra. These articular processes are attached to the vertebral body by the pedicles so that the spaces between the processes form the articular pillar. The transverse processes form a gutter and contain a transverse foramen for passage of the vertebral artery (see Figure 8-1). The two lamina, which are oblique inferiorly and laterally, meet at the midline to form

the bifid spinous process.[2] In the upper cervical spine complex, the articular surfaces of the OA and AA joints are in a horizontal plane, but C2-C3 articular processes or facets have an abrupt frontal oblique slope.[17]

Motion of the C2-C3 Segment

Motion of the C2-C3 segment is representative of the typical cervical vertebral segment, with an intervertebral disc and eight plane articulations, including four articular (apophyseal) facets and four uncovertebral joints (joints of von Luschka). The axis of motion passes through the nucleus pulposus and allows freedom of movement in all three planes. Because of the orientation of the articular facets, sidebending and rotation occur concomitantly in the same direction.[2] Because of this concomitant motion, pure rotation or pure sidebending is impossible. Sliding of the joint surface depends on the rotation perpendicular to the axis. The relative amount of rotation or sidebending that occurs depends on the obliquity of the articular surfaces in the frontal plane. The more horizontal the joint surface, the more rotation will occur; the more vertical the joint surface, the more sidebending will occur. At the second cervical vertebra, 2 degrees of coupled axial rotation occurs for every 3 degrees of sidebending.[18] The most abrupt change in joint obliquity occurs at the C2-C3 facet. Grieve[17] noted that all cervical facet joints are oriented so that the cervical facet joint surfaces converge in the region of the eyes.

Motion of the C3-C7 Segments

The midcervical spine allows the greatest ranges of motion in the neck (Table 8-3). The inclination of the facet surfaces of these vertebrae is 45 degrees to the horizontal plane. The lower segments are steeper than the upper segments. As in the C2-C3 segment, sidebending and rotation occur concomitantly in the same direction because of the oblique plane of the articular surfaces. However, at each motion segment, opposite gliding of the articular surfaces is seen. For example, with right rotation or right sidebending, the left superior articular facet glides superiorly and anteriorly, while the right superior articular facet glides posteriorly and inferiorly, both on their adjoining inferior articular surfaces.[1] The total amount of sidebending in this region is 35 to 37 degrees, and total rotation is 45 degrees. With pure flexion and extension, both superior facets at each motion segment glide in the same direction. With flexion, both facets move superiorly; with extension, both move inferiorly. Total range of flexion and extension in the lower cervical column is 100 to 110 degrees.[2] At the seventh cervical vertebra, 1 degree of coupled axial rotation is seen for every 7.5 degrees of sidebending.[18]

UPPER THORACIC SPINE

The upper thoracic spine must be included in any discussion of the cervical spine because movement of the lower cervical spine occurs in conjunction with movement of the upper

Table 8-3	Limits and Representative Values of Ranges of Rotation of the Middle and Lower Cervical Spine					
	Combined Flexion-Extension ($\pm x$-axis rotation)		One-Side Lateral Bending (z-axis rotation)		One-Side Axial Rotation (y-axis rotation)	
Interspace	Limits of Ranges, degrees	Representative Angle, degrees	Limits of Ranges, degrees	Representative Angle, degrees	Limits of Ranges, degrees	Representative Angle, degrees
Middle						
C2-C3	5-16	10	11-20	10	0-10	3
C3-C4	7-26	15	9-15	11	3-10	7
C4-C5	13-29	20	0-16	11	1-12	7
Lower						
C5-C6	13-29	20	0-16	8	2-12	7
C6-C7	6-26	17	0-17	7	2-10	6
C7-T1	4-7	9	0-17	4	0-7	2

Data from White A, Panjabi MM: Clinical biomechanics of the spine, ed 2, Philadelphia, 1990, Lippincott, Williams, and Wilkins.

thoracic spine. Gross cervical spine movements include upper thoracic spine motion as a result of distal attachment of the cervical muscles to as low as T6 in the case of the splenius, longissimus, and semispinalis cervicis and semispinalis capitis muscles.[19] To accommodate the more frontal orientation of the thoracic articular facets, the seventh cervical vertebra makes a transition in its plane of facet motion. Besides having all the characteristics of a typical vertebra, a thoracic vertebra has specific characteristics that distinguish it from a cervical vertebra. Thoracic vertebrae have no uncovertebral joints, bifid spinous processes, or intertransverse foramina. The attachments of the ribs to the thoracic vertebral bodies allow stability at the expense of mobility, with motion of the facet articulations occurring to a greater extent in the frontal plane. The spinous processes incline inferiorly.[2]

Ribs

The first two ribs are atypical in that they have only one facet. The first rib is the most curved and usually is the shortest rib. This rib slopes obliquely downward and forward from the vertebra toward the sternum. Because of the costovertebral orientation, primarily in the transverse plane, movements occur in a superior-inferior direction, with a resultant "pump-handle" effect, with secondary movement in the medial-lateral direction described as "bucket-handle" movement. The second rib is about twice as long the first but has a similar curvature. The first rib is the site of insertion for the anterior and middle scalene muscles and the site of origin for the subclavius and the first digit of the serratus anterior. The second rib is the site of origin for the serratus anterior and the site of insertion for the posterior scalene and serratus posterior superior muscles.[19]

A typical rib has two articulations with adjacent vertebrae; the costovertebral joint articulates with demifacets on the vertebral bodies, and the costotransverse joint articulates between the rib tubercle and the transverse process of the underlying vertebra. The costovertebral joint is a synovial joint with condyloid movement because the head of the rib is convex and moves on the concave costal facets of the vertebra. The costotransverse joint is a simple synovial joint that allows a gliding movement. Both of these joints are reinforced by strong ligaments.[19,20]

During breathing, the axis of the costovertebral joints of the upper ribs lies close to the frontal plane, allowing an increase in the anteroposterior diameter of the thorax. Because of the fiber orientation of the scalene muscles superior to the first two ribs, these muscles can elevate these ribs and influence rib motion.[20]

VERTEBRAL ARTERY

The vertebral artery enters the costotransverse foramen of C6 (sometimes that of C5) and traverses to the axis through the costovertebral foramina of the individual vertebrae. After entering the costotransverse foramen of the atlas, the artery exits and penetrates the atlanto-occipital membrane and the dura mater in the region of the foramen magnum at the occiput.[19] Functionally, the vertebral artery is important because the decreased blood supply in the basilar region of the brain stem reduces one of the main blood supplies to the brain. Selecki[21] observed that after 30 degrees of rotation, kinking of the contralateral vertebral artery occurs first as the vertebral artery exits from the transverse foramina. It becomes more marked as the angle of rotation is increased. At 45 degrees of neck rotation, the ipsilateral artery also begins to kink.[21] Typical neurologic symptoms of vertebrobasilar artery insufficiency include dizziness, tinnitus, visual disturbances, and nausea.[22,23] Occlusion of the vertebral artery may occur at the suboccipital region or at the C6 level.[24]

THORACIC INLET

Clinicians usually refer to the thoracic inlet as the thoracic outlet; however, from a strictly anatomical point of view, the thoracic outlet is the opening at the inferior portion of the rib cage and the diaphragm.[19] The thoracic inlet is the superior opening of the rib cage, bounded posteriorly by the first thoracic vertebra, anteriorly by the superior border of the manubrium, and laterally by the first ribs. The structures that pass through the inlet include, centrally, sternohyoid muscle, sternothyroid muscles, thymus, trachea, esophagus, and thoracic ducts. Behind these ducts and just in front of the vertebral column are the longus colli muscles and the anterior longitudinal ligament. Laterally, the inlet contains the upper lung and neurovascular structures, which join the lowest trunk of the brachial plexus. Within the thoracic inlet, the vagus nerve deserves special attention because this nerve provides parasympathetic innervation to the pharynx and visceral organs.[19] The complex anatomy of the thoracic inlet and the intimate relationship of the bony, soft tissue, and neurovascular structures within the inlet provide multiple opportunities for compression. The term *thoracic inlet (outlet) syndrome* refers to the compression of neurovascular structures to include arteries, veins, and/or the upper or lower trunk of the brachial plexus.[25]

Musculoskeletal Dysfunction and Trauma

POSTURAL ABNORMALITY

The most common postural deviation affecting the cervical spine is forward head posture. This posture involves increased kyphosis of the thoracic spine, with resultant increased lordosis of the cervical spine and increased backward bending in the upper cervical complex.[26] Over time, persons with forward head posture adjust their head position and decrease the midcervical lordosis.[27] Increased backward bend of the upper cervical complex results from the body's attempt to keep the eyes horizontal.[17] In doing so, the head is anterior to the vertical plumbline (the ideal postural alignment). This postural deviation puts abnormal stress on the soft tissues and changes the weight-bearing surfaces of the vertebrae, especially in the suboccipital and cervicothoracic areas. Forward head posture causes muscle length adaptation, which results in altered biomechanics such that normal motions produce abnormal strain.[28] The muscles most often affected are the levator scapulae, upper trapezius, sternocleidomastoid, scalene, and suboccipital muscles.

Factors that contribute to forward head posture include poor postural habits and pain. We acquire these poor postural habits at a young age when we learn that slumping the upper back requires no energy expenditure. Adolescent girls who are taller and more developed than their peers also develop this posture. In older patients, this posture may be related to working at an incorrect height or in poor lighting. The second factor that contributes to this posture is pain. Many patients with chronic cervical pain compensate by thrusting their head forward in an attempt to move away from the pain. Along with a forward

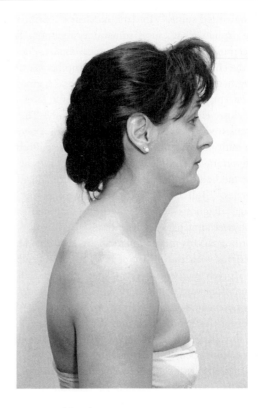

Figure 8-5 Forward head posture.

head posture, patients present with associated postural changes in the head, neck, trunk, and shoulder region, such as a retruded mandible, rounded shoulders, and protracted scapulae with tight anterior muscles and stretched posterior muscles. Because of this direct relationship between pain and posture, postural correction is an appropriate treatment goal for most patients with chronic cervical pain (Figure 8-5).[28]

SOMATIC DYSFUNCTION

By far, the most common cervical pathology seen by manual therapists is vertebral motion restriction or somatic dysfunction. The term *somatic dysfunction* is used by the osteopathic profession to refer to altered function of components of the musculoskeletal system. Many terms such as *loss of joint play,*[29] *chiropractic vertebral subluxation,*[30] *joint dysfunction,*[29] *joint blockage,*[31] and *acute facet lock*[32] describe restrictions of vertebral motion. The osteopathic profession has adopted somatic dysfunction terminology to represent a specific joint restriction in three dimensions. Specifically describing loss of joint movement in terms of its location in relationship to position or its lack of movement allows administration of treatment specific to the restriction.[33,34]

Many theories attempt to explain vertebral motion restriction. These theories range from entrapment of the synovial material[35] or a meniscoid,[36] to hypertonic contracted or contractured musculature,[37] to changes in nervous reflex activity such as sympathicotonia[38] or gamma bias,[39] to abnormal stresses on an unguarded spine.[40] To date, no clear scientific evidence exists to explain what causes somatic dysfunction. However, one conceptual model, the biomechanical model, does help to explain the clinically observable relationship between two vertebral segments or within a group of vertebral segments. This model conceptually defines the inability of the facet joints to open or close, either individually or bilaterally. The method allows consistency between patients for a single examiner and between multiple examiners for the same patient. Probably the most important reason for using this model is that it is an excellent method for distinguishing structural and functional asymmetries.[33] Jull et al[41] have demonstrated the accuracy of manual diagnosis for identifying symptomatic cervical zygapophyseal joint pain syndromes.

According to this manual medicine model, if some pathology interferes with the ability of both the right and the left facet of a given segment to open, that segment will exhibit restriction of forward bending movement. Conversely, if some pathology prevents both facets from closing, backward bending restriction of that segment occurs. If only one facet is unable to open, forward bending movement will be restricted because the facet cannot open, but sidebending movement to the contralateral side also will be limited. In determination of segmental vertebral motion, if both facets are functioning symmetrically, the excursion of paired transverse processes should be symmetrical through forward and backward bending.[42]

CERVICAL SPONDYLOSIS

Cervical spondylosis is the result of wear and tear on the weight-bearing structures of the cervical spine. This degenerative process generally is considered to occur first in the articular cartilage, but it is not limited to the cartilage. Bland[43] uses cervical osteoarthritis to describe all joint involvement, including all secondary manifestations in vertebrae, tendons, ligaments, capsules, muscles, and hyaline cartilage, without the overall assumption that the primary disorder begins in the cartilage. This wear-and-tear phenomenon is attributed to repetitive microtrauma to cartilage caused by sustained impact loading on the bone.[43-46] Changes first occur in the deepest, calcified layer of cartilage, where subchondral bone hyperplasia begins as an irregular advance of ossification into the cartilage. This change becomes evident radiographically as increased bone density and sclerosis. At the vascular borders, where cartilage, bone, synovium, and periosteum meet, a proliferation of bone formation begins, concentrated at the edges of the articular cartilage. These intra-articular osteophytes grow outward and tend to increase the lateral dimensions of the bone ends, thus increasing the joint cavity and stretching the capsule. These bony rims may trespass on pain-sensitive structures. Peripheral osteophytes are covered by a layer of fibrocartilage and are larger than they appear on radiographs because of this radiotranslucent covering. Typically, degeneration occurs at uncovertebral joints (joints of von Luschka), facets, intervertebral discs, vertebral bodies, and hyaline cartilage plates.[17,47]

RIB DYSFUNCTION

Dysfunction of the upper costovertebral joints may cause pain in the cervical spine in the posterior triangle region. Greenman[20] stated that the first and second ribs, because they are atypical, can contribute to pain in the cervicothoracic region. Costovertebral motion allows both pump-handle and bucket-handle movements, as described earlier. If the first and second ribs cannot complete a normal range of motion, several patterns of restriction are possible. The most common dysfunctions are inhalation and exhalation restrictions. If the first rib is not able to complete its anteroposterior range of motion, the motion of all underlying ribs will be restricted. Most often, a rib becomes dysfunctional as a result of the position assumed when a thoracic vertebra is restricted asymmetrically. The result is slight rotation of a rib, with rotation of the corresponding thoracic vertebra related to its inability to follow the rib in a straight plane. With rotation of the thoracic vertebra, the rib also rotates because of the attachment of the ligaments and intercostal muscles above and below the rib. If the vertebra remains rotated, soft tissue around the rib will compensate and adapt to this abnormal position, so the rib becomes hypomobile. If motion is restored to the vertebra, the rib may not return to its normal position because of this soft tissue adaptation. This situation is called *torsional rib dysfunction.*[34]

The first rib also can subluxate superiorly because no structures are present above it to limit its superior excursion. This dysfunction can contribute to a myriad of symptoms, including cervicothoracic pain, difficulty with deep breathing, restricted cervical rotation and sidebending, and possibly, numbness, tingling, and vascular complaints as seen with thoracic inlet syndrome. Often the fibromyositis described in the upper trapezius muscle is accompanied by dysfunction of the first and second ribs.

THORACIC INLET SYNDROME

As was mentioned earlier, thoracic outlet syndrome should be termed *thoracic inlet syndrome* for it to be anatomically correct in describing the superior opening of the thoracic cavity. This syndrome includes a multitude of symptoms involving the neck and upper extremities that are believed to be caused by proximal compression of the subclavian artery and vein and the brachial plexus. Probable causes of compression of the neurovascular structures include a cervical rib, a subluxated first thoracic rib, a shortened anterior scalene muscle, and anomalous fibromuscular bands. Other structures that may be involved in compression include any bony or soft tissue abnormality such as malunion of a fractured clavicle, Pancoast's tumor of the apex of the lung, altered posture, tight pectoralis minor muscles, and anomalous thoracic vertebral transverse processes. Secondary causes associated with thoracic inlet syndrome include trauma, occupational stress, obesity, and pendulous breasts.[25]

VERTEBROBASILAR INSUFFICIENCY

The vertebrobasilar arterial system supplies the spinal cord, meninges and nerve roots, plexuses, muscles, and joints of the cervical spine. Intracranially, the basilar portion supplies the medulla, cerebellum, and vestibular nuclei.[19] This arterial system can be compromised at several points during its course: as it passes through the transverse foramina of the upper six cervical vertebrae; as it winds around the articular pillar of the atlas; as it pierces the posterior OA membrane; and as it enters the foramen magnum to unite with the basilar artery. Blood flow can be diminished by a variety of mechanical disorders, which may be classified as intrinsic or extrinsic. The most common intrinsic disorder is atherosclerosis. The basilar artery is the most commonly affected component, followed by the cervical portion of the vertebral artery. Usually seen as a complication of atherosclerosis, thrombosis of the vertebrobasilar arteries can result from an embolus that usually lodges in the distal branches of the system, particularly the posterior cerebral artery.[17]

An extrinsic disorder compromises a blood vessel, restricting flow by compressing its external wall and thereby narrowing its lumen. This compression can result from the following:

1. An anomalous origin of the vertebral artery from the subclavian, causing the vertebral artery to become kinked and occluded during rotation of the neck.
2. Constriction of the vertebral artery by bands of the deep cervical fascia during rotation of the neck.
3. An anomalous divagation of the vertebral artery from its course through muscle and transverse foramina of the vertebrae, or compression or angulation caused by projecting osteophytes. Compression most commonly occurs at the C5-C6 level, with a lower incidence at the C6-C7 level. When this system is compromised, patients present with nystagmus, vertigo, blurred vision, giddiness, nausea, pallor, dysphagia, pupil dilation, and cervical pain.[17,22,23] Because compromise of the vertebral artery can occur both in the craniovertebral region and in the area where the artery passes through the transverse foramen, all patients who present with cervical pain should be screened for vertebrobasilar artery insufficiency. Manual therapists emphasize the need to test this system in patients with upper cervical complaints; however, serious compromise can occur with damage to the middle and lower cervical regions.[17,24,48] A vertebral artery test for assessing vertebrobasilar insufficiency, described under the objective portion of the examination, always must be performed before any manual therapy for the cervical spine is attempted.

CERVICAL DISC

Cervical disc disease may produce symptoms similar to those of facet involvement and/or neurologic signs caused by root or cord compression. The typical history involves insidious onset after a relatively minor physical activity is performed or a prolonged position is maintained, for example, taking a long car trip, sleeping in an uncomfortable hotel bed, holding the phone with one's shoulder, or working overhead. The pain is usually unilateral and may be felt anywhere in the cervical or scapular area.[45,46,49]

Cloward[50] described the typical referred pain pattern of cervical disc involvement. The pain usually starts in the cervical area and then diminishes and quickly extends to the scapula, shoulder, upper arm, and possibly the forearm and hand.[50] The symptoms of a cervical disc lesion are provoked in a manner similar to those in a restricted facet joint, in that certain cervical movements are painful and others are pain free; however, the pattern of painful and pain-free movements does not follow the pattern for a restricted joint.[51]

Painful or restricted neck movements may be intermittent over several months. Initially, the patient may experience only a paresthesia, but when the nerve root becomes involved, the pain is better defined and can be reproduced with extreme neck movement. Sustained holding of these neck positions will exacerbate arm paresthesia and pain.[43,45] Clinical presentation of root involvement has been described as acute radiculopathy from a posterolateral bulging disc, acute disc extrusion, or exacerbation or preexisting trespass in patients with radiographic evidence of spondylosis. Besides nerve root symptoms, the tendon reflex may be depressed or absent, or muscle weakness may be noted within the myotome. If the disc material is extruded and occupies enough of the spinal canal to put pressure on the cord, the patient may show myelopathic signs such as spasticity, a positive plantar response, clonus, and spastic quadriparesis or paraparesis.[46]

TRAUMA

All patients who present with a history of trauma to the cervical region should have radiographs taken to rule out fractures. Aside from fractures, discussion of which is beyond the scope of this chapter, a common clinical presentation of patients with cervical trauma is *the whiplash syndrome*. This term was introduced to describe the total involvement of the patient with whiplash injury and its effects.[32,52,53] The typical mechanism of injury involves flexion-extension injuries of the cervical spine that result from sudden acceleration and deceleration collision forces on a vehicle in which the patient is riding. The magnitude of this collision force is determined by the mass of the vehicle and its rate of change of velocity. The shorter the impact time, the greater is the rate of change of velocity or acceleration. As the acceleration becomes greater, the force of the impact likewise increases. The faster a vehicle is moving at the time of impact, the greater are the impact forces.[54]

A head-on collision causes deceleration injuries, with the head and neck first moving into hyperflexion and terminating when the chin touches the chest. In keeping with Newton's third law, the head and cervical spine rebound into extension after hyperflexion. These reciprocal flexion-extension movements continue until the forces are finally dissipated.

Side-on collisions cause lateral flexion of the cervical spine, with movement ceasing as the ear hits the shoulder. In rear-end collisions, the car accelerates forward, causing the front seat to be pushed into the trunk of the occupant. This force causes the trunk to be thrust forward. The unrestrained head stays at rest and moves into relative backward bending as the trunk moves forward. This backward bending of the head and cervical spine continues until the occiput strikes the headrest or the thoracic spine. Many patients describe the impact as being so great that their car seat was broken, or their glasses or dentures were thrown into the back seat, or the movement into hyperextension was so great that they came to rest facing the rear of the vehicle. Rebound into flexion occurs after the car stops accelerating and is complemented by contraction of the flexor muscles.[54]

The amount of actual damage that occurs to anatomical structures depends on the position of the head in space at the time of impact, the forces generated, and the histologic makeup of the tissues. In experimental studies simulating rear-end automobile accidents, the following lesions occurred:

1. Tearing of the sternocleidomastoid and longissimus colli muscles
2. Pharyngeal edema and retropharyngeal hematoma
3. Hemorrhage of the muscular layers of the esophagus
4. Damage to the cervical sympathetic plexus
5. Tearing of the anterior longitudinal ligament
6. Separation of the cartilaginous end plate of the intervertebral disc
7. Tearing of the facet joint capsules
8. Hemorrhage about the cervical nerve roots and spinal cord, with possible cerebral injury. The extent of damage seen in hyperflexion (head-on collision) injuries is similar. Damage may include tears of the posterior cervical musculature, sprains of the ligamentum nuchae and posterior longitudinal ligament, facet joint disruption, and posterior intervertebral disc injury with nerve root hemorrhage.[17,54]

Depending on the magnitude and direction of forces at the time of impact, patients may present with any combination of these hyperflexion and hyperextension injuries, as well as damage to the thoracic, lumbar, and temporomandibular joint (TMJ) regions. Whiplash symptoms usually begin within 24 hours after the accident. The patient may describe headache, posterior neck pain, and referred scapular pain. Pain may radiate down the arm, mimicking thoracic inlet syndrome. Other complaints include upper thoracic and pectoral pain, weakness, dysphagia, dyspnea, TMJ dysfunction, and cerebral complaints such as insomnia, fatigue, nervousness, tenseness, decreased concentration span and memory, and hyperirritability. Many patients describe dizziness, which may be associated with a high-frequency hearing loss. They also may have tinnitus and visual disturbances.[17] Because of the complexity of this syndrome, if patients are not evaluated thoroughly and treated appropriately, they may develop postural adaptations, psychogenic overlay, and chronic manifestation of any of the above symptoms.

MYOFASCIAL PAIN SYNDROME

Myofascial pain disorders are not well understood because of the use of a variety of terms to describe similar clinical findings. The different terms used may have the same, similar, or totally different meanings. Myofascial pain syndrome, also referred to as *myofascial syndrome* and *myofasciitis,* involves pain and/or autonomic responses referred from active myofascial trigger points with associated dysfunction. Other terms such as myositis, fibrositis, myalgia, and fibromyositis have multiple meanings.[55] Some authors use these terms to identify myofascial trigger points; others use them to label clinical manifestations.[56] To avoid further confusion, the definition of myofascial pain syndrome used here refers to the trigger point, as described by Travell and Simons.[56] A myofascial trigger point is a hyperirritable spot, usually within a taut band of skeletal muscle or in the fascia of the muscle, that is painful on compression and that can give rise to characteristic referred pain, tenderness, and autonomic phenomena. Normal muscle does not have these trigger points.[56]

A clinical manifestation of myofascial trigger points is a typical referred pain pattern from the trigger point. On examination, findings include local spot tenderness (the trigger point) and a palpably tense band of muscle fibers within a shortened and weak muscle. The trigger point also may respond to rapid changes in pressure; this has been described as the pathognomonic local twitch response. Direct pressure over a trigger point will reproduce referred pain patterns. Travell and Simons[56] contend that a myofascial trigger point begins with muscular strain and later becomes a site of sensitized nerves, increased local metabolism, and reduced circulation. A myofascial trigger point is to be distinguished from a trigger point in other tissues such as skin, ligament, and periosteum. Myofascial trigger points are classified as active or latent. An active trigger point causes pain, whereas a latent trigger point causes restriction of movement and weakness of the affected muscle and may persist for years after apparent recovery from an injury. However, a latent trigger point is predisposed to acute attacks of pain because minor overstretching, overuse, or chilling of the muscle may cause a latent trigger point to become active. These symptoms are not found in normal muscle.[56]

REFERRED PAIN

Pain that is perceived in a location other than its source is termed *referred pain.*[57] Nearly all pain is referred pain. It is referred segmentally, as in a dermatomal distribution, or is specific to the tissue involved, as in left upper extremity pain with myocardial infarction. Recognition of the embryologic derivation of tissues from the same somite is important in identifying many of the segmentally referred pain patterns. For example, as the upper limb bud grows, it draws the lower cervical and upper thoracic segments out into itself. Thus, the scapula and its muscles are derived from the middle and lower cervical segments, whereas the skin overlying the scapula and ribs is formed from the thoracic segments; therefore, pain perceived in the upper posterior thoracic region may have a cervical origin. Also, tissues other than visceral organs may have a specific reference pattern of pain that cannot be ascribed to a segmental distribution.[51] Most practitioners are familiar with patients who complain of suboccipital headache and describe a reference pattern at the frontal region of the cranium.

Although clinical expectation is based on the assumption that a somatic nerve goes to a specific anatomical region, pain in that peripheral distribution can be due only to abnormalities of the spinal segment associated with that nerve. This assumption may be true; however, other pain patterns have been identified. Miller[58] suggested that pain does not really occur in the hands, feet, or head, but rather in the patient's conscious image of his or her hands, feet, or head. This theory suggests that pain and referred pain are central phenomena. A classic example is the phantom pain experienced by some amputees. Supporting this idea of referred pain as a central phenomenon, Harman[59] found that anginal pain referred to the left arm was not abolished by a complete brachial plexus block with local anesthesia. Referred pain has been evoked experimentally in areas previously anesthetized by regional nerve block.[60] Bourdillon[61] suggests that the central mechanism involves both the spinal cord and higher centers.

According to Cyriax,[51] if pain is referred segmentally, a lesion at a cervical level will produce pain in all or part of that cervical dermatome. For example, a C5 nerve root compression may produce pain in the neck, midneck, shoulder, and/or lateral upper arm. All these areas are supplied by the C5 dermatome. Although this relationship appears clear-cut, some research and clinical experience show that the pain reference appears to be segmental in nature yet does not always correspond to dermatome or myotome distributions.[17,62-64] Because some referred pain patterns are not easily ascribed to particular segments, the clinician must perform a detailed, specific examination to determine the source of the pain. Experienced therapists are familiar with specific reference patterns that have several separate possible sources. An example is the clinical presentation of unilateral pain along the trapezial ridge (yoke area), which may be produced by dysfunction of the OA joint, the C4-C5 segment, or the joints of the first rib. Treatment for these dysfunctions may relieve the symptoms; however, any two or all three sites may have to be treated before the signs and symptoms are eliminated.[61] Dwyer et al[65] produced pain patterns from the cervical zygapophyseal joints in normal volunteers; this further substantiates the view that the cervical joints are sources of referred pain. Feinstein et al[60] described patients with frontal headache referred from the OA joint.

Some general characteristics of segmentally referred pain are that the pain usually is referred distally from the cervical spine; the pain never crosses the midline; and the extent of pain is controlled by the size of the dermatome and the location of the tissue involved. A tissue that does not follow segmental reference is the dura mater. Again with consideration of the C5 dermatome, a lesion at the nerve root level can result in a larger dermatomal reference pattern than a lesion of C5-derived tissue at the shoulder level.[51] A lesion at the cervical level may cause

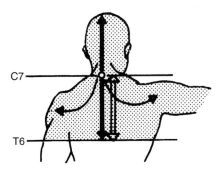

Figure 8-6 Extrasegmental reference of the dura mater.

pain anywhere from the head to the midthorax, and this pain often pervades several dermatomal levels. Symptoms are usually central or unilateral (Figure 8-6).[51,57]

OTHER PATHOLOGIES

This discussion of cervical pathologies is by no means all-inclusive; other pathologies of nonmusculoskeletal origin also can elicit cervical pain. Some of these disorders, if not recognized, can have serious consequences. The clinical picture seen in these disorders differs significantly from symptoms of musculoskeletal origin. These differences include the presence of night pain, as seen with metastatic disease; cord signs such as Lhermitte's sign, the positive plantar response, and ankle clonus, as seen in myelopathies; nuchal rigidity, as seen in spinal meningitis or subarachnoid hemorrhage; and brachial plexus tension signs, as seen in brachial plexus neuritis or stretch injuries. Unrelenting, pulsating pain may be seen in a patient with an aortic aneurysm. Patients with advanced rheumatoid arthritis may present with the neck in the characteristic "cocked robin" position because of unilateral subluxation of the AA joint. Systemic infections may enlarge the lymph nodes and cause neck pain, as is seen in sinusitis, pharyngitis, otitis media, mediastinitis, and dental abscess. Other symptoms not usually seen with pain of musculoskeletal origin include unrelenting pain, severe symptoms after a trivial insult, and neurologic symptoms such as blurred vision, visual field deficit, and loss of motor control.[66,67]

History and Physical Examination

PATIENT HISTORY

The importance of careful and precise history taking cannot be overemphasized. The clinician ultimately will base a treatment plan on the patient's presenting signs and symptoms. The history should always precede the evaluation because areas of emphasis during the examination will be determined by the history. Hoppenfeld[68] stated that this selective examination, based on a good history, produces the highest yield of information about clinical disease in the shortest time.

Asking concise, clinically relevant questions is a far more complex skill than the actual techniques of physical examination. Learning how to ask those questions by reading textbooks or listening to lectures is difficult. Good history taking is both an art and a science. A closed-end question asks for a yes or no answer. Many practitioners, in an attempt to hurry the interview, will guide the patient in answering by the way they ask the questions. A yes or no response may reflect only a portion of what the patient may really want to say. The questioning process should use open-ended rather than closed-ended questions, to allow the patient to answer in his or her own words. Instead of asking "Do you have pain?" the questioner could phrase the question as "Where do you have discomfort?" The second question requires the patient to formulate his or her own answer and probably will yield more useful information than the first question. This approach helps keep the examiner from jumping to conclusions and forces the examiner to attend to the patient as a person rather than as a disease entity.

While taking the history and performing the evaluation, the clinician should record the findings in a format that is easy to interpret and familiar to other health professions. The "subjective, objective, assessment, and plan" (SOAP) note format meets these criteria. It can be used for initial evaluations, progress notes, and discharge summaries. Although notes are important for communicating with other professionals, this record is also invaluable to the clinician as a quick reference on each patient.

The patient's chief complaint or complaints should be documented carefully. Initially, the patient should be allowed to tell his or her own story for several minutes without interruption; otherwise, important details may be pushed aside in his or her mind. The clinician then may have to guide the patient's comments with a question such as, "How did your neck problem begin?" to get a chronologic picture of the symptoms. The clinician should ask open-ended questions to find out important details about the symptoms, such as the time of day they occur, the location of the pain, and the relation of symptoms to other events. In evaluating the cervical and upper thoracic spine, the clinician should follow the general rule of evaluating the joints above and below the joint being examined and should ask the patient questions about the cranium, TMJ, and shoulder. Actual analysis of the patient's symptoms follows a logical sequence for any musculoskeletal evaluation.

Identifying the Patient's Complaints

Identifying the patient's cervical complaint is a logical introduction to establishing rapport between the therapist and the patient. Documenting the chief complaint includes noting the location of the symptoms and how the patient describes the symptoms.[69] The total area in which the patient has pain must be documented. Therefore, the area and depth of symptoms should be mapped out on a body chart for future reference. The patient also should be questioned about the nature of the pain. Typically, superficial electric shock–like pain is derived from a dermatomal reference; deep, aching, diffuse pain may come from a myotomal or sclerotomal reference.[51] Upper extremity

numbness or tingling may help the clinician pinpoint the involvement of a specific nerve root.

Present History

The patient's current history should be established before the past history is taken. The examiner should consider precipitating factors related to the onset of current symptoms. Again, the patient should have the opportunity to say what he or she thinks may have caused the problem before the clinician begins to conduct systematic questioning. If a specific injury occurred, the clinician should try to determine the exact mechanism of injury. The clinician also should ask about the onset (whether immediate or delayed) and degree of pain. This information will assist the practitioner in implicating specific tissues. For example, injured muscle or vascular tissue will cause immediate pain, whereas injury to noncontractile structures may cause delayed onset of symptoms.[70] This information allows the clinician to focus on selecting special tests that are appropriate to perform during the examination.

Behavior of Symptoms

Asking the patient to describe his or her symptoms over a 24-hour period is valuable in establishing which activities aggravate or relieve symptoms, and how long the symptoms last. It also provides a baseline for future comparison. The clinician must know about the frequency and duration of the patient's symptoms (i.e., whether they are constant or intermittent). If dysfunction is present, specific movements should exacerbate or relieve the symptoms, and rest should decrease them. Answers to the clinician's questions will reveal the positions, movements, and activities that exacerbate or relieve symptoms and will provide additional information about the nature of the problem, the tissue source of irritation, and the severity of the condition. If rest does not relieve the symptoms, and the patient describes them as constant and unrelenting, the cause of the problem may not be musculoskeletal.

Past History

If the patient has experienced similar symptoms in the past, this information is vital to the examiner. Clear information about the frequency and onset of symptoms, the recovery period, and treatment provided for previous episodes will help establish the correct diagnosis and treatment plan. Other details of the patient's past medical history such as cardiac problems, trauma, and surgeries, as well as bony pathologies such as arthritis and osteoporosis, may be pertinent and may affect treatment plans. The patient's social history is another important consideration (Table 8-4).

REVIEW OF SYSTEMS

The patient's current symptoms can be influenced easily by visceral or neurologic involvement; therefore, the clinician

Table 8-4	Review of Systems			
Symptom		**Yes**	**No**	**Comments**
1. Fever/chills/sweats				
2. Unexplained weight loss				
3. Fatigue/malaise				
4. Change in physical features				
5. Bruising/bleeding				
6. Vertigo/dizziness				
7. Dyspnea				
8. Nausea/vomiting				
9. Change in bowel habits				
10. Dysuria				
11. Urinary frequency changes				
12. Numbness/tingling				
13. Night pain				
14. Syncope				
15. Weakness				
16. Sexual dysfunction				
17. History of smoking				
18. History of substance abuse				
19. History of illness				
20. History of surgery				
21. Medications				
22. Family medical history				
23. Change in lifestyle				

should ask questions about gastrointestinal function, including recent weight loss, abdominal pain, change in bowel habits, or blood in the stool. Questions about the genitourinary system involve asking about polyuria, dysuria, blood in the urine, and problems with sexual function or menses. Questions pertaining to the cardiopulmonary systems include asking about ease of breathing, coughing, palpitations, hemoptysis, and chest pain. To rule out central nervous system disorders, the clinician should ask about lack of coordination, seizures, dizziness, tremors, and headaches (see Table 8-4).

All of this information will give the practitioner a general idea about the patient's cervical problems. However, some specific questions, including the following, not only will provide information about the problem but will help the clinician to rule out more serious pathologies:

1. Is the patient experiencing any headaches? Several disorders can cause headache. However, headaches from cervical spine problems usually present with specific referral patterns. Problems at the first cervical level usually cause headaches in a characteristic pattern at the base and top of the head. The second cervical level tends to refer ipsilateral pain retro-orbitally in the temporal region. Lower cervical problems frequently are referred to the base of the occiput.[70]

2. Is the patient experiencing dizziness, especially on rotation or extension of the spine? These symptoms may be due to vertebral artery occlusion or inner ear disorders.[71] Disorders of the cervical spine also can cause vertigo.[72]

3. Is the patient experiencing bilateral numbness or tingling of the hands or feet? Bilateral symptoms should lead the

therapist to suspect a large space-occupying lesion pressing on the spinal cord or a systemic disorder causing neuropathies, such as diabetes or alcohol abuse.[66]

4. Does the patient experience difficulty in swallowing? Anterior space-occupying lesions can cause retropharyngeal compromise. With a history of trauma, swelling may be the space-occupying lesion.[66,67]

5. Does the patient experience any electric shock–like pain? If the head is flexed and the patient experiences such pain down the spine, the therapist should consider the possibility of inflammation or irritation of the meninges (Lhermitte's sign).[49,66]

6. What kind of pillow does the patient sleep on? Cervical symptoms often are increased when a foam or very firm pillow is used, as a result of loss of cervical lordosis or abnormal pressure placed against the neck caused by lack of support.[17]

Objective Testing

Besides findings of the upper quarter screening examination (Table 8-5), the clinician needs specific objective information about the cervical spine. This information allows the practitioner to confirm the subjective findings and to identify the area that is the source of the patient's symptoms. Further, more specialized objective testing will help to isolate the structure or structures at fault. As was mentioned in the section on patient history, according to the upper quarter screen format, TMJ, shoulder, and thoracic spine joints should be cleared during the cervical spine examination. The neurologic examination should include muscle stretch reflexes; sensation testing that incorporates light touch, pinprick, and two-point discrimination; and specific muscle testing if weakness was found during the screening examination. The following special tests should be performed only if warranted by the patient's history or findings obtained during the upper quarter screen (Table 8-6).

Range-of-Motion Assessment

Observation of active cervical range of motion will give the clinician a general impression of movement dysfunction. For example, active sidebending that is restricted in the first few degrees from neutral position suggests a restriction in the upper cervical complex. In contrast, restriction at the end range of sidebending suggests a restriction in the mid- to lower cervical region.[73] If active movements are full and pain free, introduce overpressure to stress structures further, to clear that specific range of motion.

When range of motion is restricted, establishing an objective and reliable baseline assessment of the limitation of motion is important. Objective measurement of active range of motion of the neck can be performed through a variety of techniques, including the use of electrogoniometers, bubble and gravity goniometers, protractors, radiographs, and computed tomography.[74] Some of these techniques are more readily available

Table 8-5   Upper Quarter Screening Examination

Standing	• Posture • Gait • Reverse hands overhead • Hands behind back	Cervical spine (cont'd)	• Sidebending • Flexion • Backward bending • Quadrant • Compression/distraction • Resisted motions (all three planes)

Sitting	• Vital signs (temperature, pulse, blood pressure)
	• Observation of lips, nails, hair, lesions
	• Head:
	  • Eyes: Observation, acuity, visual fields, pupillary reaction, near reaction
	  • Ears: Observation, palpation, acuity
	  • Nose: Observation, breathing, sinuses, smell
	  • Mouth: Gums, teeth, tongue, gag reflex
		Scapula
		
		Shoulder/elbow/
		wrist/hand
		Neurologic
			• Active elevation/protraction/retraction/depression
			• Resisted elevation
			• Active range of motion
			• Overpressure
			• Resisted myotomes
			• Shoulder abduction C5-C6 (axillary nerve)
			• Elbow flexion C5-C6 (musculocutaneous nerve)

Neck	• Observation • Soft tissue and lymph node palpation • Salivary glands • Carotid pulses • Trachea/thyroid gland		• Elbow extension C7 (radial nerve) • Wrist extension C6 (radial/ulnar nerves) • Thumb extension C8 (radial nerve) • Finger abduction/adduction T1 (radial/median nerves)
Upper extremity	• Skin • Pulses • Lymph node—epitrochlear • Muscle tone/definition		• Reflexes • Muscle stretch reflexes • Biceps C5-C6 • Brachioradialis C6
Thorax	• Breathing/respiration • Axillary lymph nodes • Auscultation/palpation/percussion		• Triceps C7 • Pathologic (Hoffmann's) • Cutaneous sensation
Temporomandibular joint	• Open/close/lateral movement • Jaw reflex	Supine	• Palpation
Cervical spine	• Active range of motion: • Rotation		• Passive mobility testing C-spine • Inhalation/exhalation rib cage testing

Table 8-6   Schematic for Objective Examination of the Cervical and Upper Thoracic Spine

Range-of-Motion Tests	Special Tests	Thoracic Inlet Syndrome Tests
Active ROM of cervical and upper thoracic spine	Cervical distraction	Adson's
Functional occipitoatlantal range of motion	Cervical compression	Costoclavicular
Functional atlantoaxial range of motion	Vertebral artery	Hyperabduction
Foraminal closure	Layer palpation	3-Minute elevated arm exercise
Upper cervical	Transverse process	
Mid- and lower cervical	Spatial orientation, upper thoracic spine	
Passive mobility	Trigger points	
Translation occipitoatlantal, atlantoaxial, midcervical	Neurologic examination	
Transverse process positioning through flexion/ extension in upper thoracic spine	Motor testing	
Spring testing or ribs	Sensation testing	
Active respiratory motion	Muscle stretch reflexes	
	Radiographs	

and are easier to use than others and have high reliability. One technique that meets all three of these criteria is the cervical range-of-motion device (CROM) (Figure 8-7). The CROM is a plastic device that is affixed to the patient's head and aligned according to the three planes of movement. Sagittal and frontal plane motions are measured with the use of gravity goniome-ters. The transverse plane measurement involves a compass goniometer and a shoulder-mounted magnetic yoke.[74] Several studies have addressed the reliability of the CROM and have found it to be satisfactory.[75,76] The CROM also has been used to establish normal cervical range-of-motion values (Table 8-7).

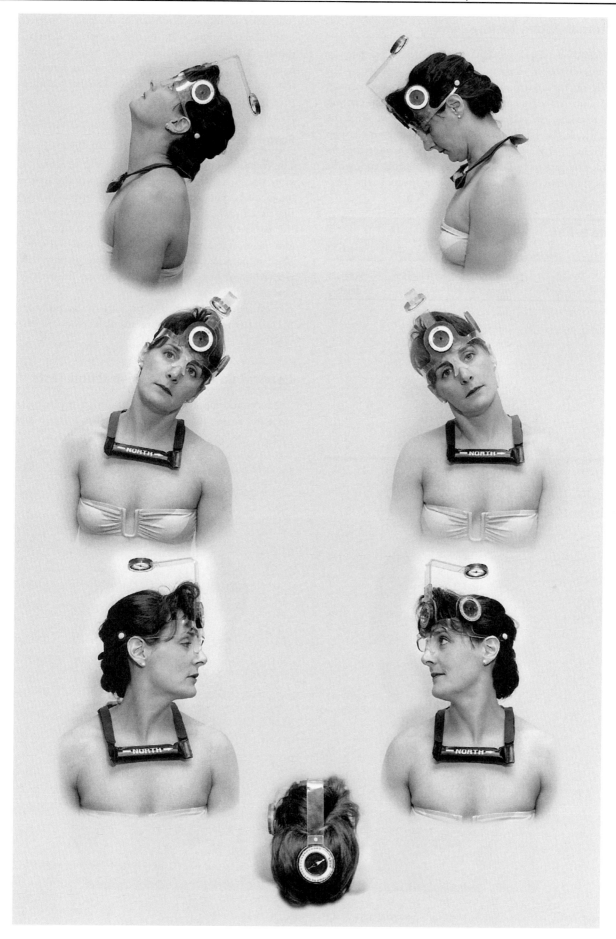

Figure 8-7 Active cervical range of motion using the CROM device.

Functional Active Testing

Several combined active movements can alert the practitioner to regions of the cervical spine that may be restricted. For example, in assessing movement of the upper cervical spine, the OA joint can be tested grossly by fully rotating the cervical spine and asking the patient to nod his or her head while the clinician looks for asymmetrical movement between the two sides (Figure 8-8, A, B). A gross test of the AA joint consists of asking the patient to sidebend as far as possible and, while sidebent, to rotate the head in the opposite direction; the clini-cian looks for restricted movement (R. Erhard, personal communication) (Figure 8-9). To test motion in the midcervical spine, ask the patient to sidebend the head and, while maintaining that range, to introduce flexion and extension. These tests tell the practitioner only whether further mobility testing is required.

Foraminal Closure Tests

The combination of cervical rotation and sidebending to the same side together with extension narrows the intervertebral foramen and puts the mid- and lower cervical facet joints in the closed-packed position.[4,40,73] If this maneuver reproduces the patient's symptoms (i.e., neck, interscapular, or upper arm pain), the cervical spine is implicated (Figure 8-10). With respect to referred pain, the more distally the pain is referred from the cervical spine, the longer the neck is held in normal lordosis while the patient actively bends the upper cervical complex backward and maintains that position (Figure 8-11).[73] If the patient's symptoms are reproduced, the test is positive.

Cervical Compression/Distraction Tests

The cervical compression test is performed by placing the head in slight flexion and sidebending and exerting a downward compressive force through the head (Figure 8-12).[68] To further test the integrity of bony and soft tissue relationships, place the neck into a combined movement pattern of sidebending,

Table 8-7	Normal Values of Cervical Range of Motion Using the CROM			
Age, years	Flexion, degrees	Extension, degrees	Lateral Flexion, degrees	Rotation, degrees
10	67	86	49	76
20	64	81	46	72
30	61	76	43	68
40	58	71	40	65
50	55	66	36	62
60	52	62	33	58
70	49	58	30	55
80	46	54	27	52
90	43	49	24	49

CROM, Cervical range-of-motion device.

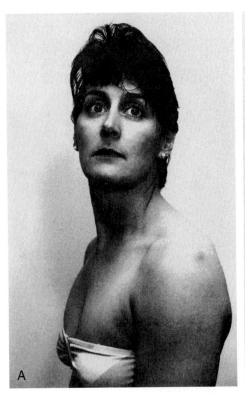
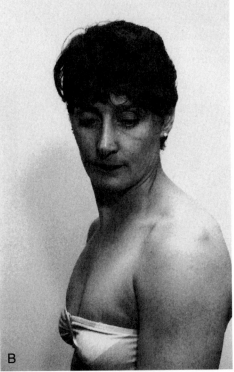

Figure 8-8 Functional active testing of the occipitoatlantal joint. **A,** Extension. **B,** Flexion.

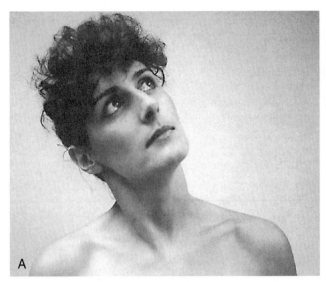 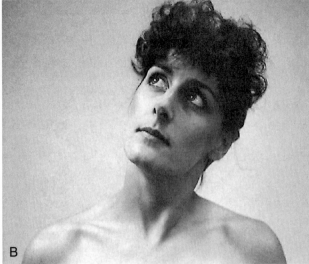

Figure 8-9 A and **B,** Functional active testing of the atlantoaxial joint.

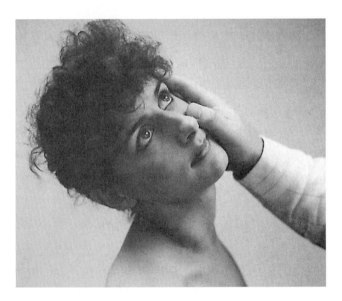

Figure 8-10 Mid- and lower cervical foraminal closure test.

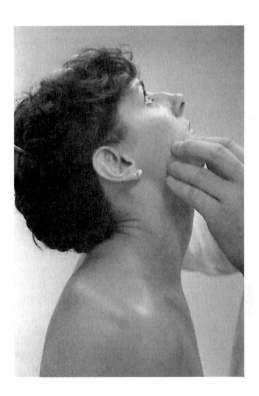

Figure 8-11 Upper cervical foraminal closure test.

extension, and rotation in the same direction, and exert a compression force. This variation is done if the first procedure has not produced any symptoms. If no symptoms are produced by placing the neck in a closed-packed position and then exerting a compression force, the clinician can be satisfied that no major musculoskeletal pathology exists. By approximating the articular surfaces, the compression test assesses foraminal patency and joint relationships. If a motion segment loses its normal anatomic spatial relationships, pain-sensitive tissue may be compromised. Therefore, the compression test is positive if this maneuver elicits articular or neural signs. Conversely, a distraction force, which separates the joint surfaces and stretches adjacent soft tissues, should decrease symptoms caused by a tissue that was being compromised by compression. A cervical distraction test is performed by having the seated patient lean

against the clinician, who stands behind the patient. The clinician slightly grasps the patient's head over the mastoid processes and, while maintaining the head and neck in a neutral position, lifts the patient's head so that the patient's body weight provides the distraction. This distraction test is positive when the patient's symptoms are decreased (Figure 8-13).[70]

Vertebral Artery Test

Provocative testing of vertebrobasilar sufficiency is necessary if the head is going to be moved through extremes of motion.

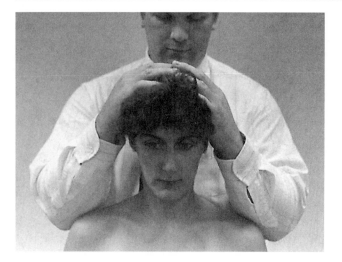

Figure 8-12 Cervical compression test.

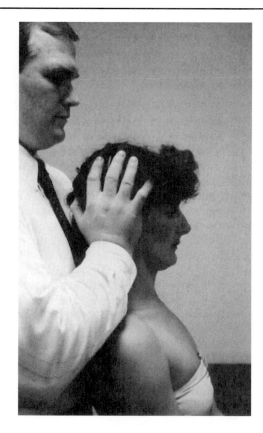

Figure 8-13 Cervical distraction test.

The vertebral artery should be tested in both a weight-bearing and a non–weight-bearing position.[24] The weight-bearing position is done with the patient seated; place the patient's head in a neutral position, and have the patient actively rotate the head to both sides (Figure 8-14). If no symptoms are produced, place the head and neck in extension, and have the patient go through active rotation. If active movement does not produce symptoms, the examiner slowly moves the head passively, asking the patient to report any symptoms experienced during the test. The non–weight-bearing test is performed with the patient supine and the head supported by the examiner off the edge of the table. From this position, the head is passively extended and rotated to either side (Figure 8-15). This position of extension and rotation is maintained for 10 to 15 seconds while the examiner observes the patient's eye movements (nystagmus) and looks for asymmetrical pupil changes. Patient reports of any unusual sensations such as dizziness, giddiness, light-headedness, or visual changes are also positive test findings.[1,24] A variation of this test is to have the patient count backward out loud. If the patient has diminished blood flow, he or she usually will stop talking before other symptoms are manifested.

Upper Limb Tension Test

Elvey[77] demonstrated on cadavers during autopsy that movement of and tension on cervical nerve roots, their investing sheaths, and the dura occur with movement of the arm in certain planes. Maximum tension on the brachial plexus and on C5, C6, and C7 nerve root complexes occurs with glenohumeral joint horizontal abduction and external rotation, elbow and wrist extension, forearm supination, shoulder girdle depression, and sidebending of the cervical spine to the opposite side. Butler[78] advocated the use of four upper limb tension tests (ULTTs):

1. ULTT1—median nerve dominant tension test that uses shoulder abduction

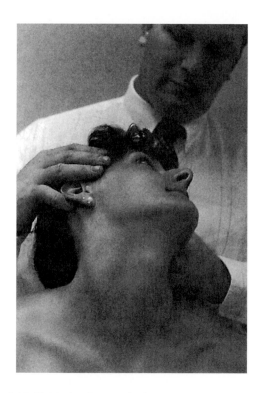

Figure 8-14 Weight-bearing vertebral artery test.

2. ULTT2a—median nerve dominant tension test that uses shoulder girdle depression and external rotation of the shoulder

3. ULTT2b—radial nerve dominant tension test that uses shoulder girdle depression and internal rotation of the shoulder

4. ULTT3—ulnar nerve dominant tension test that uses shoulder abduction and elbow flexion

Tension tests are powerful nervous system tensioning maneuvers that bias to a particular nerve trunk. The ULTT1 positions the patient supine, with the shoulder girdle held in

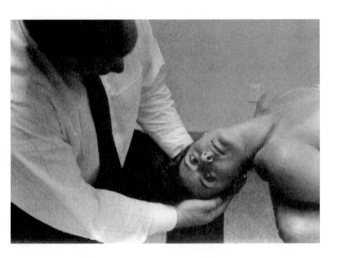

Figure 8-15 Non–weight-bearing vertebral artery test.

neutral position, the arm abducted to 110 degrees, the forearm supinated, and the wrist and fingers extended. The shoulder is rotated externally, and then the elbow is extended. With this position maintained, cervical sidebending first away from and then toward the limb that is being tested is added (Figure 8-16). Margarey[79] reported that in performing this test, when sidebending of the neck was toward the side of the arm being tested, the patient's symptoms decreased 70% of the time. This test assists the clinician in identifying the source of vague or recalcitrant shoulder or upper arm pain. If this maneuver reproduces the patient's arm pain, the test can be broken down into its parts to see which component actually insults the brachial plexus.[78,80]

ULTT2a is a predominantly median nerve bias tension test. The patient lies supine, with the scapula free of the table. The examiner's thigh rests against the patient's elbow. The patient's shoulder girdle is depressed, the shoulder is abducted 10 degrees, the elbow is extended, and then the arm is rotated externally. This position is maintained, and the patient's wrist/fingers/thumb are extended. The most common sensitizing addition is shoulder abduction (Figure 8-17).

The ULTT2b radial nerve bias test has the same starting position as the ULTT2a test; the difference consists of adding internal rotation of the entire arm (also involving forearm pronation). At this point, the position is held while the patient's wrist is flexed; this is followed by thumb flexion and ulnar deviation (Figure 8-18).

The ULTT3 is an ulnar nerve biased tension test. ULTT3 differs from ULTT1 and ULTT2 in that it introduces elbow flexion followed by wrist/finger extension (Figure 8-19).[78]

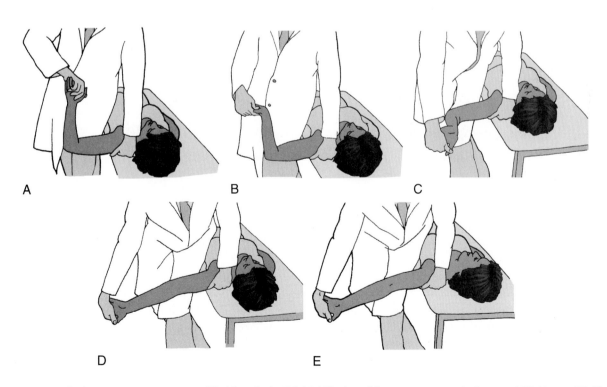

A   B   C

D   E

Figure 8-16 Upper limb tension test (ULTT1). (Modified from Butler DS: Mobilisation of the nervous system. In Cameron MH, Monroe LB: Physical rehabilitation: evidence-based examination, evaluation, and intervention, St. Louis, 2008, Saunders.)

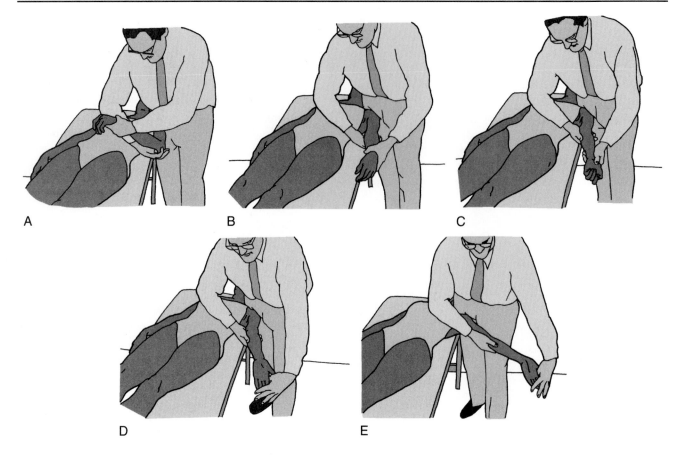

Figure 8-17 Upper limb tension test (ULTT2a). (Modified from Butler DS: Mobilisation of the nervous system. In Cameron MH, Monroe LB: Physical rehabilitation: evidence-based examination, evaluation, and intervention, St. Louis, 2008, Saunders.)

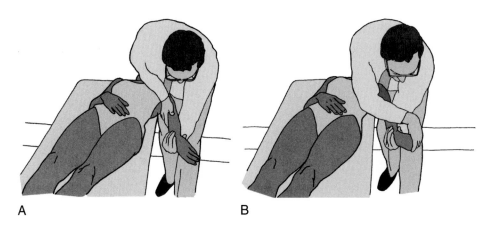

Figure 8-18 Upper limb tension test (ULTT2b). (Modified from Butler DS: Mobilisation of the nervous system. In Cameron MH, Monroe LB: Physical rehabilitation: evidence-based examination, evaluation, and intervention, St. Louis, 2008, Saunders.)

Passive Mobility Testing

Besides physical examination of the cervical spine, the clinician must assess passive motion from a manual medicine viewpoint. To enhance understanding of the passive movement of the cervical spine, a review of spinal mechanics is appropriate.

Vertebral motion is described by facet function; however, the intervertebral disc and the soft tissues also participate in motion. Available motion was described by Fryette[81] in terms of three basic laws of motion. The first law states that when the anteroposterior curve is in a neutral position (where facets are not engaged), bending to one side is accompanied by rotation to the opposite side. This law is in effect in typical thoracic and lumbar spines. The second law states that when the anteroposterior curve is flexed or extended, sidebending and rotation occur in the same direction. This law is seen in the typical cervical spinal segment and is in effect in the typical thoracic and lumbar spine. Fryette's third law states that when motion

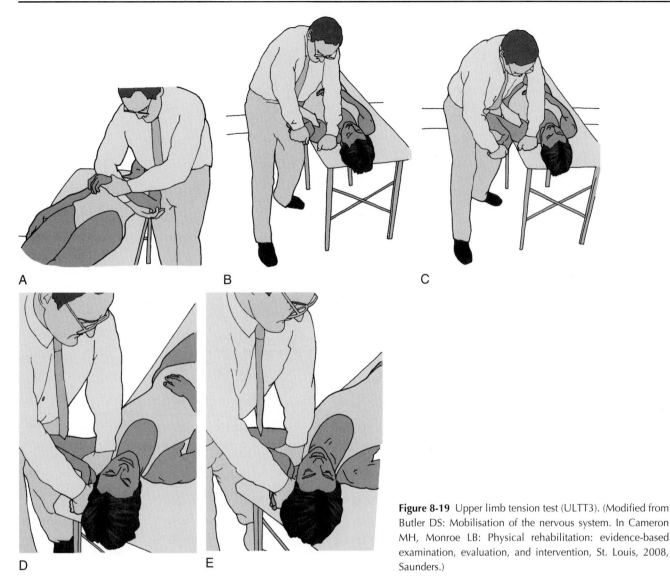

A   B   C

D   E

Figure 8-19 Upper limb tension test (ULTT3). (Modified from Butler DS: Mobilisation of the nervous system. In Cameron MH, Monroe LB: Physical rehabilitation: evidence-based examination, evaluation, and intervention, St. Louis, 2008, Saunders.)

is introduced in one direction, motion in all other directions is restricted. This law is evident when rotation in a forward head posture is compared with rotation with the head aligned over the trunk. Even though rotation occurs in the horizontal plane, rotation is restricted with a forward head posture because of accentuation of flexion of the lower cervical spine and extension of the upper cervical spine.[33,34]

Motion can be described in terms of the superior vertebra moving on the inferior vertebra during a motion segment. In the cervical spine, passive movement can be evaluated by using translation in the frontal plane. By side gliding a cervical vertebra, the clinician imparts a sidebending force. For example, with a left side glide of C4 on C5, a right sidebending movement occurs. Because sidebending and rotation occur concomitantly, the clinician also is assessing rotation to the right. This translation maneuver allows the operator to assess the quantity of movement, as well as end-feel resistance. Because rotation and sidebending occur in the same direction in the midcervical spine, according to Fryette's second law, the ability to sidebend and rotate must be determined both in flexion and in extension.

By comparing translation to the right versus to the left, the clinician can assess the total movement available at that segment.[82,83]

Restricted motion can be described either by the location of the superior segment in space or by the motion that is restricted. The location or position of the superior segment is described using the past participle (e.g., extended, flexed, rotated, sidebent). The suffixes used for physiologic motion restriction are extension, flexion, rotation, and sidebending. For example, in C4 vertebral motion on C5 for right sidebending, the right inferior articular process of C4 biomechanically glides inferiorly and posteriorly on the superior articular process of C5. At the same time, the left inferior articular process of C4 glides anteriorly and superiorly on the superior articular process of C5 (Figure 8-20). If right sidebending is restricted, the superior segment (C4) is left sidebent or in a relative position of left sidebending. The positional diagnosis is described in terms of restriction in three planes. If right sidebending is restricted, right rotation at that segment also will be restricted, because rotation and sidebending are

NECK EXTENDED TO LEVEL

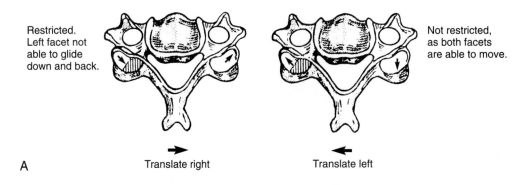

Restricted. Left facet not able to glide down and back.

Not restricted, as both facets are able to move.

A

Translate right   Translate left

NECK FLEXED

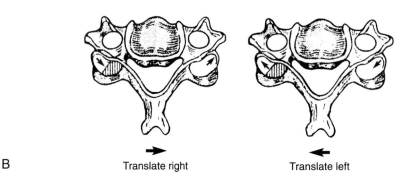

B

Translate right   Translate left

Figure 8-20 Translation of C4 on C5, illustrating a motion barrier. Arrows indicate the direction of the superior facet moving on the inferior facet. Diagonal lines indicate areas of joint restriction (loss of range). The facets in the open position are able to glide freely in both directions.

concomitant movements in the midcervical spine. The motion in the sagittal plane that causes the superior segment to glide down and back is extension.

At this point, the clinician who is assessing a patient with a right sidebending restriction at C4-C5 would not be able to ascertain whether the restriction is at the right or the left facet. However, by testing active movements, the clinician may be able to determine which facet is restricted. For example, a patient who has restricted and painful right sidebending probably also has restricted and painful right rotation. Evaluating extension and flexion will help determine right or left involvement. If the right facet is unable to go through its full active range of motion, extension movement also will be restricted; however, if the left facet is unable to glide up and forward, flexion will be restricted and painful. In theory, this presentation is plausible; however, patients do not always present in this classic mode because accommodation for loss of active movement can be accomplished at adjacent segments.[42]

When the loss of passive mobility is discerned, assessing the end-feel resistance will assist the examiner in determining which tissue or structure may be limiting the range of motion. Describing the end-feel as a barrier that is restricting motion may be helpful. This restriction may be due to one or more factors: skin, fascia, muscle, ligament, joint capsule, joint

surface, or loose bodies. The examiner must be able to differentiate normal from abnormal barriers. A normal barrier at the limit of active motion will have resilience to passive movement that is caused by stretching of muscle and fascia. If the examiner imparts a passive stretch to the anatomical limits of the tissue, a harder end-feel will be noted. Passive stretch beyond the anatomical limits will result in violation of the tissue—a ligamentous tear, a fracture, or a dislocation. By learning to recognize normal restriction of passive movement, the examiner can identify resistance within the normal limits of cervical range of motion. With practice, the examiner can assess and quantify this resistance objectively.[83,84]

For the purpose of passive motion testing, the cervical spine can be divided into atypical cervical joints (i.e., the OA and AA joints) and typical cervical joints from the inferior surface of C2 to C7. In testing the OA joint, the examiner holds the patient's head between his or her palms and thenar muscles while using the index fingers to palpate for movement of the atlas. This position will assure the operator that movement is localized between the occiput and the atlas. With the introduction of translatory movement, sidebending now can be assessed. If the OA joint is localized in flexion by acutely tipping the head forward, translation can be performed both to the right and to the left. Flexion of the neck and right translatory move-

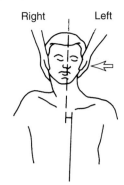
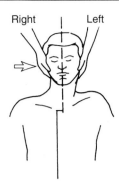
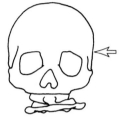
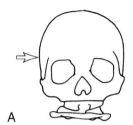

A

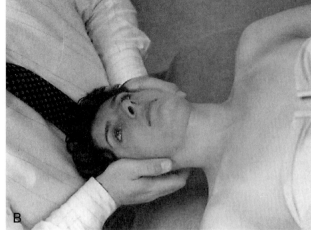

B

Figure 8-21 A, Occipitoatlantal joint translation. **B,** Translation of the occipitoatlantal joint in extension.

ment of the head test for restriction of flexion, left sidebending, and right rotation. Motion restriction is felt when resistance is encountered during the translatory movement. To test for backward bending restriction, the OA joint is localized by acutely tipping the head upward, making sure that extension has not occurred below the level of the atlas. From this position, translatory movement is introduced to both sides (Figure 8-21). The examiner is testing the ability of the OA joint to produce extension together with sidebending/rotation movement to opposite sides. Backward bending and translation to the left tests for extension, right sidebending, and left rotation movement of the occiput at the atlas. These four maneuvers, that is, translating the head to the right and left in both flexed and extended positions, test for all the motion restrictions found within the OA joint.[82,83]

Because rotation is the primary motion available at the AA joint, passive mobility evaluation of this joint will be confined to testing rotation.[6] When rotation at C1-C2 is tested, the head is flexed in an attempt to block as much rotational movement as possible in the typical cervical spine, and rotation then is introduced to the right and to the left until resistance is encountered. If resistance is encountered before the expected end range, a presumptive diagnosis of limited rotation of the atlas on the axis can be made.[82,83]

To test for movement of the typical cervical segments (C2-C7), translation is performed in the flexed and extended positions. For testing purposes, the examiner palpates the articular pillars of the segment to be tested. Then the cervical spine is flexed or extended to the level that is being tested; this is followed by translation to the right or the left. With the examiner's palpating fingers on the articular pillows of C2, the head is carried into extension, and right translation is introduced until C3 begins to move under the examiner's finger. This tests the ability of the left C2-C3 facet joint to close (extension, left

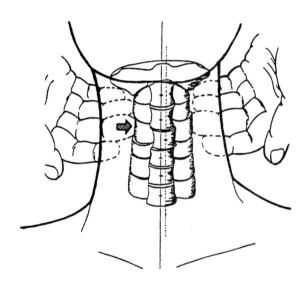

Figure 8-22 Hand positioning for translation of the midcervical spine (C3 and C4).

sidebending, and left rotation). The segment also is evaluated in flexion with right and left translation (Figure 8-22). These translatory movements can be repeated at all remaining cervical segments.[82]

The upper thoracic spine can be assessed for motion restriction by locating the transverse processes of a vertebral segment and determining their position in space through full flexion and extension. With use of the second thoracic vertebra, the examiner's thumbs are placed on each transverse process, and during forward and backward bending, the excursion of the paired transverse processes is assessed. If, during forward bending, the examiner notes that the right transverse becomes more prominent and, with backward bending, the two

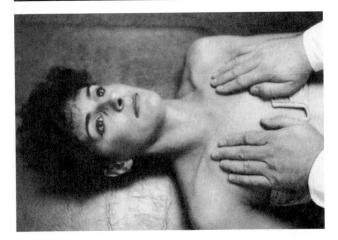

Figure 8-23 Assessing upper rib cage pump-handle motion.

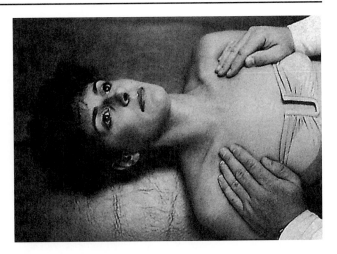

Figure 8-24 Assessing upper rib cage bucket-handle motion.

transverse processes become more equal, the right facet is closed and cannot open. When the right facet is restricted in the closed position and is unable to open, that segment exhibits restriction of forward bending, left sidebending, and left rotation.[34,83]

The upper ribs also can be assessed for their ability to move symmetrically. If the thoracic spine has been assessed and has been determined to be moving normally, any asymmetrical motion of the ribs would be considered rib dysfunction. Two methods used to assess restricted rib motion are springing of the rib cage and evaluation of rib motion during full inspiration and expiration. Springing of the thoracic cage is a gross measure of mobility; resistance to spring alerts the examiner to dysfunction within that area of the rib cage. The second method involves determining the key rib that is limiting the ability of the rib cage to produce an anteroposterior (pump-handle) and a mediolateral (bucket-handle) excursion. In performing this test, the examiner places both open hands over the anterior chest wall, with the index fingers touching the clavicles. The patient is instructed to take a deep breath, and the examiner assesses the ability of the rib cage to move symmetrically throughout the pump-handle motion (Figure 8-23). If one side of the rib cage stops moving before the other, the restricted side is the dysfunctional side. To assess the bucket-handle motion, the examiner places both cupped hands inferior to the clavicle but superior to the nipple line. Again, asymmetrical motion is assessed during inspiration, and the side that stops first is considered the restricted side (Figure 8-24). Although pump-handle movement is the main motion in the upper rib cage, restrictions of bucket-handle movement will be greater and easier to detect than restrictions of pump-handle movement.[34,83] Then the examiner's fingers are placed on the first rib to determine whether that segment is restricting inhalation. Each segment is assessed until the level of asymmetry is found. This identified level is considered the key rib-limiting motion (Figure 8-25). Exhalation is assessed in the same manner; the side that stops moving first is considered restricted; the key rib then is identified, starting inferiorly and moving superiorly.[34,83]

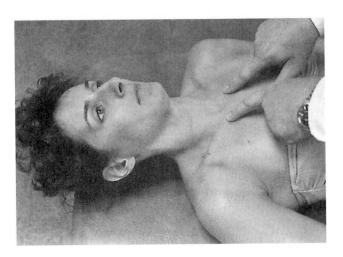

Figure 8-25 Determining the key rib resistor in pump-handle movement.

Thoracic Inlet Tests

Many tests used to assess compromise of the thoracic inlet have been described. The following provocative tests—Adson's test and the costoclavicular, hyperabduction, and 3-minute elevated arm exercise tests—have been identified as the most sensitive in locating the site of the compromise. Adson's test evaluates the role of the anterior scalene muscle in compression of the subclavian artery. This test is performed by holding the arm parallel to the floor, and turning the head first away and then toward the arm while holding a deep breath. Meanwhile, the examiner monitors the radial pulse; a positive test is indicated by an obliteration or decrease in the pulse rate, as well as by reproduction of the patient's symptoms (Figure 8-26).[85] A variation of Adson's test involves sitting erect with the chin tucked in, with the arm being tested in extension and grasping the edge of the table. The head is sidebent and rotated away. The radial pulse is monitored while the patient holds a deep breath (C. Steele, personal communication) (Figure 8-27).

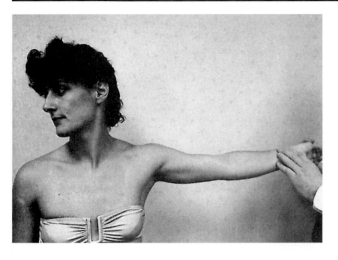

Figure 8-26 Adson's test for thoracic inlet syndrome.

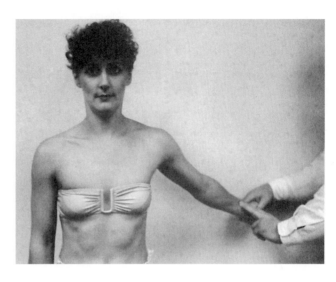

Figure 8-28 Costoclavicular test for thoracic inlet syndrome.

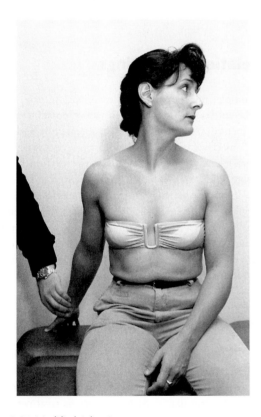

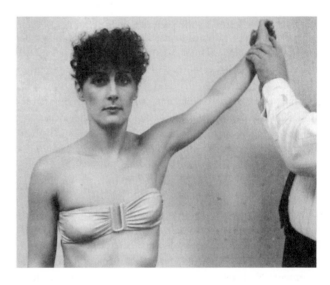

Figure 8-29 Hyperabduction maneuver for thoracic inlet syndrome.

Figure 8-27 Modified Adson's test.

The costoclavicular test, or exaggerated military position, has been described as compressing the subclavian vessels and/or the brachial plexus in the narrow space between the first rib and the clavicle. When this test is performed, the patient is seated with the arms held comfortably at the sides; the shoulder girdle then is retracted and depressed. Simultaneously, the examiner monitors for a change in the radial pulse. A positive test is indicated by obliteration of or a decrease in pulse rate and/or onset of symptoms (Figure 8-28).[86]

The hyperabduction maneuver involves passive circumduction of the upper extremity overhead while the examiner moni-

tors the radial pulse. Similar to Adson's test, this test is considered positive if the pulse rate changes and/or symptoms are elicited (Figure 8-29).[87] The 3-minute elevated arm exercise test is performed with the patient seated, arms abducted and elbows flexed 90 degrees, and the shoulder girdle slightly retracted. The patient is asked to open and close the fists slowly and steadily for a full 3 minutes. The examiner watches for dropping of the elevated arms or a decreased exercise rate before the patient's symptoms begin. Roos[88] stated that this test evaluates involvement of all neurovascular structures, and a positive test is indicated by the patient's inability to complete the full 3 minutes, as well as by the onset of symptoms (Figure 8-30).

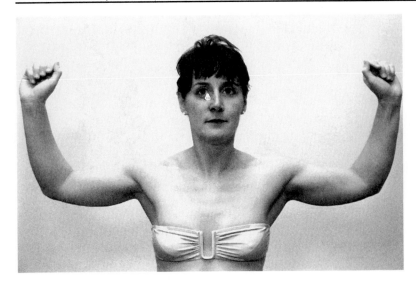

Figure 8-30 Three-minute elevated arm exercise test for thoracic inlet syndrome.

Palpation

Cyriax[51] has advocated doing palpation as the last part of an examination to preclude premature conclusions and incomplete examinations. However, in testing passive cervical mobility, the examiner is also gathering information on tissue tensions and specific structures. A thorough knowledge of cervical anatomy is necessary to perform a complete palpation examination. The examiner must view the anatomy in three dimensions before palpating any anatomical structure. Structures should be palpated from their origin to their insertion. Many structures cannot be differentiated when tissues are healthy; however, pathologically altered tissue usually can be distinguished. The ability to palpate anatomical structures, especially in the cervical spine, takes hours of practice and concentration. The examiner should always palpate by layers, identifying every structure in one layer before attempting to palpate deeper structures. If the examiner has a good mental picture of all the muscles, ligaments, and soft tissues in the cervical area, he or she can identify individual structures.[1]

Palpation gives the examiner information about the size, consistency, temperature, and location of a structure, and about swelling, bony changes, or soft tissue changes such as nodules or scar tissue. Crepitus of bony surfaces can be detected easily, and temperature changes can be appreciated. All these clinical findings represent important objective information. Palpation and point tenderness are viewed in terms of the patient's sensation, but more important, the objective sensation of the examiner (what the examiner "feels") should be guided by sound anatomical knowledge and by adequate application of pressure with regard to area, force, and direction. The clinician must remember, however, that point tenderness of a structure also may provide misinformation. Palpation should be done only after the tissue at fault has been identified by testing of its function. Treating point tenderness without identifying and treating the cause of the symptom is not an acceptable treatment approach.[51]

Correlation of Findings

After completing the objective examination, the clinician should be able to make assumptions about possible pathology or movement dysfunction that are corroborated by both subjective and objective findings. The evaluation process depends on the clinician's ability to make inferences based on his or her knowledge and experience, as well as on the information obtained from the patient history and from the examination. The clinician's inferences serve as the basis for appropriate clinical decision making. With information received from the patient and from the objective examination, the clinician now is able to establish meaningful short- and long-term goals, and to plan treatment to meet these goals.

TREATMENT

A complete, detailed description of treatment procedures for all cervical spine problems is beyond the scope of this chapter. Instead, the intent is to alert the clinician to the different treatment procedures available. Although specific treatment procedures are addressed, treatment should always include patient education on posture, neck hygiene, and recreational and workplace ergonomics. This patient education and patient responsibility for self-care form an integral part of any successful intervention.

Modalities

The decision to use physical agents must be based on appropriate treatment goals; however, the use of physical agents alone will rarely alleviate the cause of the patient's complaints. Mennell[29] stated that the only problems "cured" by physical therapy are rickets treated with ultraviolet therapy and joint dysfunction treated with joint mobilization.[68] As with the rest of the spine, heat is still the treatment of choice for acute cervical problems, when in fact, cryotherapy is more effective in acute situations for decreasing pain, swelling, and muscle spasm.[89] Aside from these acute situations, any modality, including superficial and deep heat, electricity, and cold laser, can be used as adjunctive therapy to decrease pain, promote relaxation, or prepare the tissues before other therapeutic procedures are performed.

Traction

Mechanical or manual traction of the cervical spine separates the vertebrae of the cervical spine, affecting both articular and periarticular structures. Mechanical traction allows the clinician to give a specific poundage of traction over a given time, whereas manual traction allows the therapist to better localize the traction to the vertebral segments affected and requires less time for treatment. In setting up cervical traction, the therapist must be aware of several factors: the weight of the head, the angle of pull, the position of the patient, and the poundage of the traction pull. Accurate knowledge of these components is necessary to control the stress that is being applied in a particular direction to the cervical spine and soft tissues.[90,91] As a precaution, traction usually is initiated at a relatively low poundage and is directed to the vertebral segments involved; therefore, a standard position of the cervical spine for traction is not appropriate. Because most movement is achieved when a joint is positioned at its midrange, actual distraction will vary, depending on the segment being treated. OA and AA joints should be treated in a neutral or a slightly extended head and neck position.[92] By introducing increased flexion, lower cervical spine segments can be isolated.[90]

Research reveals that traction forces greater than 20 lb separate the vertebrae by 1 to 1.5 cm per space, with the greatest separation occurring posteriorly as flexion is increased. Normal cervical lordosis is eradicated with traction forces of 20 to 25 lb. At a constant angle, a traction force of 50 lb produces greater separation than 30 lb, but the amount of separation is not significantly different at 7, 30, or 60 seconds.[91] Intermittent traction produces twice as much separation as sustained traction. If separation of vertebral bodies is desired, high traction forces applied for short periods of time will achieve that goal. When traction forces are removed, restoration of normal dimensions is four to five times quicker in posterior structures than in anterior structures. As would be expected, less separation occurs in 50-year-olds than in normal 20-year-olds.[93-95]

The behavior of the patient's symptoms during traction is important, especially if the symptoms decrease. Even if traction reduces the symptoms, there is no guarantee that symptoms will remain relieved after treatment has ceased. However, relief of symptoms during treatment is a sign that traction will benefit that particular patient.

Soft Tissue Mobilization

Regardless of cervical spine pathology, the clinician must always consider the soft tissue component of the problem. If body parts have maintained an abnormal relationship for some time, according to Wolff's law,[96] soft tissue will adapt accordingly (see Chapter 1). All soft tissues—skin, fascia, capsule, and muscle—must be recognized. Several soft tissue mobilization procedures, including stretching, myofascial release, Fluori-Methane spraying and stretching, rolfing, deep massage, strain-counterstrain,[97] and craniosacral therapy, are available.[98]

Joint Mobilization

Indications for joint mobilization include loss of active and passive range of motion, joint asymmetry, and tissue texture abnormality. Passive mobility testing during evaluation will reveal the joints to be treated. Chapter 9 discusses specific techniques such as oscillations, articulations, and muscle energy techniques. Indirect techniques such as strain-counterstrain, functional technique, and craniosacral therapy also are available.

Therapeutic Exercise

Active rehabilitation is of vital importance for restoration of function; however, patients cannot typically "work out" neck pain. An appropriate treatment plan should include restoration of normal, painless joint range of motion followed by correction of muscle weakness or imbalance, resumption of normal activities, and prevention of recurrent problems. Too often, treatment ends after normal, pain-free motion is restored. Exercise restores adequate control of movement, and increased muscle strength provides increased dynamic support to the spine.

The choice of specific exercises is just as important as the decision to initiate cervical exercises. The spinal musculature, which is composed mainly of slow twitch oxidative muscle fibers, has a role in maintaining body relationships. After restoration of normal muscle length, appropriate strengthening exercises should include isometric and endurance activities.

Supports

Cervical collars and supports do have their place in treatment program planning; however, they are appropriate only in acute conditions and in segmental instability. The amount of external support needed should be dictated by findings of the objective examination.

CASE STUDY 8-1

Rarely does the clinical presentation of cervical pain have a single underlying cause. The following case study describing an actual patient is a typical example of this point.

Subjective Examination

A 32-year-old woman presented to physical therapy with complaints of cervicothoracic pain referring into the left upper extremity. She had been working as a word processing secretary; her symptoms started 6 months previously. She reported no specific incident that might have brought on her symptoms, except for sitting at a computer terminal 5 hours a day.

The patient's chief complaints included stiffness and pain in the posterior neck that traveled along the trapezial ridge into the left superior and lateral shoulder. She described numbness along the lateral upper arm, the forearm, and the ulnar side of the left hand. Symptoms in her left upper extremity were aggravated when she attempted to lift a heavy object or to use her arms overhead. Her upper back pain was aggravated when she sneezed. She described difficulty sleeping at night, with an inability to find a comfortable position; she was using a down feather pillow.

During a 24-hour period, the patient noticed stiffness on awakening in the morning. As the day progressed, she experienced discomfort only if she was very active or sat too long (35 minutes or longer) at the computer terminal without getting up.

Her history revealed a similar episode of pain in 1978, which lasted for longer than 18 months after the patient began working at a word processing machine. When she was promoted and no longer worked at a word processor, her symptoms disappeared. She had experienced no neck symptoms since that initial episode until this episode occurred. She related a history of trauma to the cervicothoracic region that occurred 11 years previously, when she fell off a motorcycle, landing directly on her buttocks. Ten months previously, she had fallen down one flight of stairs, with minimal musculoskeletal complaints. She denied having any history of bowel or bladder dysfunction, headaches, dizziness, difficulty swallowing, weight loss, or pregnancy.

The patient was not currently being treated for any other medical condition, although she had had an epigastric hernia repair 6 years before presentation. She reported that stress played an important role in determining how she felt; she noticed a direct relationship between increased stress and exacerbation of her symptoms. In her current job, she noticed less cervical pain after her boss bought her a Pos Chair (Congleton Workplace Systems, Inc., College Station, Texas), which improved her head and neck alignment.

Objective Examination

The patient presented in no acute distress but with guarded upper quarter movement. She had a forward head posture, with rounding of the shoulder girdle complex. Active range of motion of both upper extremities was within normal limits; however, extreme elevation of the arms increased discomfort in the cervicothoracic region. Active range of motion of the cervical spine was restricted in left rotation (30%) and left sidebending (25%). Right rotation was full but produced pain along the left upper trapezius ridge. Backward bending was within normal limits but produced discomfort in the posterior neck region. Forward bending was restricted, with two fingerbreadths of distance between the chin and the anterior chest wall at maximum flexion. Right sidebending was full and pain free.

Neurologic testing revealed 2+ muscle stretch reflexes in both upper extremities. Sensation to light touch, pinprick, and two-point discrimination was intact in the upper quarter. Gross muscle testing revealed weakness in the following muscles: left biceps brachii, good minus (4/5); and left triceps brachii, good (4/5). The triceps muscle contraction appeared to give way as the result of pain felt by the patient in the cervicothoracic region.

Several special tests revealed positive findings. The foraminal closure test (quadrant) was positive for the lower cervical spine on the left and produced pain along the upper trapezius; on the left side, pain was reproduced in the right neck region. The left upper limb tension test was slightly positive, with reproduction of neck and shawl pain. The cervical compression test was negative. The cervical distraction test decreased the patient's neck and shoulder pain. A vertebral artery test was negative. Clearing tests for the TMJ shoulder, elbow, wrist, and hand were unequivocal.

Radiographs taken at the time of examination revealed flattening of lordosis at the midcervical spine and posterior spurring of the vertebral body at the C4-C5 level, with foraminal encroachment at C4-C5 greater on the right than on the left (Figure 8-31).

Passive mobility testing demonstrated restrictions at the left OA joint with translation to the left in flexion (extended, rotated right, sidebent left). The right AA joint was restricted with passive rotation to the right with the neck bent fully forward (rotated left). Translation of the cervical spine from C2 to C7 revealed restriction at the C2-C3, C4-C5, C5-C6, and C6-C7 levels. Translation of the C2-C3 level to the left in extension (flexed, rotated left, sidebent left) was diminished. The C4-C5, C5-C6, and C6-C7 levels were restricted in translation to the right in extension (flexed, rotated right, sidebent right). Asymmetry of the upper thoracic region was revealed by palpation of the transverse processes at the T1-T2 and T2-T3 levels. The transverse process at T1 was more posterior on the left in flexion of the head and upper trunk (extended, rotated left, sidebent left) than when the neck and trunk were placed in extension. The T2 transverse process was more prominent on the right in flexion (extended, rotated right, sidebent right). Inhalation/exhalation testing of the anterior rib cage showed less movement on inhalation on the left, with the left first and second ribs revealing the greatest restriction.

CASE STUDY 8-1—cont'd

Palpation revealed tightness in the posterior cervical musculature, suboccipital muscles, scalene muscles, trapezius, and levator scapulae muscles. Flexibility testing revealed tightness of the levator scapulae, pectoralis major, and scalene muscles. A trigger point was identified in the midsubstance of the upper trapezius muscle.

Assessment

Findings were consistent with cervical spondylosis with left C5 radiculopathy, upper cervical dysfunction, forward head posture, and upper rib and thoracic dysfunction.

Diagnostic classification: Musculoskeletal 4D: Late effects of dislocation (905.6)

Treatment Plan

Treatment goals included decreasing the patient's symptoms, improving her posture, and increasing range of motion in the cervical and thoracic spine and upper ribs. Other important treatment goals included patient education about work simplification, awareness of the need for lifetime postural correction, and avoidance of potentially harmful activities.

To accomplish these goals, the following treatment plan was administered:

1. Intermittent supine cervical traction using a Saunders 28 harness at 16 lb, 30-second pull, followed by 12 lb, 10-second pull, for a total treatment time of 20 minutes (static traction with intermittent increases)
2. High-voltage electrical stimulation massage of the upper trapezius, upper thoracic, and posterior cervical regions for 10 minutes
3. Postural instruction in correct head and neck alignment during all activities
4. Basic instruction in proper sleeping postures; encouragement of continued use of a down feather pillow
5. Soft tissue mobilization of the paracervical, suboccipital, levator scapulae, scalene, and upper trapezius muscles
6. Joint mobilization of the upper thoracic spine with the patient supine and the head supported; muscle energy technique to decrease upper cervical spine joint restrictions

Treatment Progression

The patient was seen every other day, three times a week, for a total of six treatments. Initial treatment included traction and high-voltage massage and posture education. Subsequent treatments focused on soft tissue and joint dysfunctions. After this treatment regimen was completed, the patient was asymptomatic and resumed her normal activities. Because this was the patient's first episode of radicular referred symptoms, home cervical traction would not be recommended unless the symptoms recurred.

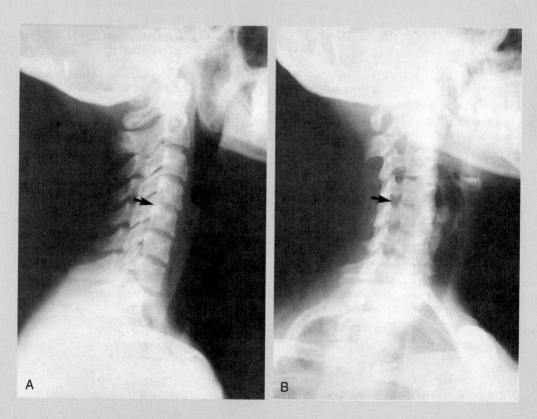

Figure 8-31 Cervical radiographs. **A,** Lateral view. Arrow shows C4-C5 spurring. **B,** Oblique view. Arrow shows bony encroachment at the C4-C5 intervertebral foramen.

CASE STUDY 8-2

This chapter has discussed the importance of performing a thorough examination, not only to determine whether a patient is a candidate for physical therapy, but also to provide appropriate treatment according to the signs and symptoms noted during the evaluation. This case study stresses the importance of taking a thorough history before starting treatment. With the advent of direct access, a physical therapist or any other health practitioner no longer should rely on another person's interpretation of subjective and objective findings in a patient. Obtaining a complete, correct clinical picture allows the clinician to design an appropriate treatment plan.

Subjective Examination

This case study describes a 53-year-old businessman who presented to our clinic with complaints of left shoulder pain and left upper extremity burning and numbness. He had been referred to our clinic by a general practitioner with a diagnosis of left cervical radiculopathy. The prescription for physical therapy treatment read "Evaluate and treat."

The patient reported a gradual onset of intermittent superior left shoulder pain for the past 4 months. His symptoms began as a diffuse ache in the left shoulder, which increased progressively in intensity. The patient recalled no specific incident or unusual activity that could have contributed to his current symptoms. He started to notice the pain traveling along the inside of his left upper extremity to his fourth and fifth digits, with numbness in the same distribution. He began to feel achiness along the medial aspect of the left scapula. Occasionally, he felt discomfort along the left trapezial ridge. He denied having any neck pain. While eating, he often noticed the feeling that something was stuck in his throat. He reported having difficulty sleeping for the past 2 months; for the past 2 weeks, he reported having to get out of bed to find relief for his left upper extremity numbness and pain.

The patient reported that his physician ordered cervical spine radiographs, which revealed moderate degenerative disc and joint disease at the C5-C6, C6-C7, and C7-T1 levels bilaterally, with minimal intervertebral foramina osteophytosis encroachment at the C5-C6 level on the left and the C6-C7 level on the right. The patient was given a nonsteroidal anti-inflammatory medication, which did not relieve his pain. Holding the left upper extremity in an awkward position usually aggravated his symptoms, mainly the numbness in the medial hand. He had difficulty grasping heavy objects with his nondominant left hand, especially his briefcase. The patient had been smoking one pack of cigarettes per day since the age of 15. He drank wine at every dinner and several six-packs of beer on the weekend. His typical work week traditionally had been 55 hours long, but for the past month, he has been working only 35 hours

weekly because of increased pain. His medical history revealed no major sickness, an appendectomy at age 15, and a negative family history.

Objective Examination

Objective examination found an older man who appeared to be in distress. He was holding his left arm against his rib cage and was trying not to move the left upper extremity. He had increased thoracic kyphosis, rounded shoulders, protracted scapulae, and a forward head posture. His blood pressure taken while sitting was 162/84 mm Hg; pulse was 82; respiration was 20; and oral temperature was 98.8° F. Active range of motion of the cervical spine showed restriction of movement in all three cardinal planes. Cervical range of motion measured with the CROM inclinometer revealed 28 degrees right sidebending with pain referred along the left medial brachium and forearm to the medial hand. Left sidebending was 34 degrees. Cervical rotation was 44 degrees right and 42 degrees left. Cervical forward bending was 40 degrees; cervical forward bending was 40 degrees; cervical backward bending was painful and diminished at 48 degrees. Active range of motion of left shoulder flexion was 155 degrees, and shoulder abduction was 152 degrees. Neck palpation revealed swelling in the left posterior triangle, with tenderness on pressure. Palpation of other soft tissues demonstrated tightness and tenderness of the following muscles: sternocleidomastoid, anterior and middle scalenes, upper trapezius, levator scapulae, left splenius capitis and cervicis, and suboccipital muscles. The left cervical foraminal encroachment test increased his left lateral trapezial pain. Compression and distraction tests of the cervical spine were unremarkable. Manual muscle testing revealed weakness in the following muscles: left interossei dorsales (3+/5), left interossei palmares (3+/5), lumbricales I and II (4/5) and III and IV (3+/5), flexor digiti minimi (3+/5), opponens digiti minimi (3+/5), abductor digiti minimi (3+/5), left pronator teres (4/5), left flexor digitorum superficialis I and II (4/5) and III and IV (3+/5), flexor pollicis longus (4/5), abductor pollicis brevis (4+/5), flexor pollicis brevis (4/5), adductor brevis (3+/5), opponens pollicis (4/5), shoulder external rotation right (4/5) and left (4/5), and grip strength using a handheld dynamometer (right, 95 lb; left, 35 lb). Symmetrical hyporeflexive muscle stretch reflexes were in the upper quarter. The patient's sensation to pinprick was significantly reduced along the ulnar distribution of the left hand. Hoffman's sign was negative bilaterally. The left upper limb tension test was positive with sidebending of the head to the right without placement of the left arm in a stretched position.

With the significant clinical features of a history of smoking, difficulty swallowing, lower trunk brachial plexopathy, sleep disturbance, and severe pain in the shoul-

CASE STUDY 8-2—cont'd

der and scapula, it was suggested that the patient return for further evaluation by the referring physician. The physician was telephoned with the findings. It was obvious from this discussion that a short, scanty evaluation had been performed by the physician. A chest radiograph and possibly a computed tomography scan were suggested.

The patient was sent for a chest radiograph (Figure 8-32, *A*), which revealed a large tumor in the superior pulmonary sulcus. It was diagnosed by computed tomography scan as a Pancoast's tumor (Figure 8-32, *B*).

Diagnostic classification: Musculoskeletal 4I: ACL tear (717.8)

Summary of Case Study

This case study illustrates the importance of performing a thorough examination on every patient. Given the findings of the examination, this patient was not a proper candidate for physical therapy. He should have been sent to a specialist immediately instead of to a physical therapist. A proper initial examination would have directed the patient to proper medical attention. The literature[99] has reported Pancoast's tumors presenting as cervical radiculopathy. However, the clinical features of this patient's history and physical examination warranted further study.

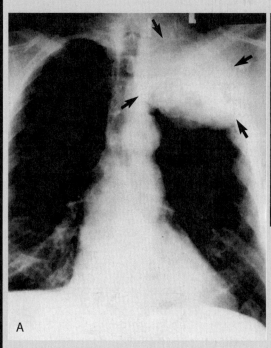
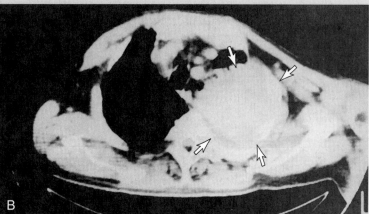

Figure 8-32 A, Chest radiograph showing Pancoast's tumor *(arrows)*. **B,** Computed tomography scan demonstrating tumor *(arrows)* in the superior pulmonary sulcus.

SUMMARY

A complete evaluation of the cervical spine must begin with a thorough understanding of its functional anatomy and biomechanics. With this background, the examiner will have a clear mental picture of the structures and the interdependency of the structures being examined. However, this mental image is sharpened and honed only with study, practice, and experience. The clinician must address all potential sources of the patient's complaints, which may go beyond physical sources. Physiologic and psychosocial factors can play an important role in the patient's symptoms. A detailed discussion of all cervical and upper thoracic spine pathology is beyond the scope of this chapter; however, the clinician must always remember that not all cervical symptoms are musculoskeletal in origin. Those patients whose pain is not musculoskeletal in origin should be referred to the appropriate physician for further evaluation.

The cervical and upper thoracic spine is indeed complex, and no two patients are alike. Each patient who presents with cervical and upper thoracic pain must be evaluated according to his or her own signs and symptoms.

REFERENCES

1. Dvorak J, Dvorak V: Manual medicine diagnostics, New York, 1984, Thieme-Stratton.
2. Kapandji I: Physiology of the joints, ed 2, vol III, The trunk and vertebral column, Edinburgh, 1974, Churchill Livingstone.
3. Werne S: Studies in spontaneous atlas dislocation, Acta Orthop Scand 23(suppl):1, 1957.
4. Kaltenborn FM: Mobilization of the extremity joints: examination and basic treatment techniques, ed 3, Oslo, 1980, Olaf Norlis Bokhandel.

5. Ingelmark BE: Ueber den craniocervicalen Uebergang bei Menschen, Acta Anat 23(suppl):1, 1957.

6. Fielding JW: Cineroentgenography of the normal cervical spine, J Bone Joint Surg 39(A):1280, 1957.

7. Fielding JW, Hawkins RJ, Hensinger RN, et al: Deformities, Orthop Clin North Am 9:955, 1978.

8. White A, Panjabi MM: The basic kinematics of the human spine, Spine 3:13, 1978.

9. Penning L: Functional pathology of the cervical spine, Amsterdam, 1968, Excerpta Medica Foundation.

10. Clark CR, Goel VK, Galles K, et al: Kinematics of the occipito-atlanto-axial complex, Trans Cervical Spine Res Soc 10:210, 1986.

11. Dvorak J, Panjabi MM, Gerber DG, et al: Functional diagnostics of the rotatory instability of the upper cervical spine: an experimental study in cadavers, Spine 12:197, 1987.

12. Panjabi M, Dvorak J, Duranceau J, et al: Three dimensional movements of the upper cervical spine, Spine 13:726, 1988.

13. Dupreux R, Mestdagh H: Anatomic functionelle de l'articulation sousoccipitale, Lille Med 19:122, 1974.

14. Lewit K: Blockierung von Atlas-Axis und Atlas-Occiput im Robild und Klink, Z Orthop 108:43, 1970.

15. Jirout J: Changes in the atlas-axis relations on lateral flexion of the head and neck, Neuroradiology 6:215, 1973.

16. White A, Panjabi MM: Clinical biomechanics of the spine, ed 2, Philadelphia, 1990, Lippincott.

17. Grieve GP: Common vertebral joint problems, Edinburgh, 1979, Churchill Livingstone.

18. Lysell E: Motion in the cervical spine, Acta Orthop Scand 123(suppl):69, 1969.

19. Warwick R, Williams PL, editors: Gray's anatomy, 35th British ed, Philadelphia, 1973, Saunders.

20. Greenman PE: Manipulative therapy for the thoracic cage, Osteop Ann 140:63, 1977.

21. Selecki BR: The effects of rotation of the atlas on the axis: experimental work, Med J Aust 1:1012, 1969.

22. Tatlow TWF, Bammer HG: Vertebral artery compression syndrome, Neurology 7:331, 1957.

23. Coman WB: Dizziness related to ENT conditions. In Grieve GP, editor: Modern manual therapy of the vertebral column, Edinburgh, 1986, Churchill Livingstone, p 303.

24. Grant ER: Clinical testing before cervical manipulation—can we recognize the patient at risk? Paper presented at the World Confederation of Physical Therapy, Sydney, Australia, 1987.

25. Howell JW: Evaluation and management of the thoracic outlet syndrome. In Donatelli R, editor: Physical therapy of the shoulder, New York, 1987, Churchill Livingstone, p 133.

26. Kendall FP, Kendall-McCreary E: Muscles: testing and function, ed 3, Baltimore, 1983, Williams & Wilkins.

27. Rocabado M: Diagnosis and treatment of abnormal craniocervical and craniomandibular mechanics, Rocabado Institute, Knoxville, Tenn, 1981.

28. Saunders HD: Evaluation, treatment and prevention of musculoskeletal disorders, ed 2, Minneapolis, 1985, Viking Press.

29. Mennell JM: Joint pain, Boston, 1964, Little, Brown.

30. Schafer RC: Chiropractic management of sports and recreational injuries, Baltimore, 1982, Williams & Wilkins.

31. Lewit K: Manipulative therapy in rehabilitation of the motor system, Boston, 1985, Butterworths.

32. Seimon LP: Low back pain: clinical diagnosis and management, East Norwalk, Conn, 1983, Appleton-Century-Crofts.

33. Greenman PE: Vertebral motion, Mich Osteopath J 6:31, 1983.

34. Mitchell FL, Moran PS, Pruzzo NA: An evaluation and treatment manual of osteopathic muscle energy procedures. Institute for Continuing Education in Osteopathic Principles, Valley Park, Md, 1979.

35. Bogduk N, Engel R: The menisci of the lumbar zygapophyseal joints: a review of their anatomy and clinical significance, Spine 9:454, 1984.

36. Kos J, Wolf J: Die "Menisci" der Zwischenwirbelgelenke und ihre mogliche Role bei Wirbelblockierung, Manuelle Med 10:105, 1972.

37. Janda V: Muscles, central nervous regulation and back problems. In Korr IM, editor: Neurobiologic mechanisms in manipulative therapy, New York, 1978, Plenum Press, p 27.

38. Korr IM: Sustained sympathicotonia as a factor in disease. In Korr IM, editor: Neurobiologic mechanisms in manipulative therapy, New York, 1978, Plenum Press, p 229.

39. Korr IM: Proprioceptors and somatic dysfunction, J Am Osteopath Assoc 74:638, 1975.

40. Calliet R: Neck and arm pain, Philadelphia, 1981, FA Davis.

41. Jull G, Bogduk N, Marsland A: The accuracy of manual diagnosis for cervical zygapophyseal joint pain syndromes, Med J Aust 148:233, 1988.

42. Greenman PE: Restricted vertebral motion, Mich Osteopath J 7:31, 1983.

43. Bland JH: Disorders of the cervical spine: diagnosis and medical management, Philadelphia, 1987, Saunders.

44. Hirsh LF: Cervical degenerative arthritis: possible cause of neck and arm pain, Postgrad Med 74:123, 1983.

45. Bateman JE: The shoulder and neck, ed 2, Philadelphia, 1978, Saunders.

46. Brain WR, Northfield D, Wilkinson M: The neurological manifestations of cervical spondylosis, Brain 75:187, 1952.

47. Cyriax JH: Cervical spondylosis, London, 1971, Butterworths.

48. Grieve GP: Manipulation therapy for neck pain, Physiotherapy 65:136, 1979.

49. Cloward RB: Cervical discography: a contribution to the etiology and mechanism of neck, shoulder and arm pain, Ann Surg 150:1052, 1959.

50. Cloward RB: The clinical significance of the sinuvertebral nerve, J Neurol Neurosurg Psychiatr 23:321, 1960.

51. Cyriax JH: Textbook of orthopaedic medicine, ed 8, vol I, Diagnosis of soft tissue lesions, London, 1983, Bailliere Tindall.

52. McNab I: The whiplash syndrome, Orthop Clin North Am 2:389, 1971.

53. Hohl M: Soft tissue injuries of the neck in automobile accidents, J Bone Joint Surg 56(A):1675, 1974.

54. Bower KD: The pathophysiology and symptomatology of the whiplash syndrome. In Grieve GP, editor: Modern manual therapy of the vertebral column, Edinburgh, 1986, Churchill Livingstone, p 342.

55. Yunus M, Masi AT, Calabro JJ, et al: Primary fibromyalgia (fibrositis): clinical study of 50 patients with matched normal controls, Semin Arthritis Rheum 11:151, 1981.

56. Travell JH, Simons DG: Myofascial pain and dysfunction: trigger point manual, Baltimore, 1983, Williams & Wilkins.

57. Cyriax JH, Cyriax PJ: Illustrated manual of orthopaedic medicine, Boston, 1983, Butterworths.

58. Miller J: How do you feel? Listener 100:665, 1978.

59. Harman JB: Angina in the analgesic limb, Br Med J 2:521, 1951.

60. Feinstein B, Langton JNK, Jameson RM, et al: Experiments on pain referred from deep somatic tissues, J Bone Joint Surg 36(A):981, 1954.

61. Bourdillon JR: Spinal manipulation, ed 3, London, 1982, Butterworth-Heinemann.

62. Inman VT, Saunders JB: Referred pain from skeletal structures, J Nerv Ment Dis 90:660, 1944.

63. Campbell DG, Parsons CM: Referred head pain and its concomitants, J Nerve Ment Dis 99:544, 1944.

64. Wall PD: The mechanisms of pain associated with cervical vertebral disease. In Hirsch C, Zotterman Y, editors: Cervical pain, Oxford, 1971, Pergamon Press, p 201.

65. Dwyer A, Aprill C, Bogduk N: Cervical zygapophyseal joint pain patterns I: a study in normal volunteers. Spine 15:453, 1990.

66. Collins RD: Dynamic differential diagnosis, Philadelphia, 1981, JB Lippincott.

67. D'Ambrosia RD: Musculoskeletal disorders, regional examination and differential diagnosis, ed 2, Philadelphia, 1986, JB Lippincott.

68. Hoppenfeld S: Physical examination of the spine and extremities, New York, 1976, Appleton-Century-Crofts.

69. Boissonnault WG: Examination in physical therapy practice: screening for medical disease, New York, 1991, Churchill Livingstone.

70. Gould JA, Davies GJ, editors: Orthopaedic and sports physical therapy, St. Louis, 1985, Mosby.

71. Bogduk N: Cervical causes of headache. In Grieve GP, editor: Modern manual therapy of the vertebral column, Edinburgh, 1986, Churchill Livingstone, p 289.

72. Ryan GM, Cope S: Cervical vertigo, Lancet 2:1355, 1955.

73. Maitland GD: Vertebral manipulation, ed 4, London, 1977, Butterworths.

74. Youdas JW, Garrett TR, Suman VJ, et al: Normal range of motion of the cervical spine: an initial goniometric study, Phys Ther 72:770, 1992.

75. Rheault W, Albright B, Byers C, et al: Intertester reliability of the cervical range of motion device, J Orthop Sports Phys Ther 15:147, 1992.

76. Youdas JW, Carey JR, Carrett TR: Reliability of measurements of cervical spine range of motion: comparison of three methods, Phys Ther 71:98, 1991.

77. Elvey RL: The investigation of arm pain. In Grieve GP, editor: Modern manual therapy of the vertebral column, Edinburgh, 1986, Churchill Livingstone, p 530.

78. Butler DS: Mobilisation of the nervous system, Melbourne, 1991, Churchill Livingstone.

79. Margarey ME: Examination of the cervical spine. In Grieve GP, editor: Modern manual therapy of the vertebral column, Edinburgh, 1986, Churchill Livingstone, p 503.

80. Kenneally M: The upper limb tension test: an investigation of responses amongst normal asymptomatic subjects. Unpublished thesis, School of Physiotherapy, South Australia Institute of Technology, 1983.

81. Fryette HH: Principles of osteopathic technique, Carmel, Calif, 1954, Academy of Applied Osteopathy.

82. Greenman PE: Motion testing the cervical spine, Mich Osteopath J 8:32, 1983.

83. Greenman PE: Principles of manual medicine, Baltimore, 1989, Williams & Wilkins.

84. Greenman PE: Barrier concepts and structural diagnosis, Mich Osteopath J 3:28, 1982.

85. Hirsch LF, Thanki A: The thoracic outlet syndrome: meeting the diagnostic challenge, Postgrad Med 77:197, 1985.

86. Falconer MA, Weddell G: Costoclavicular compression of the subclavian artery and veins, Lancet 2:539, 1943.

87. Wright IS: The neurovascular syndrome produced by hyperabduction of the arms, Am Heart J 29:1, 1945.

88. Roos DB: Congenital anomalies associated with thoracic outlet syndrome, Am J Surg 132:171, 1976.

89. Knight KL: Cryotherapy: theory, technique, and physiology, Chattanooga, Tenn, 1985, Chattanooga Corp.

90. Colachis SC, Strohm BR: A study of tractive forces and angle of pull on vertebral interspaces in the cervical spine, Arch Phys Med Rehabil 46:820, 1965.

91. Colachis SC, Strohm BR: Cervical traction: relationship of traction time to varied tractive force with constant angle of pull, Arch Phys Med Rehabil 46:815, 1965.

92. Daugherty RJ, Erhard RE: Segmentalized cervical traction. In Kent BE, editor: International Federation of Orthopaedic Manipulative Therapists Proceedings, Vail, Colo, 1977, p 189.

93. Valtonen EJ, Moller K, Wiljasalo M: Comparative radiographic study of the effect of intermittent and continuous traction on elongation of the cervical spine, Ann Med Int Fenn 57:143, 1968.

94. Colachis SC, Strohm BR: Effect of duration of intermittent cervical traction on vertebral separation, Arch Phys Med Rehabil 47:353, 1966.

95. Valtonen EJ, Kiurn E: Cervical traction as a therapeutic tool: a clinical analysis based on 212 patients, Scand J Rehabil Med 2:29, 1970.

96. Glimcher MJ: On the form and function of bone: from molecules to organs—Wolff's law revisited. In Veis A, editor: The chemistry and biology of mineralized connective tissues, New York, 1981, Elsevier/North Holland, p 617.

97. Jones LH: Strain and counterstrain. American Academy of Osteopathy, Colorado Springs, Colo, 1981.

98. Upledger JE, Vredevoogd JD: Craniosacral therapy, Seattle, 1983, Eastland Press.

99. Vargo MM, Flood KM: Pancoast tumor presenting as cervical radiculopathy, Arch Phys Med Rehabil 71:606, 1990.

Differential Diagnosis and Mobilization of the Cervical and Upper Thoracic Spine

Differential diagnosis of the cervical and thoracic spine demands the careful attention of the clinician to isolate the patient's true dysfunction and render it beneficial.[1] Differential diagnosis involves appropriate tests and measures and superior clinical reasoning capabilities, including the requirement of understanding pertinent clinical findings.[2] Subsequently, the purposes of this chapter are as follows:

1. Outline the effective clinical reasoning processes used during differentiation of the cervical and thoracic spine
2. Present a description of a differential assessment between the cervical spine and the thoracic spine
3. Present methods for mobilization of the cervical and upper thoracic spine.

DIFFERENTIAL DIAGNOSIS

Differential diagnosis is the process of weighing the probability of one disease, movement dysfunction, or pain generator vs. the probability of another.[3] This process is performed during a clinical examination by analyzing the signs and symptoms of the patient and determining the most relevant criteria associated with the pathologic process of the patient.[4] Differential diagnosis is necessary to direct treatment, whatever the mode, at the source of the patient's true disorder.

For the physical therapist, differentiation usually is required when (1) the physician has rendered a nonspecific diagnosis, (2) the diagnosis appears to be in question, and/or (3) the therapist decides that the patient's disorder may be multistructural and/or multisegmental. Physical therapists must weigh each element of the clinical findings, including the subscribed diagnosis, patient history, and physical examination. Findings from tests and measures must be analyzed for pertinence, applicability, and guilt in identifying a pattern within the patient's symptoms. Differentiation demands an understanding of the values of tests and measures, recognition of essential aspects of patient history, and sophisticated clinical reasoning during and after the examination process.[5]

Differential diagnosis involves two elements of the examination process: screening and confirmation.[5] Screening generally is performed early in the examination process and includes differentiation testing to identify a serious pathology that may not be treatable by a physical therapist.[6] Screening requires tests and measures with high levels of sensitivity, generally 90 or higher, and can guide the clinician toward the appropriate use of tests with higher specificity, such as imaging, biopsy, and other more invasive methods.[7] Several clinical tests such as reflex testing and sensibility testing are used frequently as screening tools, but they actually demonstrate poor sensitivity and may not yield useful information during an examination.[6]

Confirmatory tests are used near the end of an examination and include tests and measures that demonstrate moderate to high levels of sensitivity and higher levels of specificity.[5] Strong confirmatory tests and measures should be focused and precise, and should isolate the targeted region of interest. Confirmatory tests and measures are used to substantiate a diagnosis or to confirm the guilt regarding a specific body region, tissue, or movement dysfunction.

CLINICAL REASONING

Similar to differential diagnosis, clinical reasoning involves higher-level recognition of pertinent clinical findings that assist in driving care-related decisions.[8,9] Clinical reasoning involves assessing the probability of selected disorders and being able to discriminate among several hypotheses at any given time. Successful clinical reasoning requires the marriage of data extracted from the patient interaction and selection of the treatment technique.[10,11]

During the patient interaction, *evaluation*, as defined by the *Guide to Physical Therapist Practice*,[12] is related intimately to how the term *assessment* is used in clinical reasoning; it is the cornerstone of effective clinical practice. However, unlike evaluation, assessment involves a more fluid, continuous process that includes intangible elements of the patient interaction model. We advocate three types of assessment: (1) daily clinical assessment, (2) analytical assessment, and (3) differential assessment.

†Deceased.

DAILY CLINICAL ASSESSMENT

Daily clinical assessment is an unremitting process that includes the considerations and contributions of the patient, techniques, tests and measures, clinicians, and care patterns. For the patient history, an effective format for facilitating the flow of the clinical assessment consists of (1) the nature and kind of the disorder, (2) the area or areas of the symptoms, (3) the behavior of the symptoms, (4) pertinent present and past history, and (5) special questions.

The nature and kind of the disorder reflect the depiction of the disorder. *Nature* reflects the overall description of the patient's assessment of his or her current problem defined as an annoyance, an impairment, or a disabling condition, whereas *kind* may relate to whether the condition manifests as pain, stiffness, weakness, instability, or poor coordination. Area(s) of symptoms is an outline of the origination and progression of the patient's disorder based on his or her description. Behavior of symptoms reflects changes in the condition throughout the progression of the day, during activities, or during a given time frame. Pertinent present and past history may add useful information toward the care and understanding of the patient's condition. Special questions may include spontaneous, scripted, or response-specific queries designed to gain useful information that would not normally distill during conventional interaction.

For the physical examination (PE), an effective format comprises (1) screening tests, (2) active physiologic movement tests, (3) passive physiologic movement tests, (4) passive accessory movement tests, and, if needed, (5) confirmatory tests. Further explanation is provided throughout the chapter.

ANALYTICAL ASSESSMENT

Analytical assessment is the cognitive foundation of the clinical reasoning processes. Analytical assessment is a continuous process that enhances all effective clinical functions; it is in a sense the thinking about our thinking, the reason why we do what we do. It is a series of accumulating thoughts that result in overt acts by therapists. The acts are heard as questions in the patient history, are seen as objective tests in the PE, and finally are seen as treatment. Analytical assessment is a process of thinking, planning, and executing, to prove or disprove a hypothesis. This process is the key to self-improvement and is essential for furthering knowledge and quality of care. Without analytical assessment, progression of quality stagnates, current theories and dogma are accepted without question, and new and better ideas are not developed.

DIFFERENTIAL ASSESSMENT

Differential assessment is largely hypothesis testing, which takes place before, during, and after all phases of the patient's visit. Differential assessment primarily involves weighing physical signs and symptoms and response patterns seen in tests and measures and with techniques of treatment. A differential assessment can be completed in at least four ways: (1) prognostic epidemiologic tables, (2) traditional diagnostic tests, (3) questioning and examining during the patient history, PE, and treatment, and (4) physical differentiation.

Prognostic epidemiologic tables, such as diagnostic values and reliability measures,[13,14] may add some elements of knowledge but may not provide useful information for the particular patient at hand. Prognostic epidemiologic tables may list, compare, or discuss signs and symptoms of various disorders and are readily available in textbooks and journals. Traditional diagnostic tests, such as radiographs or magnetic resonance imaging (MRI), may be available for study. Results of these tests may be helpful in determining the source of the patient's disorder but may be misleading in selected circumstances.[15]

Questioning and examining during the patient history, PE, and treatment form the nexus of strong clinical reasoning and are discussed further in this chapter. Mark Jones defines *physical differentiation* as that which "involves altering the pain provoking position, or movement in such a way, that one structure is implicated as the source, while another is eliminated from contention."[16] The purpose of physical differentiation is to so stress one area that symptoms are produced from that area alone; thus, the other area(s) is (are) ruled out as a source of the disorder.

CRITICAL ELEMENTS IN THE CLINICAL REASONING PROCESS

Critical elements in the clinical reasoning process are designed to improve the outcome of the patient interaction. Germane to these processes are (1) types of clinical decision-making processes, (2) recognition of the source of the disorder, (3) recognition of clinical hypothesis contributors, and (4) correct use and understanding of terminology.

Types of Clinical Decision Making

The process of making clinical decisions involves both vertical and lateral thinking. Vertical thinking is characterized by logical, sequential, predictable, and what might be called conventional thinking. Lateral thinking is not necessarily sequential, and it is unpredictable. Lateral thinking involves restructuring, an escape from old patterns and the creation of new ones; it is concerned with the generation of new ideas, and with looking at things in a different way. Although vertical thinking stays within a problem space, lateral thinking tends to restructure the problem space. Vertical thinking is hindered by the necessity to be right at each stage of the thought process and by the attempt to rigidly define everything. Lateral thinking is based on the notion that premature formation and expression of an idea may inhibit its natural development.

Recognition of the Source of the Disorder

In uncomplicated presentations, the source of the disorder is clarified during the patient history, and an initial hypothesis is formed. This hypothesis is confirmed, rejected, or modified during the PE and/or during treatment. In complicated presentations, clarification of the source of the disorder often is delayed until treatment; the hypothesis then is tested at subsequent visits. The questioning techniques in the patient history, the examination techniques in the PE, and the techniques used for treatment all may influence the outcomes of the differential assessment.

Recognition of Clinical Hypothesis Contributors

Clinical hypothesis categories, as described by Jones,[17-19] provide a guideline for all types of assessment. In essence, clinical hypothesis categories are elements that may contribute to overall patient presentation, outcomes, and well-being. These categories include (1) the source of the patient's symptoms, (2) factors contributing to the disorder, (3) precautions and contraindications, (4) management, (5) prognosis, and (6) mechanisms of the symptoms. These categories are tested consistently during the patient history, during the PE, and during treatment.[17-22]

Correct Use and Understanding of Terminology

Two relevant terms, which may require clarification, are *comparable sign* and *asterisks*. The comparable sign "refers to a combination of pain, stiffness, and spasm, which the examiner finds on examination and considers comparable with the patient's symptoms."[23,24] The comparable sign may be thought of as both a comparable sign and a comparable symptom, and it is verified by the patient as being the complaint that has prompted him or her to seek diagnosis and treatment.[25] The sign is visible to or palpable by the therapist, and the symptom is felt by the patient. A comparable joint or neural sign refers to any combination of pain, stiffness, and spasm that the examiner finds on examination and considers comparable with the patient's symptoms.

Although the comparable sign is queried during the patient history, this phenomenon is also a physical response detected during the objective examination. Investigation demands inspection during the physical assessment and requires further examination throughout the length of the intervention. The comparable sign often is used as a litmus test to identify both mechanical and pain-related changes over time.[25]

Asterisks (*) "are not mandatory for treatment by passive movement to be quickly successful. The only purpose of the asterisk is to highlight the important aspects that can be used to guide the assessment of the effectiveness of the treatment—to speed up the assessment process."[23]

CERVICAL AND THORACIC SPINE ANATOMY AND BIOMECHANICS

This chapter focuses on the cervical and thoracic spine. The cervical spine is divided appropriately into the upper cervical spine and the lower cervical spine. The upper cervical segments are formed by the articulation of the occiput on C1 (OA joint) and the articulation of C1 on C2 (AA joint).[26] This region includes unique joints and ligaments and does not include an intervertebral disc.[27] The lower cervical segments are more homogenous and include the vertebral levels of C2-3 to C7-T1. All segments exhibit intervertebral discs, uncinate processes, and spinous processes.[28]

Key features of the upper cervical spine include the sacrifice of stability for increased mobility. The primary planar motion at C0-1 is flexion/extension, characterized by total segmental range-of-motion values of approximately 25 degrees.[28] Unilateral lateral flexion is limited to 5 degrees, as is unilateral rotation.[28] The axial-atlanto (AA) joint is responsible for 50% of all cervical rotation motion,[28] whereas the occipital atlantal joint (OA) accounts for 50% of flexion and extension of the complete cervical spine.[29]

Cook et al[30] reviewed the coupling characteristics of the upper cervical spine and found variations among multiple biomechanical studies. During manual therapy, coupling is used to lock joints, a term identified as *apposition*.[31] Inconsistency in coupling patterns among subjects suggests that coupling patterns of the upper cervical spine are variable and may not be useful for technique application or during assessment.

The lower cervical spine and the upper thoracic spine both demonstrate lesser range-of-motion values when compared with the upper cervical spine, and they have similar values of plane-based ranges. Segments C2-3, C3-4, C6-7, and C7-T1 display the lowest segmental combined flexion/extension ranges, and C4-5 and C5-6 exhibit the highest values.[28] Unilateral side flexion progressively declines from cephalad to caudal, dropping from a peak of 10 to 11 degrees at C2-3, C3-4, and C4-5 to a low of 4 degrees at C7-T1. Unilateral rotation is greatest at C3-4 to C6-7, with nearly comparative values throughout. One exception is the lowest recorded value for unilateral rotation at C7-T1, with a reported range of 0 to 7 degrees.

The upper thoracic spine demonstrates a combined 3 to 5 degrees of flexion or extension that is reduced to 2 to 7 degrees at T5 to T6 and further increases to 6 to 20 degrees at T12 to L1. Overall, greater range of motion is available in flexion than in extension. The combined side flexion of the thoracic spine is also bimodal, with approximately 5 degrees of motion in the upper thoracic region, slipping to 3 to 10 for the levels of T7 to T11, then progressing to 5 to 10 at T12-L1. Finally, combined rotation is purported to be 14 degrees at T1-2, which progressively declines to 2 to 3 degrees when combined at T12-L1, mimicking the movement available in the lumbar spine.

Outside of a similar reduction in range-of-motion values, the lower cervical spine and the upper thoracic spine demonstrate significant differences. Cook et al[30] reported consistent cervical coupling motion from C2-3 to C8-T1, whereas in contrast, Sizer et al[32] acknowledged significant variations in coupling of the upper thoracic region of the spine and throughout all regions of the thoracic spine. The thoracic spine harbors the rib cage and the corresponding connections to the spine. In addition to intervertebral and zygopophyseal joints, the thoracic has costovertebral joints, costotransverse joints, and costosternal joints. The costotransverse joints articulate in two regions with the transverse processes and may act as a pain generator.[33] The rib head of the costovertebral joint articulates with the lateral aspect of the intervertebral disc, in addition to the two separate vertebral connections,[34] and may be involved during acute costovertebral pain.[35]

An additional variation within the thoracic spine is the presence of the 12 sympathetic nervous system ganglia, which play an important part in pain autoregulation and perception. Although the preponderance of the sympathetic nervous system is present in the thoracic spine, stimulation of the cervical and thoracic spine has led to upper extremity changes in pain response (pressure-pain) and a measurable neurophysiologic effect.[36-38]

ASSESSMENT PRINCIPLES

Patient History

Skillful assessment separates the successful clinician from the technician. Without assessment, treatment is the blind application of techniques without guidelines; success may be a matter of luck rather than skill. Without skillful assessment, planning and progression are haphazard and lack direction, and the therapist and the patient often are confused about the purpose or the expected outcome of treatment.

A quality patient history involves more than a regimented checklist of questions. Although the information is collected by talking with the patient, as opposed to measuring objective changes, the quality of the information needed far exceeds that gathered by the recording of simple facts. For example, the accurate completion of a pain drawing or a body chart on a patient with an assortment of neck, head, upper extremity, and upper thoracic symptoms may consume 10 minutes of skilled questioning and clarification. The relationships, if any, among the different symptoms must be sorted out. The present and past histories of the disorder have yet to be addressed.

As was mentioned earlier in the section on daily clinical assessment, the patient history consists of five major elements: (1) the nature and kind of the disorder, (2) the area of symptoms, (3) the behavior of the symptoms, (4) the past and present history, and (5) special questions. Accurate definition of the area of symptoms includes the precise location on the body chart of all the patient's abnormal sensations, including depth, surface location, and extent and direction of spread peripherally. It often is helpful, when the therapist has completed the body chart, to clarify where the symptoms stop—for example, by asking, "You mean that, below your elbow, your right forearm feels the same as your left forearm—there are no abnormal sensations in either forearm?" Clarification of the distal extent of the symptoms will allow the therapist to refer to the elbow symptoms as the barometer for determining a centralization response.

Symptom behavior, both diurnal and nocturnal, provides the therapist with an understanding of the nature of the problem. Questions such as, "Are the symptoms constant or intermittent?" and, "If constant, do they vary in intensity?" are useful. If symptoms caused by mechanical deformation are completely abolished during certain periods of the day, the mechanical deformation has been removed. Once symptoms appear to be mechanical, the effects of movement and posture on these symptoms can be established. For example, are the symptoms better or worse when the patient is sitting, moving, lying, or standing? Ask the patient to compare symptoms in the morning vs. symptoms in the evening. Is sleep disturbed? If so, to what extent? For example, "Are you unable to fall asleep, or is your sleep disturbed?" If so, "How frequently are you awakened?" Pain at night may reflect inflammatory problems, other medical problems, or poor sleeping posture in need of correction. Coughing and sneezing increase intrathoracic pressure, and the behavior of symptoms during those maneuvers constitutes essential information. If the patient's responses to questions about the behaviors of symptoms are not clear, possibly because of the chronic nature of the complaints or the minor nature of the problem, the relative worsening of symptoms may be ascertained. It may be necessary to rephrase or repeat questions to get a clear picture.

The past or previous history, as compared with the recent history of current neck pain, requires establishment. For recurrent problems, it is important to clarify the severity and frequency of past bouts to determine whether the problem is progressive. Repeated progressive bouts with exacerbations in the absence of trauma strongly suggest a discogenic syndrome. It is helpful for the therapist to know the condition of the region before the most recent bout occurred. If repeated insults from intrinsic or extrinsic trauma have occurred, it is possible that recovery may be delayed, or treatment may yield lesser outcomes.

Previous treatment for the same or earlier conditions, as well as the efficacy of the prior treatment, may provide a clue as to what will be successful this time. It also is helpful to know what, if anything, has been done for the present problem and its effects, if any. Patients frequently report that they derive limited benefit from a particular exercise, and on further investigation, it is found that fine tuning of the exercise produces a more positive treatment effect. For example, the direction of the self-treatment, discovered by the patient, may have been correct, but the depth of movement or the frequency of exercise was insufficient.

Questions regarding special diagnostic tests such as radiography, computed tomography (CT), and MRI should be unbiased; simply ask, for example, "Have you had recent x-rays?" The therapist would like to know the results and where the radiographs may be located so he or she can ascertain whether problems for which certain treatments are unsuitable have been ruled out. Routinely, poor positive correlation is noted between findings on radiography and the clinical state of the patient.[39]

The patient's general health is explored to discover serious pathology that may have been undetected by the referring physician, and to determine the relevance of known health problems. Does the patient look unwell, and has a recent unplanned weight loss occurred? Does the patient have a history of rheumatoid arthritis, which may suggest laxity of the transverse ligament? Are there any systemic diseases, including recent surgery and cardiorespiratory disease, that will restrict the patient's ability to perform active exercises? Are symptoms of vertebral artery disease apparent?

Questions regarding medications, including steroids, are asked, so that the effects of the medications on the patient's pain can be determined and any systemic effects of the drugs can be estimated. The occasional use of mild analgesics that eliminate the pain suggests a moderately painful condition, whereas regular use of strong analgesics that only reduce the pain suggests a more painful condition. Long-term use of steroids may weaken the connective tissue. Patients who report suspected osteoporosis require more cautious treatment, especially in the thoracic spine.

On completion of the patient history, the therapist has gleaned extensive and relevant information in an efficient manner to the extent that the therapist is able to establish, in many cases, a tentative conclusion. When questions and answers flow in a fluid and logical manner, a particular structure is often implicated. The assessment has been successful to this point. A summary of the patient history is presented in Table 9-1.

Physical Examination

The PE is a series of appropriate active and passive movement tests aimed at collecting additional data that will confirm or deny the therapist's tentative hypotheses reached during the patient history. A typical PE consists of active physiologic movements, passive physiologic movements, passive accessory movements, and special tests, as needed.

Table 9-1	Treatment Modes Related to Reactivity and Stages of Scar Tissue Formation	
Stages	**Reactivity**	**Treatment**
Inflammation	Pain, then resistance	Rest Immobilization Grade I and II movements
Granulation fibroplastic (healing)	Pain and resistance, simultaneous	Active range-of-motion exercises Grade I and II movements
Maturation	Resistance, then pain	Passive range-of-motion exercises Grade III, IV, and V movements

Adapted from Paris SV: Extremity dysfunction and mobilization, Atlanta, 1980, Institute Press.

The PE can confirm, deny, or modify the therapist's tentative hypotheses. For example, headaches are well known to be associated with lower cervical spondylosis and upper cervical joint arthrosis.[39-42] Empirical evidence favors the upper joints as being at fault.[40] Many patients will complain of a stiff neck and a morning headache at the base of the occiput or late-day headaches behind the ipsilateral eye or on the vertex of the head. Subsequent movement tests and palpations are aimed at reproducing the pain of the stiff neck and a very small portion of the headache symptoms. It is most possible that the stiff neck and the headache are related, but it is also possible that they are two separate entities. If the relationship was not clarified during the patient history, it most likely will be clarified during the PE.

Many hypotheses regarding the proximate cause of lower cervical lesions have been put forth. Ligamentous lengthening with periosteal lifting, chronic lower cervical spine flexion deformation with weakening of the posterior annular wall, osteophyte formation, and alteration of the length and tone of the cervical musculature are the explanations most frequently suggested.

Regardless of the treatment approach favored by the therapist, it is important to address posture in sitting, standing, and lying. Few patients, except in the acute state of a disorder, are unable to benefit from a reduction in chronic forward head posture. Many patients report significant relief from their symptoms after postural correction alone.

Purpose

The general purpose of the PE is to assess movement and symptom behavior, that is, limitations, deviations, aberrations, and the effects, if any, of movement on the patient's symptoms. Any deviation from normal movement and all symptom changes are noted. Future changes in the patient's condition then can be measured against the benchmarks of objective signs and patient history–generated symptoms. Movement loss may be graded as major, moderate, minor, or none. This loss also may be expressed as a percentage of normal or may be expressed in degrees.

Besides assessing movement, a second purpose of the PE, especially when stiffness is treated, is to reproduce the patient's comparable sign. For example, if the patient's chief complaint is a moderate midcervical pain, and this same pain is reproduced by overpressure into the quadrant position, the quadrant position may be used later to assess the effects of treatment.[43]

A third purpose of the PE is to determine the preferred direction of treatment movements. Repeated movements that reduce, centralize, and eliminate the patient's symptoms should be used in treatment for discogenic syndromes. Repeated movements that temporarily produce, but do not worsen, the patient's symptoms are the movements that should be used in treatment for stiffness. If no movements, either passive or active, can be found that produce the desirable effect on the patient's symptoms, the patient may not be a good candidate for that treatment, or the examination may be faulty.

Instructions to Patients

The relative vigor and extent of the PE depend on the irritability of the patient's symptoms. If the cervical or thoracic spine is judged to be irritable, the examination must be gentle and limited to a few necessary movements. The patient with an acute nerve root irritation, with symptoms extending below the elbow, deserves a gentle examination. However, a nonirritable and moderately painful condition will require a more vigorous and extensive examination. Few patients require inclusion of all test movements to satisfy the purpose of the examination.

The therapist must know the status of the patient's symptoms immediately before starting the examination and at the conclusion of each test movement. Thus the patient is asked to describe pretest symptoms and to report clearly any change in symptoms during and immediately after each test movement. It is also important for the patient to understand that, in most circumstances, some test movements may make the symptoms worse, and others may make them better. The more accurately the patient is able to convey any changes to the therapist, the more informative the examination will be, and, quite likely, the more effective the treatment will be.

Special Tests Before the Physical Examination

If symptoms extend below the elbow, a neurologic examination should be completed before the PE is conducted.[6,25] If red flags are suspected, tests with high sensitivity may help to rule out the presence of a serious disorder.[6] If the patient complains of dizziness or other associated symptoms, an essential part of the examination should consist of tests that estimate the integrity of the vertebrobasilar and the internal carotid artery system.[44] When these tests are performed before the PE, the effects, if any, of the examination itself may be assessed at the conclusion of the examination. Without a pretest, there is no benchmark from which to measure.

Several cervical artery dysfunction testing methods have been defined within the literature. Sustained end-of-range rotation of the cervical spine, first described by Maitland in 1968,[45,46] has long been suggested as the most effective method for vertebrobasilar insufficiency (VBI) assessment of the upper cervical spine, and it is currently recommended in the premanipulation guidelines for the cervical spine[45,47-49] that are used by physiotherapists and other manual therapists. In addition, the practice of placing an individual in the premanipulative position before the procedure is performed, so the patient's tolerance to the position can be assessed, is advocated.[50]

Because use of the testing method introduces some risk for a positive VBI, it may be advisable to avoid performing the test or providing treatment in cases where subjective symptoms are commonly reported, or past tests have demonstrated positive findings. In the event of a positive VBI during testing, treatment should be stopped immediately and appropriate medical assistance obtained.[47]

Dizziness and reflex disorders of posture and movement also may be caused by degenerative, inflammatory, or traumatic disorders of the joints and muscles of the cervical spine. These structures are richly supplied with proprioceptive nerve endings.[51-53] Thus dizziness is not always vertebrobasilar or internal carotid in origin.

Proper radiographic evaluation of suspected atlantoaxial instability is imperative before any vigorous objective assessment is attempted. Afflictions of this joint do occur, especially in Down syndrome, rheumatoid arthritis, ankylosing spondylitis, psoriatic arthritis, and posttraumatic conditions. Tests and measures such as the alar ligament stability test, the Sharp Purser test, and others may be beneficial during assessment but have yet to be proven unequivocally to be effective in identifying patients with instability.[5] Vigorous examinations or treatment, where instability exists, have led to disastrous complications, dating back to early reports by Blaine.[54] When instability is expected, radiographic testing may serve as a beneficial tool, specifically when transverse ligament instability is the source of the dysfunction.[55]

THE EXAMINATION

Observation

Observation is designed to provide introspective and external findings associated with posture, attitude, compliance, and appearance. Sitting the patient on the narrow end of the treatment table enables the therapist to observe from either side and from the front. The clinician should note the general sitting posture, static deformity, asymmetry, and the condition of the skin, and should acknowledge the patient's willingness to move.

Test Movements

Before any test movements are assessed, the present symptoms noted in the sitting position must be recorded. For each test movement, the clinician should estimate movement loss and the relationship between the patient's symptoms and range. It is helpful, for the sake of consistency in recording data, for the therapist to establish a routine sequence. A routine in the order of testing movements also helps to avoid omissions.

The appropriate method used during active movement is to test a movement once and then to repeat the same test movement several times. Active movements may be sustained or oscillated to produce the desired effect. For the sake of patient education, it often is necessary to ask the patient to repeat a movement that makes him or her worse, and then to repeat a movement that makes him or her better. Movements must be sufficiently far into the range to produce a valid response to the test. A sequence of testing for the cervical spine may involve protraction, flexion, retraction, retraction and extension, bilateral sidebend, and bilateral rotation. Thoracic spine movements may include plane-based movements, as well as combined movements.

Another method of testing active physiologic movements is to have the patient move toward the pain (when treating pain) or to move toward the limit (when treating stiffness). It is important to clarify and accurately record the relationship between range and pain. A sequence of testing in balanced posture consists of flexion, extension, lateral flexion, and bilateral rotation. Movements also may be tested in different parts of the flexion/extension range.

Movements may be sustained and overpressured as needed. The quadrants (a combination of extension with sidebending and rotation to the same side) for the upper and lower cervical spines may be tested if previous tests have been negative. Compression and distraction are used when necessary. Passive physiologic movements also may be tested in the supine position. Tests of the pain-sensitive structures in the intervertebral canal and static tests for muscle pain are performed as applicable.

The patient is placed in a prone position for palpation tests, including temperature and sweating, soft tissue palpation, positions of the vertebrae, and passive accessory intervertebral movement tests. Passive accessory intervertebral movements are described later in the section on treatment procedures and techniques. The therapist marks important findings on the chart with an asterisk. The effects of the examination then are assessed both subjectively and objectively by retesting of one or two movements. The patient's chart is reviewed for reports of relevant medical tests.

For treating pain, the technique that reduces (and in some cases centralizes and eliminates) the pain is chosen as the treatment technique. For treating stiffness, the technique that produces the comparable sign but does not make it worse is selected as the treatment technique. A concurrent increase in range is a desirable treatment outcome when stiffness is treated. After treatment, the patient is reassessed. The patient then is warned of possible exacerbations, is asked to report details of the behaviors of symptoms as noted between now and the next visit, and is given instructions regarding neck and thoracic care.

For both approaches, complete objective assessment involves testing other joints, including the glenohumeral joints, which may be responsible for the production of the patient's symptoms. A summary of the physical examination is presented in Box 9-1.

DIFFERENTIAL ASSESSMENT OF THE CERVICAL AND THORACIC SPINE

The Need for Differentiation

Pain in the cervical and thoracic spine is a common but nonspecific presentation.[56] Somatic referred pain from these regions may present from the occiput, into the shoulder, toward the paramedian neck region, and into the parascapular region.[57] Somatic referred pain can radiate into the jaw and cause headaches.[57] Radicular pain may refer into the upper extremities and into the scapular region. Myelopathic symptoms generally are initiated as motor deficits first, but they also may demonstrate pain or sensory changes, if chronic.

> ### BOX 9-1   Summary of Subjective Assessment*
>
> - Type of disorder (pain, stiffness, weakness, etc.)
> - Location of the patient's symptoms, including extent of peripheralization (recorded on the body or pain chart)
> - Nature of the symptoms, including frequency, original location, and degree of disability
> - Cause of the problem, if known (trauma, systemic disease; insidious)
> - Behavior of the symptoms over a 24-hour period, including the effects of different postures
> - Effects of changes in intrathoracic pressure
> - Present or recent history
> - Past history, including treatment, if any
> - Patient's general health, results of any medical tests, and medications and their effects
> - Other relevant information peculiar to the patient

*It is assumed that the patient has already completed a brief medical history, and that this information has been reviewed by the therapist.

Although biomechanically and structurally discrete, the cervical and thoracic spine is so heavily influenced by convergence that physical differentiation is often necessary to discriminate the origin of the pain generator. Cervical and thoracic referred pain is common and frequently overlaps in presentation.[58] Cervical or thoracic pain can be felt in an undamaged part of the body, away from the actual point of injury or disease.[59] Thus, for focal and targeted care, it may be necessary to examine the cervical and thoracic spine individually.

For presentation of cervical-thoracic differentiation in this chapter, the sections to refer to are labeled "Cervical (Doubtful Thoracic)" and "Thoracic (Doubtful Cervical)." *Her* is used to refer to the therapist, and *he* is used to refer to the patient, for convenience. No gender bias is intended.

Cervical (Doubtful Thoracic)

Nature and Kind of Disorder

If he knows the source of his symptoms, he will implicate the cervical spine. In general, chronic symptoms are more difficult for him to describe accurately than are acute symptoms. Recently, Cook et al[60] described a number of findings associated with patient history and physical examination in patients with chronic clinical instability. Findings were associated with lack of perceived segmental control and with findings of giving way and/or slipping out.[60] Words like *tired* and *fatigue* suggest weakness associated with instability and may warrant anterior and posterior cervical strength testing.[61]

An acute history of trauma may suggest instability of the upper C-spine. Use of Canadian C-spine rules may assist in determining who benefits from a radiograph.[62] Tests and measures such as the alar ligament stability test, the Sharp Purser test, and others may be useful for identifying ligamentous laxity.[5] Ligamentous damage is common after motor vehicle accidents and may persist for several months.[63]

Symptoms associated with clumsiness of the lower extremities and hands may reflect myelopathic changes,[64-71] whereas difficulty walking with immediate relief upon cessation of activity suggests spinal intermittent claudication.[72] Cervical spine myelopathy (CSM) involves spinal cord compression or injury and is considered a serious finding. CSM is associated with physiologic narrowing of the sagittal diameter of the spinal canal caused by congenital or degenerative changes.[73] The compression associated with cervical CSM may progress to spinal cord ischemia, leading to histopathologic changes of the spinal cord, often termed *myelomalacia*.[74]

A painful neck is a common complaint; however, pain is frequently a secondary consequence associated with loss of range of motion. Degenerative conditions are ubiquitous in the aging population and can lead to joint stiffness, muscle spasm, and other related problems.[56] When stiffness associated with the patient's dysfunction is addressed, pain often is no longer the dominant factor; when movement is restored, pain subsides.[75]

Area of Symptoms

Cervical symptoms are often ipsilateral, referring into the medial scapular area, the supraspinatus fossa, and/or the posterior arm, forearm, and/or hand. Cervicogenic headaches, which often have an origin at C3 or above, are commonly described.[76] Nonetheless, headaches also may originate from C6 through T4.[77] Variations in the sites of headache may be due to referral from the dura and/or from the muscles.[78]

Symptoms caused by a deformed cervical disc are felt deeply, and symptoms from an apophyseal joint(s) are felt relatively superficially. The patient often can point to the site of apophyseal pain with accuracy, but not to the site of discogenic pain. Acute cervical pain is often, but not always, worse distally. Paresthesia is common but is not always recognized as significant by the patient. Ocular dysfunctions such as visual accommodation, visual convergence, and disorders of pupil function may be present in patients with cervical disorders.[79]

Behavior of Symptoms

Neck movements, especially sustained or quick movements, usually increase symptoms associated with cervical radiculopathy. Symptoms sometimes are relieved by reaching overhead or by lifting up the ipsilateral elbow.[80] At times, neck posture alters upper extremity symptoms.[81] Upper limb tension tests often reproduce cervical symptoms but are not considered specific tools for diagnosis or implication of a specific tissue lesion.[5,82] Patients with cervical disorders usually prefer to sleep on the affected side.

History of Symptoms

For stiffness or somatic-type dysfunctions, stiffness is noticed before pain onset. Both gradual and sudden onsets are common.

Patients, if questioned thoroughly, often recall previous bouts of neck stiffness. Patients with a discogenic neck disorder often awaken with their neck pain, as opposed to those with a cervical "lock," who often are awakened by their neck pain.[83,84] No history of trauma is reported in cervical lock, in contrast to the history of a neck sprain.[85] The history of many cervical disorders reveals repetitive microtrauma to the cervical spine from chronic poor posture or from patterns of postural activity.[86,87]

Physical Examination

For Cervical (Doubtful Thoracic) symptoms, the goal of the PE is to reproduce symptoms from the cervical spine and clear the thoracic spine. Active physiologic, passive physiologic, and passive accessory test movements are used to examine the cervical and thoracic spine. Later, one of these test movements probably will be used as a treatment technique; the treatment logically evolves from the examination.

Reproduction of the comparable sign is desirable but is not mandatory, especially in the irritable patient. Irritable patients may have intense symptoms, symptoms that are produced or made worse by mild activity, constant symptoms, or long-lasting, intermittent symptoms that settle slowly. In the nonirritable patient, it may be necessary to add vigor to the examination to reproduce the comparable sign—for example, upper and lower cervical quadrants, axial compression, and/or axial distraction. Compression may implicate weight-bearing structures (intervertebral disc or the apophyseal joints); axial distraction may implicate ligaments and/or muscles believed to be under stretch.[88]

Agreement between the objective findings of the therapist and the subjective responses of the patient is important for verifying the source of the disorder. If the features of the examination do not fit, that is, if no subjective and objective agreement is noted, then the examination may be faulty. After PE of the cervical spine has been performed, signs should be reassessed so the effects of the examination can be determined; the cervical signs should change.

The thoracic spine is cleared with appropriate overpressures in flexion, extension, bilateral sidebending, and bilateral rotations. Reassessment of the thoracic spine after the PE reveals no change, unless thoracic signs are cervical in origin.

Hypothesis Testing and Treatment

If the Cervical (Doubtful Thoracic) hypothesis is true, signs in the cervical spine are comparable and reproducible. Thoracic signs are minimal and are not comparable. Initially, treat the most comparable cervical sign; then reassess both areas. To confirm the cervical hypothesis, both the cervical spine and the thoracic spine should improve if thoracic signs are cervical in origin. If the cervical spine improves and clears and the thoracic spine does not, then reject the Cervical (Doubtful Thoracic) hypothesis and treat the thoracic spine; both areas are at fault.

Thoracic (Doubtful Cervical)

Nature and Kind of Disorder

Within the spine, the thoracic spine is the area least understood by most therapists and least investigated by researchers. The overall size of the thoracic spine requires subdivision into three separate sections: (1) upper, (2) middle, and (3) lower. The lower thoracic spine (thoracolumbar) is the most frequently injured region of the spine. What is less apparent is the injury rate of other regions such as the mid and upper thoracic spine. The overall size of the thoracic spine permits development of a number of unrelated disorders, some of which are more prevalent to selected regions (i.e., upper, middle, or lower).

Disorders range from trivial complaints to serious, disabling disorders. Pain, stiffness, and weakness are among the most common complaints. Findings of palpation are often easy to find and interpret.[89] The patient's own words provide extremely useful information regarding the kind and nature of the patient's problem.

Area(s) of Symptoms

In addition to soft, neural, and muscle tissues, seven joints are present at each level of the thoracic spine.[90] Sometimes symptoms are visceralogenic (heart, lungs, diaphragm) and/or vertebralogenic.[91] The thoracic spine houses the sympathetic nervous system, except for lumbar levels 1 and 2, and the costovertebral joints and other tissues are adjacent to the sympathetic trunks; thus, mechanically induced sympathetic symptoms are possible.[91,92] Hyperhidrosis, hypotrophic changes, and other symptoms are evident in chronic cases.[79]

Thoracic symptoms occur (1) in the anterior and posterior chest wall, (2) in the groin and the posterior thigh (T10-T12), (3) along the ribs, and (4) in the anterior and posterior arm (T1). Midthoracic symptoms are often neurogenic, most likely from the dura, nerve root, and/or nerve root sleeves. The terms *cervical spine* and *thoracic spine* both refer into the interscapular area. Levels T2 to T7 may produce a vertex headache.

Deep central back pain that radiates through the chest, producing central anterior chest pain, appears to arise from the intervertebral disc if the pain is neuromuscular in origin.[93] Unilateral thoracic pain, which radiates horizontally around the chest wall, is probably due to unilateral joint structures: zygapophyseal, costovertebral, and/or costotransverse joints. Unilateral thoracic pain that radiates along the line of the rib usually originates from the nerve root and, if acute, is likely to be worse either laterally on the chest wall or anteriorly in the distal part of the affected dermatome.[94]

Behavior of the Symptoms

Patients with mechanical rib dysfunction may complain of difficulty breathing, especially on inspiration. Activities involving thoracic rotation and extension frequently produce symptoms. To a lesser extent, activities requiring stabilization of the thoracic spine are informative.

History of Symptoms

Insidious onset, specifically in the elderly, is common. It often is attributed to intrinsic forces of chronic poor posture, including disuse, misuse, and overuse. Obvious causal factors are (1) motor vehicle accidents, (2) postsurgical condition, and (3) excessive physical activity. Visual disturbances, probably resulting from mechanical deformation or from chemical irritation of the sympathetic chain, may be present. Adverse neural tension signs are common, especially in chronic cases.

Physical Examination

The vigor of the PE is determined by the outcome of the patient history. Active physiologic, combined physiologic, passive physiologic, passive accessory, and neurotension tests are informative. The slump test is sensitive but not specific and produces pain in 90% of normal subjects at the T8 and T9 levels.[91] The long-sitting position usually isolates the thoracic spine better than does sitting on the edge of the treatment table. The sympathetic slump test purportedly assesses disorders of the autonomic nervous system.[95,96]

For a physiologic differentiation test, rotate the cervical spine without rotating the thoracic spine; then add only thoracic rotation to the cervical rotation. Assess the symptoms at each interval of change, and then reverse the order of the tests to confirm or reject the results. For an accessory test, the intent is to try to move one segment locally.[91] For a thoracic segment to be rotated significantly, the transverse processes and the spinous process of the segment should show asymmetry; deviation of the spinous process alone may reflect normal asymmetry. Deep-set and high-set spinous processes may be considered suspicious.[91] Reproduction of the comparable sign, coupled with significant palpation abnormalities, strengthens the hypothesis of local thoracic injury.

Suspicion of thoracic cord myelopathy suggests the need for reflex tests, clonus tests, and tests of lower limb coordination, although the merits of these tools for detection of myelopathy are unknown.[5] To reproduce an evasive comparable sign, the slump test in the long-sitting position may prove useful by applying thoracic sidebending away from the disorder coupled with a deep inspiration.[95] For indirect neural tension tests of the thoracic spine, use straight leg raise, passive neck flexion, and prone knee bend. Other authors have written extensively on the subject of nerve tension tests and glides.[82,95,97-99]

Hypothesis Testing and Treatment

If the Thoracic (Doubtful Cervical) hypothesis is true, signs in the thoracic spine are comparable and reproducible. Cervical signs are minimal and not comparable. Initially, treat the most comparable thoracic sign; then reassess both areas. For confirmation of the thoracic hypothesis, both the thoracic spine and the cervical spine should improve if cervical signs are thoracic in origin. If the thoracic spine improves and clears and the cervical spine does not, then reject the Thoracic (Doubtful Cervical) hypothesis and treat the cervical spine; both areas are at fault. Assessment of outcomes at the next visit (day 2 assessment) is useful in chronic thoracic cases, especially if the transverse accessory test provokes symptoms.[91]

Evidence for Mobilization

The constructs behind the use of mobilization and manipulation are similar, and it is most important to note that the application of each treatment method results in similar functional outcomes and similar hypothesized effects.[100] The term *manipulation* has a multitude of meanings, and there is little agreement in the literature that could lead to universal acceptance. In this chapter, *manipulation* is defined in its broadest sense, which includes the use of refined motion performed either by the therapist (technique) or by the patient (procedure). These hypothesized effects are categorized frequently as biomechanical, muscular reflexogenic, and neurophysiologic.[101-103]

Biomechanical Effects

It is established that new remodeling tissue can be influenced by movement applied at the appropriate time in the proper direction. Both Evans[104] and Cummings et al[105] have described the beneficial effects of remodeling new collagen. It also is possible that hypomobile joints that have been underexercised for an extended time can be influenced positively by movement. One possible mechanism involves stretching or rupture of abnormal cross-links that were formed between fibers. Cross-links between collagen-based fibers inhibit normal connective tissue gliding that can lead to restricted joint movement[106] and corresponding loss of range of motion. Evidence suggests that mobilization and/or manipulation techniques solicit joint displacement[107] and cause temporary increases in the degree of displacement that is produced with force due to hysteresis effects.[108]

A number of studies have demonstrated the biomechanical effects of increased extensibility and gains in range of motion upon the use of stretching, muscle energy techniques, mobilization, or manipulation.[25] Although most of the literature demonstrating biomechanical benefit describes only marginal quality, in nearly all cases a demonstrable range of motion changed immediately for short-term gains.[25]

Muscle Reflexogenic

Practitioners of manual therapy have long purported reflexogenic benefits associated with select directed manual therapy techniques.[101,109-111] The thrust-like forces incurred during a manipulation[112-119] or repeated oscillatory forces used during mobilization[110,113,114] are hypothesized to reduce pain through reflex inhibition of spastic muscles.[25] Muscle reflexogenic inhi-

bition is a consequence of stimulation of skin, muscle, and articular joint receptors.

According to Wyke,[120] three types of mechanoreceptors are known. Type I receptors, in the superficial layers of the fibrous capsule of the joints, are stimulated by end-range movements of the joints. Type II receptors are found in the deeper layers of the fibrous capsule of the joints and are stimulated by midrange movements of the joints. Type IV receptors are nociceptive afferents and are responsible for producing the unpleasant emotional experience commonly called pain.

The stimulation of either type I or type II mechanoreceptors, through an involved network of neural connections, is believed to be capable of modulating the experience of pain. Repeated movements, either active or passive, when performed at the end of the range or in the midrange, are capable of reducing pain and allowing for increased movement.

Neurophysiologic Effects

Appropriate movements may have a positive effect on the neurophysiologic activity of the tissues.[121] Passive mobilization forces arouse descending inhibitory systems that originate in the lateral periaqueductal grey matter of the brain stem[122] and exert segmental postsynaptic inhibition on dorsal horn pain pathway neurons.[122] Pain may be inhibited for up to 15 minutes after a manipulation is performed.[116] Investigators have found similar short-term effects with manipulation[118,119] and mobilization forces.[123,124] Although it is unsuitable to identify these responses as "short term," it does appear that this response decreases incrementally over 1 to 6 days. At 6 days, threshold changes were no longer reported.[125]

Moderate evidence supports that manual therapy, specifically consisting of an anteroposterior glide and a lateral glide,[126] provides an excitatory effect on sympathetic nervous system activity.[122,127,128] An excitatory effect on the sympathetic nervous system occurs concurrently with a reduction in hypoanalgesia and may parallel the effects of stimulation of the dorsal periaqueductal grey area of the midbrain.[129] Stimulation of the cervical spine has demonstrated upper extremity changes in pain response (pressure-pain) and a measurable sympathoexcitatory effect.[130,131]

Finally, the gate-control mechanism,[132] neural hysteresis, and release of endogenous opioids may represent the benefits associated with manual therapy. Small-diameter nociceptors are theorized to open the "gate," thus facilitating the perception of pain, whereas larger-diameter fibers tend to close the gate of pain.[25] Gating of pain is a mechanism whereby afferent and descending pathways modulate sensory transmission through inhibitory mechanisms within the central nervous system.[25]

THEORIES FOR MOBILIZATION OF THE CERVICAL AND THORACIC SPINE

Mobilization of the cervical and upper thoracic spine, with the intent of relieving pain or increasing range of motion, or both, may be performed actively or passively with a variety of procedures and techniques. The use of mobilization dates back to the days of Hippocrates.[133] According to Cyriax,[134] orthopaedic medicine was born in 1929. Orthopaedic manual therapy first became popular in Europe and Australia in the middle of the 20th century, largely as a result of the work of Freddy Kaltenborn, John Mennell, and Geoffrey Maitland.[135] Robin McKenzie[136] first published his theories in 1972. Stanley Paris is thought by many physical therapists to be largely responsible for introducing mobilization concepts in the United States during the 1960s.

It has been only recently that literature has been published to support the use of mobilization and/or manipulation. Recent meta-analyses have shown that mobilization and/or manipulation when combined with exercise is a useful treatment option.[137] Other studies have shown that cervical and thoracic manipulation, when targeted to patients with mechanical neck pain, leads to comparable and beneficial outcomes.

One reason that mobilization and manipulation are useful when combined with exercise is the multidimensional nature of the cervical spine. It is recognized that not all lesions of the upper spine are related to the articulations alone. Thus an effective program of treatment often will include other techniques for the soft tissues, including strengthening.[137] It also is acknowledged that not all lesions of the upper spine are mechanical. Thus, an effective program of treatment frequently will include physical agents or rest and analgesics as treatment for the chemical or inflammatory component of the patient's pain.[138]

Generally speaking, a physical therapist may elect one of three approaches to assess a patient. One approach is to conduct a patient history and a series of objective tests with the intent of reaching a tentative diagnosis, which may lead to the identification of a suspected structure at fault. From an academic and clinical point of view, physical therapists must understand diagnoses and pathologies. The stages of repair, referenced more thoroughly later in this chapter, are clearly related to proper management. Treatment then is aimed at this suspected structure. The therapist feels very comfortable and secure in addressing the problem in such a definite manner. Through this approach, usually called the *diagnostic approach,* the techniques used in treatment help to confirm or deny the diagnosis.

The second approach is to respect the medical diagnosis rendered by the referring physician, with appropriate precautions, and then to conduct a patient history and a series of objective tests with the intent of recording changes in the patient's signs and symptoms. No specific structure is designated as being at fault, and the treatment rendered is adjusted according to the patient's individual response. It is permissible to hypothesize about what is at fault, but the nature and progression of the treatment depend on the clinical behavior of the patient's problem. This approach has been called the *signs-and-symptoms approach,* the nonpathologic approach, and more recently, the *patient-response approach.*[25] Evidence indicates that the patient-response approach yields greater within- and between-session improvements when compared with non–patient-response methods.[139-141]

A third approach uses treatment that is based on a classification of signs and symptoms. This approach combines choices One and Two, but it allows treatment based on clinical prediction rules or other pertinent findings in the examination.[138] Findings from the examination require distillation into one of several categories for a specific or a nonspecific treatment.[142] It is likely that a clinician will use a variety of all three choices during treatment decision making. In this chapter, emphasis is placed on the patient-response approach, with some references made to the other selections when appropriate.

Patient-Response Approach

The patient-response approach allows signs and symptoms and findings of the examination to drive the treatment of the patient. A patient-response–based approach offers several advantages, including adaptability to each patient, specific treatment techniques, decreased reliance on untested or invalid theories, ease of use, and ability to change with patient presentation.[25] Nonetheless, the method is time intensive in that patient examination and treatment are not easily compartmentalized into common criteria, the model requires dedicated communication between the clinician and the patient, and the approach will fail without the concerted effort of both.[25]

Three Categories: Pain, Stiffness, and the Centralization Phenomenon

In the patient-response approach, in which changes in clinical signs and symptoms, with due respect for the medical diagnosis and contraindications, are used to select techniques and to determine the progression of treatment, obvious principles and theories underlie the clinical assessments and treatments. One useful method during treatment for the cervical and thoracic spine involves an understanding of the three classifications of *pain, stiffness,* and the *centralization phenomenon.*

Pain is not a primary sensation, like vision, hearing, and smell, but rather it is an abnormal affective state that is accurately described as an unpleasant emotional state. This emotional state is aroused by unusual patterns of activity within the nociceptive receptor system and is subject to different degrees of facilitation and inhibition.[143] The nociceptive receptor system is sensitive to mechanical and chemical tissue activity. Thus, if this largely inactive receptor system is stimulated by the application of sufficient mechanical forces to stress, deform, or damage it, mechanical pain is produced. However, if the system is irritated by sufficient concentrations of chemical substances such as lactic acid or potassium ions, chemical pain is produced. Thus, in a clinical situation, it is possible for the patient to have chemical pain, mechanical pain, or both concurrently.

Pain

Chemical or inflammatory pain is constant and is not much affected by movement or position. Seldom is chemical pain reduced by passive or active movement, because movement has little positive effect on the chemical irritants. Chemical pain often is increased by movement and reduced by rest. Chemical pain also may respond to medications that reduce the inflammatory process. For example, if a patient has active cervical arthritis and the main complaint is a constant burning ache together with reduced range of motion, even gentle attempts to increase this range through movement may increase the ache and may have no effect on the range or may reduce it.

Through the patient-response method, most notably identified by the Maitland approach, the therapist is obligated to decide, among other possibilities, whether she is treating the patient's pain or the patient's stiffness, with respect for the pain. This decision is based on many subjective and objective assessment variables, including joint irritability, the patient's perception of the nature of the problem, the relationship between range and pain, and the effects of passive movement during treatment. If pain is the dominant factor of concern to the patient, and if pain rather than resistance or stiffness prevents full range of motion, then the therapist elects to treat the patient's pain. Thus the success or failure of the treatment is based on its ability to reduce, centralize (where applicable), and eliminate the pain. This is not meant to imply that treatment for pain in the cervical spine is limited to cases in which the pain is produced by deformation of the intervertebral disc. Structures other than the disc are commonly capable of producing sufficient pain to warrant treatment for the pain alone.

Stiffness

Generally, mechanical pain is constant and variable or intermittent and often is affected by movement or position. Movements, either passive or active, that reduce the mechanical deformation also reduce the patient's symptoms. Patients whose problem is mechanical usually report that there is some time during the day or night when they are symptom free, or when their symptoms are significantly reduced or increased. Careful questioning by the therapist will frequently reveal that pain reported by the patient to be constant is, in fact, intermittent.

Two patients may demonstrate the same medical diagnosis associated with pain, correctly rendered. One individual may exhibit pain indirectly associated with movement, whereas another may report a main complaint of intermittent pain coupled with reduced range. Attempts to increase the second patient's range of movement in the proper direction will decrease the pain and often will increase the range concurrently. A patient with a cervical spine stiffness problem often complains of increased symptoms, potentially including occipital headache on arising in the morning. Symptoms often are limited to the first hour on awakening in the morning. Further, the patient will report that these symptoms are decreased or eliminated with movement, and frequently he or she experiences pain only after periods of inactivity.

Both Pain and Stiffness

It is acknowledged that most patients have both a chemical and a mechanical element to their dysfunction and present with both pain and stiffness. It is suggested that the two components of their pain, chemical and inflammatory, are closely related and interdependent (i.e., the chemical component may be the cause of the mechanical component). When both mechanical and chemical components are present, the therapist must make a therapeutic decision to treat either one component or both. It is possible that reduction of one component will have a positive effect on the other. For example, gentle low-grade movements applied to an apophyseal joint that is mechanically deformed may reduce the deformation and consequently the mechanical pain. The movements have no obvious effects on the chemical irritation, but at least the chemical irritation is not increased. Because the mechanical component of pain has been reduced, the range is increased, and the patient regains function without an exacerbation of the pain.

In this example, the therapist has chosen to treat the stiffness caused by mechanical deformation and, concurrently, to respect (by not increasing) the patient's inflammatory pain. Provided that the patient retains some of the increased function, it is reasonable to assume that the same treatment should be repeated until the patient's progress plateaus. It is suggested that to treat only one component may result in an incomplete recovery. For example, treating only the chemical component of the patient's pain with physical agents may have no effect, or an incomplete effect, on the mechanical component. Thus, the stage is set for recurrent bouts of the same problem caused by a likely regression of the patient's condition.

Centralization Phenomenon

McKenzie[144] described the centralization phenomenon as movement of pain from the periphery toward the midline of the spine. This mechanical pain, which originates from the spine and is referred distally, centralizes as a result of certain repeated movements or the assumption of certain positions. Movements that cause this phenomenon then may be used to eliminate radiating and referred symptoms. Centralization occurs only in the derangement syndrome during reduction of mechanical deformation. This centralization of pain in patients whose symptoms are of recent origin may occur within a few minutes. When centralization takes place, a significant increase in central spinal pain is often noted. For example, decreased arm pain is traded for a temporary increase in neck pain.

Although the centralization phenomenon has been substantially reported as associated with a positive outcome for treatment of patients with low back disorders,[145-148] little evidence supports its use in the cervical spine.[149] At present, no clinical trials have assessed the effectiveness of a treatment approach for the cervical spine driven by the centralization phenomenon, and no comparative trials have addressed this response mechanism.

*Not all these tests are performed on every patient. The therapist determines the extent of the examination on the basis of information gleaned during the subjective assessment.

SUMMARY

In summary, active, acute inflammatory pain in the cervical spine, as elsewhere, often requires rest, immobilization, and physical agents. As the healing process progresses and scar tissue forms, the area requires appropriate active or passive movement in proper doses. As the chemical pain abates and the patient presents with dominant mechanical pain, the area requires more vigorous movement. Excellent and detailed discussions of the relationships among the healing processes and treatment modes may be found in writings by Cummings et al[105] and Evans.[104] A summary of the relationships among the stages of healing, joint reactivity to movement, and treatment modes is presented in Box 9-2.

The centralization phenomenon is likely best used during treatment for both pain and stiffness. Because a number of cervical and thoracic conditions can lead to referred pain, centralizing movements may be useful during movement-related treatment for appropriate outcomes.

TREATMENT TECHNIQUES AND PROCEDURES

Technique Philosophy

The purpose of treatment is to apply purposeful techniques that reduce, centralize, or abolish the patient's signs and symptoms. A clinician's examination is completed by performing movements that alter the patient's report of signs and symptoms, a procedure defined as the *patient-response method.* The patient-response method requires a diligent effort of the patient and the clinician to determine the behavior of the patient's pain and/or impairment by analyzing comparable movements and the response of the patient's pain to repeated or applied movements.

Treatment methods are derived from the patient history and the physical examination. The comparable sign identified by the patient during the history and the repeated or sustained movements performed during the examination, which positively or negatively alter the signs and symptoms of the patient, deserve the highest priority for treatment selection and should be similar in construct to comparable examination movements. Examination methods that fail to elicit the patient response

may offer nominal or imprecise value, as do methods that focus solely on treatment decision making based on a single diagnostic label.

Active procedures are those movements performed by the patient. They are similar to active exercises, but not identical, because some active procedures may be largely passive. In the cervical spine, retraction and extension performed in the supine position, coupled with small rotations at the limit, are assisted by gravity and may require little or no active muscle action. If the patient applies overpressure, an active component is introduced into the procedure. In the lumbar spine, the press-up movement is mainly a passive procedure, without active involvement of the erector spinae or gluteal muscles. With active muscle contractions, full available range may not be obtained, and the assessment may become distorted. Side-bending or lateral flexion of the head performed in the sitting position is assisted by gravity, and relaxation of the muscles within the cervical spine often enhances a positive treatment effect.

Therapists must instruct the patient carefully in the proper method of performing active procedures. It is often necessary to demonstrate the exact movement desired. Instruct the patient to report any changes in symptom behavior that take place during and immediately after the procedure. The precise status of symptoms before the procedure is required for proper assessment. The consistency of test-retest (assessment) is affected by the patient's pretest posture.

Extension of the cervical spine usually is performed while starting in a retracted position. If consistency of the starting position (i.e., proper retraction) is not maintained, the assessment may be inaccurate. A potentially successful procedure that is thought to be ineffective, when inaccurate instruction was provided by the therapist, is wrongly abandoned or, worse yet, the approach is faulted.

Therapists' techniques are those movements performed on the patient by the therapist. They are passive and, in most respects, consist of mobilization achieved through passive physiologic or passive accessory techniques. Therapists' techniques, in contrast to active procedures, provide an extrinsic force, whereas active procedures provide an intrinsic force generated by the patient. Because the patient may, in part, be responsible for his own problem, as the result of chronic poor posture or other self-inflicted abuse, it is the patient's responsibility to treat his own problem by using active procedures. It is believed that a well-educated patient who understands the problem, including the mechanical model, most likely will be able to prevent or reduce future bouts of spinal pain. Thus, the patient stands a reasonable chance of ending or reducing a recurrent cycle of repeated bouts of spinal pain.

Therapists' techniques usually are performed as oscillating or repeated movements in a preferred direction. Movements may be sustained when a sustained position produces desirable effects. Sustained movements also may be used as provocative tests in an attempt to reproduce the patient's comparable sign. Endless variations in the speed, direction, and/or rhythm of a technique are possible.

Direction of a Procedure or Technique

Few, if any, absolutes or correct techniques or procedures are based on theory. General guidelines and contraindications provide the clinician with reasonably logical methods for selecting techniques or procedures. General guidelines and contraindications may be used in determining the desirable direction of forces. In general, these guidelines are based on current knowledge of pathology, known mechanical disorders of the vertebral column, the medical diagnosis, and changes in symptoms and signs. For the cervical and thoracic spine, Maitland[91] provides guidelines for the sequence of techniques and primary uses for mobilizing techniques. He recommends the use of cervical traction for an acute cervical condition in which severe arm pain is accompanied by markedly limited neck movement to the painful side. Once the pain has been brought under control with the use of traction, the therapist may elect to change techniques to address the residual stiffness, with respect for the pain. This is not meant to imply that techniques are used only to treat stiffness, because low-grade techniques (grades I and II) are used frequently and effectively to treat pain. Treatment for pain with passive movement is thoroughly described by Maitland.[91]

One of the advantages of the Maitland approach may be its efficacy in treating pain. For example, passive accessory movements are used frequently in the part of the range that is totally free of pain or discomfort. As the patient's pain decreases and signs of movement improve, the technique can be taken further through the range, and the amplitude of the technique increased. Gentle rotation movements of the cervical spine, often performed away from the painful side in the painless part of the range, produce significant improvements in pain behavior and range on the painful side. The patient often will report only a feeling of mild strain on the painful side during application of the technique. As this strain is reduced, active movement toward the painful side increases when it is assessed after treatment or between episodes of therapy. Stretching of the painful side in a carefully controlled manner by rotation away from the painful side is described elsewhere.[84,150]

Guidelines for determining the preferred direction of a technique are provided by the McKenzie[151] approach. These guidelines are reasonable, practical, and clinically effective. In a recent study by Long et al,[141] patients were randomized into three groups based on directional preferences elicited during the examination. Results demonstrated that those who performed exercises associated with reduction of pain during movement and centralization of symptoms performed much better than did comparative groups.

Besides providing guidelines for the preferred direction of a technique, the teachings of McKenzie[151] provide a reasonable and logical rationale for the progression of a technique. The direction of a gentle therapeutic movement in advance of more vigorous techniques has been determined to be proper. For example, in treating a patient who is demonstrating centralizing behavior, if movement in the direction of flexion of the lower cervical spine increases the patient's peripheral symptoms, this most likely is the wrong direction. However, if movement in the direction of extension of the lower cervical spine decreases and centralizes the patient's symptoms, this is most likely the preferred direction. Provocation and reduction of symptoms generate useful information. If movement is provided in the preferred direction, the patient will get better, regardless of the underlying theories.

Technique Principles

Treatment procedures or techniques usually are selected during the PE. Confirmation or denial of the original selection takes place at the second visit. It may be necessary to fine tune the procedure by, for example, correcting flaws in the patient's performance of the procedure. If the patient has made significant progress, both objectively and subjectively, there is no need to modify the procedure at the second visit. However, if the patient is the same or worse at the second visit, the therapist is obligated to reevaluate the tentative conclusion reached at the initial visit and to revise the treatment as needed. The patient with derangement should be seen daily until his pain is controlled by active procedures.

The following general principles will help guide the therapist in the selection of techniques or procedures, in the progression of treatment, and in the estimation of expected progress.

1. Use procedures to reduce the symptoms of a patient who demonstrates centralizing behavior or to produce the symptoms of dysfunction, with the knowledge that the patient understands the purpose of the procedures. The symptoms of a patient who is demonstrating centralizing behavior are expected to be reduced quickly, and the symptoms of dysfunction are expected to be reduced slowly. In centralizing behavior, once the symptoms are reduced, the next three phases of treatment consist of maintenance of the reduction, restoration of function, and prevention of recurrence.

2. Postural educational assessment is essential to the success of a treatment program. The patient who continues to use poor posture habits, which perpetuate chronic mechanical deformation, will only delay recovery or will promote treatment failure.

3. The use of a therapist's technique may promote dependence on the therapist. Techniques are needed when the application of procedures has been exhausted, or when the patient's progress has plateaued.

4. Regardless of the approach selected, active exercise performed by the patient on a regular and continuing basis is one of the keys to preventing recurrent spinal pain and/or aborting future attacks of spinal pain. This involves the implementation of a strong and appropriate home exercise program. It is reasonable to expect that most patients are able and willing to do about four different exercises on a regular basis, if they can see the benefits of the exercise.

5. In very general terms, it is reasonable to expect that most patients will retain, from one treatment session to another, about 50% of the gain that was achieved at a treatment session. Optimally, this gain will represent both a subjective and an objective improvement. The actual rate of improvement achieved by individual patients will vary, but

the average gain for each patient is useful in determining the prognosis. Patients are more secure and satisfied with their treatment program when they are aware of the expected outcome.

6. Not all patients are suitable candidates for physical therapy. All approaches have their limitations, and it is the therapist's responsibility to identify unsuitable candidates, to offer a reasonable explanation, and to recommend viable alternatives.

7. The true success of an approach is not measured by the date of return to work or by symptom-free behavior. The true success of an approach is measured, in part, by the effectiveness of the approach in preventing or reducing the severity of recurrent bouts of spinal pain.

8. Physical therapists have been guilty of seeing patients too often but not long enough. Once the patient has gained control of the symptoms, the frequency of visits may be significantly reduced. However, if one is to be confident that an effective program of prevention is actually working, it is necessary to see the patient for rechecks over a reasonable period of time. In other words, simple relief of pain is not sufficient evidence for discharging a patient.

Manual Therapy Treatment Techniques

Thousands of procedures and techniques may be used. Maitland and McKenzie have described most of those that follow within this chapter. They have contributed enormously to the delivery of effective and efficient assessment and treatment. The techniques presented here are not intended to be comprehensive or exclusive. Although proper application of procedures or techniques contributes to the success of treatment, the relative importance of proper assessment far exceeds the importance of proper technique. There are no limits on the nature and variation of procedures and techniques, and what may work for one therapist may be ineffective for another.

Books and journal articles are poor methods for learning procedures or techniques because the communication between teacher and learner is one-way. Techniques and procedures are learned most effectively either well-supervised workshops or in supervised clinical practice, where instant feedback is provided. Practicing techniques on an experienced therapist, who understands the intent of the technique, is an excellent teaching and learning situation. Treating patients under supervision is also invaluable.

Treatment Procedures for the Cervical Spine

The procedures illustrated in Figures 9-1 to 9-3 and in Figures 9-6 to 9-13 are described by McKenzie.[152,153]

Typical Slumped Posture

In the typical slumped posture (Figure 9-1), the patient sits in an unbalanced posture with loss of lumbar lordosis, increased thoracic kyphosis, and a forward head posture. Such posture is believed to cause deformation of the spine. Correction of this

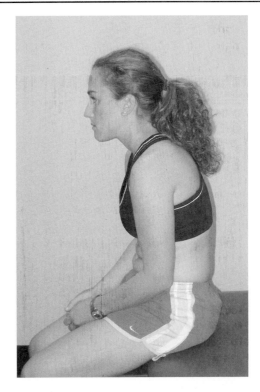

Figure 9-1 Typical slumped posture with extended upper cervical and flexed lower cervical spine. Note also the absence of lumbar lordosis, the markedly forward head, and the protracted shoulders.

poor posture, including restoration of normal lumbar lordosis, normal cervical lordosis, and normal thoracic kyphosis, is an essential part of the treatment program for all but a very few patients.

Teaching Proper Sitting Posture (Lumbar Lordosis)

The therapist assists the patient, either from in front or from the side, to attain normal lumbar lordosis (Figure 9-2). This balanced lumbar posture provides a foundation on which proper cervical and thoracic postures can be established. Use of the slump overcorrection exercise, as described by McKenzie,[151] helps the patient become aware of his posture deficit. Removing the forces that cause mechanical deformation is key to successful treatment for mechanical spine pain. Restore the hollow, and help the patient sit with a normal lordosis.

Cervical Retraction

Cervical retraction, dorsal glide, or posterior glide (Figure 9-3) is performed to help reduce the forward head posture. It is normal for the patient to have difficulty learning this procedure, probably because of poor muscle control; therefore, the therapist often must demonstrate the proper method for doing the procedure and must reinforce proper execution of the exercise at subsequent visits. The patient may add overpressure to the movement by pushing on the maxilla or the mandible in

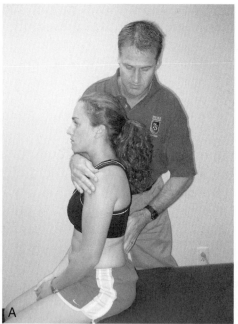
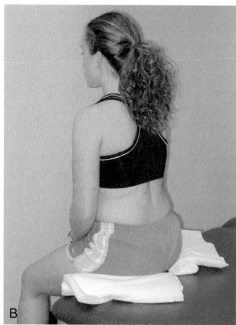

Figure 9-2 **A,** Teaching the patient proper lumbar lordosis, which for most people is about 10% off the end-range of extension. **B,** Teaching the patient proper lumbar lordosis by enhancing an anterior pelvic tilt. An awareness of this tilt is important in learning proper posture.

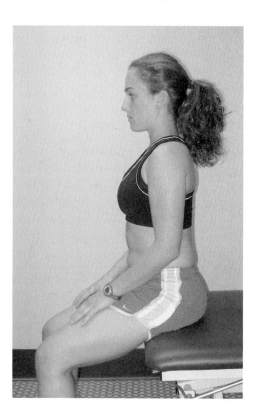

Figure 9-3 Cervical retraction added to the proper sitting posture of normal lumbar lordosis.

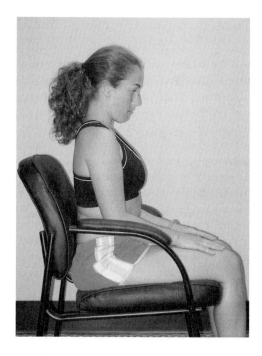

Figure 9-4 Flexion of the upper cervical spine added to retraction movement. The patient nods the head to stretch the upper cervical spine.

a posterior direction. Cervical retraction often is combined with extension of the lower cervical spine and flexion of the upper cervical spine as a procedure for treating stiffness or reducing pain. Cyriax[134] described retraction as anteroposterior glide.

Flexion of the Upper Cervical Spine

Flexion of the upper cervical spine (Figure 9-4) usually is performed with the head in the retracted position. The purpose of this procedure is to stretch the upper cervical spine. The patient is able to provide overpressure by pushing on the maxilla or mandible in the direction of flexion. This procedure is used often to treat flexion dysfunction of the upper cervical spine. This procedure, like many other procedures, may be performed

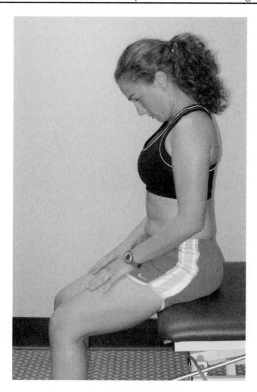

Figure 9-5 Flexion of the lower cervical and upper thoracic spine performed in sitting position. The patient brings the chin toward the sternum, with the mouth closed, whereas in flexion of the upper cervical spine, the chin is moved in the direction of the neck (nodding).

lying prone, with or without support (cervical roll) of the lower cervical spine.

Flexion of the Lower Cervical Spine

Flexion of the lower cervical spine (Figure 9-5), in combination with flexion of the upper cervical spine, is performed by having the patient move his chin toward the sternum. This procedure is used to treat flexion dysfunction of the lower cervical and upper thoracic spine. Theoretically, it also is used to reduce the pain in an anterior derangement and to restore flexion movement after the reduction of a posterior derangement. When treating the lack of flexion movement with a stable posterior derangement, flexion of the lower cervical spine must be followed by retraction and extension movements to prevent recurrence of the posterior derangement. When flexion procedures are instituted, the expected strain-pain of dysfunction should not remain worse as a result of the procedure.

Sidebending or Lateral Flexion in Sitting

The patient performs generalized sidebending (Figure 9-6), usually in the retracted position, as a physiologic movement. This movement may be used as a treatment procedure for sidebending dysfunction or to reduce and centralize the pain of derangement. Often, but not always, symptoms of lower cervical spine derangement can be reduced by sidebending to

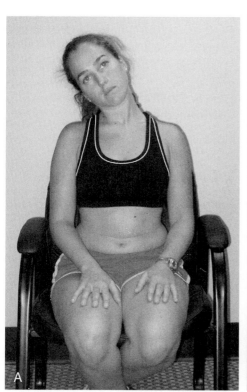
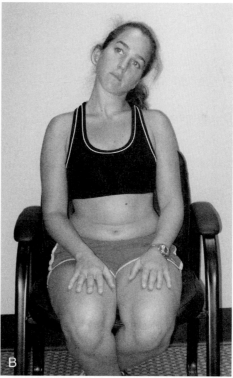

Figure 9-6 Sidebending or lateral flexion of the cervical spine. The patient is instructed to bend sideways and bring the ear toward the shoulder, as opposed to rotation movement, whereby the patient turns the nose toward the shoulder.[36] The curve of the neck, on the side away from movement, is of superior quality in left **(B)** compared with right **(A)** sidebending. Assessment of sidebending and rotation often yields similar results; therefore, it is not always necessary to assess both movements.

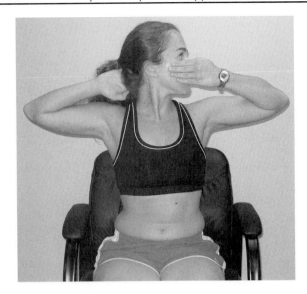

Figure 9-7 Rotation overpressure to the left. The patient applies the end-range movement using both hands. The patient's left hand is placed on the maxilla in an attempt to reduce stress on the temporomandibular joint. It is also important for the patient to keep the elbows in the position shown to facilitate feedback regarding the vigor of the overpressure. Movement of the upper cervical spine often can be enhanced by having the patient place the hands on the upper portion of the trapezius muscle to stabilize the middle and lower cervical spine (not illustrated).

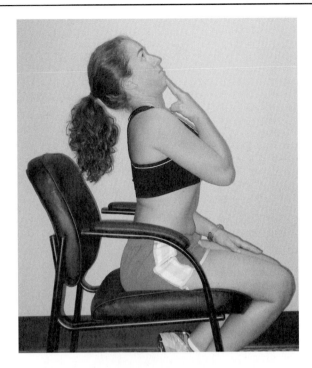

Figure 9-8 Lower cervical spine extension performed in the retracted position. The patient is holding a finger on the chin as a reminder to retain the retraction while moving into extension. A high-backed chair, which stabilizes the middle thoracic spine, helps the patient to do this procedure correctly.

the painful side. Likewise, symptoms of dysfunction can be produced by sidebending away from the painful side. However, the direction of a procedure is always dictated by careful assessment of the changes in signs and symptoms. Sidebending also may be performed while lying supine.

Rotation With Overpressure

The patient applies overpressure in the direction of rotation, usually with the head retracted[152,153] (Figure 9-7). This general physiologic movement often is restricted in the upper cervical spine by arthrosis, and in the lower cervical spine by spondylosis. Generally, rotation is most effective in producing movement in the upper cervical spine, and sidebending is most effective in producing movement in the lower cervical spine.

Lower Cervical Spine Extension Performed in Retraction

The patient first retracts the head and then moves into extension (Figure 9-8). One or both of these movements frequently are blocked in derangement. Retraction performed in different positions of flexion, as needed, may be a required variation before extension is possible. This procedure is used to reduce posterior derangement. For extension dysfunction, retraction is used to help restore lost movement into extension. Testing of the vertebral arteries often is required before this procedure is

used. The procedure also may be performed supine. The patient should be encouraged to reach the full limit of the range, and to perform small rotations at the limit of extension.[153]

Lower Cervical Spine Extension Performed in Lying

In the lying position, the effects of gravity are reduced compared with effects in the sitting position (Figure 9-9). The method used for performing the procedure and the uses for the procedure are similar to those for extension performed in retraction in the sitting position (see Figure 9-8).

Retraction in Lying

Retraction in lying (Figure 9-10) is used mainly as treatment for neck pain. This procedure, as well as others, may be performed with a sustained position and/or oscillations with appropriate precautions.

Sidebending or Lateral Flexion in Lying

Sidebending in lying must be a pure sidebending, but it may be performed at different angles of flexion for reduction and centralization of unilateral symptoms in derangement (Figure 9-11). The patient usually has better control of this movement when lying rather than sitting. When dysfunction is treated, movement usually occurs away from the painful side. At times,

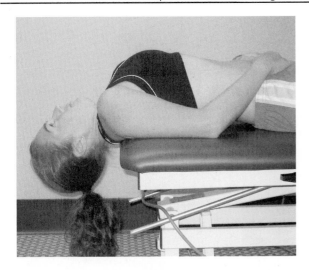

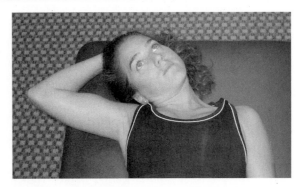

Figure 9-11 Right sidebending in lying. The head is usually moved toward the desired side without allowing any rotation. The right arm is used, as illustrated, to provide overpressure when needed.

Figure 9-9 Lower cervical spine extension performed in a lying position. This procedure usually follows retraction in a lying position and usually includes rotations performed at the limit of extension.[39,67] It is important for the edge of the table to be at the level of T4 to allow for movement in the upper thoracic spine. When returning from extension to neutral position, the patient should lift the head with the hand and should not perform the return movement actively. The patient also should rest in the neutral position on the table for about 30 seconds before sitting up. In sitting up, the patient should turn onto one side and sit up sideways to avoid neck flexion, instead of sitting straight forward.

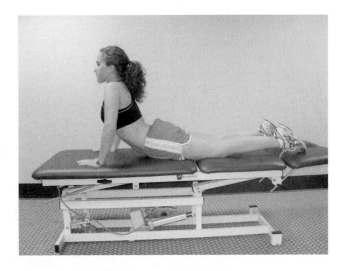

Figure 9-12 Extension in the lying position with cervical retraction. This combined procedure is best taught in parts. The patient first perfects the lumbar procedure and then adds the cervical and thoracic procedures. Many patients extend their upper cervical spine when doing this exercise, sometimes with reckless abandon. Substitution of cervical retraction for upper cervical extension is helpful in preventing treatment soreness.

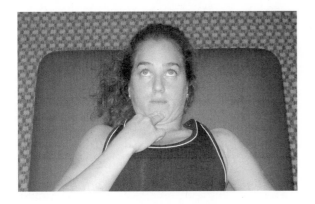

Figure 9-10 Retraction in lying. The patient is lying flat on the table. Upper cervical spine flexion may be performed in this position. Patients who are unable to gain any positive treatment effects by doing this procedure while sitting may benefit from following this procedure in a lying position.

this procedure will result in increased active flexion or extension movement.

Extension in Lying With Cervical Retraction

Cervical retraction and extension may produce movement down to T4, and repeated extension in lying may produce movement up to T4 (Figure 9-12). Combining these procedures into one exercise is most useful in treating extension dysfunction of the spine.

Patient Procedures for the Thoracic Spine

Thoracic Rotations in Sitting

To perform thoracic rotations in sitting (Figure 9-13), the patient sits straddling the end of the table, facing the table. The intent of the procedure is to produce rotation in the thoracic spine, not to rotate the cervical or lumbar spine. This procedure is used for unilateral pain and stiffness. Often the patient rotates toward the painful side when pain is treated, and away from the painful side when stiffness is treated. Thoracic spine disorder as a cause of angina-like pain has been described by Lindahl and Hamberg.[154]

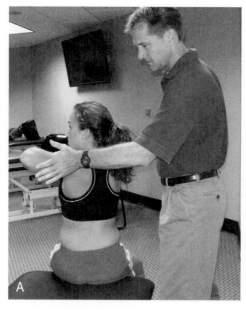
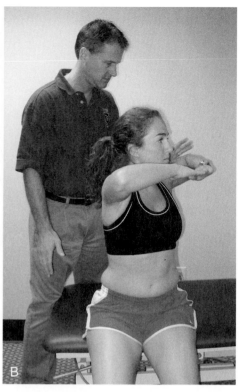

Figure 9-13 Thoracic rotation in sitting. **A,** Rotation to the left. **B,** Rotation to the left *(front view)*. The patient in **(B)** straddles the end of the treatment table, while facing the table. To reduce cervical rotations, the patient's head moves with the thoracic spine instead of facing forward. The patient must keep the chin in line with the hands, as shown in **(B).** End-range is accomplished by asking the patient to hit the therapist's hand with the elbow.

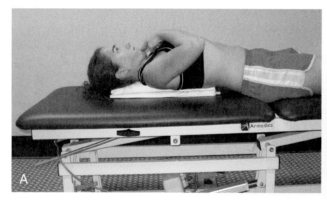
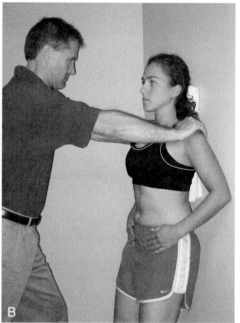

Figure 9-14 Thoracic extension performed **(A)** while lying and **(B)** while standing. In **(A),** the patient is lying supine on a firm surface with a bolster under the affected area. A bench press table (not illustrated) is most efficient because it is narrow and allows the patient to move into the posture correction position of shoulder horizontal extension. The patient should inhale when moving into horizontal extension. The same exercise may be performed by standing at the edge of a doorway **(B).** A bolster between the scapulae helps to localize the force. Overpressure may be added by the therapist or by a spouse by pushing on the patient's shoulders bilaterally.

Thoracic Extension in Lying or Standing

The intent of thoracic extension in lying or standing (Figure 9-14) is to enhance extension of the thoracic spine by using the weight of the body against a bolster.

Klapp's Crawling Position (Prayer Position)

The crawling or prayer position (Figure 9-15), when performed properly, is a passive extension of the thoracic spine performed

in the prone position. The force is provided by the weight of the body. This procedure is used as an alternative or supplement to those described previously (see Figure 9-14).

Therapist's Techniques for Cervical Spine Palpation in Supine

The upper cervical spine is palpated with the patient lying supine, if possible (Figure 9-16). In the neutral posture, with the patient supine, the therapist can feel abnormalities of tissue

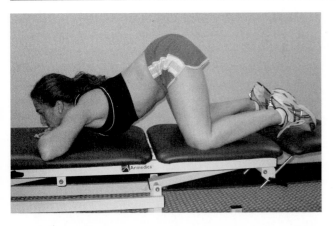

Figure 9-15 Klapp's crawling position (modified). The patient's hands are placed under the chin instead of reaching out forward. The modified position places more force on the cervical spine than does the unmodified, or prayer, position. The thighs should be kept vertical, and an extension strain should be felt in the middle thoracic spine.

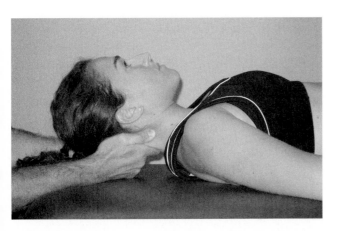

Figure 9-16 Palpation in the supine position. The patient's head is comfortably supported by the therapist over the edge of the treatment table. Palpation for abnormal joint and muscle signs may be performed in the supine or the prone position (see Figures 9-22 through 9-27). Passive physiologic intervertebral movements also may be performed in this position.

tension and joint restriction. The cervical spine also may be palpated in the prone-lying position.

Manual Cervical Traction

Cervical traction, or longitudinal movement cephalad, may be applied manually or mechanically (Figure 9-17). Manual traction is used frequently when very gentle movement is required and/or to help determine the force, position, and mode (sustained or intermittent) of mechanical traction.

Retraction and Extension in Lying

Retraction and extension in lying are used in treating posterior derangements (Figure 9-18). If tolerated, it is desirable to start the extension movement from the retracted position and/or

often to precede the retraction movement with static traction. End-range extension is required, and overpressure is applied in small rotary movements.

Sidebending in Sitting

The therapist stands behind the patient, who is sitting erect on a firm chair. The intent of the technique is to localize sidebending at a particular level of the cervical spine. Figure 9-19 illustrates sidebending left of C7 on T1. A variation of the technique, designed to improve stabilization, is for the patient to sit on a treatment table with the therapist standing behind him. The therapist then places her foot on the treatment table adjacent to the patient's hip on the side of the intended movement. The patient rests his arm on the therapist's thigh (not illustrated).

This technique is useful when full-range sidebending is needed in treatment for dysfunction. Because the spinous process of C7 moves left in normal right rotation, the technique is also useful in treating rotation dysfunction of the lower cervical spine. For example, to help restore right rotation, the spinous process of C7 at first is stabilized on the right, and the neck is sidebent to the right while the spinous process of C7 is moved left.

Sidebending in Lying on a Pillow

The patient lies supine, with his head on a pillow (Figure 9-20). The therapist stands at the head of the table and supports the patient's neck from both sides. Positioning the head on a pillow allows the therapist to perform very gentle movements into sidebending while allowing the pillow to slide on the table. This technique is useful in treating pain when other positions are not tolerated.

Grade II and IV Rotations

The patient's head is cradled properly, and the therapist stands at the head of the treatment table (Figure 9-21). Maitland[154] states that rotation is one of the most useful techniques for the cervical spine. It is most useful in treating unilateral stiffness, with movement usually in the direction away from the painful side. It is possible that restrictions that cause the stiffness are being stretched when the painful side is being opened by rotation away from the pain. Grade II movements are useful in the reduction of treatment soreness, and grade IV movements are useful in treatment for stiffness, with respect for the patient's pain. Grade I and grade III movements also are useful methods for treatment. (That grades I and III are not illustrated is not meant to imply lack of use of these techniques.)

Selected passive accessory intervertebral movements, as described by Maitland,[51] are presented in Figures 9-22 through 9-28. Further information about these and other techniques is presented by Maitland in his many writings. Selected techniques that provide a brief introduction to the approach are presented. Examples are offered of how these techniques are used in concert with patient procedures. Skillful transfer

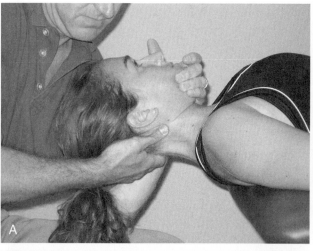
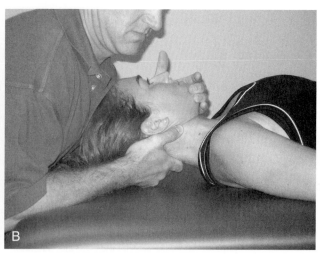
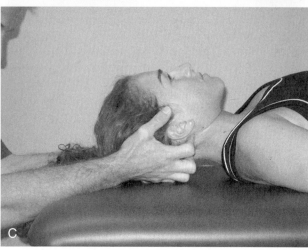

Figure 9-17 Manual cervical traction performed in the horizontal position by three different methods: **(A)** with the patient's head over the edge of the table; **(B)** with the patient lying on the table; and **(C)** with the use of pivotal traction. In **A,** the therapist provides the force by leaning backward. In **B,** the force comes from flexion of the therapist's elbows. In **C,** force is generated by the patient's head pushing against the therapist's fingers.

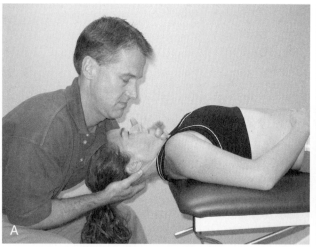
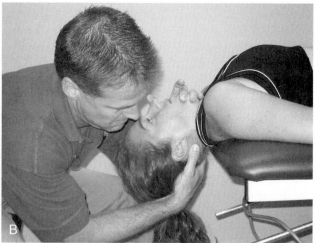

Figure 9-18 Retraction and extension in the lying position. The patient is unsupported to about T4. **A,** A traction force is applied and held, and then the neck is retracted. **B,** While in the retracted position, the neck is slowly extended. Small rotary movements are frequently applied in overpressure. Continuous assessment of changes in symptoms is essential.

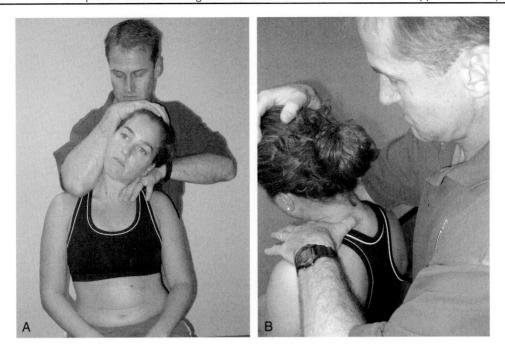

Figure 9-19 Sidebending in the sitting position. The patient's neck is near or at the end of retraction. In left sidebending **(A)**, the patient's head is sidebent to the limit of the available range, and force is applied by the therapist's right hand. **B,** The spinous process of T1 is stabilized by the therapist's left thumb. It is important for the therapist to hold her shoulders abducted, with elbows out to the side **(A)**, to obtain optimum tactile feedback from the patient.

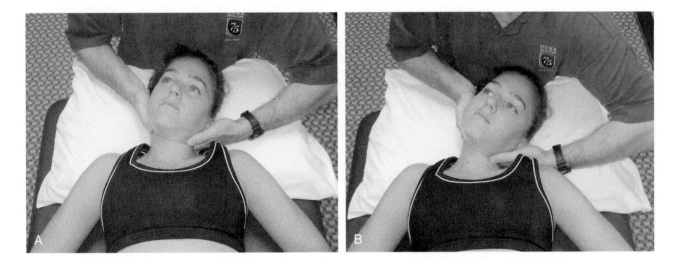

Figure 9-20 Sidebending while lying on a pillow. **A,** Left sidebending. **B,** Further left sidebending. The patient is lying supine on a pillow, and the therapist stands at the head of the treatment table. The patient's neck is supported from both sides. The therapist's left hand may act as a fulcrum for the sidebending. The force for movement comes from the therapist's right hand. The left side is closed down, and the right side is opened or stretched.

between use of the therapist's techniques and use of the patient's procedures is always challenging.

For the techniques presented in Figures 9-22 to 9-28, the patient lies prone, with the forehead resting on the overlapped and supinated hands. The therapist uses the tips or the pads of the thumbs to provide an oscillating movement in the desired direction. The movement force is generated by movement of the therapist's shoulders and/or trunk, and this force is transmitted through the arms to the thumbs, which act as eccentric springs. No intrinsic muscle action should take place in the therapist's thumbs or hands because accurate feedback from the patient is destroyed by such action.

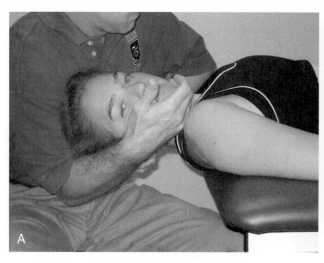
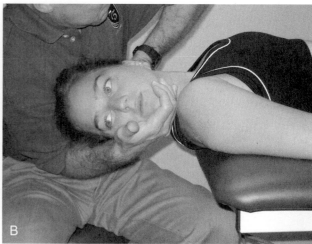

Figure 9-21 Rotations of **(A)** grade II and **(B)** grade IV. The therapist cradles the patient's head at the occiput and at the chin. Grade II is a mid-range rotation, and grade IV, an end-range rotation. The therapist should be able to perform this technique with one hand at a time if the position is correct. Note that the patient's head is in contact with the therapist's chest and with the anterior surface of the shoulder. Gentle oscillations are given at the proper position of the range. The angle of flexion or extension may be varied to produce an optimum treatment effect.

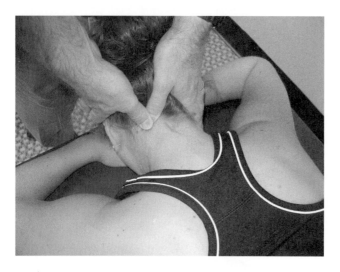

Figure 9-22 Posteroanterior unilateral vertebral pressure to C0-C1 (ap). Force is applied in the direction of the patient's ipsilateral eye. Therefore, the therapist must lean over the patient's head. The therapist's thumbs are placed on, above, or below the joint. Medial and lateral inclinations are other variations.

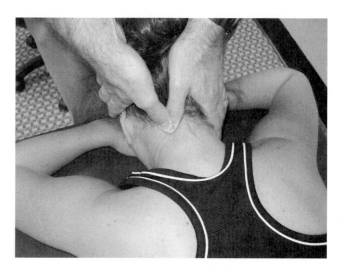

Figure 9-23 Posteroanterior unilateral vertebral pressure to C2-C3 (ap). Force is applied on the left articular pillar of C2 to move C2-C3. The patient's head is in neutral rotation. The therapist's arms are directed about 30 degrees medially to prevent the thumbs from slipping off the articular pillar. (From Maitland,[25] with permission.)

The Nelson Technique

The Nelson technique for traction and improved extension of the cervical-thoracic junction and upper thoracic spine (Figure 9-29) is taught as part of the McKenzie approach.[151] The Nelson technique is used only after premanipulative testing for providing extrinsic reductive or stretching forces in the lower cervical and upper thoracic spine is confirmed. Other procedures or techniques, if required, are used before this technique is performed, to obtain and/or retain centralization of symptoms. This procedure cannot be performed on patients with significant shoulder pathology because of the discomfort pro-

duced when the shoulders are moved into end-range horizontal extension and external rotation. It is very difficult to position well-muscled persons properly. This technique is described by Laslett.[155]

Extension Mobilizations

The intent of the extension mobilization technique (Figure 9-30), also taught in the McKenzie approach, is to provide central posteroanterior movement of the involved segment and gentle distraction. It is used on C2 through T4 to effect an extension movement. Asymmetrical variations are used often

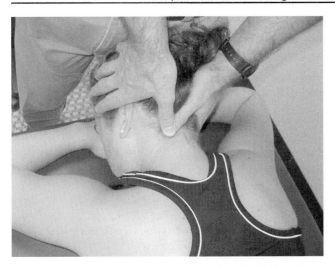

Figure 9-24 Posteroanterior unilateral vertebral pressure to C1-C2 (ap in 30 degrees of rotation left). Force is applied as in Figure 9-23, except that the patient's head is turned 30 degrees to the left. Rotation at C1-C2 is enhanced in this rotated position. (From Maitland,[25] with permission.)

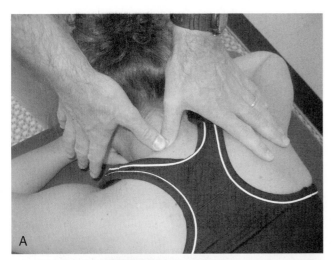

A

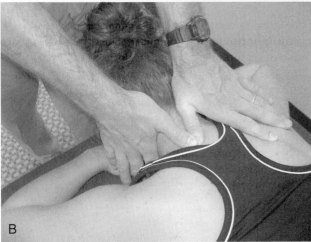

B

Figure 9-25 A, Posteroanterior unilateral vertebral pressure to C5-C6. These techniques also may be directed medially and laterally, or **(B)** cephalad and caudad as variations.

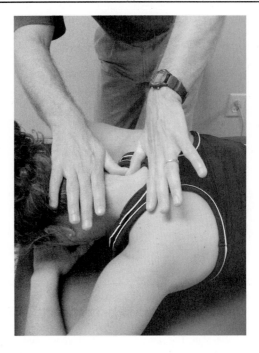

Figure 9-26 Transverse vertebral pressures to C7. Force is applied on the lateral surface of the spinous process of C7. Here, the force is applied through the therapist's right thumb to the nonactive left thumbnail. The pad, not the tip, of the nonactive thumb is used for the patient's comfort. The therapist's right forearm should be held nearly parallel to the surface of the treatment table, to provide movement in the desired direction. Often in treatment for stiffness, the patient rotates the neck to the limit of the available range. The technique then is performed at the pathologic limit (not illustrated).

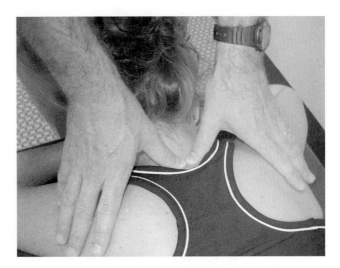

Figure 9-27 Posteroanterior central vertebral pressures directed on C7. The therapist's two thumbs, often in contact with each other, cradle the spinous process; for gentle techniques, the tips of the thumbs may be used to localize movement. If the technique is to be applied in the pain-free range, the neck may have to be placed in slight flexion. Prominent spinous processes are often the source of the patient's complaint.

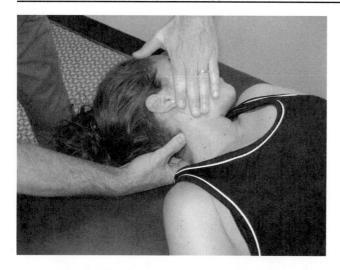

Figure 9-28 A combined technique using left rotation and unilateral posteroanterior pressures on the right side of C2. Shown is an example of a physiologic and an accessory movement performed simultaneously. It frequently is necessary to combine movements to reproduce the comparable sign. The same movements then are used as a treatment technique to reduce pain and/or increase the range. In general, the technique performed at the lowest grade that produces the desired treatment effect is preferred. The lowest grade provides for smooth, controlled rather than rough, random movement.

to treat unilateral or asymmetrical pain or stiffness. This technique is described by Laslett.[155]

Thoracic Spine Techniques for Transverse Vertebral Pressure to T4

The technique for applying transverse vertebral pressure to T4 is similar to the technique shown for transverse vertebral pressure on C7 (Figure 9-31). This technique usually is directed toward the side of pain. When dysfunction is being treated, the patient's comparable sign is reproduced, and the range of physiologic movements often is increased. Although accessory movement occurs in a frontal plane, physiologic movements in the sagittal plane (i.e., flexion or extension) often are improved.

Posteroanterior Central Vertebral Pressure to T4

The technique for applying posteroanterior central vertebral pressure to T4 (ap) is similar to that shown for posteroanterior central vertebral pressure to C7, except that in this case, the force usually is not directed laterally (Figure 9-32). This technique is used commonly for central or symmetrical symptoms and may be used for vague or generalized unilateral symptoms.[50] It is one of the most useful techniques for the thoracic spine and often is followed by a more vigorous technique, which is illustrated later.

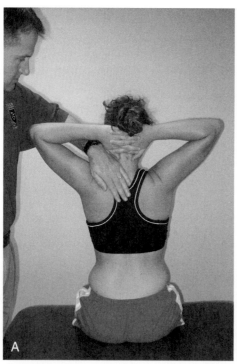
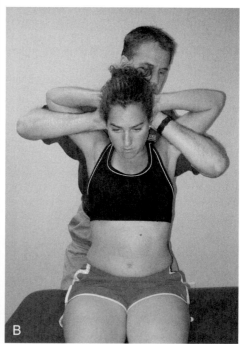

Figure 9-29 The Nelson technique for traction and improved extension of the cervical-thoracic junction and the upper thoracic spine. **A,** The index and middle fingers of the therapist's left hand are placed over the spinous process of C7. The same two fingers of the therapist's right hand then are placed on top of these fingers. A posteroanterior force is directed cephalad by the therapist's arms and hands through the index and middle fingers of both hands. This force is generated by pushing on C7 and pulling the patient's shoulders into horizontal extension. The traction force is applied by attempting to lift the patient off the table. At the peak of the traction force, the therapist applies the extension force. **B,** Note that the shoulders of the therapist and the shoulders of the patient are at the same level.

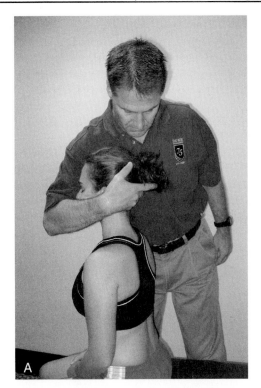
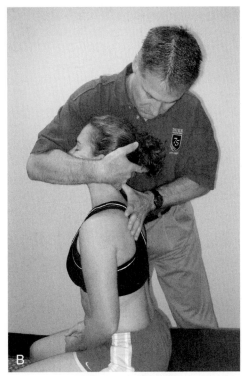

Figure 9-30 Extension mobilization. The patient should be sitting in a high-backed chair (not illustrated). **A,** The patient's head is cradled by the therapist's left hand and forearm against the therapist's chest. The therapist's little finger is placed on the spinous process of the appropriate vertebra. **B,** The therapist's right thumb, or right pisiform-hamate groove, is placed securely on her left little finger. The movement desired is gentle traction, provided by the therapist's left arm, combined with posteroanterior central vertebral pressures, provided by the thumb or hand. The patient's head should remain stable.

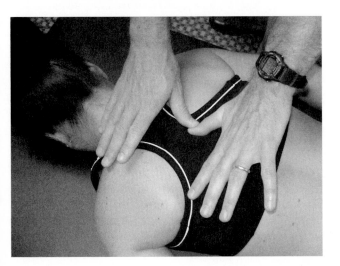
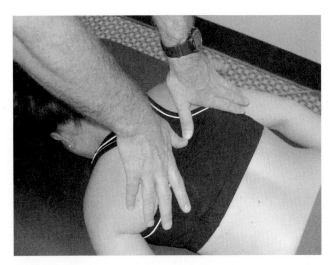

Figure 9-31 Transverse vertebral pressures to T4. Force is applied on the lateral surface of the spinous process of T4. The force is applied through the therapist's right thumb to the nonactive left thumbnail. The pad, not the tip, of the nonactive thumb is used for the patient's comfort. Note that the patient's arms are at the sides to enhance relaxation of the thoracic spine.

Intervertebral Rotatory Posteroanterior Movements of T1-T4

The technique for intervertebral rotatory posteroanterior movements of T1-T4 provides a method for producing desirable

Figure 9-32 Posteroanterior central vertebral pressures (ap) to T4. The therapist's two thumbs, often in contact with each other, cradle the spinous process. For gentle techniques, the tips of the thumbs may be used to localize movement.

movement without direct contact with the spinous processes (Figure 9-33). It is suggested that localized movement, depending on placement of the hands, may be produced in the costotransverse joints, the costovertebral joints, the intervertebral (apophyseal) joints, and the intervertebral junction. It is common for even gentle techniques to produce local sounds of release, and for the patient to gain rapid relief from symptoms through this technique.

Thoracic Rotations

Thoracic rotations may be tested with the patient standing (mostly lower movement), sitting (Figure 9-34), and lying. For stretching of stiff structures, rotation often is performed in the direction away from the symptomatic side. Assessment of the individual patient and his response to movement tests dictate the proper direction.

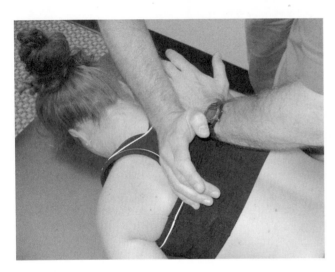

Figure 9-33 Intervertebral rotatory posteroanterior movements of T1-T4. Force is applied bilaterally through the therapist's hypothenar eminences to the spaces between the spinous processes and the medial borders of the scapulae. A combination of clockwise and counterclockwise movements is applied in a posteroanterior direction. The force also may be directed cephalad, caudad, and laterally.

Longitudinal Movement and Extension in Sitting

The generalized technique of longitudinal movement and extension may be performed with the patient sitting (Figure 9-35) or standing. Because of the nonspecific nature of the technique, it is most useful in treating generalized stiffness of the middle thoracic spine. Greater specificity may be achieved with the technique described next.

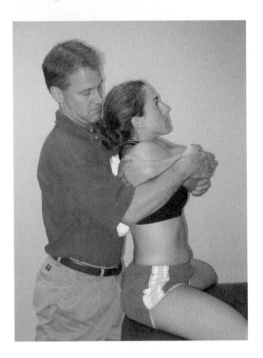

Figure 9-35 Longitudinal movement and extension in sitting. The patient sits straddling the end of the treatment table. Longitudinal movement is provided by partially lifting the patient off the table. Extension movement is provided when the therapist leans backward and applies overpressure (when desired) through her chest.

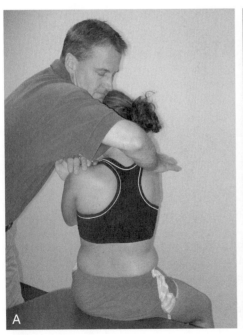

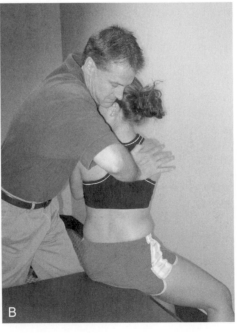

Figure 9-34 Thoracic rotation to the left. **A,** Generalized thoracic rotation. The patient sits straddling the end of the treatment table, with the arms folded in front of the chest. **B,** More localized overpressure in the middle thoracic spine.

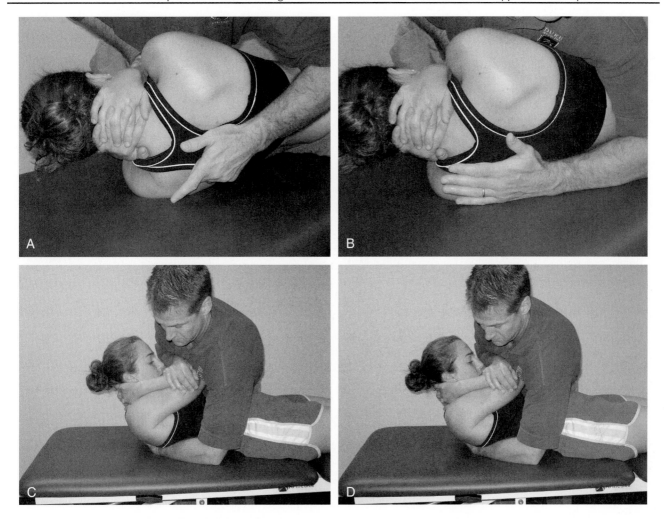

Figure 9-36 Posteroanterior manipulation (ap) of T4. **A,** The therapist's hand placement for the central technique. **B,** The therapist's hand placement for the unilateral technique. **C,** Positioning of the patient in neutral flexion and extension for the level to be treated. **D,** Application of force through the patient's elbows. At this point, the patient exhales. The hand of the therapist under the patient provides localization for the technique. In **C** and **D,** the therapist's right hand is underneath the patient.

Posteroanterior Manipulation of T4

Posteroanterior manipulation of T4 (ap), which must be learned and practiced under the supervision of an experienced therapist, is one of the most useful techniques for the upper and middle thoracic spine (Figure 9-36). When successful, the patient experiences dramatic relief. It is suggested not only that stiff joints are loosened but that thoracic spine derangements may be reduced by selected use of this technique. Reduction, if achieved, must be retained through consistent use of the patient's procedures.

Thoracic spine disorders as a cause of angina-like pain have been described by Lindahl and Hamberg.[154] This technique has been useful in treating this type of disorder. The technique is described in detail by Maitland,[51] McGuckin,[156] and Flynn.[157]

CASE STUDY 9-1

The use of passive movement techniques coupled with active exercise is the main emphasis of this case study.

Initial Assessment
Patient History

The patient was a 33-year-old female factory worker who spent most of her time operating a forklift. She had a headache in the occipital region and neck pain extending from C1 to T4, which spread bilaterally and equally to the area of the glenohumeral joints. She had no upper extremity symptoms. Initially, her symptoms were constant but variable. They were worsened by sitting, driving a forklift, and doing housework. They were reduced by lying in the fetal position and by taking a hot bath. The patient's sleep was disturbed because she had increased pain when turning her head from side to side. Both coughing and sneezing increased her symptoms temporarily.

Her symptoms commenced as a result of shoveling cullet (broken glass). She was first seen for this examination 18 months after the initial injury but had never been symptom free for longer than a few hours since the original injury. Radiographs were negative. She had received chiropractic treatment and physical therapy elsewhere. She was fully employed at the time of these treatments.

Physical Examination

The patient's general cervical flexion was limited to 50% of normal. Lower cervical extension was blocked by pain at 15 degrees. Left cervical rotation was 55 degrees, and right cervical rotation was 65 degrees. Extension reproduced the patient's comparable sign in the C7 area centrally.

The patient's posture was poor, with a marked forward head on a long neck with a definite cervical-thoracic kyphus. Her upper thoracic spine was held in excessive flexion, and she had forward shoulders bilaterally.

Repeated test movements into protraction of the head made her C7 pain worse. Repeated retractions of the head increased her headache and increased her C7 pain, both temporarily. She was very stiff in both of these movements (i.e., she had great difficulty performing test movements except in the early part of the ranges).

Passive accessory movements and passive physiologic movements revealed the following:
1. The C7 spinous process was rotated to the patient's left. Attempted correction by pushing the spinous process to the patient's right (in a transverse grade II pl passive movement) reproduced her C7-area symptoms.
2. Her headache was reproduced by passive posteroanterior pressures in the suboccipital muscles bilaterally.
3. The upper thoracic spine was very stiff and painful locally at each level, especially in extension-type articulations.

4. Overpressure in left cervical rotation also reproduced the C7-area pain.
5. Extension of the lower cervical spine was blocked at the C7 level.

Interpretation

This patient presented with marked hypomobility secondary to known trauma. Her poor posture, coupled with excessive stiffness, suggested that she may have had a posture problem before the trauma. Her main complaints were reproduced with passive accessory movements and/or passive physiologic movements. It was suggested that she had marked hypomobility caused by shortening of joint structures and soft tissue secondary to the trauma.

Diagnostic classification: Musculoskeletal 4B: Impaired posture (781.92)

Treatment

The primary goals of treatment were to eliminate the patient's headache, restore normal movement to her cervical and upper thoracic spine, and restore other functional components such as strength and endurance. Treatment consisted of posture correction, passive mobilization, and active exercises, as well as an explanation of the rationale to the patient. She remained fully employed.

1. The patient was seen twice the first week. C7 was passively mobilized transversely to the right on both days to increase left rotation and possibly extension. The patient was taught upper cervical spine flexion to reduce her suboccipital headache. She was also taught the slump/overcorrection to correct her posture.

   Left rotation increased from 55 to 70 degrees. The patient's posture started to improve, especially her body awareness. She tolerated the active exercises and was able to reduce but not eliminate her headache.

2. The patient was also seen twice this week. The upper thoracic spine was mobilized vigorously, and the C7 transverse pressures were continued. Retraction, extension, and rotation of the cervical spine performed actively in lying were initiated.

   The patient's headache disappeared. Cervical rotations were near normal limits, and active lower cervical spine extension increased from the initial 15 degrees to about 60 degrees. The patient was very encouraged and highly motivated. Her pain of hypomobility decreased.

3. The patient was seen once this week. All active exercises were continued, and T4 was vigorously mobilized centrally but was not manipulated.

   The patient was progressing well in all areas, except that T4 was painful locally and very stiff. She probably needed to be manipulated unless active exercises reduced the dysfunction at T4.

CASE STUDY 9-1—cont'd

4. The patient was seen twice, and T4 was manipulated at the first visit. All active exercises were rechecked and progressed as tolerated.

   Cervical-thoracic extension improved to near normal limits, but right rotation of the upper thoracic spine was limited by 10 degrees. Active right rotation exercises for the thoracic spine were added.

5. The patient was seen once. Thoracic rotations were near normal limits. Cervical-thoracic extension was clear. A manual muscle test of the neck and shoulder girdle revealed a fair plus lower trapezius on the right. Strengthening exercises were initiated. Upper limb tension tests and the slump test were normal.

   Range of movement for the cervical and upper thoracic spine was normal. Posture was good. Isolated lower trapezius weakness was the only known deficit.

6. Recheck of the weak trapezius showed a good plus. All exercises were rechecked. The patient was to be seen only as needed. She remained symptom free and was discharged.

CASE STUDY 9-2

The use of passive movement techniques and active exercises used to eliminate a cervical headache is the focus of this case study.

Initial Assessment
Patient History

The patient was a 53-year-old domestic laundry worker. Her main complaint was an intermittent, severe upper cervical headache with spread to the right temporal region, coupled with feelings of light-headedness and dizziness. The symptoms, when present, usually lasted for about 2 hours. The patient's headache commenced for no apparent reason, and at times her pain, when at its worst, involved her whole head.

Her headache was worsened by cold air, bending her head forward as when ironing, and, most significantly in her mind, 2 to 5 minutes after she entered a store. Her headache was reduced or eliminated by wearing a soft cervical collar. Her sleep was not disturbed, and coughing and sneezing signs were negative. Previous treatment consisted of the neck collar, isometric exercises, and anti-inflammatory medications. The medications did not help. The isometric exercises, at times, reduced the patient's headache.

A CT scan showed that the patient had degenerative disc disease of C6-C7. She reportedly had high blood pressure under control with medication. She also claimed to have a nervous disorder and prior heart disease, with no symptoms at this time. She was referred for evaluation and treatment.

Physical Examination

Cervical range of movement was within normal limits, and there was no reproduction of symptoms with these test movements. The patient did have a moderate forward head, with extension of the upper cervical spine and flexion of the lower cervical spine. Palpation of her neck using passive accessory movements reproduced her headache by right unilateral vertebral pressures on the articular pillar of C2, moving C2 on C1.

Treatment

1. The patient was seen twice the first week and was taught active postural exercises to reduce her forward head. Upper cervical flexion with partial retraction was chosen because the patient reported, at her first visit, that this exercise reduced her headache. She was instructed to do the exercise frequently and to stop or reduce the exercise if any of her symptoms were aggravated. At the second visit, her neck was palpated in detail, and C1-C2 on the right was mobilized using grade II for three bouts. Joint resistance diminished, and local pain was eliminated.

   At her second visit, the patient stated that her exercises were helpful, but she believed that the headache was unchanged because she had to use the collar as usual. She responded well to the passive accessory movement on C1-C2.

2. At her third visit, the patient reported that she had not worn the collar for 1 week and that her headache was well controlled by her exercises. She had created a modification of her exercise that she believed stretched her headache area. Essentially, she had combined upper cervical flexion (her original exercise) with left sidebending to produce a desirable stretch at C1-C2 on the right.

3. At her fourth visit, the patient reported that her headache was no problem because the symptoms were less frequent, less severe, and did not spread beyond the local area of C1-C2. Her neck was palpated and appeared to be normal for her age, with no reproduction of symptoms beyond normal local pressure/strain. She was discharged with instructions to continue her exercise program and was advised to report if her exercises did not eliminate her headache.

REFERENCES

1. Cyriax J: Examination of the spinal column, Physiotherapy 56(1):2-6, 1970.
2. Gifford L: Acute low cervical nerve root conditions: symptom presentations and pathobiological reasoning, Man Ther 6(2):106-115, 2001.
3. Richardson SW et al: Users' guides to evidence based medicine, JAMA 281:1214-1219, 1999.
4. Dans AL, Dans LF, Guyatt GH, Richardson S: Users' guides to the medical literature: XIV. How to decide on the applicability of clinical trial results to your patient. JAMA 279:545-549, 1998.
5. Cook C, Hegedus E: Orthopedic physical examination tests: an evidence based approach, Upper Saddle River, NJ, 2007, Prentice-Hall Publishing.
6. Sizer PS, Brismee JM, Cook C: Medical screening for red flags in the diagnosis and management of musculoskeletal spine pain, Pain Pract 7(1):53-71, 2007.
7. Obuchowski NA, Graham RJ, Baker ME, et al: Ten criteria for effective screening: their application to multislice CT screening for pulmonary and colorectal cancers, Am J Roent 176:1357-1362, 2001.
8. Guyatt GH, Sackett DL, Cook DJ, for the Evidence-Based Medicine Working Group: Users' guides to the medical literature: II. How to use an article about therapy or prevention: A. Are the results of the study valid? JAMA 270:2598-2601, 1993.
9. Guyatt GH, Sackett DL, Cook DJ, for the Evidence-Based Medicine Working Group: Users' guides to the medical literature: II. How to use an article about therapy or prevention: B. What are the results and will they help me in caring for my patients? JAMA 271:59-63, 1994.
10. Pauker SG, Kassirer JP: The threshold approach to clinical decision making, N Engl J Med 302:1109-1117, 1980.
11. Tversky A, Kahneman D: Judgment under uncertainty: heuristics and biases, Science 185:1124-1131, 1974.
12. American Physical Therapy Association: Guide to physical therapist practice, ed 2, Alexandria, Va, 2001, pp 9-744.
13. Jaeschke R, Guyatt GH, Sackett DL, for the Evidence-Based Medicine Working Group: Users' guides to the medical literature: III. How to use an article about a diagnostic test: A. Are the results of the study valid? JAMA 271:389-391, 1994.
14. Jaeschke R, Guyatt GH, Sackett DL, for the Evidence-Based Medicine Working Group: Users' guides to the medical literature: III. How to use an article about a diagnostic test: B. What are the results and will they help me in caring for my patients? JAMA 271:703-707, 1994.
15. Aouba A et al: Crowned dens syndrome misdiagnosed as polymyalgia rheumatica, giant cell arteritis, meningitis or spondylitis: an analysis of eight cases, Rheumatology (Oxford) 43(12):1508-1512, 2004.
16. Jones M, Jones H: Cervical-shoulder differentiation (course handout), Trumansburg, NY, 1993, Cayuga Professional Education Association.
17. Jones M: Clinical reasoning in physical therapy, Phys Ther 72:875-884, 1992.
18. Jones M: Clinical reasoning process in manipulative therapy. In Boyling J (ed): Grieve's Modern Manual Therapy, New York, 1994, Churchill Livingstone, pp 471-490.
19. Jones M, Christensen N, Carr J: Clinical reasoning in orthopaedic manual therapy. In Grant R, editor: Physical therapy of the cervical and thoracic spine, New York, 1994, Churchill Livingstone, p 89.
20. Anderson M, et al: Cervical spine. In Myers R, editor: Saunders manual of physical therapy practice, Philadelphia, 1995, Saunders, pp 727-788.
21. Higgs J, Jones M, editors: Clinical reasoning in the health professions, Boston, 1995, Butterworth-Heinemann, pp 35-104.
22. Tichenor C, Davidson J, Jensen G: Cases as shared inquiry: model for clinical reasoning, J Phys Ther Ed 9 (2):57-62, 1995.
23. Maitland G: Peripheral manipulation, Oxford, 1991, Butterworths.
24. Laslett M et al: Diagnosing painful sacroiliac joints: a validity study of a McKenzie evaluation and sacroiliac provocation tests, Aust J Physiotherapy 49:89-97, 2003.
25. Cook C: Orthopedic manual therapy: an evidence based approach, Upper Saddle River, NJ, 2007, Prentice-Hall Publishing.
26. Malanga GA: The diagnosis and treatment of cervical radiculopathy, Med Sci Sports Exerc 29(7 Suppl):S236-S245, 1997.
27. Penning L: Normal movements of the cervical spine, Am J Roentgenology 130:317-326, 1978.
28. White A, Panjabi M: Clinical biomechanics of the spine, Philadelphia, 1990, JB Lippincott Co.
29. Cook C et al: Identifiers suggestive of clinical cervical spine instability: a Delphi study of physical therapists, Phys Ther 85(9):895-906, 2005.
30. Cook C et al: Coupling behavior of the cervical spine: a systematic review of the literature, J Manipulative Physiol Ther 29(7):570-575, 2006.
31. Hartman L: Handbook of osteopathic technique, ed 2, San Diego, Calif, 1985, Singular Pub Group.
32. Sizer PS, Brismee JM, Cook C: Coupling behavior of the thoracic spine: a systematic review of the literature, J Manipulative Physiol Ther 30(5):390-399, 2007.
33. Daffner SD, Vaccaro AR: Managing disorders of the cervicothoracic junction, Am J Orthop 31(6):323-327, 2002.
34. Lee D: Rotational instability of the mid thoracic spine: assessment and management, Man Ther 1:234-241, 1996.
35. Erwin WM, Jackson PC, Homonko D: Innervation of the human intercostals joint: implications for clinical back

pain syndromes, J Manip Physiol Ther 23:395-403, 2000.

36. Cleland J et al: Short-term effect of thoracic manipulation on lower trapezius muscle strength, J Man Manip Ther 12(2):82-90, 2004.

37. Vicenzino B et al: Specific manipulative therapy treatment for chronic lateral epicondylalgia produces uniquely characteristic hypoalgesia, Man Ther 6:205-212, 2001.

38. Simon R, Vicenzino B, Wright A: The influence of an anteroposterior accessory glide of the glenohumeral joint on measures of peripheral sympathetic nervous system function in the upper limb, Man Ther 2(1):18-23, 1997.

39. Jull G: Use of high and low velocity cervical manipulative therapy procedures by Australian manipulative physiotherapists, Aust J Physiother 48(3):189-193, 2002.

40. Jull G: Management of cervical headache, Man Ther 2(4):182-190, 1997.

41. Zito G, Jull G, Story I: Clinical tests of musculoskeletal dysfunction in the diagnosis of cervicogenic headache, Man Ther 11(2):118-129, 2006.

42. Zwart JA: Neck mobility in different headache disorders, Headache 37(1):6-11, 1997.

43. Bogduk N: Cervical causes of headache and dizziness. In Grieve G, editor: Modern manual therapy of the vertebral column, Edinburgh, 1986, Churchill Livingstone, p 289.

44. Lyle MA et al: Relationship of physical examination findings and self-reported symptom severity and physical function in patients with degenerative lumbar conditions, Phys Ther 85(2):120-133, 2005.

45. Rivett DA: Adverse events and the vertebral artery: can they be averted? Man Ther 11(4):241-242, 2006.

46. Grant R: Vertebral artery testing—the Australian Physiotherapy Association Protocol after 6 years, Man Ther 1(3):149-153, 1996.

47. Zaina C et al: The effect of cervical rotation on blood flow in the contralateral vertebral artery, Man Ther 8(2):103-109, 2003.

48. Barker WH et al: Effect of contralateral occlusion on long-term efficacy of endarterectomy in the asymptomatic carotid atherosclerosis study (ACAS): ACAS Investigators, Stroke 10:2330-2334, 2000.

49. Grant R: Physical therapy of the cervical and thoracic spine, ed 3, New York, 2002, Churchill Livingstone.

50. Magarey ME, et al: Pre-manipulative testing of the cervical spine review, revision and new clinical guidelines, Man Ther 9(2):95-108, 2004.

51. Maitland GD: Maitland's vertebral manipulation, ed 6, London, 2001, Butterworth-Heinemann.

52. Jansen J, Sjaastad O: Cervicogenic headache: Smith/Robinson approach in bilateral cases, Funct Neurol 21(4):205-210, 2006.

53. Wyke B: Articular neurology: a review, Physiotherapy 58:94, 1972.

54. Blaine E: Manipulative (chiropractic) dislocation of the axis, JAMA 1356, 1925.

55. Dvorak J et al: CT-functional diagnostics of the rotary instability of the upper cervical spine, Spine, 12(suppl 3):197, 1987.

56. Rao R: Neck pain, cervical radiculopathy, and cervical myelopathy: pathophysiology, natural history, and clinical evaluation, J Bone Joint Surg Am 84:1872-1881, 2002.

57. Grubb SA, Kelly CK, Bogduk N: Cervical discography: clinical implications form 12 years of experience, Spine 25:1382-1389, 2000.

58. Jordan SE, Machleder HI: Diagnosis of thoracic outlet syndrome using electrophysiologically guided anterior scalene blocks, Ann Vasc Surg 12(3):260-264, 1998.

59. Cruz-Martinez A, Arpa J: Electrophysiological assessment in neurogenic thoracic outlet syndrome, Electromyogr Clin Neurophysiol 41(4):253-256, 2001.

60. Cook C, et al: Identifiers suggestive of clinical cervical spine instability: a Delphi study of physical therapists, Phys Ther 85(9):895-906, 2005.

61. Falla D, et al: An endurance-strength training regime is effective in reducing myoelectric manifestations of cervical flexor muscle fatigue in females with chronic neck pain, Clin Neurophysiol 117(4):828-837, 2006.

62. Steill IG, et al: The Canadian C-spine rule versus the NEXUS low-risk criteria in patients with trauma, N Engl J Med 349(26):2510-2518, 2003.

63. Guez M: Chronic neck pain: an epidemiological, psychological and SPECT study with emphasis on whiplash-associated disorders, Acta Orthop Suppl 77(320):preceding 1, 3-33, 2006.

64. Montgomery DM, Brower RS: Cervical spondylotic myelopathy: clinical syndrome and natural history, Orthop Clin North Am 23:487-493, 1992.

65. Chiles BW 3rd, et al: Cervical spondylotic myelopathy: patterns of neurological deficit and recovery after anterior cervical decompression, Neurosurgery 44:762-769; discussion 769-770, 1999.

66. Clark CA, Barker GJ, Tofts PS: Magnetic resonance diffusion imaging of the human cervical spinal cord in vivo, Magn Reson Med 41:1269-1273, 1999.

67. Good DC, Couch JR, Wacaser L: "Numb, clumsy hands" and high cervical spondylosis, Surg Neurol 22:285-291, 1984.

68. Kadanka Z, Bednarik J, Vohanka S, et al: Conservative treatment versus surgery in spondylotic cervical myelopathy: a prospective randomised study, Eur Spine J. 9:538-544, 2000.

69. MacFadyen DJ: Posterior column dysfunction in cervical spondylotic myelopathy, Can J Neurol Sci 11:365-370, 1984.

70. Nurick S: The natural history and the results of surgical treatment of the spinal cord disorder associated with cervical spondylosis, Brain 95:101-108, 1972.

71. Rowland LP: Surgical treatment of cervical spondylotic myelopathy: time for a controlled trial, Neurology 42:5-13, 1992.

72. Kikuchi S, Watanabe E, Hasue M: Spinal intermittent claudication due to cervical and thoracic degenerative disease, Spine 21(3):313-318, 1996.

73. Gross J, Benzel E: In Camins MD, editor: Techniques in neurosurgery, Philadelphia, 1999, Lippincott Williams & Wilkins, pp 162-176.

74. Young WF: Cervical spondylotic myelopathy: a common cause of spinal cord dysfunction in older persons, Am Fam Physician 62:1064-1070, 1073, 2000.

75. Isaacs E: Should physical therapists diagnose?: a neurologist's viewpoint, J Phys Ther Ed 9(2):63-64, 1995.

76. Schoensee S, et al: The effect of mobilization on cervical headaches, J Orthop Sports Phys Ther 21(4):184-196, 1995.

77. Butler D: Mobilization of the nervous system, New York, 1991, Churchill Livingstone.

78. Hack G, et al: Anatomic relation between the rectus capitis posterior minor muscle and the dura mater, Spine 20(23):2484-2486, 1995.

79. Brown S: Ocular dysfunction associated with whiplash injury, Aust Physiother 41(1):59, 1995.

80. Davidson R, Dunn E, Metzmaker J: The shoulder abduction test in the diagnosis of radicular pain in cervical extradural compression monoradiculopathies, Spine 6:441-445, 1981.

81. Pascarelli EF, Hsu YP: Understanding work-related upper extremity disorders: clinical findings in 485 computer users, musicians, and others, J Occup Rehabil 11(1):1-21, 2001.

82. Butler DS: The sensitive nervous system, Adelaide Australia, 2000, Noigroup Publications.

83. Maitland G: Acute locking of the cervical spine, Aust J Physiother 24:103-109, 1978.

84. Sprague R: The acute cervical joint lock, Phys Ther 63(9):1439-1444, 1983.

85. Saunders D: Evaluation, treatment, and prevention of musculoskeletal disorders, Eden Prairie, Minn, 1985, Educational Opportunities.

86. Demetra J: Pathologies of the cervical spine. Orthopedic physical therapy home study course 96-1, pp 1-17, Washington, DC, 1996, Orthopedic section, American Physical Therapy Association.

87. Grant R, Forrester C, Hides J: Screen-based keyboard operation: the adverse effects on the nervous system, Aust Phys Ther 41(2):99-107, 1995.

88. Reif R: Evaluation and differential diagnosis of the cervical spine. Orthopedic physical therapy home study course 96-1, pp 1-26, Washington, DC, 1996, Orthopedic and sports section, American Physical Therapy Association.

89. Corrigan B, Maitland G: Practical orthopedic medicine, Oxford, 1983, Butterworths.

90. Blair J: Examination of the thoracic spine. In Grieve G, editor: Modern manual therapy: the vertebral column, New York, 1986, Churchill Livingstone, p 536.

91. Maitland G: Vertebral manipulation, Oxford, 1986, Butterworths.

92. Grieve G: The autonomic nervous system in vertebral pain patterns. In Boyling J, editor: Grieve's modern manual therapy, New York, 1994, Churchill Livingstone, pp 293-308.

93. Slater H, Butler D, Shacklock M: The dynamic central nervous system: examination and assessment using tension tests. In Boyling J, editor: Grieve's modern manual therapy, New York, 1994, Churchill Livingstone, pp 587-606.

94. Magarey M: Examination of the cervical and thoracic spine. In Grant R, editor: Physical therapy of the cervical and thoracic spine, New York, 1994, Churchill Livingstone, p 109.

95. Butler D, Slater H: Neural injury in the thoracic spine: a conceptual basis for manual therapy. In Grant R, editor: Physical therapy of the cervical and thoracic spine, New York, 1994, Churchill Livingstone, p 313.

96. Slater H, Vicenzino B, Wright A: "Sympathetic slump": the effects of a novel manual therapy technique on peripheral sympathetic nervous system function, J Man Manip Ther 2(4):156-162, 1994.

97. Butler D, Shacklock O, Slater H: Treatment of altered nervous system mechanics. In Boyling J, editor: Grieve's modern manual therapy: the vertebral column, New York, 1994, Churchill Livingstone, pp 693-704.

98. Shacklock M: Improving application of neurodynamic (neural tension) testing and treatments: a message to researchers and clinicians, Man Ther 10(3):175-179. Epub, 2005.

99. Hall T, Quintner J: Responses to mechanical stimulation of the upper limb in painful cervical radiculopathy, Aust J Physiother 42(4):277-285, 1996.

100. Hurwitz EL, et al: University of California-Los Angeles. A randomized trial of medical care with and without physical therapy and chiropractic care with and without physical modalities for patients with low back pain: 6-month follow-up outcomes from the UCLA low back pain study, Spine, 27(20):2193-2204, 2002.

101. Potter L, McCarthy C, Oldham J: Physiological effects of spinal manipulation: a review of proposed theories, Phys Ther Reviews 10:163-170, 2005.

102. Arkuszewski Z: (abstract). Joint blockage: a disease, a syndrome or a sign, Man Med 3:132-134, 1988.

103. Nyberg R: Role of physical therapists in spinal manipulation. In Basmajian J, editor: Manipulation, traction and massage, ed 3, Baltimore, 1985, Williams & Wilkins, p 36.

104. Evans P: The healing process at the cellular level: a review, Physiotherapy 66:256, 1980.

105. Cummings G, Crutchfield C, Barnes M: Orthopedic physical therapy series: soft tissue changes in contractures. vol 1, Atlanta, 1983, Stokesville Publishing.

106. Donatelli R, Owens-Burkhart H: Effects of immobilization on the extensibility of periarticular connective tissue, J Orthop Sports Phys Ther 3:67-72, 1981.

107. Cramer G, et al: Effects of side-posture positioning and side-posture adjusting on the lumbar zygopophyseal

joints as evaluated by magnetic resonance imaging: a before and after study with randomization, J Manipulative Physiol Ther 23:380-394, 2000.

108. Herzog W: Clinical biomechanics of spinal manipulation, London, 2000, Churchill Livingstone.

109. Haldeman S: The clinical basis for discussion of mechanisms of manipulative therapy. In Korr I, editor. The neurobiologic mechanisms in manipulative therapy, New York, 1978, Plenum.

110. Farfan H: The scientific basis of manipulation procedures. In Buchanan W, Kahn M, Rodnan G, editors: Clinics in rheumatic diseases, London, 1980, Saunders.

111. Giles L: Anatomical basis of low back pain, Baltimore, 1989, Williams and Wilkens.

112. Collaca C, Keller T, Gunzberg R: Neuromechanical characterization of in vivo lumbar spinal manipulation. Part 2. Neurophysiologic response, J Manipulative Physiol Ther 26:579-591, 2003.

113. Randall T, Portney L, Harris B: Effects of joint mobilization on joint stiffness and active motion of the metacarpal-phalangeal joint, J Orthop Sports Phys Ther 16:30-36, 1992.

114. Shamus J et al: The effect of sesamoid mobilization, flexor hallucis strengthening, and gait training on reducing pain and restoring function in individuals with hallux limitus: a clinical trial, J Orthop Sports Phys Ther 34:368-376, 2004.

115. Raftis K, Warfield C: Spinal manipulation for back pain, Hosp Pract 15:89-90, 1989.

116. Glover J, Morris J, Khosla T: Back pain: a randomized clinical trial of rotational manipulation of the trunk, Br J Physiol 150:18-22, 1947.

117. Denslow JS: Analyzing the osteopathic lesion—1940, J Am Osteopath Assoc 101(2):99-100, 2001.

118. Terrett AC, Vernon H: Manipulation and pain tolerance: a controlled study of the effect of spinal manipulation on paraspinal cutaneous pain tolerance levels, Am J Phys Med 63(5):217-225, 1984.

119. Vernon H, et al: Spinal manipulation and beta-endorphin: a controlled study of the effect of a spinal manipulation on plasma beta-endorphin levels in normal males, J Manipulative Physiol Ther 9:115-123, 1986.

120. Wyke B: Neurology of the cervical spine, Physiotherapy, 65(suppl. 10):72, 1979.

121. Peterson B, editor: The collection of papers of Irivin M. Korr, Colorado Springs, Colo, 1979, American Academy of Osteopathy.

122. Zusman M: Mechanisms of musculoskeletal physiotherapy, Physical Therapy Reviews 9:39-49, 2004.

123. Wright A, Thurnwald P, Smith J: An evaluation of mechanical and thermal hyperalgesia in patients with lateral epicondylalgia, Pain Clin. 1992;5:199-282.

124. Wright A, Thurbwald P, O'Callaghan J: Hyperalgesia in tennis elbow patients, J Musculoskel Pain 2:83-89, 1994.

125. Butler D, Slater H: Neural injury in the thoracic spine: a conceptual basis for manual therapy. In Grant R, editor: Physical therapy of the cervical and thoracic spine, New York, 1994, Churchill Livingstone, p 313.

126. Vicenzino B, Collins D, Wright A: Sudomotor changes induced by neural mobilization techniques in asymptomatic subjects, J Manual Manip Ther 2:66-74, 1994.

127. Lovick T: Interactions between descending pathways from the dorsal and ventrolateral periaqueductal gray matter in the rat. In Depaulis A, Bandler R, editors: The midbrain periaqueductal gray matter, New York, 1991, Plenum Press.

128. Sterling M, Jull G, Wright A: Cervical mobilization: concurrent effects on pain, sympathetic nervous system activity, and motor activity, Man Ther 6:72-81, 2001.

129. Wright A: Pain-relieving effects of cervical manual therapy. In Grant R: Physical therapy of the cervical and thoracic spine, ed 3, New York, 2002, Churchill Livingstone.

130. Vicenzino B, et al: Specific manipulative therapy treatment for chronic lateral epicondylalgia produces uniquely characteristic hypoalgesia, Man Ther 6:205-212, 2001.

131. Simon R, Vicenzino B, Wright A: The influence of an anteroposterior accessory glide of the glenohumeral joint on measures of peripheral sympathetic nervous system function in the upper limb, Man Ther2(1):18-23, 1997.

132. Melzack R, Wall P: Pain mechanisms: a new theory. Science 150:971-979, 1965

133. Basmajian J, editor: Manipulation, traction, and massage, ed 3, Baltimore, 1985, Williams & Wilkins.

134. Cyriax J: Textbook of orthopedic medicine, ed 6, Baltimore, 1975, Williams & Wilkins.

135. Cookson JC, Kent B: Orthopedic manual therapy: an overview. II. The spine, Phys Ther 59:259, 1979.

136. McKenzie R: Manual correction of sciatic scoliosis, NZ Med J 76:484, 1972.

137. Gross AR, et al: A Cochrane review of manipulation and mobilization for mechanical neck disorders, Spine 29(14):1541-1548, 2004.

138. Fritz JM, Brennan G: Preliminary examination of a proposed treatment-based classification system for patients receiving physical therapy interventions for neck pain, Phys Ther 87(5):513-524, 2007.

139. Tuttle N: Do changes within a manual therapy treatment session predict between-session changes for patients with cervical spine pain? Aust J Physiother 51(1):43-48, 2005.

140. Hahne A, Keating J, Wilson S: Do within-session changes in pain intensity and range of motion predict between-session changes in patients with low back pain? Aust J Physiotherapy 50:17-23, 2004.

141. Long A, Donelson R, Fung T: Does it matter which exercise? A randomized control trial of exercise for low back pain, Spine 29(23):2593-2602, 2004.

142. Childs JD, et al: Proposal of a classification system for patients with neck pain, J Orthop Sports Phys Ther 34(11):686-696; discussion 697-700, 2004.

143. Wyke B: The neurology of low back pain. In Jayson M, editor: The lumbar spine and back pain, ed 3, New York, 1987, Churchill Livingstone, p 56.

144. McKenzie R: The lumbar spine, Waikanae, New Zealand, 1981, Spinal Publications.

145. Berthelot JM, et al: Contribution of centralization phenomenon to the diagnosis, prognosis, and treatment of diskogenic low back pain, Joint Bone Spine 2007;74:319-323.

146. Werneke M, Hart D: Centralization: association between repeated end-range pain responses and behavioral signs in patients with acute non-specific low back pain, J Rehabil Med 37(5):286-290, 2005.

147. George SZ, Bialosky JE, Donald DA: The centralization phenomenon and fear-avoidance beliefs as prognostic factors for acute low back pain: a preliminary investigation involving patients classified for specific exercise, J Orthop Sports Phys Ther 35(9):580-588, 2005.

148. Skytte L, May S, Petersen P: Centralization: its prognostic value in patients with referred symptoms and sciatica, Spine 30(11):E293-E299, 2005.

149. Aina A, May S, Clare H: The centralization phenomenon of spinal symptoms: a systematic review, Man Ther 9(3):134-143, 2004.

150. McNair J: Acute locking of the cervical spine. In Grieve G, editor: Modern manual therapy of the vertebral column, Edinburgh, 1986, Churchill Livingstone, p 357.

151. McKenzie R: The lumbar spine, Waikanae, New Zealand, 1981, Spinal Publications.

152. McKenzie R: The cervical and thoracic spine, Waikanae, New Zealand, 1990, Spinal Publications.

153. McKenzie R: Treat your own neck, Lower Hut, New Zealand, 1983, Spinal Publications.

154. Lindahl O, Hamberg J: Thoracic spine disorders as a cause of angina-like pain, Pract Cardiol, 10(suppl 2):62, 1984.

155. Laslett M: The rationale for manipulative therapy in the treatment of spinal pain of mechanical origin. Unpublished workshop manual. Mark Laslett. 211-213, White Swan Rd., Mt. Rosekill, Auckland, New Zealand, 1986.

156. McGuckin N: The T4 syndrome. In Grieve G, editor: Modern manual therapy of the vertebral column, Edinburgh, 1986, Churchill Livingstone, p 370.

157. Flynn T: The thoracic spine and rib cage, Boston, 1996, Butterworth-Heinemann.

The Shoulder

The shoulder is a complex and highly mobile joint that requires a detailed understanding of its inherent anatomy and biomechanics to enable the clinician to perform a comprehensive evaluation and to formulate an optimal treatment program. The exceptional degree of mobility and the requirement for dynamic stabilization, coupled with the repetitive nature of human shoulder function in daily activities and sports, produce challenges for the clinician during rehabilitation. This chapter will review anatomical and biomechanical concepts to provide the framework for the presentation of key clinical evaluation methods, to allow for the development of evidence-based treatment progressions for the patient with shoulder dysfunction.

ANATOMICAL AND BIOMECHANICAL CONCEPTS OF THE SHOULDER

Several key inherent anatomical and biomechanical concepts of the human shoulder have significant ramifications for evaluation and treatment. These are presented here to provide a framework for later discussion of clinical evaluation methods and treatment guidelines. These concepts include scapular plane, force couple, and glenohumeral resting position.

One of the key concepts in upper extremity rehabilitation is the *scapular plane concept.* The scapular plane has ramifications in treatment, in evaluation, and even in functional activity in sports. According to Saha, the scapular plane is defined as being 30 degrees anterior to the coronal or frontal plane of the body.[1] This plane is formed by the retroversion of the humeral head, which averages 30 degrees relative to the shaft of the humerus, coupled with the native anteversion of the glenoid, which is also 30 degrees.[2,3] It is important for clinicians to recognize this relationship during humeral head translation testing and exercise positioning because of the inherent advantages of this position. With the glenohumeral joint placed in the scapular plane, bony impingement of the greater tuberosity against the acromion does not occur because of the alignment of the tuberosity and the acromion in this orientation.[1] In addition to the optimal bony congruency afforded in the scapular plane, this position decreases stress on the anterior capsular components of the glenohumeral joint, and enhances activation of the pos-

terior rotator cuff through length-tension enhancement compared with function in the coronal plane.[1,2] Placement of the glenohumeral joint in the scapular plane optimizes the osseous congruity between the humeral head and the glenoid and is widely recommended as an optimal position for the performance of various evaluation techniques and for use during many rehabilitation exercises.[1,4]

Another important general concept of relevance for this chapter is that of muscular force couples. One of the most important biomechanical principles in shoulder function is the deltoid rotator cuff force couple.[5] This phenomenon, known as a *force couple,* can be defined as two opposing muscular forces working together to enable a particular motion to occur, with these muscular forces being synergists or agonist/antagonist pairs.[5] The deltoid muscle provides force primarily in a superior direction when it contracts unopposed during arm elevation.[6] The muscle tendon units of the rotator cuff must provide a compressive force, as well as an inferiorly or caudally directed force, to minimize superior migration and to minimize contact or impingement of the rotator cuff tendons against the overlying acromion.[5] Failure of the rotator cuff to maintain humeral congruency leads to glenohumeral joint instability, rotator cuff tendon pathology, and labral injury.[7] Imbalances in the deltoid rotator cuff force couple, which primarily occur during inappropriate and unbalanced strength training, as well as during repetitive overhead sports activities, can lead to development of the deltoid without concomitant increases in rotator cuff strength and can increase the superior migration of the humeral head provided by the deltoid, leading to rotator cuff impingement.

Additionally, the serratus anterior and trapezius force couple is the primary muscular stabilization and prime mover of upward rotation of the scapular during arm elevation. Bagg and Forrest have shown how the upper trapezius and the serratus anterior function during the initial 0 to 80 degrees of arm elevation, providing upward scapular rotation and stabilization.[8] Because of a change in the lever arm of the lower trapezius that occurs during the lateral shift of the scapulothoracic instantaneous center of rotation with arm elevation, the lower trapezius and the serratus anterior function as the primary scapular stabilizer in phases II and III (80 to 140 degrees) of elevation.[8] Knowledge of the important muscular force couples in the human shoulder and scapulothoracic region is imperative and can lead to proper evaluation and ultimately treatment provided via strengthening and monitoring of proper strength balance in these important muscular pairings.

Finally, the concept of glenohumeral resting position deserves discussion in this section of the chapter because of its relevance both in evaluation of the shoulder and in the application of treatment, specifically mobilization and interventions performed to improve glenohumeral motion. The resting position of the human glenohumeral joint generally is considered to be the position where there is maximum range of motion (ROM) and laxity, caused by minimal tension or stress in the supportive structures surrounding the joint.[9] This position has been referred to as the *loose-pack* position of the joint as well. Kaltenborn and Magee both have reported that the resting position of the glenohumeral joint ranges between 55 and 70 degrees of abduction (trunk humeral angle) in the scapular plane.[10,11] This loose-pack position is considered to be a "mid-range" position, but only recently has it been subjected to experimental testing.

Hsu et al measured maximal anterior posterior displacements and total rotation ROM in cadaveric specimens, with altering positions of glenohumeral joint elevation in the plane of the scapula.[9] Their research identified the loose-pack position, where maximal anterior posterior humeral head excursion and maximal total rotation ROM occurred within the proposed range of 55 to 70 degrees of humeral elevation in the scapular plane (trunk-humeral angle) at a mean trunk-humeral angle of 39.33 degrees. This corresponded to 45% of the available ROM of the cadaveric specimens. Anterior posterior humeral head translations and maximal total rotation ranges of motion were significantly less at 0 degrees of abduction and near 90 degrees of abduction, respectively, in the plane of the scapula, and were greatest near the experimentally measured resting position of the glenohumeral joint (39.3 degrees). This study provides key objective evidence for the clinician to obtain the maximal loose-pack position of the glenohumeral joint by using the plane of the scapula and approximately 40 degrees of abduction. This information is important to clinicians who wish to evaluate the glenohumeral joint in a position of maximal excursion or translation, to determine the underlying accessory mobility of the joint.

CLINICAL EXAMINATION OF THE SHOULDER

Although it is beyond the scope of this chapter to completely discuss examination of the shoulder complex, several key areas of the examination process deserve mention and form the platform for the development of an evidence-based treatment program. The reader is referred to more complete references for thorough presentations of the shoulder examination process.[11]

Posture and Scapular Examination

Evaluation of posture for the patient with shoulder dysfunction begins with shoulder heights evaluated in the standing posi-

tion, as well as use of the hands-on-hips position to evaluate the prominence of the scapula against the thoracic wall. Typically, the dominant shoulder is significantly lower than the nondominant shoulder in neutral, nonstressed standing postures, particularly in unilaterally dominant athletes like baseball and tennis players.[12] Although the exact reason for this phenomenon is unclear, theories include increased mass in the dominant arm, leading the dominant shoulder to be lower secondary to the increased weight of the arm, as well as elongation of the periscapular musculature on the dominant or preferred side secondary to eccentric loading.

In the standing position, the clinician can observe the patient for symmetrical muscle development and, more specifically, focal areas of muscle atrophy. One of the positions recommended, in addition to observing the patient with the arms at the sides in a comfortable standing posture, is the hands-on-hips position, which simply places the patient's shoulders in approximately 45 to 50 degrees of abduction with slight internal rotation. The hands are placed on the iliac crests of the hips such that the thumbs are pointed posteriorly. Placement of the hands on the hips allows the patient to relax the arms and often enables the clinician to observe focal pockets of atrophy along the scapular border, and more commonly over the infraspinous fossa of the scapula. Thorough visual inspection using this position can often identify excessive scalloping over the infraspinous fossa, which may be present in patients with rotator cuff dysfunction and in patients with severe atrophy who may have suprascapular nerve involvement. Impingement of the suprascapular nerve can occur at the suprascapular notch and the spinoglenoid notch and from paralabral cyst formation commonly found in patients with superior labral lesions.[13] Figure 10-1 shows the isolated atrophy present in the infraspinous fossa of an overhead athlete who presented with anterior shoulder pain. Further diagnostic testing of the patient with extreme wasting of the infraspinatus muscle is warranted to rule out suprascapular nerve involvement.

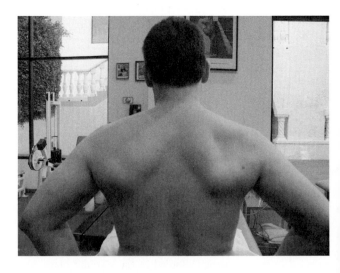

Figure 10-1 Posterior view of a patient in the hands-on-hips position showing extensive infraspinatus muscle atrophy.

Examination of the scapulothoracic joint is an extremely important part of the comprehensive clinical examination process for the patient with shoulder dysfunction. It entails several component parts. Understanding the normal and abnormal movement patterns of the scapula is imperative. Although many variations in normal scapular position do exist, resting scapular orientation is 30 degrees anteriorly rotated with respect to the frontal plane as viewed from above.[14] Additionally, the scapula is rotated approximately 3 degrees upward (superiorly), as viewed from the posterior orientation.

Scapulothoracic movement was initially described in clinical terms as "scapulo-humeral rhythm" by both Codman and Inman.[5,15] Inman stated that "the total range of scapular motion is not more than 60 [degrees]," and that the total contribution from the glenohumeral joint is not greater than 120 degrees. The scapulohumeral rhythm was described for the total arc of elevation of the shoulder joint to contain 2 degrees of glenohumeral motion for every degree of scapulothoracic motion.[5] In addition to this ratio of movement, Inman identified what he termed a *setting phase*, which occurred during the first 30 to 60 degrees of shoulder elevation. Inman described this setting phase as when "the scapula seeks, in relationship to the humerus, a precise position of stability which it may obtain in one of three ways":

1. The scapula may remain fixed, with motion occurring solely at the glenohumeral joint until a stable position is reached.
2. The scapula may move laterally or medially on the chest wall.
3. In rare instances, the scapula may oscillate until stabilization is achieved.

Once 30 degrees of abduction and 60 degrees of flexion have been reached, the relationship of scapulothoracic to glenohumeral joint motion remains remarkably constant.[5] Observation of early motion of the scapula during arm elevation based on these early descriptions of scapular mechanics usually indicates glenohumeral hypomobility and/or force couple imbalance and leads the clinician to a more detailed examination of both the scapulothoracic and glenohumeral joints.

Later research using three-dimensional analysis and other laboratory-based methods has confirmed Inman's early descriptions of scapulohumeral rhythm.[8,16] These studies have provided more detailed descriptions of the exact contributions of the scapulothoracic and glenohumeral joints during arm elevation in the scapular plane. Doody et al[16] found that the ratio of glenohumeral to scapulothoracic motion changes from 7.29 : 1 in the first 30 degrees of elevation to 0.78 : 1 at between 90 and 150 degrees. Bagg and Forrest found similar differences based on the ROM examined.[8] In the early phase of elevation, 4.29 degrees of glenohumeral joint motion occurred for every 1 degree of scapular motion, with 1.71 degrees of glenohumeral motion occurring for every 1 degree of scapular motion between the functional arc of 80 and 140 degrees.

Bagg and Forrest also clearly identified the instantaneous center of rotation (ICR) of the scapulothoracic joint at various points in the ROM.[8] Figure 4.1 in the study shows the ICR of the scapulothoracic joint at 20 degrees of elevation, and Figure 4.2 in the study shows the ICR of the scapulothoracic joint

at approximately 140 degrees of elevation. The ICR moves from the medial border of the spine of the scapula, with the shoulder at approximately 20 degrees of elevation very near the side of the body, and migrates superolaterally to the region near the acromioclavicular (AC) joint at approximately 140 degrees. Bagg and Forrest's research also identified an increased muscular stabilization role of the lower trapezius and serratus anterior force couple at higher, more functional positions of elevation.

Typical movement of the scapula occurs in the coronal, sagittal, and transverse planes. Brief descriptions here provide a framework for the classification of scapular dysfunction. Primary movements consist of three rotations: upward/downward, internal/external, and anterior/posterior, along with two translations: superior/inferior and protraction/retraction (Figure 10-2).

Movements of upward and downward rotation occur in the coronal or frontal plane. The angle typically used to describe the position of scapular rotation is formed between the spine and the medial border of the scapula. Poppen and Walker[17] reported normal elevation of the acromion to be approximately 36 degrees from the neutral position to maximum abduction. Sagittal plane motion of the scapula is referred to as *anterior/ posterior tilting*. The angle of scapular tilting is formed by a vector passing via C7 and T7 and a vector passing via the inferior angle of the scapula and the root of the spine of the scapula.[18] Transverse plane movement of the scapula is referred to as *internal and external rotation*. The angle used to describe internal/external rotation of the scapula is formed by the coronal (frontal) plane of the body and a vector passing via the

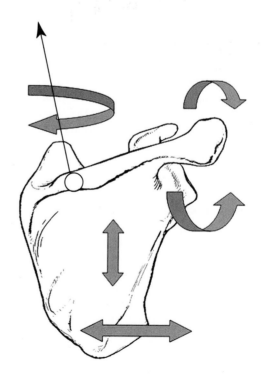

Figure 10-2 Representation of scapular motion showing three rotations and two translations.

transverse plane projection of the root of the spine of the scapula and the posterior angle of the scapula.[18] Abnormal increases in the internal rotation angle of the scapula lead to changes in the orientation of the glenoid. This altered position of the glenoid, referred to as "antetilting," allows for opening up of the anterior half of the glenohumeral articulation.[19] The antetilting of the scapula has been shown by Saha to be a component of the subluxation/dislocation complex in patients with microtrauma-induced glenohumeral instability.[1] Further biomechanical study has shown increased scapular internal rotation in patients with atraumatic glenohumeral joint instability.[20] Results of this study support the use of exercise programming directed at improving the strength of synergistic function of the serratus anterior and trapezius to stabilize the scapula and address malpositioning of the scapula in patients with glenohumeral joint instability.

The movement of protraction and retraction occurs literally around the curvature of the thoracic wall.[21] Retraction typically occurs in a curvilinear fashion around the wall, while protraction may proceed in a slightly upward or downward motion, depending on the position of the humerus relative to the scapula.[21] Depending on the size of the individual and the vigorousness of the activity, translation of the human scapula during protraction and retraction can occur over distances of 15 to 18 cm.[21] The scapula also can move in the coronal plane along the thoracic wall superiorly and inferiorly in movements typically called *elevation* and *depression*, respectively. Evaluation of the patient with rotator cuff weakness often identifies excessive early scapular elevation as a compensatory movement to optimize humeral movement.[21]

Several studies have measured the movement of the scapulothoracic joint while providing reference information for clinicians that is relevant during the observation phase of the examination. Normal scapulothoracic motion during arm elevation includes the following key components: upward rotation, external rotation, and posterior tilting. Bourne et al[22] reported the following during arm elevation: 49 degrees of upward rotation, 27 degrees of external rotation, and 44 degrees of posterior tilting. Similarly, McClure et al[23] found 50 degrees, 24 degrees, and 30 degrees for those important scapular movement components, respectively.

The most widely described and overused term pertaining to scapular pathology is *scapular winging*. Scapular winging is a term that is used to describe gross disassociation of the scapula from the thoracic wall.[24] It is typically very obvious to a trained observer who is simply viewing a patient from the posterior and lateral orientation, and it becomes even more pronounced with active or resistive movement to the upper extremities. True scapular winging occurs as the result of involvement of the long thoracic nerve.[24] Isolated paralysis of the serratus anterior muscle with resultant "winged scapula" was first described by Velpeau in 1837. Winged scapula is peripheral in origin and ultimately is derived from involvement of the fifth, sixth, and seventh spinal cord segments.[24] Isolated serratus anterior muscle weakness due to nerve palsy will create a prominent superior medial border of the scapula and depressed acromion, and isolated trapezius muscle weakness due to nerve palsy will create a protracted inferior border of the scapula and an elevated acromion.[21]

Although it is possible that some patients with shoulder pathology may present with true scapular winging, most patients with shoulder pathology present with less obvious and less severe forms of scapular dysfunction. Clinicians traditionally have had little nomenclature and few objective descriptions for scapular dysfunction; this has led to the use of numerous terms to describe nonoptimal or abnormal scapular positions and movement patterns.[21] Kibler has defined scapular dysfunction as encompassing abnormal motion and position of the scapula. Therefore, evaluation of the scapula must involve both static and dynamic methods.[25]

Kibler has developed a more specific scapular classification system for clinical use that allows clinicians to categorize scapular dysfunction based on common clinical findings obtained via visual observation of both static posture and dynamic upper extremity movements.[21,25] Kibler has identified three specific scapular dysfunctions or patterns. These scapular dysfunctions are termed *Inferior* or *Type I*, *Medial* or *Type II*, and *Superior* or *Type III*; each is named for the area of the scapula that is visually prominent during clinical evaluation. In the Kibler classification system, normal symmetrical scapular motion characterized by symmetrical scapular upward rotation "such that the inferior angles translate laterally away from the midline and the scapular medial border remains flush against the thoracic wall with the reverse occurring during arm lowering."[25]

In the type I or inferior angle classification of scapular dysfunction, the primary external visual feature is the prominence of the inferior angle of the scapula (Figure 10-3). This pattern of dysfunction involves anterior tilting of the scapula in the sagittal plane, which produces the prominent inferior angle of the scapula. No other abnormality is typically present with this dysfunction pattern; however, the prominence of the inferior angle of the scapula does increase oftentimes in the hands-on-hips position, as well as during active flexion, scaption, or

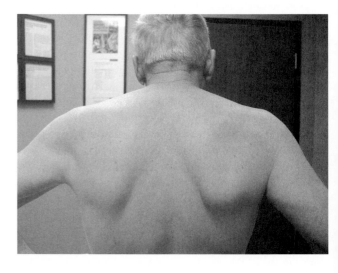

Figure 10-3 Patient with Kibler Type I, inferior border scapular dysfunction.

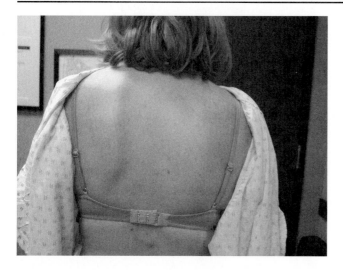

Figure 10-4 Patient with Kibler Type II, medial border scapular dysfunction.

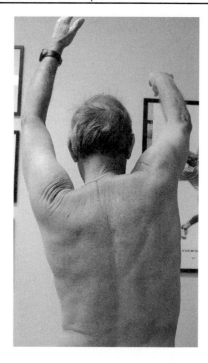

Figure 10-5 Patient with Kibler Type III, superior scapular dysfunction.

abduction movements of the shoulder, particularly during eccentric lowering of the extremity from the overhead position. According to Kibler, inferior angle dysfunction or prominence is most commonly found in patients with rotator cuff dysfunction. Anterior tilting of the scapula places the acromion in a position closer to the rotator cuff and humeral head, thus compromising the subacromial space.[25]

In the type II or medial border classification of scapular dysfunction, the primary external visual feature is the prominence of the entire medial border of the scapula (Figure 10-4). This pattern or dysfunction involves internal rotation of the scapula in the transverse plane. Internal rotation of the scapula produces a prominent medial border of the scapula. Similar to the inferior or inferior angle dysfunction, the medial or medial border dysfunction often increases in the hands-on-hips position, as well as during active movements of the upper extremity, particularly during eccentric lowering from overhead motion. According to Kibler, Saha, and Von Eisenhart-Rothe, medial border scapular dysfunction most often occurs in patients with instability or rotator cuff dysfunction caused by glenohumeral joint instability.[1,20,25] Previous discussions in this chapter outlined the opening up of the anterior aspect of the glenoid that occurs with scapular antetilting, which would be a characteristic of this medial border scapular dysfunction.

Superior scapular dysfunction or Type III scapular dysfunction is characterized by excessive and early elevation of the scapula during arm elevation (Figure 10-5). This has been referred to as a *shoulder shrug*, or "hiking" of the shoulder girdle by clinicians, and it is most often seen with rotator cuff dysfunction and deltoid–rotator cuff force couple imbalances.[5] This superior movement of the scapula is thought to occur as a compensatory movement pattern to assist with arm elevation.

The specific sequence recommended for scapular evaluation includes both static and dynamic aspects. Both are critical for obtaining the clinical cues that allow the clinician to determine the often subtle scapular dysfunction present in patients with shoulder pathology. Evaluation of the patient, as mentioned earlier, occurs in the standing position, with arms held comfortably against the sides of the body. The clinician should note the outline of the scapula and compare the scapulae bilaterally. Although many variations in standing posture are seen, the clinician should be particularly discriminating when bilateral differences in scapular posture are present and, most notably, when the greater prominence of the scapula is present on the involved side. Bilateral symmetry, with respect to scapular position and scapular prominence in the patient with unilateral shoulder dysfunction, is not necessarily an indicator of scapular dysfunction.

After examination of the patient with the arms in complete adduction at the sides of the body, the patient is examined in the hands-on-hips position. Following the static examination, the patient is asked to bilaterally elevate the shoulders using a self-selected plane of elevation. The clinician should be directly behind the patient, to best observe the movement of the scapula during concentric elevation and especially during eccentric lowering. Excessive superior movement of the scapula during concentric arm elevation, as well as inferior angle and medial border prominence during the eccentric phase, is commonly encountered in patients with scapular dysfunction. Repeated bouts of arm elevation to confirm initial observations, as well as to determine the presence and locations of symptoms (location in/on the shoulder, as well as the ROM where symptoms occur), are recommended. Additionally, the effect of repeated movements is of critical importance for assessing the effects of fatigue on scapular stabilization. In the patient with subtle symptom presentation, 1 pound to 1 kilogram weights may be added to further provoke the scapula and provide additional loading.

Additional tests are recommended for examination of the scapula. These include the lateral scapular slide test, the scapular assistance test, the scapular retraction test, and the flip sign. The lateral scapular slide test (LSST) was developed by Kibler as a semidynamic test, to evaluate scapular position and scapular stabilizer strength on injured and noninjured sides, in relationship to a fixed point on the spine, as varying amounts or loads and movement are superimposed on the supporting musculature.[19,21] The lateral scapular slide test is not a true dynamic test, and it relies on static positions to assess scapular muscle stabilization.[21] The test involves measuring the distance between the inferior angle of the scapula and the corresponding vertebral spinous process in the transverse plane in three positions; neutral resting posture with arms at the sides, hands on hips position, and 90 degrees of abduction in the coronal plane with full internal rotation. The distance is measured in centimeters and is compared bilaterally. A difference of 1.5 cm or more between sides indicates a positive test. Patients with a positive Kibler lateral scapular slide test (bilateral difference of greater than 1.5 cm) may have deficits in dynamic scapular stabilization or may have postural adaptations that produce significant differences in scapular positioning identified with this test. These patients are candidates for rehabilitative exercise to promote scapular stabilization. Several studies have reported test-retest reliability of the LSST. Intraclass correlation coefficients (ICCs) ranged between 0.69 and 0.96 for intratester reliability.[21,26,27] The validity of the Kibler LSST has been tested on patients with impingement and instability.[28,29] It is important to note, however, that this test is just one part of the clinical examination process and simply records the degree of lateral slide or movement away from the midline. Positive findings must be correlated with other key parts of the scapular and glenohumeral evaluation.

The scapular assistance test (SAT) reported by Kibler involves independent elevation of the shoulder by the patient to determine ROM and pain provocation.[21] After baseline motion and pain responses are established, the patient is asked to again elevate the shoulder while the examiner "assists" with upward rotation of the scapula by manually providing a generous upward rotation force during arm elevation (Figure 10-6). Negation or lessening of the symptoms of pain provocation and/or improved elevation in ROM indicate a positive scapular assistance test. The improved scapular control and upward rotation provided by the examiner's hands indicate the need for scapular stabilization interventions in rehabilitation and indicate a scapular causation or component to the patient's shoulder dysfunction.[21] Rabin et al[30] tested the intertester reliability of the SAT and found coefficient of agreements ranging from 77% to 91% for the scapular and sagittal planes, respectively. They concluded that the SAT demonstrates moderate interrater reliability acceptable for clinical use.

Another scapular test similar to the SAT is the scapular retraction test (SRT).[21] This test again uses manual repositioning of the scapula by the examiner's hands (Figure 10-7) achieved by retracting and externally rotating the scapula. The movement of glenohumeral internal and external rotation in 90 degrees of abduction is often targeted for baseline testing

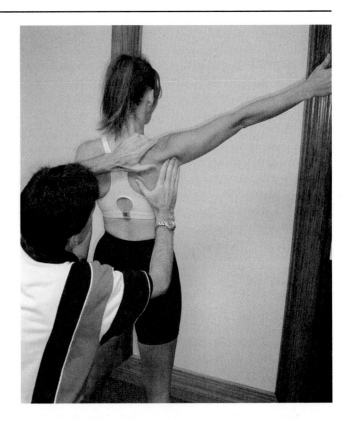

Figure 10-6 Kibler scapular assistance test. (From Ellenbecker T: Clinial examination of the shoulder, Philadelpha, 2005, Saunders.)

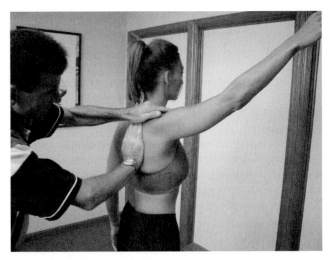

Figure 10-7 Kibler scapular retraction test. (From Ellenbecker T: Clinial examination of the shoulder, Philadelpha, 2005, Saunders.)

and retesting with manual repositioning of the scapula. The negation or lessening of symptoms in the retracted, externally rotated scapular position again indicates the need for inclusion of scapular stabilization exercise in the treatment program.

Finally, the scapular "flip sign" has been reported by Kelley et al.[31] This sign, initially observed in patients with spinal accessory nerve lesions, is brought about by simply performing an external rotation manual muscle test maneuver with the shoulder at the side of the body (Figure 10-8). Provocation of the medial and inferior borders of the scapula away from the thorax under the load of the manual muscle test force of exter-

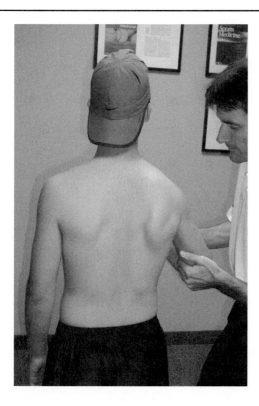

Figure 10-8 Patient with positive "flip" sign showing prominence of the inferior medial border during external rotation manual muscle testing.

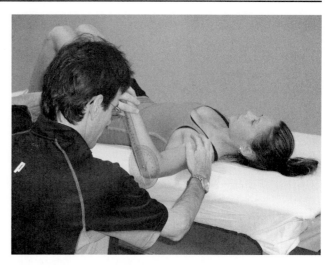

Figure 10-9 Recommended technique for measurement of internal rotation at 90 degrees of glenohumeral joint abduction with scapular stabilization.

nal rotation constitutes a positive flip sign. Initially reported in patients with spinal accessory nerve lesions, this test has been noted by the authors of this chapter to be positive in patients with scapular dysfunction, including overhead athletes, and has proved to be a useful tool for identifying subtle scapular dysfunction. The inability of the scapular stabilizers (serratus anterior and trapezius) to adequately control scapular position during an external rotation load is an important finding worth documenting. This test can be used along with the other scapular tests to gain an improved understanding of the ability of the scapula and its dynamic stabilizers to function during both glenohumeral positioning and dynamic loading.

Range of Motion Measurement

Discussing the complete methodology for range-of-motion testing in depth is beyond the scope of this chapter; however, the measurement of one of the most important movement patterns (humeral rotation) will be covered, along with the concept of total rotation ROM. Thorough objective documentation of the cardinal movements of the glenohumeral joint is recommended, and the reader is referred to two texts for a more complete discussion.[32,33]

Several important principles should be discussed to optimize the measurement of humeral rotation in the patient with shoulder dysfunction. One of these is the contribution of the scapulothoracic joint to glenohumeral motion, which has been widely documented.[5,34] This is one of the variables that can lead to extensive variation of rotational measurement in the human

shoulder. In a study by Ellenbecker et al,[35] active rotational ROM measures were taken bilaterally in 399 elite junior tennis players using two differing measurement techniques and a universal goniometer. Two hundred fifty-two subjects were simply measured in the supine position for internal and external rotation with 90 degrees of glenohumeral joint abduction and with no attempt made to stabilize the scapula. One hundred forty-seven elite junior tennis players were measured for internal and external rotation active ROM in 90 degrees of glenohumeral joint abduction using scapular stabilization. This stabilization was provided by a posteriorly directed force applied by the examiner's hand placed over the anterior aspect of the shoulder, over the anterior acromion and coracoid process (Figure 10-9). Results from the two groups showed significantly less internal rotation ROM when the measurement technique was used with scapular stabilization (18% to 28% reduction in ROM). Changes in external rotation ROM were smaller between groups, with 2% to 6% reductions in active ROM measured.

One common finding confirmed in this research is the finding of significantly less (approximately 10 to 15 degrees) dominant arm glenohumeral joint internal rotation in elite junior tennis players.[34,35] The significance of this present research, however, lies in the fact that this difference between extremities in internal rotation ROM was identified only in the condition in which the scapula was stabilized. Failure to stabilize the scapula did not produce glenohumeral joint internal rotation ROM measurements that identified a deficit. Only measuring this population with scapular stabilization identified the characteristic ROM limitation in internal rotation. This study clearly demonstrates the importance of using consistent measurement techniques when documenting ROM of glenohumeral joint rotation.

Reinold et al[36] used three methods to measure internal rotation with 90 degrees of abduction in asymptomatic baseball pitchers. These methods included (1) visual observation to determine when scapular motion occurred with no physical stabilization of the scapula; (2) scapular stabilization achieved by placing a hand over the humeral head; and (3) scapular stabilization achieved by placement of the examiner's hand over the coracoid process and acromion. Significantly less dominant arm internal rotation was found with all three methods of internal rotation measurement when compared with similar measures on the nondominant extremity. Significant differences also were seen in the amount of internal rotation measured through the three methods of internal rotation measurement. The least motion was measured with humeral head support, and the most internal rotation was seen with no physical stabilization and only visual observation. On the basis of these study results, the authors of this chapter highly recommend the use of scapular stabilization during measurement of humeral rotation to obtain more isolated and representative values of shoulder rotation. Consistent use of a method outlined in this chapter that describes stabilization directly on the scapula is recommended.

One final concept to be discussed in this section on ROM measurement is the total rotation ROM concept. This concept simply combines the glenohumeral joint internal and external rotation ROM measures by summing the two numbers to obtain a numeric representation of the total rotation ROM available at the glenohumeral joint. Recent research by Kibler et al[37] and Roetert et al[38] has identified decreases in the total rotation ROM arc in the dominant extremity of elite tennis players correlated with increasing age and number of competitive years of play. Most recently, Ellenbecker et al[39] measured bilateral total rotation ROM in professional baseball pitchers and elite junior tennis players. Findings of this study showed the professional baseball pitchers to have greater dominant arm external rotation and significantly less dominant arm internal rotation, when compared with the contralateral nondominant side. Total rotation ROM, however, was not significantly different between extremities in professional baseball pitchers (145 degrees dominant arm, 146 degrees nondominant arm). This research shows that, despite bilateral differences in actual internal or external rotation ROM, or both, in the glenohumeral joints of baseball pitchers, the total arc of rotational motion should remain the same.

In contrast, Ellenbecker et al[39] tested 117 elite male junior tennis players. Among these tennis players, significantly less internal rotation ROM was found on the dominant arm (45 versus 56 degrees), and significantly less total rotation ROM was seen on the dominant arm (149 versus 158 degrees). Total rotation ROM did differ slightly between extremities. Approximately 10 degrees less total rotation ROM can be expected in the dominant arm of the uninjured elite junior tennis player, as compared with the nondominant extremity. Utilization of normative data from population-specific research, such as this study, can assist clinicians in interpreting normal ROM patterns and in identifying when sport-specific adaptations or clinically significant maladaptations are present.

Clinical application of the total rotation ROM concept is best demonstrated by a case presentation of a unilaterally dominant upper extremity athlete. If, during the initial evaluation

of a high-level baseball pitcher, the clinician finds an ROM pattern of 120 degrees of external rotation and only 30 degrees of internal rotation, some uncertainty may exist as to whether this represents an ROM deficit in internal rotation that requires rehabilitative intervention via muscle tendon unit stretching and possibly via the use of specific glenohumeral joint mobilization. However, if measurement of that patient's nondominant extremity rotation reveals 90 degrees of external rotation and 60 degrees of internal rotation, the current recommendation based on the total rotation ROM concept would be to avoid extensive mobilization and passive stretching of the dominant extremity because the total rotation ROM in both extremities is 150 degrees (120 degrees external rotation + 30 degrees internal rotation = 150 degrees dominant arm total rotation, and 90 degrees external rotation + 60 degrees internal rotation = 150 degrees total rotation nondominant arm). In elite level tennis players, the total active rotation ROM can be expected to be up to 10 degrees less on the dominant arm before clinical treatment to address internal rotation ROM restriction would be recommended or implemented.

This total rotation ROM concept can be used as illustrated to guide the clinician during rehabilitation, specifically in the area of application of stretching and mobilization, to best determine which glenohumeral joint requires additional mobility, and which extremity should not have additional mobility, because of the obvious harm induced by increases in capsular mobility and increases in humeral head translation during aggressive upper extremity exertion. Burkhart et al[7] describe this loss of internal rotation ROM as glenohumeral internal rotation deficit (GIRD).

Several definitions of GIRD have been proposed and are used to guide clinicians in the identification of a patient with significant internal rotation ROM loss.[7,39,40] These definitions include the following:

- Loss of 20 degrees or more internal rotation on the dominant arm compared with the contralateral side
- Loss of 25 degrees or more internal rotation on the dominant arm compared with the contralateral side
- Loss of 10% of the total rotation ROM of the contralateral side

For this example, a total rotation ROM of 150 degrees on the contralateral side would result in a definition of GIRD occurring when greater than 15 degrees of internal rotation ROM loss was present in the dominant extremity. Further research is needed to identify critical levels of internal rotation loss in overhead athletes and to improve the interpretation of this important measure.

The loss of internal rotation ROM is significant for several reasons. The relationship between internal rotation ROM loss (tightness in the posterior capsule of the shoulder) and increased anterior humeral head translation has been scientifically identified.[41] The increase in anterior humeral shear force reported by Harryman et al[42] was manifested by a horizontal adduction cross-body maneuver, similar to that incurred during follow-through of the throwing motion or tennis serve. Tightness of the posterior capsule also has been linked to increased superior migration of the humeral head during shoulder elevation.[43]

Recent research by Koffler et al[44] and Grossman et al[45] examined the effects of posterior capsular tightness in a functional position of 90 degrees of abduction and 90 degrees or more of external rotation in cadaveric specimens. In the presence of posterior capsular tightness, the humeral head will shift in an anterior-superior direction, as compared with a normal shoulder with normal capsular relationships, during which the humeral head translates in a posterior-inferior direction with arm cocking at 90 degrees of abduction. With more extensive amounts of posterior capsular tightness, the humeral head was found to shift posterosuperiorly. These effects of altered posterior capsular tensions experimentally representing in vivo posterior glenohumeral joint capsular tightness highlight the clinical importance of using a reliable and effective measurement method to assess internal rotation ROM during examination of the shoulder.

Special Tests for the Shoulder

Discussion of several types of manual orthopaedic tests is warranted as their inclusion in the comprehensive examination sequence gives the clinician the ability to determine the underlying cause or causes of shoulder dysfunction. Tests discussed in this chapter include impingement tests, instability tests, and labral tests.

Impingement Tests

Tests to identify glenohumeral impingement primarily involve the re-creation of subacromial shoulder pain using maneuvers that are known to reproduce and mimic functional positions in which significant subacromial compression is present. These motions involve forcible forward flexion (Neer's impingement sign),[46] forced internal rotation in the scapular plane (Hawkins' impingement sign),[47] forced internal rotation in the sagittal plane (coracoid impingement test),[48] and cross-arm adduction.[11] These tests all involve passive movement of the glenohumeral joint. Yocum's test involves the active combination of elevation with internal rotation and can provide a valuable understanding of the patient's ability to control superior humeral head translation during active arm elevation in a compromised position.[49] Valadie et al[50] has provided objective evidence of the degree of encroachment and compression of the rotator cuff tendons against the coracoacromial arch during several impingement tests. These tests can be used effectively to reproduce a patient's symptoms of impingement and to give important insight into positions that should be avoided in the exercise progressions used during treatment following evaluation. Use of exercises that simulate impingement positions is not recommended.[4,51]

Instability Tests

Another type of clinical test that must be included during the examination of the shoulder is instability testing. Two main types of instability tests are used: humeral head translation tests and provocation tests. Each is presented here.

Several authors believe that the most important tests used to identify shoulder joint instability are humeral head translation tests.[56,57] These tests attempt to document the amount of movement of the humeral head relative to the glenoid through the use of carefully applied directional stresses to the proximal humerus. Harryman et al[58] measured the amount of humeral head translation in vivo in healthy, uninjured subjects using a three-dimensional spatial tracking system. They found a mean of 7.8 mm of anterior translation and 7.9 mm of posterior translation when an anterior and posterior drawer test was used. Translation of the human shoulder in an inferior direction was evaluated with a multidirectional instability (MDI) sulcus test. During in vivo testing of inferior humeral head translation, an average of 10 mm of inferior displacement was measured. Results from this detailed laboratory-based research study indicate that approximately a 1:1 ratio of anterior-to-posterior humeral head translation can be expected in normal shoulders with manual humeral head translation tests. No definitive interpretation of bilateral symmetry in humeral head translation is available from this research.

One key test used to evaluate the stability of the athlete's shoulder is the MDI sulcus test. This test is the primary test used to identify the patient with MDI of the glenohumeral joint. Excessive translation in the inferior direction during this test most often indicates a forthcoming pattern of excessive translation in an anterior or posterior direction, or in both anterior and posterior directions. This test, when performed in the neutral adducted position, directly assesses the integrity of the superior glenohumeral ligament and the coracohumeral ligament.[59] These ligaments are the primary stabilizing structures against inferior humeral head translation in the adducted glenohumeral position.[60] To perform this test, it is recommended that the patient be examined in the seated position with the arms in neutral adduction and resting gently in the patient's lap. The examiner grasps the distal aspect of the humerus using a firm but unassuming grip with one hand, while several brief, relatively rapid downward pulls are exerted to the humerus in an inferior (vertical) direction (Figure 10-10). A visible "sulcus sign" (tethering of the skin between the lateral acromion and the humerus from the increase in inferior translation of the humeral head and the widening subacromial space) is usually present in patients with MDI (Figure 10-11).[61]

Gerber and Ganz[57] and McFarland et al[56] believe that testing for anterior and posterior shoulder laxity is best performed with the patient in the supine position because of greater inherent relaxation of the patient. This test allows the patient's extremity to be tested in multiple positions of glenohumeral joint abduction, thus selectively stressing specific portions of the glenohumeral joint anterior capsule and capsular ligaments. Figure 10-12 shows the authors' preferred technique for assessing and grading the translation of the humeral head in both anterior and posterior directions. It is important to note that the direction of translation must be along the line of the glenohumeral joint, with an anteromedial and posterolateral direction used because of the 30 degree version of the glenoid.[1] This is accomplished by ensuring that the examiner places the

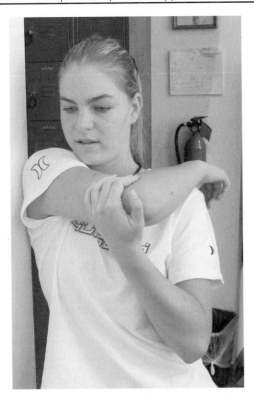

Figure 10-10 Multidirectional instability (MDI) sulcus test.

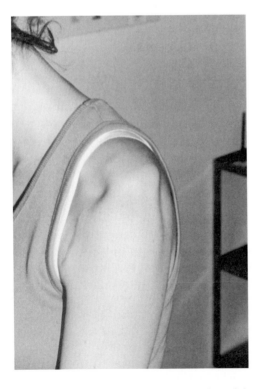

Figure 10-11 Patient with a positive multidirectional instability (MDI) sulcus test.

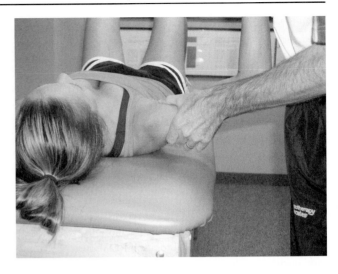

Figure 10-12 Supine humeral head translation test measured at 90 degrees of glenohumeral joint abduction in the scapular plane.

patient's glenohumeral joint in the scapular plane as pictured (see Figure 10-12). Testing for anterior translation is performed in the range between 0 and 30 degrees of abduction, between 30 and 60 degrees of abduction, and at 90 degrees of abduction to test the integrity of the superior, middle, and inferior glenohumeral ligaments, respectively.[59,60] Posterior testing typically is performed at 90 degrees of abduction because no distinct thickenings of the capsule are noted, with the exception of the posterior band of the inferior glenohumeral ligament complex.[60] Grading (assessing the translation) for this test is performed using the classification of Altchek and Dines.[62] This classification system defines grade I translation as humeral translation within the glenoid without edge loading or translation of the humerus over the glenoid rim. Grade II represents translation of the humeral head up over the glenoid rim with spontaneous return on removal of the stress. The presence of grade II translation in an anterior or posterior direction without symptoms does not indicate instability but instead merely represents laxity of the glenohumeral joint. Unilateral increases in glenohumeral translation in the presence of shoulder pain and disability can ultimately lead to the diagnosis of glenohumeral joint instability.[63,64] Grade III translation, which is not seen clinically in orthopaedic and sports physical therapy, involves translation of the humeral head over the glenoid rim without relocation upon removal of stress. Ellenbecker et al[65] tested the intrarater reliability of humeral head translation tests and found improved reliability when using the main criterion of whether the humeral head traverses the glenoid rim. The use of end-feel classification and other estimators decreases intrarater reliability and interferes with the interpretation of findings from glenohumeral translation testing.[65]

The last and possibly the most important test used to identify subtle anterior instability in the overhead-throwing athlete or the individual with symptoms in overhead positions is the subluxation/relocation test. This test is a form of provocation test that does not measure humeral head translation. Originally described by Jobe,[66] the subluxation/relocation test is designed to identify subtle anterior instability of the glenohumeral joint. Credit for the development and application of this test is also given to Dr. Peter Fowler.[67] Fowler described the diagnostic quandary of microinstability (subtle anterior instability) versus rotator cuff injury or both in swimmers and advocated the use of this important test to assist in the diagnosis. The subluxation/relocation test is performed with the patient's shoulder held and stabilized in the patient's maximal end-range of external rotation at 90 degrees of abduction. The examiner then provides a mild anterior subluxation force (Figure 10-13, A). The patient is asked if this subluxation reproduces his or her symptoms. Reproduction of patient symptoms of anterior or posterior shoulder pain with subluxation leads the examiner to reposition his or her hand on the anterior aspect of the patient's shoulder and perform a posterior-lateral directed force, using a soft, cupped hand to minimize anterior shoulder pain from the hand/shoulder (examiner/patient) interface (see Figure 10-13, B). Failure to reproduce the patient's symptoms with end-range external rotation and 90 degrees of abduction leads the examiner to reattempt the subluxation maneuver with 110 degrees and 120 degrees of abduction. This modification has been proposed by Hamner et al[68] to increase the potential for contact between the undersurface of the supraspinatus tendon and the posterior superior glenoid. In each position of abduction (90 degrees, 110 degrees, and 120 degrees of abduction), the same sequence of initial subluxation and subsequent relocation is performed as described previously.

Reproduction of anterior or posterior shoulder pain with the subluxation portion of this test, with subsequent diminution or disappearance of anterior or posterior shoulder pain with the relocation maneuver, constitutes a positive test. Production of apprehension with any position of abduction during the anteriorly directed subluxation force phase of testing would indicate occult anterior instability. The primary ramifications of a positive test would indicate subtle anterior instability and secondary glenohumeral joint impingement (anterior pain) or posterior or internal impingement in the presence of posterior

pain with this maneuver. A posterior type II superior labrum anterior to posterior (SLAP) lesion has also been implicated in patients with a positive subluxation/relocation test.[69]

Labral Testing

Many tests have been proposed to assess the integrity of the glenoid labrum. A brief discussion of the glenoid labrum and its injury patterns and characteristics will enable the clinician to better understand how clinical examination maneuvers for the glenoid labrum can be applied.

The glenoid labrum serves several important functions, including deepening the glenoid fossa to enhance concavity and serving as the attachment for the glenohumeral capsular ligaments. Injury to the labrum can compromise the concavity compression phenomena by as much as 50%.[70] Individuals with increased capsular laxity and generalized joint hypermobility have increased humeral head translation, which can subject the labrum to increased shear forces.[71] In the throwing athlete, large anterior translational forces are present at levels up to 50% of body weight during arm acceleration of the throwing motion, with the arm in 90 degrees of abduction and external rotation.[72] This repeated translation of the humeral head against and over the glenoid labrum can lead to labral injury. Labral injury can occur as tearing or as actual detachment from the glenoid.

Labral Tears

Terry et al[73] arthroscopically evaluated tears of the glenoid labrum in 83 patients. They classified labral tears into several types, including transverse tears, longitudinal tears, flap tears, horizontal cleavage tears, and fibrillated tears. Additionally, Terry et al[73] reported the distribution of the location of these labral tears in the 83 patients they evaluated arthroscopically. Primary tears of the glenoid labrum occurred most commonly in the anterior-superior (60%) or the posterior-superior part of

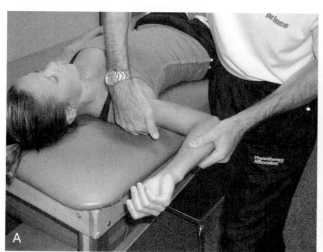
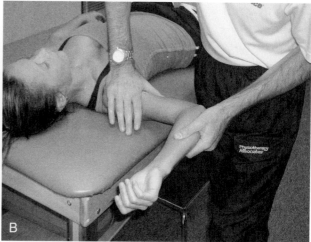

Figure 10-13 Jobe subluxation/relocation test. **A,** End-range external rotation in the coronal plane with subluxation force at 90 degrees of glenohumeral joint abduction. **B,** Relocation of the humeral head during the latter portion of this test.

the shoulder (18%). Only 1% of tears occurred in the anterior-inferior part of the shoulder. Finally, tears were located in more than one location 22% of the time in the patients studied by Terry et al.[73]

The role of the labrum in the hypermobile shoulder was studied clinically by Altchek et al.[74] In a 3-year follow-up of 40 overhead athletes who underwent arthroscopic labral debridement, 72% initially reported relief of symptoms during the first year after surgery. At the 2-year follow-up, only 7% of patients reported symptom relief, with consistent generalized deterioration occurring over time. These authors concluded that arthroscopic labral debridement is not an effective long-term solution for labral tears and postulated that the underlying instability of the shoulder that led to labral injury in these overhead athletes must be addressed to effectively return function and symptomatic relief to the patient over the long term.

Labral Detachment

In addition to the tearing that can occur in the labrum, actual detachment of the labrum from the glenoid rim has been reported. The two most common labral detachments encountered clinically are the Bankart lesion and the SLAP lesion. Perthes[75] in 1906 was the first to describe the presence of a detachment of the anterior labrum in patients with recurrent anterior instability. Bankart[76,77] initially described a method for surgically repairing this lesion that now bears his name.

A Bankart lesion, which is found in as many as 85% of dislocations,[78] is described as a labral detachment that occurs at between 2 o'clock and 6 o'clock on a right shoulder, and between the 6 and 10 o'clock positions on a left shoulder. This anterior-inferior detachment decreases glenohumeral joint stability by interrupting the continuity of the glenoid labrum and compromising the glenohumeral capsular ligaments.[67] Detachment of the anterior-inferior glenoid labrum creates increases in anterior and inferior humeral head translation—a pattern commonly seen in patients with glenohumeral joint instability.[67]

In addition to labral detachment in the anterior-inferior aspect of the glenohumeral joint, similar labral detachment can occur in the superior aspect of the labrum. SLAP lesions are defined as superior labrum anterior posterior. Snyder et al[79] classified superior labral injuries into four main types (Figure 10-14). Type I shows labral degenerative changes and fraying at the edges, but no distinct avulsion. Type II, the most commonly reported superior labral injuries,[69] have been described as complete labral detachment from the anterosuperior to the posterosuperior glenoid rim with instability of the biceps long head tendon noted. Morgan et al[69] have further subclassified the type II superior labral lesion into type II anterior, type II posterior, and type II anterior and posterior. Of significance is the increased (three times greater) likelihood of type II posterior SLAP lesions in throwing athletes, as well as the finding of the Jobe subluxation/relocation test as the most accurate and valuable test for identifying the type II posterior lesion.[69] Type II anterior SLAP lesions are most commonly

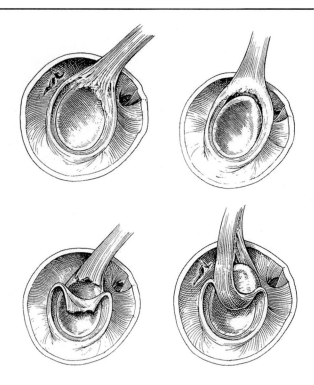

Figure 10-14 Superior labral tear classification. (From Snyder SJ: Karzel RP, Del Pizzo W, et al: SLAP lesions of the shoulder, Arthroscopy 6:274-279, 1990.)

associated with trauma and are less likely to be found in overhead athletes. A type III labral injury involves the displacement of the free margin of the labrum into the joint in a bucket-handle–type fashion, with no instability of the biceps long head tendon noted. A type IV labral lesion is similar to a type III lesion with a bucket-handle displacement of the glenoid labrum; however, in contrast, a type IV lesion involves a partial rupture in the direction of its fibers of the biceps long head tendon.[79]

One of the consequences of a superior labral injury is the involvement of the biceps long head tendon and the biceps anchor in the superior aspect of the glenoid. This compromise of the integrity of the superior labrum and loss of the biceps anchor lead to significant losses in the static stability of the human shoulder.[80] Cheng and Karzel[80] demonstrated the important role the superior labrum and biceps anchor play in glenohumeral joint stability by experimentally creating a SLAP lesion at between 10 and 2 o'clock positions. They found an 11% to 19% decrease in the ability of the glenohumeral joint to withstand rotational force, as well as a 100% to 120% increase in strain on the anterior band of the inferior glenohumeral ligament. This demonstrates a significant increase in the load on the capsular ligaments in the presence of superior labral injury.

One final area of discussion before the actual clinical tests used to evaluate glenoid labral injury are described is the proposed mechanism of injury for superior labral injury. This is particularly relevant as it will help the clinician to understand the positions used and maneuvers recommended to test for superior labral injury. Andrews and Gillogly[81] first described labral injuries in throwers and postulated tensile failure at the biceps insertion as the primary mechanism of failure. The Andrews theory was based on the important role the biceps plays in decelerating the extending elbow during the follow-through phase of pitching, coupled with the large distractional forces present during this violent phase of the throwing motion. Recent hypotheses have been developed based on the finding by Morgan et al[69] of a more commonly located posterior type II SLAP lesion in the throwing or overhead athlete. This posteriorly based lesion can best be explained by the "peel back mechanism" as described by Burkhart and Morgan (Figure 10-15).[82] The torsional force created when the abducted arm is brought into external rotation is thought to "peel back" the biceps and posterior labrum. Several of the tests discussed in this chapter that are used to identify the patient with a superior labral injury utilize the position of abduction. External rotation similar to this position is described by Burkhart and Morgan[82] for the peel back mechanism. Kuhn et al[83] compared load versus failure of the superior labrum after repair was performed cadaverically using both distractional and peel back simulation models in the throwing motion. They found significantly lower load to failure for the peel back pathomechanical model than is seen with distraction, indicating the vulnerability of the superior labrum and of subsequent labral repair to this type of loading.

Tests given to assess the glenoid labrum can be general or location specific. Many general labral tests such as the clunk test, circumduction test, compression rotation, and crank test utilize a long axis compression exerted via the humerus to scour the glenoid and to attempt to trap the torn or detached labral fragment between the humeral head and the glenoid, much like a mortar and pestal type mechanism.[81,84-86] Other tests that specifically utilize muscular tension exerted in the bicep long head to tension the superior labrum are specifically designed to identify superior labral injury. These tests include the O'Brien Active Compression test, the Mimori test, the biceps load test, and the external rotation supination test, which specifically mimics the peel back mechanism.[84,87,88] Diagnostic data from clinical labral maneuvers and tests and particularly show the variability in reported research for each of these tests. Of particular importance is the difficulty involved when independent researchers report psychometric indices comparable to those reported in the literature by the originator of each test. One important variable in the interpretation of these tests for clinical application is the ability of virtually any examiner to reproduce the exceptional diagnostic accuracy reported in these tests.

Pandya et al[89] and Hegedus et al[90] provide recent reviews of the diagnostic accuracy of clinical labral tests. Each of these studies ultimately compared the effectiveness of the clinical examination maneuver versus findings obtained at arthroscopic surgery or with magnetic resonance imaging (MRI). Noncontrast MRI has been reported in previous studies to have shown sensitivities ranging from 42% to 98% and specificity of 71% for the diagnosis of SLAP lesions.[91] Improved diagnostic accuracy has been reported with the use of contrast MRI or an MRI arthrogram with sensitivities ranging between 67% and 92% and specificities of 42% to 91%.[92] Further research will assist the clinician in the utilization of clusters of labral tests to obtain the most efficient and effective evaluation of the glenoid labrum.

PATHOPHYSIOLOGY OF ROTATOR CUFF INJURY

For many clinicians, the main understanding of the mechanism underlying rotator cuff disease is the impingement progression outlined by Neer.[93,94] Although this concept has greatly influenced treatment philosophies and surgical management of patients with rotator cuff injury, several other important mechanisms of rotator cuff injury have been proposed and tested. Understanding how each of these injury mechanisms affects the rotator cuff can lead to a more complete and global understanding of rotator cuff injury and can facilitate the development of evidence-based strategies to treat this important injury. Box 10-1 lists the main etiologic factors discussed in this chapter

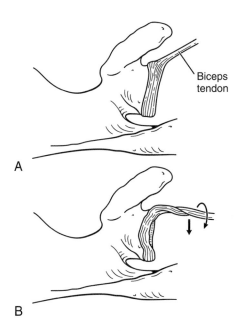

A

B

Figure 10-15 Peel back mechanism for superior labral injury. (From Burkhart SS, Morgan CD, Kibler WB: The disabled throwing shoulder: Spectrum of pathology, Part I: pathoanatomy and biomechanics. Arthroscopy 19:404-20, 2003.)

Biceps tendon

BOX 10-1	Etiologic Factors: Rotator Cuff Injury

- Primary impingement
- Secondary impingement
- Tensile overload
- Macrotraumatic tendon failure
- Undersurface impingement

for rotator cuff injury before the section on nonoperative treatment for rotator cuff injury is presented.

Primary Compressive Disease (Primary Impingement)

Primary compressive disease or impingement is a direct result of compression of the rotator cuff tendons between the humeral head and the overlying anterior third of the acromion, coracoacromial ligament, coracoid, or acromioclavicular joint.[93,94] The physiologic space between the inferior acromion and the superior surface of the rotator cuff tendons is termed the *subacromial space*. It has been measured with the use of anteroposterior radiographs and was found to be 7 to 13 mm in patients with shoulder pain[95] and 6 to 14 mm in those with normal shoulders.[96]

Biomechanical analysis of the shoulder has produced theoretical estimates of the compressive forces against the acromion with elevation of the shoulder. Poppen and Walker[97] calculated this force at 0.42 times body weight. Peak forces against the acromion were measured at between 85 and 136 degrees of elevation.[98] The positions of the shoulder in forward flexion, horizontal adduction, and internal rotation during the acceleration and follow-through phases of the throwing motion are likely to produce subacromial impingement due to abrasion of the supraspinatus, infraspinatus, or biceps tendon.[72] These data provide a scientific rationale for the concept of impingement or compressive disease as a cause of rotator cuff pathology.

Neer[93,94] outlined three stages of primary impingement as it relates to rotator cuff pathology. Stage I, *edema and hemorrhage*, results from mechanical irritation of the tendon by the impingement incurred with overhead activity. This is characteristically observed in younger patients who are athletic and is described as a reversible condition with conservative physical therapy. The primary symptoms and physical signs of this stage of impingement or compressive disease are similar to those of the other two stages and consist of a positive impingement sign, a painful arc of movement, and varying degrees of muscular weakness.

The second stage of compressive disease outlined by Neer is termed *fibrosis and tendonitis*. This occurs from repeated episodes of mechanical inflammation and may include thickening or fibrosis of the subacromial bursae. The typical age range for this stage of injury is 25 to 40 years. Neer's stage III impingement lesion, termed *bone spurs and tendon rupture*, is the result of continued mechanical compression of the rotator cuff tendons. Full-thickness tears of the rotator cuff, partial-thickness tears of the rotator cuff, biceps tendon lesions, and bony alterations of the acromion and the acromioclavicular joint may be associated with this stage. In addition to bony alterations that are acquired with repetitive stress to the shoulder, the native shape of the acromion is of relevance.

The specific shape of the overlying acromion process, termed *acromial architecture*, has been studied in relation to full-thickness tears of the rotator cuff. Bigliani et al[99] described three types of acromions: type I (flat), type II (curved), and type III (hooked). A type III or hooked acromion was found in 70% of cadaveric shoulders with a full-thickness rotator cuff tear, and type I acromions were associated with only 3%.[99] In a series of 200 clinically evaluated patients, 80% with a positive arthrogram had a type III acromion.[100]

Secondary Compressive Disease (Secondary Impingement)

Impingement or compressive symptoms may result from underlying instability of the glenohumeral joint.[101,102] Attenuation of static stabilizers of the glenohumeral joint, such as the capsular ligaments and the labrum from excessive demands incurred with throwing or overhead activities, can lead to anterior instability of the glenohumeral joint. Because of increased humeral head translation, the biceps tendon and the rotator cuff can become impinged as the result of the ensuing instability.[101,102] A progressive loss of glenohumeral joint stability is created when the dynamic stabilizing functions of the rotator cuff are diminished through fatigue and tendon injury.[102] The effects of secondary impingement can lead to rotator cuff tears as instability and impingement continue.[101,102]

Tensile Overload

Another etiologic factor in rotator cuff pathology is repetitive intrinsic tension overload. The heavy, repetitive eccentric forces incurred by the posterior rotator cuff musculature during the deceleration and follow-through phases of overhead sport activities can lead to overload failure of the tendon.[102,103] The pathologic changes referred to by Nirschl as *angiofibroblastic hyperplasia* occur in the early stages of tendon injury and can progress to rotator cuff tears caused by continued tensile overload.[102,103]

Recent research conducted by Kraushaar and Nirschl[104] in a histologic study of the extensor carpi radialis brevis, the primary tendon involved in lateral humeral epicondylitis, has identified specific characteristics inherent in the injured tendon. Based on their histopathologic study, these investigators recommended that the term *tendinosus* rather than *tendonitis* should be used to more accurately describe tendon injury. Histopathologic study reveals that tendons taken from areas of chronic overuse in the human body do not contain large numbers of macrophages, lymphocytes, or neutrophils. "Rather, tendonosis appears to be a degenerative process that is characterized by the presence of dense populations of fibroblasts, vascular hyperplasia, and disorganized collagen."[104] Kraushaar and Nirschl point out that it is unknown why tendinosus is painful, given the absence of acute inflammatory cells, nor is it known why the collagen fails to mature.

Tensile stresses incurred by the rotator cuff during the arm deceleration phase of the throwing motion to resist joint distraction, horizontal adduction, and internal rotation are reported to be as high as 1090 N with biomechanical study of highly skilled pitchers.[72] The presence of acquired or congenital capsular laxity, as well as labral insufficiency, can greatly increase tensile stresses to the rotator cuff muscle tendon units.[101,102]

Macrotraumatic Tendon Failure

Unlike the previously mentioned rotator cuff classifications, cases involving macrotraumatic tendon failure usually entail a previous or single traumatic event in the clinical history.[102] Forces encountered during the traumatic event are greater than the normal tendon can tolerate. Full-thickness tears of the rotator cuff with bony avulsions of the greater tuberosity can result from single traumatic episodes. According to Cofield,[105] normal tendons do not tear, as 30% or more of the tendon must be damaged to produce a substantial reduction in strength. Although a single traumatic event that resulted in tendon failure is often reported by the patient in the subjective examination, repeated microtraumatic insults and degeneration over time may have created a substantially weakened tendon that ultimately failed under the heavy load involved in the specific event described by the patient. Full-thickness rotator cuff tears require surgical treatment and aggressive rehabilitation to achieve a positive functional outcome.[61,94] Further specifics of rotator cuff surgical treatment are discussed later in this chapter.

Posterior, Undersurface, or Internal Impingement

One additional cause of the undersurface tear of the rotator cuff in the young athletic shoulder is termed *posterior, inside* or *internal*, or *undersurface impingement*.[106,107] This phenomenon was originally identified by Walch[107] during shoulder arthroscopy with the shoulder placed in the 90/90 position. Placement of the shoulder in a position of 90 degrees of abduction and 90 degrees of external rotation causes the supraspinatus and infraspinatus tendons to rotate posteriorly. This more posterior orientation of the tendons aligns them such that the undersurface of the tendons rubs on the posterior-superior glenoid lip, and becomes pinched or compressed between the humeral head and the posterosuperior glenoid rim.[107] Individuals who present with posterior shoulder pain brought on by positioning of the arm in 90 degrees of abduction and 90 degrees or more of external rotation, typically from overhead positions in sport or industrial situations, may be considered as potential candidates for undersurface impingement.

Anterior translation of the humeral head with maximal external rotation and 90 degrees of abduction, which has been confirmed arthroscopically during the subluxation/relocation test, can produce mechanical rubbing and fraying on the undersurface of the rotator cuff tendons. Additional harm can be caused by the posterior deltoid if the rotator cuff is not functioning properly. The posterior deltoid's angle of pull pushes the humeral head against the glenoid, accentuating the skeletal, tendinous, and labral lesions.[106] Walch et al[107] arthroscopically evaluated 17 throwing athletes with shoulder pain during throwing and found undersurface impingement that resulted in 8 partial-thickness rotator cuff tears and 12 lesions in the posterosuperior labrum. Impingement of the undersurface of the rotator cuff on the posterosuperior glenoid labrum may be a cause of painful structural disease in the overhead athlete.

Additional research confirming the concept of posterior or undersurface impingement in the overhead athlete has been published. Halbrecht et al[108] confirmed, via MRI performed in the position of 90 degrees of abduction and 90 degrees of external rotation, contact of the undersurface of the supraspinatus tendon against the posterior-superior glenoid in baseball pitchers with arm placed in 90 degrees of external rotation and 90 degrees of abduction. Ten collegiate baseball pitchers were examined, and in all 10 pitchers, physical contact was encountered in this position. Paley et al[109] also published a series on arthroscopic evaluation of the dominant shoulder of 41 professional throwing athletes. With the arthroscope inserted into the glenohumeral joint, they found that 41 of 41 dominant shoulders evaluated had posterior undersurface impingement between the rotator cuff and the posterior superior glenoid. Among these professional throwing athletes, 93% had undersurface fraying of the rotator cuff tendons, and 88% showed fraying of the posterosuperior glenoid.

NONOPERATIVE REHABILITATION GUIDELINES FOR ROTATOR CUFF PATHOLOGY

The information discussed in this chapter, including anatomical and biomechanical concepts, evaluation methods, and the pathophysiology of rotator cuff injury, can be integrated to develop an effective treatment program for the patient with shoulder dysfunction. The application of specific treatment progressions is based on these principles and is discussed here.

Although complete discussion of the complex and comprehensive evaluation methods used specifically is beyond the scope of this chapter, a detailed and systematic approach to shoulder and upper extremity evaluation must be undertaken to identify the specific type of rotator cuff pathology involved and to identify specifically the often subtle underlying cause or causes. Additionally, in all types of rotator cuff pathology listed in the previous section, scapular dysfunction can be the underlying cause or can greatly exacerbate the disease or injury process, with altered scapular kinematics measured in patients with both rotator cuff instability and impingement.[21,110,111] Initial rehabilitation begins with protection of the rotator cuff from stress but not function.

Protection of the rotator cuff against mechanical compression by the overlying coracoacromial arch or the posterior glenoid must be undertaken by modifying ergonomic, sport-specific, and activities of daily living (ADL) postures and movement patterns. Modalities such as electrical stimulation, ultrasound, and iontophoresis can be applied to promote improved blood supply and to decrease pain levels; however, present research is lacking regarding the identification of a clearly superior modality or sequence of modalities for the early management of tendon pathology in the human shoulder. One study highlights the importance of early submaximal exercise in increasing local blood flow. Jensen et al[112] studied the effects of submaximal (5% to 50% maximal voluntary contraction [MVC]) contractions in the supraspinatus tendon measured with laser Doppler flowmetry. Results showed that even submaximal contractions increased perfusion during all 1-minute contractions but produced a postcontraction latent hyperemia following the muscular contraction. These findings have provided a rationale for the early use of internal and external rotation isometrics or submaximal manual resistance in the scapular plane with low levels of elevation to prevent any subacromial contact early in the rehabilitation process.

A key component of the early management of rotator cuff pathology is scapular stabilization. Manual techniques are recommended to directly interface the clinician with the patient's scapula, to bypass the glenohumeral joint and allow for repetitive scapular exercise without undue stress to the rotator cuff in the early phase. Figure 10-16 shows the specific technique used by this author to manually resist scapular retraction. Solem-Bertoft et al[113] have shown the importance of scapular retraction posturing with reports of a reduction in the width of the subacromial space when scapular protraction posturing was compared with scapular retraction. Activation of the serratus anterior and lower trapezius force couple is imperative to enable scapular upward rotation and stabilization during arm elevation.[8] Rhythmic stabilization applied to the proximal aspect of the extremity, progressing to distal with the glenohumeral joint in 80 to 90 degrees of elevation in the scapular plane, can be initiated to provide muscular co-contraction in a functional position. Additionally, with this technique, a protracted scapular position can be utilized to enhance the activation of the serratus anterior,[114,115] because several studies have identified decreased muscular activation of this muscle in patients given a diagnosis of glenohumeral impingement and instability.[111,116]

In addition to the early scapular stabilization and submaximal rotator cuff exercise, ROM and mobilization may be indicated according to the underlying mobility status of the patient. Use of examination procedures to assess anterior and posterior humeral head translation, as discussed earlier in this chapter, and to determine the accessory mobility of the glenohumeral joint is of critical importance in guiding this portion of the treatment. Patients with secondary rotator cuff impingement and tensile overload injury due to underlying instability should not undergo accessory mobilization techniques to increase mobility, as this would only compound their existing capsular laxity. However, patients who present with primary impingement often present with underlying capsular hypomobility and are definite candidates for specific mobilization techniques performed to improve glenohumeral joint arthrokinematics. One specific area that has received a great deal of attention in the scientific literature is the presence of internal rotation ROM limitation, particularly in the overhead athlete with rotator cuff dysfunction.[7,39] To determine the optimal course of treatment for the patient with limited internal rotation ROM, clinical assessment strategies must be employed, to identify whether the limitation and the subsequent treatment strategy selected to address the limitation in glenohumeral joint internal rotation should be targeted for the muscle tendon unit, or the posterior capsule.

To determine tightness of the posterior glenohumeral joint capsule, an accessory mobility technique is recommended to assess the mobility of the humeral head relative to the glenoid. This technique most often is referred to as the *posterior load and shift* or the *posterior drawer test*.[56,63] Figure 10-12 shows the recommended technique for this examination maneuver whereby the glenohumeral joint is abducted 90 degrees in the scapular plane (note the position of the humerus 30 degrees anterior to the coronal plane). The examiner is careful to utilize a posterior-lateral directed force along the line of the glenohumeral joint. The examiner then feels for translation of the humeral head along the glenoid face. Patients who present with a limitation in internal rotation ROM who have grade II translation should not have posterior glide accessory techniques applied to increase internal rotation ROM because of the hypermobility of the posterior capsule made evident during this important passive clinical test.

It should be pointed out that incorrect use of this posterior glide assessment technique may lead to the false identification of posterior capsular tightness. A common error in this examination technique is the use of the coronal plane for testing, as well as the use of a straight posterior directed force by the examiner's hand, rather than the recommended posterior-lateral force. The straight posterior force compresses the humeral head into the glenoid, because of the anteverted position of the glenoid, and this would inaccurately lead to the assumption by the examining clinician that limited posterior capsular mobility is present.

The second important test used to determine the presence of internal rotation ROM limitation is the assessment of physiologic ROM. Several authors recommend measurement of glenohumeral internal rotation with the joint in 90 degrees of abduction in the coronal plane.[117-119] Care must be taken to stabilize the scapula with measurement taking place with the

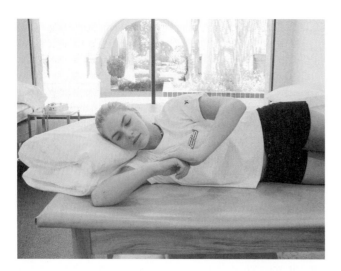

Figure 10-16 Manual scapular retraction exercise in sidelying.

patient in the supine position so that the patient's body weight can minimize scapular motion. In addition, a posteriorly directed force is used by the examiner on the anterior aspect of the coracoid and shoulder during internal rotation ROM measurement (see Figure 10-9). Internal rotation ROM is compared bilaterally with careful interpretation of isolated glenohumeral motion.

One common finding present during the examination of the overhead athlete is the rather consistent finding of increased dominant arm external rotation and reduced dominant arm glenohumeral joint internal rotation.[39,119-121] As mentioned earlier in this chapter, Ellenbecker et al[35] identified that this consistent relationship could occur only in a condition where glenohumeral joint rotation was measured with the scapula stabilized. Several proposed mechanisms have been discussed to attempt to explain this glenohumeral ROM relationship of increased external rotation and limited internal rotation.[39,122,123] Tightness of the posterior capsule, tightness of the muscle tendon unit of the posterior rotator cuff, and humeral retroversion all have been described as structures that limit internal glenohumeral joint rotation. Crockett et al[122] and others[124-126] have shown unilateral increases in humeral retroversion in throwing athletes, which would explain the increase in external rotation noted with accompanying internal rotation loss. Recent research by Reinold et al[127] demonstrated the acute effects of pitching on glenohumeral ROM. Sixty-seven professional baseball pitchers were measured for glenohumeral joint rotational ROM with the use of scapular stabilization before and immediately after 50 to 60 pitches at full intensity. Results show a loss of 9.5 degrees of internal rotation and 10.7 degrees of total rotation ROM during this short-term response to overhead throwing. This study shows significant decreases in internal rotation and total rotation ROM of the dominant glenohumeral joint in professional pitchers following an acute episode of throwing. Reinold et al[127] suggest that muscle tendinous adaptations from eccentric loading likely are implicated in this ROM adaptation following throwing. This musculotendinous adaptation occurs in addition to the osseous and capsular mechanisms previously reported.[127]

Careful measurement of glenohumeral rotational measurement using the total rotation concept outlined earlier in this chapter guides the progression of either physiologic ROM and light stretching used in rehabilitation or the inclusion of specific mobilization techniques used to address capsular deficiencies. The total rotation ROM concept can be used as illustrated to guide the clinician during rehabilitation, specifically in the area of application of stretching and mobilization, to best determine what glenohumeral joint requires additional mobility and which extremity should not have additional mobility, because of the obvious harm induced by increases in capsular mobility and increases in humeral head translation during aggressive upper extremity exertion. This extensive section outlining the importance of accurate ROM measurement and clinical decision making based on the latest scientific evidence can guide the clinician through the rehabilitation process, since a large spectrum of mobility can be encountered when one is treating the patient with glenohumeral impingement. To

further illustrate the role of ROM and passive stretching during this phase of the rehabilitation, Figures 10-17 and 10-18 show versions of clinical internal rotation stretching positions that utilize the scapular plane, and that can be performed in multiple and varied positions of glenohumeral abduction. Each inherently possesses an anterior hand placement used to give varying degrees of posterior pressure to minimize scapular compensation, and also to provide a checkrein against anterior humeral head translation during the internal rotation stretch because of the effects of obligate translation. These stretches can be used in a proprioceptive neuromuscular facilitation (PNF) contract-relax format of following a low-load prolonged stretch-type paradigm to facilitate the increase in ROM.[128,129] Additionally, Figures 10-19 and 10-20 are examples of home stretches given to patients to address internal

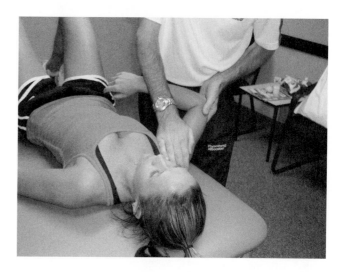

Figure 10-17 "Figure 4" stretch position used to increase internal rotation ROM. The forearm is used to obtain overpressure, while the examiner's hand limits anterior humeral head translation by exerting a posteriorly directed force.

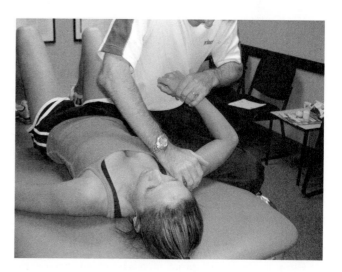

Figure 10-18 Internal rotation stretch position to allow for stabilization of the scapula and limitation of obligate anterior humeral head translation during the stretch.

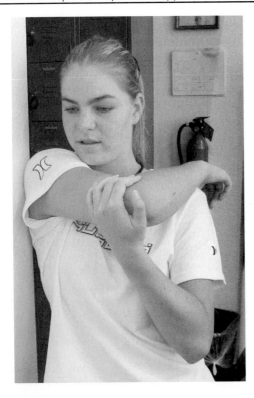

Figure 10-19 Cross-arm adduction stretch.

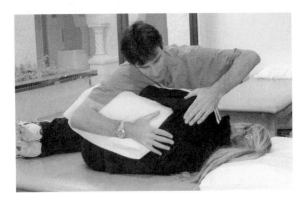

Figure 10-20 Sleeper stretch performed in sidelying position.

rotation ROM deficiency. Note the inherent means of scapular stabilization in both methods, which are necessary to optimize the value of the stretching procedure. Recent research[130] has compared the effects of the cross-arm stretch vs. the sleeper stretch in a population of recreational athletes, some with significant glenohumeral internal rotation ROM deficiency. Four weeks of stretching produced significantly greater internal rotation gains in the group performing the cross-body stretch as compared with the sleeper stretch. Further research is clearly needed to better define the optimal application of these stretches; however, studies have shown improvement in internal rotation ROM with a home stretching program.[130]

Goals in the initial phase of rehabilitation include the following:

1. Decrease in pain to allow for initiation of submaximal rotator cuff and scapular exercise

2. Normalization of capsular relationships through the use of specific mobilization and stretching techniques
3. Early submaximal rotator cuff and scapular resistance training

Total Arm Strengthening/Kinetic Chain Exercise Application

This phase is dominated by strength and local muscle endurance training of the rotator cuff and scapular stabilizers. Although the entire kinetic chain, including the lower extremity, pelvis, and trunk segments, are also critically important, it is beyond the scope of this chapter to completely list the broad scope of all kinetic chain exercises indicated. However, this section of the chapter reviews the use of an evidence-based progression of a resistive exercise program. The primary goals are to elicit high levels of rotator cuff and scapular muscular activation using movement patterns and positions that do not create subacromial contact, or undue stress to the static stabilizers of the glenohumeral joint. Figure 10-21 shows the progression used by this author for rotator cuff strengthening. These exercises are based on electromyographic (EMG) research showing high levels of posterior rotator cuff activation,[131-135] and they place the shoulder in positions well tolerated by patients with rotator cuff and scapular dysfunction. Sidelying external rotation and prone extension with an externally rotated (thumb out) position are utilized first, with progressions to prone horizontal abduction and prone external rotation with scapular retraction following a demonstrated tolerance to the initial two exercises. Prone horizontal abduction is used at 90 degrees of abduction to minimize the effects resulting from subacromial contact.[98] Research has shown that this position creates high levels of supraspinatus muscular activation,[132,133,135] making it an alterative to the widely used empty can exercise, which often can cause impingement through the combined inherent movements of internal rotation and elevation. Three sets of 15 to 20 repetitions are recommended to create a fatigue response and improve local muscular endurance.[136,137] The efficacy of these exercises in a 4-week training paradigm has been demonstrated, and 8% to 10% increases have been noted in isokinetically measured internal and external rotation strength in healthy subjects. These isotonic exercises are coupled with an external rotation oscillation exercise (Figure 10-22), which uses 30 second sets and elastic resistance to provide a resistance bias to the posterior rotator cuff during this phase of the rehabilitation process.

All exercises for external rotation strengthening in standing are performed with the addition of a small towel roll placed in the axilla as pictured (see Figure 10-22). In addition to assisting in isolation of the exercise and controlling unwanted movements, this towel roll application has been shown to elevate muscular activity by 10% in the infraspinatus muscle when compared with identical exercises performed without towel placement.[133] Another theoretical advantage of the use of a towel roll to place the shoulder in approximately 20 to 30 degrees of abduction is that it prevents the "wringing out" phenomena proposed in cadaverically based microvascularity

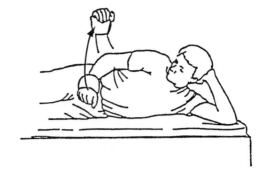

1. Side-lying external rotation:
Lie on uninvolved side, with involved arm
at side, with a small pillow between arm
and body. Keeping elbow of involved arm bent
and fixed to side, raise arm into external
rotation. Slowly lower to starting position
and repeat.

2. Shoulder extension:
Lie on table on stomach, with involved arm
hanging straight to the floor. With thumb
pointed outward, raise arm straight back into
extension toward your hip. Slowly lower
arm and repeat.

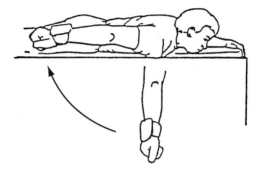

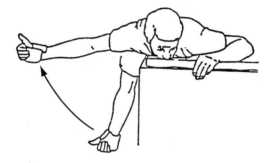

3. Prone horizontal abduction:
Lie on table on stomach, with involved arm
hanging straight to the floor. With thumb
pointed outward, raise arm out to the side,
parallel to the floor. Slowly lower arm,
and repeat.

4. 90/90 external rotation:
Lie on table on stomach, with shoulder
abducted to 90 degrees and arm supported
on table, with elbow bent at 90 degrees.
Keeping the shoulder and elbow fixed,
rotate arm into external rotation, slowly
lower to start position, and repeat.

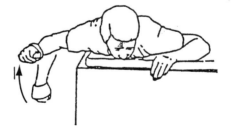

Figure 10-21 Isotonic rotator cuff strengthening program. (From Ellenbecker T: Shoulder rehabilitation: non-operative treatment, New York, 2007, Thieme.)

research. Rathburn and McNab[138] showed enhanced blood flow in the supraspinatus tendon when the arm was placed in slight abduction as compared with complete adduction. Finally, another research study has further supported the use of a towel roll or pillow between the humerus and the torso under the axilla during a humeral rotational training exercise. Graichen et al[139] studied 12 healthy shoulders using MRI at 30, 60, 90, 120, and 150 degrees of abduction. A 15 Newton force was performed, which resulted in an abduction isometric contrac-

tion or an adduction isometric contraction. Adduction isometric muscle contraction produced a significant opening or increase in the subacromial space in all positions of glenohumeral joint abduction. No change in scapular tilting or scapulohumeral rhythm was encountered during abduction or adduction isometric contractions. Results from this research can be applied for the patient with impingement during humeral rotation exercise. Use of the towel roll can facilitate an adduction isometric contraction in patients who may need

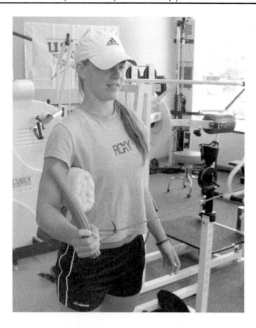

Figure 10-22 External oscillation exercise.

enhanced subacromial intervals during the humeral rotation exercise.[139]

Recent research has provided guidance regarding the use of resistive exercise in shoulder rehabilitation[140] and has measured EMG activity of the infraspinatus and middle and posterior deltoid during external rotation exercise in healthy subjects. Muscular activity was monitored during external rotation exercise at 10%, 40%, and 70% activation levels (percentage of maximal). This important study found increased relative infraspinatus activity when the resistive exercise level was at 40% of maximal effort, indicating more focused activity from the infraspinatus and less compensatory activation of the deltoid. This study confirms the use of lower-intensity strengthening exercise to optimize activation from the rotator cuff and to de-emphasize input from the deltoid and other prime movers, which often occurs with higher-intensity resistive loading.

Scapular stabilization exercises are progressed to include external rotation with retraction (Figure 10-23), an exercise shown to recruit the lower trapezius at a rate 3.3 times greater than the upper trapezius, and to utilize the important position of scapular retraction.[141] Multiple seated rowing variations, continued manual scapular protraction/retraction resistance exercise (see Figure 10-16), and the 90 degree abducted external rotation exercise in prone (see Figure 10-21, *D*) are used to facilitate the lower trapezius and other scapular stabilizers during this stage of the rehabilitation.[131,133,142]

Closed-chain exercise using the "plus" position, which is characterized by maximal scapular protraction, has been recommended by Moesley et al[143] and Decker et al[115] for its inherent maximal serratus anterior recruitment. Closed-chain step-ups (Figure 10-24), quadruped position rhythmic stabilization, and variations of the pointer position (unilateral arm and ipsilateral leg extension weight bearing) all are used in endurance-oriented formats (timed sets of 30 seconds or more) to enhance scapular stabilization.[144] Uhl et al[145] have demonstrated the

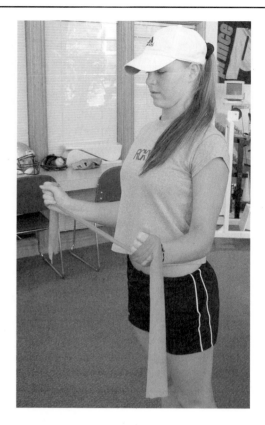

Figure 10-23 External rotation with scapular retraction exercise with elastic resistance.

effects of increased weight bearing and of successive decreases in the number of weight-bearing limbs on muscle activation of the rotator cuff and scapular musculature, and have provided guidance regarding closed-chain exercise progression in the upper extremity.

Progression to the functional position of 90 degrees of abduction in the scapular plane to simulate the throwing and overhead patterning inherent in many sport activities, such as serving in tennis and volleyball, and daily functions is based on tolerance of the initial rotator cuff and scapular exercise progression as listed earlier in this chapter. Basset et al[146] have shown the importance of training the muscle in the position of function based on the change in muscular lever arms and subsequent function in the 90/90 position. Rhythmic stabilization (i.e., pertubations applied to the proximal and distal aspects of the upper extremity) against a therapy ball (Figure 10-25) is one example of an early abducted exercise performed with therapist guidance. The scapular plane position is chosen as an optimal position for this exercise and other exercises in lower planes of elevation in the earlier phase of rehabilitation, as well with humeral elevation to 90 degrees during this phase, for several important reasons. The inherent optimal bony congruency between the humeral head and the glenoid,[1] as well as the mathematically derived research finding that the rotator cuff is best able to maintain glenohumeral stability with the glenohumeral joint positioned 29.3 degrees anterior to the coronal plane of the body, makes the scapular plane position an optimal position for rehabilitative exercise.[147]

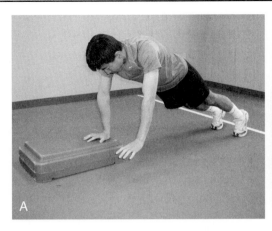
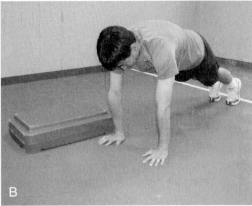

Figure 10-24 Closed-chain step-up exercise with emphasis on scapular protraction phase of the exercise.

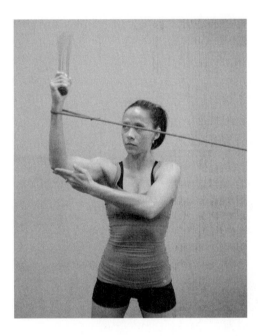

Figure 10-25 Statue of Liberty oscillation exercise with elastic resistance providing additional resistance bias to the posterior rotator cuff.

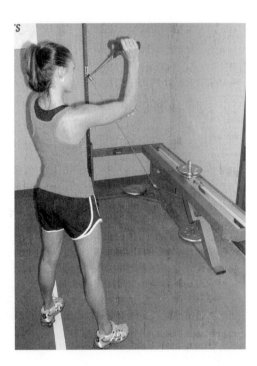

Figure 10-26 Impulse trainer (source) for the provision of eccentric training of the posterior rotator cuff in the 90 degree elevated position in the scapular plane.

Additional applications of the 90/90 position include the external oscillation or "statue of liberty" exercise (see Figure 10-25) and use of the impulse inertial exercise trainer (Impulse Training Systems; Newnan, Georgia) (Figure 10-26) to provide external rotation eccentric overload training in a position of 90 degrees of elevation in the scapular plane and 90 degrees of external rotation, simulating the functional position used during serving in tennis[148] or throwing in baseball.[72] The importance of external rotation fatigue resistance training has ramifications for the proper biomechanical function of the entire upper extremity kinetic chain. Tsai et al[149] demonstrated significant scapular positional changes during the early and middle phases of arm elevation, specifically, decreases in posterior scapular tilting and scapular external rotation following fatigue of the glenohumeral external rotators. In a similar study, Ebaugh et al[150] used an external rotation fatigue protocol to fatigue the posterior rotator cuff. Following fatigue of the

external rotators, this study found less posterior tilting during subsequent arm elevation, indicating scapular compensations and abnormal movement patterns resulting from rotator cuff fatigue. These studies provide an evidence-based rationale for the significant use of external rotation–based training for the patient with shoulder dysfunction.

As the patient tolerates isotonic exercise with 2 to 3 pounds and also can perform rotational training without pain using elastic resistance, isokinetic rotational exercise is initiated in the modified base position. This position places the glenohumeral joint in 30 degrees of flexion and 30 degrees of abduction, and it uses a 30 degree tilt of the dynamometer relative to the horizontal Figure 10-16.[151,152] This position is well tolerated and allows the patient to progress from submaximal to more maximal levels of resistance at velocities ranging between 120 and 210 degrees per second for nonathletic patient populations, and between 210 and 360 degrees per second during later stages of rehabilitation in more athletic patients. Use of the isokinetic dynamometer is also important to quantify objectively muscular strength levels and most critically muscular balance between the internal and external rotators.[151,152] Achieving a level of internal and external rotation strength equal to that of the contralateral extremity is an acceptable initial goal for many patients; however, unilateral increases in internal rotation strength of 15% to 30% have been reported in many descriptive studies of overhead athletes[153-156]; thus greater rehabilitative emphasis may be required to achieve this level of documented "dominance."

A predominance of internal/external rotation patterning is used during isokinetic training. This internal/external rotation focus is based on an isokinetic training study by Quincy et al,[157] who showed that internal/external rotation training for a period of 6 weeks not only can produce statistically significant gains in internal and external rotation strength, but can improve shoulder extension/flexion and abduction/adduction strength as well. Training in the patterns of flexion/extension and abduction/adduction over the same 6 weeks produces only strength gains specific to the direction of training. This overflow of training allows for a more time-efficient and effective focus in the clinic during isokinetic training.

Muscular balance indicated by the external/internal rotation ratio provides objective information for the clinician to ensure that proper balance is present between the anterior and poste-

rior dynamic stabilizers. Ratios in normal, healthy shoulders have been reported at 66%.[151,158,159] Emphasis on the development of external rotators (posterior rotator cuff) in rehabilitation for anterior instability has led to the concept of a "posterior dominant" shoulder—a shoulder that essentially has a unilateral strength ratio greater than 66% with a goal of attaining a ratio of 75% to 80%.[158] Careful monitoring of muscular strength with the use of a dynamometer allows the clinician to specifically observe and focus the rehabilitation program in such a way as to promote the return of muscular balance.

During the end stage of rotator cuff rehabilitation, individuals returning to overhead activities and sports are candidates for advanced isokinetic training using functionally specific rotational training at 90 degrees of abduction in the scapular plane (Figure 10-27), with several studies reporting increases in rotator cuff strength and functional overhead sport enhancement following 6 weeks of isokinetic training with 90 degrees of glenohumeral joint abduction.[158,160] Additionally, a plyometric exercise progression is initiated at this time in the rehabilitation progression. Several studies reported in the literature show increases in upper extremity function with plyometric exercise variations.[161-163] The functional application of the eccentric prestretch followed by a powerful concentric muscular contraction closely parallels many upper extremity sport activities and serves as an excellent exercise modality for transitioning the active patient to the interval sport return programs.

Carter et al[163] studied the effects of an 8-week training program of plyometric upper extremity exercise and external

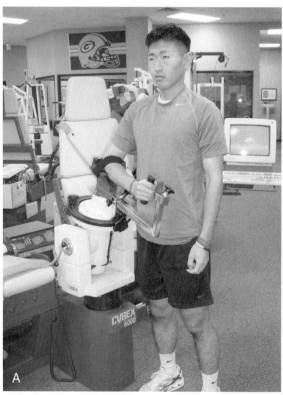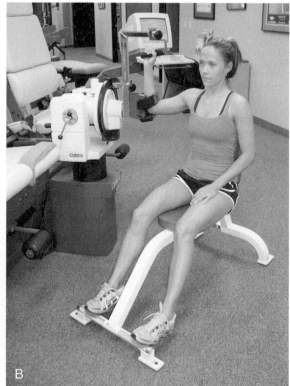

Figure 10-27 Cybex modified base position **(A)** and 90 degree abducted scapular plane position **(B)**.

rotation strengthening with elastic resistance. They found increased eccentric external rotation strength, concentric internal rotation strength, and improved throwing velocity in collegiate baseball players, thus showing the positive effects of plyometric and elastic resistance training in overhead athletes. Figure 10-28 shows a prone 90/90 plyometric that can be used with the athlete maintaining a retracted scapular position with the shoulder in 90 degrees of abduction and 90 degrees of external rotation. The plyo ball is rapidly dropped and caught over a 2 to 3 inch (3 to 6 cm) movement distance for sets of 30 to as much as 40 seconds, to address local muscular endurance.[136] Figure 10-29 shows a reverse catch plyometric exercise that is performed again with the glenohumeral joint in the 90/90 position. The ball is tossed from behind the patient to load eccentrically the posterior rotator cuff (external rotators) with a rapid concentric external rotation movement performed as the patient throws the ball back to keep the abducted position of the shoulder with 90 degrees of elbow flexion. These one-arm plyometric exercises can be preceded by two-arm catches over the shoulder to determine readiness for one-arm loading. Small (0.5 kg), 1 pound medicine balls or soft weights

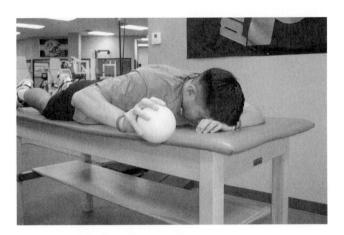

Figure 10-28 Prone 90/90 plyometric exercise.

(Thera-Band, Hygenic Corporation, Akron, OH) are used initially with progression to 1 to 1.5 kg as the patient progresses in both skill and strength development.

Ellenbecker et al[164] studied plyometric exercises (prone 90/90 plyometric and reverse catch plyometric) using surface EMG to quantify muscular activation levels during exercise. The prone 90/90 plyometric showed 85% to 102% maximum voluntary isometric control (MVIC) activity for the infraspinatus, and 118% to 131% activity for the lower trapezius, using 0.5 and 1 kg medicine balls. Activity levels in the reverse catch plyometric included 71 to 73 MVIC for the infraspinatus, and 79% to 81% MVIC for the lower trapezius. This study provides objective evidence of the degree of muscular activation in the rotator cuff and in scapular stabilizers during these recommended plyometric exercises.

A multifaceted approach is recommended for determining when the patient is ready for progression to an interval-based sport return program and ultimately to be considered for discharge from formal physical therapy. Areas for consideration include normalization of previously positive manual special tests, ROM, strength, and functional status.

The use of manual orthopaedic tests to originally diagnose the patient with rotator cuff pathology should be revisited, and ultimately they should not be used when progression to advanced activities and discharge is considered.[4] Negative traditional impingement tests (e.g., Neer's, Hawkins', and Yocum's) all compromise the subacromial space using specific prevocational movement patterns encountered during ADLs and functional activities, and can provide valuable insight into the patient's ability to tolerate these functional positions. Additionally, provocation tests such as the subluxation/relocation test[66] can be very important for determining the patient's competency and stability in the abducted, externally rotated position.

Evaluation of glenohumeral joint ROM is another important discharge parameter. A premature return of the patient to overhead throwing activity with significant external rotation ROM limitation may further compromise both shoulder func-

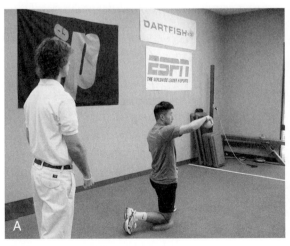
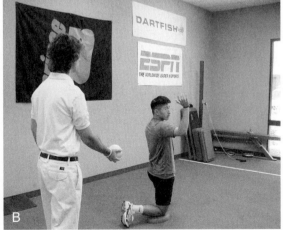

Figure 10-29 Reverse catch plyometric exercise.

tion and distal elbow loading.[165] Normalization of glenohumeral capsular relationships resulting in the restoration of optimal glenohumeral internal and external rotation ROM is of critical importance and has been described at length in this chapter.

Additionally, an evaluation of muscular strength is of critical importance in terms of discharge planning. Although an isokinetic or computerized device cannot always be available in all settings and applications, the use of even manual muscle testing to determine bilateral symmetry of key components of the deltoid rotator cuff force couple[5,166] and of scapular stabilizers[167] is warranted. In many applications, significantly greater dominant arm strength can be expected and required before the return to overhead athletic function.[154-156] The external/internal rotation unilateral strength ratio is emphasized in this author's discharge planning because of the importance of muscular balance and optimal posterior rotator cuff stabilization required for pain-free shoulder function. Ratios of 66% to 75% are targeted and can be measured by means of isokinetic or isometric dynamometry.[152]

Finally, functional indexes or rating scales are used to include the patient's perception of shoulder function in the clinical decision-making process. Research has shown that commonly used rating scales such as American Shoulder Elbow Surgeons (ASES), UCLA, and Rowe scales can be used in athletic populations and can provide valuable information regarding the perception of function.[63,168,169] The numeric nature of these scales can facilitate longitudinal comparison if they are used throughout the rehabilitation process, or comparison vs. normative levels.[168,169]

REHABILITATION FOLLOWING ARTHROSCOPIC ROTATOR CUFF REPAIR

Significant changes and advances in the surgical approach to repair a torn rotator cuff tendon or tendons have allowed accelerated rehabilitation following surgery because of decreased tissue morbidity and enhanced surgical fixation methods. A basic understanding of rotator cuff tears and some of the surgical principles of arthroscopic rotator cuff repair will facilitate the development of safe and effective postsurgical rehabilitation progressions.

One of the factors that affect the progression of resistive exercise and ROM is tear type. The degree of rotator cuff tear, partial or full thickness, and tear size are important determinants of rehabilitative progression. Several primary types of rotator cuff tears are commonly described in the literature. Full-thickness tears in the rotator cuff consist of tears that comprise the entire thickness (from top to bottom) of the rotator cuff tendon or tendons. Full-thickness tears are often initiated in the critical zone of the supraspinatus tendon and can extend to include the infraspinatus, teres minor, and subscapularis tendons.[202] Often associated with a tear in the subscapularis tendon is subluxation of the biceps long head tendon from the intertubercular groove, or partial or complete tears of the biceps tendon.

A second type of rotator cuff tear is an incomplete or partial-thickness tear. Partial-thickness tears can occur on the superior surface (bursal side) or the undersurface (articular side) of the rotator cuff. Although both bursal and articular side tears are partial-thickness tears of the rotator cuff, significant differences in etiology are proposed for each.[102]

Neer[93,94] and Fukoda et al[203] have emphasized that superior surface (bursal side) tears in the rotator cuff are the result of subacromial impingement. In the classification scheme listed earlier in this chapter, tears on the superior or bursal side of the rotator cuff are generally associated with both primary and secondary compressive disease, as well as with macrotraumatic tendon failure. Progression of mechanical irritation on the superior surface can produce a partial-thickness tear that can ultimately progress to a full-thickness tear.

Partial-thickness tears on the undersurface or the articular side of the rotator cuff generally are associated with tensile loads and glenohumeral joint instability.[102,170] Tears on the undersurface of the rotator cuff are commonly found in overhead throwing athletes, in whom anterior instability, capsular and labral insufficiency, and dynamic muscular imbalances are often reported. To further understand the differing origins of rotator cuff tears, Nakajima et al[170] performed a histologic and biomechanical study of rotator cuff tendons. Biomechanically, their results showed greater deformation and tensile strength on the bursal side of the supraspinatus tendon.

One of the factors that predicates the rate at which a patient can be rehabilitated following a rotator cuff repair is tear size.[171] Full-thickness rotator cuff tears can be classified by actual size, with small tears measuring less than 1 cm across the full-thickness defect, medium tears ranging between 1 and 3 cm, large ranging between 3 and 5 cm, and massive tears measuring larger than 5 cm. Inspection of the patient's operative report most often will provide an estimate of tear size, which can be used to estimate the amount of tissue repair, mobilization, and subsequent damage found at the time of surgery. These factors all have implications when a rehabilitation program is designed, starting with the amount of immobilization (larger tears immobilized for a longer period of time typically than smaller tears) and ultimately influencing the rate at which ROM and strength are progressed. Knowledge of this classification system will assist the clinician in understanding the operative report and communicating with the patient and physician regarding the size of the rotator cuff tear and subsequent repair.

Principles of Operative Management of Full-Thickness Rotator Cuff Tears

Efficacious operative treatment for complete rotator cuff tears is based on several principles: tear pattern recognition, secure fixation, and restoration of the footprint. Proper tear pattern recognition is crucial. Many repairs fail because of lack of proper recognition, so a nonanatomical repair is attempted, with increased tension and poor restoration of anatomy.[172]

Complete tear patterns can be broadly divided into two types: crescent shaped and U-shaped (with several variations). Crescent-shaped tears do not usually retract far from the greater tuberosity and usually are directly repaired back to the greater tuberosity. Their greatest extent is most frequently in a transverse direction to the longitudinal axis of the tendon. They must be débrided to allow high-quality tissue attachment. Adhesion formation usually occurs on both surfaces; these need to be removed to allow complete mobilization and to decrease tension on the repair.

U-shaped tears frequently have their greatest extent in a longitudinal direction to the tendon. The medial point of the tear does not represent retraction, but represents the shape that an L-shaped or T-shaped tear assumes with muscle contraction. Mobilization of the two leaves of the tendon by release of the subacromial and intra-articular adhesions will allow better recognition of the tear pattern. The longitudinal component can be repaired by margin convergence, and the transverse component, now a crescent-shaped tear, can be repaired to the bone. Margin convergence by longitudinal side-to-side closure of the leaves of the tear progressively decreases the strain on the lateral margins of the tear, so that the resulting strain on the lateral transverse margin is within the tolerance for repair.[172]

Suture placement in the tendon is the subject of much study.[173,174] The types of suture placement may be categorized as simple, mattress, or combination (modified Mason-Allen). Although there is literature favoring each type of suture placement, it is probably more important how securely the sutures are tied (proper loop security of tendon to bone and knot security within the throws of the knot) and how much load is carried across each suture. Fixation placement should result in proper position of the cuff to bone and optimum pullout strength of the fixation device or construct. Suture anchors should be placed at a 45 degree angle to increase the anchor's resistance to pullout. For single-row repairs, they are placed within 4 to 5 mm of the articular margin. Lately, double-row repairs have been advocated to maximize suture placement and load per suture and to maximize fixation placement. The rows consist of medial suture anchors and lateral bone tunnels, or medial and lateral suture anchors.[174] Clinical reports demonstrate good results with either of these techniques. Figure 10-30 shows a double-row rotator cuff repair technique. The double-row repairs also appear to result in the closest reapproximation of the total geometry of the rotator cuff footprint. Most repairs replicate the width, but not the size, of the original insertion. By allowing a larger, more physiologic area of contact, these double-row repairs have a theoretical ability to increase healing potential and ultimate tensile strength of the repair construct.

REHABILITATION FOLLOWING ARTHROSCOPIC ROTATOR CUFF REPAIR

The previous paragraphs of this chapter have outlined several important concepts of arthroscopic rotator cuff repair, which have significant ramifications in postsurgical rehabilitation. Key factors such as tear size, tear type, chronicity of the tear, fatty infiltration, and fixation of the torn tendon all must be taken into account when progression rates are developed fol-

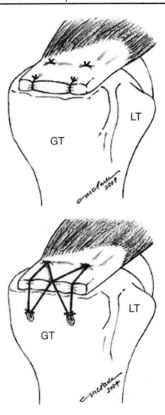

Figure 10-30 Arthroscopic rotator cuff repair using a double-row suture anchor fixation method. (From Park MC, Idjadi JA, El Attrache NS, et al: The effect of dynamic external rotation comparing two footprint-restoring rotator cuff repair techniques, Am J Sports Med 36:893-900, 2008.)

lowing rotator cuff repair. Box 10-2 lists a postsurgical rehabilitation protocol following arthroscopic rotator cuff repair. The following discussions are meant to further clarify the ROM and strength progressions specific to the patient following arthroscopic rotator cuff repair.

Initial postsurgical rehabilitation focuses on ROM to prevent capsular adhesions while protecting surgically repaired tissues. Some postsurgical rehabilitation protocols have specific ROM limitations to be applied during the first 6 weeks of rehabilitation. Several basic science studies have been published that provide a rationale for the safe application of glenohumeral joint ROM and the movements that allow joint excursion, as well as capsular lengthening, yet safe and protective inherent tensions are produced in the repaired tendon. Hatakeyama et al[175] used a cadaveric model to repair 1 × 2 cm supraspinatus tears and studied the effects of humeral rotation ROM on tension in the supraspinatus at 30 degrees of elevation in the coronal, scapular, and sagittal planes. Results show that compared with tension in a position of neutral rotation, 30 degrees and 60 degrees of external rotation actually showed a decrease in tension within the supraspinatus muscle tendon unit. In contrast, 30 degrees and 60 degrees of internal rotation showed increases in tension within the supraspinatus tendon. This study provides important insight into the ability to

BOX 10-2   Postoperative Rehabilitation Protocol for Arthroscopic Rotator Cuff Repair (Medium-Sized Tear)

General Guidelines

1. Progression of resistive exercise and ROM is dependent on patient tolerance.
2. Resistance exercise should not be performed with specific shoulder joint pain or pain over the incision site.
3. A sling is provided to the patient for support as needed with daily activities and to wear at night. The patient is weaned from the sling as tolerated.
4. Early home exercises are given to the patient following surgery, including stomach rubs, sawing, and gripping activity.
5. Progression to active range of motion (AROM) against gravity and duration of sling use are predicated on the size of the rotator cuff tear and the quality of the tissue and fixation.

Postop Weeks 1 and 2

1. Early passive range of motion (PROM) to patient tolerance during the first 4 to 6 weeks:
   - Flexion
   - Scapular and coronal plane abduction
   - Internal rotation/external rotation (IR/ER) with 90 to 45 degrees abduction
2. Submaximal isometric IR/ER, flexion/extension, and adduction.
3. Mobilization of the glenohumeral joint and the scapulothoracic joint. Passive stretching of elbow, forearm, and wrist to terminal ranges.
4. Sidelying scapular protraction/retraction resistance to encourage early serratus anterior and lower trapezius activation and endurance.
5. Home exercise instruction:
   - Instruction in PROM and active assistive range of motion (AAROM) home exercises with T-bar, pulleys, or opposite arm assistance in supine position using ROM to patient tolerance.
   - Weight-bearing (closed-chain) Codman's exercise instruction over a ball or countertop/table.
   - Theraputty for grip strength maintenance

Postop Week 3

1. Continue above shoulder ROM and isometric strength program to patient tolerance. Progress patient to active assistive ROM.
2. Add upper body ergometer (UBE) if available.
3. Begin active scapular strengthening exercises and continue sidelying manual scapular stabilization exercise:
   - Scapular retraction
   - Scapular retraction with depression
4. Begin resistive exercise for total arm strength using positions with glenohumeral joint completed support, including the following:
   - Bicep curls
   - Tricep curls
   - Wrist curls—flexion, extension, radial and ulnar deviation
5. Begin submaximal rhythmic stabilization using the balance point position (90 to 100 degrees of elevation) in supine position to initiate dynamic stabilization.

Postop Week 5/6

1. Initiate isotonic resistance exercise focusing on the following movements:*

   - Sidelying ER
   - Prone extension
   - Prone horizontal abduction (limited range to 45 degrees)
   - Supine IR
   - Flexion to 90 degrees
2. Progression to full PROM and AROM in all planes, including ER and IR, in neutral adduction progressing from the 90 degree abducted position used initially postop
3. External rotation oscillation (resisted ER with towel roll under axilla and oscillation device)
4. Home exercise program for strengthening the rotator cuff and the scapular musculature with isotonic weights and/or elastic tubing (Thera-Band)

Postop Week 8

1. Begin closed-chain step-ups and quadruped rhythmic stabilization exercise.
2. Initiate upper extremity plyometric chest passes and functional two-hand rotation tennis groundstroke or golf swing simulation using small exercise ball and progressing to light medicine ball as tolerated.

Postop Week 10

1. Initiation of submaximal isokinetic exercise for IR/ER in the modified neutral position; criteria for progression to isokinetic exercise:
   - Patient has IR/ER ROM greater than that used during isokinetic exercise.
   - Patient can complete isotonic exercise program pain-free with a 2- to 3-pound weight or medium-resistance surgical tubing or Thera-Band.
2. Progression to 90 degree abducted rotational training in patients returning to overhead work or sport activity
   - Prone external rotation
   - Standing external/internal rotation with 90 degree abduction in the scapular plane
   - Statue of Liberty (external rotation oscillation)

Postop Week 12 (3 months)

1. Progression to maximal isokinetics in IR/ER and isokinetic testing to assess strength in modified base 30/30/30 position. Formal documentation of AROM, PROM, and administration of shoulder rating scales.
2. Begin interval return programs if criteria below have been met:
   - IR/ER strength minimum of 85% of contralateral extremity
   - ER/IR ratio 60% or higher
   - Pain-free ROM
   - Negative impingement and instability signs during clinical examination

Postop Week 16 (4 months)

1. Isokinetic reevaluation, documentation of AROM, PROM, and Shoulder Rating Scales
2. Progression continues for return to full upper extremity sport activity (e.g., throwing, serving in tennis)
3. Preparation for discharge from formal physical therapy to home program phase

From Manske RC: Sports rehabilitation: knee and shoulder, St. Louis, 2006, Mosby.

*A low-resistance/high-repetition (i.e., 30 reps) format is recommended with no resistance used initially (e.g., weight of the arm).

perform early passive range of motion (PROM) in the directions of external rotation following rotator cuff repair. Additionally, because most patients are placed in positions of internal rotation following surgery during the period of immobilization, movement of the shoulder into internal rotation is performed despite the increased tension identified by Hatakeyama et al.[175] One final aspect of clinical relevance in the study by Hatakeyama et al[175] was the comparison of the intrinsic tensile load in the repaired supraspinatus tendon between the frontal or coronal plane, the scapular plane, and the sagittal plane during humeral rotation. Significantly higher loading was present in the supraspinatus tendon during humeral rotation in the sagittal plane as compared with both the frontal and scapular planes. Therefore, based on this important basic science study, early PROM is performed into the directions of both external and internal humeral rotation using the scapular plane position to minimize tensile loading in the repaired tendon.[175]

One additional basic science study provides guidance for ROM application in the early postoperative phase. Muraki et al[176] studied the effects of passive motion on tensile loading of the supraspinatus tendon in cadavers, in a study similar to the one conducted by Hatakeyama et al.[175] They found no significant increases in strain during the movement of cross-arm adduction in either the supraspinatus or the infraspinatus tendon at 60 degrees of elevation. However, internal rotation performed at 30 degrees and 60 degrees of elevation did place increased tension in the inferior-most portion of the infraspinatus tendon over the resting or neutral position. This study provides additional guidance for clinicians in the selection of safe ROM positions following surgery. It also shows the importance of knowing the degree of tendon involvement and repair as posteriorly based rotator cuff repairs (those involving the infraspinatus and teres minor) may be subjected to increased tensile loads if early internal rotation is applied during postoperative rehabilitation. Therefore, communication between the surgeon and the treating therapist is of vital importance, to ensure that optimal ROM is performed following repair.

One area of initial concern in the rehabilitation process following rotator cuff repair lies in the progression from passive-based ROM applications to active assistive and active ROM. Some disagreement as to the degree of muscular activation that occurs during commonly used rehabilitation activities; this can be clarified by a review of the appropriate literature. Research by McCann et al[177] provides clear delineation of the degree of muscular activation of the supraspinatus during supine assisted ROM and seated elevation with the use of a pulley. Although both activities arguably produce low levels of inherent muscular activation in the supraspinatus, the upright pulley activity produces significantly more muscular activity as compared with the supine activities studied by McCann and colleagues.

Additionally, research by Ellsworth et al[178] has quantified levels of muscular activation during Codman's pendulum exercise. Their study shows minimal levels of muscular activation in the rotator cuff musculature during Codman's pendulum

exercise; however, the exercise cannot be considered passive because the musculature is truly activated, especially in individuals with shoulder pathology. Additionally, although many therapists, including the authors of this chapter, do not recommend the use of weight application in the hand during pendulum exercises because of the potential for unwanted anterior translation, Ellsworth et al[178] found that muscular activity in the rotator cuff musculature was not changed between the performance of pendulum exercises with and without weight application. Pendulum exercises without weight have the same effect on muscular activity as those performed with weight application; thus the use of pendulum exercises in the early postsurgery phase may be questioned in cases in which only passive movements may be indicated.

These studies provide objective guidance for the early application of assisted ROM activities that can be applied safely in early postsurgical rehabilitation following rotator cuff repair. As further research becomes available, clinicians will be able to make evidence-based decisions regarding the appropriateness of specific rehabilitation exercises according to their inherent muscular activation. Rehabilitation in the first 2 to 4 weeks following rotator cuff repair typically consists of the use of truly passive, as well as several minimally active or active assistive, exercises for the rotator cuff such as active assisted elevation, overhead pulleys, and pendulums. Additionally, the balance point position (90 degrees of shoulder flexion) is used in the supine position, where the patient is queued to perform small active motions of flexion/extension from the 90 degree starting position to recruit rotator cuff and scapular muscular activity. These exercises coupled with early scapular stabilization via manual resistance techniques emphasizing direct hand contacts on the scapula are recommended to bypass force application to the rotator cuff and to optimize trapezius, rhomboid, and serratus anterior muscular activation (see Figure 10-16). Kibler[179] has published EMG quantification of low-level closed-chain exercise such as weight-shifting on a rocker board and highlighted the low levels (<10%) of activation of the rotator cuff and the scapular musculature during application.

Finally, new research has studied the effects of simulated active ROM on the integrity of a cadaveric supraspinatus repair performed with the use of transosseous tunnels or suture anchors.[180] Results showed no difference between repair constructs following repetitive loading, indicating that the ability of an arthroscopically based suture anchor fixation model to withstand active loading is similar to that seen in transosseous repair and during mini-open and open rotator cuff repair. Additionally, this study did show significant gapping and repair failure in both types of rotator cuff repair (transosseous tunnel and suture anchor) following low-level physiologic load application.

Progression to resistive exercise for the rotator cuff and the scapular musculature typically occurs in a time interval approximating 6 weeks following surgery, when early theoretical healing is assumed in the repaired tissues. Significant variation exists in the time course for this initiation of resistive exercise in the literature.[99,171,181] and it is based on several factors. These factors include but are not limited to tear size, tear type, tissue quality, concomitant surgical procedures, and patient health status and age.

Clinical application of resistive exercise during this critical stage of rehabilitation is guided both by published literature detailing the level of muscular activity within individual muscles of the rotator cuff and scapular stabilizers and by patients who demonstrate exercise tolerance.* These studies provide the rationale behind the determination of optimal exercise movement patterns to produce the desired level of muscular activation in the rotator cuff and scapular stabilizers. The application of very low resistance levels in a repetitive format is recommended for safety and for relative protection of the repaired tissues, as well as to improve local muscular endurance. Multiple sets of 15 to 20 repetitions have been recommended and described in several studies to improve muscular strength in the rotator cuff and scapular stabilizing musculature.[137,184,185] Exercise patterns using shorter lever arms, and maintaining the glenohumeral joint in positions of less than 90 degrees of elevation and anterior to the coronal plane of the body are theorized to reduce the risks of both compressive irritation and capsular loading/attenuation during performance.[4] Additionally, early focus on the rotator cuff and scapular stabilizers without emphasis on larger prime mover muscles such as the deltoid, pectorals, and upper trapezius is recommended to minimize unwanted joint shear and inappropriate arthrokinematics, in addition to attempting to optimize external/internal rotation muscle balance.[185,186] An understanding of the deltoid/rotator cuff force couple of Inman et al[5] provides a theoretical platform for the exercise emphasis on the compressive and depressive ability of the rotator cuff and de-emphasis on the deltoid and larger prime movers during rehabilitation.

One specific exercise that has been described extensively in the literature is the empty can exercise (scapular plane elevation with an internally rotated [thumb down] extremity position). Although EMG studies have shown high levels of activation of the supraspinatus during the empty can exercise,[31,134,183] the combined movements of elevation and internal rotation have produced clinically disappointing results in practical application, as well as the common occurrence of patterns of substitution and improper biomechanical execution.[187] Increases in scapular internal rotation and anterior tilting have been shown when the empty can is compared with the full can (scapular plane elevation with external rotation) exercise using motion analysis. Movement patterns characterized by scapular internal rotation and anterior tilting theoretically decrease the subacromial space and could jeopardize the ability for application of repetitive movement patterns required for strength acquisition needed during shoulder rehabilitation.[187]

Specific exercise application for the scapular stabilizers focuses on the lower trapezius and serratus anterior musculature. Donatelli and Ekstrom[188] and others[114,115] have summarized the upper extremity exercise movement patterns that elicit high levels of activation of these important force couple

components responsible for scapular stabilization.[8] Progression from early manual resistive patterns to exercise patterns with elastic resistance and light dumbbells is an important part of the rehabilitation protocol following rotator cuff and labral repair. Wang et al[184] have shown improvements in muscular strength and positive changes in scapulohumeral rhythm following 6 weeks of training using elastic resistance exercise. The use of resistive exercise patterns emphasizing scapular retraction and external humeral rotation is emphasized to optimize scapular stabilization and promote muscular balance during shoulder rehabilitation.

Short-term follow-up of patients following both mini-open and all-arthroscopic rotator cuff repair shows the return of nearly full range of active and passive motion, with deficits in muscular strength ranging from 10% to 30% in internal and external rotation compared with the uninjured extremity.[171] Greater deficits following mini-open and all-arthroscopic rotator cuff repair have been reported in the posterior rotator cuff (external rotators), despite particular emphasis being placed on these structures during postsurgical rehabilitation.

REHABILITATION FOLLOWING SUPERIOR LABRAL (SLAP) REPAIR

Box 10-3 lists the protocol used by the authors of this chapter for rehabilitation following superior labral (SLAP) repair. The progression of ROM and strength is again predicated on physiologic healing limitations, and on early ROM and strengthening. Several key guidelines are applied during rehabilitation following superior labral repair.

In most protocols,[156,164] early passive, active assistive, and active ROM and glenohumeral joint mobilization are recommended following superior labral repair. Although individual surgeon preference may vary, few limitations in the initial ROM are typically recommended unless capsular plication or concomitant procedures were performed. Basic science research has provided guidance on the provision of early ROM for patients following superior labral repair. Morgan et al[69] have identified the concept of the "peel back" mechanism (see Figure 10-15). The peel back mechanism occurs with the glenohumeral joint in 90 degrees of abduction and external rotation in a position simulating the throwing motion. In this position, the biceps tendon force vector has been found to assume a more vertical and posterior direction, creating the peel back of the superior labrum. In the first 6 weeks following surgery, this ROM (external rotation in 90 degrees of abduction) is limited and no aggressive attempts at end ROM are recommended to protect the superior labral repair and to minimize any shear force applied via the bicep from ROM in this position. Glenohumeral external rotation ROM and stretching are initially performed in more neutrally abducted positions (0 to 45 degrees of abduction) during the initial 6 to 8 weeks following superior labral repair.

Few published reports detail the return of ROM following superior labral repair. Ellenbecker et al[164] studied 39 patients with a mean age of 43 years who underwent arthroscopic supe-

BOX 10-3   Arthroscopic Superior Labral (SLAP) Repair Postoperative Protocol

- *Note:* Specific alterations in postoperative protocol if SLAP repair is combined with thermal capsulorrhaphy, capsular plication, rotator interval closure, or repair of full-thickness rotator cuff repair
- Sling use as needed for precarious activities and to minimize biceps muscle activation during initial postoperative phase. Duration and degree of sling use determined by physician at postop recheck.
- Early use of stomach rubs, sawing, and wax-on/wax-off exercise recommended to stimulate home-based motion between therapy visits

Phase I: Early Motion (Weeks 1 to 3)*

1. Passive ROM of the glenohumeral joint in movements of flexion, scapular and coronal plane abduction, cross-arm adduction, and internal rotation in multiple positions of elevation. External rotation performed primarily in the lower ranges of abduction (<60 degrees) to decrease stress on the repair from peel-back mechanism. Cautious use of glenohumeral joint accessory mobilization unless specific joint hypomobility identified on initial postoperative examination. Use of pulleys and supine active assistive elevation with a cane applied according to patient tolerance to initial passive ROM postop
2. Patient to wear sling for comfort as needed
3. ROM of elbow, forearm, and wrist
4. Manual resistive exercise for scapular protraction and retraction, minimizing stress to glenohumeral joint
5. Initiation of submaximal internal and external rotation resistive exercise, progressing from manual resistance to very light isotonic and elastic resistance based on patient tolerance, using a position with 10 to 20 degrees of abduction in the scapular plane
6. Manual resistance for elbow extension/flexion, forearm pronation/supination, and wrist flexion/extension, as well as the use of theraputty or ball squeezes for grip strengthening*
7. Modalities to control pain in shoulder as indicated

Phase II: Progression of Strength and ROM (Weeks 4 to 6)

1. Continue with above exercise guidelines.
2. Begin to progress gentle PROM of the glenohumeral joint with 90 degrees of abduction to terminal ranges with full ER, with 90 degrees of abduction expected between 6 and 8 weeks postop. All other motions continue as in Phase I, with continued use of both physiologic and accessory mobilization as indicated by the patient's underlying mobility status.

3. Initiate rotator cuff progression using movement patterns of sidelying external rotation, prone extension, and prone horizontal abduction using a lightweight and/or elastic resistance.
4. Initiate upper body ergometer for scapular and general upper body strengthening.
5. Perform rhythmic stabilization in 90 degrees of shoulder elevation with limited flexion pressure application to protect SLAP repair.

Phase III: Total Arm Strength (Weeks 6 to 10)

1. Initiation of elbow flexion (biceps) resistive exercise
2. Initiation of seated rowing variations for scapular strengthening
3. Advancement of rotator cuff and scapular progressive resistive exercise using oscillation-based exercise to increase local muscular endurance. Initiation of 90 degrees abducted exercise in scapular plane for internal and external rotation if patient is an overhead athlete or requires extensive overhead function at work
4. Progression to closed-chain exercises by week (8), including step-ups, quadruped rhythmic stabilization, and progressive weight bearing on unstable surface (baps/bosu)
5. Initiation of upper extremity (two arm) plyometric program, progressing from Swiss ball to weighted medicine balls as tolerated

Phase IV: Advanced Strengthening (Weeks 10 to 12/16)

1. Begin isokinetic exercise in the modified neutral position at intermediate and fast contractile velocities. Criteria for progression to isokinetics include the following:
   - Completion of isotonic exercise with a minimum of a 3-pound weight or medium-resistance Thera-Band/theratubing
   - Pain-free ROM in the isokinetic training movement pattern
2. Isokinetic test performed after two to three successful sessions of isokinetic exercise; modified neutral test position
3. Progression to 90 degree abducted isokinetic and functional plyometric strengthening exercises for the rotator cuff (shoulder IR/ER) based on patient tolerance
4. Continue with scapular strengthening and ROM exercises listed in earlier stages.

Phase V: Return To Full Activity

1. Return to full activity is predicated on physician's evaluation, isokinetic strength parameters, functional ROM, and tolerance to interval sport return programs.

Note: No elbow flexion resistance or biceps activity for the first 6 weeks postop to protect the superior labral repair.

rior labral repair and subsequent rehabilitation in keeping with the protocol provided in this chapter (see Box 10-3). At 12 weeks after surgery, mean shoulder flexion, abduction, and external rotation ranges of motion were 2 to 6 degrees greater than those of the contralateral extremity. Deficiencies of 10 degrees in internal rotation ROM were measured compared with the contralateral extremity. This deficiency in internal rotation ROM recovery may be explained in part by the patient population, which included many overhead athletes with ROM adaptations.[41]

Resistive Exercise: (Strengthening Progression)

The importance of regaining dynamic stabilization following SLAP repair has been elucidated in basic science research by Burkart et al,[7] who identified inadequate and incomplete return of glenohumeral joint stability and restoration of normal amounts of translation following repair of the superior labrum alone. Repair of the labral lesion alone did not return normal joint arthrokinematics and points to the important role that dynamic stabilization plays in rehabilitation following superior labral repair.

The information outlined earlier in this chapter highlighting the evidence-based approach to rotator cuff and scapular stabilization applies to the patient after superior labral repair. The return of essential dynamic stabilization by these structures, as well as the optimal positioning of the scapula during upper extremity sport and nonsport use, is of critical importance. One specific issue pertaining to the strengthening sequences and rehabilitation protocol following superior labral repair involves protection of the bicep anchor during the initial postoperative period. Typically, no resistive bicep exercise is used during the initial 6 to 8 weeks following surgery. This specifically pertains to resisted elbow flexion exercises and lifting activities. Exercises and activities that use the movement of shoulder flexion against gravity or during resistance can be integrated gradually. The use of shoulder flexion initially in an active assistive role and then in an active and eventually resisted role is warranted based on the work of Yamaguchi et al and Levy et al.[189,204] These studies have shown minimal levels (1.7% to 3.6% MVC) of muscle activation of the biceps long head during multiple directions of shoulder movement such as scapular plane elevation and glenohumeral rotational movement. This basic science research helps to differentiate early exercise and active ROM patterns for clinicians to use while protecting the repaired superior labrum/biceps long head anchor. Resistive exercise for the elbow flexors is delayed until between 6 to 8 weeks postoperatively and is applied in the form of rowing variations, upper body ergometry, and isolated elastic and isotonic resistance exercise.

The application of resistive exercise to strengthen the rotator cuff and the scapular stabilizers is warranted during rehabilitation following superior labral repair. Progression from the initial patterns used to recruit high levels of rotator cuff and scapular muscle activation to positions at 90 degrees of glenohumeral joint elevation in the scapular plane forms an important part of the end stage strengthening performed before the patient can return to activities such as throwing and serving in the overhead position.

Research specifically outlining the return of rotator cuff strength following superior labral repair is sparse at the present time. Ellenbecker et al[164] measured glenohumeral internal and external rotation strength in 30 patients following superior labral repair. Deficits of approximately 10% were found in the internal and external rotators at 12 weeks post surgery following the strength progression outlined in the protocol presented in Box 10-3. This finding shows that continued strengthening is needed even 12 weeks following surgery before full functional recovery and progression to interval sport return programs can be carried out safely.

REHABILITATION FOLLOWING ARTHROSCOPIC BANKART RECONSTRUCTION

Many of the same principles apply to postsurgical rehabilitation following arthroscopic Bankart reconstruction as were listed previously for the patient following rotator cuff and superior labral repair. Early protected ROM is one of the most specific progressions followed during the initial 4 to 6 week period after surgery. Specifically, this protected ROM progression involves the limitation of external rotation ROM to minimize tensile stress to the anterior inferior aspect of the labrum, which was repaired during the Bankart reconstruction. Research guides the use of a specific ROM of external rotation and the performance of that external rotation in positions of abduction that specifically limit stress to the anterior-inferior joint capsule and labrum.

Black et al[155] studied capsular tension in Bankart repairs in cadavers at 0 degrees of abduction in the coronal plane. They identified a "low-tension zone," which occurred in the first 46.5 degrees of external rotation in this position. After 45 degrees of external rotation, researchers found a significant rise in tension in the anterior capsule. This research helps the clinician to understand the internal capsular ramifications of limited external rotation ROM. Using this initial range of external rotation allows the patient to perform a functional ROM without jeopardizing the labral repair by exposing it to increased tensile loading. Changes in anterior capsular tension were reported in conditions of capsular shortening (e.g., plication, shifting) and may indicate further protection of external rotation ROM during the initial rehabilitation period.

In addition to the actual amount of external rotation used in the initial rehabilitation, the position of abduction used during external rotation ROM is important. Both Pagnani et al[59] and O'Brien et al[60] have eloquently performed basic science research that identifies which portions of the anterior glenohumeral capsule are under tension based on the position of glenohumeral abduction. During 90 degrees of abduction, these studies have identified the inferior glenohumeral ligament as the primary restraint to anterior translation. This directly stresses the capsule where the Bankart repair has occurred. External rotation in the first 30 degrees of abduction at the patient's side places more specific tensile loading near the superior glenohumeral ligament and superior capsular structures.[59] These basic science studies provide much of the specific information applicable to rehabilitation of the patient following Bankart reconstruction. Adherence to these ROM guidelines along with rotator cuff and scapular stabilization serves as the primary basis for postsurgical rehabilitation following arthroscopic Bankart reconstruction.

REHABILITATION FOLLOWING SHOULDER ARTHROPLASTY

Several important concepts are imperative for clinicians who perform rehabilitation following shoulder arthroplasty. These include the concepts of obligate translation, balance of dynamic muscle forces, and subscapularis precautions. A brief discussion of the primary indications for shoulder arthroplasty will be undertaken before the expanded text covers these postsurgical rehabilitation concepts.

Degenerative osteoarthritis of the glenohumeral joint is less common than in weight-bearing joints (i.e., hip, knee) of the lower extremity, accounting for only 3% of all osteoarthritis lesions.[190] Osteoarthritis of the glenohumeral joint (GHOA) can be classified as primary or secondary. Primary usually presents with no apparent antecedent cause, and secondary generally results from a preexisting problem such as previous fracture, avascular necrosis, "burned-out" rheumatoid arthritis, or crystalline arthropathy.

Wear patterns in the human shoulder vary based on the type of underlying arthritic condition that is present and its cause. Characteristic wear of the subchondral bone and the glenoid cartilage in the shoulder with degenerative osteoarthritis occurs posteriorly, often leaving an area anterior of intact cartilage.[191] The cartilage of the humeral head is typically eroded in a pattern of central baldness, the so-called Friar Tuck pattern. This differs from the pattern of humeral head wear in cuff tear arthropathy, wherein a chronic large rotator cuff defect subjects the uncovered humeral head to abrasion against the acromion and the coracoacromial arch, resulting in superior rather than central wear patterns.

Another important diagnosis for which shoulder arthroplasty is performed is capsulorrhaphy arthropathy.[192] This has resulted in a more common finding of shoulder arthritis in young active patients and often leads to early shoulder arthroplasty.[193] Neer et al[195] initially reported glenohumeral arthritis after anterior shoulder instability, and in 1982 reported on an initial series of 26 patients who underwent shoulder arthroplasty had who had had prior anterior or posterior instability. Many of the patients in this series had undergone prior stabilization surgery. Samilson and Prieto[194] later developed the term *dislocation arthropathy* after presenting their series of 74 patients with glenohumeral arthritis with previous anterior and posterior instability.

Neer[195] further reported on the association of osteoarthritis with glenohumeral instability by finding subluxation of the humerus in the direction opposite of the initial instability due to excessive tightening at the time of initial stabilization surgery. Matsen et al[196] coined the term *capsulorrhaphy arthropathy* to refer to patients who develop osteoarthritis as a consequence of overly tightened soft tissue structures during treatment for glenohumeral joint instability. Buscayret et al[197] reported the incidence of glenohumeral osteoarthritis to range between 12% and 62% following operative treatment of shoulder instability. Factors specific to stabilization procedures that may contribute to the development of glenohumeral arthritis include encroachment on the articular cartilage by hardware, laterally placed bone block in a Bristow or Latarjet procedure, and excessive soft tissue tensioning imparted by a Putti-Platt procedure.[198]

CONCEPT OF OBLIGATE TRANSLATION

The concept of obligate translation has been applied extensively in orthopaedic and sports physical therapy and in orthopaedics in general since the publication of the study by Harryman et al,[199] identifying an increase in anterior humeral head translation and shear following a controlled posterior capsular plication in cadaveric specimens. Obligate translation,

defined as the translation of the humeral head in the direction opposite of the tight capsule and soft tissue structures, has been a paramount concept applied in treatment of the overhead athlete with subtle anterior glenohumeral joint instability secondary to adaptive posterior rotator cuff and posterior capsule tightness.[4,200] Harryman et al[199] also reported the presence of obligate translation in flexion, internal and external rotation, and maximal elevation with shoulder arthroplasty following insertion of an oversized humeral head prosthesis. Shoulder arthroplasty can tend to cause global capsular restriction due to substitution of a humeral head prosthesis for a degenerative and collapsed humeral head. This overstuffing can prohibit return of optimal ROM unless adequate capsular release and early postoperative physical therapy to address capsular tightness are performed.[191] Figure 10-31 demonstrates the concept of obligate translation.

In general, surgical considerations must first include anatomic joint reconstruction with a well-fixed, stable implant. This is done with a cementless humeral head resurfacing implant or a third- or fourth-generation stemmed implant. The ultimate goal is to match the native humeral version with inclination, offset, and height. The glenoid then can be resurfaced with a prosthesis, or it can be managed with a number of nonimplant resurfacing techniques such as interpositional arthroplasty.[164] Finally, the soft tissues must be released, balanced, and repaired to allow for adequate restoration of long-term function.

Although every surgeon may have his preference, we have used resurfacing primarily in those patients who desire to return to high-demand activity such as strength training, collision sports (skiing, football, mountain biking, etc.), tennis, basketball, and martial arts.[193] We also have chosen to avoid placing a glenoid component in these individuals, so as to avoid the potential pitfalls of loosening and revision.[201] Other alternatives that we have utilized include microfracture, reaming the glenoid to restore version and bone graft of cysts and defects with biological covering of the glenoid surface (with autograft or allograft tissue).

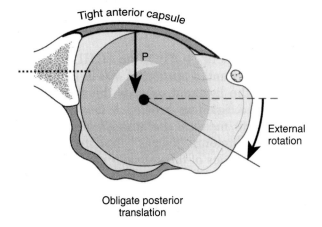

Figure 10-31 Obligate translation showing posterior translation in the presence of a tight anterior capsular component. (From Rockwood CA, Matsen FA, Wirth MA: The shoulder, ed 4, Philadelphia, 2009, Saunders.)

Key to the success of arthroplasty in any patient, but especially in those who desire to return to more demanding sports, is restoring soft tissue tension. Specifically, a complete 360 degree subscapularis release is needed to increase excursion and restore external rotation. Lengthening the tendon is not needed and ultimately will weaken this structure with the potential for delayed rupture. This release will allow the humeral head to return to the center of the glenoid and will permit the normal obligate translation that occurs with rotational motion. This, in turn, helps to restore normal forces across the glenohumeral joint and leads to decreased pain and improved strength and function.

Rehabilitation considerations must take into account the amount of motion obtained under anesthesia after subscapularis closure. This information should be communicated to the patient and the therapist. The goal is to obtain normal motion, and this can be achieved in almost all cases. The subscapularis repair must be sound and protected for the first 6 weeks (limit external rotation to 30 to 45 degrees). If a larger rotator cuff repair is performed, these precautions should be instituted according to the surgeon's confidence in the repair. Full passive motion can be performed immediately, with rapid progression to active assisted and active motion during the initial 6 weeks.

The surgical exposure used during shoulder arthroplasty has significant ramifications for the immediate postoperative management of these patients. Two approaches are typically used: the deltopectoral approach and the anterior-superior or Mackenzie approach.[189] The skin incision for the anterior-superior approach extends distally in a straight line from the acromioclavicular joint for a distance of 9 cm. The anterior deltoid fibers are split for a distance of not more than 6 cm to protect the axillary nerve. The acromial attachment of the deltoid is detached to expose the anterior aspect of the acromion. The subscapularis is completely released and is held by stay sutures and detached. The long head of the biceps can be dislocated posteriorly over the humeral head as the humeral head is dislocated anteriorly.[189] Complete release and detachment of the subscapularis through this approach is required to gain exposure for preparation of the humeral head during hemiarthroplasty, as well as during total shoulder arthroplasty.

Subscapularis Precautions

For the first 6 weeks, specific subscapularis precautions must be followed to protect this important structure postoperatively. This entails limitation of passive or active external rotation ROM, with no active resistive exercise for internal rotation. Although gentle attempts at passive external rotation can occur to as far as 30 to 45 degrees of external rotation beyond neutral, techniques that place increased or undue tension on the anterior capsule and subscapularis are avoided for the first 6 weeks following surgery. Additional precautions may be needed, depending on the repair of additional rotator cuff tendons at the time of surgery, as well as whether bicep tenolysis, tenodesis, or tenotomy has been performed. Specifically, resistive exercise for the biceps brachii is not performed for the first 6 weeks postoperatively if a release of the biceps long head or

tenodesis has been performed to minimize the chance of rerupture and reappearance of a "Popeye" deformity. Since it is beyond the scope of this chapter to completely discuss the entire rehabilitation process following shoulder arthroplasty, complete details of the authors' postoperative protocol are summarized in Box 10-4.

The restoration of optimal muscle balance is imperative during rehabilitation of all shoulder injuries and pathologies; however, it is particularly important following shoulder arthroplasty. Figure 10-32 shows the effects of unbalanced muscular forces during shoulder muscular contraction and volitional movement. Unbalanced internal rotation strength or dominant anterior muscular strength development can lead to anterior translation of the humeral head relative to the glenoid.[186] Likewise, excessive posterior development could accentuate posterior subluxation from an eroded posterior glenoid and overly tight anterior structures (obligate translation) and may produce posterior instability.

Optimal muscle balance between external and internal rotators has been reported and recommended in the range between 66% and 75% ER/IR.[159,158] This can be assessed with a hand-held dynamometer or through isometric function of an isokinetic dynamometer system to ensure proper restoration of

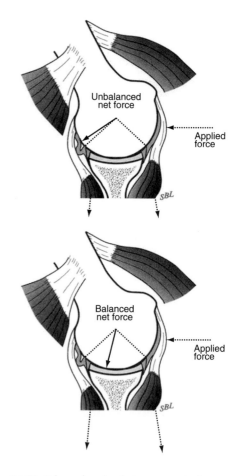

Figure 10-32 Balanced and unbalance muscle force representation. (From Rockwood CA, Matsen FA, Wirth MA, et al: The shoulder, ed 4, Philadelphia, 2010, Saunders.)

BOX 10-4 Rehabilitation After Glenohumeral Joint Arthroplasty

General Guidelines

- Sling use and duration directed by surgeon in postoperative instructions
- Immediate postoperative passive and active assistive range of motion consisting of stomach rubs, sawing movements, and elbow range of motion instructed following hospital discharge

Postop Weeks 1 to 4

1. Modalities to decrease pain and inflammation
2. Passive ROM initiated with no limitation in flexion, abduction, or internal rotation. NO EXTERNAL ROTATION stretching against tension or anterior capsular mobilization in this rehabilitation phase to protect the subscapularis repair; movement and ROM (ROM) into 30 to 40 degrees of external rotation allowed with 30 to 45 degrees abduction by the therapist, provided it is not against tension
3. Elbow, wrist, and forearm ROM/stretching
4. Manually applied scapular resistive exercise for protraction/retraction and submaximal biceps/triceps manual resistance with shoulder in supported position supine
5. Ball approximation (closed-chain Codman's) using Swiss ball or tabletop

Postop Weeks 2 to 4

1. Initiation of active assistive ROM using pulley for sagittal plane flexion and scapular plane elevation

Postop Weeks 4 to 6

1. Continuation of above program
2. Initiation of submaximal multiple-angle isometrics and manual resistive exercise for shoulder external rotation, ab/adduction, flexion/extension
3. Upper body ergometer (UBE)

4. External rotation isotonic exercise using pulley or weight/tubing with elbow supported and glenohumeral joint in scapular plane and at 10 to 20 degrees of abduction (towel roll or pillow under axilla)

Postop Weeks 6 to 8

1. Initiation of passive external rotation ROM and stretching beyond neutral rotation position
2. Initiation of internal rotation submaximal resistive exercise progression
3. Traditional rotator cuff isotonic exercise program
   - Sidelying external rotation
   - Prone extension
   - Prone horizontal abduction (limited from neutral to scapular plane position initially with progression to coronal plane as ROM improves)
4. Biceps/triceps curls in standing with glenohumeral joint in neutral resting position
5. Oscillation exercise with resistance bar or body blade
6. Rhythmic stabilization in open and closed kinetic chain environments

Postop Weeks 8 to 12

1. Continuation of resistive exercise and ROM progressions
2. Addition of ball dribbling and upper body plyometrics with small Swiss ball

Postop Weeks 12 to 24

1. Continuation of rehabilitation
2. Isometric internal/external rotation strength testing/assessment in neutral scapular plane position
3. Subjective rating scale completion
4. Range of motion assessment

---

this optimal muscle balance.[32,34] Patients frequently present with overly dominant anterior muscular strength, which can jeopardize glenohumeral mechanics and lead to complications and functional impairment. Figure 10-33 shows the "rocking horse" phenomenon, which can lead to implant loosening, one of the most frequently encountered complications following total shoulder arthroplasty.[191,201] Restoration of proper muscular balance via monitoring and addressing the ER/IR strength ratio, as well as use of ROM and glenohumeral mobilization techniques during postoperative rehabilitation, ensure proper capsular excursion and minimize the effects of obligate translation, thereby forming the essential tenets of postsurgical management of the patient's condition following shoulder arthroplasty.

SUMMARY

This chapter has provided an overview of the anatomy and biomechanics of the shoulder and has applied this information to the clinical examination and to the development of treatment progressions for patients with shoulder dysfunction. The

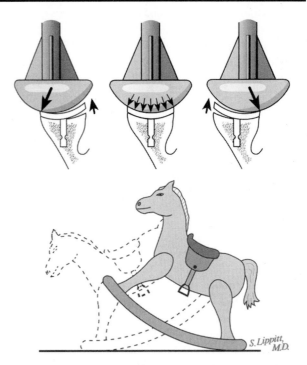

Figure 10-33 Rocking horse phenomenon. (From Rockwood CA, Matsen FA, Wirth MA, et al: The shoulder, ed 4, Philadelphia, 2010, Saunders.)

evidence-based guidelines provided highlight the importance of applying basic science and clinical research to clinical practice to optimize identification of pathology and ultimately to design treatment programs to address the pathology. A "total arm" or "total extremity" approach has been presented to show the importance of proximal stabilization and input of the scapulothoracic joint for human shoulder function.

REFERENCES

1. Saha AK: Mechanism of shoulder movements and a plea for the recognition of "zero position" of glenohumeral joint, Clin Orthop 173:3-10, 1983.
2. Neumann DA: Kinesiology of the musculoskeletal system: foundations for physical rehabilitation, St Louis, 2002, Mosby.
3. Kapandji IA: The physiology of the joints: upper extremity, Philadelphia, 1985, Churchill Livingstone.
4. Ellenbecker TS: Shoulder rehabilitation: non-operative treatment, New York, 2006, Thieme.
5. Inman VT, Saunders JB, Abbott LC: Observations on the function of the shoulder joint, J Bone Joint Surg 26(1):1-30, 1944.
6. Weiner DS, MacNab I: Superior migration of the humeral head, J Bone Joint Surg Br 52:524-527, 1970.
7. Burkhart SS, Morgan CD, Kibler WB: The disabled throwing shoulder: spectrum of pathology. Part I: pathoanatomy and biomechanics, Arthroscopy 19(4):404-420, 2003.
8. Bagg SD, Forrest WJ: A biomechanical analysis of scapular rotation during arm abduction in the scapular plane, Arch Phys Med Rehabil 238-245, 1988.
9. Hsu AT, Chang JH, Chang CH: Determining the resting position of the glenohumeral joint: a cadaver study, J Orthop Sports Phys Ther 32(12):605-612, 2002.
10. Kaltenborn FM: Manual mobilization of the extremity joints, Oslo, Norway, 1989, Olaf Norlis Bokhandel.
11. Magee DJ: Orthopaedic physical assessment, ed 5, St. Louis, 2009, Saunders.
12. Priest JD, Nagel DA: Tennis shoulder, Am J Sports Med 4(1):28-42, 1976.
13. Piatt BE, Hawkins RJ, Fritz RC, et al: Clinical evaluation and treatment of spinoglenoid notch ganglion cysts, J Shoulder Elbow Surg 11:600-604, 2002.
14. Kibler WB, McMullen J: Scapular dyskinesis and its relation to shoulder pain, J Am Acad Orthop Surg 11:142-151, 2003.
15. Codman EA: The shoulder, Boston, 1934, privately printed.
16. Doody SG, Freedman L, Waterland JC: Shoulder movements during abduction in the scapular plane, Arch Phys Med Rehabil 595-604, 1970.
17. Poppen NK, Walker PS: Forces at the glenohumeral joint in abduction, Clin Orthop 135:165, 1978.
18. Lukasiewicz AC, McClure P, Michener L, et al: Comparison of 3-dimensional scapular position and orientation between subjects with and without shoulder impingement, J Orthop Sports Phys Ther 29(10):574-586, 1999.
19. Kibler WB: Role of the scapula in the overhead throwing motion, Contemporary Orthopaedics 22(5):525-532, 1991.
20. Von Eisenhart-Rothe R, Matsen FA, Eckstein F, et al: Pathomechanics in atraumatic shoulder instability, Clin Orthop Rel Research 433:82-89, 2005.
21. Kibler WB: The role of the scapula in athletic shoulder function, Am J Sports Med 26(2):325-337, 1998.
22. Bourne DA, Choo AM, Regan WD, et al: Three-dimensional rotation of the scapula during functional movements: an in vivo study in healthy volunteers, J Shoulder Elbow Surgery, 16(2):150-162, 2007.
23. McClure PW, Michener LA, Sennett BJ, et al: Direct 3-dimensional measurement of scapular kinematics during dynamic movements in vivo, J Orthop Sports Phys Ther 10(3):269-277, 2001.
24. Zeier FG: The treatment of winged scapula, Clin Orthop Rel Res 91:128-133, 1973.
25. Kibler WB, Uhl TL, Maddux JWQ, et al: Qualitative clinical evaluation of scapular dysfunction: a reliability study, J Shoulder Elbow Surg 11:550-556, 2002.
26. Gibson MH, Goebel GV, Jordan TM, et al: A reliability study of measurement techniques to determine static scapular position, J Orthop Sports Phys Ther 21(2):100-106, 1995.
27. T'Jonck L, Lysens R, Gunther G: Measurement of scapular position and rotation: a reliability study, Physiother Res Int 1(3):148-158, 1996.
28. Litchfield DG, Jeno S, Mabey R: The lateral scapular slide test: is it valid in detecting glenohumeral impingement syndrome? Physical Therapy 78(5):S29, 1998.
29. Odom CJ, Taylor AB, Hurd CE, et al: Measurement of scapular asymmetry and assessment of shoulder dysfunction using the lateral scapular slide test: a reliability and validity study, Phys Ther 81(2):799-809, 2001.
30. Rabin A, Irrgang JJ, Fitzgerald GK, et al: The intertester reliability of the scapular assistance test, J Orthop Sports Phys Ther 36(9):653-660, 2006.
31. Kelley MJ, Kane TE, Leggin BG: Spinal accessory nerve palsy: associated signs and symptoms, J Orthop Sports Phys Ther 38(2):78-86, 2008.
32. Berryman-Reese N, Bandy WD: Joint range of motion and muscle length testing, Philadelphia, 2002, Saunders.
33. Norkin CC, White DJ: Measurement of joint motion: a guide to goniometry, ed 2, Philadelphia, 1995, FA Davis.
34. Mallon WJ, Herring CL, Sallay PI, et al: Use of vertebral levels to measure presumed internal rotation at the shoulder: a radiographic analysis, J Shoulder Elbow Surg 5:299-306, 1996.
35. Ellenbecker TS, Roetert EP, Piorkowski PA: Shoulder internal and external rotation range of motion of elite junior tennis players: a comparison of two protocols, J Orthop Sports Phys Ther 17(1):65, 1993 (Abstract).

36. Reinold, MM, Wilk KE, Macrina LC, et al: Intratester and intratester reliability of a new method of measuring glenohumeral internal rotation range of motion: a comparison of three methods, J Orthop Sports Phys Ther 36(1):A70, 2006.

37. Kibler WB, Chandler TJ, Livingston BP, et al: Shoulder range of motion in elite tennis players, Am J Sports Med 24(3):279-285, 1996.

38. Roetert EP, Ellenbecker TS, Brown SW: Shoulder internal and external rotation range of motion in nationally ranked junior tennis players: a longitudinal analysis, J Strength Cond Res 14(2):140-143, 2000.

39. Ellenbecker TS, Roetert EP, Bailie DS, et al: Glenohumeral joint total rotation range of motion in elite tennis players and baseball pitchers, Med Sci Sports Exerc 34(12):2052-2056, 2002.

40. Myers JB, Laudner KG, Pasquale MR, et al: Glenohumeral range of motion deficits and posterior shoulder tightness in throwers with pathologic internal impingement, Am J Sports Med 34(3):385-391, 2006.

41. Gerber C, Werner CML, Macy JC, et al: Effect of selective capsulorrhaphy on the passive range of motion of the glenohumeral joint, J Bone Joint Surg 85-A(1):48-55, 2003.

42. Harryman DT, Sidles JA, Clark MJ, et al: Translation of the humeral head on the glenoid with passive glenohumeral motion, J Bone Joint Surg 72-A:1334-1343, 1990.

43. Matsen FA III, Artnz CT: Subacromial impingement. In Rockwood CA Jr, Matsen FA III, editors: The shoulder, Philadelphia, 1990, Saunders.

44. Koffler KM, Bader D, Eager M, et al: The effect of posterior capsular tightness on glenohumeral translation in the late-cocking phase of pitching: a cadaveric study. Abstract (SS-15) presented at Arthroscopy Association of North America Annual Meeting, Washington, DC, 2001.

45. Grossman MG, Tibone JE, McGarry MH, et al: A cadaveric model of the throwing shoulder: a possible etiology of superior labrum anterior-to-posterior lesions, J Bone Joint Surg 87-A:824-831, 2005.

46. Neer, CS, Welsh, RP: The shoulder in sports, Orthop Clin North Am 8:583-591, 1977.

47. Hawkins RJ, Kennedy JC: Impingement syndrome in athletes, Am J Sports Med 8:151-158, 1980.

48. Davies GJ, DeCarlo MS: Examination of the shoulder complex: current concepts in rehabilitation of the shoulder, LaCrosse, Wis, 1995, Sports Physical Therapy Association Home Study Course.

49. Yocum LA: Assessing the shoulder, Clin Sports Med 2:281-289, 1983.

50. Valadie AL, Jobe CM, Pink MM, et al: Anatomy of provocative tests for impingement syndrome of the shoulder, J Shoulder Elbow Surg 9(1):36-46, 2000.

51. Ellenbecker TS: Rehabilitation of shoulder and elbow injuries in tennis players, Clinics in Sports Med 14(1):87-109, 1995.

52. Leroux JL, Thomas E, Bonnel F, et al: Diagnostic value of clinical tests for shoulder impingement syndrome, Rev Rhum 62(6):423-428, 1995.

53. Post M, Cohen J: Impingement syndrome: a review of late stage II and early stage III lesions, Clin Orthop Rel Res. 207:127-132, 1986.

54. Calis M, Akgun K, Birtane M, et al: Diagnostic values of clinical diagnostic tests in subacromial impingement syndrome, Ann Rheum Dis 59:44-47, 2000.

55. Sackett DL, Straus SE, Richardson WS, et al: Evidence based medicine, ed 2, Edinburgh, 2000, Churchill Livingstone.

56. McFarland EG, Torpey BM, Carl LA: Evaluation of shoulder laxity, Sports Med 22:264-272, 1996.

57. Gerber C, Ganz R: Clinical assessment of instability of the shoulder with special reference to anterior and posterior drawer tests, J Bone Joint Surg Br 66(4):551-556, 1984.

58. Harryman DT, Sidles JA, Harris SL, et al: Laxity of the normal glenohumeral joint: in-vivo assessment, J Shoulder Elbow Surg 1:66-76, 1992.

59. Pagnani MJ, Warren RF: Stabilizers of the glenohumeral joint, J Shoulder Elbow Surg 3:73-90, 1994.

60. O'Brien SJ, Beves MC, Arnoczky SJ, et al: The anatomy and histology of the inferior glenohumeral ligament complex of the shoulder, Am J Sports Med 18:449-456, 1990.

61. Hawkins RJ, Mohtadi NGH: Clinical evaluation of shoulder instability, Clin J Sports Med 1:59-64, 1991.

62. Altchek DW, Dines DW: The surgical treatment of anterior instability: selective capsular repair, Op Tech Sports Med 1:285-292, 1993.

63. Ellenbecker TS: In Clinical examination of the shoulder, Philadelphia, 2004, Saunders.

64. Hawkins RJ, Schulte JP, Janda DH, et al: Translation of the glenohumeral joint with the patient under anesthesia, J Shoulder Elbow Surg 5:286-292, 1996.

65. Ellenbecker TS, Bailie DS, Mattalino AJ, et al: Intrarater and inter-rater reliability of a manual technique to assess anterior humeral head translation of the glenohumeral joint, J Shoulder Elbow Surg 11(5):470-475, 2002.

66. Jobe FW, Bradley JP: The diagnosis and nonoperative treatment of shoulder injuries in athletes, Clin Sports Med 8:419-437, 1989.

67. Speer KP, Hannafin JA, Altchek DW, et al: An evaluation of the shoulder relocation test, Am J Sports Med 22(2):177-183, 1994.

68. Hamner DL, Pink MM, Jobe FW: A modification of the relocation test: arthroscopic findings associated with a positive test, J Shoulder Elbow Surg 9:263-267, 2000.

69. Morgan CD, Burkhart SS, Palmeri M, et al: Type II SLAP lesions: three subtypes and their relationships to superior instability and rotator cuff tears, Arthroscopy 14:553-565, 1998.

70. Matsen FA, Harryman DT, Sidles JA: Mechanics of glenohumeral instability, Clin Sports Med 10:783, 1991.

71. Kvitne KS, Jobe FW, Jobe CM: Shoulder instability in the overhead or throwing athlete, Clin Sports Med 14(4):917, 1995.

72. Fleisig GS, Andrews JR, Dillman CJ, et al: Kinetics of baseball pitching with implications about injury mechanisms, Am J Sports Med 23:233, 1995.

73. Terry GC, Friedman SJ, Uhl TL: Arthroscopically treated tears of the glenoid labrum: factors influencing outcome, Am J Sports Med 22(4):504-512, 1994.

74. Altchek DW, Warren RF, Wickiewicz TL, et al: Arthroscopic labral debridement: a three year follow-up study, Am J Sports Med 20(6):702-706, 1992.

75. Perthes G: Ueber Operationen der habituellen Schulterluxation, Deutsche Ztschr Chir. 85:199, 1906.

76. ASB Bankart: Recurrent or habitual dislocation of the shoulder joint, BMJ 2:1132-1133, 1923.

77. ASB Bankart: The pathology and treatment of recurrent dislocation of the shoulder joint, BMJ 26:23-29, 1938.

78. Gill TJ, Micheli LJ, Gebhard F, et al: Bankart repair for anterior instability of the shoulder, J Bone Joint Surg 79-A:850-857, 1997.

79. Snyder SJ, Karzel RP, Del Pizzo W, et al: SLAP lesions of the shoulder, Arthroscopy 6:274-279, 1990.

80. Cheng JC, Karzel RP: Superior labrum anterior posterior lesions of the shoulder: operative techniques of management, Op Tech Sports Med 5(4):249-256, 1997.

81. Andrews JR, Gillogly S: Physical examination of the shoulder in throwing athletes. In Zarins B, Andrews JR, Carson WG, editors: Injuries to the throwing arm, Philadelphia, 1985, Saunders.

82. Burkhart SS, Morgan CD: The peel-back mechanism: its role in producing and extending posterior type II SLAP lesions and its effect on SLAP repair rehabilitation, Arthroscopy 14:637-640, 1998.

83. Kuhn JE, Bey MJ, Huston LJ, et al: Ligamentous restraints to external rotation in the humerus in the late-cocking phase of throwing: a cadaveric biomechanical investigation, Am J Sports Med 28:200, 2000.

84. Ellenbecker TS: Etiology and evaluation of rotator cuff pathologic conditions and rehabilitation. In Donatelli RA, editor: Physical therapy of the shoulder, ed 4, Philadelphia, 2004, Churchill Livingstone.

85. Liu SH, Henry MH, Nuccion S: A prospective evaluation of a new physical examination in predicting glenoid labrum tears, Am J Sports Med 24(6):721-725, 1996.

86. Stetson WB, Templin K: The crank test, the O'Brien test, and routine magnetic resonance imaging scans in the diagnosis of labral tears, Am J Sports Med 30(6):806-809, 2002.

87. O'Brien SJ, Pagnani MJ, Fealy S, et al: The active compression test: a new and effective test for diagnosing labral tears and acromioclavicular joint abnormality, Am J Sports Med 26(5):610-613, 1998.

88. Myers TH, Zemanovic JR, Andrews JR: The resisted supination external rotation test: a new test for the diagnosis of superior labral anterior posterior lesions, Am J Sports Med 33(9):1315-1320, 2005.

89. Pandya NK, Colton A, Webner D, et al: Physical examination and magnetic resonance imaging in the diagnosis of superior labrum anterior-posterior lesions of the shoulder: a sensitivity analysis, Arthroscopy 24(3):311-317, 2008 Mar.

90. Hegedus EJ, Goode A, Campbell S, et al: Physical examination tests of the shoulder: a systematic review with meta-analysis of individual tests, Br J Sports Med 42(2):80-92, 2008 Feb.

91. Reuss BL, Schwartzberg R, Ziatkin MB, et al: Magnetic imaging accuracy for the diagnosis of superior labrum anterior-posterior lesions in the community setting: eighty-three arthroscopically confirmed cases, J Shoulder Elbow Surg 15:580-585, 2006.

92. Jee WH, McCauley TR, Katz LD, et al: Superior labral anterior posterior (SLAP) lesions of he glenoid labrum: reliability and accuracy of MR arthrography for diagnosis, Radiology 218:127-132, 2001.

93. Neer CS: Impingement lesions, Clin Orthop 173:70-77, 1983.

94. Neer CS: Anterior acromioplasty for the chronic impingement syndrome in the shoulder, J Bone Joint Surg Am 54:41-50, 1972.

95. Golding FC: The shoulder: the forgotten joint, Br J Radiol 35:149, 1962.

96. Cotton RE, Rideout DF: Tears of the humeral rotator cuff: a radiological and pathological necropsy survey, J Bone Joint Surg 46-B:314, 1964.

97. Poppen NK, Walker PS: Forces at the glenohumeral joint in abduction, Clin Orthop 135:165, 1978.

98. Wuelker N, Plitz W, Roetman B: Biomechanical data concerning the shoulder impingement syndrome, Clin Orthop 303:242, 1994.

99. Bigliani LU, Ticker JB, Flatow EL et al: The relationship of acromial architecture to rotator cuff disease, Clin Sports Med 10:823, 1991.

100. Zuckerman JD, Kummer FJ, Cuomo JF et al: The influence of coracoacromial arch anatomy on rotator cuff tears, J Shoulder Elbow Surg 1:4, 1992.

101. Jobe FW, Kivitne RS: Shoulder pain in the overhand or throwing athlete: the relationship of anterior instability and rotator cuff impingement, Orthop Rev 28:963, 1989.

102. Andrews JR, Alexander EJ: Rotator cuff injury in throwing and racquet sports, Sports Med Arthroscop Rev 3:30, 1995.

103. Nirschl RP: Shoulder tendonitis. In Pettrone FP, editor: Upper extremity injuries in athletes, American Academy of Orthopaedic Surgeons Symposium, Washington, DC, 1988, Mosby.

104. Kraushaar BS, Nirschl RP: Current concepts review: tendinosus of the elbow (tennis elbow): clinical features and findings of histological, immunohistochemical, and electron microscopy studies, J Bone Joint Surgery 81-A(2):259, 1990.

105. Cofield R: Current concepts review of rotator cuff disease of the shoulder, J Bone Joint Surg 67-A:974, 1985.

106. Jobe FW, Pink M: The athlete's shoulder, J Hand Ther (April June):107, 1994.

107. Walch G, Boileau P, Noel E, et al: Impingement of the deep surface of the supraspinatus tendon on the postero-superior glenoid rim: an arthroscopic study, J Shoulder Elbow Surg 1:238, 1992.

108. Halbrecht JL, Tirman P, Atkin D: Internal impingement of the shoulder: comparison of findings between the throwing and nonthrowing shoulders of college baseball players, Arthroscopy 15(3):253-258, 1999.

109. Paley KJ, Jobe FW, Pink MM, et al: Arthroscopic findings in the overhand throwing athlete: evidence for posterior internal impingement of the rotator cuff, Arthroscopy 16(1):35-40, 2000.

110. Warner JJP, Micheli LJ, Arslanian LE, et al: Scapulothoracic motion in normal shoulders and shoulders with glenohumeral instability and impingement syndrome: a study using Moire Topographic Analysis, Clin Orthop Rel Research 285:191-199, 1991.

111. Ludewig PM, Cook TM: Alternations in shoulder kinematics and associated muscle activity in people with symptoms of shoulder impingement, Phys Ther 80(3):276-291, 2000.

112. Jensen BR, Sjogaard G, Bornmyr S, et al: Intramuscular laser-Doppler flowmetry in the supraspinatus muscle during isometric contractions, Eur J Appl Physiol 71:373-378, 1995.

113. Solem-Bertoft E, Thuomas K, Westerberg C: The influence of scapula retraction and protraction on the width of the subacromial space, Clin Orthop 266:99-103, 1993.

114. Mosely JB, Jobe FW, Pink M: EMG analysis of the scapular muscles during a shoulder rehabilitation program, Am J Sports Med 20:128-134, 1992.

115. Decker MJ, Hintermeister RA, Faber KJ, et al: Serratus anterior muscle activity during selected rehabilitation exercises, Am J Sports Med 27:784-791, 1999.

116. McMahon PJ, Jobe FW, Pink MM, et al: Comparative electromyographic analysis of shoulder muscles during planar motions: anterior glenohumeral instability versus normal, J Shoulder Elbow Surgery 5:118-123, 1996.

117. Awan R, Smith J, Boon AJ: Measuring shoulder internal rotation range of motion: a comparison of 3 techniques, Arch Phys Med Rehabil 83:1229-1234, 2002.

118. Boon AJ, Smith J: Manual scapular stabilization: its effect on shoulder rotational range of motion, Arch Physi Med Rehab 81(7):978-983, 2000.

119. Ellenbecker TS, Roetert EP, Piorkowski PA, et al: Glenohumeral joint internal and external rotation range of motion in elite junior tennis players, J Orthop Sports Phys Ther 24(6):336-341, 1996.

120. Ellenbecker TS: Shoulder internal and external rotation strength and range of motion in highly skilled tennis players, Isok Exercise Science 2:1-8, 1992.

121. Brown LP, Neihues SL, Harrah A, et al: Upper extremity range of motion and isokinetic strength of the internal and external shoulder rotators in major league baseball players, Am J Sports Med 16:577-585, 1988.

122. Crockett HC, Gross LB, Wilk KE, et al: Osseous adaptation and range of motion at the glenohumeral joint in professional baseball pitchers, Am J Sports Med 30:20-26, 2002.

123. Meister K, Day T, Horodyski MB, et al: Rotational motion changes in the glenohumeral joint of the adolescent little league baseball player, Am J Sports Med 33(5):693-698, 2005.

124. Reagan KM, Meister K, Horodyski MB, et al: Humeral retroversion and its relationship to glenohumeral rotation in the shoulder of college baseball players, Am J Sports Med 30(3):354-360, 2002.

125. Osbahr DC, Cannon DL, Speer KS: Retroversion of the humerus in the throwing shoulder of college baseball pitchers, Am J Sports Med 30(3):347-353, 2002.

126. Chant CB, Litchfield R, Griffin S, et al: Humeral head retroversion in competitive baseball players and its relationship to glenohumeral rotation range of motion, J Orthop Sports Phys Ther 37(9):514-520, 2007.

127. Reinold MM, Macrina LC, Wilk KE, et al: Electromyographic analysis of the supraspinatus and deltoid muscles during 3 common rehabilitation exercises, J Athletic Training 42(4):464-469, 2007.

128. Sullivan PE, Markos PD, Minor MD: An integrated approach to therapeutic exercise: theory and clinical application, Reston, 1982, Reston Publishing Co.

129. Zachezewski JE, Reischl S: Flexibility for the runner: specific program considerations, Top Acute Care Trauma Rehab 1:9-27, 1986.

130. McClure P, Balaicuis J, Heiland D, et al: A randomized controlled comparison of stretching procedures in recreational athletes with posterior shoulder tightness, J Orthop Sports Phys Ther 35(1):A5, 2005 Abstract.

131. Ballantyne BT, O'Hare SJ, Paschall JL et al: Electromyographic activity of selected shoulder muscles in commonly used therapeutic exercises, Phys Ther 73:668, 1993.

132. Blackburn TA, McLeod WD, White B et al: EMG analysis of posterior rotator cuff exercises, Athletic Training 25:40, 1990.

133. Reinhold MM, Wilk KE, Fleisig GS, et al: Electromyographic analysis of the rotator cuff and deltoid musculature during common shoulder external rotation exercises, J Orthop Sports Phys Ther 34(7):385-394, 2004.

134. Townsend H, Jobe FW, Pink M et al: Electromyographic analysis of the glenohumeral muscles during a baseball rehabilitation program, Am J Sports Med 19:264, 1991.

135. Malanga GA, Jenp YN, Growney ES, et al: EMG analysis of shoulder positioning in testing and strengthening the supraspinatus, Med Sci Sports Exercise 28(6):61-664, 1996.

136. Fleck SJ, Kraemer WJ: Designing resistance training programs, Champaign, Ill, 1987, Human Kinetics Publishers.

137. Moncrief SA, Lau JD, Gale JR, et al: Effect of rotator cuff exercise on humeral rotation torque in healthy individuals, J Strength Conditioning Research 16(2):262-270, 2002.

138. Rathburn JB, MacNab I: The microvascular pattern of the rotator cuff, J Bone Joint Surgery (Br) 52-B:540, 1970.

139. Graichen H, Hinterwimmer S, von Eisenhart-Roth RVR, et al: Effect of abducting and adducting muscle activity on glenohumeral translation, scapular kinematics and subacromial space width in vivo, J Biomechanics 38(4):755-760, 2005.

140. Bitter NL, Clisby EF, Jones MA, et al: Relative contributions of infraspinatus and deltoid during external rotation in healthy shoulders, J Shoulder Elbow Surgery 16(5):563-568, 2007.

141. McCabe RA, Tyler TF, Nicholas SJ, et al: Selective activation of the lower trapezius muscle in patients with shoulder impingement, J Orthop Sports Phys Ther 31(1):A-45, 2001 (Abstract).

142. Englestad ED, Johnson RL, Jeno SHN, et al: An electromyographical study of lower trapezius muscle activity during exercise in traditional and modified positions, J Orthop Sports Phys Ther 31(1):A-29-A-30, 2001 (Abstract).

143. Moesley JB, Jobe FW, Pink M: EMG analysis of the scapular muscles during a shoulder rehabilitation program, Am J Sports Med 20:128, 1992.

144. Ellenbecker TS, Davies GJ: Closed kinetic chain exercise: a comprehensive guide to multiple joint exercises, Champaign, Ill, 2001, Human Kinetics.

145. Uhl TL, Carver TJ, Mattacola CG, et al: Shoulder musculature activation during upper extremity weightbearing exercise, J Orthop Sports Phys Ther 33(3):109-117, 2003.

146. Basset RW, Browne AO, Morrey BF, et al: Glenohumeral muscle force and moment mechanics in a position of shoulder instability, J Biomechanics 23:405-415, 1994.

147. Happee R, VanDer Helm CT: The control of shoulder muscles during goal directed movements, an inverse dynamic analysis, J Biomechanics 28(10):1179-1191, 1995.

148. Elliott B, Marsh T, Blanksby B: A three dimensional cinematographic analysis of the tennis serve, Int J Sport Biomechanics 2:260-271, 1986.

149. Tsai NT, McClure PW, Karduna AR: Effects of muscle fatigue on 3-dimensional scapular kinematics, Arch Phys Med Rehabil 84:1000-1005, 2003.

150. Ebaugh DD, McClure PW, Karduna AR Scapulothoracic and glenohumeral kinematics following an external rotation fatigue protocol, J Orthop Sports Phys Ther 36(8):557-571, 2006.

151. Davies GJ: A compendium of isokinetics in clinical usage, LaCrosse, Wis, 1992, S & S Publishers.

152. Ellenbecker TS, Davies GJ: The application of isokinetics in testing and rehabilitation of the shoulder complex, J Athletic Training 35(3):338-350, 2000.

153. Ellenbecker TS: Shoulder internal and external rotation strength and range of motion in highly skilled tennis players, Isok Exerc Sci 2:1-8, 1992.

154. Ellenbecker TS, Roetert EP: Age specific isokinetic glenohumeral internal and external rotation strength in elite junior tennis players, J Science Med Sport 6(1):63-70, 2003.

155. Black KP, Lim TH, McGrady LM, et al: In vitro evaluation of shoulder external rotation after a Bankart reconstruction, Am J Sports Med 25(4):449-453, 1997.

156. Wilk KE, Andrews JR, Arrigo CA, et al: The strength characteristics of internal and external rotator muscles in professional baseball pitchers, Am J Sports Med 21:61-66, 1993.

157. Quincy RI, Davies GJ, Kolbeck KJ, et al: Isokinetic exercise: the effects of training specificity on shoulder strength development, J Athletic Training 35:S64, 2000.

158. Ellenbecker TS, Davies GJ, Rowinski MJ: Concentric versus eccentric strengthening of the rotator cuff: objective data versus functional test, Am J Sports Med 1988.

159. Ivey FM, Calhoun JH, Rusche K, et al: Isokinetic testing of shoulder strength: normal values, Arch Phys Med Rehabil 66:384-386, 1985.

160. Mont MA, Cohen DB, Campbell KR, et al: Isokinetic concentric versus eccentric training of the shoulder rotators with functional evaluation of performance enhancement in elite tennis players, Am J Sports Med 22:513-517, 1994.

161. Vossen JE, Kramer JE, Bruke DG, et al: Comparison of dynamic push-up training and plyometric push-up training on upper-body power and strength, J Strength Cond Res 14(3):248-253, 2000.

162. Schulte-Edelmann JA, Davies GJ, Kernozek TW, et al: The effects of plyometric training of the posterior shoulder and elbow, J Strength Cond Res 19(1):129-134, 2005.

163. Carter AB, Baminski TW, Douex AT Jr, et al: Effects of high volume upper extremity plyometric training on throwing velocity and functional strength ratios of the shoulder rotators in collegiate baseball players, J Strength Cond Res 21(1):208-215, 2007.

164. Ellenbecker TS, Bailie DS, Lamprecht D: Interpositional case study, JOSPT 2008-04-29.

165. Marshall RN, Elliott BC: Long-axis rotation: the missing link in proximal to distal sequencing, J Sports Science 18:247-254, 2000.

166. Kelly BT, Kadrmas WH, Speer KP: The manual muscle examination for rotator cuff strength: an electromyographic investigation, Am J Sports Med 24:581-588, 1996.

167. Donatelli R, Ellenbecker TS, Ekedahl SR, et al: Assessment of shoulder strength in professional baseball

pitchers, J Orthop Sports Phys Ther 30(9):544-551, 2000.

168. Ellenbecker TS, Nazal F, Roetert EP, et al: Shoulder rating scale data from healthy unilaterally dominant overhead sports, J Orthop Sports Phys Ther 35(1):A-79, 2005 (Abstract).

169. Romeo AA, Bach BR, O'Halloran KL: Scoring systems for shoulder conditions, Am J Sports Med 24:472-476, 1996.

170. Nakajima T, Rokumma N, Kazutoshi H, et al: Histologic and biomechanical characteristics of the supraspinatus tendon: reference to rotator cuff tearing, J Shoulder Elbow Surgery, 3:79, 1994.

171. Ellenbecker ES, Bailie DS, Kibler WB: Rehabilitation after mini-open and arthroscopic repair of the rotator cuff. In Manske RC: Postsurgical orthopedic sports rehabilitation: knee and shoulder, St Louis, 2007, Mosby.

172. Burkhart SS, Danaceau SM, Pearce CE Jr: Arthroscopic rotator cuff repair: analysis of results by tear size and by repair technique: margin convergence versus direct tendon-to-bone repair, Arthroscopy 17:905-912, 2001.

173. Burkhart SS: A stepwise approach to arthroscopic rotator cuff repair based on biomechanical principles, Arthroscopy 16:82-90, 2000.

174. Fealy S, Kingham P, Altchek DW: Mini-open rotator cuff repair using a 2 row fixation technique: outcomes analysis in patients with small, moderate, and large rotator cuff tears, Arthroscopy 18:665-670, 2002.

175. Hatakeyama, Y, Itoi, E, Urayama, M, et al: Effect of superior capsule and coracohumeral ligament release on strain in the repaired rotator cuff tendon, Am J Sports Medicine 29:633-640, 2001.

176. Muraki T, Aoki M, Uchiyama E, et al: The effect of arm position on stretching of the supraspinatus, infraspinatus, and posterior portion of deltoid muscles: a cadaveric study, Clin Biomech 21(5):474-480, 2006 Jun.

177. McCann PD, Wooten ME, Kadaba MP, et al: A kinematic and electromyographic study of shoulder rehabilitation exercises, Clin Orthop Rel Research 288:178-189, 1993.

178. Ellsworth AA, Mullaney M, Tyler TF, et al: Electromyography of selected shoulder musculature during unweighted and weighted pendulum exercises, North Am J Sports Phys Ther 1(2):73-79.

179. Kibler WB: Specificity and sensitivity of the anterior slide test in throwing athletes with superior glenoid labral tears, Arthroscopy 11(3):296-300, 1995.

180. Tashjian RZ, Levanthal E, Spenciner DB, et al: Initial fixation strength of massive rotator cuff tears: in vitro comparison of single-row suture anchor and transosseous tunnel constructs, Arthroscopy 23(7):710-716, 2007.

181. Timmerman LA, Andrews JR, Wilk KE: Mini open repair of the rotator cuff. In Andrews JR, Wilk KE: The athlete's shoulder, Philadelphia, 1994, Churchill Livingstone.

182. Reinold MM, Macrina LC, Wilk KE, et al: Electromyographic analysis of the supraspinatus and deltoid muscles during 3 common rehabilitation exercises, J Athl Train 42(4):464-469, 2007 Oct-Dec.

183. Malanga GA, Jemp YN, Growney E, et al: EMG analysis of shoulder positioning in testing and strengthening the supraspinatus, Med Sci Sports Exercise 28:661-664, 1996.

184. Wang CH, McClure P, Pratt NE, et al: Stretching and strengthening exercises: their effect on three-dimensional scapular kinematics, Arch Phys Med Rehabil 80:923-929, 1999.

185. Malliou PC, Giannakopoulos K, Beneka AG, et al: Effective ways of restoring muscular imbalances of the rotator cuff muscle group: a comparative study of various training methods, Br J Sports Med 38(6):766-772, 2004 Dec.

186. Lee SB, An KN: Dynamic glenohumeral stability provided by three heads of the deltoid muscle, Clin Orthop Rel Research 400:40-47, 2002.

187. Thigpen CA, Padua DA, Morgan N, et al: Scapular kinematics during supraspinatus rehabilitation exercise: a comparison of full-can versus empty-can techniques, Am J Sports Med 34(4):644-652, 2006.

188. Donatelli RA, Ekstrom RA: Surface electromyographic analysis of exercises for the trapezius and serratus anterior muscles, J Orthop Sports Phys Ther 33(5):247-258, 2003.

189. Levy O, Funk L, Sforza G, et al: Copeland surface replacement arthroplasty of the shoulder in rheumatoid arthritis, J Bone Joint Surgery 86-A(3):512-518, 2004.

190. Badet R, Boileau P: Arthrography and computed arthrotomography study of seventy patients with primary glenohumeral osteoarthritis, Expansion Scientifique Francaise 62(9):555-562, 1995.

191. Rockwood CA, Wirth MA, Lippitt SB: Glenohumeral arthritis and its management. In Rockwood CA, Matsen FA, editors: The shoulder, ed 3, Philadephia, 1998, Saunders.

192. Parsons M, Campbell B, Titelman RM, et al: Characterizing the effect of diagnosis on presenting deficits and outcomes after total shoulder arthroplasty, J Shoulder Elbow Surgery 14(6):575-584, 2005.

193. Bailie DS, Llinas PJ, Ellenbecker TS: Cementless humeral resurfacing arthroplasty in active patients less than fifty-five years of age, J Bone Joint Surgery 90-A(1):110-117, 2008.

194. Samilson RL, Prieto V: Dislocation arthropathy of the shoulder, J Bone Joint Surg 65-A:456-460, 1995.

195. Neer CS: Shoulder reconstruction, Philadelphia, 1990, Saunders, pp 208-212.

196. Matsen FA, Rockwood CA, Wirth MA, et al: Glenohumeral arthritis and its management. In Rockwood CA, Matsen FA, editors: The shoulder, ed 3, Philadephia, 1998, Saunders, pp 879-888.

197. Buscayret F, Edwards TB, Szabo I, et al: Glenohumeral arthrosis in anterior instability before and after surgical treatment, Am J Sports Med 32(5):1165-1172, 2004.

198. Matsoukis J, Tabib W, Guiffault P, et al: Shoulder arthroplasty in patients with a prior anterior shoulder

dislocation, J Bone Joint Surg 85-A(8):1417-1423, 2003.

199. Harryman DT, Sidles JA, Harris SL, et al: The effect of articular conformity and the size of the humeral head component on laxity and motion after glenohumeral arthroplasty: a study in cadavera, J Bone Joint Surg Am 77(4):555-563, 1995 Apr.

200. Grossman MG, Tibone JE, McGarry MH, et al: A cadaveric model of the throwing shoulder: a possible etiology of superior labrum anterior-to-posterior lesions, J Bone Joint Surg 87-A:824-831, 2005.

201. Bohsali KI, Wirth MA, Rockwood CA: Complications of total shoulder arthroplasty, J Bone Joint Surgery 88-A:2279-2292, 2006.

202. Ianotti JP. Lesions of the rotator cuff: pathology and pathogenesis. In Matsen FA, Fu FH, Hawkins RJ, editors: The shoulder: a balance of mobility and stability, Rosemont, Ill, 1993, American Academy of Orthopaedic Surgeons.

203. Fukoda H, Hamada K, Nakajima T, et al: Pathology and pathogenesis of the intratendinous tearing of the rotator cuff viewed from en bloc histologic sections, Clin Orthop 304:60, 1994.

204. Yamaguchi K, Riew KD, Galatz LM, et al: Biceps activity during shoulder motion: an electromyographic analysis, Clin Orthop Relat Res Mar;(336):122-129, 1997.

CHAPTER

11

Todd S. Ellenbecker,
Brian Shafer,
and Frank W. Jobe

Dysfunction, Evaluation, and Treatment of the Elbow

Dr. Bernard Morrey[1] termed the elbow *the unforgiving joint*. As such, it requires early recognition of injury, a thorough evaluation, and comprehensive upper extremity rehabilitation strategies to ensure optimal treatment. The purpose of this chapter is to overview the unique anatomic structures and biomechanic concepts of the elbow joint, as well as to provide physical evaluation and treatment guidelines for some of the common injuries incurred in the human elbow joint.

FUNCTIONAL ANATOMY

Anatomically, the elbow joint is comprised of three joints. The humeroulnar joint, humeroradial joint, and the proximal radioulnar joint are the articulations that make up the elbow complex (Figure 11-1). The elbow allows for flexion, extension, pronation, and supination movement patterns about the joint complex. The bony limitations, ligamentous support, and muscular stability help to protect it from vulnerability of overuse and resultant injury.

The elbow complex is comprised of three bones: the distal humerus, proximal ulna, and proximal radius. The articulations between these three bones dictate elbow movement patterns.[2] The appropriate strength and function of the upper quarter (cervical spine to the hand, including the scapulothoracic joint) needs to be addressed when evaluating the elbow specifically. The elbow complex has an intricate articulation mechanically between the three separate joints of the upper quarter to allow for function to occur.

The joint capsule plays an important role in the elbow. The capsule is continuous between the three articulations and highly innervated.[1] This is important not only for support of the elbow joint complex but also for proprioception of the joint. The capsule of the elbow will function as a neurologic link between the shoulder and the hand. This has an effect on upper-quarter activity and an obvious aspect of the rehabilitation process if injury does occur.

Humeroulnar Joint

The humeroulnar joint is the articulation between the distal humerus medially and the proximal ulna. The humerus has distinct features distally. The medial aspect has the medial epicondyle and an hourglass-shaped trochlea, located anteromedial on the distal humerus.[3,4] The trochlea extends more distal than the lateral aspect of the humerus. The trochlea will articulate with the trochlear notch of the proximal ulna.

Because of the more distal projection of the humerus medially, the elbow complex will demonstrate a carrying angle that is essentially an abducted position of the elbow in the anatomic position. The normal carrying angle in female subjects is 10 degrees to 15 degrees. In male subjects, it is 5 degrees.[5]

Radiocapitellar Joint (Humeroradial Joint)

The radiocapitellar or humeroradial joint is the articulation of the distal lateral humerus and the proximal radius. The lateral aspect of the humerus has the lateral epicondyle and the capitellum, which is located anterolateral on the distal humerus. With flexion, the radius is in contact with the radial fossa of the distal humerus, whereas in extension the radius and the humerus are not in contact.

Proximal Radioulnar Joint

The proximal radioulnar joint is the articulation between the radial notch of the proximal lateral aspect of the ulna, the radial head, and the capitellum of the distal humerus. The proximal and distal radioulnar joints are important for supination and pronation. Proximally, the radius articulates with the ulna by the support of the annular ligament, which attaches to the ulnar notch anteriorly and posteriorly. This ligament circles the radial head for support. The interosseous membrane is the connective tissue that functions to complete the interval between the two bones. When a fall on the outstretched arm occurs, the interosseous membrane can transmit some forces off the radius, the main weight-bearing bone to the ulna. This can help prevent the radial head from having forceful contact with the

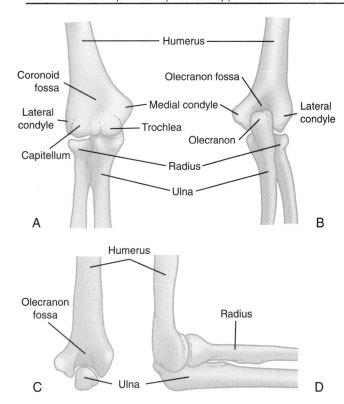

Figure 11-1 Bony anatomy of distal humerus and elbow region. **A,** Anterior view. **B,** Posterior view. **C,** Posterior view, 90-degree flexion. **D,** Lateral view. Right elbow is shown. (Modified from Connolly JF: DePalma's management of fractures and dislocations. In Marx JA: Rosen's emergency medicine: concepts and clinical practice, ed 6, St Louis, 2004, Mosby.)

capitellum. Distally, the concave radius will articulate with the convex ulna. With supination and pronation, the radius will move on the more stationary ulna.

LIGAMENTOUS STRUCTURES

The stability of the elbow starts with the joint capsule and excellent bony congruity inherent in the three articulations of the human elbow. The capsule is loose anteriorly and posteriorly to allow for movement in flexion and extension.[6] The joint capsule is taut medially and laterally because of the added support of the collateral ligaments.

The medial ulnar collateral ligament (MUCL) is fan-shaped in nature and has three bands (Figure 11-2). The anterior band of the MUCL is the primary stabilizer of the elbow against valgus loads when the elbow is near extension.[3,6] The posterior band of the MUCL becomes taut after 60 degrees of elbow flexion and assists in stabilizing against valgus stress when the elbow is in a flexed position. The oblique band of the MUCL does not technically cross the elbow joint and does not provide extensive stabilization to the medial elbow like the anterior and posterior bands.

The lateral elbow complex consists of four structures. The radial collateral ligament attachments are from the lateral

epicondyle to the annular ligament. The lateral ulnar collateral ligament (UCL) is the primary lateral stabilizer and passes over the annular ligament into the supinator tubercle. It reinforces the elbow laterally, as well as reinforcing the humeroradial joint.[3,7] The accessory lateral collateral ligament passes from the tubercle of the supinator into the annular ligament. The annular ligament, as previously stated, is the main support of the radial head in the radial notch of the ulna. The interosseous membrane is a syndesmotic condition that connects the ulna and the radius in the forearm. This structure prevents the proximal displacement of the radius on the ulna.

Dynamic Stabilizers of the Elbow Complex

The elbow flexors are the biceps brachii, brachialis, and brachioradialis muscles. The biceps brachii originate via two heads proximally at the shoulder; the long head originates from the supraglenoid tuberosity of the scapula, and the short head originates from the coracoid process of the scapula. The insertion is from a common tendon at the radial tuberosity and lacertus fibrosus to origins of the forearm flexors. The biceps brachii function is flexion of the elbow and supination of the forearm.[8] The brachialis originates from the lower two thirds of the anterior humerus to the coronoid process and tuberosity of the ulna. It functions to flex the elbow. The brachioradialis, which originates from the lower two thirds of the lateral humerus and attaches to the lateral styloid process of the distal radius, functions as an elbow flexor and as a weak pronator and supinator of the forearm.

The elbow extensors are the triceps brachii and the anconeus muscles. The triceps brachii has a long, medial and lateral head origination. The long head originates at the infraglenoid tuberosity of the scapula, the lateral and medial heads to the posterior aspect of the humerus. The insertion is via the common tendon posteriorly at the olecranon. Through this insertion along with the anconeus muscle that assists the triceps, extension of the elbow complex is accomplished.

Biomechanics of the Elbow

Normal elbow function is vital to the participation in most simple daily activities, as well as for higher-level actions such as sports. In particular the art of throwing or pitching a baseball requires coordination and sequential activation of various body parts including the elbow to result in maximal velocity at the time of ball release. Peak elbow accelerations have been shown to be as high as 3000 degrees per second[9,10] Major stresses occur at the elbow during acceleration and follow-through that require normal functioning musculature to prevent excess load from being transmitted through the articular and ligamentous stabilizers of the elbow. The biomechanics of the elbow can be more easily understood by dividing the pitch into six phases.[11] During the cocking phase contraction of the wrist flexor-pronator group generates a varus torque to counter the valgus extension load on the medial collateral ligament (MCL).[12] In addition, the anconeus and triceps compress

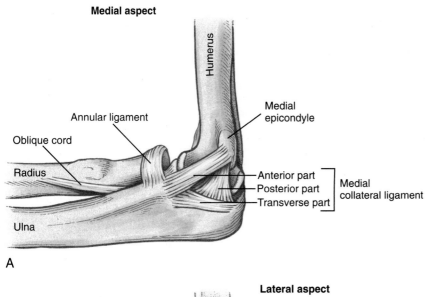

Medial aspect

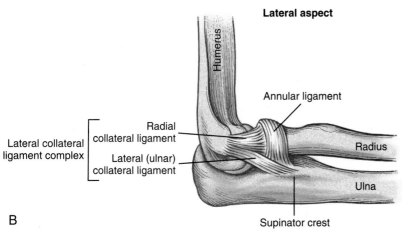

Lateral aspect

Figure 11-2 A, The components of the medial collateral ligament (MCL) of the right elbow. **B,** The components of the lateral collateral ligament of the right elbow. (From Neumann DA: Kinesiology of the musculoskeletal system: foundations for physical rehabilitation, St Louis, 2003, Mosby.)

the joint to assist with taking pressure off of the MCL. During acceleration, triceps activity increases and biceps force decreases. As the deceleration phase begins, biceps, triceps, wrist flexor, and wrist extensor muscular contraction intensity is increased. The trunk and lower extremity also act to dissipate the force during follow-through, illustrating the kinetic chain concept and its integral role in the throwing motion. These complex actions must be thoroughly understood to develop the proper throwing mechanics, muscle strength, and coordination required to prevent or rehabilitate injuries of the elbow that occur during throwing.

CLINICAL EXAMINATION OF THE ELBOW

Structural inspection of the patient's elbow must include a complete and thorough inspection of the entire upper extremity and trunk.[13] The heavy reliance on the kinetic chain for power generation and the important role of the elbow as a link in the kinetic chain necessitates the examination of the entire upper extremity and trunk in the clinical evaluation.[13,14]

However, because many overuse injuries occur in athletic individuals, structural inspection of the patient or athlete with an injured elbow can be complicated by a lack of bilateral symmetry in the upper extremities. Adaptive changes are commonly encountered during clinical examination of the athletic elbow, particularly in the unilaterally dominant upper extremity athlete. In these athletes, use of the contralateral extremity as a baseline is particularly important to determine the degree of actual adaptation that may be a contributing factor in the patient's injury presentation. A brief overview of the common adaptations that have been reported in the literature can provide valuable information to assist the clinician during the structural inspection of the patient with an active or athletic background.

Before discussing the special tests used during a thorough elbow evaluation, specific anatomic adaptations in the areas of range of motion, muscular strength, osseous and ligamentous are presented. Each are presented in the context of the clinical examination of the patient with elbow dysfunction, with an emphasis on the clinical application of how each adaptation can be applied to the clinical examination.

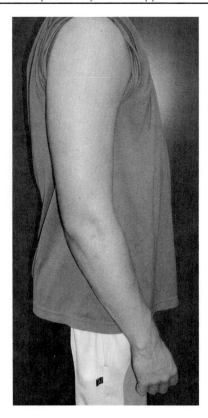

Figure 11-3 Flexion contracture of the dominant arm of an elite tennis player.

Range of Motion Adaptations

King et al.[15] initially reported on elbow range of motion in professional baseball pitchers. Fifty percent of the pitchers they examined were found to have a flexion contracture of the dominant elbow, with 30% of subjects demonstrating a cubitus valgus deformity. Chinn et al.[16] measured world-class professional adult tennis players and reported significant elbow flexion contractures on the dominant arm, but no presence of a cubitus valgus deformity. Figure 11-3 shows the dominant elbow of an elite tennis player revealing the degree of flexion contracture compared with the nondominant extremity.

More recently Ellenbecker et al.[17] measured elbow flexion contractures averaging 5 degrees in a population of 40 healthy professional baseball pitchers. Directly related to elbow function was wrist flexibility, which Ellenbecker et al.[17] reported as significantly less in extension on the dominant arm because of tightness of the wrist flexor musculature, with no difference in wrist flexion range of motion between extremities. Wright et al.[119] reported on 33 throwing athletes before the competitive season. The average loss of elbow extension was 7 degrees, and the average loss of flexion was 5.5 degrees. Ellenbecker and Roetert[18] measured senior tennis players 55 years and older and found flexion contractures averaging 10 degrees in the dominant elbow, as well as significantly less wrist flexion range of motion. The higher use of the wrist extensor musculature is likely the cause of limited wrist flexor range of motion among the senior tennis players, as opposed to the reduced wrist exten-sion range of motion from excessive overuse of the wrist flexor muscles inherent in baseball pitching.[19,20]

More proximally, measurement of range of motion of humeral rotation in the older overhead athlete is also recommended. Several studies have shown consistent alterations of shoulder rotational range of motion in the overhead athlete.[21-23] Ellenbecker et al.[21] has shown statistically greater dominant shoulder external rotation and less internal rotation in a sample of professional baseball pitchers. Despite these differences in internal and external rotation range of motion, the total rotation (IR + ER) between extremities remained equal, such that any increases in external rotation range of motion were matched by decreases in internal rotation range of motion in this uninjured population. Elite-level tennis players had significantly less internal rotation and no significant difference in external rotation on the dominant arm, as well as an overall decrease in total rotation range of motion on the dominant arm of approximately 10 degrees. Careful monitoring of proximal glenohumeral joint range of motion is recommended for the athlete with an elbow injury.

Based on the findings of these descriptive profiles, the finding of an elbow flexion contracture and limited wrist flexion or extension range of motion, as well as reduced glenohumeral joint internal rotation, can be expected during the examination of an athlete from a unilaterally dominant upper extremity sport. Careful measurement during the clinical examination is recommended to determine baseline levels of range of motion loss in the distal upper extremity. This careful measurement serves to determine if rehabilitative interventions are needed, as well as to assess progress during rehabilitation.

Osseous Adaptation

In a study by Priest et al.,[24] 84 world-ranked tennis players were studied using radiography, and an average of 6.5 bony changes were found on the dominant elbow of each player. Additionally, they reported two times as many bony adaptations, such as spurs, on the medial aspect of the elbow as compared with the lateral aspect. The coronoid process of the ulna was the number one site of osseous adaptation or spurring. An average of 44% increase in thickness of the anterior humeral cortex was found on the dominant arm of these players, with an 11% increase in cortical thickness reported in the radius of the dominant tennis-playing extremity. Additionally, in a magnetic resonance imaging (MRI) study, Waslewski et al.[25] found osteophytes at the proximal or distal insertion of the UCL in 5 of 20 asymptomatic professional baseball pitchers, as well as posterior osteophytes in 2 of 20 pitchers.

Ligamentous Laxity

Manual clinical examination of the human elbow to assess medial and lateral laxity can be challenging, given the presence of humeral rotation and small increases in joint opening that often appear with UCL injury. Ellenbecker et al.[17] measured medial elbow joint laxity in 40 asymptomatic professional baseball pitchers, to determine if bilateral differences in medial elbow laxity exist in healthy pitchers with a long history of repetitive overuse to the medial aspect of the elbow. A Telos stress radiography device was used to assess medial elbow joint opening, using a standardized valgus stress of 15 kPa (kilopaschals), with the elbow placed in 25 degrees of elbow flexion and the forearm in a supinated position. The joint space between the medial epicondyle and coronoid process of the ulna was measured using anterior-posterior radiographs by a musculoskeletal radiologist and compared bilaterally, with and without the application of the valgus stress. Results showed significant differences between extremities with stress application, with the dominant elbow opening 1.20 mm and the nondominant elbow opening 0.88 mm. This difference, although statistically significant, averaged 0.32 mm between the dominant and nondominant elbow (and would be virtually unidentifiable with manual assessment). Previous research by Rijke et al.[26] using stress radiography had identified a critical level of 0.5 mm increase in medial elbow joint opening in elbows with UCL injury. Thus the results of the study by Ellenbecker et al.[17] do support this 0.5 mm critical level, because asymptomatic professional pitchers in their study exhibited less than this 0.5 mm of medial elbow joint laxity.

Muscular Adaptations

Several methods can be used to measure upper extremity strength in athletic populations. These can range from measuring grip strength with a handgrip dynamometer to the use of isokinetic dynamometers to measure specific joint motions and muscular parameters. Increased forearm circumference was measured on the dominant forearm in world-class tennis players,[16] as well as in the dominant forearm of senior tennis players.[27]

Isometric grip strength measured using a handgrip dynamometer has revealed unilateral increases in strength in elite adult and senior tennis players as well. Increases ranging from 10% to 30% have been reported using standardized measurement methods.[13,16,27,28]

Isokinetic dynamometers have been used to measure specific muscular performance parameters in elite-level tennis players and baseball pitchers.[13,28,29,30] Specific patterns of unilateral muscular development have been identified by reviewing the isokinetic literature from different populations of overhead athletes.

STRENGTH PROFILES IN ELITE-LEVEL TENNIS PLAYERS

Ellenbecker[28] measured isokinetic wrist and forearm strength in mature adult tennis players who were highly skilled and found 10% to 25% greater wrist flexion and extension, as well as forearm pronation strength on the dominant extremity as compared with the nondominant extremity. Additionally, no significant difference between extremities in forearm supination strength was measured. No significant difference between extremities was found in elbow flexion strength in elite tennis players, but dominant-arm elbow extension strength was significantly stronger than the nontennis-playing extremity.[29]

STRENGTH PROFILES IN ELITE-THROWING ATHLETES

Research on professional throwing athletes has identified significantly greater wrist flexion and forearm pronation strength on the dominant arm by as much as 15% to 35% compared with the nondominant extremity,[13] with no difference in wrist extension strength or forearm supination strength between extremities. Wilk et al[31] reported 10% to 20% greater elbow flexion strength in professional baseball pitchers on the dominant arm, as well as 5% to 15% greater elbow extension strength as compared with the nondominant extremity.

These data help to portray the chronic muscular adaptations that can be found in the overhead athlete who may have an elbow injury, as well as help to determine realistic and accurate discharge strength levels after rehabilitation. Failure to return the stabilizing musculature to its often-dominant status (10% to as much as 35%) on the dominant extremity in these athletes may represent an incomplete rehabilitation and prohibit the return to full activity.

ELBOW EXAMINATION SPECIAL TESTS

In addition to the examination methods outlined in the previous section, including accurate measurement of both distal and proximal joint range of motion, radiographic screening, and muscular strength assessment, several other tests should be included in the comprehensive examination of the elbow of the older active patient. Although it is beyond the scope of this chapter to completely review all of the necessary tests, several are highlighted based on their overall importance. The reader is referred to Morrey,[1] Ellenbecker et al.,[17] and Magee[32] for more complete resources solely on examination of the elbow.

Clinical testing of the joints proximal and distal to the elbow allows the examiner to rule out referral symptoms and ensure that elbow pain is from a local musculoskeletal origin. Overpressure of the cervical spine in the motions of flexion and extension and lateral flexion and rotation, as well as quadrant or Spurling test[33] combining extension with ipsilateral lateral flexion and rotation, are commonly used to clear the cervical spine and rule out radicular symptoms.[34] Tong et al.[33] tested the Spurling maneuver to determine the diagnostic accuracy of this examination maneuver. The Spurling test had a sensitivity of 30% and specificity of 93%. Caution therefore must be used when solely basing the clinical diagnosis on this examination maneuver. The test is not sensitive but is specific for cervical radiculopathy and can be used to help confirm a cervical radiculopathy.

In addition to clearing the cervical spine centrally, clearing the glenohumeral joint is important as well. Determining the presence of concomitant impingement or instability is also highly recommended.[13] Use of the Sulcus sign[35] to determine the presence of multidirectional instability of the glenohumeral joint, along with the subluxation and relocation sign[36] and load and shift test, can provide valuable insight into the status of the glenohumeral joint. The impingement signs of Neer[37] and Hawkins and Kennedy[38] are also helpful to rule out proximal tendon pathologic condition.

In addition to the clearing tests for the glenohumeral joint, full inspection of the scapulothoracic joint is recommended. Removal of the patient's shirt or examination of the patient in a gown with full exposure of the upper back is highly recommended. Kibler et al.[39] has recently presented a classification system for scapular pathologic conditions. Careful observation of the patient at rest and with the hands placed on the hips, as well as during active overhead movements, is recommended to identify prominence of particular borders of the scapula, as well as a lack of close association with the thoracic wall during movement.[40,41] Bilateral comparison forms the primary basis for identifying scapular pathologic conditions; however, in many athletes, bilateral scapular pathologic conditions can be observed.

The presence of overuse injuries in the elbow occurring with proximal injury to the shoulder complex or with scapulothoracic dysfunction is widely reported,[1,13,42-44] and thus a thorough inspection of the proximal joint is extremely important in the comprehensive management of pathologic conditions of the elbow.

Several tests specific for the elbow should be performed to assist in the diagnosis of elbow dysfunction. These include Tinel's test, varus and valgus stress tests, Milking test, valgus extension overpressure test, bounce home test, provocation tests, and the moving valgus test. The Tinel's test involves tapping of the ulnar nerve in the medial region of the elbow, over the cubital tunnel retinaculum. Reproduction of paresthesias or tingling along the distal course of the ulnar nerve indicates irritability of the ulnar nerve.[1]

The valgus stress test is used to evaluate the integrity of the UCL. The position used for testing the anterior band of the UCL is characterized by 15 to 25 degrees of elbow flexion and forearm supination (Figure 11-4). The elbow flexion position is used to unlock the olecranon from the olecranon fossa and decreases the stability provided by the osseous congruity of the joint. This places a greater relative stress on the MUCL.[3] Reproduction of medial elbow pain, in addition to unilateral increases in ulnohumeral joint laxity, indicates a positive test. Grading the test is typically performed using the American Academy of Orthopaedic Surgeons (AAOS) guidelines of 0 to 5 mm, grade I; 5 to 10 mm, grade II; and greater than 10 mm, grade III.[17] Use of greater than 25 degrees of elbow flexion will increase the amount of humeral rotation during performance of the valgus stress test and result in misleading information. The test is typically performed with the shoulder in the scapular plane, but it can be performed with the shoulder in the coronal plane to minimize compensatory movements at the shoulder during testing. Safran et al.[45] studied the effect of forearm rotation during performance of the valgus stress test of the elbow. They found that laxity of the ulnohumeral joint

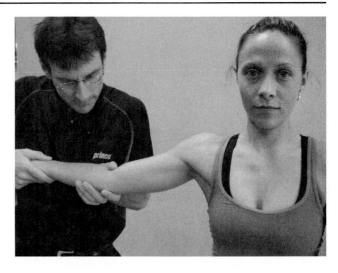

Figure 11-4 Valgus stress test clinical examination maneuver.

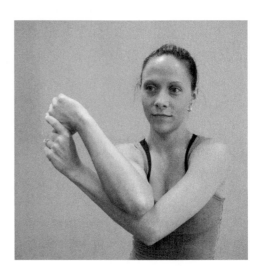

Figure 11-5 Milking sign clinical examination maneuver.

was always greatest when the elbow was tested with the forearm in neutral rotation as compared with either the fully pronated or supinated position. This study suggests testing in the neutral forearm condition to uniformly identify laxity in the UCL.

The milking sign is a test the patient performs on himself or herself, with the elbow in approximately 90 degrees of elbow flexion (Figure 11-5). By reaching under the involved elbow with the contralateral extremity, the patient grasps the thumb of their injured extremity and pulls in a lateral direction, thus imposing a valgus stress to the flexed elbow. Some patients may not have enough flexibility to perform this maneuver, and the examiner can impart a valgus stress to mimic this movement, which stresses the posterior band of the UCL.[3]

The varus stress test is performed using similar degrees of elbow flexion and shoulder and forearm positioning. This test assesses the integrity of the lateral UCL, and it should be performed along with the valgus stress test to completely evaluate the medial and lateral stability of the ulnohumeral joint.

Andrews et al.[46] has reported use of the valgus extension overpressure test to determine whether posterior elbow pain is caused by a posteromedial osteophyte abutting the medial margin of the trochlea and the olecranon fossa. This test is performed by passively extending the elbow while maintaining a valgus stress to the elbow. The action is meant to simulate the stresses imparted to the posterior medial part of the elbow during the acceleration phase of the throwing or serving motion. Reproduction of pain in the posteromedial aspect of the elbow indicates a positive test.

The use of provocation tests can be applied when screening the muscle tendon units of the elbow. Provocation tests consist of manual muscle tests to determine pain reproduction. The specific tests used to screen the elbow joint of a patient with suspected elbow pathologic condition include wrist and finger flexion and extension, as well as forearm pronation and supination.[42] These tests can be used to provoke the muscle tendon unit at the lateral or medial epicondyle. Testing of the elbow at or near full extension can often recreate localized lateral or medial elbow pain secondary to tendon degeneration.[47] Reproduction of lateral or medial elbow pain with resistive muscle testing (provocation testing) may indicate concomitant tendon injury at the elbow and would direct the clinician to perform a more complete elbow examination.

One of the more recent elbow special tests reported in the literature is the moving valgus test.[48] This test is performed with the patient's upper extremity in approximately 90 degrees of abduction. The elbow is maximally flexed, and a moderate valgus stress is imparted to the elbow to simulate the late cocking phase of the throwing motion (Figure 11-6).[12] Maintaining the modest valgus stress at the elbow, the elbow is extended from the fully flexed position. A positive test for UCL injury is confirmed when reproduction of the patient's pain occurs and is maximal over the MUCL between 120 and 70 degrees in what the authors have termed the *shear angle* or *pain zone.* O'Driscoll et al.[48] used the moving valgus test to examine 21 athletes with a primary complaint of medial elbow pain from MCL insufficiency or other valgus overload abnormality. This test was found to be highly sensitive (100%) and specific (75%) when compared with arthroscopic exploration of the MUCL. The mean angle of maximum pain reproduction in their study was 90 degrees of elbow flexion. This test can provide valuable clinical input during the evaluation of the patient with medial elbow pain.

These special examination techniques are unique to the elbow. When combined with a thorough examination of the upper extremity kinetic chain and cervical spine, they can result in an objectively based assessment of the patient's pathologic condition and enable the clinician to design a treatment plan based on the examination findings.

REHABILITATION TECHNIQUES FOR SPECIFIC INJURIES

Overuse injuries constitute most of the elbow injuries seen in many orthopaedic and sports physical therapy clinics. In addi-

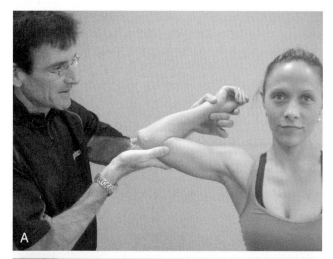
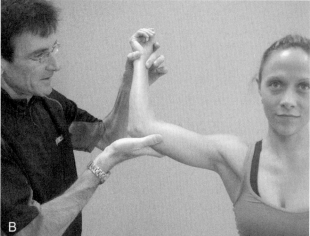
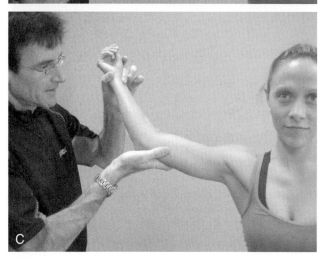

Figure 11-6 Moving valgus clinical examination maneuver.

tion to the incidence of overuse injury in the general population and industry, the athletic elbow patient also displays this classification of injury. One of the most common overuse injuries typically seen is in the outpatient setting is humeral epicondylitis.[13,44,49] The repetitive overuse reported as one of the primary causative factors is particularly evident in the history of many athletic patients with elbow dysfunction. Epidemiologic research on adult tennis players reports incidences of humeral epicondylitis ranging from 35% to 50%.[50-54] This incidence is actually far greater than that reported in elite junior players (11% to 12%).[55,56]

Pathomechanics: Cause of Humeral Epicondylitis

Runge[57] reported humeral epicondylitis, or "tennis elbow" as it is more popularly known, in the literature as early as 1873. Since then, many authors have extensively studied the condition. In 1936, Cyriax[58] listed 26 causes of tennis elbow, whereas an extensive study of this overuse disorder by Goldie,[59] in 1964, reported hypervascularization of the extensor aponeurosis and an increased quantity of free nerve endings in the subtendinous space. More recently, Leadbetter[60] described humeral epicondylitis as a degenerative condition consisting of a time-dependent process including vascular, chemical, and cellular events that lead to a failure of the cell-matrix healing response in human tendon. This description of tendon injury differs from earlier theories in which an inflammatory response was considered as a primary factor; hence the term *tendonitis* was used as opposed to the term recommended by Leadbetter,[60] and Nirschl.[43]

Nirschl[43] and Morrey[44] have defined humeral epicondylitis as an extraarticular tendinous injury characterized by excessive vascular granulation and an impaired healing response in the tendon, termed *angiofibroblastic hyperplasia*. In the most recent and thorough histopathologic analysis, Nirschl et al.[47] studied specimens of injured tendon obtained from areas of chronic overuse and reported that they do not contain large numbers of lymphocytes, macrophages, and neutrophils. Instead, tendinosus appears to be a degenerative process characterized by large populations of fibroblasts, disorganized collagen, and vascular hyperplasia.[47] It is not clear why tendinosus is painful, given the lack of inflammatory cells, and it is also unknown why the collagen does not mature.

Structures Involved in Humeral Epicondylitis

Nirschl[43] has described the primary structure involved in lateral humeral epicondylitis as the tendon of the extensor carpi radialis brevis. Approximately one third of cases involve the tendon of the extensor communis.[47] Additionally, the extensor carpi radialis longus and extensor carpi ulnaris can be involved. The primary site of medial humeral epicondylitis is the flexor carpi radialis, pronator teres, and flexor carpi ulnaris tendons.[43,44]

Recent research has described in detail the anatomy of the lateral epicondylar region.[61,62] The specific location of the extensor carpi radialis brevis tendon lies inferior to the tendinous origin of the extensor carpi radialis longus, which can be palpated along the anterior surface of the supracondylar ridge just proximal or cephalad to the extensor carpi radialis brevis tendon on the lateral epicondyle.[61] Greenbaum et al.[62] describe the pyramidal slope or shape of the lateral epicondyle and show how both the extensor carpi radialis brevis and the

extensor communis originate from the entire anterior surface of the lateral epicondyle. These specific relationships are important for the clinician to bear in mind when palpating for the region of maximal tenderness during the clinical examination process. Although detailed recent reports are not present in the literature regarding the medial epicondyle, careful palpation can be used to discriminate between the muscle tendon junctions of the pronator teres and flexor carpi radialis. Additionally, palpation of the MUCL, which originates from nearly the entire inferior surface of the medial epicondyle and inserts into the anterior medial aspect of the coronoid process of the ulna, should be performed. Understanding the involved structures, as well as a detailed knowledge of the exact locations where these structures can be palpated, can assist the clinician in better localizing the painful tendon or tendons involved.

Dijs et al.[63] reported on 70 patients with lateral epicondylitis. They reported the area of maximal involvement in these cases, which identified the extensor carpi radialis longus in only 1% and the extensor carpi radialis brevis in 90%. The body of the extensor carpi radialis tendon was cited in 1% of cases, and 8% were over the muscle tendon junction over the most proximal part of the muscle of the extensor carpi radialis brevis.

Epidemiologic Examination of Humeral Epicondylitis

Nirschl[43] and Morrey[44] report that the incidence of lateral humeral epicondylitis is far greater than that of medial epicondylitis in recreational tennis players and in the leading arm (left arm in a right-handed golfer), although medial humeral epicondylitis is far more common in elite tennis players and throwing athletes (because of the powerful loading to the flexor and pronator muscle tendon units during the valgus extension overload inherent in the acceleration phase of those overhead movement patterns). Additionally, the trailing arm of the golfer (right arm in a right-handed golfer) is reportedly more likely to have medial symptoms than lateral symptoms.

Valgus Extension Overload Injuries

Repeated activities such as overhead throwing, tennis serving, or throwing the javelin can lead to characteristic patterns of osseous and osteochondral injury in the elbows of older active patients and adolescents. These injuries are commonly referred to as *valgus extension overload injuries*.[64]

Pathomechanics

As a result of the valgus stress incurred during throwing or the serving motion, traction placed via the medial aspect of the elbow can create body spurs or osteophytes at the medial epicondyle or coronoid process of the elbow.[65-67] Additionally, the valgus stress during elbow extension creates impingement, which leads to the development of osteophyte formation at the posterior and posteromedial aspects of the olecranon tip,

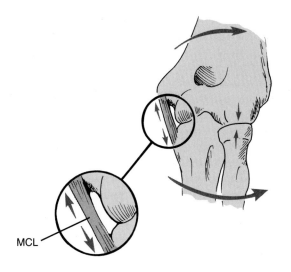

Figure 11-7 Valgus overload depiction showing medial tensile overload and lateral compressive forces. (From Shankman G: Fundamental orthopaedic management for the physical therapist assistant, ed 2, St Louis, 2004, Mosby.)

causing chondromalacia and loose body formation.[64] The combined motion of valgus pressure with the powerful extension of the elbow leads to posterior osteophyte formation because of impingement of the posterior medial aspect of the ulna against the trochlea and olecranon fossa. Joyce et al[68] has reported the presence of chondromalacia in the medial groove of the trochlea, which often precedes osteophyte formation. Erosion to subchondral bone is often witnessed when olecranon osteophytes are initially developing.

Figure 11-7 shows the valgus loading of the athletic elbow and site of medial tension injury or valgus tensile overload response. Injury to the UCL and medial muscle-tendon units of the flexor-pronator group can also occur with this type of repetitive loading.[66,69]

During the valgus stress that occurs to the human elbow during the acceleration phase of both throwing and serving motions, lateral compressive forces occur in the lateral aspect of the elbow, specifically at the radiocapitellar joint. Of great concern in the immature pediatric throwing athlete is osteochondritis dissecans (OCD) and Panner's disease.[13,68] Although the incidence of OCD and Panner's disease is low, the importance of obtaining radiographs in the thorough evaluation of the pediatric elbow cannot be understated. The presence of OCD and Panner's disease, although not common, should be ruled out in every case.[70] The characteristics of Panner's disease are the presence of fissuring and increased density of the capitellum.[70] The most common onset age of both Panner's disease and OCD is less than 10 years. Both conditions occur most commonly in male subjects and typically in the dominant arm.[71] In the older adult elbow, the radiocapitellar joint can be the site of joint degeneration and osteochondral injury from the compressive loading.[66] This lateral compressive loading is increased in the elbow with MUCL laxity or ligament injury.[13]

REHABILITATION PROGRESSION: HUMERAL EPICONDYLITIS

After the detailed examination, a total extremity rehabilitation program can commence. Three main stages of rehabilitation can conceptually be applied for the patient, which include protected function, total arm strength, and the return-to-activity phase. Each is discussed in greater detail in this section of the chapter, with specific highlights on the therapeutic exercises used during each stage of the rehabilitation process.

Protected-Function Phase

During this first phase in the rehabilitation process, care is taken to protect the injured muscle tendon unit from stress but not from function. Nirschl[43] and Morrey[44] caution against the use of an immobilizer or sling because of the further atrophy of the musculature and negative effects on the upper extremity kinetic chain. Protection of the patient from offending activities is recommended, however, with cessation of throwing and serving for medial-based humeral symptoms. Allowing the patient to bat or hit two-handed backhands allows for continued activity while minimizing stress to the injured area. Very often, however, all sport activity must cease to allow the muscle tendon unit time to heal and, most importantly, to allow formal rehabilitation to progress. Continued work or sport performance can severely slow the progression of resistive exercise and other long-term treatments in physical therapy.

Use of modalities is very helpful during this time; however, agreement on a clearly superior modality or sequence of modalities has not been substantiated in the literature.[61,72] A meta-analysis of 185 studies on treatment of humeral epicondylitis showed glaring deficits in the scientific quality of the investigations, with no significantly superior treatment approach identified. Although many modalities or sequences of modalities have anecdotally produced superior results, a tremendous need occurs for prospective, randomized controlled clinical trials to better identify optimal methods for initial treatment. Modalities such as ultrasound,[49,73] electrical stimulation and ice, cortisone injection,[49,51] nonsteroidal antiinflammatory drugs (NSAIDs),[74] acupuncture,[75] transverse friction massage,[76] and dimethyl sulfoxide (DMSO) application[77] have all been reported to provide varying levels of effectiveness historically in the literature. Boyer and Hastings,[61] in a comprehensive review of the treatment of humeral epicondylitis, reported no significant difference with the use of low-energy laser, acupuncture, extracorporeal shockwave therapy, or steroid injection.

The use of cortisone injection has been widely reported in the literature during the pain reduction phase of treatment of this often-recalcitrant condition. Dijs et al.[63] compared the effects of traditional physical therapy and cortisone injection in 70 patients diagnosed with humeral epicondylitis. In their research, 91% of patients who received the cortisone injection reported initial relief, as compared with 47% who reported relief from undergoing physical therapy. However, the recurrence rate in their study after only 3 months, showed 51% in the cortisone injection group and only 5% in the physical therapy group had a return of primary symptoms. Similar findings were reported in a study by Verhaar et al.[78] that compared physical therapy consisting of Mills manipulation and cross-friction massage with corticosteroid injection in a prospective randomized controlled clinical trial in 106 patients with humeral epicondylitis. At 6 weeks, 22 of 53 subjects reported a complete relief from the cortisone injection, although only three subjects had complete relief from this type of physical therapy treatment. At 1 year, no differences between treatment groups were seen regarding the course of treatment. This study shows the short-term benefit from the corticosteroid injection, as well as the ineffectiveness of physical therapy using manipulation and cross-friction massage.

Several additional studies deserve further discussion, because they also can be used to direct clinicians in the development of appropriate interventions. Nirschl et al.[79] studied the effects of iontophoresis with dexamethasone in 199 patients with humeral epicondylitis. Results showed 52% of the subjects in the treatment group reported overall improvement on the investigators' improvement index, with only 33% of the placebo group reporting improvement 2 days after the series of treatments with iontophoresis. One month after the treatment, no statistical difference was seen in the overall improvement in the patients in the treatment group versus the control group. One additional finding from this study that has clinical relevance was the presence of greater pain relief in the group that underwent six treatments in a 10-day period, as opposed to subjects in the treatment group who underwent treatment over a longer period of time. Although this study does support the use of iontophoresis with dexamethasone, it does not report substantial benefits during follow-up.

Haake et al.[80] studied the effects of extracorporeal shock wave therapy in 272 patients with humeral epicondylitis in a multicenter prospective randomized control study. They reported that extracorporeal shock wave therapy was ineffective in the treatment of humeral epicondylitis. Similarly, Basford et al.[81] used low-intensity Nd:YAG laser irradiation at seven points along the forearm three times a week for 4 weeks and also reported it to be ineffective in the treatment of lateral humeral epicondylitis.

Based on this review of the literature, it appears that no standardized modality or modality sequence has been identified in the literature that is clearly statistically more effective than any other at the present time. Clinical reviews by Nirschl,[43] Morrey,[44] and Ellenbecker and Mattalino[13] advocate the use of multiple modalities, such as electrical stimulation and ultrasound, as well as iontophoresis with dexamethasone, to assist in pain reduction and encourage increases in local blood flow. The copious use of ice or cryotherapy after increases in daily activity is also recommended. The use of therapeutic modalities and also cortisone injection, if needed, can only be seen as one part of the treatment sequence, with increasing evidence being generated favoring progressive resistive exercise.

Exercise is one of the most powerful modalities used in rehabilitative medicine. Research has shown increases in local blood flow after isometric contraction of the musculature at levels as submaximal as 5% to 50% of maximum voluntary contraction (MVC), both during the contraction and for periods of up to 1 minute postcontraction.[82] Several studies have shown superior results in the treatment of humeral epicondylitis using progressive resistive exercise compared with ultrasound.[83] Additionally, a study by Svernl and Adolffson,[84] monitored 38 patients with lateral humeral epicondylitis who were randomly assigned to a contract-relax stretching or eccentric exercise treatment group. Results of their study showed a 71% report of full recovery in the eccentric exercise group, as compared with the group that performed contract-relax stretching, which only found 39% of the subjects rating themselves as fully recovered. Finally, Croisior et al.[85] compared the effectiveness of a passive standardized treatment in patients diagnosed with chronic humeral epicondylitis (nonexercise control) to a program that included eccentric isokinetic exercise. After training, the patients in the eccentric exercise group had a significant reduction in pain intensity, an absence of bilateral strength deficit in the wrist extensors and forearm supinators, improved tendon imaging, and improved disability status with rating scales. This study supports the use of eccentric exercise over the typical passive treatment in patients with chronic humeral epicondylitis. These studies support the heavy reliance on the successful application of progressive resistive exercise in the treatment of humeral epicondylitis.

Total Arm Strength Rehabilitation

Early application of resistive exercise for the treatment of humeral epicondylitis mainly focuses on the important principle that states that "proximal stability is needed to promote distal mobility."[86] The initial application of resistive exercise actually consists of specific exercises to strengthen the upper extremity proximal force couples.[87] The rotator cuff (deltoid and serratus anterior) lower trapezius force couples are targeted to enhance proximal stabilization using a low-resistance, high-repetition exercise format (i.e., three sets of 15 repetition maximum [RM] loading). Specific exercises such as side-lying external rotation, prone horizontal abduction and prone extension (both with externally rotated humeral positions and prone external rotation) all have been shown to elicit high levels of posterior rotator cuff activation during electromyography (EMG) research.[88-90] Additionally, exercises such as the serratus press and the use of manual scapular protraction and retraction resistance directly applied by the therapist can be safely applied without stress to the distal aspect of the upper extremity during this important phase of rehabilitation. The use of cuff weights allows some of the rotator cuff and scapular exercises to be performed with the weight attached proximal to the elbow to further minimize overload to the elbow and forearm during the earliest phases of rehabilitation (if needed for some patients).

The initial application of exercise to the distal aspect of the extremity follows a pattern that stresses the injured muscle-tendon unit last. For example, the initial distal exercise sequence for the patient with lateral humeral epicondylitis would include wrist flexion and forearm pronation, which provides most of the tensile stress to the medially inserting tendons that are not directly involved in lateral humeral epicondylitis. Gradual addition of wrist extension and forearm supination, as well as radial and ulnar deviation exercises, are added as signs and symptoms allow. Additional progression is based on the elbow position used during distal exercises. Initially, most patients tolerate the exercises in a more pain-free fashion, with the elbow placed in slight flexion, with a progression as signs and symptoms allow to more extended and functional elbow positions. These exercises are performed with light weights, often as little as 1 lb or 1 kg, as well as a tan or yellow Theraband, emphasizing both the concentric and the eccentric portions of the exercise movement. According to the research by Svernl and Adolffson[84] and Croisier et al.,[85] the eccentric portion of the exercise may actually have a greater benefit than the concentric portion. However, more research is needed before a greater and more clear understanding of the role isolated eccentric exercise plays in the rehabilitation of degenerative tendon conditions is fully understood. Multiple sets of 15 to 20 repetitions are recommended to promote muscular endurance.

Once the patient can tolerate the most basic series of distal exercises (wrist flexion and extension, forearm pronation and supination, and wrist radial and ulnar deviation), exercises are progressed to include activities that involve simultaneous contraction of the wrist and forearm musculature with elbow flexion and extension range of motion. These include exercises such as exercise ball dribbling (Figure 11-8, A), Body Blade (Hymanson, TX), Boing (OPTP, Minneapolis, MN), Theraband (Hygenic Corporation, Akron, OH) resistance bar external oscillations (Figure 11-8, B) (which combine wrist and forearm stabilization with posterior rotator cuff and scapular exercise), and seated rowing and other types of scapular retraction resistive exercise. Additionally, the use of closed kinetic chain exercise such as quadruped rhythmic stabilization for the upper extremity are added to promote cocontraction and mimic functional positions with joint approximation in athletes, as well as in industrial patients who bear weight on their upper extremities for job-specific functioning.[91]

In addition to the resistive exercise, the use of gentle passive stretching to optimize the muscle tendon unit length is indicated. Combined stretches with the patient in the supine position are indicated to elongate the biarticular muscle tendon units of the elbow, forearm, and wrist using a combination of elbow, wrist, and forearm positions (Figure 11-9, A and B). Additionally, stretching the distal aspect of the extremity in varying positions of glenohumeral joint elevation is also indicated.[13] Mobilization of the ulnohumeral joint can also be effective in cases where significant flexion contractures exist. Use of ulnohumeral distraction (Figure 11-9, C) with the elbow near full extension will selectively tension the anterior joint capsule.[92]

As the patient tolerates the distal isotonic exercise progression pain-free at a level of 3 to 5 lb or medium-level elastic tubing or bands, as well as demonstrates a tolerance to the oscillatory type of exercises in this phase of rehabilitation, he or she is progressed to the isokinetic form of exercise. Advantages of isokinetic exercise are the inherent accommodative resistance and use of faster, more functional contractile velocities, in addition to providing isolated patterns to elicit high levels of muscular activation. The initial pattern of exercise used anecdotally has been wrist flexion and extension (Figure 11-10), with forearm pronation and supination added after successful tolerance of a trial treatment of wrist flexion and extension. Contractile velocities ranging between 180 to 300 degrees per second, with six to eight sets of 15 to 20 repetitions, are used to foster local muscular endurance[93] in athletic patients with slower contractile velocities ranging from 120

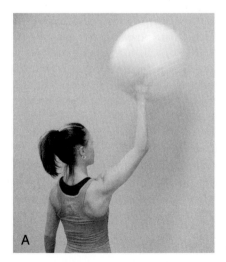

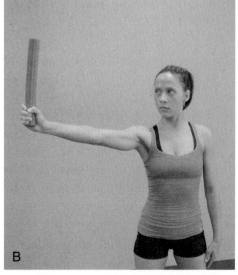

Figure 11-8 A, Ball-dribbling exercise used to increase forearm and wrist strength and local muscular endurance. **B,** Flex-bar oscillation exercise.

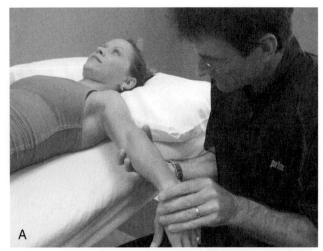

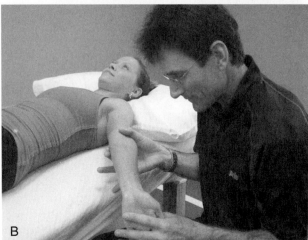

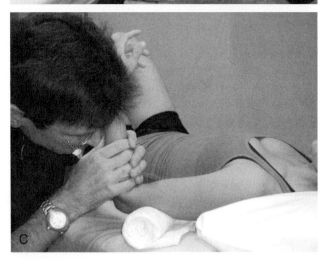

Figure 11-9 A, Range-of-motion stretch position to stretch the forearm supinators and wrist extensors. **B,** Range-of-motion stretch position to stretch the forearm pronators and wrist flexors. **C,** Ulnohumeral distraction joint mobilization technique.

degrees per second to 210 degrees per second for less active and nonathletic patients. In addition to the isokinetic exercise, plyometric wrist snaps (Figure 11-11, *A* and *B*) and wrist flips (Figure 11-11, *C* and *D*) are used to begin to train the active elbow for functional and sport-specific demands.

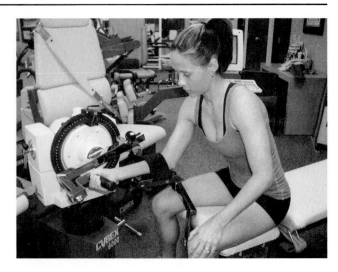

Figure 11-10 Isokinetic wrist flexion-extension exercise.

Return-to-Activity Phase

Of the three phases in the rehabilitation process for humeral epicondylitis, return to activity is the one that is most frequently ignored or cut short, resulting in serious consequences for reinjury and the development of a "chronic" status for this injury. Objective criteria for entry into this stage include the following: tolerance of the previously stated resistive exercise series, objectively documented strength equal to the contralateral extremity with either manual assessment (manual muscle testing [MMT]) or preferably isokinetic testing and isometric strength, distal grip strength measured with a dynamometer, and a functional range of motion. It is important to note that often in the elite athlete with chronic musculoskeletal adaptations, the full elbow range of motion is not always attainable (secondary to the osseous and capsular adaptations discussed earlier in this chapter).

Characteristics of interval sport return programs include alternate-day performance, as well as gradual progressions of intensity and repetitions of sport activities. For the interval tennis program, for example, using low-compression tennis balls such as the Pro-Penn Star Ball (Penn Racquet Sports, Phoenix, AZ) or Wilson Gator Ball (Wilson Sporting Goods, Chicago, IL) during the initial contact phase of the return to tennis decreases impact stress and increases tolerance to the activity. Additionally, performing the interval program under supervision, either during therapy or with a knowledgeable teaching professional or coach, allows for the biomechanic evaluation of technique and guards against overzealous intensity levels, which can be a common mistake in well-intentioned, motivated patients. Using the return program on alternate days, with rest between sessions, allows for recovery and decreases reinjury.

The interval tennis program is contained in Appendix 1. This program specifically outlines the progression for the patient after an upper extremity injury. Often, throwing athletes are seen for medial humeral epicondylitis. Similar concepts are used in the interval throwing program contained in

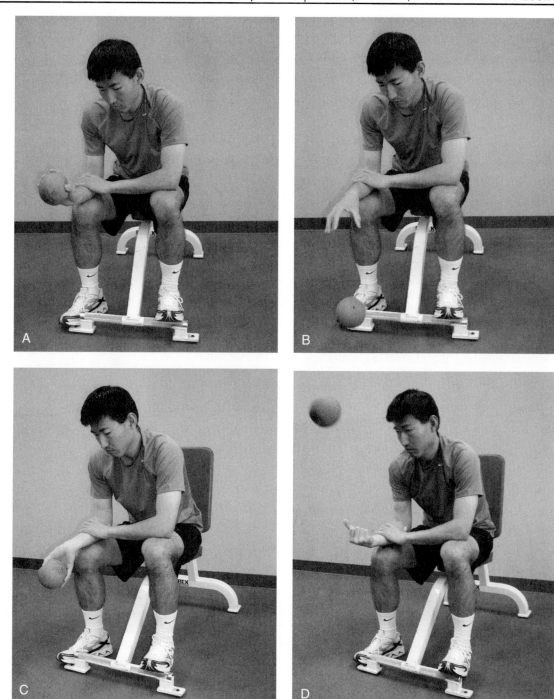

Figure 11-11 A-B, Plyometric wrist "snaps" exercise. **C-D,** Plyometric wrist "flips" exercise.

Appendix 2. Again, having the patient's throwing mechanics evaluated using video (and by a qualified coach or biomechanist) is a very important part of the return-to-activity phase of the rehabilitation process.

Two other important aspects of the return to sport activity are the continued application of resistive exercise and the modification or evaluation of the patient's equipment. Continuation of the total arm strength rehabilitation exercises using elastic resistance, medicine balls, and isotonic or isokinetic resistance

is important to continue to enhance not only strength but also muscular endurance. Inspection and modification of the patient's tennis racquet or golf clubs is also important. For example, lowering the string tension several pounds and ensuring that the player use a more resilient or softer string such as a coreless multifilament synthetic string or gut, is widely recommended for tennis players with upper extremity injury histories.[43,44,49] Grip size is also very important, with research showing changes in muscular activity with alteration of handle or grip size.[94] Measurement of proper grip size has been described as corresponding to the distance between the distal tip of the ring finger along the radial border of the finger to the proximal palmar crease.[44] Researchers have also recommended the use of a counterforce brace to decrease stress on the insertion of the flexor and extensor tendons during work or sport activity.[95]

Postoperative Rehabilitation Progression: Humeral Epicondylitis

In a study of over 3000 cases of humeral epicondylitis, Nirschl[43] has reported that 92% respond to nonoperative treatment. Characteristics of patients who often require surgical correction for this condition are failure of nonoperative rehabilitation programs, minimal relief with corticosteroid injection, and intense pain in the injured elbow even at rest. Surgical treatment for lateral humeral epicondylitis, as reported by Nirschl,[43] involves a small incision from the radial head to 1 inch proximal to the lateral epicondyle. Through this incision, the surgeon removes the pathologic tissue termed *angiofibroblastic hyperplasia*, without disturbing the attachment extensor aponeurosis to preserve stability of the elbow.[43] Vascular enhancement is afforded by drilling holes into the cortical bone in the anterior lateral epicondyle to cancellous bone level. Postoperative immobilization is brief (i.e., 48 hours), with early motion of the wrist and fingers on postoperative day 1, progressing to elbow active assistive range of motion during the first 2 to 3 weeks. Resistive exercise is gradually applied after the third postoperative week, with a return to normal daily activities expected at 8 weeks postoperatively and a return to sport activity several months thereafter.[43,44]

REHABILITATION AFTER ELBOW ARTHROSCOPY

Repetitive stresses to the athletic elbow often result in loose body formation and osteochondral injury, in addition to the more commonly reported tendon injury resulting in humeral epicondylitis. Andrews and Soffer[96] report the most common indications for elbow arthroscopy are loose body removal and removal of osteophytes. Posteromedial decompression includes the excision of osteophytes, with or without resection of additional posteromedial bone from the proximal olecranon (Fig. 11-12).[97] Early emphasis on regaining full extension range of motion is possible because of the minimally invasive arthroscopic procedure. (The author's postoperative protocol after arthroscopic procedures of the elbow is presented in Appendix 3.) Progressive application of resistive exercise to increase both strength and local muscle endurance forms the bulk of the rehabilitation protocol. Use of early shoulder and scapular stabilization is also recommended in these patients to prepare them to return to overhead activities and aggressive functional activity after discharge.

Oglive-Harris et al.[98] reported outcomes after elbow arthroscopy for posteromedial osteophyte and loose body

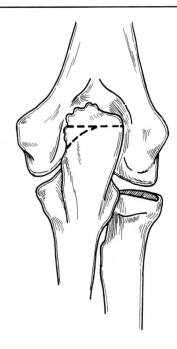

Figure 11-12 Posterior medial osteophyte excision during elbow arthroscopy. (From Andrews JR, Soffer SR: Elbow arthroscopy, St Louis, 1994, Mosby.)

removal. In their study, 21 patients were monitored for an average of 35 months postoperatively, rendering good and excellent results in seven and 14 patients, respectively. O'Driscoll and Morrey[99] reported that arthroscopic removal of loose bodies was of benefit in 75% of all patients; however, when loose bodies were not secondary to some other intraarticular condition, 100% of patients rated the procedure as beneficial. Andrews and Timmerman[100] reviewed the results of 73 cases of arthroscopic elbow surgery in professional baseball pitchers. Eighty percent of players were able to return to full activity, pitching at their preinjury level for at least one season. Further review of these patients found that 25% returned for additional surgery, often requiring stabilization and reconstruction of the UCL because of valgus instability. This important study shows the close association between medial elbow laxity and posterior medial osteochondral injury. In addition, it highlights the importance of identifying subtle instability in the athletic elbow.

Reddy et al.[101] retrospectively reviewed a sample of 172 patients who underwent elbow arthroscopy and had a mean follow-up of 42 months. Fifty-six percent of patients had an excellent result, which allowed them a full return to activity, with 36% having a good result. A 1.6% complication rate was reported, with an overall conclusion that this procedure is both safe and efficacious for the treatment of osteochondral injury of the elbow.

Ellenbecker and Mattalino[13] measured muscular strength at a mean of 8 weeks postoperatively in eight professional baseball pitchers after arthroscopic removal of loose bodies and posteromedial olecranon spur resection. Results showed a complete return of wrist flexion and extension strength and forearm pronation and supination strength at 8 weeks after arthroscopy. This allows for a gradual progression to interval sport return programs between 8 and 12 weeks postoperatively.

Ulnar Collateral Ligament Injury

Attenuation of the UCL can produce valgus instability of the elbow, which can lead to medial joint pain, ulnar nerve compromise, and lateral radiocapitellar and posterolateral osseous dysfunction, which is a severely restricting injury to the throwing or racquet sport athlete. The repetitive valgus loading that occurs in the elbow during the acceleration phase of the throwing or serving motion can attenuate this UCL. Sprains and partial-thickness tears of the MUCL can occur and can progress to complete tears and avulsions of the ligament from its bony attachments.[102]

Nonoperative rehabilitation of the athlete with a MUCL sprain also involves the primary stages outlined in the rehabilitation of humeral epicondylitis listed earlier in this chapter. During the initial stage of rehabilitation, immobilization of the elbow is often a characteristic part of the process to decrease pain and enhance healing. Either an immobilizer or hinged brace is used to limit end ranges of elbow extension and flexion. Modalities are again used to assist in the healing process, as is gentle range of motion and submaximal isometric and manual resistance of both wrist and forearm midrange movements.

Use of a total arm strength rehabilitation protocol is indicated to facilitate both muscular strength and endurance to the elbow, forearm, and wrist. In addition to previously mentioned exercises, particular attention is given to eccentric muscle work of the wrist flexors and forearm supinators to attempt to dynamically support the attenuated UCL. Because of the intimate association between the flexor carpi ulnaris and the ulnar collateral ligament, early strengthening in the pattern of wrist flexion and ulnar deviation may provoke symptoms; however, later in rehabilitation the repeated use of exercises to strengthen the muscles directly overlying the injured ligament to provide dynamic stabilization is highly recommended (Figure 11-13).[103]

Progression to plyometric exercises that impart a submaximal, controlled valgus stress to the medial aspect of the elbow, such as a 90/90 shoulder and elbow medicine ball toss in later stages of rehabilitation, attempt to simulate loads placed on the medial elbow. Use of the isokinetic dynamometer for distal strengthening is also recommended, with additional training focused on the shoulder for internal and external rotation with the arm abducted 90 degrees and elbow flexed 90 degrees. Use of this position imparts a controlled valgus stress to the elbow, in addition to strengthening the rotator cuff, and subjects the medial elbow to a controlled loading process during the later stages of rehabilitation.[104]

A complete return of range of motion and isokinetically documented elbow, forearm, and wrist strength is required before an interval program is initiated. Reoccurrence of pain, feelings of instability, or neural irritation with throwing or

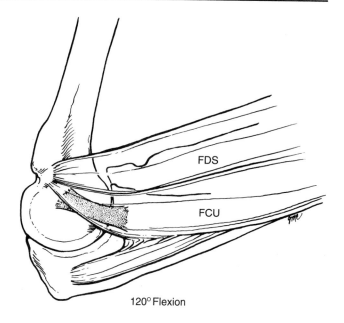

120° Flexion

Figure 11-13 Anatomic association between the flexor carpi ulnaris and flexor digitorum superficialis and the ulnar collateral ligament (UCL). (From Davidson PA, Pink M, Perry J et al: Functional anatomy of the flexor pronator muscle group in relation to the medial collateral ligament of the elbow, Am J Sports Med 23(2):245-250, 1995.)

functional activity identify the patient as a potential candidate for a UCL repair or reconstruction.

Postoperative Rehabilitation: Ulnar Collateral Ligament Reconstruction

Operative procedures for the athlete with valgus instability of the elbow have focused on direct primary repair of the ligament,[105] as well as use of an autogenous graft for reconstruction of the medial elbow.[102,106,107] Regan et al.[108] reported that the palmaris tendon used as the autogenous graft harvested from the ipsilateral forearm, fails at higher loads (357 N) and is four times as strong as the anterior band of the UCL, which fails at 260 N.

In a retrospective study of 71 throwing athletes by Conway et al.[102] who underwent either surgical repair or reconstruction of the MUCL, 87% were found to have a midsubstance tear of the UCL, 10% had a distal ulnar avulsion, and only 3% avulsed from the medial epicondyle. Thirty-nine percent of these athletic elbows had calcification and scar formation in the UCL, with 16% demonstrating an osteophyte to the posteromedial olecranon (most likely from the increased valgus extension overload secondary to UCL attenuation).

The clinical evaluation of these patients preoperatively resulted in a positive valgus stress test in eight of the 14 patients who underwent a UCL repair, and 33 of 56 patients who underwent autogenous reconstruction. Valgus stress radiographs were also used in the preoperative evaluation, with greater emphasis placed on the subjective and clinical evaluation.[102] Fifty percent of these athletes demonstrated a flexion contracture that limited full elbow extension.

Surgical Technique: Ulnar Collateral Ligament Reconstruction

Conway et al.,[102] Jobe et al.,[106] and Jobe and ElAttrache[109] extensively described the surgical technique used to reconstruct the UCL. A 10 cm medial incision over the medial epicondyle is used to provide exposure, with careful dissection and protection of the ulnar nerve carried out before the UCL is addressed. If a primary repair is performed, then adequate normal-appearing ligamentous tissue is required to allow for direct repair. However, primary repair has been shown to have poorer results compared with reconstruction.[100,102] Additional exposure is required to perform the reconstruction, which can be obtained by detaching the flexor and pronator tendinous origin.

This has important ramifications with respect to rehabilitation. The removal of this tendinous origin results in a greater amount of time required for healing, as well as a longer period before resistive exercise of the flexor and pronator muscles and forearm supination and wrist extension range of motion can be performed. Modifications of the original technique for reconstruction have also been described more recently that do not involve detachment of the flexor and pronator mass.[110,111] These techniques involve elevating or splitting the tendon rather than detaching it from its origin on the medial epicondyle. Obviously, these modifications would have important consequences on timing of rehabilitation because of the preservation of the flexor pronator origin.

Calcification within the ligament and surrounding soft tissues is also removed, with relocation of the ulnar nerve performed by removing it from the cubital tunnel. The ulnar nerve is mobilized from the level of the arcade of Struthers to the interval between the two heads of the flexor carpi ulnaris. The attachment sites of the anterior band of the UCL are identified, and tunnels are drilled in the medial epicondyle and proximal ulna to approximate the anatomic location of the original ligament. The graft taken from the ipsilateral palmaris longus (if available) is then placed in a figure-eight fashion through the tunnels. The ulnar nerve is carefully transposed, either submuscularly or subcutaneously, so that no impingement or tethering occurs. Reattachment of the flexor pronator origin is then performed in those cases in which it has been detached. Other recent modifications have described including slightly different tunnel position in the proximal limb that allows for an anatomic graft placement without necessitating an ulnar nerve transposition.[111] An additional modification termed the *docking technique* has also been described. This technique alters the way the graft is fixed proximally to the medial epicondyle. It allows for the graft to be pulled through a single tunnel and sutured over the medial epicondyle rather than weaved through three drill holes in a figure- eight fashion.[112] The DANE procedure has also recently been described that involves this docking technique for proximal fixation and interference screw fixation distally in the ulna.[107] The elbow is immobilized postoperatively in a position of 90 degrees of flexion, neutral forearm rotation, with the wrist left free to move.

Postoperative Rehabilitation After Ulnar Collateral Ligament Reconstruction

After UCL reconstruction, the elbow remains immobilized for the first 10 days after surgery, with gentle gripping exercises allowed to prevent further disuse atrophy. Active and passive range of motion of the elbow, wrist, and shoulder are performed at 10 days postoperatively. Close monitoring of the ulnar nerve distribution in the distal upper extremity is recommended because of the transposition of the nerve that frequently accompanies surgical reconstruction of the MUCL. As discussed in the previously cited surgical summary, care is taken to protect the graft by gradually progressing elbow extension range of motion to 30 degrees by week 2 and, finally, to terminal ranges of elbow extension by 4 to 6 weeks after surgery. Protection of the graft from large stresses is recommended, even though loss of extension range of motion is an undesirable postoperative result. Therefore progressive increases in elbow extension range of motion and the use of gentle joint mobilization such as ulnohumeral distraction and posterior glides of the ulna on the distal humerus in addition to contract-relax stretching techniques are warranted to achieve timely, optimal elbow extension range of motion. Because of the reattachment of the flexor pronator tendinous insertion, limited range of motion into wrist extension and forearm supination is performed for the first 6 weeks until healing of the flexor-pronator insertion takes place.

Rehabilitation of the postoperative elbow should also include activities to restore proprioceptive function to the injured joint. Kinesthesia is the perceived sensation of the position and movement of joints and muscles and is an important part in the coordination of movement patterns in the peripheral joints. Simple use of exercises such as angular replication and end-range reproduction can be used early in rehabilitation, without visual assistance, to stimulate mechanoreceptors in the postoperative joint. These procedures are used early in the rehabilitation process concomitant with range of motion and joint mobilization. Smith and Brunolli[113] have objectively identified kinesthetic awareness in the upper extremity after injury.

The postoperative protocol used for rehabilitation after UCL reconstruction is included in Appendix 4. The progression of resistive exercise follows those previously discussed for humeral epicondylitis, beginning with multiple-angle isometrics at week 2 and submaximal isotonics during the fourth postoperative week. Use of the total arm strength concept is followed, with proximal weight attachment for glenohumeral exercises to prevent stresses placed across the elbow. No glenohumeral joint internal or external rotation strengthening for at least 6 weeks to as many as 16 weeks postoperative is allowed because of the valgus stress placed on the elbow with this movement pattern. During 8 to 12 weeks after surgery, both concentric and eccentric exercises are performed in the elbow extensors and flexors, as well as a continued total arm strengthening emphasis, with all distal movement patterns described in nonoperative rehabilitation of humeral epicondylitis being applied. Plyometric exercises, ball dribbling, and closed-chain exercises are also used during this time frame.

Isokinetic training is introduced at 4 months postoperative, with isokinetic testing applied to identify areas needing specific emphasis.[31,114] Progression of isokinetic training patterns by these authors again follows from wrist extension and flexion to forearm pronation and supination, and finally elbow extension and flexion. The isokinetic dynamometer is also used at 4 to 6 months postoperative for shoulder internal and external rotation strengthening with 90 degrees of abduction and 90 degrees of elbow flexion to impart a gentle, controlled valgus stress to the elbow. At 4 months postoperative, throwing athletes begin an interval throwing program to prepare the elbow for the stresses of functional activity.

The duration of rehabilitation postoperatively is often 6 months to 1 year. A slow revascularization of the graft through a sheath of granulation tissue that grows from the tissue adjacent to the site of implantation encircles the graft and is the rationale provided by Jobe et al.[106] for their time-based rehabilitation program. They are convinced that at least 1 year is required for the tendon graft and its surrounding tissues to develop sufficient strength and endurance to function as a ligament in the medial elbow.

In their series of 56 reconstructed elbows, Conway et al.[102] reported baseball players return to throwing a distance of 15 feet by 4.5 months, with competition at 12.5 months postoperative. The average throwing athlete with a repaired UCL performed throwing activities of 15 feet at 3 months and competed at 9 months. Overall, an excellent result was achieved in 64% of the elbows operated on (achieving a level of activity equal to or greater than preinjury) in elite athletes by Conway et al.[102] Bennet et al.[115] reported improved stability in 13 of 14 cases of UCL reconstruction in an active adult and working population, with improved stability reported in all cases of direct repair by Kuroda and Sakamaki.[105] A flexion contracture was reported in as many as 50% of the athletes at a mean of 6 years after an autogenous UCL reconstruction.[102] Conway et al.[102] did not feel that this finding limits performance, because elbow range of motion during throwing ranges from 120 degrees to 20 degrees, although conscious effort during rehabilitation is given to regain as much extension as possible during the time-based rehabilitation program.

Dines et al.[107] report on the 36 month mean follow-up of 22 patients who underwent the DANE TJ UCL reconstruction technique. This technique, which consisted of a proximal docking procedure at the humerus and distal interference screw fixation in the ulna, was performed with only four complications among the 22 patients. These complications included two with range of motion loss that required lysis of adhesions and two with ulnar neuritis that did go on to excellent long-term results. Nineteen of the 22 patients were found to have excellent modified Conway scores at follow-up. This study shows comparable results to earlier methods of UCL reconstruction in overhead athletes. Vitale and Ahmad[116] have provided the most extensive review of the literature on this topic, publishing a systematic review of UCL reconstruction. An overall successful outcome (excellent result by subjective rating) was reported in 83% of cases reviewed in this comprehensive study.

Dealing With Range of Motion of the Elbow

Elbow range of motion may not be completely regained after traumatic injury, surgery, or immobilization. Morrey[70] has termed the elbow the *unforgiving joint* because of its reluctance and inability to respond to treatment for range-of-motion loss. Decreased range of motion may be caused by osseous structures in some cases, but it is usually the result of an injury to the joint capsule or soft tissue structures (i.e., muscles, tendons, ligaments) surrounding the elbow complex. As with any injury, the viscoelastic properties of soft tissue must be considered during treatment to regain range of motion. These properties include strain rate dependency, creep, stress relaxation, elastic deformation, and plastic deformation. Strain rate is the dependence of material properties on the rate or speed that a load is applied. Rapidly applied forces will cause stiffness and elastic deformation, whereas gradually applied forces will result in plastic deformation.

Creep is defined as the continued deformation with the application of a fixed head (e.g., traction and dynamic splinting). Stress relaxation is the reduction of forces, over time, in a material that is stretched and held at a constant length (e.g., serial casting, static splinting). Elastic deformation is the elongation produced by loading that is recovered after the load is removed. No long-term effect on tissues occurs. Plastic deformation is the elongation produced under loading that will remain after the removal of a load, resulting in a permanent increase in length.[117]

A study by Bonutti et al.[117] evaluated the effectiveness of a patient-directed static progressive stretch therapy in the treatment of elbow contractures. Subjects had elbow contractures for 1 month to 42 years that did not respond to previous treatment consisting of physical therapy, dynamic splinting, serial casting, surgery, or a combination of these treatments. The orthosis providing a static progressive stretch was worn for 30 minutes, with the patient increasing the amount of stretch every 5 minutes as tolerated. Separate 30-minute sessions were used in patients requiring flexion and extension improvement. Results showed an average improvement of 17-degree extensions and 14-degree flexions. Improved results were seen in 4 to 6 weeks, with continued improvement in patients using the orthotic device 3 months or more. There was no change in range of motion in subjects 1 year after discontinuation of the orthosis, suggesting plastic deformation of soft tissue occurred and the elongation of tissue was maintained over time.

According to Morrey et al.,[118] several features of the anatomy of the elbow predispose it to range of motion loss and stiffness after injury. These factors include the congruity and conformity of the ulnohumeral joint, as well as the fact that the anterior aspect of the elbow is traversed by muscle (i.e., brachioradialis) rather than tendons. Additionally, the elbow capsule has a unique response to trauma, resulting in thickening and contracture. The functional arc of motion at the elbow for activities of daily living (ADL) is reported to be between 30 degrees of extension to 130 degrees of flexion.[118]

Manual rehabilitation techniques for improving elbow range of motion include active range of motion, active assisted range of motion, passive range of motion, and joint mobilizations. Elbow joint mobilizations may be used to restore joint arthrokinematics. These include ulnohumeral and radioulnar joint distraction, posterior glides of the ulna, medial and lateral ulnohumeral glides, and dorsal and ventral glides of the proximal radioulnar joint.[13] Shoulder passive range of motion should also be performed early in the rehabilitation process to prevent glenohumeral capsular hypomobility, especially if the injury required prolonged immobilization.

SUMMARY

A complete understanding of the elbow joint's unique anatomy and biomechanics forms the basis for clinical evaluation and formulation of thorough and comprehensive treatment program for patients with elbow dysfunction. The information in this chapter includes key elements of the clinical evaluation, as well as treatment techniques for the entire upper extremity kinetic chain. Integration of these concepts with those outlined in other chapters in this book covering the scapulohumeral and glenohumeral joints ensure a complete rehabilitation effort for all patients with elbow injury.

REFERENCES

1. Morrey BF: The elbow and its disorders, ed 2, Philadelphia, 1993, Saunders.
2. Stroyan M, Wilk KE: The functional anatomy of the elbow complex, J Orthop Sport Phys Ther 17:279-288, 1993.
3. Morrey B, An KN: Articular and ligamentous contributions to the stability of the elbow joint, Am J Sports Med 11:315-319, 1983.
4. Guerra JJ, Timmerman LA: Anatomy, histology, and pathomechanics: elbow injuries in throwing athletes, Oper Tech Sports Med 4(2):69-76, 1996.
5. Andrews JR, Wilk KE, Groh G: Elbow rehabilitation. In Brotzman SB, editor: Clinical orthopaedic rehabilitation, Philadelphia, 1996, Mosby, pp 67-71.
6. Tullos HS, Ryan WJ: Functional anatomy of the elbow. In Zarins B, Andrews JR, Carson WD, editors: Injuries to the throwing arm, Philadelphia, 1985, Saunders.
7. Olsen BS, Søjbjerg JO, Dalstra M, et al: Kinematics of the lateral ligamentous constraints of the elbow joint, J Shoulder Elbow Surg 5:333-341, 1996.
8. Warfel JH: The extremities: muscles and motor points, Philadelphia, 1993, Lea & Febiger.
9. Pappas AM, Zawacki RM, Sullivan TJ: Biomechanics of baseball pitching: a preliminary report, Am J Sports Med 13(4):216-222, 1985.
10. Cain EL, Dugas JR, Wolf RS, et al: Elbow injuries in throwing athletes: a current concepts review, Am J Sports Med 31(4):621-635, 2003.
11. Meister K: Injuries to the shoulder in the throwing athlete. Part I: biomechanics, pathophysiology, classification of injury, Am J Sports Med 28:265-275, 2000.
12. Fleisig GS, Andrews JR, Dillman CJ, et al: Kinetics of baseball pitching with implications about injury mechanisms, Am J Sports Med 23:233, 1995.
13. Ellenbecker TS, Mattalino AJ: The elbow in sport, Champaign, Ill, 1997, Human Kinetics.
14. Kibler WB: Clinical biomechanics of the elbow in tennis: implications for evaluation and diagnosis, Med Sci Sports Exerc 26:1203-1206, 1994.
15. King JW, Brelsford HJ, Tullos HS: Analysis of the pitching arm of the professional baseball pitcher, Clin Orthop Relat Res 67:116-123, 1969.
16. Chinn CJ, Priest JD, Kent BE: Upper extremity range of motion, grip strength, and girth in highly skilled tennis players, Phys Ther 54:474-482, 1974.
17. Ellenbecker TS, Mattalino AJ, Elam EA, et al: Medial elbow laxity in professional baseball pitchers: a bilateral comparison using stress radiography, Am J Sports Med 26(3):420-424, 1998.
18. Ellenbecker TS, Roetert EP: Data from the USTA on range of motion of the elbow and wrist in senior tennis players, Unpublished material, 1994.
19. Glousman RE, Barron J, Jobe FW, et al: An electromyographic analysis of the elbow in normal and injured pitchers with medial collateral ligament insufficiency, Am J Sports Med 20:311-317, 1992.
20. Rhu KN, McCormick J, Jobe FW, et al: An electromyographic analysis of shoulder function in tennis players, Am J Sports Med 16:481-485, 1988.
21. Ellenbecker TS, Roetert EP, Bailie DS, et al: Glenohumeral joint total rotation range of motion in elite tennis players and baseball pitchers, Med Sci Sports Exerc 34(12):2052-2056, 2002.
22. Roetert EP, Ellenbecker TS, Brown SW: Shoulder internal and external rotation range of motion in nationally ranked junior tennis players: a longitudinal analysis, J Strength Cond Res 14(2):140-143, 2000.
23. Kibler WB, Chandler TJ, Livingston BP, et al: Shoulder range of motion in elite tennis players, Am J Sports Med 24(3):279-285, 1996.
24. Priest JD, Jones HH, Nagel DA: Elbow injuries in highly skilled tennis players, J Sports Med 2(3):137-149, 1974.
25. Waslewski GL, Lund P, Chilvers M, et al: MRI evaluation of the ulnar collateral ligament of the elbow in asymptomatic, professional baseball players. Paper presented at the AOSSM Meeting, Orlando, Fla, 2002.
26. Rijke AM, Goitz HT, McCue FC: Stress radiography of the medial elbow ligaments, Radiology 191:213-216, 1994.
27. Kulund DN, Rockwell DA, Brubaker CE: The long term effects of playing tennis, Phys Sportsmed 7:87-92, 1979.
28. Ellenbecker TS: A total arm strength isokinetic profile of highly skilled tennis players, Isokinet Exerc Sci 1:9-21, 1991.

29. Ellenbecker TS, Roetert EP: Isokinetic profile of elbow flexion and extension strength in elite junior tennis players, J Orthop Sports Phys Ther 33(2):79-84, 2003.

30. Ellenbecker TS, Roetert EP: Age specific isokinetic glenohumeral internal and external rotation strength in elite junior tennis players, J Sci Med Sport 6(1):63-70, 2003.

31. Wilk KE, Arrigo CA, Andrews JR: Rehabilitation of the elbow in the throwing athlete, J Orthop Sports Phys Ther 17:305-317, 1993.

32. Magee DJ: Orthopedic physical assessment, ed 3, Philadelphia, 1997, Saunders.

33. Tong HC, Haig AJ, Yamakawa K: The Spurling test and cervical radiculopathy, Spine 27(2):156-159, 2002.

34. Gould JA: The spine. In Gould JA, Davies GJ, editors: Orthopaedic and sports physical therapy, St Louis, 1985, Mosby.

35. McFarland EG, Torpey BM, Carl LA: Evaluation of shoulder laxity, Sports Med 22:264-272, 1996.

36. Jobe FW, Kivitne RS: Shoulder pain in the overhand or throwing athlete, Orthop Rev 18:963-975, 1989.

37. Neer CS: Impingement lesions, Clin Orthop 173:70-77, 1983.

38. Hawkins RJ, Kennedy JC: Impingement syndrome in athletes, Am J Sports Med 8:151-158, 1980.

39. Kibler WB, Uhl TL, Maddux JWQ, et al: Qualitative clinical evaluation of scapular dysfunction: a reliability study, J Shoulder Elbow Surg 11:550-556, 2002.

40. Kibler WB: Role of the scapula in the overhead throwing motion, Contemp Orthop 22(5):525-532, 1991.

41. Kibler WB: The role of the scapula in athletic shoulder function, Am J Sports Med 26(2):325-337, 1998.

42. Ellenbecker TS: Rehabilitation of shoulder and elbow injuries in tennis players, Clin Sports Med 14(1):87-110, 1995.

43. Nirschl RP: Elbow tendinosus/tennis elbow, Clin Sports Med 11:851-870, 1992.

44. Morrey BF: The elbow and its disorders, ed 2, Philadelphia, 1993, Saunders.

45. Safran MR, McGarry MH, Shin S, et al: Effects of elbow flexion and forearm rotation on valgus laxity of the elbow, J Bone Joint Surg Am 87(9):2065-2074, 2005.

46. Andrews JR, Wilk KE, Satterwhite YE, et al: Physical examination of the thrower's elbow, J Orthop Sport Phys Ther 6:296-304, 1993.

47. Kraushaar BS, Nirschl RP: Tendinosus of the elbow (tennis elbow): clinical features and findings of histopathological, immunohistochemical and electron microscopy studies, J Bone Joint Surgery Am 81:259-278, 1999.

48. O'Driscoll SW, Lawton RL, Smith AM: The "moving valgus stress test" for medial collateral ligament tears of the elbow, Am J Sports Med 33(2):231-239, 2005.

49. Nirschl R, Sobel J: Conservative treatment of tennis elbow, Phys Sportsmed 9:43-54, 1981.

50. Carroll R: Tennis elbow: incidence in local league players, Br J Sports Med 15:250-255, 1981.

51. Kamien M: A rational management of tennis elbow, Sports Med 9:173-191, 1990.

52. Kitai E, Itay S, Ruder A, et al: An epidemiological study of lateral epicondylitis in amateur male players, Ann Chir Main 5:113-121, 1986.

53. Hang YS, Peng SM: An epidemiological study of upper extremity injury in tennis players with particular reference to tennis elbow, J Formos Med Assoc 83:307-316, 1984.

54. Priest JD, Jones HH, Tichenor CJC, et al: Arm and elbow changes in expert tennis players, Minn Med 60:399-404, 1977.

55. Winge, S, Jorgensen U, Nielsen AL: Epidemiology of injuries in Danish championship tennis, Int J Sports Med 10:368-371, 1989.

56. Roetert EP, Ellenbecker TS: Complete conditioning for tennis, Champaign, Ill, 2007, Human Kinetics.

57. Runge F: Zur genese unt behand lung bes schreibekramp fes, Berl Klin Woschenschr 10:245, 1873.

58. Cyriax JH, Cyriax PJ: Illustrated manual of orthopaedic medicine, London, 1983, Butterworth.

59. Goldie I: Epicondylitis lateralis humeri, Acta Chir Scand Suppl 339:1, 1964.

60. Leadbetter WB: Cell matrix response in tendon injury, Clin Sports Med 11:533-579, 1922.

61. Boyer MI, Hastings H: Lateral tennis elbow: is there any science out there? J Shoulder Elbow Surg 8:481-491, 1999.

62. Greenbaum B, Itamura J, Vangsness CT, et al: Extensor carpi radialis brevis, J Bone Joint Surg Br 81(5):926-929, 1999.

63. Dijs H, Mortier G, Driessens M, et al: A retrospective study of the conservative treatment of tennis elbow, Acta Belg Med Phys 13:73-77, 1990.

64. Wilson FD, Andrews JR, Blackburn TA: Valgus extension overload in the pitching elbow, Am J Sports Med 11(2):83-88, 1983.

65. Bennett GE: Elbow and shoulder lesions of baseball players, Am J Sur 98:484-492, 1959.

66. Indelicato PA, Jobe FW, Kerlan RK, et al: Correctable elbow lesions in professional baseball players: a review of 25 cases, Am J Sports Med 7:72-75, 1979.

67. Slocum DB: Classification of the elbow injuries from baseball pitching, Am J Sports Med 6:62, 1978.

68. Joyce ME, Jelsma RD, Andrews JR: Throwing injuries to the elbow, Sports Med Arthrosc 3:224-236, 1995.

69. Wolf BR, Altchek DW: Elbow problems in elite tennis players, Tech Shoulder Elbow Surg 4(2):55-68, 2003.

70. Morrey BF: The elbow and its disorders, Philadelphia, 1998, Elsevier.

71. Kobayashhi K, Burton KJ, Rodner C, et al: Lateral compression injuries in the pediatric elbow: Panner's disease and osteochondritis dissecans of the capitellum, J Am Acad Orthop Surg 12(4):246-254, 2004.

72. Labelle H, Guibert R, Joncas J, et al: Lack of scientific evidence for the treatment of lateral epicondylitis of the elbow, J Bone Joint Surg 74-B:646-651, 1992.

73. Bernhang AM, Dehner W, Fogarty C: Tennis elbow: a biomechanical approach, Am J Sports Med 2:235-260, 1974.

74. Rosenthal M: The efficacy of flurbiprofen versus piroxicam in the treatment of acute soft tissue rheumatism, Curr Med Res Opin 9:304-309, 1984.

75. Brattberg G: Acupuncture therapy for tennis elbow, Pain 16:285-288, 1983.

76. Ingham K: Transverse cross friction massage, Phys Sportsmed 9(10):116, 1981.

77. Percy EC, Carson JD: The use of DMSO in tennis elbow and rotator cuff tendinitis: a double blind study, Med Sci Sports Exerc 13:215-219, 1981.

78. Verhaar JAN, Walenkamp GHIM, Kester ADM, et al: Local corticosteroid injection versus Cyriax-type physiotherapy for tennis elbow, J Bone Joint Surg Br 77:128-132, 1995.

79. Nirschl RP, Rodin DM, Ochiai DH, et al: Iontophoretic administration of dexamethasone sodium phosphate for acute epicondylitis: a randomized, double blind, placebo controlled study, Am J Sports Med 31(2):189-195, 2003.

80. Haake M, Konig IR, Decker T, et al: Extracorporeal shock wave therapy in the treatment of lateral epicondylitis: a randomized multi-center study, J Bone Joint Surg 84:1982-1991, 2002.

81. Basford JR, Sheffield CG, Cieslak KR: Laser therapy: a randomized, controlled trial of the effects of low intensity Nd:YAG laser irradiation on lateral epicondylitis, Arch Phys Med Rehabil 81:1504-1510, 2000.

82. Jensen BR, Sjogaard G, Bornmyr S, et al: Intramuscular laser-Doppler flowmetry in the supraspinatus muscle during isometric contractions, Eur J Appl Physiol 71:373-378, 1995.

83. Gam AN, Warming S, Larsen LH, et al: Treatment of myofascial trigger points with ultrasound combined with massage and exercise: a randomized controlled trial, Pain 77(1):73-79, 1998.

84. Svernl AB, Adolfsson L: Non-operative treatment regimen including eccentric training for lateral humeral epicondylalgia, Scand J Med Sci Sports 11(6):328-334, 2001.

85. Croisior JL: An isokinetic eccentric program for management of chronic lateral epicondylar tendinopathy, Br J Sports Med (91)4: 2007.

86. Sullivan PE, Markos PD, Minor MD: An integrated approach to therapeutic exercise: theory and clinical application, Reston, VA, 1982, Reston Publishing Company.

87. Inman VT, Saunders JB de CM, Abbot LC: Observations on the function of the shoulder joint, J Bone Joint Surg Am 26:1-30, 1944.

88. Townsend H, Jobe FW, Pink M, et al: Electromyographic analysis of the glenohumeral muscles during a baseball rehabilitation program, Am J Sports Med 19:264-272, 1992.

89. Ballentyne BT, O'Hare SJ, Paschall JL, et al: Electromyographic activity of selected shoulder muscles in commonly used therapeutic exercises, Phys Ther 73:668-682, 1993.

90. Blackburn TA, McLeod WD, White B, et al: EMG analysis of posterior rotator cuff exercises, J Athl Train 25:40-45, 1990.

91. Ellenbecker TS, Davies GJ: Closed kinetic chain exercise, Champaign, Ill, 2001, Human Kinetics.

92. Bowling RW, Rockar PA: The elbow complex. In Davies GJ, Gould JA, editors: Orthopaedic and sports physical therapy, St Louis, 1985, Mosby, pp 476-496.

93. Fleck SJ, Kraemer WJ: Designing resistance training programs, Champaign, Ill, 1987, Human Kinetics.

94. Adelsberg S: An EMG analysis of selected muscles with rackets of increasing grip size, Am J Sports Med 14:139-142, 1986.

95. Groppel JL, Nirschl RP: A biomechanical and electromyographical analysis of the effects of counter force braces on the tennis player, Am J Sports Med 14:195-200, 1986

96. Andrews JR, Soffer SR: Elbow arthroscopy, St Louis, 1994, Mosby.

97. Andrews JR, Heggland EJH, Fleisig GS, et al: Relationship of ulnar collateral ligament strain to amount of medial olecranon osteotomy, Am J Sports Med 29(6):716-721, 2001.

98. Oglive-Harris DJ, Gordon R, MacKay M: Arthroscopic treatment for posterior impingement in degenerative arthritis of the elbow, Arthroscopy 11(4):437-443, 1995.

99. O'Driscoll SW, Morrey BF: Arthroscopy of the elbow, J Bone Joint Surg 74-A:84-94, 1992.

100. Andrews JR, Timmerman LA: Outcome of elbow surgery in professional baseball players, Am J Sports Med 23:407-4134, 1995.

101. Reddy AS, Kvitne RS, Yocum LA, et al: Arthroscopy of the elbow: a long-term clinical review, Arthroscopy 16(6):588-594, 2000.

102. Conway JE, Jobe FW, Glousman RE, et al: Medial instability of the elbow in throwing athletes, J Bone Joint Surg 74:A(1):67-83, 1992.

103. Davidson PA, Pink M, Perry J, et al: Functional anatomy of the flexor pronator muscle group in relation to the medial collateral ligament of the elbow, Am J Sports Med 23(2):245-250, 1995.

104. Ellenbecker TS, Davies GJ, Rowinski MJ: Concentric versus eccentric isokinetic strengthening of the rotator cuff: objective data versus functional test, Am J Sports Med 16:64-69, 1988.

105. Kuroda S, Sakamaki K: Ulnar collateral ligament tears of the elbow joint, Clin Orthop Rel Res 208:266-271, 1986.

106. Jobe FW, Stark H, Lombardo SJ: Reconstruction of the ulnar collateral ligament in athletes, J Bone Joint Surg 68A:1158-1163, 1986.

107. Dines JS, ElAttrache NS, Conway JE: Clinical outcomes of the DANE TJ technique to treat ulnar collateral liga-

ment insufficiency of the elbow, Am J Sports Med 35:2039-2044, 2007.

108. Reagan WD, Korinek SL, Morrey BF, et al: Biomechanical study of the ligaments around the elbow joint, Clin Orthop 271:170-179, 1991.

109. Jobe FW, ElAttrache NS: Diagnosis and treatment of ulnar collateral ligament injuries in athletes. In Morrey BF, editor: The elbow and its disorders, ed 2, Philadelphia, 1993, Saunders, pp. 566-572.

110. Azar FM, Andrews JR, Wilk KE, et al: Operative treatment of ulnar collateral ligament injuries of the elbow in athletes, Am J Sports Med 28:16-23, 2000.

111. Thompson WH, Jobe FW, Yocum LA, et al: Ulnar collateral ligament reconstruction in athletes: muscle-splitting approach without transposition of the ulnar nerve, 10:152-157, 2001.

112. Rohrbough JT, Altchek DW, Hyman J, et al: Medial collateral ligament reconstruction of the elbow using the docking technique, Am J Sports Med 30:541-548, 2002.

113. Smith RL, Brunolli J: Shoulder kinesthesia after anterior glenohumeral joint dislocation, Phys Ther 69(2):106-112, 1989.

114. Wilk KE, Azar FM, Andrews JR: Conservative and operative rehabilitation of the elbow in sports, Sports Med Arthrosc 3:237-258, 1995.

115. Bennett JB, Green MS, Tullos HS: Surgical management of chronic medial elbow instability, Clin Orthop Rel Res 278:62-68, 1992.

116. Vitale MA, Ahmad CS: The outcome of elbow ulnar collateral ligament reconstruction in overhead athletes: a systematic review, Am J Sports Med 36:1193-1205, 2008.

117. Bonutti PM, Windau JE, Ables BA, et al: Static progressive stretch to reestablish elbow range of motion, Clin Orthop Rel Res 303:128-134, 1994.

118. Morrey BF, Askew LJ, An KN: A biomechanical study of normal functional elbow motion, J Bone Joint Surg 63A:872-877, 1981.

119. Wright RW, Steger-May K, Wasserlawf BL, et al: Elbow range of motion in professional baseball pitchers, Am J Sports Med 34(2):190-193, 2006.

11-1

Interval Tennis Program*

INTERVAL TENNIS PROGRAM GUIDELINES

- Begin at stage indicated by your therapist or physician.
- Do not progress or continue program if joint pain is present.
- Always stretch your shoulder, elbow, and wrist before and after exercise during the interval program, and perform a whole-body dynamic warm-up before performing the interval tennis program.
- Play on alternate days, giving your body a recovery day between sessions.
- Do not use a wallboard or backboard because it leads to exaggerated muscle contraction without rest between strokes.
- Ice your injured arm after each stage of the interval tennis program.
- It is highly recommended to have your stroke mechanics formally evaluated by a United States Professional Tennis Association (USPTA) tennis teaching professional.

- Do not attempt to impart heavy topspin or underspin to your ground strokes until later stages in the interval program.
- Contact your therapist or physician if you have questions or problems with the interval program.
- Do not continue to play if you encounter localized joint pain.

Preliminary Stage: Foam ball impacts beginning with ball feeds from a partner. Perform 20 to 25 forehands and backhands, assessing initial tolerance to ground strokes only. Presence of pain or abnormal movement patterns in this stage indicates that the patient is not ready to progress to the actual interval tennis program. In this case continued rehabilitation should be emphasized.

Interval Tennis Program: Perform each stage [X] times before progressing to the next stage. Do not progress to the next stage if you have pain or excessive fatigue on your previous outing. Instead, remain at the previous stage or level until you can perform that part of the program without fatigue or pain.

---

*From Ellenbecker TS, Wilk KE, Reinold MM, et al: Use of interval return programs for shoulder rehabilitation. In Ellenbecker TS: Shoulder rehabilitation: non-operative treatment. New York, 2006, Theime.

Stage 1	A. Have a partner feed 20 forehand ground strokes to you from the net. (Partner must use a slow, looping feed that results in a waist-high ball bounce for player contact.)
	B. Have a partner feed 20 backhand ground strokes as in stage 1A.
	C. Rest 5 minutes.
	D. Repeat 20 forehand and backhand feeds as previously described.
Stage 2	A. Begin as in stage 1, with partner feeding 10 forehands and 10 backhands from the net.
	B. Rally with partner from baseline, hitting controlled ground strokes until you have hit 50 to 60 strokes. (Alternate between forehand and backhand and allow 20 to 30 seconds to rest after every two to three rallies.)
	C. Rest 5 minutes.
	D. Repeat stage 2B.
Stage 3	A. Rally ground strokes from the baseline for 15 minutes.
	B. Rest 5 minutes.
	C. Hit 10 forehand and 10 backhand volleys, emphasizing a contact point in front of body.
	D. Rally ground strokes for 15 additional minutes from the baseline.
	E. Hit 10 forehand and 10 backhand volleys as previously described.
Preserve interval: (perform before stage 4)	(Note: This can be performed off court and is meant solely to determine readiness for progression into stage 4 of the interval tennis program.)
	A. After stretching, with racquet in hand, perform serving motion for 10 to 15 repetitions without a ball.
	B. Using a foam ball, hit 10 to 15 serves without concern for performance result (only focusing on form, contact point, and the presence or absence of symptoms).
Stage 4	A. Hit 20 minutes of ground strokes, mixing in volleys using a 70% ground strokes/30% volleys format.
	B. Perform 5 to 10 simulated serves without a ball.
	C. Perform 5 to 10 serves using a foam ball.
	D. Perform 10 to 15 serves using a standard tennis ball at approximately 75% effort.
	E. Finish with 5 to 10 minutes of ground strokes.
Stage 5	A. Hit 30 minutes of ground strokes, mixing in volleys using a 70% ground strokes/30% volleys format.
	B. Perform 5 to 10 serves using a foam ball.
	C. Perform 10 to 15 serves using a standard tennis ball at approximately 75% effort.
	D. Rest 5 minutes.
	E. Perform 10 to 15 additional serves as in stage 5C.
	F. Finish with 15 to 20 minutes of ground strokes.
Stage 5A	A. Repeat stage 5 (listed previously) increasing the number of serves to 20 to 25 instead of 10 to 15.
	B. Before resting between serving sessions, have a partner feed easy short lobs to attempt a controlled overhead smash.
Stage 6	Before attempting match play, complete stages 1 to 5 without pain or excess fatigue in the upper extremity. Continue to progress the amount of time rallying with ground strokes and volleys in addition to increasing the number of serves per workout until 60 to 80 overall serves can be performed interspersed throughout a workout. Remember that an average of up to 120 serves can be performed in a tennis match; therefore be prepared to gradually increase the number of serves in the interval program before full competitive play is engaged.

11-2

Interval Throwing Program for Baseball Players*

PHASE I: FLAT GROUND THROWING FOR BASEBALL PITCHERS		
45-foot phase	Step 1	A. Warm-up throwing
		B. 45 feet (25 throws)
		C. Rest (5 to 10 minutes)
		D. Warm-up throwing
		E. 45 feet (25 throws)
	Step 2	A. Warm-up throwing
		B. 45 feet (25 throws)
		C. Rest (5 to 10 minutes)
		D. Warm-up throwing
		E. 45 feet (25 throws)
		F. Rest (5 to 10 minutes)
		G. Warm-up throwing
		H. 45 feet (25 throws)
60-foot phase	Step 3	A. Warm-up throwing
		B. 60 feet (25 throws)
		C. Rest (5 to 10 minutes)
		D. Warm-up throwing
		E. 60 feet (25 throws)
	Step 4	A. Warm-up throwing
		B. 60 feet (25 throws)
		C. Rest (5 to 10 minutes)
		D. Warm-up throwing
		E. 60 feet (25 throws)
		F. Rest (5 to 10 minutes)
		G. Warm-up throwing
		H. 60 feet (25 throws)
90-foot phase	Step 5	A. Warm-up throwing
		B. 90 feet (25 throws)
		C. Rest (5 to 10 minutes)
		D. Warm-up throwing
		E. 90 feet (25 throws)
	Step 6	A. Warm-up throwing
		B. 90 feet (25 throws)
		C. Rest (5 to 10 minutes)
		D. Warm-up throwing
		E. 90 feet (25 throws)
		F. Rest (5 to 10 minutes)
		G. Warm-up throwing
		H. 90 feet (25 throws)

*From Reinold MM, Wilk KE, Reed J, et al: Interval sport programs: guidelines for baseball, tennis, and golf, J Orthop Phys Ther 32:293-298, 2002.

PHASE I: FLAT GROUND THROWING FOR BASEBALL PITCHERS—cont'd

120-foot phase	Step 7	A. Warm-up throwing
		B. 120 feet (25 throws)
		C. Rest (5 to 10 minutes)
		D. Warm-up throwing
		E. 120 feet (25 throws)
	Step 8	A. Warm-up throwing
		B. 120 feet (25 throws)
		C. Rest (5 to 10 minutes)
		D. Warm-up throwing
		E. 120 feet (25 throws)
		F. Rest (5 to 10 minutes)
		G. Warm-up throwing
		H. 120 feet (25 throws)
150-foot phase	Step 9	A. Warm-up throwing
		B. 150 feet (25 throws)
		C. Rest (5 to 10 minutes)
		D. Warm-up throwing
		E. 150 feet (25 throws)
	Step 10	A. Warm-up throwing
		B. 150 feet (25 throws)
		C. Rest (5 to 10 minutes)
		D. Warm-up throwing
		E. 150 feet (25 throws)
		F. Rest (5 to 10 minutes)
		G. Warm-up throwing
		H. 150 feet (25 throws)
180-foot phase	Step 11	A. Warm-up throwing
		B. 180 feet (25 throws)
		C. Rest (5 to 10 minutes)
		D. Warm-up throwing
		E. 180 feet (25 throws)
	Step 12	A. Warm-up throwing
		B. 180 feet (25 throws)
		C. Rest (5 to 10 minutes)
		D. Warm-up throwing
		E. 180 feet (25 throws)
		F. Rest (5 to 10 minutes)
		G. Warm-up throwing
		H. 180 feet (25 throws)
	Step 13	A. Warm-up throwing
		B. 180 feet (25 throws)
		C. Rest (5 to 10 minutes)
		D. Warm-up throwing
		E. 180 feet (25 throws)
		F. Rest (5 to 10 minutes)
		G. Warm-up throwing
		H. 180 feet (20 throws)
		I. Rest (5 to 10 minutes)
		J. Warm-up throwing
		K. 15 throws progressing from 120 to 90 feet
	Step 14	Return to respective position or progress to step 14 (following).

All throws should be on an arc with a crow hop.

Warm-up throws consist of 10 to 20 throws at approximately 30 feet.

Throwing program should be performed every other day, three times per week unless otherwise specified by your physician or rehabilitation specialist.

Perform each step [X] times before progressing to next step.

PHASE I: FLAT GROUND THROWING FOR BASEBALL PITCHERS—cont'd

	Step 14	A. Warm-up throwing
		B. Throw 60 feet (10 to 15 throws)
		C. Throw 90 feet (10 throws)
		D. Throw 120 feet (10 throws)
		E. Throw 60 feet (flat ground) using pitching mechanics (20 to 30 throws)
	Step 15	A. Warm-up throwing
		B. Throw 60 feet (10 to 15 throws)
		C. Throw 90 feet (10 throws)
		D. Throw 120 feet (10 throws)
		E. Throw 60 feet (flat ground) using pitching mechanics (20 to 30 throws)
		F. Throw 60 to 90 feet (10 to 15 throws)
		G. Throw 60 feet (flat ground) using pitching mechanics (20 throws)
	Step 16	Progress to phase II—Throwing off the mound
		45 feet = 13.7 meters
		60 feet = 18.3 meters
		90 feet = 27.4 meters
		120 feet = 36.6 meters
		150 feet = 45.7 meters
		180 feet = 54.8 meters

Interval Throwing Program: Phase II—Throwing Off the Mound*

Stage 1—fastballs only	Step 1	Interval throwing
		15 throws off mound 50%†
	Step 2	Interval throwing
		30 throws off mound 50%
	Step 3	Interval throwing
		45 throws off mound 50%
		Use interval throwing 120 feet (36.6 meters) phase as warm-up
	Step 4	Interval throwing
		60 throws off mound 50%
	Step 5	Interval throwing
		70 throws off mound 50%
	Step 6	45 throws off mound 50%
		30 throws off mound 75%
	Step 7	30 throws off mound 50%
		45 throws off mound 75%
	Step 8	10 throws off mound 50%
		65 throws off mound 75%
Stage 2—fastballs only	Step 9	60 throws off mound 75%
		15 throws in batting practice
	Step 10	50 to 60 throws off mound 75%
		30 throws in batting practice
	Step 11	45 to 50 throws off mound 75%
		45 throws in batting practice
Stage 3	Step 12	30 throws off mound 75% warm-up
		15 throws off mound 50% (begin breaking balls)
		45 to 60 throws in batting practice (fastball only)
	Step 13	30 throws off mound 75%
		30 breaking balls 75%
		30 throws in batting practice
	Step 14	30 throws off mound 75%
		60 to 90 throws in batting practice (gradually increase breaking balls)
	Step 15	Simulated game progressing by 15 throws per workout (pitch count)

*Important: All throwing off the mound should be done in the presence of your pitching coach or sport biomechanist to stress proper throwing mechanics. Use a speed gun to aid in effort control.
†Percentage effort.

Postoperative Protocol for Elbow Arthroscopy and Removal of Loose Bodies

Acute phase	Primary goals:
	1. Reduce pain and postoperative edema.
	2. Regain joint range of motion and muscle length.
	3. Initiate submaximal resistive exercise as tolerated.
Postoperative days 1 and 2	A. Removal of bulky postoperative dressing and replace with Ace wrap.
	B. Use electric stimulation and ice to decrease pain and inflammation.
	C. Initiate range-of-motion exercise for the glenohumeral joint, elbow, forearm, and wrist.
	D. Initiate submaximal strengthening exercises including the following:
	1. Putty
	2. Isometric elbow and wrist flexion and extension
	3. Isometric forearm pronation and supination
Postoperative days 2 to 7	A. Perform range-of-motion and joint mobilization to terminal ranges for the elbow, forearm, and wrist. (Avoid overaggressive elbow extension passive range of motion.)
	B. Begin progressive-resistance exercise program with 0 to 1 lb weight and three sets of 15 repetitions.
	1. Wrist flexion curls
	2. Wrist extension curls
	3. Radial deviation
	4. Ulnar deviation
	5. Forearm pronation
	6. Forearm supination
	C. Upper body ergometer
Intermediate phase	Primary goals:
	1. Begin total arm strength training program.
	2. Emphasize full elbow range of motion.
Postoperative day 7 to week 3	A. Continue progressive resistance exercise program adding the following:
	1. Elbow extension
	2. Elbow flexion
	3. Isolated rotator cuff program (Jobe exercises)
	4. Seated row
	5. Manual and isotonic scapular program
	6. Closed chain upper extremity program
Advanced/return-to-activity phase	Primary goals:
	1. Begin advance strengthening progression of distal upper extremity.
	2. Prepare patient for return to functional activity with simulation of joint angles and muscular demands inherent in intended sport activity.

Postoperative weeks 4 to 8

    A. Introduce isokinetic exercise using wrist flexion and extension and forearm pronation and supination movement patterns.

    B. Add upper extremity plyometrics with medicine balls.

    C. Perform isokinetic test to formally assess distal strength.

    D. Begin interval sport return program.

    1. Criterion for advancement:

    a. Full, pain-free range of motion

    b. Return of muscle strength at 85% to 100%

    c. No provocation of pain on clinical examination

    E. Perform upper extremity strength and flexibility maintenance program.

Postoperative Rehabilitation After Chronic Ulnar Collateral Ligament Reconstruction Using Autogenous Graft

Immediate postoperative phase weeks 0 to 3	Primary goals:
	1. Protect healing tissue.
	2. Decrease pain and inflammation.
	3. Retard muscular atrophy.
Postoperative week 1	1. Use posterior splint at 90-degrees elbow flexion.
	2. Perform wrist active range-of-motion extension and flexion.
	3. Wear elbow compression dressing (2 to 3 days).
	4. Perform exercises such as gripping exercises, wrist range of motion, shoulder isometrics (except shoulder external rotation), and biceps isometrics.
	5. Apply cryotherapy.
Postoperative week 2	1. Apply functional brace (300 to 1000).
	2. Initiate wrist isometrics.
	3. Initiate elbow flexion and extension isometrics.
	4. Continue all exercises previously described.
Postoperative week 3	1. Advance the brace 150 to 1100 (gradually increase range of motion; 50 extension/100 flexion per week).
Intermediate phase weeks 4 to 8	Goals:
	1. Gradually increase range of motion.
	2. Promote healing of repaired tissue.
	3. Regain and improve muscular strength.
Postoperative week 4	1. Set functional brace at (100 to 1200).
	2. Begin light resistance exercises for arm (1 lb) (i.e., wrist curls, wrist extensions, wrist pronation and supination, elbow extension and flexion).
	3. Progress shoulder program; emphasize rotator cuff strengthening. (Avoid external rotation until week 6 [for 1 hour per week].)
Postoperative week 6	1. Set functional brace at (00 to 1300); active range of motion should be 00 14V (without brace).
	2. Progress elbow-strengthening exercises.
	3. Initiate shoulder external rotation strengthening.
	4. Progress shoulder program.
Advanced strengthening phase weeks 9 to 13	Goals:
	1. Increase strength, power, and endurance.
	2. Maintain full elbow range of motion.
	3. Gradually initiate sporting activities.
Postoperative week 9	1. Initiate eccentric elbow flexion and extension.
	2. Continue isotonic program (forearm and wrist).
	3. Continue shoulder program (Throwers Ten Program).
	4. Practice manual-resistance diagonal patterns.
	5. Initiate plyometric exercise program.

Postoperative week 11	1. Continue all exercises listed previously.
	2. Consider beginning light sport activities (e.g., golf, swimming).
Return to activity phase weeks 14 to 26	Goals:
	1. Continue to increase strength, power, and endurance of upper extremity musculature.
	2. Gradually return to sport activities.
Postoperative week 14	1. Initiate interval throwing program (immediate postoperative phase).
	2. Continue strengthening program.
	3. Place emphasis on elbow and wrist strengthening and flexibility exercises.
Postoperative weeks 22 to 26	1. Return to competitive throwing.

Dysfunction, Evaluation, and Treatment of the Wrist and Hand

Prehensile function of the hand is interdependent on the shoulder complex, joint stability of the wrist and upper arm, efficient tendon gliding, and accurate feedback from the nerve. The same principles of stability and mobility and rhythm and balance in the shoulder complex also apply to the wrist and hand. The restoration of function requires the knowledge of these complex anatomic relationships and the application of skilled rehabilitative efforts.

This chapter focuses on special considerations of the articular, the musculotendinous, the neurovascular, and the lymphatic systems of the wrist and hand. Abnormal postural observations are compared with normal resting postures and with changes with dynamic movement. Specific clinical tests are described that contribute to the validation of these clinical observations. General principles of assessing wrist and hand dysfunction are reviewed, and a classification system for hand imbalances is discussed. Finally, two case studies are provided to explain wrist and hand pathologic condition and intervention. The medical diagnosis, careful history intake, and the soft tissue response to the condition, seen as abnormal postures, are discussed as paramount to guiding the therapeutic intervention.

ARTICULAR STRUCTURES

Kinematic effects from muscle loading affect the stability and mobility of each ascending and descending joint. For example, activities that involve reaching and lifting require proximal joint stabilization and in turn affect the quantity of distal joint mobility. Conversely, the distal function of grasping and holding large objects affects the response of the proximal joints to elevate and lift.

Clinical Tip
Hand strength requires proximal shoulder stability as seen in the case of diminished grip strength on the same side of those patients with a rotator cuff injury or humeral fracture.

Anatomic positions at rest are influenced by the skeletal architecture and its corresponding neuromuscular system. The skeletal design of convexity and concavity contributes to the amount of joint stability. The orientation and matrix of the capsular fibers also contribute to joint stability. When the joint is congruous, a high degree of stability occurs and the need for extraarticular stability is reduced. The relationship of bone length, size, and joint configuration determines the shape and structure of the hand. Three arches comprise the overall structure. The 27 bones and corresponding joints define the arches and direct the complex movements that contribute to manipulation and prehension. One arch is longitudinal, and two are transverse (Figure 12-1).

The transverse arches produce the palmar concavity or cupping of the hand. The proximal transverse arch is located at the distal carpal row, is somewhat fixed, and has the capitate as the central landmark. The distal transverse arch passes through the metacarpal heads and is more mobile. The arches are connected by the fixed longitudinal arch that passes through the central carpus and the second and third metacarpals distal to the middle digits.[1] The specific joint arrangement and the inherent soft tissue mobility contribute to movement around an axis, and each joint has a profound effect on the kinematic chain. That is, the combined motions of multiple joints working together are influenced by the flexibility of each individual joint. Some joints have more innate mobility and extensive range of motion; those with less mobility have smaller arcs of motion. These relationships create an expected rhythm and balance that are predicable and consistent. As seen in an isolated joint injury, the normal patterns of movement change and the surrounding proximal and distal joints will compensate. The kinematic chain of the upper extremity is easily altered when the adjacent joints overcompensate to accommodate for the primary joint restriction. The musculotendinous system contracts and moves the joints in the path of least resistance, compensating for the loss of an isolated joint motion in an effort to accomplish the desired function. The principles of mobility and stability, along with musculotendinous accommodation to the path of least resistance, contribute to the concept of imbalance. When postural imbalance is identified,

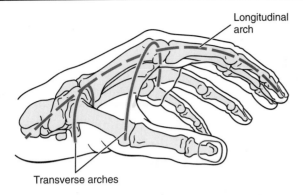

Figure 12-1 Transverse and longitudinal arches of the hand (lateral view). (From Magee DJ: Orthopaedic physical assessment, ed 5, St Louis, 2008, Saunders.)

the evaluation can be directed to a specific joint within the imbalanced kinematic chain. The identified joint can be the starting position or the set point of change to assess the possible contributors of dysfunction.

> ### Clinical Tip
> The presence of a hyperextended metacarpal-pha-langeal (MP) joint during dynamic activity may be a result of proximal interphalangeal (PIP) stiffness and the compensation for the tip of the finger to clear an object.

Distal Radial-Ulnar Joint

With the hand at rest and the forearm on the table, observable landmarks exist. The ulnar styloid is the most prominent protuberance on the dorsum of the proximal forearm. Distal to the styloid is the ulnar carpal fovea. This small hollow depression can be palpated to determine the tenderness of the extensor carpi ulnaris (ECU) and ulnotriquetral ligament structures. The more medial aspect of the ulnar styloid is the depression between the radius and ulna. Pain in the middle of the distal wrist during activity maybe an indication of pathologic condition of the radioulnar ligament.

The radioulnar joint is a biaxial ellipsoid joint and has two supporting ligaments described as the dorsal and volar radio-ulnar ligaments (Figure 12-2). The radius and ulna move in relationship to the carpus. During supination and pronation, the radius pivots around the ascending and descending glide of the ulna. In extreme supination, the ulna descends and the styloid is absent.

The triangular fibrocartilage complex (TFCC) is comprised of the articular disc and ligament connections from the ulna to the radius and ulnar carpus (Figure 12-3). The ulnocarpal portion of the TFCC is composed of the discus articularis and the ulnar-lunate and ulnar-triquetral ligaments. Frequently, the two ligaments are referred to the *disk carpal ligaments.* The

floor of the ECU tendon sheath broadly connects with the TFCC and provides a continuous gliding surface across the entire distal face of the radius and ulna, allowing for flexion-extension and translational movements (Figure 12-4).

Abnormal postures should be examined by comparing asymmetries between both hands and wrists. During assessment of the dorsal forearm, an excessive prominent ulnar head, ulnar sag, or ECU displacement are indications of pathologic condition of soft tissue supports. The dysfunctional arthro-kinemechanics of the distal radioulnar joint and the TFCC can limit the range of motion for supination and pronation, as well as the load shift and stabilization required for torque tasks. Common patient complaints are pain on the ulnar side of the wrist and forearm, as well as joint clicking during pinch, grip, and carry tasks.

Radiocarpal Joint

The radial head and styloid are palpable. Lister's tubercle can be located and palpated on the dorsum of the distal radius. In the moving hand, the dorsal wrist creases are observed at rest. During active wrist extension, the creases appear as skinfolds that run across the wrist and correspond with the underlying carpal anatomy.

The radiocarpal (RC) joint is a condyloid articulation of the radial head and the corresponding scaphoid and lunate. The radial head has a separate fossa for the scaphoid and lunate. Wrist flexion, extension, radial and ulnar deviation, and the forearm pronation and supination are controlled by the contraction of extrinsic muscles. Radial deviation results in flexion of the scaphoid and the trapezium. The scaphoid flexes about 15 degrees and influences the lunate to palmarly flex because of the attachments of the scapholunate ligament. The lunate moves in an ulnar direction until it rests on the TFCC. The entire proximal row rotates into flexion and shortens to allow radial deviation of the wrist.

In ulnar deviation of the wrist, the scaphoid dorsiflexes and is pulled into a longitudinal direction. Simultaneously, the lunate extends approximately 20 degrees. The hamate rotates to an inferior position and influences the triquetrum to move in a dorsiflexed position. The lunate is in a suspended state of dynamic antagonistic balance between the scaphoid and triquetrum. When the balance is interrupted, the lunate will flex toward the direction of the intact ligament. In the event of injury to the ulnar supports from the triquetrum, the lunate has a tension bias to move toward the scaphoid. With an injury to the scapholunate ligament, the lunate flexes in the direction of the triquetrum.

The balance of the wrist and hand occurs when the third metacarpal is aligned with the longitudinal line of the radius. Imbalances can be seen with bony malunion of the radius as the longitudinal and transverse arches will deviate. A silver fork deformity is seen in a Colles' fracture in which the wrist or forearm has a curve like that of the back of a fork. In the anterior-posterior view, the carpus dips below the radial head and contributes to the abnormal curve. In the lateral view, the longitudinal line is radially deviated. A Maisonneuve's sign is

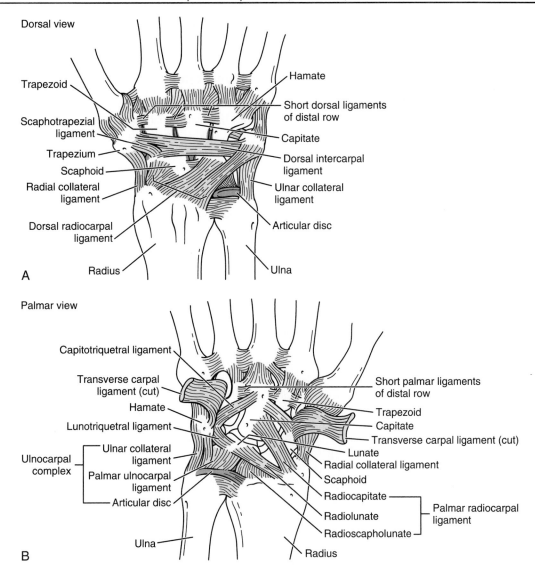

Figure 12-2 Ligaments of the wrist. **A,** Dorsal aspect of the right wrist. **B,** Palmar aspect of the right wrist. The transverse carpal ligament has been cut and reflected to show the underlying ligaments. (Redrawn from Neumann DA: Kinesiology of the musculoskeletal system: foundations for physical rehabilitation, St Louis, 2002, Mosby.)

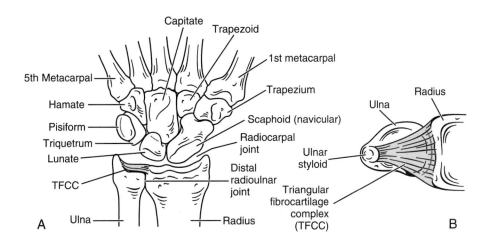

Figure 12-3 Bones and triangular fibrocartilage complex (TFCC). **A,** Palmar view. **B,** End view of TFCC and radius and ulna. (From Magee DJ: Orthopaedic physical assessment, ed 5, St Louis, 2008, Saunders.)

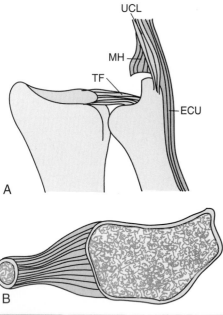

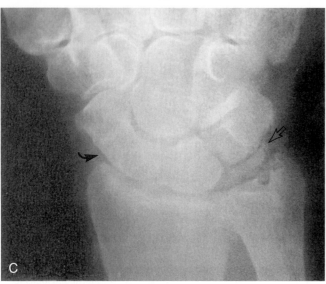

Figure 12-4 Triangular fibrocartilage complex (TFCC). **A,** This complex includes the triangular fibrocartilage (articular disc, TF), the meniscus homolog (MH), the ulnar collateral ligament (UCL), and the dorsal and volar radioulnar ligaments (not shown). The extensor carpi ulnaris (ECU) tendon is shown. **B,** The TF (dotted area) attaches to the ulnar border of the radius and the distal ulna. The triangular shape is evident on this transverse section through the radius and ulnar styloid. The volar aspect of the wrist is at the top. **C,** Chondrocalcinosis. Heavy calcification of the articular cartilage (curved arrow) and area of the TF complex (open arrow) is seen. (From Weissman BNW, Sledge CB: Orthopaedic radiology, Philadelphia, 1986, Saunders.)

found when hyperextension of the fingers occurs with attempts at wrist extension. The cause of this imbalance is the articular misalignment of the radius, other carpal dysfunctions, and/or extrinsic muscle elongation that may contribute to motor inefficiency of the wrist extensors. The extensor digitorum communis (EDC) will compensate for poor wrist extension resulting

in hyperextension of the MP joint of the fingers and flattening of the transverse arches.

Carpal Joints

Wrist kinematics is a complex pattern of movement that begins with the distal radial head and the seating of the scaphoid and lunate. Radial head inclination, tilt, and angulations have a profound effect on the subsequent motion of the carpus. Eight carpal bones exist: four bones in the distal row and four bones in the proximal row (see Figure 12-3). Each carpal bone has six surfaces except for the pisiform. They are synovial joints, and their opposing surfaces provide only a small amount of gliding movement.

The distal row of carpal bones consists of the trapezium, the trapezoid, the capitate, and the hamate. Moving from radial to ulnar deviation, the distal row translates from a palmar to a dorsal position. Total flexion and extension motion of the wrist is divided equally between RC and midcarpal joints.

The proximal row of carpal bones consists of the scaphoid, the lunate, and the triquetrum. More motion occurs in the proximal row than the distal row of the carpal bones. Moving from radial to ulnar deviation, the proximal row moves from flexion to extension, whereas the distal row translates in a palmar to dorsal direction and rotates radial to ulnar.

The tubercles of the scaphoid and the pisiform can be palpated on the volar aspect of the wrist. The two protuberances are observable in most people. The carpus adds length from the radius and ulna to the base of the MP joints of the hand. The carpal bones cannot be seen from the dorsum of the hand but can be envisaged just proximal to the expanse of the hand.

The loss of normal carpal motion and degenerative joint disease can be acquired primarily from direct trauma or secondarily over time from an articular or ligament injury. Carpal collapse can lead to further hand deformity and functional limitations. Scapholunate advanced collapse (SLAC) refers to a specific pattern of osteoarthritis and subluxation that results from untreated chronic scapholunate dissociation or from chronic scaphoid nonunion. Intercalated segment instability, either dorsally (DISI) or volarly (VISI), are deformities that occur from scapholunate or lunate-triquetral ligament loss. These conditions will generally have limited painful range of motion.

Clinical tests can be used to identify potential wrist pathologic conditions in the acute and subacute stages. The scapholunate ballottement test, the lunotriquetral ballottement test, and the Kleinman shear test are performed by holding one of the carpal bones with the thumb and index fingers and pushing the articulating carpal bone in a dorsal or volar direction. Testing should be done on both wrists, and a positive finding occurs with the client reporting associated pain. The Watson scaphoid shift test is performed by stabilizing the scaphoid tubercle on the dorsal surface in the anatomic snuffbox and the scapholunate ligament at the base of the thumb on the volar surface (Figure 12-5). A positive finding occurs when a painful click is palpated with radial deviation of the wrist.

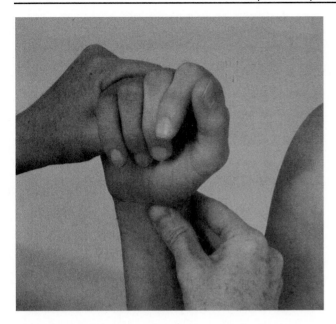

Figure 12-5 Watson scaphoid shift test. (From Magee DJ: Orthopaedic physical assessment, ed 5, St Louis, 2008, Saunders.)

Table 12-1	Thumb CMC Movements*	
CMC	**Acceptable Terms**	**Common Descriptions**
Extension	Radial abduction, radial extension	Hitchhiking position
Flexion	Palmar flexion	Touching the base of the little finger
Abduction	Palmar abduction	Away from the palm
Adduction	Adduction	Lateral pinch
Circumduction	Opposition, pronation	Thumb rotation

CMC, Carpal-metacarpal.

*The planes of motion are in relation to the palm, flexion-extension movements are parallel, and abduction-adduction movements are perpendicular.

Carpal-Metacarpal Joints

Five carpal-metacarpal (CMC) joints are found in each hand. The first and fifth joints have the most motion, whereas the second through fourth joints are stable posts for manipulating objects. In a healthy hand, the base of the first metacarpal can be palpated as only a slight prominence of the CMC joint. The thenar eminence extends over the metacarpal bone on the palmar surface; the web space fills the expanse between the first and the second metacarpals. On the volar surface the thenar eminence is the largest muscle wad in the hand and covers the entire metacarpal bone.

The first CMC joint is a saddle joint formed by the trapezium and metacarpal bones. It is a biaxial joint with opposing surfaces shaped like a saddle. The concave and convex articulations permit movement in two different planes. Because many variations in the names of CMC joint motions exist, it will be described as the relationship between the first and second metacarpals rather than describing their movements by anatomic planes. The movements of the CMC joint are extension in a radial direction, flexion in an ulnar direction, abduction away from the palm or the same direction as wrist flexion, and adduction toward the palm. Axial rotation, commonly referred to as *circumduction* or *opposition,* is observed when the thumb is flexed and abducted across the palm toward a digit. Circumduction movement is a combination of planar movements directed by the supportive ligamentous structures. It can be observed by watching the thumbnail pronate during CMC abduction and flexion. The names of the CMC joint movements are provided in Table 12-1.

Important ligament attachments to the CMC joint of the thumb include three oblique capsular ligaments. The anterior, posterior, and radial capsular ligaments attach the first meta-carpal to the trapezium. The anterior capsular ligament is the strongest of the three and is taut in CMC extension and lax in CMC flexion. Laxity in these capsular ligaments allows for circumduction and rotation of the CMC joint. The laxity on one side of the capsule during extrinsic muscle pull leads to a tightening of another portion of the capsule. The taut aspect of the capsule pulls on the base of the metacarpal and it shifts to opposite the tightness and forces a rotation. The capsular pattern guides and modifies the action of the extrinsic forces that are exerted by the muscles. This complex combination of extrinsic and intrinsic movements permits the intricate fine-motor prehension observed in the thumb.[2]

The first and fifth CMC joints have similar joint characteristics. The thumb has more motion and is a major contributor to grasp and prehension. The fifth CMC joint is mobile and is most pronounced during a tight composite grasp. The meta-carpal bone descends as the CMC flexes and the transverse distal arch becomes more curved. Lack of CMC joint motion limits the mobility of the fifth metacarpal bone and compromises the distal transverse arch. As a result, the timing and the ability of the small finger to completely flex or extend will alter.

The CMC joint of the thumb is the most common arthritic joint of the hand. It is present in a majority of postmenopausal women, and one third of women older than 40 years have radiographic changes.[3] Initial resting imbalances of the first CMC joint show joint laxity, imbalance of the surrounding ligament and abnormal tension from the extrinsic tendons. When the joint capsule becomes permanently weakened by joint disease, the direction of instability will be posterior; this is most often observed with the abnormal prominent head of the proximal metacarpal near the wrist. The posterior CMC joint subluxation over time will forwardly tilt the metacarpal. The lack of stability at the CMC joint alters the forces at the MP joint and increases volar capsule laxity. With the loss of MP dynamic stabilizers during pinch, the joint cascades into hyperextension and simultaneous interphalangeal (IP) flexion. This zigzag resting posture is classified as a *swan neck deformity.* If this posture is observed during active pinch it is called *Jeanne sign,* which indicates the presence of adductor pollicis weakness. The final result can be seen in the chronic imbalance and fixed position of MP hyperextension and IP flexion.[4,5]

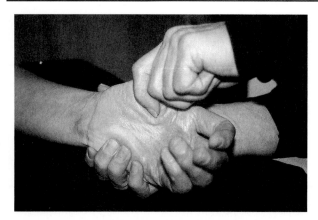

Figure 12-6 The grind test for crepitus at the carpometacarpal joint involves compressing the joint while gently rotating the metacarpal at the carpometacarpal joint. (From Biese J: Therapist's evaluation and conservative management of rheumatoid arthritis in the hand and wrist. In Mackin EJ, Callahan AD, Skirven TM et al, editors: Rehabilitation of the hand and upper extremity, ed 5, St Louis, 2002, Mosby.)

The CMC joint of the thumb can be assessed for degenerative articular changes. The grind test identifies mild to severe disease by compressing and rotating the first metacarpal bone on the trapezium (Figure 12-6). A positive finding occurs when the patient has crepitation and increased pain with this maneuver.

Several deformities of the CMC joint of the thumb have been associated with rheumatoid arthritis.[6,7] Type 1 is referred to as a *Boutonniere deformity* in which the MP joint is flexed and the IP joint is hyperextended (Figure 12-7, *A*). The pathologic condition originates at the MP joint with synovitis, dorsal hood disruption, and subluxation of the extensor pollicis longus (EPL) tendon ulnarly. The distal phalanx is drawn into extension as the proximal phalanx subluxes dorsally. A type 1 deformity is the most common thumb abnormality in persons with rheumatoid arthritis. Type 2 results in hyperextension of the MP with CMC joint subluxation. Type 3 is a swan neck deformity in which the MP joint is hyperextended and the IP joint is flexed (Figure 12-7, *B*). This is the second most common type of thumb disfigurement in persons with rheumatoid arthritis. CMC joint synovitis initiates the subluxation of the first metacarpal radially and dorsally. The first metacarpal adducts and, in combination with volar plate laxity, results in hyperextension of the MP joint. Shortening of the lateral bands and additional pull from the flexor pollicis longus (FPL) draws the distal phalanx into flexion. Type 4 is analogous to skier's thumb or gamekeeper's thumb. The MP joint synovitis initiates the pathologic condition, resulting in laxity of the ulnar collateral ligament (UCL) and possible adduction of the first metacarpal. Type 5 is similar to type 3 deformities, except the adduction of the first metacarpal does not occur. Type 5 is initiated at the MP joint, fostering volar plate laxity, subsequent MP hyperextension, and IP joint flexion. Type 6 involves isolated IP joint and/or MP joint destruction with subluxation, as a result of bone resorption and destruction.

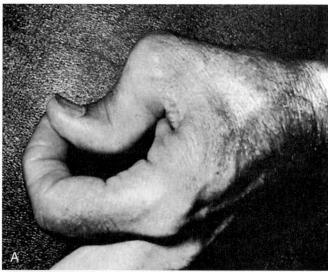

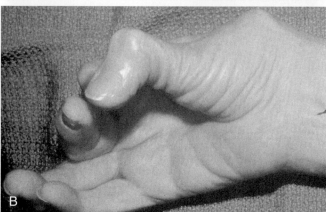

Figure 12-7 A, The type I deformity with metacarpophalangeal joint flexion and distal joint hyperextension. **B,** Swan neck deformity of the thumb with hyperextension at the metacarpophalangeal joint and a flexion deformity of the interphalangeal joint. (From Mackin EJ, Callahan AD, Skirven TM et al: Rehabilitation of the hand and upper extremity, ed 5, St Louis, 2002, Mosby.)

Metacarpal-Phalangeal Finger Joints

The MP joints of the digits are condyloid joints where the rounded head of the metacarpal bone articulates in the shallow elliptical cavity of the proximal phalanx. This type of joint permits all planes of movements except axial rotation. In addition to the head, the distal ends of the metacarpal bones have two tubercles for attachment of the transverse ligament. The metacarpal head has a large bony prominence. Between each metacarpal head are valleys that are easily identifiable in flexion. In some individuals the extensor tendon is visible over the central aspect of each joint. The metacarpal heads and palmar crease lie proximal to the MP joint. This is important when stabilizing the metacarpals and when allowing full motion of the MP joint.

Collateral and transverse metacarpal ligaments attach to the volar aspect of the MP joints and are thick, dense, and fibrous structures. The collateral ligaments are strong, rounded cords

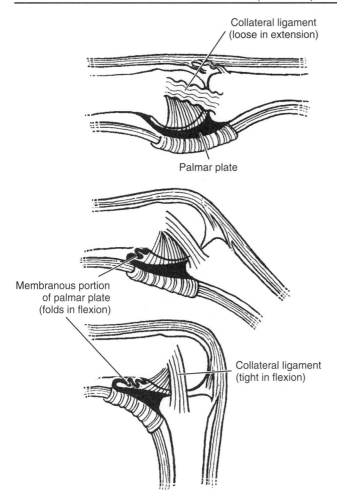

Collateral ligament
(loose in extension)

Palmar plate

Membranous portion
of palmar plate
(folds in flexion)

Collateral ligament
(tight in flexion)

Figure 12-8 Finger metacarpophalangeal collateral ligaments. (Modified from Wynn Parry CB et al: Rehabilitation of the hand, ed 3, London, 1973, Butterworth.)

that are found on each side of the joint and are attached to the posterior tubercle of the metacarpal head.[8] The direction of the ligaments is lateral and oblique. The collateral ligaments are lax when the MP joint is in extension and taut in flexion (Figure 12-8). The MP joint of the fingers are capable of flexion, extension, abduction, and adduction. Abduction and adduction occurs in MP joint extension when the collateral ligaments are lax. The orientation and properties of the collateral ligaments are the basis for positioning and splinting the MP joint in flexion to prevent joint contracture in the injured hand.

Abnormalities of the finger MP joints at rest and in dynamic postures are created by imbalances from articular and soft tissue disease. Fractures to the metacarpal bones account for 30% to 50% of all hand fractures, and the fifth metacarpal fracture is the most common fracture. Described as a boxer's fracture, the pathogenesis occurs from direct compression of a fisted hand.[9] The injury involves a displaced metacarpal shaft, which results in shortening of the anatomic bone. As a result, the proximal transverse and longitudinal arch are disrupted. Reduced grip strength occurs from the change in the bony architecture,

alterations from the pull of the soft tissues, and rerouting of deforming forces along the kinetic chain. In the resting hand, these variations result in less prominent, absent, or sunken metacarpal heads, and they are best observed when the fingers are flexed.

Metacarpal-Phalangeal Thumb Joints

The collateral ligaments, accessory collateral ligaments, palmar plate, and dorsal capsule provide the stability of the first MP joint. These are considered static restraints that respond to the tension and pull of extensor and flexor extrinsic muscles. An intrinsic muscle, the adductor pollicis, has a superficial insertion into the extensor mechanism of the thumb and aids in ulnar stability of the MP joint.

An injury to the first metacarpal can affect 50% of overall hand function and the kinematics of the CMC and MP joints of the thumb.[10] A Bennett's fracture is an intraarticular fracture dislocation of the CMC joint. A Rolando's fracture is a comminuted fracture at the base of the metacarpal, with major fragments in the metacarpal shaft and into the articular surface.

Injury to the MP joint can result in either an avulsion fracture or ligament strain followed by instability of the collateral ligament. A gamekeeper's fracture is a displaced bony fragment from the base of the thumb phalanx. Gamekeeper's lesion is a spectrum of UCL instabilities that produces MP joint laxity. Dynamic instability broadens with repeated injuries, laxity to the volar plate of the MP joint, and injury to the adductor aponeurosis. Evaluating for imbalances or joint laxities should begin with observation and comparison of both thumbs. A supination deformity of the joint is usually associated with palmar subluxation of the proximal phalanx. With repeated UCL stresses, the dorsal expansion may attenuate, allowing the EPL to shift ulnarly and compromising the ability to extend the MP joint. At rest, the MP joint is in flexion and has difficulty or is unable to actively extend to neutral.

A test to load the joint is used to assess the quality of ligamentous stability. The MP joint is placed in slight flexion, and a valgus stress is applied. Frequently, the test is performed in conjunction with radiographs and should be evaluated by the physician because of the potential for further injury. Point tenderness is present on the lateral border of the proximal phalanx, especially with ligamentous tears.[11] Clinical testing with tip pinch and self-report of painful prehensile activity can help to confirm the diagnosis.

Interphalangeal Joints

The PIP joints of the fingers and the distal interphalangeal (DIP) joints of the fingers and thumb are hinge joints, with 1 degree of freedom available for flexion and extension. The heads of each joint are convex, and the bases of the corresponding joints are concave. The collateral joints pass directly through the axis of rotation and provide lateral stability. When the joint is moving from extension to flexion, the collateral ligaments maintain constant tension. The ligaments have an attachment

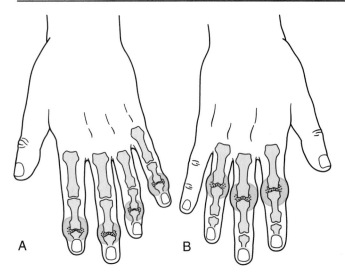

Figure 12-9 A, Osteoarthritic enlargement of the distal interphalangeal (DIP) joints (Heberden's nodes) is present. The metacarpophalangeal joints are not affected. **B,** Osteoarthritic enlargement of the proximal interphalangeal joints (Bouchard's nodes) is present. The metacarpophalangeal joints are not affected. (From Magee DJ: Orthopaedic physical assessment, ed 5, St Louis, 2008, Saunders.)

to the palmar plate that is a strong cartilage structure on the volar joint surface. The palmar plate serves as a checkrein because of its bony attachments and limits hyperextension and dorsal dislocation. The extensor tendon provides dorsal capsular support.

The interphalangeal joints have corresponding skinfolds that originate dorsally and proximally to the actual joint. On the volar surface, the joints have creases that deepen with flexion. After injury and inflammation, the PIP joints will prefer flexion and the creases become absent. In chronic cases of joint destruction, the joints may rotate or angle depending on the amount of laxity and the pull of the tendons that cross the joint.

Nodules may appear at the interphalangeal joints in response to degenerative inflammatory disease. Heberden's nodes, found at the DIP joints, are caused by spurs of the articular cartilage of the joint (Figure 12-9, *A*). Typically, they develop during middle age, beginning with chronic swelling of the affected joints or a sudden onset of pain, redness, numbness, and loss of manual dexterity. The initial inflammation and pain eventually subside, and the patient is left with a permanent bony outgrowth that causes deviation of the fingertip. Bouchard's nodes are similar bony growths but occur in the middle joints of the fingers and are also associated with osteoarthritis (Figure 12-9, *B*). These nodes compromise the mobility of the hand and inspire complaints of disfigurement.

MUSCULOTENDINOUS STRUCTURES

Upper extremity function requires the knowledge of muscle rhythm and balance. The smooth, coordinated, and effortless movement of successful task performance is a highly complex coordination of extrinsic and intrinsic muscle function, agonists and antagonists, and eccentric and concentric contractions all working on a stable skeletal frame. The quality of muscle extensibility has a starting point and a level of motor efficiency that is predetermined. Muscle tendon length and joint ligamentous structures are biomechanically designed to control the skeleton, constantly adjusting to gravitational and environmental demands. The starting point of motor activity is understood as a resting balance posture of normal muscle tone.

Muscle tone is in constant adjustment and is a variable of the gravitational pull on the skeleton. Muscle changes in direction and intensity are determined by the body's position in space. "Unconscious nerve impulses maintain the muscles in a partially contracted state."[12] If a sudden pull or stretch occurs, the body responds by automatically increasing the muscle's tension, a reflex that helps to guard against danger and to maintain balance.

The presence of near-continuous innervation describes tonus as a *default* or *steady-state condition.* For the most part, no actual "rest state" exists other than in the place where movement begins. In terms of skeletal muscle, both the extensor and the flexor muscles use the term *tonus* to describe rest or normal innervation that maintains the positions of the bones.

Resting Tone of the Wrist and Hand

Predictable resting positions of the fingers occur with wrist extension. In the neutral position, the muscles are balanced and are in the best position to control muscle tension and contraction.[12] Wrist extension increases the mechanical advantage of the digital flexors that originate in the forearm and cross multiple joints. With the wrist positioned in neutral and slight flexion, the muscle tension of the long finger flexors is decreased, resulting in limited composite range of motion and grip strength. These positions can be used to assess the balance of the extrinsic flexor and extensor systems.

Several observations can be made for balanced hand postures at rest. When a normal arm is pronated (Figure 12-10, *A*) or supinated (Figure 12-10, *B*) and supported on a table, the wrist is positioned in slight extension. The middle finger is aligned with the radius, creating the need for some ulnar deviation of the wrist. The MP, the PIP, and DIP joints of the hand are flexed. A natural progression of finger flexion occurs, starting with less flexion of the index finger and increasingly more flexion with the middle, ring, and little fingers. Similarly, PIP flexion is greater than MP or DIP flexion. The base of the thumb is extended, but the remaining portion of the thumb is parallel with the radius. The majority of the nail can be observed. In observing the same position from an ulnar view, similar observations can be made about the wrist, the fingers, and the thumb (Figure 12-10, *C*). However, in this position more of a natural cascade of finger flexion is present.

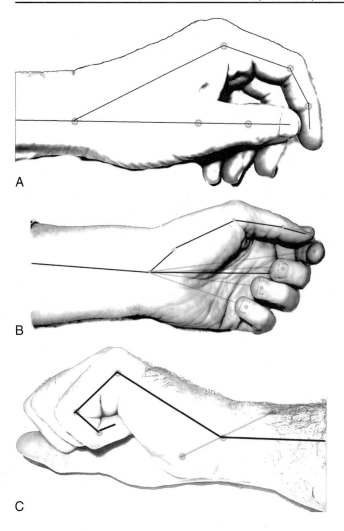

A

B

C

Figure 12-10 A, Resting hand lateral view: a normal arm supported on a table in forearm pronation. **B,** Resting hand palmer view: a normal arm supported on a table in forearm supination. **C,** Resting hand ulnar view: a normal arm supported on a table in neutral forearm rotation.

> ### Clinical Tip
> When resting imbalances of the wrist, the hand, or the digits are observed, further assessments of the articular, musculotendinous, and neurovascular structures are necessary.

The position of the wrist can dictate the tone and position of the fingers and thumb. This relationship is called *tenodesis* and is created from the manipulative position of the digits in response to wrist motion. When the forearm is pronated and the wrist is allowed to passively flex, the fingers extend and abduct and the base and terminal joints of the thumb extend. However, when the wrist is passively extended while the forearm is supinated, the fingers flex at each joint and the thumb approximates the tip of the index finger.

> ### Clinical Tip
> Tenodesis of the hand is useful to assess the influence of the wrist position on the fingers and the thumb. In the absence of active finger and thumb motion, patients can learn or compensate using wrist extension and flexion to enhance grip and pinch objects.

The purpose of this section is to present the dynamic relationships of the musculotendinous system of the wrist and hand. Muscle function is reviewed by describing common origins, whether the muscle is extrinsic or intrinsic, and the influence of musculotendinous extensibility on the multiple joints it may cross. Tendon function is reviewed by examining their relationship to supporting structures at various levels and how their activity changes throughout different locations. Postural observations are provided because intact ligamentous structures modify the direction of forces exerted by the muscles.[2] Finally, common clinical tests are included for both the wrist and the hand.

> ### Clinical Tip
> The extrinsic and intrinsic muscles of the hand are responsible for movement of the wrist and hand, but the axis of rotation and all of the accessory joint movements are determined by the arrangement of the ligaments.

Muscles

Muscles that originate proximal to the wrist crease and that have tendons that cross the wrist joint are considered to be extrinsic muscles. The actions of these muscles are influenced by the different positions of the wrist. Intrinsic muscles are those muscles that originate within the hand and that have tendons that cross the joints of the fingers. The actions of these muscles are influenced by the different position of the MP, PIP, and DIP joints rather than changes in wrist position. Fifteen extrinsic and eighteen intrinsic muscles control the wrist, the fingers, and the thumb. All but one finger extrinsic muscle originates from the epicondyles of the humerus, whereas the majority of extrinsic muscles for the thumb originate on the long bones of the forearm.

An appreciation for the influence of the wrist on hand function is critical to intervention. Familiarity of muscles with common origins is important to understand the positions that achieve full passive extensibility of the musculotendinous unit and to understand the influence of multiple joint positions. For example, full passive stretch of the EDC, an extrinsic muscle originating from the lateral epicondyle, occurs with elbow extension, forearm pronation, wrist flexion, and fisted fingers and thumb. Similarly, the flexor digitorum superficialis (FDS) is an extrinsic muscle originating from the medial epicondyle that requires elbow extension, forearm supination, wrist extension, and finger extension to provide full passive stretching.

In a similar way, positions of the MP joints can influence the movements acting on the PIP and DIP joints. For example, full passive stretch of the intrinsic muscles requires complete MP extension with PIP and DIP flexion. This is a clinical test called the *Bunnell-Littler test*. Similarly, the position of the PIP joints can influence the movement of the DIP joint. The Retinacular test is a clinical test that checks the full passive stretch of the extensor mechanism at the PIP joint. A normal finding is present when full DIP flexion occurs when the PIP joint is held in extension.

Extrinsic muscles do not represent all of the muscles that originate from the epicondyles of the humerus. Four additional muscles (the anconeus, the brachioradialis, the supinator, and the pronator) originate from the lateral and medial epicondyles, but their tendons do not cross the wrist. Because the epicondyles are a common origin for many extrinsic muscles and are a common site for tendonitis, anatomic information is provided by identifying common origins, whether the muscle is extrinsic or not, the action, and the position for achieving full passive stretch (Tables 12-2 through 12-4). Similar data are provided for the intrinsic muscles of the hand and the thumb (Tables 12-5 and 12-6).

> ### Clinical Tip
> Length tension tests for extrinsic flexor and extensors are based on full passive range of motion (PROM) of muscles from common origins that ensure full mobility across multiple joints and the contractile power of the agonist and antagonist muscles.

Tendons

Twenty-four tendons are associated with 15 extrinsic muscles. Each of the muscles has one tendon except the flexor digitorum profundus (FDP), the FDS, and the EDC, which has four tendons for one muscle belly. Likewise, each of the 20 intrinsic muscles has one tendon. Proximal to the wrist, the tendons from the extrinsic muscles are not constrained. Once they cross the wrist joint, a variety of supportive structures channel the direction of their movement and their ability to glide independently. To examine these relationships, tendons are classified by zones for the extensor and flexor tendons.

Table 12-2   Origin of Muscles From the Lateral Epicondyle

Origin	Name	Action	Position for Full Musculotendinous Flexibility
Not an extrinsic muscle	Anconeus	Primary: extension of the elbow	Elbow flexion, forearm pronation
	Brachioradialis	Primary: flexion of the elbow in neutral forearm rotation	Elbow extension, forearm pronation
	Supinator	Primary: supination of the forearm	Elbow extension, forearm pronation
Extrinsic muscles	Extensor carpi radialis longus (ECRL)	Primary: extension of the wrist in a radial direction Secondary: flexion of the elbow	Elbow extension, forearm pronation, wrist flexion in an ulnar direction
	Extensor carpi radialis brevis (ECRB)	Primary: extension of the wrist Secondary: radial deviation of the wrist	Elbow extension, forearm pronation, wrist flexion
	Extensor carpi ulnaris (ECU)	Primary: extension of the wrist in a ulnar direction	Elbow extension, forearm pronation, wrist flexion in an radial direction
	Extensor digitorum communis (EDC)	Primary: extension of the metacarpalphalangeal (MP) of the second through fifth digits; in conjunction with the lumbricals and interossei, extension of the proximal interphalangeal (PIP) of the second through fifth digits Secondary: abduction of the index, ring, and little fingers; extension of the wrist in a radial direction	Elbow extension; forearm pronation; wrist flexion; MP, PIP, and distal interphalangeal (DIP) flexion of the fingers
	Extensor digiti minimi (EDM)	Primary: extension of the MP of the fifth digit; in conjunction with the lumbricals and interossei, extension of the PIP of the fifth digit Secondary: abduction of the fifth finger	Elbow extension; forearm pronation; wrist flexion; MP, PIP, and DIP flexion of the little finger

Table 12-3 **Origin of Muscles From the Medial Epicondyle**

Origin	Name	Action	Position for Full Musculotendinous Flexibility
Not an extrinsic muscle	Pronator	Primary: pronation of the forearm Secondary: flexion of the elbow	Elbow extension, forearm supination
Extrinsic muscles	Flexor carpi radialis (FCR)	Primary: flexion of the wrist in a radial direction Secondary: pronation of the forearm and flexion of the elbow	Elbow extension, forearm supination, wrist extension in an ulnar direction
	Palmaris longus	Primary: tensing of the palmar fascia; flexion of the wrist Secondary: flexion of the elbow	Elbow extension, forearm supination, wrist extension
	Flexor carpi ulnaris (FCU)	Primary: flexion of the wrist in an ulnar direction Secondary: flexion of the elbow	Elbow extension, forearm supination, wrist extension in an radial direction
	Flexor digitorum superficialis (FDS)	Primary: flexion of the proximal interphalangeal (PIP) of the second through fifth digits Secondary: flexion of the wrist and the metacarpal-phalangeal (MP) of the second through fifth digits	Elbow extension; forearm supination; wrist extension; MP, PIP, and distal interphalangeal (DIP) extension of the fingers
	Flexor pollicis longus (FPL)	Primary: flexion of the interphalangeal (IP) of the thumb Secondary: MP and carpal-metacarpal (CMC) flexion of the thumb; may assist with flexion of the wrist	Elbow extension; forearm supination; wrist extension; CMC, MP, and IP extension of the thumb

Table 12-4 **Origin of Muscles From the Forearm Bones**

Origin	Name	Action	Position for Full Musculotendinous Flexibility
Radius, extrinsic muscles	Extensor pollicis brevis (EPB)	Primary: extension of the metacarpal-phalangeal (MP) of the thumb, abduction of and extension of the carpal-metacarpal (CMC) of the thumb Secondary: radial deviation of the wrist	Forearm pronation, wrist flexion in an ulnar direction, CMC adduction, MP flexion of the thumb
Ulna, extrinsic muscles	Flexor digitorum profundus (FDP)	Primary: flexion of the distal interphalangeal (DIP) of the second through fifth digits Secondary: proximal interphalangeal (PIP) and MP flexion and flexion of the wrist	Forearm supination; wrist extension; MP, PIP, and DIP extension
	Extensor indicis proprius (EIP)	Primary: extension of the MP of the index finger; in conjunction with the lumbricals and interossei, extension of the PIP and DIP of the index finger Secondary: adduction of the index finger	Forearm pronation; wrist flexion; MP, PIP, and DIP flexion of the index finger
	Extensor pollicis longus (EPL)	Primary: extension of the IP of the thumb, assists with extension of the MP of the thumb, extension of the CMC of the thumb Secondary: extension of the wrist in a radial direction	Forearm pronation, wrist flexion in an ulnar direction, CMC adduction, MP and IP flexion of the thumb
	Abductor pollicis longus (APL)	Primary: abduction of and extension of the CMC of the thumb, flexion of the wrist in a radial direction	Forearm pronation, wrist flexion in an ulnar direction, CMC adduction

Table 12-5 | **Origin of Hand Muscles**

Origin	Name	Action	Position for Full Musculotendinous Flexibility
Soft tissue, carpal and metacarpal bones—intrinsic muscles	Dorsal interossei (4)	Primary: abduction of the metacarpal-phalangeal (MP) of the index, middle, and ring fingers Secondary: flexion of the MP for the index, middle, and ring fingers; extension of the proximal interphalangeal (PIP) and distal interphalangeal (DIP) for the index, middle, and ring fingers; and the first dorsal interossei in adduction of the carpal-metacarpal (CMC) for the thumb	MP extension of the index, middle, and ring fingers; PIP and DIP flexion of the index, middle, and ring fingers; CMC extension of the thumb
	Palmar interossei (3)	Primary: adduction of the MP of the thumb, index, ring, and little fingers Secondary: flexion of the MP for the thumb, index, ring, and little fingers; PIP and DIP extension for the index, ring, and little fingers	MP extension of the index, ring, and little fingers; PIP and DIP flexion of the index, index, ring, and little fingers
	Lumbricals (4)	Primary: flexion of the MP of the second through fifth digit; extension of the PIP and DIP of the second through fifth digit	MP extension of the second through fifth fingers, PIP and DIP flexion of the second through fifth fingers
	Abductor digiti minimi	Primary: abduction of MP of the little finger Secondary: circumduction and flexion of the MP of the little finger, PIP and DIP extension	CMC extension of the little finger, MP extension of the little finger, PIP and DIP flexion of the little finger
	Flexor digiti minimi	Primary: flexion of the MP of the little finger Secondary: circumduction of the CMC of the little finger	CMC extension of the little finger, MP extension of the little finger
	Opponens digiti minimi	Primary: circumduction of the CMC of the little finger	CMC extension of the little finger

Table 12-6 | **Origin of Thumb Muscles**

Origin	Name	Action	Position for Full Musculotendinous Flexibility
Soft tissue, carpal and metacarpal bones—intrinsic muscles	Adductor pollicis	Primary: adduction of the carpal-metacarpal (CMC) of the thumb Secondary: flexion of the metacarpal-phalangeal (MP) of the thumb, circumduction of the CMC of the thumb, extension of the interphalangeal (IP) of the thumb	CMC and MP extension of the thumb, IP flexion of the thumb
	Abductor pollicis brevis	Primary: abduction of the CMC of the thumb, extension of the IP of the thumb Secondary: MP flexion, circumduction of the CMC of the thumb	
	Flexor pollicis brevis	Primary: flexion of the MP and CMC of the thumb Secondary: circumduction of the CMC of the thumb, extension of the IP of the thumb	
	Opponens pollicis	Primary: circumduction of the CMC of the thumb	CMC extension of the thumb

Extensors

Extensor tendon zones define the tendons on the dorsum of the hand. Seven zones (I-VII) organize the finger tendons and five zones (T1-5) organize the thumb tendons (Figure 12-11, A). In the most proximal extensor tendon zones, VII and T5, the deep layers of the dorsal fascia maintain the tendons. Six dorsal compartments are created by the extensor retinaculum and direct the excursion of the tendons (Figure 12-11, B). The first compartment contains the tendons from the abductor pollicis longus, the extensor pollicis brevis, and their lubricating synovial sheaths. Inflammation of the contents in this compartment can result in deQuervain's syndrome. The Finkelstein's test is a clinical procedure for this disorder in which point tenderness exists over the anatomic snuffbox and increased pain with thumb circumduction and ulnar deviation of the wrist (Figure 12-12). The second compartment contains the extensor carpi radialis and brevis, which can be palpated over the second and third metacarpal. Because the wrist prefers to move in a diagonal pattern, radial wrist extension, motored by these tendons, is important to hand function. The third compartment contains the EPL. The tendon is easy to palpate when the thumb is abducting toward a hitchhiking position. The fourth compartment contains five tendons; four from the EDC and one from the extensor indicis proprius (EIP). The EDC simultaneously extends the MP joints of the fingers, whereas the EIP must cross the EDC to extend the MP joint to the index finger. The fifth compartment contains the extensor digiti minimi (EDM), which can be problematic after repetitive movements of the little finger. The sixth compartment contains the ECU. Although wrist extension in an ulnar direction is not common, pain and limited excursion of this tendon suggests possible distal radioulnar joint dysfunction.

> ### Clinical Tip
> Testing the excursion of the tendons sequentially using the six dorsal compartments at the wrist provides valuable information on the mechanical efficiency of each tendon to glide through the retinaculum pulley system.

An appreciation of the tendons to the fingers and to the thumb after they cross the wrist joint highlights the complexity of extension that occurs for the terminal joints. In zone VI, the tendons of the EDC are connected by the juncturae tendinum to prevent subluxation of the tendon over the MP joint. Continuing distally, the tendons of the EDC penetrate the sagittal bands at the MP joints of the second through fifth digits and divides into medial and lateral bands (zones IV-V). The medial band inserts into the middle phalanx, becomes the central slip of the common extensor, and extends the PIP joint (zone III). The lateral bands join with the tendons of the lumbricals and interossei, insert into the distal phalanx, and extend the DIP joint (zones 1-II). Therefore digital extension is a combination of extrinsic and intrinsic muscle function (Figure 12-13). An imbalance in the extensor mechanism creates deformities of the fingers. A Boutonniere deformity (Figure 12-14, A) occurs with elongation or attenuation of the central tendon to the middle phalanx. The lateral bands change their original anatomic position from dorsal to volar to the axis of the PIP joint, and they become strong PIP flexors. Over time, the lateral bands and volar structures will shorten, causing a secondary imbalance as the DIP joint hyperextends. Similarly, a Mallet deformity (Figure 12-14, B) occurs when trauma to the terminal portion of the extensor tendon occurs. This injury frequently has a fracture fragment from the distal phalanx attached to the extensor tendon. Initially, the DIP joint will not extend. Over time, an imbalance occurs because of the intact long extrinsic flexors, tight lateral bands dorsally, and chronic stretching of the volar plate at the PIP joint. Secondarily, a swan neck deformity can result where the resting posture of the PIP joint is in hyperextension and the DIP joint is flexed.

> ### Clinical Tip
> Stabilizing the wrist and MP joints in extension accentuates extrinsic muscle power while minimizing the intrinsic muscle contribution to PIP extension. Flexing and extending the DIP joint with the PIP stabilized in extension allows for isolated intrinsic muscle function.

In the thumb an extrinsic muscle, the EPL, does the primary extension of the IP joint. However, the dorsal extensor expansion over the MP joint of the thumb joins the combined efforts of three intrinsic muscles (the adductor pollicis, the abductor pollicis brevis, and the flexor pollicis brevis). Together, the terminal extension of the thumb is a combination of extrinsic and thenar muscle functions.

Flexors

Flexor tendon zones define the tendons on the volar aspect of the hand. Five zones (I-V) organize the finger tendons and three zones (T1-3) organize the thumb tendons (Figure 12-15). Flexor tendons to the fingers that are located in zone V are proximal to the carpal canal and are not affected by the excursion of the flexor tendons once they enter the hand. Zone IV includes the contents of the carpal canal (Figure 12-16). The tendons of the FDS to the middle and ring fingers become the most superficial structures, followed by the tendons of the FDS to the index and little fingers, and finally the tendons of the FDP to the index through little fingers as the deepest structures of the carpal tunnel. In addition to these tendons, the FPL, the median nerve, and the synovium that encases the tendons are contained the carpal canal. Pain with passive extension of a digit, one of four Kanavel's signs, may suggest that the flexor tendon sheath is infected (Figure 12-17). Active tendon gliding of the FDP and the FDS at this level are important for individualized movements of each muscle group. The straight

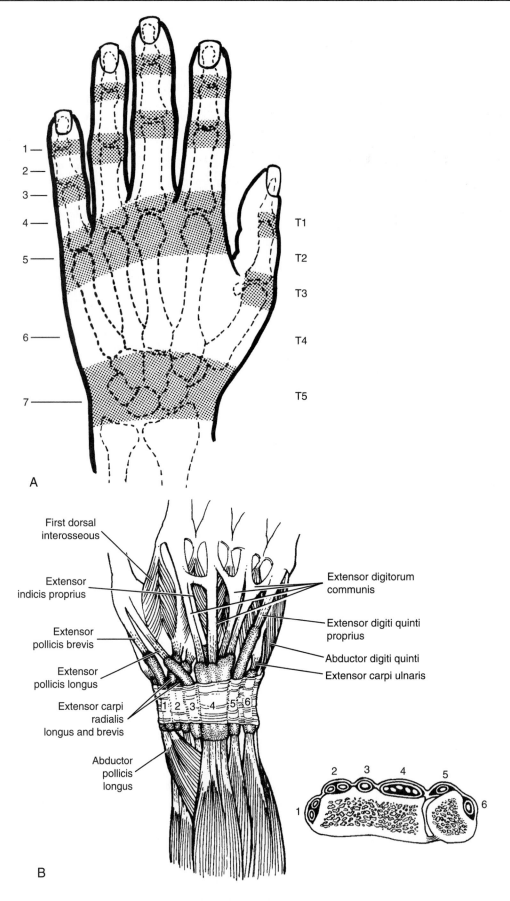

Figure 12-11 A, Extensor tendon zones as defined by the Committee on Tendon Injuries for the International Federation of the Societies for Surgery of the Hand. **B,** Arrangement of the extensor tendons in the compartments of the wrist. (**A** from Kleinert HE, Schepel S, Gill T: Surg Clin North Am 61:267, 1981. **B** from Fess E: Hand and upper extremity splinting: principles and methods, ed 3, St Louis, 2004, Mosby.)

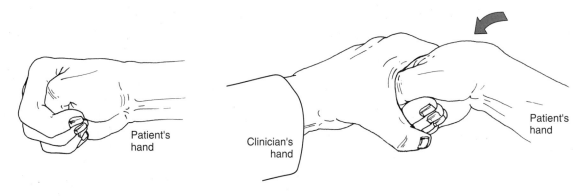

Figure 12-12 Finkelstein test for deQuervain's disease. (From Magee DJ: Orthopaedic physical assessment, ed 5, St Louis, 2008, Saunders.)

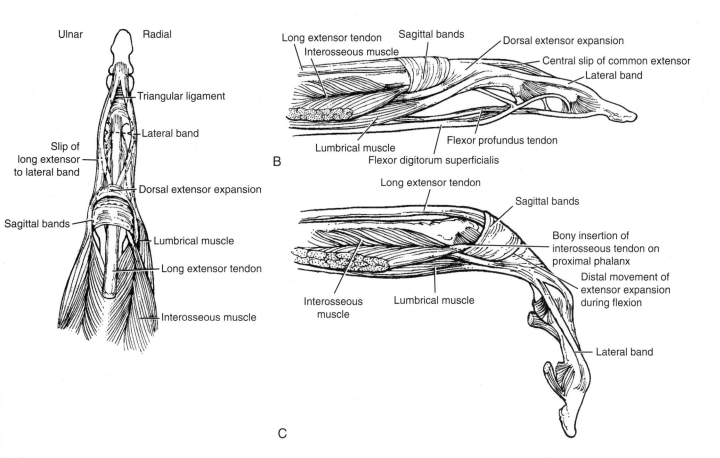

Figure 12-13 Normal extensor anatomy. (From Fess E: Hand and upper extremity splinting: principles and methods, ed 3, St Louis, 2004, Mosby.)

finger and fisted position of the fingers allows for full excursion of the FDP and FDS (Figure 12-18). The hook position represents a differential excursion between the FDP and the FDS, whereas the straight fist represents increased FDS excursion.

> **Clinical Tip**
> Four different positions of the fingers are required to ensure full active and independent tendon gliding of the fingers.

In zone III, the lumbrical muscles originate from the FDP. A lubricating sheath does not protect the flexor tendons to the fingers in this zone, and they are prone to adhesions and triggering when trauma occurs. In zone II the relationship between the FDP and the FDS changes. At the level of the proximal phalanx, the FDS splits and continues distally to insert into the middle phalanx. The tendon of the FDP begins deep to the FDS, transverses through the decussation of the FDS, and then becomes superficial to the FDS (Figure 12-19, *A*). Because the FDS has individual muscle bellies, isolated movement of each finger and tendon is important to maintain dexterity of the

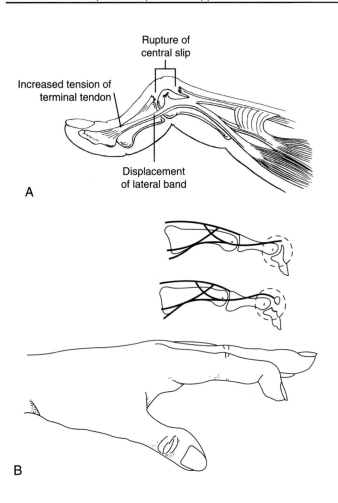

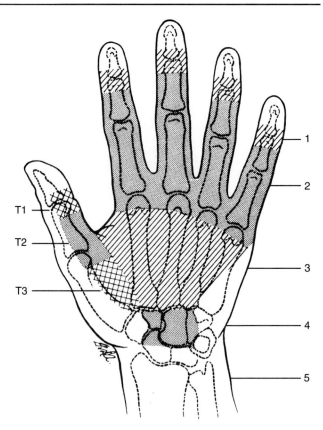

Figure 12-15 Flexor tendon zones of the hand. (From Kleinert HE, Schepel S, Gill T: Surg Clin North Am 61:267, 1981.)

Figure 12-14 A, Boutonniere deformity. **B,** Mallet finger deformity. (**A** from The hand: examination and diagnosis, ed 2, Edinburgh, 1983, Churchill Livingstone. **B** from Burke SL: Hand and upper extremity rehabilitation: a practical guide, ed 3, St Louis, 2005, Churchill Livingstone.)

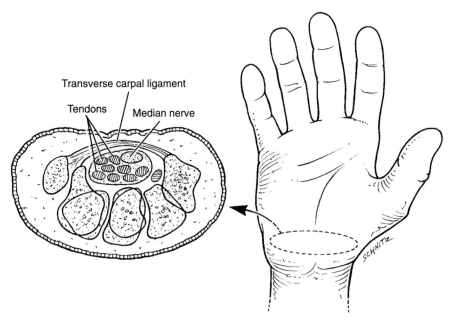

Figure 12-16 Cross-sectional anatomy of the carpal tunnel shows its anatomic boundaries. The carpus and the palmar roof formed by the transverse carpal ligament are shown, as is the position of the median nerve. An increased volume in this passageway most frequently resulting from thickening or inflammation around the nine flexor tendons can result in compression of the median nerve and the condition known as carpal tunnel syndrome (CTS). (From Fess E: Hand and upper extremity splinting: principles and methods, ed 3, St Louis, 2004, Mosby.)

finger. In zones I and II, the tendons are protected in sheaths, five annual pulleys, and three cruciate pulleys (Figure 12-19, *B*). The structures provide smooth gliding surfaces, nourishment, and close binding to the bone, which improves mechanical efficiency of the tendon.

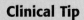

> **Clinical Tip**
> To test the individual function of the FDS in each finger, eliminate the influence of the FDP by holding the DIP joints of the untested fingers in extension and allow the PIP joint to flex.

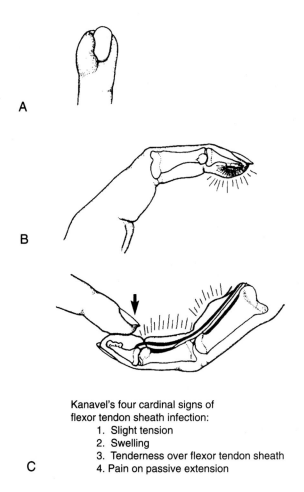

Kanavel's four cardinal signs of flexor tendon sheath infection:
1. Slight tension
2. Swelling
3. Tenderness over flexor tendon sheath
4. Pain on passive extension

Figure 12-17 Kanavel's four signs of flexor tendon sheath infection. **A,** Paronychia. **B,** Felon, **C,** Flexor tendon sheath infection. (From American Society for Surgery of the Hand: The hand: examination and diagnosis, ed 3, New York, 1990, Churchill Livingstone.)

Similarities exist between the flexor tendons to the fingers and the thumb. Intrinsic and extrinsic tendons flex the MP and IP joints of the thumb. Tendons are protected in sheaths and have pulley systems similar to the extrinsic finger flexors. Swelling in thumb zones 1 and 2 can create triggering of the FPL. This occurs when full active flexion of the MP and IP joints are possible but active extension is blocked because of the inability of the swollen flexor tendons to pass smoothly into the tendon sheath (Figure 12-20).

NEUROLOGIC STRUCTURES

The median, ulnar, and radial nerves supply the motor function and sensibility to the wrist and hand. Each peripheral nerve begins at the cervical spine, travels across many joints in the upper extremity, and pierces muscle bellies and other compact areas. Lack of normal nerve gliding, inflammation of supporting structures, or direct compression can affect the capacity of the axons to conduct electrical impulses. Therefore common areas for impingement and levels of innervation for each muscle are discussed. Sensibility and manual muscle testing (MMT) by nerve distribution is an approach to identify potential compressions, level of compression, and the resultant deformities that can occur.

Radial Nerve

The radial nerve is known as the *preparatory nerve* because of its innervation to the muscles that position the hand, stabilize the wrist, and open the fingers in anticipation of functional activity. The origin of the nerve comes from C5-T1 nerve roots that form the posterior cord of the brachial plexus.

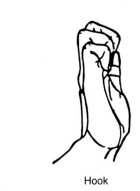
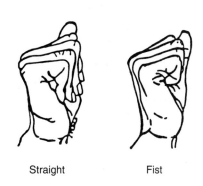

Straight   Hook   Straight   Fist

Figure 12-18 Tendon glide exercises. (From Hayes EP et al: Carpal tunnel syndrome. In Mackin E, Callahan AD, Skirven TM et al, editors: Rehabilitation of the hand and upper extremity, ed 5, St Louis, 2002, Mosby.)

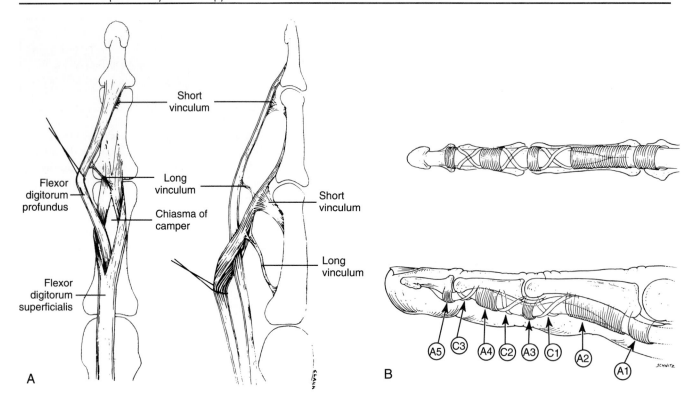

Figure 12-19 A, The flexor digitorum superficially lies volar to the flexor digitorum profundus (FDP) as the tendons enter the sheath. **B,** Five annular (A) and three cruciate (C) pulleys exist. A2 and A4 are the largest and most important. (**A** from Schneider LH: Flexor tendon injuries, Boston, 1985, Little, Brown. **B** from Cannon NM, Foltz RW, Koepfer JN et al: Manual of hand splinting, New York, 1985, Churchill Livingstone.)

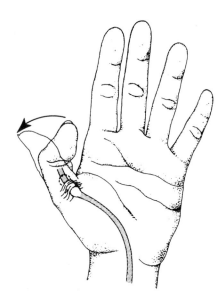

Figure 12-20 Trigger thumb. (From American Society for Surgery of the Hand: The hand: examination and diagnosis, ed 3, New York, 1990, Churchill Livingstone.)

Damage to the radial nerve can occur from limited nerve gliding at the neck and shoulder, direct trauma to the nerve, or common sites of entrapments. The most common injury to the radial nerve occurs with midhumeral fractures because of its location in the spiral groove of the humerus. Manual testing

of the muscles innervated by the radial nerve is advantageous because one may find that the triceps muscle may be spared because it frequently receives its innervation above the common sites of humeral fractures (Figure 12-21). However, the loss of elbow extension, forearm supination, as well as wrist, finger, and thumb extension results in a wrist drop deformity and in limitations in placing the arm in various planes of movement.

In addition to direct trauma, the radial nerve can be compressed in multiple locations. Complete sensory and motor function of the radial nerve can be disrupted from using crutches incorrectly. Saturday night palsy can occur when pressure is placed on the radial nerve for extended periods of time in positions such as sleeping on the upper arm. The resulting impairment of the nerve is similar to that found with midhumeral fractures and is described as *high-level lesions of the radial nerve* (Figure 12-22).

Moving distally, several low-level lesions occur. At the radial head, the radial nerve divides into two branches: the posterior motor branch and the anterior superficial sensory branch. The motor branch, called the *posterior interossei nerve,* travels between the two heads of the supinator. Motor function is spared to the radial two wrist extensors, leaving impairment in the finger and thumb extensors. In addition, the nerve can be compressed between the radial head and the supinator, resulting in radial tunnel syndrome. Motor and sensory functions are spared. However, patients complain of severe pain and burning sensations over the extensor wad musculature. It is

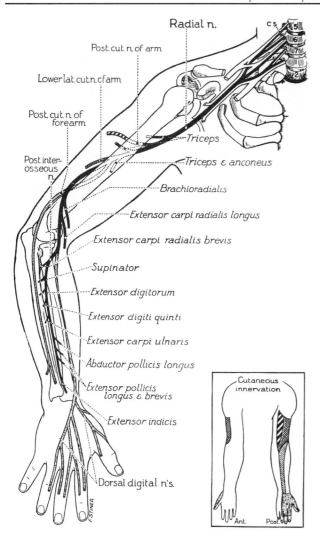

Figure 12-21 Schematic of the radial nerve. (From Haymaker W, Woodhall B: Peripheral nerve injuries: principles of diagnosis, Philadelphia, 1953, Saunders.)

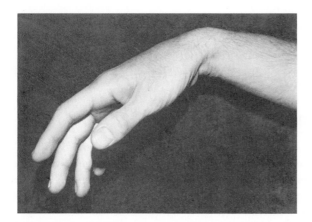

Figure 12-22 High radial nerve palsy. The patient is unable to actively extend the wrist and finger MP joints. (From Lister G: The hand: diagnosis and indication, ed 2, Edinburgh, 1984, Churchill Livingstone.)

frequently misdiagnosed as tennis elbow or lateral epicondylitis.

Loss of sensibility from the radial nerve usually does not result in significant disability. However, injury to the superficial radial sensory nerve at the wrist can occur from repeated trauma such as constriction around the wrist (e.g., handcuffs, watchbands, jewelry), scarring from external fixators used after Colles' fracture, or inflammation from CMC thumb tendonitis or arthritis. Complaints can range from mild tenderness during active wrist movements to intolerance to sleeves and air blowing across the radial side of the wrist.

Median Nerve

The median nerve is known as the *precision nerve* because of its innervation to the prehensile side of the hand. The origin of the nerve comes from C5-T1 nerve roots that form the lateral and medial cords of the brachial plexus. In addition to the potential irritation that can occur at the neck and shoulder, three additional sites of median nerve compression can occur. At the elbow the nerve can be entrapped when it passes through the two heads of the pronator teres. Moving distally, a deep motor branch of the nerve, the anterior interosseous nerve, can be compressed, causing paralysis of the FPL, the FDP to the index finger, and the pronator quadratus. The terminal end of the anterior interosseous nerve innervates the volar wrist capsule and contributes to its sensory feedback. Finally, the median nerve becomes more superficial and enters the carpal tunnel along with nine extrinsic finger flexor tendons.

Variations in the nerve, called *Martin-Gruber anastomosis,* have been estimated in 19% of the population.[13] In addition, double crush syndrome can occur to any peripheral nerve that is impinged in multiple areas along the entire length of the nerve. In spite of these possibilities, manual testing of extrinsic and intrinsic muscles based on their level of innervation can be advantageous (Figure 12-23). For example, traditional MMT of the three wrist flexors may not identify possible neuropathies because of weakness of the median innervated muscles, the flexor carpi radialis (FCR) and palmaris longus compared with the strength of the ulnar innervated nerve, the flexor carpi ulnaris (FCU). Muscle testing by nerve distribution can provide valuable information about the integrity of the nerve and the location of possible impingements.

Several clinical observations are apparent, depending on the level of impairment. A low-level lesion of the median nerve is described as *carpal tunnel syndrome* (CTS). Individuals with this syndrome have weakness in the five intrinsic muscles innervated by the median nerve. Atrophy of the thenar muscles, referred to as an *ape hand,* can be observed. However, the CMC web space of the thumb can be tight because of an imbalance between the functioning ulnar innervated muscle, the adductor pollicis, and the absence of the median innervated thenar muscles.

A high lesion to the median nerve can result in additional problems compared with those associated with a low lesion of the median nerve. Individuals with pronator syndrome frequently use shoulder abduction and gravity to compensate for

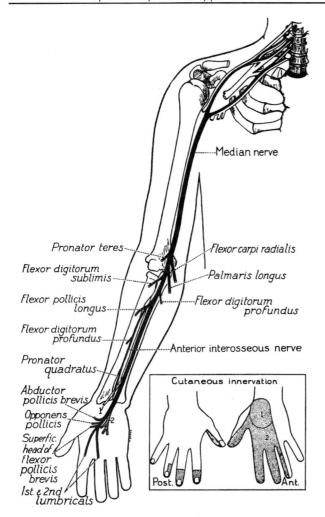

Figure 12-23 Schematic of median nerve. (From Haymaker W, Woodhall B: Peripheral nerve injuries: principles of diagnosis, Philadelphia, 1953, Saunders.)

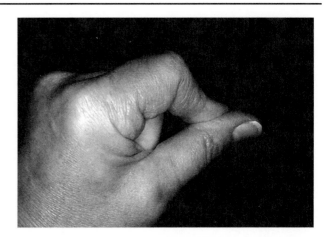

Figure 12-24 Ballentine test for high median nerve palsy. (From Colditz JC: Splinting the hand with a peripheral nerve injury. In Mackin E, Callahan AD, Skirven TM et al, editors: Rehabilitation of the hand and upper extremity, ed 5, St Louis, 2002, Mosby.)

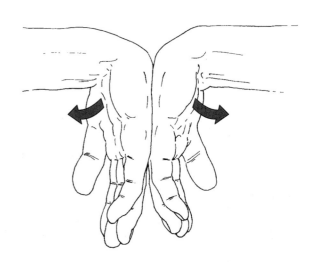

Figure 12-25 Phalen's test for median nerve sensibility. (From Magee DJ: Orthopaedic physical assessment, ed 5, St Louis, 2008, Saunders.)

poor active forearm pronation. In addition, impingement of the anterior interosseous nerve can result in difficulty making an *O* (Figure 12-24). This clinical procedure is called the *Ballentine sign.*

After identifying deficits in motor function as a result of nerve impairment, sensibility of the hand also can provide information about the integrity of the median nerve. Cutaneous distributions of the median nerve innervate the thumb, the index, the middle, and the radial half of the ring finger. The Phalen's test is a provocative test to evaluate the sensory response of the median nerve when it is placed in a position of stress. The wrist is positioned in full flexion and reproduction or exacerbation of symptoms in the median nerve distribution is considered a positive finding (Figure 12-25). Testing one extremity at a time prevents the need for full elbow flexion and confounding the test with ulnar nerve impairment at the elbow. Another differential test of the median nerve occurs when assessing the superficial sensory branch. It arises from the median nerve proximal to the carpal tunnel and innervates the thenar eminence. Therefore sensibility of this area may be spared when the median nerve is compressed in the carpal tunnel.

Ulnar Nerve

The ulnar nerve is referred to as the *power nerve* because of its innervation to the long flexors of the ring and little fingers. However, it contributes to hand coordination because of the function of the intrinsic muscles that control the thumb and the ulnar two fingers.

The origin of the nerve comes from C8-T1 nerve roots that form the medial cords of the brachial plexus. In addition to the potential irritation that can occur at the neck and shoulder, two additional sites of ulnar nerve compression can occur. At the elbow, the nerve can be entrapped in multiple locations. Most frequently, ulnar neuropathies at the elbow occur when the nerve passes around the posterior area of the medial epicondyle and through the cubital tunnel. This syndrome can be caused by direct trauma such as weight-bearing activities on the elbows as a result of weakened lower extremity and back muscles, repetitive elbow flexion as a result of weakened shoulder flexors, cubitus valgus deformities, and supracondylar fractures. The elbow flexion test is a clinical test in which the elbow is placed in full flexion. Reproduction or exacerbation of sensory changes in the cutaneous distributions of the ulnar nerve is a positive finding. In considering a high level injury to the ulnar nerve, manual muscle and sensibility testing can identify the specific impairment to the wrist, fingers, and thumb (Figure 12-26). Weakness of the ulnar wrist flexor and two DIP joints to the fingers are classical problems associated with a high-level injury to the ulnar nerve. Based on the dura-

tion of the compression to the nerve, a mild clawhand deformity, atrophy of the intrinsic muscles, and loss of arch supports can result from overpowering of the extrinsic finger extensors as they attempt to compensate for the lack of intrinsic function (Figure 12-27).

The second site for compression of the ulnar nerve occurs at the wrist when it passes between the pisiform and the hook of the hamate in the ulnar tunnel. This low-level lesion of the ulnar nerve, Guyon's canal compression, results in the loss of many intrinsic muscles to the fingers and thumb. More severe clawhand deformities result in low-level lesions (compared with high-level lesions) because of the presence of the long flexor tendons to the ring and little fingers. Several clinical procedures are suggested for testing the intrinsic muscle loss found in high and low ulnar neuropathies. The Wartenberg's sign suggests ulnar neuropathy as the little finger maintains an abducted position because of weakness of the intrinsic muscle (Figure 12-28). The ulnar and the median nerves both contribute to the motor function of the thumb (Figure 12-29). An

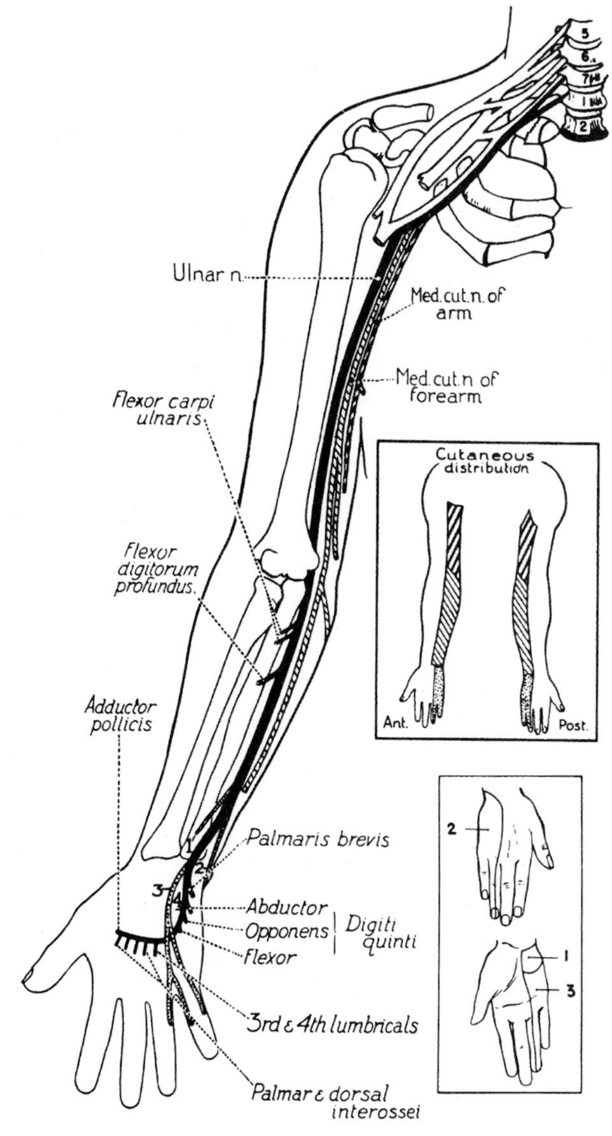

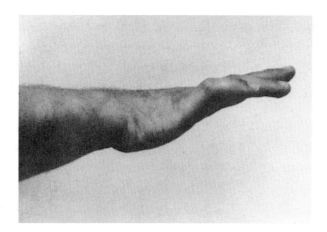

Figure 12-27 Clawhand deformity resulting from ulnar nerve palsy. (From Stanley BG, Tribuzi SM: Concepts in hand rehabilitation, Philadelphia, 1992, FA Davis.)

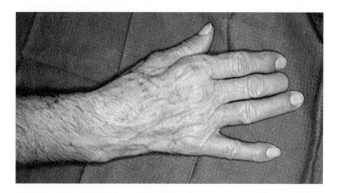

Figure 12-28 The little finger assumes an abducted position and cannot be adducted to the adjacent fingers (Wartenberg's sign). (From Townsend CM: Sabiston textbook of surgery, ed 18, St Louis, 2008, Mosby.)

Figure 12-26 Schematic of the ulnar nerve. (From Haymaker W, Woodhall B: Peripheral nerve injuries: principles of diagnosis, Philadelphia, 1953, Saunders.)

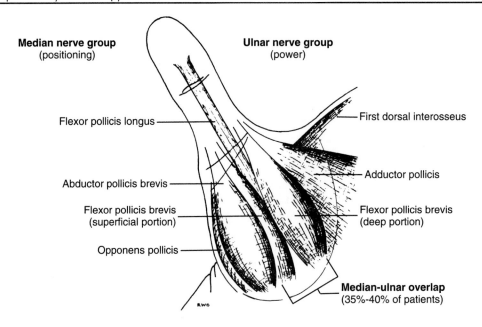

Figure 12-29 Three muscle groups are found in the thumb that lie lateral to the flexor pollicis longus (FPL) tendon and two groups that lie medial to it. (From Beasley RW: Hand injuries, Philadelphia, 1985, Saunders.)

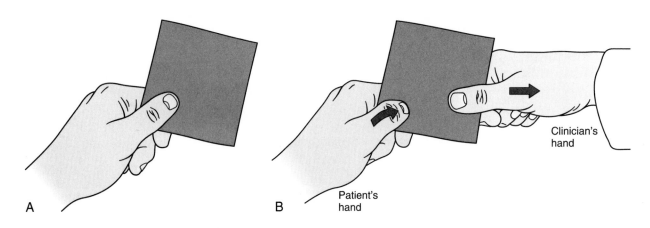

Figure 12-30 Froment's sign. **A,** Start position. **B,** Thumb flexes when paper is pulled away (positive test). (From Magee DJ: Orthopaedic physical assessment, ed 5, St Louis, 2008, Saunders.)

injury to the ulnar nerve can result in a positive Froment's sign when the lateral pinch of the thumb cannot hold a piece of paper because of weakness of the adductor pollicis or if the IP joint of the thumb overcompensates with hyperflexion (Figure 12-30).

VASCULAR STRUCTURES

The vascular structures contain vessels that carry blood and lymph throughout the body. The arterial and venous systems transport blood, deliver oxygen and nutrients, and remove waste products from the body. The lymphatic system transports fluid that contains excessive water from the tissues and fatty cells.

Arterial System

The radial and ulnar arteries that are branches from the brachial artery provide the major vascular supply to the hand. The radial artery forms the deep palmar arch that primarily supplies blood to the thumb and index finger. The ulnar artery forms the superficial palmar branch that supplies blood to the majority of the fingers. Collateral branches of the ulnar nerve connect with the radial artery superficially and deep. The modified Allen's test is used to assess the integrity of the vascular function to the hand (Figure 12-31). After occluding both arteries to the hand, repetitive grasp and release motions are done to remove the blood from the hand. A positive finding occurs when each artery is released separately and the capillary refill is slow and the color of the fingers remains ashen. Clinical

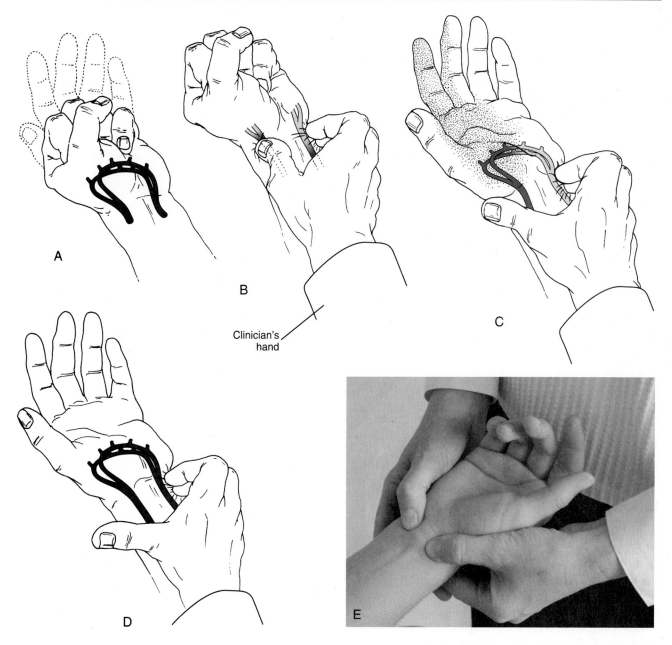

Clinician's
hand

Figure 12-31 Allen test. **A,** The patient opens and closes the hand. **B,** While the patient holds the hand closed, the examiner compresses the radial and ulnar arteries. **C,** One artery (in this case, the radial artery) is then released, and the examiner notes the filling pattern of the hand until the circulation is normal. **D,** The process is then repeated with the other artery. **E,** Alternative handhold. (From Magee DJ: Orthopaedic physical assessment, ed 5, St Louis, 2008, Saunders.)

testing of the arterial system is useful for individuals with Raynaud's Syndrome, a condition with vasoconstriction to the blood vessels in the fingers or complex regional pain syndromes such as reflex sympathetic dystrophy, a condition with significant temperature changes to the extremity, burning pain, hypersensitivity, sweating, and swelling (Figure 12-32).

Venous and Lymphatic System

The venous and lymphatic systems work together to remove waste products from the extremities. Together they form net-

works in the hand that drain on the dorsum of the hand. Anatomically, the veins are part of a continuous-loop pumping system that uses hydrostatic pressure gradients to remove smaller molecules of waste.[4] Conversely, the lymphatic system must be stimulated to activate a force pump that removes the larger waste products such as proteins, fatty acids, hormone cells, and toxins. More valves are present in the lymphatic system than in the venous systems. Filtration occurs in lymphatic nodes, and fluid enters the thoracic duct for removal. The characteristics of each system must be considered when applying techniques to reduce hand edema.

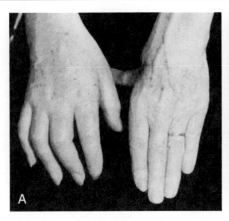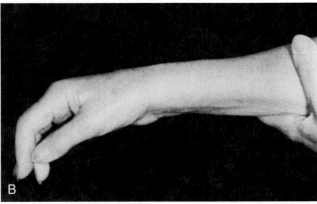

Figure 12-32 Reflex sympathetic dystrophy. (From Salter MI: Hand injuries: a therapeutic approach, Edinburgh, 1987, Churchill Livingstone.)

EVALUATION OF THE WRIST AND HAND

Positive outcomes in hand therapy begin with a personalized care assessment and an effective and efficient intervention plan. Clinical reasoning skills are needed in the initial visit to obtain an accurate medical history, to observe postural balance, to palpate abnormalities, to select objective measures that validate clinical observations, to develop plausible treatment hypotheses, and to engage the patient in a meaningful treatment program. Each of these sections are explored in more detail following. Case studies are provided that apply these principles.

History

A good patient history will guide the clinician in looking for specific postural imbalances and will assist in the development of the treatment hypotheses. Facts gathered in the patient history cannot always be discovered during a clinical examination. Without input from the patient, the type of intervention and the rehabilitation potential will be compromised. This process is initiated at registration using a written questionnaire and followed with an interview with the treating therapist. A short answer form asks the patient to describe the mechanism of injury, the date of injury, the date and type of surgery, the chief complaint, the type of pain and location, the medications being taken, other medical conditions that may affect the condition, and dominance. The therapist will read the history and sign and date the form (because it becomes a vital part of the patient chart). The interview begins with listening and comprehending the patient's understanding of his or her condition and what is it that he or she wants to achieve from treatment.

During the initial interview, the therapist directs open-ended questions that allow the patient to tell his or her story. This communication is patient-centered and generally is symptom and activity focused. Symptoms of pain, swelling, numbness, and stiffness are a few of the concerns that are easily described by the patient. The major problem or problems that brings the patient to therapy is documented as the chief complaint or complaints. If the patient has not been a part of the medical system, he or she will generally discuss activity limitations spontaneously in comparison with individuals with chronic problems, who will speak like medical professionals. However, it is important to encourage the patient to describe the condition in personal terms. When did the problem start? Was there pain initially? Where was it located? Were there any signs of swelling? Was there pain during the activity or the next day? How stiff is the patient when he or she awakes in the morning? Questions are generated from the patient's responses. The success of the therapist-patient interview depends on the ability of the professional to gather and to assemble the history. Patient histories will assist in understanding the overall status of the patient, provide the targeted limitations of specific functional performance, and serve as qualifiers of patient satisfaction.

Once the patient's story has been established, the therapist asks questions that focus on the biomechanical actions of the upper extremity. Questions that are used to understand the patient's presenting condition include those regarding the mechanism of injury, the date of injury, the length of immobilization, if any, prior therapy attempts, the patient's attempts at symptom relief, and the quality of success for those attempts. Pain descriptors provide the level of pain aggravation and general irritability. The patient history is essential to understand postural imbalances, to identify sites for further palpation, and to select measures for the objective examination.

Postural Imbalances

The kinematics of the extremity relies heavily on the contributions of the articular structure and the efficiency of the neuromuscular system. Therefore imbalances in the hand and wrist are the foundation for understanding the complex nature of hand dysfunction. Observations of these imbalances play a critical role in identifying the "real problem" and in developing the appropriate treatment plan. Postural imbalances can be observed during various dynamic movement and static postures. Over time, these imbalances can become fixed and less malleable to treatment.

Resting and dynamic imbalances can be the result of a primary or secondary orthopaedic or neuromuscular disorder. After the onset of joint and soft tissue changes, lengthening and shortening of the surrounding structures occur. The permanency and specific tissue changes can be investigated using available clinical tools and manual techniques.

Initially, the resting balance posture of a patient is observed; then the dynamic movement is assessed. Consider the individual with a posterior interosseous nerve lesion. In the resting position, the wrist may have good anatomic alignment. With the increased demands of gross grasp against resistance, the wrist becomes increasingly flexed. The weakened ECU and EDC are overpowered by the unopposed extrinsic finger and wrist flexors, resulting in wrist flexion during active effort. As the effort increases, the dynamic postural imbalance increases. Eventually the postural imbalance of increasing wrist flexion will inhibit flexion of the digit joints by virtue of the tenodesis principle. Patients report the loss of mechanical advantage as the grip loosens and objects are dropped.

> **Clinical Tip**
> As loads increase, dynamic posture imbalances become more pronounced. However, dynamic imbalance can be present when the resting posture is normal.

Classifications of Imbalances

Three types of wrist and hand imbalances have been identified. The first imbalance is described as postural resting balance (PRB). The resting postural imbalances must be compared with normal balance of the wrist and hand. Observations must be assessed in various static postures. The second type of dysfunction is observed during motion and is described as *postural dynamic balance* (PDB). The last imbalance is described as *postural fixed balance* (PFB). This type of imbalance may occur over time or may be the result of a joint derangement. As a result, the static joint position is not altered at rest or with movement. A patient may have developed one or all of the categories of postural imbalances. These imbalances will be reviewed in more depth.

Postural Resting Balance

This classification is based on the observations of a patient's forearm, hand, and digits in static, resting position. The resting position is defined as *static* because the patient makes no volitional attempt to change or consciously control the joint or anatomic part. Balance, or imbalance, is determined by the expected balanced postures described in the articular, musculotendinous, neurologic, and vascular structures of the wrist and hand. Imbalances are easier to observe with patients who have severe nerve injuries and motor denervation. For individuals with a low ulnar nerve lesion, claw deformities of the ulnar two fingers and a supinated thumb are created from the absence of finger MP flexion and IP extension (intrinsics) and adduction of the thumb.

Resting imbalances are assessed by observing the balance of intrinsic and extrinsic effects on a joint. The intrinsic effects on the joint are found in the capsular pathologic condition. For example, a resting imbalance is seen after a hyperextension injury to the PIP joint. Capsular laxity in an injured PIP palmar plate results in dorsal displacement of the lateral band. Over time this imbalance becomes a swan neck deformity.

> **Clinical Tip**
> Postural resting imbalances can result from forces directed on the joint capsule that repositions and shifts the articulation opposite to the restriction.

When the joint integrity is not altered but the extrinsic balance on the joint is interrupted, resting balance can be interrupted by the antagonist muscle that works unopposed. An example is observed in the case of a digital flexor tendon laceration or adhesion. The extrinsic extensor tendon will pull unopposed into an extended posture, and a loss of normal flexion cascade of digit position is observed (Figure 12-33).

Resting imbalances are seen in patients with neuromuscular and articular system disorders such as those seen in cases of advanced rheumatoid arthritis. As the wrist becomes unstable, intrinsic capsular support is lost, the axis of the joint changes, and the extrinsic muscle tendons will dictate the joint position. Frequently, a zigzag deformity at rest will occur with the wrist

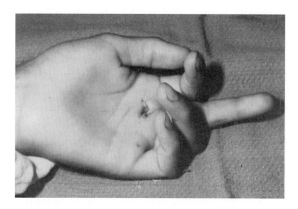

Figure 12-33 The posture of the middle finger in this anesthetized hand reveals division of both flexor tendons to that digit. (From Lister G: The hand: diagnosis and indication, ed 2, Edinburgh, 1984, Churchill Livingstone.)

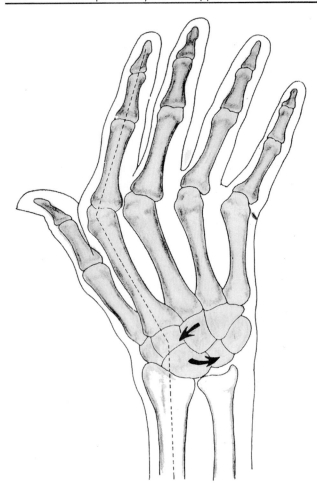

Figure 12-34 The zigzag deformity with wrist radial deviation and metacarpophalangeal joint ulnar deviation. (Redrawn from Melvin JL: Rheumatoid disease: occupational therapy and rehabilitation, ed 3, Philadelphia, 1989, FA Davis.)

in radial deviation and the MP joints of the finger in ulnar deviation (Figure 12-34).

Postural Dynamic Balance

Dynamic balance of movement is coordinated rhythmic mobility of the joints in relative effortlessness during task performance. A deficiency in PDB may originate intrinsically at an isolated joint or involve the entire kinematic chain. The motoric compensations that arise from the imbalance come from an individual's unconscious attempts to complete a task, regardless of pathologic condition.

Patterns of normal dynamic balance of the upper extremity are complex, and injury or disease may be the cause of imbalance. Postural changes may start centrally and progress distally or start distally and having a progressive effect proximally. The imbalance may begin at an isolated joint, become exaggerated after an application of stress, and alter the patterns of the one or more joints in the kinematic chain as demands from the environment increase.

"Posture is the composite of the positions of all the joints of the body at any given moment."[14] Assessment of posture for the back and shoulder complex has been well documented in the literature. Scapular stabilization and position is essential for upper extremity movement. The humerus is guided by the angle of the glenoid. The rotator cuff muscles work to balance and control the humeral head in rotation and depression. The scapula-humeral rhythm will maximize shoulder elevation, abduction, and rotation in an efficient manner. Likewise, the elbow flexors in conjunction with the forearm rotators, position and stabilize the forearm in space for wrist, hand, and digit movement. The wrist is held and repositioned throughout a task in various degrees of extension for most digit manipulation tasks.

Although core postures control the kinematic events of the distal extremity, the biomechanics of dynamic balance at successive joints requires keen observation of the smallest details in the upper extremity. Many examples of postural dynamic imbalance exist. One example occurs with overhead reaching tasks. The shoulder complex elevates (shrugs) and the trunk extends to assist in getting an object above shoulder height. Another example is with individuals who have radioulnar joint problems. Compensation by the shoulder adductors and external rotators are needed to replace limited supination of the forearm when holding and carrying a flat box. Distally the hand will supinate, the fifth metacarpal flexes, and the thumb CMC joint extends to assist with hand placement on the side of the box. A final example of dynamic imbalance is that found at an isolated joint. In the PIP palmar plate injury, laxity of the volar support results in PIP joint hyperextension and eventual lateral band dorsal displacement and subsequent distal phalanx flexion. The dynamic collapse pattern is usually provoked with fingertip pressure. Functionally, individuals will use digit tip pressure to satisfactorily grasp large objects.

The importance of dynamic balance is related to the ability to identify the primary cause of the dysfunction and not the obvious deformity. Understanding the dynamic balance of digit flexion and extension will direct the care. Clinicians may think the diagnosis of a patient is a mallet deformity because of the lag at the end joint; however, obtaining an accurate history and understanding the imbalances of the hand may uncover the true cause of the DIP joint flexion posture as PIP palmar laxity. With a true mallet deformity, the position of the PIP joint will not influence the amount of DIP flexion that is in a resting state of imbalance. However, the dynamic imbalance caused by the PIP joint pathologic condition will be observed when full DIP flexion and extension occurs (with PIP joint flexion and lack of full extension at the DIP when the PIP joint hyperextends).

In other situations, problems occur when treating specific joint injuries in the upper extremity and movement dysfunction is not assessed. In time, continued imbalances will result in permanent degenerative joint and soft tissue changes. For example, a TFCC injury can result in a patient holding the forearm in a neutral position and controlling the amount of supination as a strategy to minimize pain. The imbalance can be seen in the ulnar wrist region with a prominent ulnar styloid and fifth MP depression. The source of the problem appears to be the distal radial-ulnar joint with joint restriction. If most of the treatment is directed to the lack of supination and pronation, the weakened ECU and atrophied hypothenar eminence are missed. Their absences contribute to lack of soft tissue stabilization and ulnar carpal balance. If this situation is not treated properly, painful supination will continue and degenerative changes can occur.

> ### Clinical Tip
> The imbalance of the ulnar carpal wrist as it relates to TFCC injury frequently is the cause of limited supination.

Dynamic balance assessments occur when the wrist and hand joints are moving. Several steps are important in observing PDB. Table 12-7 includes a series of observations and possible abnormalities that suggest that imbalance issues are present.

Postural Fixed Balance

This imbalance is defined as static, fixed joint position that is not altered during active muscle activity or with passive mobilization. PFB is a restriction in the joint, soft tissue contracture, or other types of restrictive immobilization. For example, a fixed position is present when MP joint flexion and extension does not occur with simultaneous wrist motion. If the MP joint is palmarly dislocated and ulnarly deviated, as seen in an advanced case of rheumatoid arthritis, no positional changes occur at rest or with dynamic wrist motion.

PFBs are easy to assess. They occur when the joint does not move passively. As a fixed posture, direct therapeutic procedures such as progressive low-load prolonged-stretch concepts are considered, or ultimately therapy will be limited to adaptation and compensation strategies for functional activity.

PALPATION

Palpation skills add another dimension of investigation in the evaluation of hand and wrist dysfunction. The therapist can manually assess soft tissues, bone, muscle, edema, and nerves to understand their properties. The ability to palpate these structures is beneficial in identifying an isolated pathologic condition and assessing the quality of that tissue for future treatment.

Palpation of soft tissue may be used to assess the quality of joint movement, both the accessory and PROM. The accessory motion is an aspect of joint play in which pathologic condition severely restricts the arc of available motion. The anterior-posterior or side-to-side glides are mobilization techniques used to determine the flexibility of the capsular and ligamentous structures. This maneuver is called the *end-feel* and is a

Table 12-7	Examples of Dynamic Imbalance
Maneuver	**Evidence of Imbalance**
Reach behind back	Forward trunk shift with anterior humeral head positioning
Reach to ceiling	Trunk extension with humeral motion in scapular plane, superior shoulder girdle positioning (shrug)
Forearm supination/ pronation	Hand lies outside midline orientation twisting in direction of turn
Wrist extension during grasp and pinch prehension patterns	Metacarpal-phalangeal (MP) extension with wrist extension, inability to maintain small objects in palm (because the grasp pattern resembles a hook position), MP joints extend simultaneously with wrist extension
Wrist flexion and extension with fingers open and relaxed	Digits' joints do not increase in flexion with wrist extension and extend with wrist flexion, as expected with normal tenodesis
Arches during grasp and pinch patterns	Flattening of palmar and distal transverse arches occurs during extended reach and release
Digital flexion and composite fisting	Fingertips do not converge simultaneously to the distal palmar crease
Open and close fingers	Interphalangeal (IP) joints initiate action, then the MP joint motion follows during flexion, open digits abduct and extend
The position of the thumb in opposition to each finger	Terminal joint of the thumb does not flex and pronate as the thumb moves across the palm to the small finger
Thumb extension to end range	MP joint is prominent, IP joint may flex

subjective expression of available motion. The end-feel of joint capsular motion is first assessed on the noninvolved side and then is compared with the involved tissues. Soft end-feel of the joint indicates a potential for improved or normal flexibility, whereas the contrasting spectrum is a bony end-feel that indicates an unyielding quality of the joint capsule. The grading of the end-feel and the force provided is essential for purposes of documentation. Table 12-8 provides a summary of common upper extremity sites for palpation of osseous and soft tissue.[15]

Passive joint mobility is the arc of motion that is achieved when the joint is moved by an outside force. The manual technique is measured by using goniometry and is reported in degrees. A variety of methods are acceptable, and the reliability is improved with consistency of the method and the rater. Although MMT is a technique used to assess the strength of agonist and synergist muscle contractions, palpation is used to determine the quality of muscle activation in the prime mover during static joint resistance. The ability of the muscle to hold

Table 12-8	Summary of Palpations (Wrist)	
Area	Osseous Structures	Soft Tissue
Radial dorsal	Radial styloid	First dorsal extensor compartments (extensor pollicis brevis [EBP], abductor pollicis longus [APL])
	Scaphoid	Third dorsal extensor
	Scaphotrapezial joint	compartment (extensor
	Trapezium	pollicis longus [EPL])
	First carpal-metacarpal (CMC) Joint	
Central dorsal	Lister's tubercle	Second dorsal extensor
	Scapholunate joint	compartment (extensor carpi radialis longus [ECRL], extensor carpi radialis brevis [ECRB])
	Lunate	Fourth dorsal extensor
	Capitate	compartment (extensor digitorum communis [EDC], extensor indicis proprius [EIP])
	Base of second and third metacarpals	Fifth dorsal extensor compartment (extensor digiti minimi [EDM])
	CMC joints of index and middle fingers	
Ulnar dorsal	Ulnar styloid	Triangular fibrocartilage complex (TFCC)
	Distal radioulnar joint	Sixth dorsal
	Triquetrum	compartment (extensor
	Hamate	carpi ulnaris [ECU])
	Base of fourth and fifth metacarpals	
Ulnar volar	Pisiform	Flexor carpi ulnaris (FCU)
	Hook of Hamate	Ulnar nerve and artery
	Triquetrum	(Guyon's canal)
Radial volar	Tubercle of the trapezium	Palmaris longus
	Radial styloid	Carpal tunnel Flexor carpi ulnaris [FCU] Radial artery

against a resistance is a valuable tool for documentation of muscle strength.

Palpation for swelling is a way to determine the type and consistency of inflammation. Spongy-to-fibrotic feel is based on the tissue resistance to fingertip pressure. Brawny edema is characterized by firm tissue. Pitting tissue is the result of a pit that slowly fills back after fingertip pressure and is a determination of tissue flexibility and remodeling potential. The examiner's thumb is placed on the tissue for 10 seconds. When the pressure is removed, the time for the tissue to return to the original shape is an objective measurement of tissue rebound. The denseness or firmness to the tissue has not been standardized, but measures for rebound offer guidelines to determine the ability to mobilize the edema.[4]

Sensory disturbances initially can be assessed by palpation. Skin temperature can be assessed by comparing extremities. Identifying colder or warmer parts are useful when assessing vascular instability, joint irritability, or even local infection. Tapping along the path of the nerve assists the clinician in localizing the site of compression or the level of sensory nerve return in cases of denervation. Light touch and the patient's response to pain provides information about neurologic irritability. Moisture patterns (e.g., slippery, dry, normal) are important indicators of peripheral nerve function. During palpation of the joint and soft tissue structures, the therapist can assess the pain response of the patient and use this response to assess the patient's overall performance response. Excessive pain responses can overshadow all assessment results and render them inconclusive. Therapeutic use of touch is an art to understanding the complex nature of the tissue equilibrium and its response to disease and injury.

Clinical Tip
Generally the *why* (cause) of the patient condition can be derived from the physician diagnosis, the patient history, and the interview that occurs before the physical examination.

OBJECTIVE MEASURES

The first step in evaluating a patient is to identify the presence of postural imbalances, to inspect those structures using palpation, and to use patient history and medical reports for validating the potential mechanics that create the imbalances. Once the problem is identified, objective measures are selected to establish the patient's baseline performance and to demonstrate progress in resolving specific imbalances. A review of assessments for body functions and activity limitations is provided following.

Upper Extremity Screening

Functional range of motion is the observation of motion during simulated tasks such as touching the top and back of the head, reaching overhead, making contact with the small of the back, and using the thumb to pinch to each digit. The combination of motions may demonstrate an ease of motion or difficulty that will predict limitations in functional tasks. These bilateral motions also allow for screening of possible asymmetries.

The most common complaint of patients is paresthesias or pain. The pathologic condition may arise from proximal structures such as cervical or shoulder articular and neuromuscular structures. Screening of these areas is essential to recognizing the cause and source of the pathologic condition.

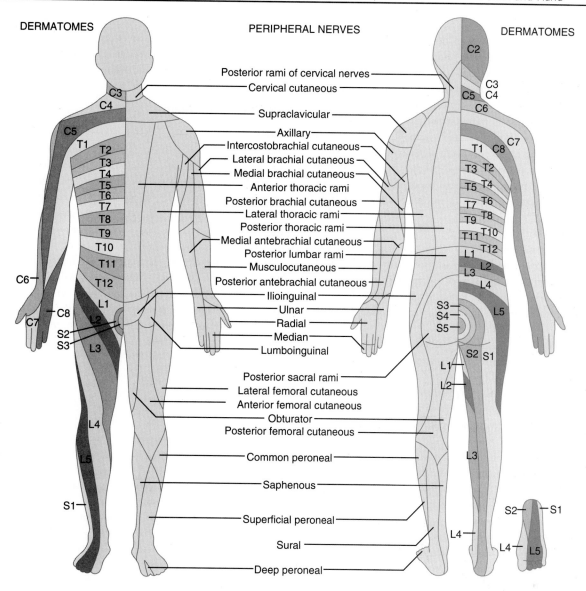

Figure 12-35 Dermatomes and cutaneous distribution of peripheral nerves. (From Lundy-Ekman L: Neuroscience: fundamentals for rehabilitation, ed 3, St Louis, 2008, Saunders.)

The cervical nerve roots, discs, facets, intrinsic soft tissues, and extrinsic soft tissues may present as trigger point pain, radiating pain, or complete sensory and motor loss of the extremity. Cervical vertebra, like all joints, may have soft tissue adhesions intrinsically or extrinsically that decrease range of motion. The worsening of symptoms while performing flexion, extension, rotation, or lateral flexion of the cervical spine is indicative of a pathologic condition. Overpressure at the end range of a structure with lesions will also provoke the symptoms. The sensory dermatomes are well established for determining nerve root pathologic condition (Figure 12-35). If a cervical condition is considered a possibility, then a complete cervical examination is recommended.

The shoulder complex represents another contributor to upper extremity pain and parenthesis. The thoracic outlet is a pathway of vascular and neural structures to the upper extrem-

ity and is divided into four regions. The sternocostovertebra, scalene, costoclavicular, and coracopectoral spaces are bordered by muscle and contain aspects of vascular and brachial plexus structures. If the spaces are compressed, the cords of the plexus and subclavian artery and vein will be affected. Patients with soft tissue restrictions in these areas will experience a variety of pain, temperature, and fatigue complaints.

Brachial plexopathies have vague symptoms and do not match the cervical or peripheral sensory and motor distributions. Patients' complaints are weakness, pain, and paresthesias that are delayed months after an injury to the shoulder or neck. The patient history may include slow progression and worsening of symptoms as the soft tissue shortens from postural imbalances that limit vascular and neural structures. Many times the patients' symptoms worsen with stretching and overhead activities.[9]

Pain

Details of a patient's pain perceptions are helpful in understanding how soft tissue responds to injury. Pain that is not grounded in a firm diagnosis requires a thorough knowledge of the upper extremity and cervical spine as the location, because the complaints of pain are not always the site of the pathologic condition. Positions and movements that exacerbate or relieve symptoms are important to plan a patient's treatment program. Referred pain is reported by the patient in an area other than would be expected with a provocative maneuver. Reproducing the pain is important in understanding the associated pathology.

In addition, the patient's perception and general response to pain can be descriptive. Many terms can create qualitative meaning about pain and a baseline for future comparison. The terms define the onset, severity, chronicity, and provocative nature of the pain complaint. Several observations and series of questions are useful in interviewing patients with pain.

1. Location. Patients can touch the location of pain at the site, or they can identify the location of pain on a body diagram.
2. Radiating. Pain that is moving proximal or distal to the original site of pain is considered radiating pain. This pain frequently is described as *shooting pain* and may be the result of nerve damage.
3. Quality. The description of a sensation is qualified with other forms of sensation. The patient may describe the pain as *throbbing, shooting, burning,* or *aching.* The McGill Pain Questionnaire is useful in measuring the subjective responses of a patient's pain response.[16]
4. Quantity. Asking the patient to describe the level of pain can help the clinician to assess the magnitude of experienced pain. Using self-report or a visual analog pain scale can quantify pain. The scale ranges from 0 to 10, with zero representing *no perception of pain* and ten attributed to *the worst pain ever experienced by the patient.*
5. Duration. The length of time that a patient's pain remains can be described in episodes and periods over time. Chronic pain is classified as *6 months or longer,* whereas acute pain is classified as *more recent,* generally after an episode of trauma or overuse. The duration is accompanied by questions regarding when the pain began and if it occurred during, before, or after activity.
6. Frequency. It may be important to know how often the pain occurs in a 24-hour period, if the painful area hurts everyday or only on workdays, and if pain increases as the day progresses.
7. Aggravation and Relief. Factors that increase or decrease symptoms can be supportive in treating patients with pain. The therapist consistently asks the patient to relate pain responses with specific activities, postures, and known pathologic condition. It also is helpful to identify aggravating factors related to nocturnal pain, such as how often the pain wakes the patient up or if the patient awakens first, then moves and the movement results in pain.
8. Associated Symptoms. Frequently, pain is associated with other symptoms such as swelling, weakness, stiffness, and changes in activity patterns. Understanding associated symptoms can identify early-warning signs of pain.

Wound Assessment

Patients who have sustained an open traumatic injury or have undergone an acute flare-up of disease will have obvious signs of the healing and inflammatory responses. Acute healing is described earlier in this chapter as the inflammatory response that progresses from the fibroplasia to the collagen-remolding phase. The phases are progressive, predictable, and overlapping. After injury, the body will undergo an inflammatory phase as macrophages clean up injured or dead cells. Then, fibroblastic activity will lay down a new matrix for the formation of collagen. The body automatically will attempt to repair injured tissue. Study of the healing phases will assist the therapist in understanding wound closure of normal healing skin tissue, as well as the phases for repair of injured bone, tendon, and other soft tissue. The healing phases provide guidelines for applying safe stresses.

A color classification exists for wound care. Wounds that have necrotic tissue are classified as *black* and will proceed to the *yellow stage* as observed with light-colored edges and semi-liquid exudate. The *red* classification is identified by granulation tissue and angiogenesis that indicates new blood vessel formation. The red wound is a healthy, progressing wound that will reepithilialize or be a candidate for surgical closure or grafting. Each classification has specific treatment suggestions. Documentation of the size, depth, odor, and type of tissue present within the wound is made for objective comparable information.

Abnormal, delayed, and excessive scar formation are all complications of the normal healing process. Wounds that remain open and heal via a secondary route may produce a type of scar that is thick, raised, and nonelastic. The scar formation at the joint or within the vicinity may restrict motion because skin mobility is essential for joint mobility. Keloid formation is excessive raised scar that exceeds the boundaries of the initial injury. Hypertrophy of scar is a healing phenomenon of tissue that is raised above the surrounding tissue. Complications of healing that forms scar both superficially and within the depth of the wounds will potentially compromise functional mobility.

Edema

The purpose of edema testing is to measure the amount of localized swelling found within a digit or the amount of generalized inflammation in an extremity. Hand swelling is the body's attempt to immobilize a part and an initial stage to healing in response to an injury or a disease process. However, edema can also occur in response to excessive repetition or resistance from everyday activities or overzealous therapy programs.[17] The amount of interstitial fluid produced in response to any trauma and the length of time it remains in the soft

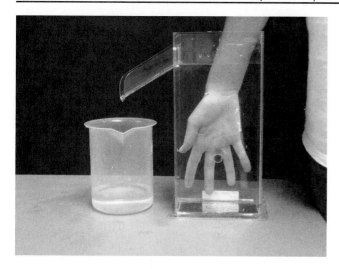

Figure 12-36 Volumetric measurement for edema. (From Cameron MH, Monroe LG: Physical rehabilitation: evidence-based examination, evaluation, and intervention, St Louis, 2007, Saunders.)

tissue leads to deformity, fibrosis, impaired cellular nutrition, risk of infection, and joint stiffening. Therefore early and continued assessment of edema is critical to reducing expected posttrauma swelling and in breaking the cycle of cumulative trauma.

Before treating localized swelling, the clinician should identify if barriers in lymphatic flow of the extremity exists. If the patient is cancer free and the edema extends beyond 21 days, proper lymphatic drainage is recommended, such as diaphragmatic breathing, opening the lymphatic channels, and adding increasing pressure gradients to the extremity. Two common assessments for edema are used: volumetric displacement and circumferential measures.[18] Commercially available hand volumeters measure the water displaced from edematous extremities (Figure 12-36). Testing is appropriate for upper limbs that are free of open wounds or external devices such as pins and fixators. The hand volumeter is placed on a level surface and is filled with tepid water until it overflows. Patients are asked to remove jewelry and dressings before testing. The hand is slowly placed into the volumeter until the middle and ring fingers straddle the inside bar. The collected runoff water is measured. If hand volumes are measured successively using the same instrument, procedure, and examiner, no more than 6 to 10 ml difference can be expected.[19] Comparison measures of the injured hand to the noninjured hand are done in the initial evaluation, and they become baseline scores during ongoing treatment. Graphing hand volumes from both extremities over time is beneficial to identify changes in the injured hand and possible overuse symptoms in the unaffected hand.[20] Although normative hand volume data are not available, a difference of 17 ml can be expected between dominant and nondominant hands.[21] Factors that effect hand volume measurements are resistive exercise,[22] increased water temperature,[23] differences in test positions,[24] time of day,[25] and stress levels.[20]

Circumferential measures are less reliable than hand volumes in measuring swelling but are useful for isolated digital swell-

ing. Consistent placement of a sturdy tape measure, caliper, or commercially available finger circumference gauge can aide the clinician in producing consistent measures. In using this assessment, poor measures can result from joints that lack full range of motion. As extension decreases, the amount of edema reduction can be overestimated.

Vascular Issues

The purpose of testing the vascular system is to identify the potential of highly traumatized tissues to heal and their appropriate response to increasing levels of resistive activity. Advances in technology have produced instruments that can monitor vascular function, and they are critical tools in the management of replant and revascularization hands and digits. For patients with fewer traumas, assessments begin with a complete patient history that includes medications, amounts of alcohol and tobacco use, comorbid conditions (e.g., diabetes; hypertension; cardiac, renal, pulmonary disease), and occupational exposures to vibration and high repetition. A hand with vascular compromise typically has color changes, poor temperature regulation, extended time to heal wounds, and trophic changes such as hair growth. Pain is reported by a majority of patients and commonly is described as *aching, cramping, tightness,* or *cold intolerance.*[18] These symptoms are usually seen at rest but are magnified with activity. As mentioned before, the modified Allen's test is useful in assessing blood flow. Other assessments can provide valuable information such as recording peripheral pulses at rest, after exercise, and in various positions such as neck rotation, scapular adduction, glenohumeral abduction, and overhead activities.

Range of Motion

The purpose of range-of-motion testing is to provide information about the arc of allowable motion and to provide measurable changes over time. Several methods are available. PROM represents the total flexibility of a joint when it is moved by external sources. The application of force must be gentle for small joints and applied in a consistent method. In cases in which objective and precise passive measurement are needed, such as in serial casting or range-of-motion measurement from different therapists, torque range of motion (TROM) has significant advantages.[26] TROM is similar to PROM except that the external force, generally 200 g, is applied to the joint by an orthotic gauge or similar torque device. In this way, reproducible measures are achieved. Active range of motion (AROM) represents the total motion that can be achieved by the patient. A difference between PROM and AROM identifies hand weakness, poor tendon excursion, swelling, nerve palsy, pain, or fear of movement.

Individual joint measurements of the hand and thumb frequently are taken at the initial evaluation. Composite scores may be calculated for each digit from these findings. Total active motion (TAM) is computed using the AROM from the MP, PIP, and DIP joints of one digit minus the extension lag at those same joints. A normal TAM is 240 degrees, with contributions from the MP joint of 90 degrees, the PIP joint of 90 degrees, and the DIP joint of 60 degrees. Variations in TAM exist based on diagnosis. For example, the TAM for a patient with a flexor tendon repair in zone II is 175 degrees.[27] Similar measures can be calculated for passive range of motion (total passive motion [TPM]).

Clinical Tip

TAM and TPM measurements are useful in identifying true progress, especially with a patient who makes improvements in flexion at the expense of losing extension.

Less precise measurements are useful in ongoing treatment sessions.

Measurement Type	Measurement Technique	Figure
Finger flexion	Distance from the fingertips to the distal palmar crease	Figure 12-37, *A*
Tightness of the intrinsic muscles	Distance from the fingertips to the base of the metacarpal heads	Figure 12-37, *B*
Thumb flexion-abduction	Distance from the pad of the thumb to the metacarpal head of the little finger	Figure 12-37, *C*
Finger and thumb extension	Distance of the digit tip to the table or, in severe cases, using the distance of the digit tip to the wrist crease	Figure 12-37, *D* and *E*

Measuring the influence of elbow and forearm position on wrist range of motion is needed. Comparison range-of-motion readings can be done in positions of slack and full tension on the musculotendinous structures. Range of motion for wrist flexion may change when elbow flexion, forearm supination, and relaxed fingers are used compared with elbow extension, forearm pronation, and fisted fingers (Figure 12-38, *A*). Range of motion for wrist extension can change when elbow flexion, forearm pronation, and relaxed fingers are used compared with elbow extension, forearm supination, and extended fingers (Figure 12-38, *B*).

Clinical Tip

Range-of-motion measurements should reflect the purpose of the assessment, whether it is to measure the function of an isolated joint or to predict the quality of movement in everyday activities.

Sensibility

The purpose of sensibility testing in the upper extremity is to determine the patient's ability to identify and discriminate sensory input. The results help to explain the diagnosis, the level and severity of the impairment, and the activity limitations that can occur.

In administering any sensibility test, several factors need to be controlled. Testing is done in a quiet, distraction-free area of the clinic. Cooler room temperatures are minimized because of their effect in decreasing sensibility. Testing is done by the same examiner to ensure reliable scores across time. Patients are instructed in the procedure with eyes open, then with vision occluded for all tests except the objective and functional pickup tests. The hand and fingers are supported adequately to avoid cueing from proprioception receptors. Patients who make good candidates for sensibility testing are adults with good cognitive abilities and who have testing sites that are not hypersensitive. Patients should clean the hands and when possible, and comparison to an unaffected area should be done. Clinical observations of burned or cut areas, differences in calluses, and trophic changes should be noted.

Many sensibility evaluations have been developed. Table 12-9 provides a summary of the most commonly used tests. They are organized in three categories: objective, threshold, and functional.[15] The method of administration is based on recommendations from the American Society of Hand Therapists.[28] The choice of testing sites depends on the neuroanatomic structures that are involved. If the patient's responses do not match a peripheral distribution, testing should include sensibility testing in respective dermatome distribution.

A complete battery of sensibility testing is not always indicated. Therefore the selection of a test depends on many factors (the type of injury, the amount of time after injury, and the expected recovery for that time period) being the foremost considerations to test patients with acute nerve injuries. When the sensibility of a patient is evaluated within 6 to 24 weeks of a nerve injury, or if a patient demonstrates problems with the function of the sympathetic nervous system, objective categories of assessment can be selected. Ninhydrin and wrinkle tests provide information about the sudomotor function, and they are easy to administer. In patients with nerve repairs, a Tinel's test can identify the level of nerve regeneration and can suggest the appropriate timing for threshold and functional tests. The Tinel's test is administered by tapping over the nerve, starting at the repair site where the first tingling sensation generally occurs, and moving distally along the nerve distribution. A positive Tinel's test occurs when the patient reports a second localized site of tingling or radiating pain. For patients with nerve compression, the site of compression can be identified by tapping the nerve distally and finding the Tinel's sign, or the point of high nerve irritability. Once the Tinel's test is negative, further sensibility testing is indicated. Starting with the threshold testing, protective sensibility and light touch can be assessed followed by functional tests and functional activities.

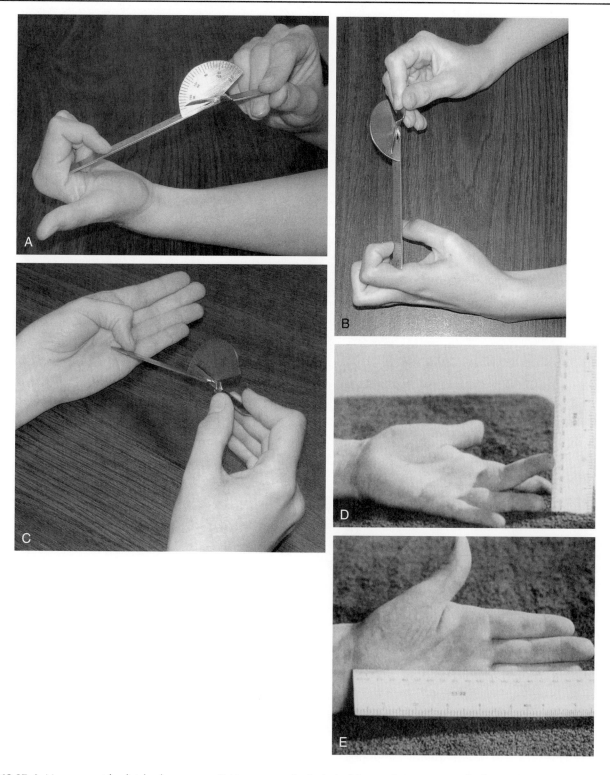

Figure 12-37 A, Measurement for distal palmar crease. **B,** Measurement for intrinsic tightness. **C,** Measurement for flexion abduction of the thumb. **D,** Distance of the fingertips from the table. **E,** Distance of the fingertips away from the scar or the wrist. (**D** and **E** from Salter MI: Hand injuries: a therapeutic approach, Edinburgh, 1987, Churchill Livingstone.)

Strength

MMT of agonist or synergist muscles are used to evaluate the impairment that results from nerve injuries or specific musculotendinous injuries. More often, instruments are used to quantify gross grasp and pinch strengths. Only after adequate healing of hand injuries, especially fractures and tendon repairs, can grip and pinch strength be evaluated. Maximum effort testing should be done only after receiving a physician release that the bone, the muscle, the tendon, or the nerve has healed and it is ready for unrestricted activity.

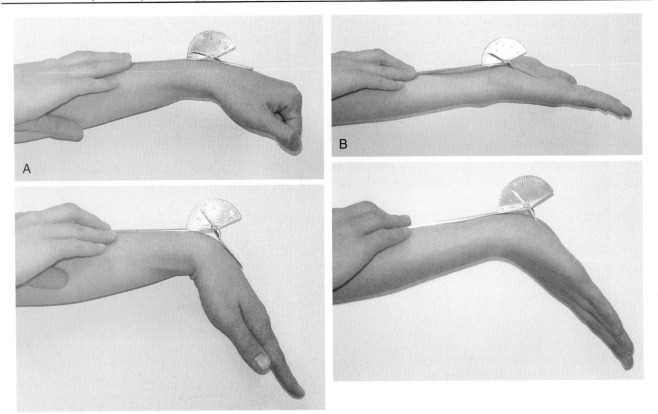

Figure 12-38 A, Comparison range-of-motion wrist flexion. **B,** Comparison range-of-motion wrist extension (1 and 3: Relaxed positions; 2 and 4: Elongated positions).

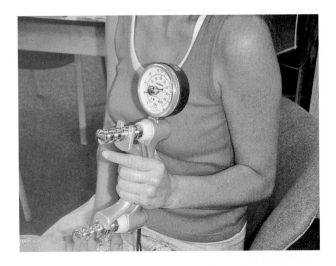

Figure 12-39 Dynamometer used to measure grip strength. (From Henderson A: Hand function in the child: foundations for remediation, ed 2, St Louis, 2006, Mosby.)

A calibrated Jamar dynamometer is recommended to measure static grip, five-level grip strength, and rapid-exchange grip.[18] Patients should be tested in a seated position, shoulder adducted, elbow flexed at 90 degrees, and forearm and wrist in neutral position (Figure 12-39). For the static test, the average score of three trials is calculated. Although

problems have been reported with normative data, the 10% rule is used. An overall difference of 10% grip strength has been validated for right hand–dominant subjects only, and equivalent hand grips are expected for left hand–dominant patients.[29] Evidence has not supported the use of the five-grip and rapid-exchange tests to determine sincerity of effort but can be used as another measure of grip force.[30] For the five-level grip test, measurements are taken at each setting, and a bell-shaped curve is expected. The rapid-exchange test requires 10 trials of alternating grips between the right and left hands. Comparison of scores for the injured and noninjured hands is made.

A calibrated pinch meter is recommended to measure tip, key or lateral, and three-point pinches. The same starting postures for grip strength testing are used for assessing pinch strength. Figure 12-40 describes the positions for each assessment. Three trials are taken, and the average scores between the injured and noninjured extremities are compared. Observations of thumb imbalances and reports of pain should be noted.

Dynamic grip and pinch strengths are desirable because functional activity requires a combination of static and dynamic strength. Unfortunately, static testing does not predict dynamic strength.[31-33] Functional testing equipment, such as the Baltimore Therapeutic Equipment, is commercially available to test strength. To date, preliminary studies have found significant amounts of error in classifying healthy

Table 12-9	Summary of Sensibility Tests				
Test		Sensation	Instrument	Method	Response
Objective	Ninhydrin	Sudomotor function—sweating	Acid-free paper and Ninhydrin spray	Hand is placed under a light for 20 minutes, fingers are rolled on paper to wick available sweat, paper is sprayed	Scale 0 to 3: 0 = absent sweating, 3 = normal sweating
	O'Riain wrinkle test	Sudomotor function—wrinkling	Sink or tub of water 108° F	Immerse both hands for 30 minutes	Scale 0 to 3: 0 = absent wrinkling 3 = normal sweating wrinkling
Threshold	Pinprick test	Pain, protective	Using a sterile needle because of deinnervated skin and risk of human immunodeficiency virus (HIV) transmission	Apply enough force to indent the skin	Correct number of responses for sharp and dull
	Temperature test	Pain, protective	Hot and cold discrimination kits with thermometer	Apply hot and cold alternately	Correct number of responses for cold and hot
	Light touch test	Pressure	Five-kit Semmes Weinstein monofilaments	Apply filament three times to the six sites beginning with 2.83 until one of three responses is accurate	Normal = 2.83 Diminished light touch = 3.61 Diminished protective sensation = 4.31 Loss of protected sensation = 6.65
	Tuning fork test	Vibration	30 and 256 CPS	Application of prong or stem	More, less, same as contralateral hand
Sensation response	Vibrometer test	Vibration	Biothesiometer	Hold in contact with tested area, gradually increase intensity until vibration perceived	More, less, same as contralateral hand
Functional	Weber static two-point test	Discriminative touch	Disk-Criminator or calipers; use of paper clips should be avoided because of single barbed end	Apply 5 mm opening longitudinally randomly, with one and two points; increase or decrease space based on patient response until seven of ten responses is accurate	Normal 0-5 mm Fair 6-10 mm Poor 10-15 mm Protective 1 point perceived Anesthetic no points perceived
	Moving two-point test	Discriminative touch	Same as static two point	Same as static two point plus the instrument is moved distally along the lateral border of the digit	Normal = 2 mm
	Localization test	Touch	Cotton ball or Semmes Weinstein monofilaments	Lightly touch a digit, identify location with eyes open	Map discrepancies
	Dellon modified pick-up test	Motor discriminative	Thirteen test items	Objects are on the table, each individual item is placed in a container with eyes open and closed	Observation only, no normative data

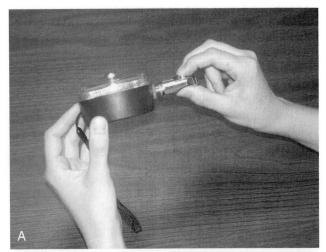

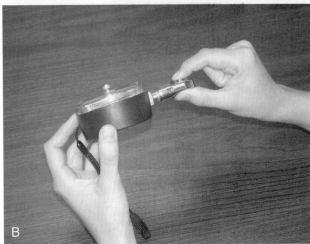

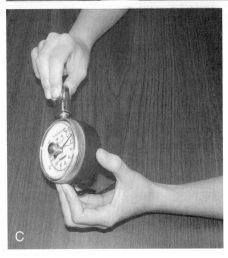

Figure 12-40 Positions for pinch strength. **A,** Tip pinch. **B,** Key (or lateral) pinch. **C,** Three-point pinch.

subjects' maximal and submaximal grip strengths.[34] Therefore dynamic strength testing should not stand alone and is recommended as an adjunct measure for static strength tests, for functional testing, and for grading treatment sessions for strengthening.

Dexterity

The purpose of assessing dexterity is to demonstrate the ability of the hands and fingers to perform more complex movements, such as turning and placing objects skillfully and manipulating small items rapidly and accurately.[35] Dexterity testing is important because measures of sensibility, range of motion, and strength do not always predict a patient's performance in everyday activities, especially for female patients.[36] Many standardized assessments have been developed to evaluate dexterity, and normative data are available for each test. Choosing one of these tests is enhanced through a classification system developed by the American Society of Hand Therapists.[37] Six categories are reported:

1. The size of the test area determines the position of the extremity and the amount of reaching required. Large test areas extend beyond 12 square inches.
2. Small test areas are contained in 12 square inches.
3. Handling involves working the whole hand to grasp and release objects smoothly.
4. Finger dexterity differs from handling in that the fingers are used to manipulate objects.
5. Tool use involves the manipulation of instruments such as wrenches, screwdrivers, or tweezers.
6. Activities of daily living (ADL) simulations involve self-care tasks such as eating, dressing, and hygiene.

A review of nine commonly used dexterity tests is provided in Table 12-10. Some of the instruments can be fabricated by the clinic, but all of the measures are commercially available.

Outcome Measures

The purpose of using outcome measures is to overcome the discrepancies that can occur between the severity of symptoms reported by patients and the limitations clinically assessed by a hand specialist.[38] For instance, patients with severe nerve impairment may report minimal carpal tunnel symptoms but have significant complaints related to their hand function. Three well-known outcome measures have been identified to measure limitations in ADL and instrumental activities of daily living (IADL) experienced by patients with hand and upper extremity disorders. They are the Levine Symptom Severity Scale, the Michigan Hand Outcomes Questionnaire, and the Disabilities of the Arm, Shoulder, and Hand (DASH). Several patient-rated evaluations have been developed. Assessments focus on the pain and the function of specific joints to include the wrist, the forearm, the elbow, and the combined issues of the wrist and hand. Another measure is the Focus on Therapeutic Outcomes (FOTO), which combines outcome data collection and documentation across the rehabilitation continuum. The Flinn Performance Screening Tool (FPST) is an outcomes measure that personalizes the functional outcomes that are important but problematic for each patient. To date, 323 photographs of daily life activities are used: 144 personal-care pictures, 157 home and outside pictures, and 22 physical capacity line drawings. Table 12-11 provides a summary of all these assessments.

Table 12-10 Classification of Dexterity Tests by Characteristics

Tests	Large Test Area	Small Test Area	Handling	Finger Dexterity	Tool Use	Activities of Daily Living (ADL)	Job Simulation
Box and blocks	x		x				
Bennett hand tool dexterity	x			x	x		x
Crawford small parts		x		x	x		x
Purdue pegboard	x			x			x
Grooved pegboard		x		x			
O'Connor finger dexterity		x		x			
Nine-hole peg		x		x			
Jebson Taylor hand function test	x		x	x		x	
Minnesota Rate of Manipulation Test	x			x			

Table 12-11 Upper Extremity Outcomes Measures

Name	Domains	Format	Reference
Symptoms severity scale	Symptoms (number of items = 11) Function (number of items = 8)	Likert	Levine D, Simmons B, Koris M et al: A self-administered questionnaire for the assessment of severity of symptoms and functional status in carpal tunnel syndrome, *J Bone Joint Surg* 75-A (11):1585-1592, 1993.
Michigan Hand Outcomes Questionnaire	Overall hand function (number of items = 10) Activities of daily living (ADL) (number of items = 17) Pain (number of items = 10) Work performance (number of items = 5) Aesthetics (number of items = 8) Patient satisfaction (number of items = 12)	Likert	Available at: http://surgery.med. umich.edu/plastic/research/index. shtml
Disabilities of the Arm, Shoulder, And Hand (DASH)	Symptoms (number of items = 9) Function (number of items = 21) Optional: Work (number of items = 4) Sports/performing arts (number of items = 4)	Likert	Available at: http://www.dash.iwh. on.ca/index.htm
Patient-Rated Wrist Evaluation (PRWE), Patient-Rated Forearm Evaluation (PRFEQ), Patient-Rated Elbow Evaluation (PREE)	Symptoms (number of items = 5) Function (number of items = 10)	Likert	Dr. Joy MacDermid, Physiotherapy Program, McMaster University School of Rehabilitation Science IAHS 1400 Main Street W, Hamilton, ON L8S 1C7
Wrist and Hand Evaluation (PRWHE)	Symptoms (number of items = 5) Function (number of items = 15)	10-Interval visual analog scale	Dr. Joy MacDermid Physiotherapy Program McMaster University School of Rehabilitation Science IAHS 1400 Main Street W, Hamilton, ON L8S 1C7
Focus on Therapeutic Outcomes (FOTO)	Pain Function/QOL Return to work Patient global assessment Patient satisfaction	Likert	Available at: http://www.fotoinc.com/ company.htm
Flinn Performance Screening Tool (FPST)	Personal care (number of items = 144) Home and outside (number of items = 157) Physical capacities (number of items = 22)	Dichotomous rating of important but poorly performed	Functional Visions Inc Donna Ventura, Product Manager 829 Bethel Road #313 Columbus, Ohio

---

BOX 12-1 **Suggestions for Patient Participation**

- The quality of collaboration between the patient and the therapist is the basis for selling the plan of care.
- Success in treatment depends on the patient's perception of meaningfulness about the clinical program.
- Therapeutic procedures are personalized based on a patient's specific functional need.
- Simulated tasks that are performed in the clinical setting encourage confidence for home programming.
- Positive adaptations will facilitate a patient's success in completing clinical tasks and home programs.
- The ability to curtail exercise and functional activity when overuse or accelerated healing occurs leads to long-term therapy compliance.
- Skillful progression of activity levels by the therapist requires an understanding of different types of compensations that may be used and maladaptive compensations that must be avoided.
- Recovery of function is the weighted exchange between a home programming of forced use, spontaneous recovery, and a complement of therapeutic exercises.

PARTICIPATION IN TREATMENT

Recovery is "a way of living a satisfying, hopeful, and contributing life, even with the limitations caused by illness."[39] Engaging individuals in the rehabilitation process is an important part of achieving successful recovery outcomes. Even though these efforts are difficult to measure, five characteristics have been associated with individuals who demonstrate positive attitudes during their healing process:

1. Having personal confidence and hope
2. Asking for help
3. Being goal and success orientated
4. Relying on others
5. Coping with symptoms[40]

Empowering patients to participate in the treatment process requires these characteristics to be reinforced with compliant patients or by modeling the behavior from the therapist when they are absent. One approach to facilitating positive recovery behaviors is through patient education on the healing process, personalized home programs that are realistic, and strategies for monitoring compliance. Suggestions to facilitate a patient's participation in hand therapy are included in Box 12-1.

Treatment Hypothesis

The development of the treatment hypothesis is the process of identifying all of the patient's problems, determining the specific therapeutic intervention, and predicting the outcome of the intervention.

Clinical Tip
The treatment hypothesis asks the following: If a problem exists, then what specific therapeutic intervention can be used to treat it, and what outcomes can be expected from that particular treatment?

Answering the question of whether or not a problem exists begins with the observation of the forearm, wrist, and hand in various resting postures. By using the normal anatomic lines of balance, the therapist can determine which joints display irregular patterns. The joint with an atypical angle may be the presenting problem but not the cause. The mechanism of imbalance occurs when a loss of supporting structures and abnormal pull from the unaffected muscles exist. Particular attention to the pathomechanics of the resting posture and the mechanism by which the soft tissue has contributed to the imbalance is fundamental to the assessment.

To explain the cause of a problem requires further investigation of the anatomic systems. The muscle can be short (adhered), long (attenuated), or weak. The capsule and ligaments can be lax (unstable) or tight (adhesive capsulitis) and be a major contributor to joint limitation. Articular structures can be misaligned, contracted, or permanently fused as a consequence of an injury or disease. For example, a patient is referred postoperatively with a primary diagnosis of distal radius fracture and subsequent open reduction and internal fixation. Observation of the resting balanced posture identifies a neutral forearm position and wrist flexion. During dynamic movements of opening and closing the hand, the wrist does not increase the extension posture. Several hypotheses can be generated. If the wrist flexors are shortened, then they will limit the ability of the wrist extensors to contract and to assist with RC mobility. If the wrist flexors are lengthened from the application of therapeutic modalities, then the wrist extensors should be able to be strengthened and improve the amount of RC joint extension. When the resting postures of the wrist and digits are normalized, grasp abilities are improved.

A treatment hypothesis is based on therapeutic evidence. Specific questions should be proposed. Does the plan of care justify stretching the adhered structures and/or strengthening the weakness? Would the imbalance require splinting for joint support or mobilizing for soft tissue changes? Does the clinician understanding the healing phases and expectations of stresses allowed at each stage of recovery? When changes in normal patterns of movement occur statically and dynamically, a disruption in the rhythmic kinematic chain occurs. Patients describe dysfunction as *pain, paresthesia, stiffness,* and *weakness.* It is important to use the patient's self-report and observable performance of essential tasks for clinical reasoning.

Once postural observations have been made and objective testing has validated the patient's problems, the therapist must substantiate the therapeutic hypothesis. In collaboration with the patient, specific limitations in activities are identified and therapeutic interventions are developed to improve task performance. Using patient self-report and direct observation of valued life activities (occupation), the effect of treatment can be substantiated. The balance of clinical improvement and functional gains are good indicators of progress and are necessary to justify therapeutic intervention. The emphasis on task performance individualizes the plan of care and personalizes the patient's participation in the therapeutic continuum. Working with skilled team members, such as occupational therapists, will improve the focus on isolated task performance of all the skills needed for ease and satisfaction of performance.

SUMMARY

Several principles are followed when working to restore full function of individuals with injured or diseased hands and wrists. Eight steps are recommended:

1. During assessment, observe the entire person during dynamic and static postures in standing, sitting, weight-bearing activities, and various reaching heights.
2. Identify the location of pain and physical complaints, but do not assume this is the cause of the pathologic condition. Use classification of imbalance as a guide for evaluation of soft tissue.
3. Theorize the imbalance link to dysfunction and prove it through examination. Use objective tools to validate observations.

4. Address the source of complaints but identify, differentiate, and treat the cause.
5. If muscles adhesions exist, the antagonist is most likely in a weakened state.
6. Identified adhesions in the muscle or capsule must be addressed early in treatment.
7. Fixed deformities have a low probability of therapeutic change. The emphasis of intervention is limiting further deformity, strengthening proximal and distal joints, providing environmental modifications, using adaptive equipment, encouraging proper body mechanics, and suggesting work simplification techniques.
8. Reassessment will validate the hypothesis and direct changes in the plan of care.

CASE STUDIES

Two case studies illustrate the principles of evaluation and treatment for common wrist and hand diagnoses. A brief history is provided for each patient, followed by the findings from the initial visit, a treatment hypothesis, and recommendations for acute and restorative treatment.

CASE STUDY 12-1: DISTAL RADIUS FRACTURE

Distal radial fractures account for approximately 14% of all fractures.[41] Impairment of bony structures, ligaments, nerves, and muscles can influence the wrist, as well as forearm and finger functions. In general, malunion of bone fragments is not a concern for patients with open reduction and plating. If the fracture had been treated conservatively by closed reduction and percutaneous pinning, imperfect length, angulations, and inclination of the radial head may effect the orientation of the scapholunate fosse and alter the articulation of the joint. If the fracture fragments heal and the length of the radius is relatively shortened in respect to the ulna, the entire wrist complex may become dysfunctional. Ligament laxity or adhesions of the carpal ligaments and joint capsule contributes to altered joint configurations. Pain during AROM can be attributed to ineffective flexor tendon gliding as it clears the sheaths. Tendinosus is a degenerative pathologic condition that produces microscopic changes within the tendon fibers and leads to chronic forms of cumulative disorder. Stenosing tenosynovitis decreased the size of the sheath, which in turn restricts tendon excursion. Tendons that become impaired as a result of the fracture are the extensor pollicis brevis (EBP) and abductor pollicis longus (APL) from the first dorsal compartment, the EPL over Lister's tubercle, and ECU over the ulnar styloid. Positive neural tension produces symptoms with glide and stretch at potential entrapment or compression sites. Atrophy of the muscles within the hand is possible from median nerve injury or forced immobilization

and is observed as loss of muscle mass. Joint arthritis of the thumb CMC may be a source of pain. As the mechanism of injury, previous osteoarthritis or postinjury inflammation can contribute to poor motion and increased pain during pinch and grasp tasks.

History

A 59-year-old right-dominant woman sustained a fall on an outstretched hand (FOOSH) at work as a full-time advertising agent. She had an open reduction internal fixation (ORIF) of a comminuted distal radial head fracture, and plating was done on the volar aspect. Her postoperative course was not significant. She was placed in a prefabricated wrist splint and referred to therapy at 2 weeks after surgery.

Diagnostic Classification: Musculoskeletal 4G: Fracture of Radius 813.4

Because of missed appointments, the patient was not seen until 4 weeks after surgery. The patient has a 15-year history of controlled diabetes mellitus, and she is postmenopausal. She eats healthy meals, does not smoke or drink, and exercises three times per week. Her work involves frequent use of a computer and household tasks such as cleaning and cooking.

Initial Visit

Postural imbalances of the wrist and hand were observed. At rest, the wrist was positioned in mild radial flexion. The MP joints of the fingers were in extension, and the PIP

Continued

CASE STUDY 12-1: DISTAL RADIUS FRACTURE—cont'd

joints remained in a flexed posture. The distal phalanx of the digit rested on the table so that the metacarpal heads were not visible. With movement, the fingers worked as one unit. Extension primarily occurred at the MP joints because of overcompensation of the EDC and poor contributions from weak wrist extensors. Wrist extension takes place in a radial plane because of the shortened extensor carpi radialis longus (ECRL) and extensor carpi radialis brevis (ECRB) and lengthened ECU. Internal rotation and adduction of the humerus, along with trunk flexion and lateral rotation, compensated for lack of forearm supination while holding a small object. Fixed postures were observed with forearm supination. PIP joints of the digits lacked 20 degrees of extension and did not change position during tenodesis movements.

Joint mobility was compared between the affected and nonaffected extremities. The right arm had less RC, radioulnar, and PIP joint mobility than the left. Palpation of the soft tissue on the back of the hand left a faint imprint, and mild pitting edema was noted. The Watson scaphoid shift test was negative.

In screening the upper extremity, the patient's neck movements were symmetrical and without pain or sensory changes. She could demonstrate full overhead movements and the ability to touch the top and back of her head without difficulty. However, she lacked the ability to touch the middle of her back and used compensatory trunk movements.

The pain intensity of the patient's wrist was 4 of 10 at rest and increased to 7 at the end of the day. A body diagram located the pain "all around" the wrist area. She reports that pain wakes her at night and limits her hand function to the point that she must use her left hand to perform many daily activities. She uses nonprescription pain medications to manage increased pain symptoms with only minimal relief.

The incision was healing as expected for this phase of diminished inflammatory response and increased collagen remodeling. The volar wrist incision was pink in color and slightly elevated. Good hand color and temperature were found. A generalized swollen appearance of the wrist, hand, and digits was present, although not serious enough to require manual lymph drainage. Based on the patient's age, history of diabetes, and type of reduction, only active, gentle passive, and light resistance was allowed. Light functional activities were limited to eating, tying shoes, and lifting less than 5 lb.

The patient reported sensibility changes in the thumb and index digits. Tinel's signs were absent along the course of the median nerve. Diminished light touch was found in the thumb, the index, and the middle fingers. Further sensibility testing was deferred for 2 weeks to allow therapy to resolve these changes. No evidence of increased sympathetic activity was observed.

AROM measurements were taken as a baseline for treatment. Significant deficits were noted in the elbow, forearm, wrist, fingers, and thumb (measurements are reported in

Table 12-12	Distal Radius Fracture Measurements	
	Right	Left
Elbow extension	−20	Within normal limits (WNL)
Forearm supination	10	WNL
Forearm pronation	75	WNL
Wrist extension	20 (Antigravity)	WNL
Wrist flexion	40 (Antigravity)	WNL
Metacarpal-phalangeal (MP) flexion	Within normal limits (WNL)	WNL
Proximal interphalangeal (PIP) extension	−25 all fingers	WNL
Finger flexion to distal palmar crease	−4 cm all fingers	WNL
Thumb to the base little finger	−2 cm	WNL

Table 12-12). Strength testing through MMT was performed on median and ulnar innervated intrinsic muscles. Weakness was found in the abductor pollicis brevis (APB), adductor pollicis (AP), flexor digiti minimi (FDM), and the first and fifth dorsal interossei (3 of 5). The use of dynamometers and pinch meters were deferred until adequate healing has been identified by the referring physician. Dexterity of this patient was assessed through tip prehension to each finger. The placement of the fingertips and the shape of the opening were observed. More pulp and less distal tip pinch was observed, and the patient could not create a round 0 shape. In addition, increased wrist flexion compensated for limited thumb opposition. Specific dexterity testing was deferred until the patient's resting and dynamic balance improved and tenodesis function was restored.

The patient participation in treatment was enhanced through personalized education on the healing times for bone and soft tissues. This timetable was applied to estimate full function in daily activities. Short-term and long-term goals were developed to recommend self-care activities, to adapt home management tasks, and to suggest gradual return-to-work strategies. The 5 lb restriction was used to recommend environmental modifications and acceptable movement compensations. A home exercise program was established that addressed edema management and mobility issues of the wrist and hand. The therapist demonstrated specific therapeutic activities that the patient then performed. Therapy visits were scheduled so that the patient could manage her work and home life and arrange transportation to therapy.

Treatment Hypothesis

Four plausible hypotheses were developed from the history and initial visit to therapy:

CASE STUDY 12-1: DISTAL RADIUS FRACTURE—cont'd

1. If the volar soft tissue on the radial side of the wrist has restrictive adhesions, then therapeutic procedures that increase soft tissue mobility for radial wrist tissues and strengthen the ulnar wrist extrinsic muscles will restore the synergistic balance of movement at the wrist.

2. If the wrist extensors are weak and the finger extensors compensate for them, then decreasing the mechanical advantage of the MP joints through increased flexion and using therapeutic procedures to strengthen the wrist extensors will restore tenodesis function.

3. If the median nerve is irritable and wrist pain and decreased sensibility of the digits exists, then therapeutic procedures that increase nerve gliding and reduce inflammation and mechanical pressure on the nerve will restore ease of motion and improve fine-motor performance.

4. If the PIP joints of the digits have palmar capsular adhesions that limit intrinsic function to extend the joint, then therapeutic procedures to decrease joint swelling and increase extensibility of the PIP joint palmar capsule will improve intrinsic strength and normal prehension.

Management

Treatment options address the initial needs of the patient followed by restorative therapy. Acute management of this patient begins with pain reduction modalities. Rest, ice, compression, and elevation (RICE) were used as the general rule in acute injury rehabilitation. These techniques were provided based on the physical symptoms and the length of time from the injury. Splinting the wrist in neutral wrist extension mobilized the shortened and adhered tissues into a balanced resting position and improved digit and thumb motion. The patient performed light activity and exercises with the splint removed and discontinued the splint once weakened wrist extensors and volar wrist joint adhesions were not problematic. An isotoner glove was added in the initial phases to assist lymphatic flow. With an improvement in wrist position and AROM, the mild edema resolved. Patient education was used to increase patient participation in the home program. It emphasized the anatomic limitations, the healing guidelines, and the expected symptoms over the course of the recovery period. Fear avoidance and self-limiting activities were addressed to prevent secondary joint problems. Instruction in healthy biomechanics limited early compensatory maladaptive patterns.

A gradual progression of therapeutic procedures increased the motion of the wrist, the fingers, and the thumb without a negative response to the tissues that were not injured. Treatment begins with progressive resistance to lengthen short and adhered tissues; then to maximize tissue gliding in the acquired range of motion. For this patient, PROM, short of pain, was started at 4 weeks. Grade 1 joint mobilization was added for pain reduction and to restrict the patient in a pain-free range of movement. Short arcs of

AROM were encouraged. Pain-free isometric exercises were provided with place and hold at the end of the ranges. Once the patient had achieved these steps, full AROM was allowed. For this patient, a progression of resistive range of motion occurred from 6 to 8 weeks, starting with eccentric loading and ending with concentric strengthening. Weight exchanges were upgraded continuously to represent corresponding ADL.

Restorative management also was used with this patient. Superficial heat modalities, such as fluid therapy, increased available wrist and digit range of motion. Exercises such as flexor tendon glides, wrist range of motion in all planes, and forearm rotation were performed during the heat treatment. After this procedure, manual stretches and joint mobilizations were applied to the restricted soft tissue. Specific attention was given to the structures that had pulled the wrist into radial deviation and wrist flexion. Deep heat modalities, such as ultrasound, were applied to the wrist capsule during the manual stretch increase soft tissue capability.

Light-grade manual mobilization of the RC and radioulnar joint were performed in specific dorsal and volar glides. Following this technique, the joint was passively taken to its end range and held for 15 seconds. The restrictive adhesions at the incision and injury site were addressed with light hand pressure to the volar wrist incision and superficial pressure and mobilization of the underlying adhesions. A small ball roll encouraged range of motion in all anatomic planes of movement. The benefit of using this therapeutic activity is the focus on the ball rather than on joint range of motion. This technique assisted the patient to move spontaneously to the end ranges of wrist and forearm motions, to stretch in all planes of movement, and to normalize her movement by writing out letters of the alphabet.

A home exercise program was provided early for self-mobilization techniques of the wrist. The patient was instructed in placing her hand and digits flat on the table and raising her elbow above the hand until a stretch was perceived on the volar surface of the wrist and in the forearm. The approach was repeated for wrist flexion by dropping the elbow below the table until a stretch was perceived on the dorsal wrist capsule and extensor forearm. Then the elbow was placed in neutral position, and she was instructed to raise and lower her arm to stretch the lateral and medial aspects of the wrist and forearm. Finally, self-mobilization of the radioulnar joint was done. The patient's right arm was at her side and the left hand was under and around the forearm. The left thenar eminence supported the ulnar styloid, and the patient was instructed in active supination of the forearm. All of these positions were maintained for 10 seconds. In addition to the self-mobilization exercises for the wrist and forearm, the PIP

Continued

CASE STUDY 12-1: DISTAL RADIUS FRACTURE—cont'd

joints required stretching because of capsular adhesions and tightness of the volar plate. The heat-and-stretch, place-and-hold, and nighttime extension positions were options for treatment.

Strengthening was used for weakened muscles that had not been used, were shortened, or were biomechanically disadvantaged. Once joint flexibility and extrinsic muscle extensibility had improved, restoration of balance was emphasized through strengthening. Specific exercises were applied for the supinator, ECRL, ECRB, and ECU. E-stimulation was applied to reeducate the muscle, and light

Thera-Band exercises were used to advance this learning. Once the balance of tenodesis was restored, therapeutic activity and simulated task performance were initiated.

Periodic measurements were taken throughout the treatment program, and the patient had continuous improvement. After 1 month of treatment, the patient had minimal pain complaints, demonstrated normal sensibility, was compliant with her home program, and had 80% of the range motion and strength compared with the left extremity. She was discharged with a home program and was encouraged to call if her progress was interrupted.

CASE STUDY 12-2: CARPAL TUNNEL SYNDROME

More than 1.9 million people have carpal tunnel syndrome, and 500,000 carpal tunnel releases (CTR) are performed annually.[42] Thirty percent of patients who receive surgical releases report continued pain and weakness 2 years after surgery.[43] Therefore this case study focuses on the management of patients who seek conservative treatment for non-surgical, milder cases of CTS.

History

A 40-year-old right-dominant female factory worker was referred for right CTS. She was not pregnant and denied having diabetes or kidney, thyroid, or inflammatory diseases such as rheumatoid arthritis. She smoked one-half pack of cigarettes per day. No previous hand and wrist injuries were reported, although her symptoms have gradually increased over the past year. During this same time, the demands of her job increased, which included large amounts of repetition and force in awkward wrist positions. The patient's chief complaints are nocturnal pain on a daily basis, morning swelling, numbness in the right hand, and clumsiness. She takes Tylenol 100 mg six times per day.

Diagnostic Classification: Peripheral Nerve Injury 5F: Carpal Tunnel Syndrome 354.0

Initial Visit

At rest the patient maintained a rounded-shoulders forward-head position (RSFH). No other postural imbalances were observed in the upper arm or forearm while standing. The resting tone of the wrist and hand suggested increased tension of the finger flexors. No atrophy of the thenar eminences was present.

In screening the upper extremity, the patient was able to correct her forward head posture without increased paresthesias to the hands. Cervical and glenohumeral movements were within normal limits (WNL). No temperature

or sensory changes were reported in either hand with sustained overhead postures of 5 minutes. No sensitivity was found when palpating the median and ulnar nerves of both hands except for a positive Tinel's sign at the right wrist. Using a modified Allen's test, the vascular responses for the right radial and ulnar arteries were found to be slower compared with the left vessels. A positive Phalen's test was present for the right hand only. The grind test was negative for both CMC joints of the thumb. No point tenderness was found over the FCR or the first dorsal compartments of either hand. The Kanavel's and Ballentine signs were negative.

Based on the Waterloo Handedness Questionnaire,[44] the patient showed a tendency to be ambidextrous for 15 of the 19 items. The findings from the Symptom Severity Scale identified mild pain (25 of 55 points) but moderate difficulty with function (29 of 40 points).

Sensibility testing was done using Semmes Weinstein monofilaments. Light touch was normal for both thenar areas of the hands. However, diminished light touch was found in the median and ulnar distributions of the right and left hands. Paresthesias were present when placing the hand in positions of full stretch on the median nerve.

Range of motion of the patient's finger flexors remained fixed with tenodesis movements. Extensibility of the musculotendinous unit of the extrinsic flexor and extensor muscle groups of both hands was significantly impaired. Pain-free, active wrist extension of both hands was 30 degrees less when full finger extension, supination, and elbow extension was added. Similarly, pain-free, active wrist flexion of both hands was 50 degrees different when full finger flexion, pronation, and elbow extension were added. Intrinsic tightness and poor tendon gliding of the FDS was present. Normal web spaces were present bilaterally. The patient was unable to complete strength and dexterity

CASE STUDY 12-2: CARPAL TUNNEL SYNDROME—cont'd

testing because of increased fatigue, symptoms, and hand volumetric measures (right 75 ml, left 50 ml) from the beginning of the session.

The patient's participation in treatment was enhanced through education on the anatomy of the carpal tunnel and the approaches to reduce ongoing cumulative trauma to structures of the upper extremity. Risk factors associated with work and nonwork activities were identified. Safe baselines of performance and adequate rest-to-activity ratios were acknowledged. Alternative techniques and temporary activity modifications were discussed. Short-term, success-oriented goals were developed collaboratively, and measurable progress and setback graphs were maintained in therapy sessions to modify active treatment plans.

Treatment Hypothesis

Three plausible hypotheses were developed from the history and initial visit to therapy:

1. If full extensibility of the nerve and musculoskeletal structures was achieved, then therapeutic procedures that address stretching, gliding, and tenodesis will restore balance to the tissues and improve stamina levels for motor function.
2. If adequate activity-to-rest ratios were known and applied, then therapeutic procedures that address morning and postactivity swelling will diminish the amount of cumulative trauma to the nerve and soft tissues of the upper extremity.
3. If unhealthy behaviors found in work and nonwork activities were eliminated, then therapeutic procedures that

address posture, smoking, and activity related risk factors will improve functional performance and reduce the number of inflammatory episodes.

Recommendations for Treatment

The recovery of individuals with CTS requires restorative therapy. The primary focus of treatment is to break the cycle of repetitive trauma to the wrist and hand structures, to address issues of chronic swelling, and to return the patient to a balanced state of rest and activity. Several treatment options are suggested.

Maintaining effective amounts of rest for the wrist and hand is paramount. The pathogenesis of CTS has been associated with chronic flexor tenosynovitis, differential excursion between the median nerve and flexor tendons to the fingers, nonneutral positions of the wrist, the retraction of lumbricals muscles into the carpal canal, and ischemia to the median nerve.[45-52] These newer models suggest that splinting the wrist and the fingers may be more efficacious than wrist-only splints for providing adequate rest to the wrist and hand. Although splint studies are plagued with methodology issues, two randomized controlled trials evaluated the effectiveness of a splint that rested the wrist and fingers and a brace maintaining the middle and ring fingers in full extension. Both studies reported decreased symptoms and improved function.[53,54] In this case study, the patient received a CTS splint that provided support of the wrist at night and during the day as needed (Figure 12-41). A removable finger trough was used at night and intermittently during the day for rest.

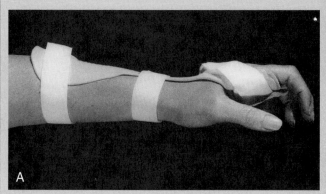
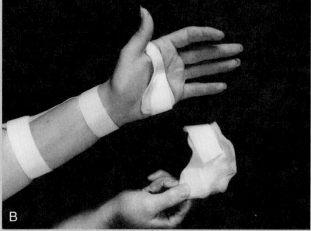

Figure 12-41 A, Index-small finger interphalangeal (IP) extension and flexion torque transmission splint, type 2 (13). **B,** Index-small finger extension and flexion torque transmission splint, type 1 (13). A removable palmar proximal interphalangeal bar allows easy changeover from a type 2 IP torque transmission splint to a type 1 finger torque transmission splint. (Courtesy Sharon Flinn, MEd, OTR/L, CHT, Cleveland, Ohio. In Cooper C: Fundamentals of hand therapy, St Louis, 2006, Mosby.)

Continued

CASE STUDY 12-2: CARPAL TUNNEL SYNDROME—cont'd

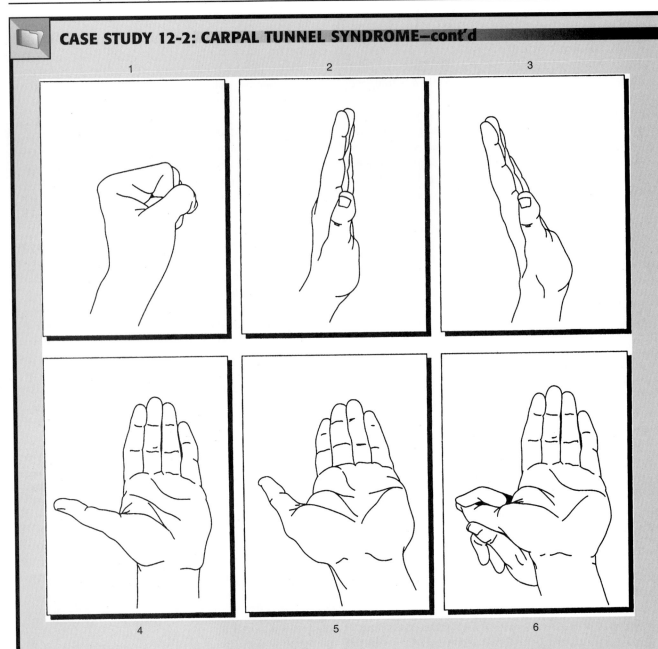

Figure 12-42 Traditional median nerve glide exercises. (Redrawn from Totten PA, Hunter JM: Hand Clin 7(3):505-520, 1991. In Mackin E, Callahan AD, Skirven TM et al, editors: Rehabilitation of the hand and upper extremity, ed 5, St Louis, 2002, Mosby.)

Full PROM of the neurovascular and musculoskeletal structures was needed to restore motor and sensory function. A graduated exercise program was used with this patient. Cervical and shoulder exercises were initiated to address RSFH. Light aerobic and nerve-gliding exercises (Figure 12-42) were used to promote blood flow to the epineurium, the vascular system of the nerve.[55] Once the neurovascular system was mobile, passive stretches were provided to elongate tight motor structures. Passive assisted tenodesis movements were used as a precursor to stretching exercises. Extrinsic muscle-tendon groups were passively ranged, based on their attachment to the medial and lateral epicon-

dyle. Intrinsic stretches addressed tight lumbrical and interossei muscles in the hand. Finally, tendon-gliding exercises were provided to ensure that the extrinsic tendons to the finger flexors moved independently and the shearing force between the FDP and the FDS was minimized (see Figure 12-18).

Lifestyle changes were suggested to modify high-risk work and nonwork activities. Repetitive and forceful activities that were performed in nonneutral wrist positions were identified from the Symptom Severity Scale and the FPST. Tasks were modified if they had high intensity, frequency, and duration cycles. Examples of

CASE STUDY 12-2: CARPAL TUNNEL SYNDROME—cont'd

valued life activities were changed to include writing, holding the phone, peeling vegetables, and wringing cloths. The client was asked to review this list quarterly for the upcoming year to modify problematic activities as needed.

Treatment was scheduled on 3 consecutive days of the week so that a day off from therapy did not provide additional recovery time between sessions. Hand volumes were graphed before and after each treatment session as a measure of overall tissue stability. Three weeks of treatment were needed to establish a suitable baseline where activity-to-rest ratios were sufficient to maintain after activity hand volumes. Once this occurred, improved sleep and range-of-motion goals were achieved. The patient reported improved stamina for functional activities at home and at work. No additional flare-ups occurred. The patient was monitored for an additional 3 months and was discharged after successful attainment of all her goals.

SUMMARY

The hand is an organ capable of delicate prehension and immense strength. When functioning properly, it is a primary contributor to self-sufficiency, overall health, and quality of human life. More than any other body part, problems occur with restoration of hand function when therapy does not address the correct pathologic condition, when therapy is too aggressive, and when therapy does not include the patient as part of the recovery solution. This chapter is designed to familiarize the reader with the issues of stability and mobility and rhythm and balance in the upper extremity. A review of basic anatomy is presented, along with common provocative tests. Evaluation and treatment strategies are discussed for individuals with wrist and hand diagnoses, and cases studies are selected to assist clinicians in managing common problems found in this population.

REFERENCES

1. Fess EE, Gettle K, Philips CA editors: Hand and upper extremity splinting principles and methods, ed 3, St Louis, 2005, CV Mosby.
2. Haines RW: The mechanisms of rotation at the first carpometacarpal joint, J Anat 78:44-46, 1944.
3. Wheeless CR, Nunley JA, Urbaniak JR: Wheeless' textbook of orthopaedics, Duke University Medical Center, Durham, North Carolina. Available at www.wheelessonline.com
4. Artzberger S: Edema reduction techniques: a biological rationale for selection. In Cooper C, editor: Fundamentals of hand therapy: clinical reasoning and treatment guidelines for common diagnoses of the upper extremity, St Louis, 2007, Mosby.
5. Swanson A: Rheumatoid arthritis. In Mackin EJ, Callahan AC, Skirven TM et al, editors: Rehab of the hand and upper extremity, ed 5, St Louis, 2002, Mosby, p. 898.
6. Nalebuff EA: Rheumatoid swan neck deformity, Hand Clin 5:209-214, 1989.
7. Ratliff AHC: Deformities of the thumb in rheumatoid arthritis, J Hand Surg Eur 3:138-143, 1971.
8. Gray H: Gray's anatomy: the classic collector's edition, rev ed 15, New York, 1989, Gramercy Books.
9. Cooper C, editor: Fundamental of hand therapy, clinical reasoning and treatment guidelines for common diagnoses of the upper extremity, St Louis, 2007, Mosby.
10. Nunley JA, Joneschild ES: Metacarpal fractures. In Koman LA, Sieler JG, Jinnah RH, editors: Orthopaedic care: medical and surgical management of musculoskeletal disorders, Towson, MD, 2006, Southern Orthopaedic Association. Available at www.orthopaediccare.net
11. Ebrahim FS, DeMaeseneer M, Jager T et al: US diagnosis of UCL tears of the thumb and Stener lesions: technique, pattern-based approach, and differential diagnosis, Radiographics 26(4):1007-1020, 2006.
12. Brand P, Hollister A: Clinical mechanics of the hand, St Louis, 1999, Mosby.
13. Leibovic SJ, Hastings H: Martin-Gruber revisited, J Hand Surg [Am] 17(1):47-53, 1992.
14. Kendall FP, McCreary EK, Provance PG et al: Muscles testing and function with posture and pain, ed 5, Baltimore, 2005, Lippincott Williams & Wilkins.
15. Gonzales-King Z, Syen D, Burgess B: Dysfunction, evaluation, and treatment of wrist and hand. In Donatelli R, Wooden M, editors: Orthopaedic physical therapy, ed 3, Philadelphia, 2001, Churchill Livingstone, p. 227.
16. Melzack R: The McGill pain questionnaire: major properties and scoring methods. Pain 1:277-299, 1975.
17. Jaffee R, Farney-Mokris S: Edema. In Casanova J, editor: Clinical assessment recommendations, ed 2, Chicago, 1992, American Society of Hand Therapists.
18. Klein L: Evaluation of the hand and upper extremity. In Cooper C, editor: Fundamentals of hand therapy: clinical reasoning and treatment guidelines for common diagnoses of the upper extremity, St Louis, 2007, Mosby.
19. Waylett-Randall J, Seibly D: A study of accuracy of a commercially available volumeter, J Hand Ther 4(1):(Jan-Mar):10-13, 1991.
20. Flinn S, Ventura D: The use of hand volumes to predict pain, stress, and fatigue in upper extremity and non-upper extremity patients, J Hand Ther 15(3):293, 2002.
21. van Velze C, Kluever I, van der Merwe C, et al: The difference in volume of dominant and non-dominant hands, J Hand Ther 4(1):(Jan-Mar):6-9, 1991.

22. McGough C, Zurwasky M: Effect of exercise on volumetric and sensory status of the asymptomatic hand, J Hand Ther 4(4):(Oct-Dec):177-180, 1991.

23. King T: The effect of water temperature on hand volume during volumetric displacement using the water displacement method, J Hand Ther 6(3):(July-Sept):202-204, 1993.

24. Stern E: Volumetric comparison of seated and standing test postures, Am J Occup Ther 45(9):801-805, 1991.

25. Devore D, Hamilton G: Volume measuring of the severely injured hand, Am J Occup Ther 22(1):16-18, 1968.

26. Breger-Lee D, Bell-Krotoski J, Bransdma J: Torque range-of-motion in the hand clinic, J Hand Ther 3(1):(Jan-March):7-13, 1990.

27. Libberecht K, Lafaire C, Van Hee R: Evaluation and functional assessment of flexor tendon repair in the hand, Acta Chir Belg 106:560-565, 2006.

28. Stone J: Sensibility. In Casanova J, editor: Clinical assessment recommendations, ed 2, Chicago, 1992, American Society of Hand Therapists.

29. Petersen P, Petrick M, Connor H et al: Grip strength and hand dominance: challenging the 10% rule, Am J Occup Ther 43(7):444-447, 1989.

30. Shechtman O, Gutierrez Z, Kokendofer E: Analysis of the statistical methods used to detect submaximal effort with five rung grip strength tests, J Hand Ther 18(1):(Jan-Mar):10-18, 2005.

31. Knapik JJ, Ramos MU: Isokinetic and isometric torque relationships in the human body, Arch Phys Med Rehabil 61(2):64-67, 1980.

32. Murphy AJ, Wilson GJ: Poor correlations between isometric tests and dynamic performance: relationship to muscle activation, Eur J Appl Physiol Occup Physiol 73(3e4):353-357, 1996.

33. Osternig LR, Bates BT, James ST: Isokinetic and isometric torque force relationships, Arch Phys Med Rehabil 58(6):254-257, 1977.

34. Shechtman O, Hope L, Bhagwant S: Evaluation of the torque velocity test of the BTE-Primus as a measure of sincerity of effort of grip strength, J Hand Ther 20(4):(Oct-Dec):326-333, 2007.

35. US Department of Labor: Selected characteristics of occupations defined in the dictionary of occupational titles, Washington DC, 1981, US Government Printing Office.

36. Harwin S, Adams J: Can pinch grip strength be used as a valid indicator of manual dexterity? Int J Ther Rehab 14(10):447-453, 2007.

37. Apfel E, Carranza J: Dexterity. In Casanova J, editor: Clinical assessment recommendations, ed 2, Chicago, 1992, American Society of Hand Therapists.

38. Hewlett S: Patients and clinicians have different perspectives on outcomes in arthritis, J Rheumatol 30(4):877-879, 2003.

39. Anthony W: Recovery from mental illness: the guiding vision of the mental health service system in the 1990s, Rehabil Psychol 16(4):11-23, 1993.

40. Corrigan P: Personal communication, July 1, 2004; Corrigan P, Salzer M, Ralph R et al: Examining the factor structure of the recovery assessment scale, Unpublished manuscript, 2004.

41. Wakefield AE, McQueen MM: The role of physiotherapy and clinical predictors of outcome after fracture of the distal radius, J Bone Joint Surg Br 82:972-976, 2000.

42. Priganc V, Henry S: The relationship among five common carpal tunnel syndrome tests and the severity of carpal tunnel syndrome, J Hand Ther 16:225-236, 2003.

43. Padua L, Padua R, Aprile I et al: Carpal tunnel syndrome: relationship between clinical and patient-oriented assessment, Clin Orthop Relat Res 395(2):128-134, 2002.

44. Bryden P, Pryde K, Roy E: A performance measure of the degree of hand preference, Brain Cogn 44:402-414, 2000.

45. Cobb T, An K, Cooney W: Effects of lumbrical muscle incursion within the carpal tunnel on carpal tunnel pressure, J Hand Surg 20(2):186-192, 1995.

46. Ettema A, Amadio P, Zhao C et al: Changes in the functional structure of the tenosynovium in idiopathic carpal tunnel syndrome: a scanning electron microscope study, Plast Reconstr Surg 118(6):1413-1422, 2006.

47. Gerritsen A, de Vet H, Scholten R et al: Splinting versus surgery in the treatment of carpal tunnel syndrome: a randomized controlled trial, JAMA 288(10):1245-1251, 2002.

48. Moore J: Biomechanical models for the pathogenesis of specific distal upper extremity disorders, Am J Ind Med 41:353-369, 2002.

49. Rempel D, Diao E: Entrapment neuropathies: pathophysiology and pathogenesis, J Electromyography and Kinesiology 14:71-75, 2004.

50. Sud V, Chu M, Freeland A: Biochemistry of CTS, Microsurgery 25:44-46, 2005.

51. Werner R, Andary M: Carpal tunnel syndrome: pathophysiology and clinical neurophysiology, Clin Neurosci 113:1373-1381, 2002.

52. Zhao C, Ettema A, Osamura N, et al: Gliding characteristics between flexor tendons and surrounding tissues in the carpal tunnel: a biomechanical cadaver study, Clin Orthod Res 25(2):185-190, 2007.

53. Brininger T, Rogers J, Holm M, et al: Efficacy of a fabricated customized splint and tendon and nerve gliding exercises for the treatment of CTS: a randomized controlled trial, Arch Phys Med Rehabil 88:1429-1435, 2007.

54. Manente G, Torrierei F, DiBlasio F, et al: An innovative hand brace for CTS, Muscle Nerve 24(8):1020-1025, 2001.

55. Moscony A: Common peripheral nerve problems. In Cooper C, editor: Fundamentals of hand therapy, clinical reasoning and treatment guidelines for common diagnoses of the upper extremity, St Louis, 2007, Mosby.

Reconstructive Surgery of the Wrist and Hand

The hand is the main manipulative organ of the human body and performs many different functions, ranging from lifting very heavy objects to repairing objects with microscopic instruments. Reconstructive surgical considerations for acquired and congenital problems of the hand and wrist pose considerable challenges for both the surgeon and the physical therapist. Attempts to correct these problems can be very satisfying to all involved; they can also prove frustrating if problems arise either in the surgical procedure or in the rehabilitation. To overcome these potential problems, a separate specialty dedicated to hand and wrist problems has been formed among both surgeons and therapists. These professionals are trained to examine all aspects of the hand, as well as to consider the lifestyle and occupation of the patient. Two patients with similar severe impairments but with different lifestyles may require different surgical procedures to restore function and to allow them to use the hand in their chosen lifestyle or occupation. Hand injuries alone, however slight, may render the patient completely unemployable in his or her normal occupation. Therefore care of hand injuries, for patients and for workers' compensation boards, can be among the most costly areas of medical care in our modern technical world.[1]

EXAMINATION

A good history should accompany any physical examination, but especially one involving the hand. Specific areas to define are (1) the onset of the problem, whether acute or insidious; (2) the length of time the problem has been present; (3) the types of movements that exacerbate the problem, as well as what seems to reduce the problem; (4) the functional limitations that are caused by the problem; and (5) associated manifestations relating either to the arm or to other parts of the body. The examination itself should include both active and passive motion of all joints, along with palpation of the joints, as indicated by swelling or a history of pain.

Any deformity of the hand should be examined in detail. The tendons about the wrist and the fingers should be palpated through the skin and their excursion appreciated on active move-

ment. The bony prominences that may be involved should be palpated, and the clinician should note whether they are in their normal position and whether any swelling or tenderness exists. The tendons and muscles should be tested separately for the wrist, as well as for each finger and each tendon or muscle for the fingers (Figure 13-1). Some trick movements can occur with intrinsic and extrinsic muscles; therefore specific testing for the radial, ulnar, and median nerves is necessary.[2] These peripheral nerves innervate the hand; occasional innervation of the dorsum of the wrist by the musculocutaneous nerve also occurs.

Once a thorough physical examination has been performed and a history has been taken, further studies may be necessary. Radiographs are valuable in evaluating the bony structures and joint spaces. Other tests for problems that are more difficult to diagnose may include bone scans, arthrograms, nerve conduction testing, tomograms, and electromyographic testing, as well as computed tomography (CT) and magnetic resonance imaging (MRI) scans.

Traumatic Injuries

Traumatic injuries account for the largest number of problems of the hand and wrist.[3] The injuries can range from simple sprains or contusions to major disruptions of hand function, including amputation. Traumatic injuries can occur in any setting, including work, home, and recreational activities. Traumatic injuries frequently seen by the hand surgeon include fractures, tendon injuries, nerve injuries, and wrist sprains (Figure 13-2).

Fractures

Fractures occur when a force of such magnitude strikes the hand or wrist that the osseous structure is interrupted, causing a bone to separate into two or more fragments. Treatment of displaced fractures includes a general realignment of the part so that, when healing takes place, the part will function in an essentially normal manner. In the hand and fingers, close anatomic approximation of the fracture surfaces is generally required to achieve this level of function.

External support, such as a cast, is usually necessary for stable fractures for several weeks to allow bony union to occur. If the fracture is not immobilized long enough to allow healing to occur, then nonunion may result (or malunion if the fracture is displaced during the healing process). The soft tissue structures should be tested at the time of initial examination to be sure that the neurovascular and muscular structures of the area are intact. If they are found to be involved, then treatment of the fracture may be altered.

The distal radius fracture, or Colles' fracture, is one of the most common fractures of the wrist and hand. It can occur in any age group but appears to be more prevalent in older patients in whom osteoporosis is a factor. This injury generally occurs, as do a large proportion of hand injuries, when the patient sustains a fall on an outstretched hand (FOOSH). Depending on the magnitude of the force and the direction in which it is applied, the fracture pattern may vary, but most commonly the fracture occurs within 1 inch of the articular surface, causing dorsal angulation of the distal fragment in the metaphyseal area of the distal radius, with or without a fracture of the ulnar styloid (Figure 13-3, *A* and *B*). In most cases this fracture can be treated by closed reduction with appropriate anesthesia to allow relaxation of the muscles. The type of cast varies from a short arm splint to a long arm cast, depending on the fracture pattern and whether comminution exists. In older individuals, the cast is retained for 3 to 4 weeks until early healing occurs. In younger patients, a longer period, closer to 6 to 8 weeks, is required for sufficient stability to start early motion. After the cast is removed, a removable splint is used to protect the fracture while early motion and strength of the healing bone are restored (Figure 13-3, *C* and *D*). If the fracture involves the articular surface or cannot be maintained by an external support such as a cast, then some type of fixation of the fracture will be necessary.

Many methods of fixation of a Colles' fracture exist. They include simple closed reduction, a pin or a rod across the fracture surface, plates and screws, or a metallic external fixator. The metallic external fixator is held in place by pins placed in the bone proximal and distal to the fracture site, holding the fracture in a reduced position (Figures 13-4 and 13-5).

Generally if this fracture can be reduced to even a marginally acceptable position in the older patient, then good function will be regained after the fracture heals and appropriate therapy is concluded. Younger patients will require close anatomic reduction for long-term painless function. During surgical reduction, visualization of the articular surface is desirable either by open incision or arthroscopically.

Another very common fracture of the wrist and hand is that of the navicular (Figure 13-6, *A*). The navicular bone has an unusual blood supply, entering from the distal pole and proceeding retrograde into the proximal pole.[4] Fractures may occur at any level in the navicular, but the more proximal the fracture, the greater the chance of avascular necrosis of the proximal fragment and nonunion of the fracture because of the loss of blood supply (Figure 13-6, *B*). Frequently, these fractures are hard to see on the initial radiograph because they have a hairline component. In addition, because of the anatomy of the bone, it is very difficult to get straight accurate anteroposterior and lateral views of the bone. The result is that these fractures are frequently missed. In this situation, when a patient has wrist trauma and pain in the anatomic snuffbox on the radial aspect of the wrist, the thumb, wrist, and forearm should be at least splinted for 10 to 14 days, when because of bone resorption in the early healing phase, the fracture can be seen better on radiograph and a reexamination is performed to determine if a fracture has, in fact, occurred. This protects the patient and should decrease the incidence of nonunion and avascular necrosis. Early immobilization is essential in this type

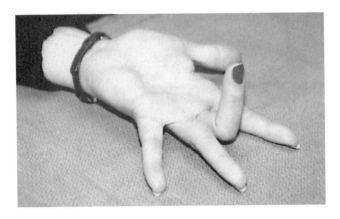

Figure 13-1 Inability to flex the distal interphalangeal (DIP) joint indicates that the flexor digitorum profundus to the finger is not functioning.

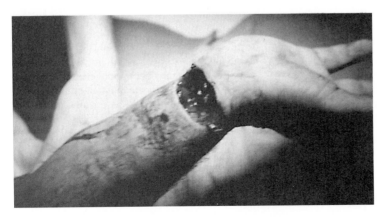

Figure 13-2 Severe laceration of the wrist disrupts the tendons and major nerves and arteries to the hand.

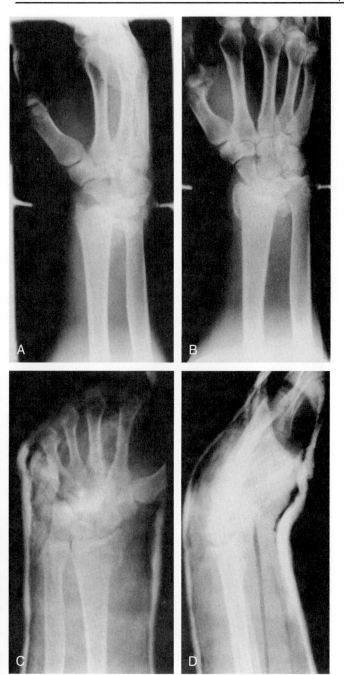

Figure 13-3 Distal radius fracture. **A-B,** Radiographs show mild displacement. **C-D,** After closed reduction and casting, acceptable alignment is seen.

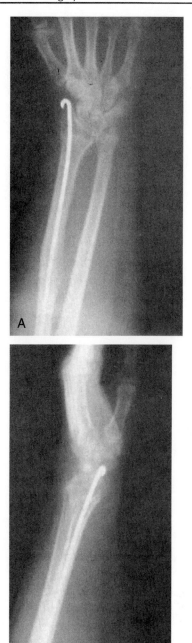

Figure 13-4 An unstable distal radius fracture is held with a Rush rod.

of fracture to reduce the incidence of these problems. Displaced fractures of the navicular may require open reduction and internal fixation (ORIF) either with crossed Kirschner wires or with a special screw made particularly for the navicular called the *Herbert screw* or one of the variations.[5] In addition, delayed union or nonunion of the fracture may require a subsequent surgical procedure for bone grafting and/or fixation of the fracture to stimulate healing.[6]

The length of time necessary for a navicular fracture to heal is variable, from a minimum of 6 weeks to as long as 9 months.

This fracture is treated with a thumb spica cast, holding the thumb in the palmar abducted position.

The wrist is generally kept in a neutral position or in some other position that will maintain reduction of the fracture, and either a short or long arm cast is used, depending on the surgeon's preference.

Fractures or dislocations of the other carpal bones may occur, and a high index of suspicion is generally needed to diagnose these problems. A careful history and a physical examination are necessary to point the clinician to the appropriate area for consideration. Frequently, multiple radiographic views and/or follow-up studies with tomograms or bone scans may

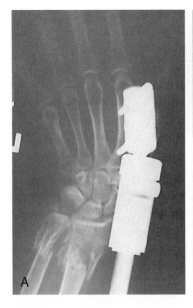
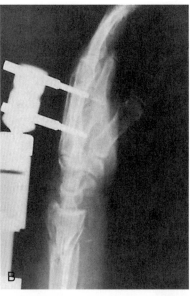

Figure 13-5 A, Comminuted displaced intraarticular distal radius fracture. **B,** After open reduction and internal fixation (ORIF) surgery with anatomic alignment.

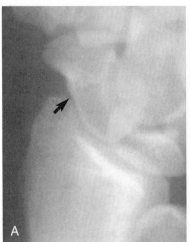
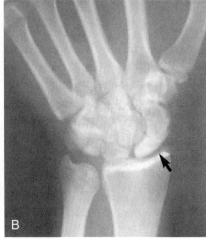

Figure 13-6 Navicular fracture. **A,** Hairline navicular fracture. **B,** Navicular fracture that progressed to avascular necrosis and nonunion.

be necessary for a definitive diagnosis. Treatment of these fractures is by closed or open reduction as necessary, including the dislocations that frequently require anatomic ligament repair and then splinting for an appropriate period of time to allow healing. Fractures of the nonarticular portions of the metacarpals and phalanges most frequently are stable injuries, and close anatomic alignment with external support will generally suffice for these injuries.

Intraarticular fractures involving the wrist or hand require anatomic alignment of the articular surfaces. The articular surface is a smooth gliding surface on which movement occurs in the wrist and fingers. If a step off or a significant gap in this smooth surface exists, then deterioration of the joint can occur very quickly. If the fracture is displaced and cannot be reduced, then ORIF must be considered to provide close to normal function when the fracture heals (Figure 13-7). In addition, fractures that are in close association with the insertion of a tendon, whether in the wrist or the fingers, are frequently unstable because of the muscle pull, which cannot be completely neutralized by casting. If the fractures cannot be brought into a

stable position by closed technique, ORIF is frequently required to align and immobilize the fracture against muscle and tendon pull.

Fractures associated with injuries to adjacent structures, such as tendon ruptures or nerve lacerations, may require more aggressive treatment, such as ORIF, to allow for appropriate repair and rehabilitation of the tendons and nerves.[7] This can allow for an earlier introduction of therapy for range of motion and gentle use of the hand for rehabilitation.

Tendon Injuries

Tendonitis is an inflammation of the tendon unit. It can be associated with either an overuse syndrome or a sprain of the muscle tendon unit resulting from a traumatic episode. Tendonitis can generally be treated with a period of immobilization to allow the initial inflammation to settle down, followed by gentle stretching and toning exercises with local therapy, such as ice, heat, and friction massage or other modalities as necessary to allow the tendonitis to subside.

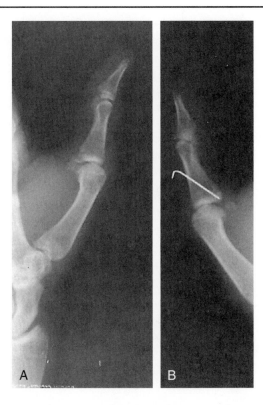

Figure 13-7 Intraarticular fracture. **A,** Displaced intraarticular fracture of the thumb metacarpophalangeal joint. **B,** After open reduction and pin fixation.

More serious tendon injuries include ruptures and lacerations. These injuries generally are treated by open repair because approximation of the tendon ends is very difficult with closed methods of treatment; therefore loss of function is likely. One condition in which rupture of a tendon can frequently be treated satisfactorily by closed methods is mallet finger.[8] In this injury the extensor tendon is avulsed at the level of the distal interphalangeal (DIP) joint, causing lack of extension of the joint (Figure 13-9). Splinting in a hyperextended position generally allows healing of the tendon and excellent function subsequently.

Most other tendon injuries are approached surgically for open repair. A tendon that does not require significant excursion with motion, such as most extensor tendons, especially the wrist extensors or the abductor of the thumb, can be treated after open repair with casting for 4 to 6 weeks and then with gentle mobilization. Adhesions in extensor tendon areas generally are not severe, and near-normal function is usually achieved. In the flexor tendons of the fingers and thumb, the excursion is much greater; therefore adhesions can significantly inhibit restoration of normal function. The repair of these tendons is very delicate, and an atraumatic method of repair is used to secure the tendon and ensure a smooth surface at the level of the cut (Figure 13-10, A). Repair of flexor tendons in "no man's land," the area in the digits where the flexor superficialis and the flexor profundus glide against one another in the fibroosseous tunnel, is the hardest area in which to gain good function. Repair of both tendons at this level is generally recommended,

as with all flexor tendon lacerations of the digits. In addition, early motion with a dynamic splint as recommended by Lister et al.[9] allows for early function and decreased problems with adhesions (Figure 13-10, B).

Repair of the pulley system of the fibroosseous tunnel is very important in decreasing the incidence of serious adhesions to a lacerated flexor tendon.[10] If adhesions do limit the range of motion and function of the finger, then tenolysis should be performed no earlier than 6 months after the original repair. This allows for settling down of the original scar tissue so that scarring is not reactivated and only the reaction to the new surgery becomes an inhibitor. With tenolysis, the fibroosseous tunnel should be repaired if possible to allow for good nourishment of the tendon, decrease of adhesions, and better mechanical function of the tendon. After tenolysis, active and active assisted range-of-motion (AAROM) exercises are initiated unless a violation of the tendon itself has occurred. Late repairs of tendon ruptures may require insertion of a Silastic rod to reestablish the synovial space in the sheath and allow for reconstruction of the pulley system before introduction of a graft tendon. Once the pulley system has been established and full passive motion is achieved in all joints, a tendon graft can be inserted from the distal stump to the distal forearm.[11] Passive range of motion (PROM) is performed over approximately 6 weeks to achieve full range. Again, early motion with a dynamic splint is recommended, with a prolonged rehabilitation time to allow for vascularization of the grafted tendon.

Nerve Injuries

Nerve injuries may occur anytime a nerve undergoes trauma. The injury may be a simple contusion, a stretch injury, or a disruption of nerve fibers secondary to a laceration. Nerve injuries are also frequently associated with fractures and particularly flexor tendon injuries, where the nerves run in close proximity to the flexor tendons, not only at the wrist but also in the fingers. Three types of nerve injury can cause nerve dysfunction. Neurapraxia occurs when an injury such as a contusion causes electrical interruption of nerve conduction but without disruption of the nerve itself and without degeneration of the axons. Recovery is generally expected within days to several weeks. The next, more serious type of injury, axonotmesis, occurs when the nerve is injured to such an extent that, although the nerve appears intact when inspected, degeneration occurs from the point of injury distally. Healing requires regrowth of the axons from the point of injury to the area of innervation. This can cause a prolonged period of nonfunction of the nerve but generally results in excellent return of function once the axons have regenerated. The most serious type of injury to the nerve is neurotmesis, in which the nerve is actually severed. Because disruption of the nerve bundles exists, even with surgical repair these bundles are very crudely realigned and return of function is variable, although with microsurgical techniques the return of function is generally fair to good and occasionally excellent.[12]

In the rehabilitation of these nerve injuries, it is very important to educate the patient as to the type of nerve injury is

Case Study 13-1: Navicular Fracture

A 20-year-old man sustained a FOOSH injury while playing rugby on the evening before evaluation. On evaluation, he was found to have swelling and deformity of the left wrist. On examination, his neurovascular function was found to be intact. The motors to the fingers appeared to be intact. Movement of the wrist was extremely painful and could not be tested. Radiographs showed a transscaphoid perilunate dislocation (Figure 13-8).

Immediately after evaluation with a Xylocaine block in the area of injury, a closed reduction of the perilunate dislocation was accomplished without problems. Postreduction radiographs showed excellent relocation of the carpus, but the fracture of the navicular remained unacceptably

displaced. The next day, the patient underwent an ORIF with a Herbert screw of the navicular fracture (see Figure 13-8, *C* and *D*). He remained in a long arm cast for 5 weeks and then in a short arm thumb spica cast for 4 weeks. At that time he was taken out of the cast, placed in a removable splint, and started on a physical therapy program for range of motion of the wrist and thumb and muscle rehabilitation. His course was complicated by avascular necrosis of the proximal pole of the navicular. With only moderate use of his wrist, he regained full range of motion and strength in the hand and wrist. The avascular necrosis completely resolved spontaneously at 9 months after injury.

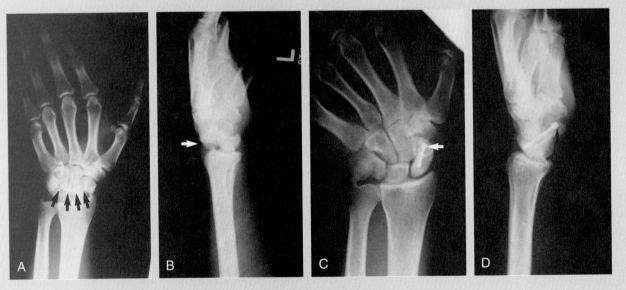

Figure 13-8 Radiographs showing **(A)** dorsal transscaphoid perilunate dislocation with overlapping of the carpal bones on the anteroposterior view *(small arrows)* and **(B)** dorsal displacement of the capitate from the lunate fossa on the lateral view *(large arrow)*. **C-D,** Anteroposterior and lateral views of the wrist after healing, with anatomic positioning of the carpal bones and healing of the fractured scaphoid with a retained Herbert screw fixation device.

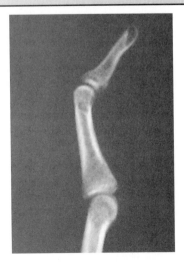

Figure 13-9 Abnormal flexion of the distal interphalangeal (DIP) joint after disruption of the extensor tendon distal to the proximal interphalangeal (PIP) joint, typical of a mallet deformity.

possible or known and the length of time that dysfunction of the nerve is expected to persist. This allows the patient to adjust his or her daily lifestyle to the dysfunction and to protect any areas of lost sensation from injury.[13]

If nerves to muscle groups are involved, splinting may be necessary to avoid contractures of joints and loss of function secondary to the temporary loss of muscle function. Nerve regeneration from axonotmesis or neurotmesis occurs at a rate of approximately 1 mm/day; thus a clinician can estimate the length of time before return of function by measuring the distance from the nerve injury to the most proximal innervation site. Depending on the nature of the injury, the healing response of the particular individual, the amount of scarring in the area of injury, and the surgical technique used for repair, this return of sensation can range from only protective sensation (against sharp objects, heat, and cold) to almost normal sensation. Muscle groups are generally the most difficult to restore to function because of the time needed for return of the

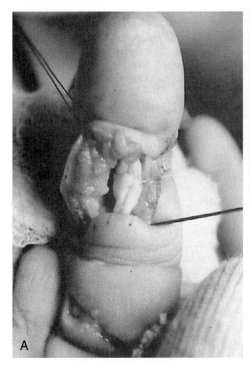

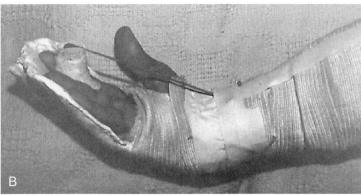

Figure 13-10 Tendon repair. **A,** Suture of the flexor digitorum profundus after laceration. **B,** Immediate dynamic splinting mobilization for early rehabilitation.

Case Study 13-2: Flexor Digitorum Profundus Tear

A 47-year-old man who is active in karate sustained a kick to his left fifth finger, with subsequent loss of the ability to flex the DIP joint of the fifth finger. He was seen 10 days later with a history as noted, and no symptoms of numbness or vascular compromise. Examination confirmed the absence of active flexion at the DIP joint of the fifth finger. The problem was complicated by the fact that the patient had sustained a fracture mallet deformity approximately 9 months previously, which was untreated. He was interested in regaining the function of flexion of the DIP joint and underwent advancement and repair of the flexor digitorum profundus, which had been disrupted at its insertion on the distal phalanx. Postoperatively, he was placed in a dynamic flexion splint with a mallet splint over the DIP joint to avoid overpull on the previously injured extensor mechanism. This splint was removed several times a day to allow for flexion of the DIP joint and pull through of the flexor digitorum profundus. The patient was taken completely out of his splint in 5 weeks and started on physical therapy. At the end of 3.5 months, he had 0 to 35 degrees of motion in the DIP joint and 0 to 95 degrees in the proximal interphalangeal (PIP) joint. At the end of 4.5 months, he still lacked 1 cm of closing the fifth finger to the distal palmar crease. He was continued on exercises but was satisfied with the result at that point. Because of his work demands, he was unable to undergo further physical therapy.

axon to the muscle. During this time, atrophy and fibrosis can occur in the muscle.

Carpal tunnel syndrome (CTS) is a very common acquired loss of nerve function, which, if encountered and treated early, whether conservatively with splinting and medication or surgically with release of the transverse carpal ligament, results in early functional return of the nerve because the injury is only neurapraxic. Prolonged carpal tunnel disease with atrophy of the thenar muscles is associated with an axonotmesis, and occasionally scarring has already occurred in the area of compression. In these cases, functional return is sometimes incomplete even after release and neurolysis. With severe chronic CTS, some return of sensation is typically achieved, but motor return is poor. Both in CTS with atrophy of the thenar muscles and in neurotmesis injuries of motor nerves about the wrist,

muscle transfers can be performed using muscles innervated by a different nerve to substitute for the muscles no longer functioning from the injured nerve. This naturally requires a period of rehabilitation for reeducation of the muscle tendon unit, as well as for mobilization of the joints that were immobilized to allow for healing of the transferred muscle tendon unit. Loss of the nerve supply without full return can also cause hypersensitivity to cold weather. Therefore repair of major nerves about the wrist and the fingers is indicated to restore satisfactory function of the hand.

Wrist Sprains

Sprains of the wrist are very common and generally mild. A sprained wrist that displays moderate to large amounts of swelling or pain inappropriate to the level of possible injury should indicate to the clinician that a more serious injury may have occurred.[14] One such injury is hairline fracture of the navicular bone, which frequently cannot be picked up on initial radiographs.

Other injuries associated with a wrist sprain that could be of clinical importance include tears of the intercarpal ligaments or of the triangular fibrocartilage complex. These injuries can be seriously debilitating and over time can cause degeneration of the wrist joints, further limiting function of the wrist and requiring more extensive and radical surgical correction. A tear of the scapholunate ligament is probably the most common symptomatic ligament tear of the wrist area. A tear of this ligament severs the connection between the proximal row of carpal bones, which includes the proximal half of the navicular, the lunate, and the triquetrum, from the distal row (Figure 13-11). The scaphoid is the interconnecting link that coordinates not only flexion and extension movements but also radial and ulnar deviation between the two rows of carpal bones. When the scapholunate ligament is ruptured, the scaphoid generally falls into a palmar flexed position; the proximal row is then an unconnected middle segment between the distal forearm and the more stable distal carpal row and the hand. This allows for subluxation in either a dorsal or a volar direction, depending on the forces transmitted, as well as any other ligamentous stretching that might have occurred at the time of the injury. The result is a painful, weak wrist, which does not respond to conservative treatment. The wrist may get over the initial soreness, but when normal use is attempted, soreness and weakness are noted.

With a high index of suspicion, the ligament tear can be diagnosed by the history and physical examination, noting tenderness and swelling dorsally over the junction of the scaphoid and the lunate; on radiographic examination a widened space between the scaphoid and Innate is observed. On the anteroposterior radiograph, the scaphoid may have the appearance of a signet ring rather than its normal oblong shape. The ligament sometimes can be repaired acutely, but it is a very short ligament, and frequently it is difficult to get adequate sutures to repair it. In this situation or in the case of chronic scapholunate dissociation, a limited intercarpal fusion such as a triscaphe fusion can stabilize the carpus. This procedure fuses the scaphoid to the trapezium and the trapezoid so that it is maintained in a reduced position in its normal dorsiflexed attitude rather than the palmar flexed attitude associated with the ligament tear (Figure 13-12). Minimal loss of motion in the wrist is associated with this limited fusion, but pain is generally relieved, advancement of degeneration can be slowed down or stopped, and strength returns.

On occasion, an intercarpal ligament tear or a tear of the triangular fibrocartilage cannot be diagnosed on clinical examination and plain radiography alone. In this situation the patient generally has a prolonged history, usually of several months' duration after a traumatic episode, complaining of persistent pain, occasional swelling, and popping or clicking in the wrist. A wrist arthrogram may be able to elucidate the torn ligament

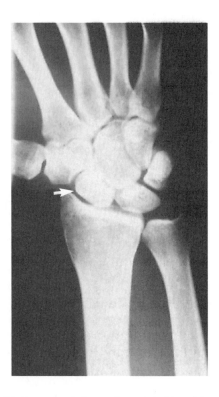

Figure 13-11 The space between the scaphoid and lunate *(arrow)* indicates scapholunate dissociation. Signet ring formation of the scaphoid indicates volar rotation of the scaphoid.

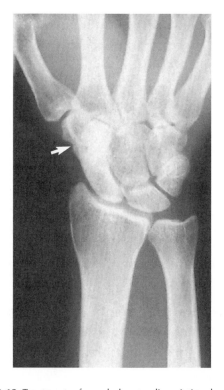

Figure 13-12 Treatment of scapholunate dissociation by triscaphe fusion *(arrow)*.

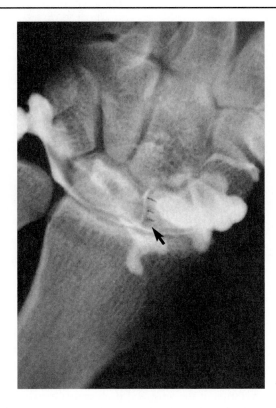

Figure 13-13 Arthrogram of the wrist showing dye leakage through the scapholunate space into the distal carpal row *(arrow)*, indicating a disruption of the scapholunate ligament.

or triangular fibrocartilage (Figure 13-13). Once the diagnosis of intercarpal ligament tear is made, a limited intercarpal fusion may solve the problem, and if a torn triangular fibrocartilage is found, then it should be repaired if possible. Arthroscopic partial débridement of the triangular fibrocartilage may be sufficient. With advanced degenerative changes from old trauma, replacement with limited intercarpal fusion to unload the prosthesis or a wrist fusion may be necessary to restore satisfactory function of the hand.

After repair of an intercarpal ligament or an intercarpal fusion, immobilization is necessary for a sufficient length of time to allow the ligament to heal or the fusion to become solid. Immobilization frequently will need to include one or several fingers besides the wrist and forearm. The time in the cast is usually no less than 6 weeks, and the wrist and hand can be very stiff once the cast is removed. Physical therapy is generally indicated to increase the range of motion both passively and actively, as well as to strengthen the wrist. Methods for reduction of swelling along with heat and ultrasound can be useful to decrease the likelihood of tendonitis associated with the prolonged immobilization.

Wrist Arthroscopy

Wrist arthroscopy has become standard for treating some conditions. Currently the indications for wrist arthroscopy are identification of problems that may be associated with unresolved wrist pain; removal of loose bodies, débridement of the

triangular fibrocartilage, synovectomy for a chronic synovitis or associated with rheumatoid arthritis, and visualization of depressed infraarticular wrist fractures during limited ORIF. This approach can limit the amount of scarring associated with this procedure and allow for more normal return of function and a more adequate reduction of the fracture under visualization.

Technique

Wrist arthroscopy has become standard for treating some conditions. The patient is given either a regional or a general anesthetic agent, the shoulder is abducted 90 degrees, and the elbow is flexed 90 degrees with the fingers suspended (usually from a finger trap device) to distract the wrist. The wrist and hand are then prepared for surgery. Arthroscopic visualization 3 mm or smaller provides the best overall view and is the least traumatic to the wrist (Figure 13-14). The arthroscope is introduced between the third and fourth extensor compartments after insufflation of the wrist joint with normal saline by injection needle.

Working instruments can be introduced either between the first and second dorsal compartment groups, more laterally between the fourth and fifth compartments, or just lateral to the sixth compartment. Visualization of the articular surfaces is usually very good, and the intercarpal ligaments between the scapholunate and lunotriquetral articulations can be evaluated (Figure 13-15). The triangular fibrocartilage and the fossa of the ulnar styloid are also visualized through the arthroscope. The midcarpal joint can also be entered between the innate and the capitate, visualizing these surfaces for occult chondromalacia and loose bodies.

Assuming that no open procedure is necessary in association with the arthroscopy, the patient is usually allowed to go home the same day with a light dressing on the wrist, and gentle range-of-motion exercises are started immediately. After the initial soreness disappears in 2 to 5 days, physical therapy can be started to increase mobility and regain strength about the wrist. When the procedure is performed under appropriate conditions, patients generally function at a normal level within at least a few weeks, and the return to normal activities is much faster than when an open procedure is used.

Overuse Syndromes

Overuse syndromes of the wrist and hand are very common in modern work conditions. Work that requires repetitive use of the hand, especially assembly line activities or clerical tasks such as key punching or invoice rectification, can produce these overuse syndromes. Heavier work such as the use of air hammers and power equipment can also cause overuse syndromes. The most common overuse entity is CTS (usually related to either repetitive microtrauma to the wrist that causes inflammation of the tissues about the median nerve in the carpal canal or inflammation secondary to flexor tendon overuse). Other overuse syndromes include wrist or digital flexor and extensor tendonitis. All of these problems can result in time lost from

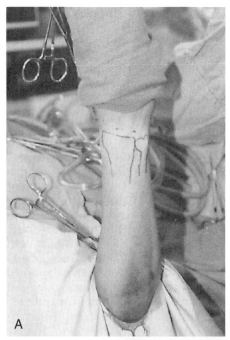

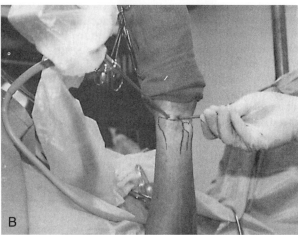

Figure 13-14 Technique of wrist arthroscopy. **A,** Primary portals for the arthroscope and working instruments are between dorsal compartments three and four and compartments four and five. **B,** Setup for wrist arthroscopy, with the arthroscope placed in the entrance portal between the third and fourth extensor groups.

work and should be treated aggressively with splinting, antiinflammatory medication, and therapy, as well as evaluation of the workplace to try to decrease the recurrence of repetitive-use trauma. Appropriate medical treatment and physical therapy can reduce the intensity and time for recovery.

Arthritis

Arthritis by definition means inflammation of a joint, but the term generally refers to a pathologic process involving inflammation that causes destruction of the joint. Many processes can cause arthritis, such as general wear and tear producing osteoarthritis; metabolic abnormalities, such as that which causes

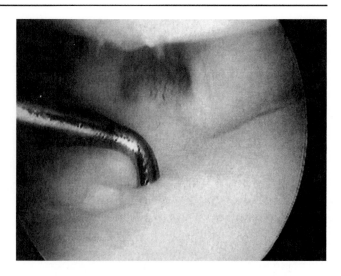

Figure 13-15 Intraarticular view of the wrist.

gouty arthritis; immune abnormalities resulting in rheumatoid arthritis or lupus arthritis; infections that can cause septic arthritis; and traumatic injuries that result in damage or unevenness of the joint surfaces, causing traumatic arthritis.

Osteoarthritis of the wrist and hand occurs mostly in the wrist, the DIP joints of the fingers, and the carpal-metacarpal (CMC) joint of the thumb. The inflammation may be controlled conservatively by using nonsteroidal antiinflammatory drugs (NSAIDs), heat, and maintenance of motion in the joints. Intermittent splinting may control developing deformities, although this is necessary only in a small proportion of patients with osteoarthritis. Surgical procedures for severe arthritis, in which uncontrolled pain, destruction of the joint on radiographic evaluation, or deformity with loss of function exists, may include simple débridement of the joint with removal of osteophytes or bone spurs and débridement of abnormal cartilage in the joint. Capsular reinforcement may also be necessary to control deformities. For more involved destruction, fusion of the joint may be necessary or, specifically in the case of the basilar thumb joint and wrist, a prosthesis or resection arthroplasty may be useful to retain function after removing the abnormal joint (Figure 13-16). Physical therapy is frequently necessary with conservative treatment for maintenance of range of motion in acutely inflamed joints by the use of gentle range-of-motion exercises, as well as heat, paraffin baths, and massage. Again, intermittent splinting may be necessary for some patients. After surgical procedures, immobilization is usually needed for a time, after which return of function is achieved through exercise and strengthening.

Rheumatoid arthritis is particularly debilitating to the hand, and treatment can be very involved. Briefly, rheumatoid arthritis not only affects the articular surfaces but also involves the soft tissues to a large extent, including the ligamentous structures and the tendinous structures about the wrist and hand. The cartilage surfaces are destroyed, and the soft tissue structures are weakened by degradation of the collagen and infiltration by the rheumatoid process. The joints most often involved are the wrist, the CMC joint of the thumb, and the

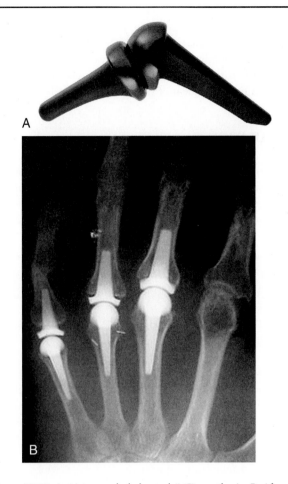

Figure 13-16 A, Metacarpal-phalangeal (MP) prosthesis. **B,** After MP replacement long ring and small fingers. (Courtesy Ascension Orthopaedics, Inc., Austin, Texas.)

metacarpophalangeal joints of the fingers. Deformity can occur simply by collapse of the joint surfaces or in combination with laxity of the surrounding capsular and ligamentous structures, causing subluxation and subsequent abnormal pull of the musculotendon units, resulting in grossly abnormal function of the hand. The tendons can also become involved, particularly the flexor tendons, and chronic uncontrolled inflammation can cause rupture of the tendons.

Treatment consists of controlling the disease process with medication, splinting to prevent stretching of the soft tissue structures and subsequent subluxation of the joints, and vigorous therapy to maintain strength and motion in the digits and the wrist. Surgical treatment in cases of minimal involvement of the articular surfaces can be accomplished by synovectomy and soft tissue reconstruction as necessary and then rehabilitation once healing of the reconstruction has occurred. In cases of more advanced destruction of the joints along with subluxation, soft tissue releases of the tight structures and reinforcement and reconstruction of the loose structures are necessary. Joint replacement of the metacarpophalangeal joints and fascial arthroplasty of the basilar joint of the thumb and the wrist may be indicated (Figure 13-17, *A* and *B*).[15] Fusion of the joints may be required for stability if severe involvement of the soft tissues exists. Reconstruction of ruptured tendons is necessary to regain function, but it will fail if control of the disease by medication or synovectomy is not achieved. Prolonged dynamic splinting after reconstruction is generally necessary, with slow return of function. However, because of the severe deformities, reconstructions of rheumatoid hands are generally very satisfying.

Septic arthritis can occur either through direct introduction of bacteria into the joint from a puncture wound or surgical

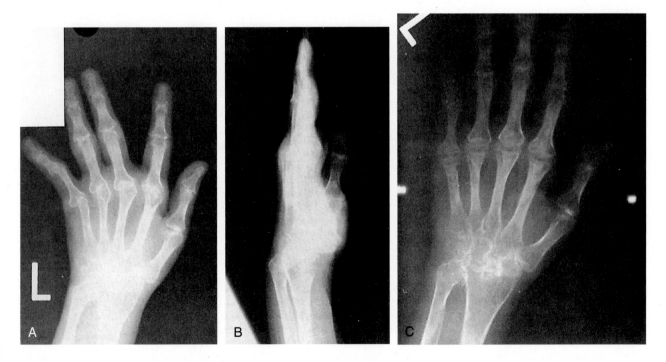

Figure 13-17 Rheumatoid arthritis. **A-B,** Severely degenerative rheumatoid hand showing degeneration and subluxation of the metacarpal-phalangeal (MP) joints and severe degeneration of the wrist. **C,** Postoperative view with Silastic MP joints in place.

procedure or via the bloodstream through hematogenous seeding of the joint with bacteria. Sepsis in a joint that is not treated early will result in destruction of the articular surfaces of the joint and cause septic arthritis.[16] Initially, control of the infection is necessary. If arthritis sets in from the septic process, then a fusion or resection arthroplasty may be indicated, depending on the joint involved. It is only with great hesitation that an artificial joint would be placed in a previously septic joint.

Traumatic arthritis can occur when any traumatic episode results in injury to the articular surface and damage to the cartilaginous covering or to the ligamentous stability of the joint that causes abnormal mechanics and motion about the joint. Once the arthritis has set in, it is approached much like osteoarthritis, with control by NSAIDs. Maintenance of joint mobility and function is important. Once the disease process had advanced past the point of control by conservative methods, arthrodesis or replacement of the joint may be indicated.

AMPUTATION

Amputations may occur for many reasons; trauma, vascular disease, surgical resection of tumors, and uncontrolled infections are some of the possible causes. Traumatic amputations or near amputations that have, because of the mechanism of

Case Study 13-3: Reconstructive Surgery for Index PIP and DIP Degenerative Joint Disease

A 60-year-old woman who worked in a cafeteria had ongoing limitation of motion and pain in both hands, but it became acutely severe in the right index and long fingers, for which she came in for consultation. The patient was found to have a severely swollen index finger DIP joint and long finger PIP joint. On examination, she was found to have limitation of motion of the index DIP joint and a large cystic mass on the long finger PIP joint with ulnar deviation at the joint. Radiographs confirmed severe degeneration of the index DIP joint and moderate degeneration with ulnar deviation at the long finger PIP joint (Figure 13-18, A and B). After examination assuring function of the neurovascular structures and all tendons, the patient underwent excision of the cyst and radial collateral ligament reconstruction of the long

finger PIP joint and fusion of the DIP joint of the index finger with a Herbert screw technique (Figure 13-18, C and D).

The patient was treated with a splint for the index finger and early range of motion for the long finger, with buddy taping to the index finger. At 4 months, she had excellent fusion of the DIP joint but still lacked some motion in the PIP joint of the index finger and the long finger. The index finger had excellent range of motion at the end of 6 months, except for the DIP joint, which was fused. The patient was able to gain motion in the long finger PIP joint to approximately 10 degrees to 90 degrees, with good function in the hand. The patient returned to work and was satisfied with her result.

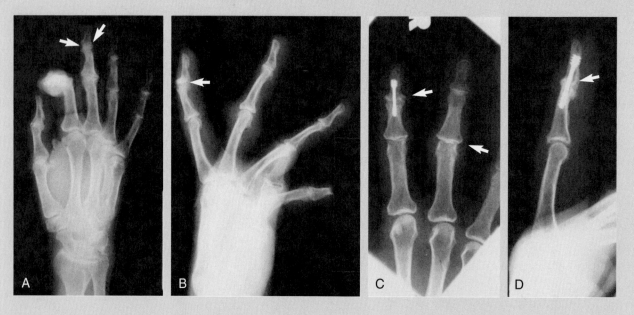

Figure 13-18 A-B, Anteroposterior and lateral views of the right hand showing a severely degenerative index finger distal interphalangeal (DIP) joint and a large cystic mass with ulnar deviation of the proximal interphalangeal (PIP) joint of the long finger. **C-D,** Anteroposterior and lateral views of the index finger showing fusion of the DIP joint with a retained Herbert screw device, decreased soft tissue swelling about the PIP joint of the long finger, and decreased ulnar deviation.

Case Study 13-4: Rehabilitation After Reconstructive Surgery of the Carpometacarpal Joint

History

A 66-year-old left-dominant woman was referred to therapy with a diagnosis of CMC basilar joint arthritis and de Quervain's tenosynovitis in her right thumb and wrist. She reported progressive pain in the basilar joint of her non-dominant right thumb that was atraumatic. The patient also reported occasional, mild discomfort in her dominant left CMC joint.

Her job as a dental hygienist included cleaning calcareous deposits, accretions, and stains from the teeth and beneath the margins of the gums using dental instruments.

The most stressful activities for the CMC joint are those that require a strong pinch, increased with applicable pressure, force, and tension. Gripping a dental instrument is an activity that requires a common pinch (tripod) associated with symptomatic complaints of basilar joint arthritis. However, the involved CMC was her nondominant right hand. Occupational speculation reveals that a strong lateral pinch is required to retract the mouth with a dental instrument. This positional pinch is also hazardous to a progressively degenerating joint, because the shearing force of the thumb metacarpal and trapezium with prolonged lateral pinch pressure exaggerate the articular wear.

Patient History

Previous symptoms include "thumb pain." This patient reported that she was diagnosed with de Quervain's tenosynovitis and given three cortisone injections in a period of 4.5 months from a previous physician with no prescription for therapy. The patient further reported that she was advised to have a "first dorsal compartment release."

Diagnostic Classification: Musculoskeletal 4E: Tenosynovitis (727.04)

Examination

The right hand had normal attitude except for deformity at the base of the first metacarpal. She had full range of motion and all tendons and nerves tested intact. She had severe pain on first CMC grind test and a positive Finkelstein's test (for de Quervain's syndrome).

Treatment (Preoperative)

She was initially positioned in a thumb spica splint to rest the CMC joint and the extensor pollicis brevis (EPB) and the abductor pollicis longus in the first dorsal compartment. The interphalangeal (IP) was left free for range of motion. Additionally, she was treated therapeutically for the tenosynovitis; once subsided, the splint was reduced to a custom CMC joint stabilization splint.

The patient's functional complaints of discomfort and weakness were mostly with grasping objects and rotation, such as doorknobs, turning a key in the car ignition, carry-ing a jug of tea or a large object that required strain to the basilar joint, and most especially, the continued pinch strain when using her dental instruments.

Supporting the fact that de Quervain's tenosynovitis is a potential diagnosis, the probable origin of this first dorsal compartment pain is most likely based on her description of acquired "contorted" wrist and thumb positions to "prevent pain in the base of the thumb" when performing her job. The patient also established that the requirement to wear latex gloves in her occupation as a dental hygienist limited her ability in wearing a splint at work to protect her joint. As a result, the de Quervain's subsided, but obviously, the CMC pain did not. The patient was discharged until surgical reconstruction (CMC arthroplasty), with a home program of splinting, joint protection techniques and a home exercise program to prevent further "flare-up" of tenosynovitis indicative with compensatory movements.

Surgery

Three months after her initial consultation, the patient underwent resection arthroplasty of the right thumb CMC. The surgery was a volar approach technique, taking down the thenar muscles on the first metacarpal. The trapezium was excised, and the metacarpal base articular surface was removed. One half of the flexor carpi radialis tendon was harvested and left attached distally at the base of the second metacarpal. The tendon graft was passed through a drill hole in the first metacarpal from the proximal cut surface and out radially and distally on the first metacarpal. Holding the metacarpal in the reduced position, the tendon transfer was attached by sutures to the fascia and periosteum on the radial aspect. With satisfactory stability, the thenar muscles were repaired and the wound was closed. Along with a sterile dressing, the patient was placed in a thumb spica splint.

The splint was removed at 2 weeks; her wound was well healed and thumb had good position. The patient was placed in a removable splint and encouraged to move the thumb in the plane of the palm two to three times per day over the next 2 weeks. She was the then given a thumb spica cock-up splint and referred for postoperative therapy (Figure 13-19).

Treatment (Postoperative)

One-Month Postoperative

The patient returned to therapy 4-weeks postoperative right thumb CMC arthroplasty and reported that she was "almost pain free" based on the constant pain she had before surgery. She arrived to therapy with a postoperative splint immobilizing the wrist, thumb metacarpal-phalangeal (MP), and leaving the IP free for movement. She was cautioned regarding her zeal and postoperative excitement to anxiously "return to life."

Case Study 13-4: Rehabilitation After Reconstructive Surgery of the Carpometacarpal Joint—cont'd

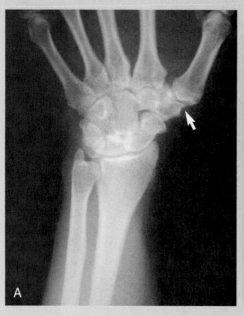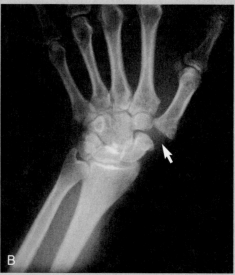

Figure 13-19 **A,** Severe first carpal-metacarpal (CMC) arthritis with subluxation *(arrow)*; **B,** after CMC resection arthroplasty *(arrow)*.

Evaluation (4-Weeks Postoperative)
- Range of motion:
  - Wrist extension-flexion: 45/0/45
  - Radial deviation and ulnar deviation: 15/0/15
  - Thumb MP: 0/20
  - Uninvolved digits (I,L,R,S): Within normal limits (WNL)
  - IP : 0/20
- Strength (gross grip and pinch): DNT (did not test) because of infancy of reconstruction
- Sensation: No hypersensitivity or deficits noted in superficial radial nerve branch
- Edema: Moderate edema noted at base of thumb and radial wrist

Treatment Goals
- Protect reconstruction
- Increase functional use for activities of daily living (ADL)
- Increase range of motion
- Increase strength
- Decrease edema

Treatment
Four-Weeks Postoperative: Initial Postoperative Evaluation
Modalities
1. Heat: Used because the main problem was stiffness. Heat was chosen because warmth increases circulation and decreases pain and stiffness.
2. Therapeutic exercises: Active assisted range of motion (AAROM) and AROM initiated to thumb and wrist

- CMC abduction, opposition to each fingertip, radial extension
- No MP flexion and opposition to base of fifth
3. Continue splinting after exercises and at night.
4. Perform moderate ADL while wearing the splint.

Six-Weeks Postoperative
1. Initiated MP flexion and opposition to the base of the fifth finger as the patient was able to oppose to each fingertip with ease and "walk" down the small finger with minimal effort to the base.
2. Reduce splint wear time; discharge at night.
3. Initiate gentle isometric thenar strengthening.

Eight-Weeks Postoperative
1. Discharged splint (CMC basilar) except when performing stressful activities.
2. Initiated gentle grip and pinch strengthening (patient is pain free).

Ten-Weeks Postoperative
1. Progress with strengthening and prolonged progressive pinching with grading resistance to mimic as much as possible the retraction of the mouth with dental instruments.
2. Continue with home exercises and performing progressive ADL.

Twelve-Weeks Postoperative: Discharge Evaluation
- Range of motion
- Wrist extension and flexion: 75/0/75
- Radial deviation and ulnar deviation: 20/0/25
- Thumb MP: 0/35
- IP: 0/60

Case Study 13-4: Rehabilitation After Reconstructive Surgery of the Carpometacarpal Joint—cont'd

- Strength

Right grip:	Pinch: (tip):	(Tripod):	(Lat):
43 #	7.5 #	9 #	10 #
Left grip:	Pinch: (tip):	(Tripod):	(Lat):
46 #	11 #	12 #	11 #

- Pain: The patient was asymptomatic and reported no pain. She reported that she was ready to return to work, and her plans were to maintain a part-time position.

Fourteen-Weeks Postoperative

The patient called to report that she was doing very well, reporting only fatigue at the end of the day, with no pain.

---

injury, maintained satisfactory tissue on either side of the amputation may lend themselves to reimplantation. This has become a specialized area within hand surgery. The reimplantation surgeon must consider many complex problems when anticipating reimplantation of a digit or hand. The length of the period of ischemia and the temperature of the divided part during that time can play a very important role in determining whether the tissue of the amputated part will survive. In addition, with longer periods of ischemia, the arterial and venous anastomoses have a lower incidence of patency after repair. The coordination of several procedures including fixation of the skeletal structure, repair of the muscle-tendon units, as well as repair of the arteries, veins, and nerves that supply the part must be taken into account. This is very tedious work, and frequently failure of one or more of these areas can cause subsequent loss of the digit. Reimplantation of digits distal to the DIP joint is rarely considered except on the thumb, and reimplantation of amputated tissue proximal to the wrist becomes much more complicated because of the amount of muscle tissue involved and the amount of myoglobin produced because of muscle necrosis, which can cause systemic complications, particularly in the kidneys.[17]

After loss of a part of the hand, if digits remain, then it is very important to provide some type of pincer mechanism for grasping. Therefore if the thumb has been lost, then one of the other digits will need to be transferred into an opposing position to the other one or two digits to produce the pincer motion.

Loss of a single digit proximal to the DIP joint from a sharp amputation can necessitate replantation for good function.[18] Loss of a single digit proximal to the PIP joint, particularly the long or ring finger, can cause dysfunction when trying to hold fairly small objects such as coins, which can fall through the gap in the fingers.[19] In these patients, ray amputation is frequently indicated to allow for more normal hand function if reimplantation is not feasible. A hand with three fingers and one thumb seems to work very satisfactorily, almost as well as a regular hand. Occasionally in a heavy laborer, maintenance of the partially amputated digit rather than ray amputation may be desirable to maintain the breadth of the hand and allow for greater grip strength. When the thumb has been amputated or when all the digits have been amputated with maintenance of some function of the thumb, a toe-to-hand transfer using free-tissue technique can restore the former pincer movement of the hand.[20] Amputation proximal to the base of the metacarpals is very difficult to reconstruct, and a prosthetic replacement may provide satisfactory function.

Rehabilitation when only a single digit is involved can be as simple as reeducating the individual in the use of the hand without the amputated digit. If a transfer of digits within the same hand or toe-to-hand transfer of digits is performed to replace the thumb, then the rehabilitation and reeducation in use of the hand can be very complex. Therapy after reimplantation is very prolonged because of scarring through the area of the amputation and repair. Consideration must be given to bone healing, the sliding and gliding motions of the tendons, and protection of the digit until sensation returns.

CRUSH INJURIES

Crush injuries to the hand and fingers frequently cause damage to a large area and can involve multiple or all structures including fractured bones, crushed or lacerated nerves and tendons, torn ligaments, crushed muscles, and macerated or avulsed skin. Thus these injuries are frequently devastating to hand function and present challenges for repair and reconstruction. Examination both in the emergency department and in the operating room will help identify damaged structures, as well as those intact and the viability of the hand and fingers.

The approach to repair is generally to restore skeletal stability, then tendon repair. These are done first to provide a stable frame and to avoid disrupting the vascular and neural repairs performed at the same surgery. Loss of digits and compromised function can now be prevented in some cases by the use of cadaver parts, including whole bones such as phalanges and tendons, especially the extensor head.

Rehabilitation from these injuries is prolonged, with the challenges of extensive scarring, slow nerve recovery, and hypersensitivity, sometimes including past traumatic sympathetic dystrophy. The approach to repair in a particular patient requires an assessment of the occupational and nonoccupational demands, as well as the psychosocial aspects of the patient's life.

REFERENCES

1. Flynn JE: Disability evaluations. In Flynn JE, editor: Hand surgery, ed 2, Baltimore, 1975, Lippincott Williams & Wilkins.

2. Lee M: Tendon injuries. In Crenshaw AH, editor: Campbell's operative orthopaedics, ed 7, St Louis, 1987, Mosby.

3. Nichols HM: Manual of hand injuries, Chicago, 1957, Year Book Medical Publishers

4. Taleisnik J, Kelly PJ: The extraosseous and intraosseous blood supply of the scaphoid bone, J Bone Joint Surg 48(A):125, 1966.

5. Herbert TJ: Use of the Herbert bone screw in surgery of the wrist, Clin Orthop 202:79, 1986.

6. Cooney WP, Dobyns JH, Linscheid RL: Fractures of the scaphoid: a rational approach to management, Clin Orthop 149:90, 1980.

7. Lee M: Fractures. In Crenshaw AH, editor: Campbell's operative orthopaedics, ed 7, St Louis, 1987, Mosby.

8. Abouna JM, Brown H: The treatment of mallet finger: the results in a series of 148 consecutive cases and a review of the literature, Br J Surg 55:653, 1968.

9. Lister GD, Kleinert HE, Kurz JE et al: Primary flexor tendon repair followed by immediate controlled mobilization, J Hand Surg 2:441, 1977.

10. Pennington DG: The influence of tendon sheath integrity and vincular blood supply on adhesion formation following tendon repair in hens, Br J Plast Surg 32:302, 1979.

11. Schneider LH, Hunter JM: Flexor tendons late reconstruction. In Green DP, editor: Operative hand surgery, ed 2, New York, 1988, Churchill Livingstone.

12. Poppen NK: Recovery of sensibility after suture of digital nerves, J Hand Surg 4:212, 1979.

13. Frykman GK, Waylet J: Rehabilitation of peripheral nerve injuries, Orthop Clin North Am 12:361, 1981.

14. Johnson RP: The acutely injured wrist and its residuals, Clin Orthop 149:33, 1980.

15. Cook SD, Beckenbaugh RD, Redondo J, et al: Long-term follow-up of pyrolytic carbon metacarpophalangeal implants, J Bone J Surg 81(A):635, 1999.

16. Neviaser RJ: Infections. In Green DP, editor: Operative hand surgery, ed 2, New York, 1988, Churchill Livingstone.

17. Urbaniak JR: Replantation of amputated parts technique, results, and indications. In AAOS surgical symposium on microsurgery: practical use in orthopaedics, St Louis, 1979, Mosby.

18. Soucacos PN, Beris AE, Touliatos AS, et al: Current indications for single digit replantation, Acta Orthop Scand (suppl 264) 266:12-15, 1995.

19. Chow SP, Ng C: Hand function after digital amputation, J Hand Surg [Br] 18:125, 1993.

20. Wei FC, el Gammal TA: Toe to hand transfer: current concepts, techniques, and research, Clin Plast Surg 23:103, 1996.

14

Bruce Greenfield,
Marie A. Johanson,
and Michael J. Wooden

Mobilization of the Upper Extremity

Joint mobilization has become an increasingly popular and important physical therapy intervention. As recently as 25 years ago, manipulation was a controversial topic, considered off-limits to any practitioners other than chiropractors or osteopaths. Thanks, however, to the dedication of many pioneers in this field, peripheral and vertebral joint mobilization has become standard fare in most physical therapy curricula.

In particular the profession is indebted to such teachers as Paris, Maitland, and Kaltenborn, themselves physical therapists, as well as to such physicians as Mennell, Cyriax, and Stoddard, who were willing to share their knowledge. Their efforts have mushroomed into such developments as continuing education courses, as well as graduate programs, residencies, and fellowships in manual therapy and orthopaedics. These programs have stimulated an increase in research, both basic and clinical. Indeed, interest in joint mobilization was the main factor leading to creation of the American Physical Therapy Association's Orthopaedic Section, which has paved the way for specialization in physical therapy.

An additional benefit has been the publication of some excellent books dealing with assessment and treatment including joint mobilization. Many are cited in the References and Suggested Readings sections of this chapter and in Chapter 26. The purpose of these two chapters is to summarize briefly the information contained in the various textbooks and to describe the peripheral joint techniques with which we have had the most success.

GENERAL PRINCIPLES

In general terms, mobilization is defined as restoration of joint motion, which can be accomplished by different forms of active or passive exercise or by such mechanical means as continuous passive motion (CPM) machines.[1]

In the context of manual therapy, however, mobilization is passive range-of-motion exercise applied to the joint surfaces, as opposed to the physiologic, cardinal plane movement of the joint as a whole. Passive movement of the joint surfaces requires knowledge of arthrokinematics, first described by Basmajian

and MacConail,[2] such as intimate movements of roll, spin, glide, compression, and distraction. These movements occur between the joint surfaces (hence the term *arthrokinematic*) and are necessary for normal, physiologic, or osteokinematic movement of bones.

To illustrate, Basmajian and MacConail[2] described movement of a convex joint surface on a concave surface (e.g., the femur on the tibia). As the convex bone rolls in any direction, it must simultaneously slide (minutely) in the opposite direction on the concave bone to keep the two surfaces approximated. Conversely, when a concave bone surface moves on a convex one (e.g., the tibia on the femur), the glide of the concave surface will occur in the same direction.

Mennell[3] elaborated on these arthrokinematic movements, labeling them *joint play*: movements that are small but precise, which cannot be reproduced by voluntary muscle control, but that are necessary for full, painless range of motion. Similarly, Paris[4] classified these movements as *accessory movements,* either joint play or component. He stressed that these movements occur not only during physiologic movement but also at end range to protect the joint from external forces. The clinician assesses end-range joint play by applying overpressure at end range to determine end-feel and the presence of pain. Kaltenborn's system[5] uses similar arthrokinematic principles.

The techniques described later in this chapter are primarily based on accessory motion concepts and are primarily osteopathic techniques. The greater the congruency of a peripheral joint is, the more likely it is that arthrokinematic principles (based on the convex-concave principles) explain the effects of the techniques. Joints that lack bony congruency, however, may not exhibit traditional arthrokinematic principles, but rather may be more influenced by changes in capsular tightness and direction of muscle forces. At the glenohumeral joint, for example, the head of the humerus glides in a superior direction during elevation of the humerus because of tightening of the inferior capsule and in a posterior direction during external rotation because of tightening of the anterior capsule.[6,7] However, techniques that "follow" arthrokinematic principles are often still used and may simply stretch portions of the capsule via direct pressure of the humeral head. Alternatively, arthrokinematic principles used to determine the direction of glide based on the desired osteokinematic movement might not always be assumed to be correct. For example, Johnson et al.[8] demonstrated that although both anterior and posterior glides increased glenohumeral external rotation range of motion, a posterior glide (usually used to increase physiologic glenohumeral internal rotation) increased external rotation more than the anterior glide for patient with adhesive capsulate. Thus further ongoing research is needed to establish the directional effects of these techniques. However, where possible, the techniques described in this chapter are linked with the physiologic movements that they theoretically enhance.

THEORIES OF MOBILIZATION

In the periphery, mobilization is used either for its effect on reducing joint restrictions (mechanical) or to relieve pain or muscle guarding (neurophysiologic). This section reviews the theoretic bases for each.

Joint Restrictions

Loss of range of motion can be caused by trauma or immobilization or, most often, a combination of the two. Picture a contracted elbow joint that has been immobilized for 6 to 8 weeks after a supracondylar fracture. Experience tells us that this elbow, despite weeks of aggressive therapy, may never regain full mobility. What are the reasons for this? The effects of trauma and immobilization on joint-related structures are discussed in detail in Chapter 1. To summarize, the most significant range limiting effects are as follows: [9-18]

1. Loss of extensibility of periarticular connective tissue structures: ligaments, capsule, fascia, and tendons
2. Deposition of fibrofatty infiltrates acting as intraarticular "glue"
3. Adaptive shortening of muscles
4. Breakdown of articular cartilage

All of these effects could contribute to abnormal limitation of movement and must be dealt with in treatment.

Muscle has been shown to be an incredibly plastic tissue, with the ability to regenerate and return to normal length even after prolonged immobilization.[14,15] However, little research has been conducted to show the direct effects of mobilization techniques per se on immobilized connective tissue. Researchers have demonstrated that passive movement does seem to maintain distance, lubrication, and mobility between collagen fibers.[10-12] During the healing of traumatized connective tissue, passive movement restores the ability of collagen fibers to glide on one another as scar tissue matures.[18] Stress to this healing connective tissue, applied as early as 3 weeks but no later than 3 to 4 months after injury, appears to reduce the formation of cross-links between and within collagen fibers.[16,17] Therefore the scar is allowed to lengthen in the direction of the stress applied as its tensile strength increases. Thus the development of joint contracture is reduced.[16,17] Finally, forceful passive

movement has been shown to rupture infraarticular adhesions that form during immobilization.[18-21]

Pain and Muscle Guarding

Wyke[22] has identified receptor nerve endings in various periarticular structures. These nerve endings have been shown to influence pain, proprioception, and muscle relaxation.

Type I (postural) and type II (dynamic) mechanoreceptors are located in joint capsules. They have a low threshold and are excited by repetitive movements including oscillations. Type III mechanoreceptors are found in joint capsules and extracapsular ligaments; they are similar to Golgi tendon organs in that they are excited by stretching and perhaps thrusting maneuvers. Pain receptors, or type IV nociceptors, are found in capsules, ligaments, fat pads, and blood vessel walls. These receptors are fired by noxious stimuli, as in trauma, and have a relatively high threshold.

Pain impulses from type IV nociceptors are conducted slowly. Impulses from type I and II mechanoreceptors are fast, conducting at a much lower threshold. The differences between types I and II and type IV conductivity may explain why oscillating a joint relieves pain. Theoretically, the faster mechanical impulses overwhelm the slower pain impulses. Whether this is achieved by "closing the gate" or perhaps by release of endorphins in the central nervous system is still under investigation.[23]

Muscle relaxation is an additional benefit of passive movement. One theory is that causing type III joint receptors and Golgi tendon organs to fire by stretching or thrusting a joint results in temporary inhibition or relaxation of muscles crossing the joint.[22] This in itself may cause an increase in range of motion and helps prepare the joint for further stretching and mobilization.

Application

Many schools of thought exist regarding the hands-on approach to manual therapy. Mobilization can be applied with osteopathic articulations, distraction of joint surfaces, oscillations, stretching, and thrust manipulations. When using stretching and oscillations, the authors favor those techniques that stress accessory motion based on arthrokinematics. These are primarily glides, distractions, and capsular stretches. Except for gentle stretching, one should avoid mobilizing, especially thrusting, in physiologic movements. Ultimately, which techniques are chosen should not matter as long as the therapist is well trained and follows a few guidelines. Most importantly, the therapist should follow Paris' four simple but critical rules before mobilizing:

1. Identify the location and direction of the limitation (e.g., In a stiff ankle, is it posterior glide of the talus that is restricted?).
2. Prepare the soft tissues (i.e., decrease swelling, pain, muscle guarding or tightness).
3. Protect neighboring hypermobilities. This is particularly important in spinal mobilization but could apply, for

example, to a shoulder dislocation that has resulted in anterior capsule laxity. In mobilizing to increase abduction and rotation, one would want to avoid anterior glide or other maneuvers that would stress the anterior capsule.

A fourth rule, really an extension of the previous three, applies to postsurgical cases.

4. Communicate with the surgeon. Find out which tissues have been cut or sacrificed and what motions to avoid at least initially.

Maitland's[24] description of the grades of joint movement has been a major contribution to manual therapy. He uses oscillatory movements of different amplitudes applied at different parts of the range of motion, either accessory or physiologic. Grade I oscillations are of very small amplitude at the beginning of the range, whereas grade II oscillations are large-amplitude oscillations from near the beginning to midrange. No tissue resistance is encountered with grade I or II movements, so they do not "mobilize" to increase range. However, they do reduce pain and induce relaxation through the mechanoreceptor mechanisms already described. The actual mobilization movements, those that are taken into tissue resistance, are grades III, IV, and V. A grade III movement uses large amplitudes from mid- to end range, hitting at end range rather abruptly. A grade IV movement also goes to end range but is of very small amplitude. Because they may be less painful and less likely to traumatize a joint, grade IV movements should be used before grade IIIs, the latter being more useful as the joint becomes less acute. A grade V movement is a small-amplitude thrust beyond end range, a so-called manipulation.

Figure 14-1, *A,* depicts Maitland's grades of movement in a normal joint. Figure 14-1, *B,* shows movements applied to a restricted joint. The reader should note that in the latter, the end range (limited) will gradually approach end range (normal) as treatment progresses. Often a restricted joint is also painful, and the therapist must decide whether to treat the pain or the stiffness. One advantage of the Maitland system is that grades of movement provide the tools for either form of therapy.

To generalize, grades I and II oscillation are used for pain; grades III, IV, and V are for stiffness. The therapist must now decide when to use them.

Mobilization With Movement

Mulligan[25] has introduced joint mobilization techniques he classified as *mobilization with movement* (MWM). These techniques combine traditional sustained passive accessory motion techniques based on arthrokinematics with active or passive physiologic movements. Mulligan's theory is that adaptive shortening does not always explain painful and restricted active movements. He believes that minor positional faults often result in painfully restricted active movements; in these cases he asserts that repositioning, rather than increasing extensibility of capsular and ligamentous structures, is the key to restoration of normal physiologic motions. MWM techniques are only performed when the technique is painless and can be followed by taping techniques or self-administered MWM techniques to maintain the positional correction.[25]

Although several case reports document good outcomes using MWM techniques,[26] few clinical trials compare these techniques with traditional accessory techniques, other interventions, or control groups. However, these clinical trials are beginning to appear in the literature. Yang et al.[27] compared

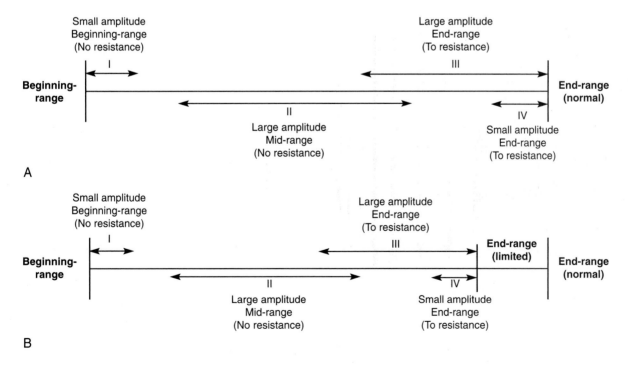

Figure 14-1 Grades of movement. **A,** In a normal joint; **B,** in a stiff joint. (Modified from Maitland GD: Maitland's vertebral manipulation, ed 7, Edinburgh, 2005, Butterworth-Heinemann.)

the effects of a MWM technique (see Figure 14-16) to accessory glides of the humeral head in midrange and at end range among patients with adhesive capsulitis on shoulder active range of motion (AROM) and scapulohumeral rhythm. The MWM technique and the accessory glides at end range both improved active shoulder elevation, active external rotation, active internal rotation, and scapulohumeral rhythm compared with the accessory glides performed in midrange. Additionally, the MWM techniques showed greater improvement in scapulohumeral rhythm than the accessory glides performed at end range. Paungmali et al.[28] compared a MWM technique (see Figure 14-26) to a sham technique and a control condition on pain-free grip strength for patients with lateral epicondylitis. These investigators reported that the MWM technique increased pain-free grip force compared with the sham technique and control. At the lower extremity, a MWM technique performed during weight bearing or nonweight bearing (see Figure 28-26) improved posterior talar glide compared with a control group receiving no intervention among patients with recurrent ankle sprains.[29]

Indications for Mobilization

After trauma, surgery, and immobilization, no predetermined schedules state when mobilization can begin. The severity of trauma, extent of surgery, complications, and length of time since onset all need to be considered. Even when no clear contraindications for rehabilitation exist, including passive exercise, experience tells us that great variability exists regarding safety and tolerance.

To reduce the chances of being too aggressive, the therapist should try to determine what stage of the healing process the injured joint is in: acute with extravasation, fibroplasia, or scar maturation (see Chapter 1). At best, this is an educated guess, but certain steps in the subjective and objective evaluation will increase accuracy.

Subjectively, one must determine the irritability of the joint, that is, how much of a particular activity increases the pain and to what extent. Consider, for example, a posttraumatic knee. At one extreme is the patient who experiences severe pain and effusion for several days after mowing the lawn. Compare this patient to the patient who reports moderate soreness for a few hours after playing two sets of tennis. Obviously, the first patient's joint is highly irritable, whereas that of the tennis player is much less so.

Subjective responses can be reinforced by assessing objectively the level of reactivity.[4] By carefully taking the joint through its passive range, the therapist monitors the sequence of pain versus resistance.[4] If the patient reports pain before tissue resistance (not muscle guarding) is felt by the therapist, then the joint is highly reactive and, theoretically, is in an acute inflammatory stage. Therefore the joint should remain protected and splinted. If necessary, then the therapist can apply grade I oscillations to reduce pain.

Moderate reactivity is assumed when pain and tissue resistance are simultaneous. The joint injury is now subacute, perhaps indicating that fibroplasia and early scar formation are underway. The patient will tolerate careful active range-of-motion exercises, as well as grade I and II oscillations to decrease pain. Actual mobilization (grades III and IV) should be delayed, however, to avoid disturbing the immature scar.

If significant tissue resistance is felt before (or in the absence of) pain, low reactivity is assumed. By now the collagen matrix has matured, and mobilization is needed to stress and remodel the scar. At this time grade III, IV, and V movements are indicated (Table 14-1). If these more aggressive maneuvers induce soreness, then the therapist can fall back on grade I and II movements to ease the pain.[24] The key to preventing overaggressiveness is to assess the patient's response to treatment and reactivity for each restriction at every session.

Some conditions that require precautions before mobilization in the periphery are moderate reactivity, osteoporosis, and recent fractures. Choose techniques that will minimize stress to a fracture site while mobilizing an adjacent joint. In addition, beware of the patient with poor tolerance of treatment (i.e., when mobilization sessions consistently increase pain and reactivity).

A few contraindications should also be considered: high reactivity, indicating the presence of acute inflammation; active inflammatory disease; malignancy; and hypermobility from trauma or disease (e.g., rheumatoid arthritis).[4,24]

Techniques

It is always difficult to determine which techniques are most effective. The References and Suggested Readings sections list volumes in which literally hundreds of techniques are described. One cannot state which ones are best for every clinician, but those discussed here are, in the authors' experience, safe, easy to apply, and effective. Each technique is either an accessory

Table 14-1	Objective Reactivity Levels		
Reactivity Level	Sequence	Stage of Healing	Treatment
High	Pain before resistance	Acute, inflammatory	Immobilize Grade I oscillations for pain
Moderate	Pain and resistance simultaneous	Fibroblastic activity	Active range of motion (AROM) Grade II oscillations for pain
Low	Resistance before pain	Scar maturation and remodeling	Passive range of motion (PROM) Grade III, IV, and V movements as indicated

motion or a specific capsular stretch and can be applied with any grade of movement. However, grade V thrust maneuvers are not discussed and should not be used without appropriate hands-on training.

The reader must realize that these are also evaluative techniques. They should first be used to determine reactivity and the need for mobilization. Besides goniometric measurement of physiologic range of motion, accessory movement testing is performed using the mobilization positions. To assess the quality and quantity of movement, the accessory motions are usually compared with those in the contralateral limb. This passive movement testing is somewhat out of context in this chapter because it is actually part of the evaluation process. The reader is referred to Chapters 10 to 14, which review other evaluation procedures for each joint. These chapters also contain information pertaining to anatomy, mechanics, and pathology.

Mobilization is difficult to teach on paper without the benefit of laboratory sessions. However, those experienced in basic manual therapy will be able to follow the figures. For each technique, the patient's position, the therapist's hand contacts, and the direction of movement are described. Table 14-2 is for reference, listing each technique with the physiologic movement it theoretically enhances.

Table 14-2   Summary of Upper Extremity Techniques

Joint	Mobilization Technique	Movement Promoted	Figure
Sternoclavicular	Superior glide	Elevation	14-2
	Inferior glide	Depression	14-3
	Posterior glide	General	14-4
Acromioclavicular	Anteroposterior glides	General	14-5, 14-6
Scapulothoracic	Distraction	General	14-7
	Superior glide	Elevation	14-8, *A*
	Inferior glide	Depression	14-8, *B*
	Upward and downward rotation	Rotation	14-9, *A* and *B*
Glenohumeral	Anteroposterior glides	Neutral	14-10
	Anterior glide	Flexion, abduction	14-11, 14-12, 14-13
	Inferior glide	Flexion, abduction	14-14, *A* and *B*; 14-15, 14-16
	Long axis distraction	General	14-17
	Lateral glide	General	14-18, *A, B,* and *C*
	Distraction in flexion	Flexion	14-19
	Anterior capsule stretch	External rotation	14-20, *A* and *B*
	Inferior capsule stretch	Abduction	14-21
	Posterior capsule stretch	Internal and external rotation Horizontal adduction	14-22, *A, B,* and *C*
Humeroulnar	Abduction	Extension	14-23
	Adduction	Flexion	14-24
	Distraction	General	14-25
	Mobilization with movement (MWM)	N/A	14-26
Radiohumeral and radioulnar	Dorsal glide radial head	Pronation	14-28, *A* and *B*
Distal radioulnar	Inward and outward roll	Pronation, supination	14-29
	Anteroposterior glides	General	14-30
Radiocarpal (RC)	Glides	Flexion, extension, deviation	14-31, *A, B, C,* and *D*
	Distraction	General	14-32, *A* and *B*
	Scaphoid glide	General	14-33
	Lunate glide	General	14-34
Ulnomeniscotriquetral	Glide	General	14-35
Pisiform	Glide	Wrist mobility	14-36, *A, B, C,* and *D*
Intercarpal	Glide	Hand mobility	14-38
Metacarpal-phalangeal (MCP)	Distraction	General	14-39
	Anteroposterior glide	Flexion, extension	14-40, *A* and *B*
	Mediolateral glide	Adduction, abduction	14-41, *A* and *B*
	Mediolateral tilt	Adduction, abduction	14-42, *A* and *B*
	Rotation		14-43
Interphalangeal (IP)	Anterior and posterior glides	Flexion and Extension	14-44
	Mediolateral glide and tilt	Adduction, abduction	14-45

Table 14-3	Specific Intercarpal and Carpometacarpal Glides
Stabilize	**Mobilize**
Scaphoid	Lunate
	Capitate
	Trapezium
	Trapezoid
Lunate	Capitate
	Triquetrum
	Hamate
Triquetrum	Hamate
Hamate	Capitate
	Base of fifth metacarpal
	Base of fourth metacarpal
Capitate	Base of third metacarpal
	Trapezoid
Trapezium	Base of first metacarpal
Trapezoid	Base of second metacarpal

Shoulder: Sternoclavicular Joint

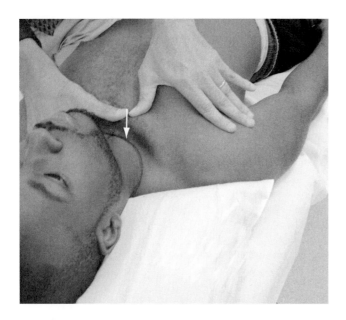

Figure 14-2 Superior glide. Patient position: supine. Contacts: both thumbs inferior to the proximal end of the clavicle. Direction of movement: push cephalad.

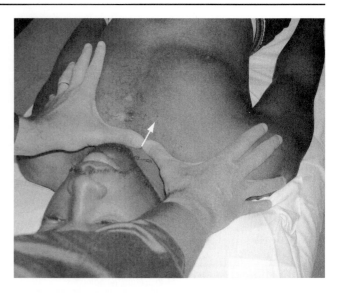

Figure 14-3 Inferior glide. Patient position: supine. Contacts: both thumbs superior to the proximal end of the clavicle. Direction of movement: push caudally and slightly laterally.

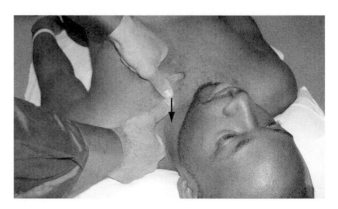

Figure 14-4 Posterior glide. Patient position: supine. Contacts: both thumbs anterior to the proximal end of the clavicle. Direction of movement: push posteriorly.

Acromioclavicular Joint

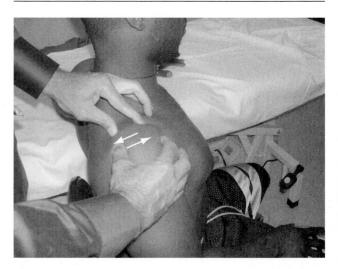

Figure 14-5 Anteroposterior glide. Patient position: sitting. Contacts: grasp the distal end of the clavicle with the thumb and forefinger of one hand; the other hand grasps the acromion process. Direction of movement: glide the acromion anteriorly and posteriorly.

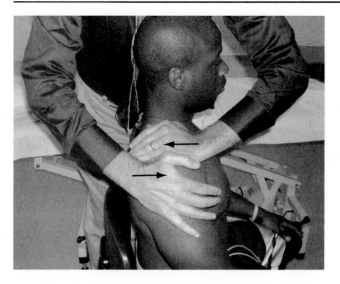

Figure 14-6 Anteroposterior glide. Patient position: sitting. Contacts: the pisiform of one hand contacts the anterior aspect of the distal end of the clavicle; the carpal tunnel of the other hand contacts the posterior aspect of the acromion. Direction of movement: hands push in opposite directions.

Scapulothoracic Joint

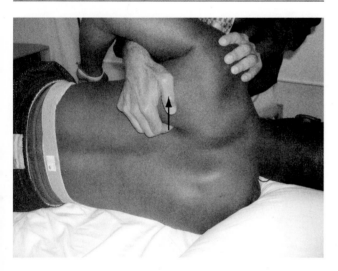

Figure 14-7 Scapular distraction. Patient position: side lying, arm supported by clinician. Contacts: pads of fingers under the medial scapular border. Direction of movement: the scapula is distracted from the thorax.

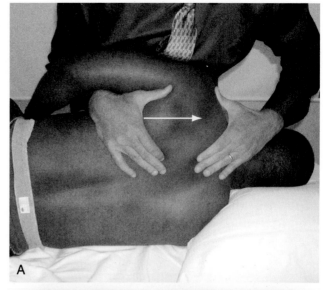

A

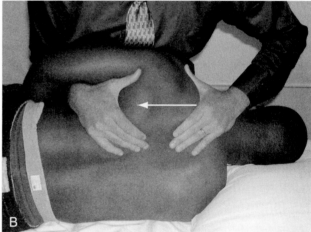

B

Figure 14-8 Superior and inferior glide. Patient position: side lying, arm supported by clinician. Contacts: **A,** web contact of one hand under the inferior scapular border; the web contact of other hand grasps the superior border. Direction of movement: superiorly **(A)** and inferiorly **(B).**

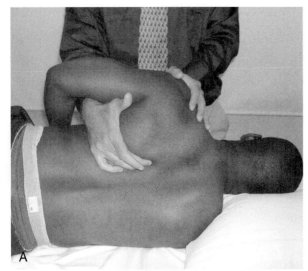

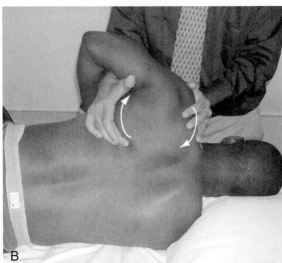

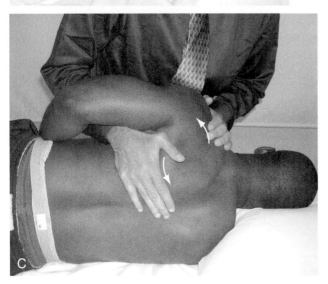

Figure 14-9 Rotation. Patient position: side lying, arm supported by clinician. Contacts: **A,** one hand hooks around inferior border of the scapula; the other hand contacts superior border of the scapula. Direction of movement: under slight distraction, rotate the scapula upward **(B)** and downward **(C).**

Glenohumeral Joint

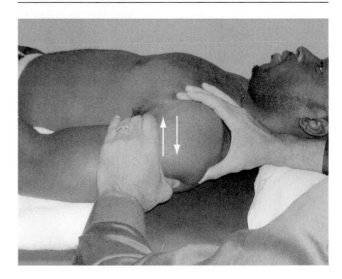

Figure 14-10 Anteroposterior glide. Patient position: supine, arm at side, elbow propped. Contacts: hands grasp the humeral head; thumbs posterior, fingers anterior. Direction of movement: glide the humeral head anteriorly and posteriorly.

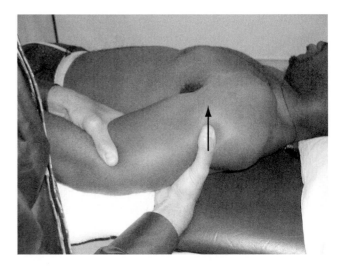

Figure 14-11 Anterior glide. Patient position: supine, arm at side. Contacts: one hand stabilizes at the lateral aspect of the elbow; the other hand grasps the humerus near the axilla. Direction of movement: glide the humeral head anteriorly.

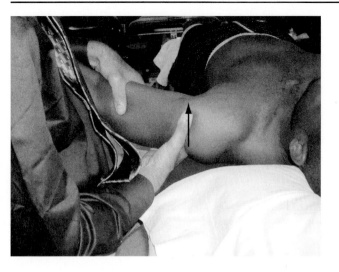

Figure 14-12 Anterior glide at 45 degrees. Patient position: supine, arm in 45 degrees of abduction. Contacts: one hand stabilizes the lateral aspect of the elbow; the other hand grasps the humerus near the axilla. Direction of movement: glide anteriorly while maintaining abduction.

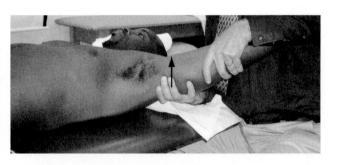

Figure 14-13 Anterior glide in full flexion. Patient position: supine, arm at end range flexion. Contacts: both hands grasp the proximal humerus, with the fingers near the axilla. Direction of movement: glide anteriorly.

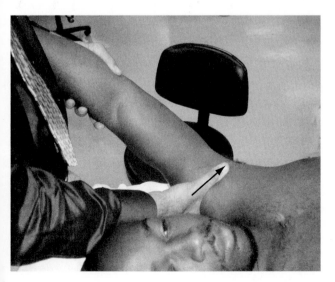

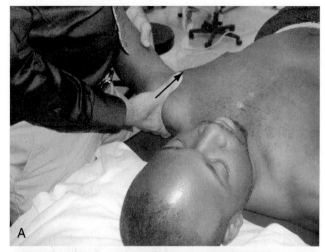

A

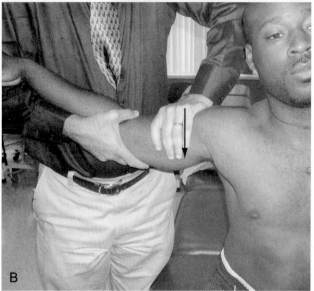

B

Figure 14-14 Inferior glide (depression) in abduction. Patient position: **(A)** supine or **(B)** sitting. Contacts: grasp the arm near the elbow to stabilize in 90 degrees of abduction; the first web space of the other hand contacts the head of the humerus. Direction of movement: depress the head of the humerus (inferiorly).

Figure 14-15 Inferior glide (depression) in full abduction. Patient position: supine, shoulder abducted to 120 degrees. Contacts: the patient's elbow is stabilized by the therapist's shoulder; hands grasp the proximal humerus, with fingers interlocked. Direction of movement: pull the humeral head inferiorly.

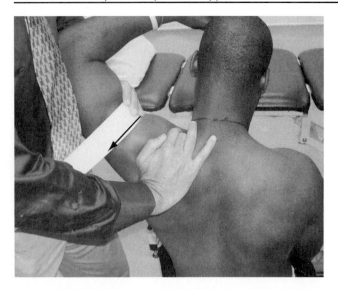

Figure 14-16 Mobilization with movement (MWM) for shoulder abduction. Patient position: sitting. Contacts: stabilize the scapula with one hand; the other hand places belt over anterior proximal humerus. Direction of movement: use trunk to provide a posterior or posterolateral glide of the humeral head.

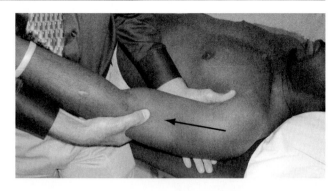

Figure 14-17 Long axis distraction. Patient position: supine. Contacts: hands grasp the humerus above the elbow. Direction of movement: pull along the long axis of the arm.

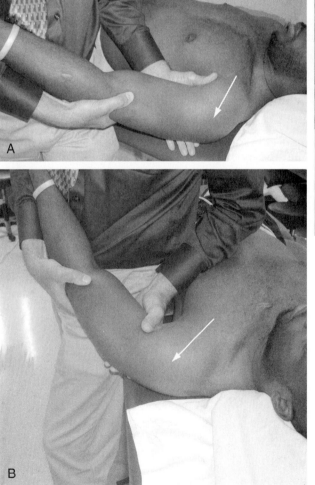

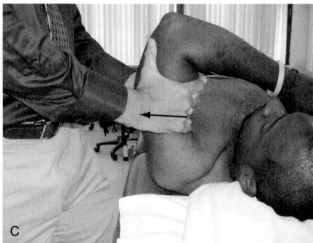

Figure 14-18 Lateral glide (distraction). Patient position: **A,** supine, arm at side; **B,** supine, arm in 45 degrees of abduction; **C,** supine, arm in 90 degrees flexion. Contacts: grasp near the elbow to stabilize; the other hand grasps the proximal humerus at the axilla. Direction of movement: distract the humeral head laterally.

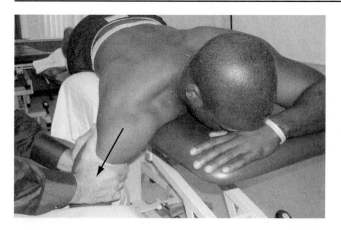

Figure 14-19 Distraction in flexion. Patient position: prone, arm in 90 degrees of flexion off the edge of the table. Contacts: hands grasp the airshaft of the humerus, with fingers interlocked. Direction of movement: distract along the long axis of the arm.

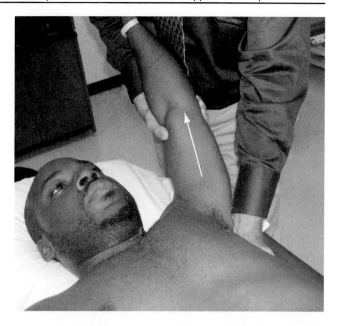

Figure 14-21 Inferior capsule stretch. Patient position: supine, arm in end range abduction. Contacts: carpal tunnel contact of one hand stabilizes the lateral border of the scapula; the other hand grasps the humerus above the elbow. Direction of movement: stretch into abduction.

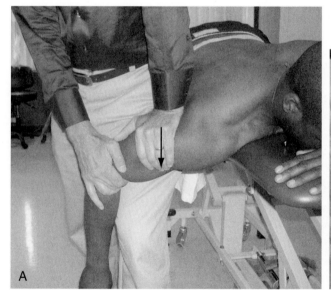

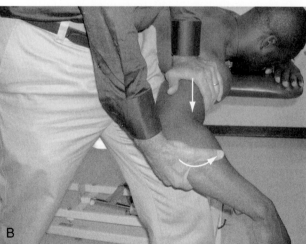

Figure 14-20 Anterior capsule stretch. Patient position: prone, near the edge of the table. Contacts: the palm of one hand stabilizes the posterior aspect of the shoulder; the other hand grasps the humerus above the elbow. Direction of movement: **A,** glide humerus anteriorly with shoulder in neutral rotation; **B,** glide humerus anteriorly while externally rotating shoulder.

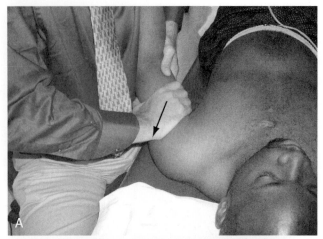

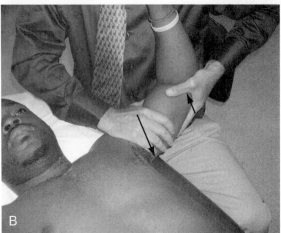

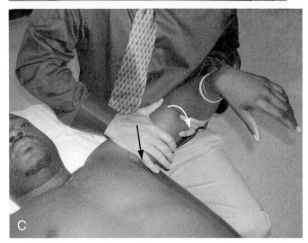

Figure 14-22 Posterior capsule stretch. Patient position: supine, arm in 45 degrees of flexion and slight abduction, elbow flexed. Contacts: stabilize the elbow contact; the other hand contacts the anterior and proximal surface of the humerus. Direction of movement: **A,** glide humerus posteriorly; **B,** glide humerus posterior in 90 degrees of abduction; **C,** glide humerus posteriorly in 90 degrees abduction while internally rotating shoulder.

Elbow: Humeroulnar Joint

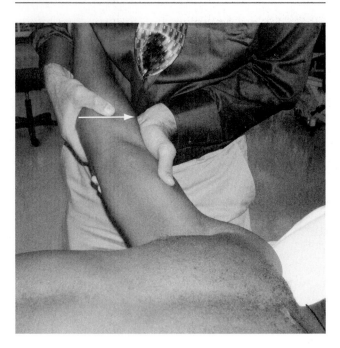

Figure 14-23 Abduction. Patient position: supine. Contacts: stabilize the distal humerus laterally; the other hand grasps the proximal forearm. Direction of movement: the forearm is abducted on the humerus.

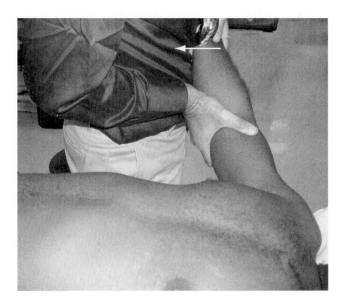

Figure 14-24 Adduction. Patient position: supine. Contacts: stabilize the distal humerus medially; the other hand grasps the radial aspect of the forearm above the wrist. Direction of movement: the forearm is adducted on the humerus.

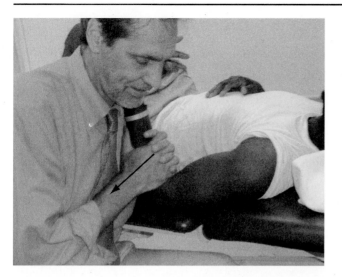

Figure 14-25 Distraction. Patient position: supine, elbow flexed to 90 degrees. Contacts: the patient's forearm is stabilized against the therapist's shoulder; the therapist's hands grasp the proximal aspect of the forearm, with fingers interlocked. Direction of movement: distract the forearm from the humerus.

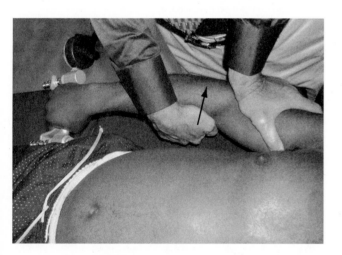

Figure 14-26 Mobilization with movement (MWM) for grip strength. Patient position: sitting, shoulder in internal rotation and forearm in pronation. Contacts: stabilize distal humerus; the other hand grasps medial aspect of proximal forearm and glide in a lateral direction.

Radiohumeral and Proximal Radioulnar Joints

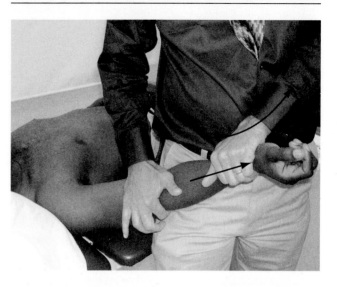

Figure 14-27 Radial distraction. Patient position: supine, arm abducted. Contacts: stabilize by holding the elbow on the treatment table; the other hand grasps the radius above the wrist. Direction of movement: pull the radius distally by rotating the body.

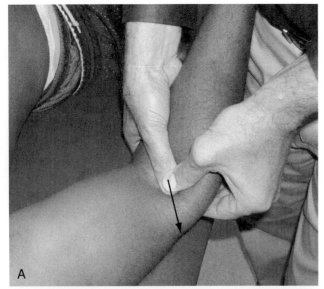

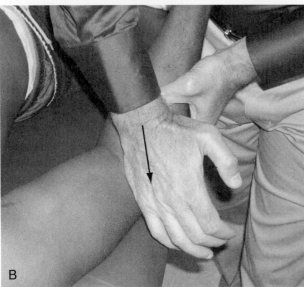

Figure 14-28 Dorsal glide of the radial head. Patient position: supine. Contacts: stabilize by holding the arm on the table; pads of both thumbs contact along volar surface of radial head. Direction of movement: **A,** glide the radially head in a dorsal direction; **B,** same position as **A** but use hypothenar contact to glide the radial head in a dorsal direction.

Wrist and Hand: Distal Radioulnar Joint

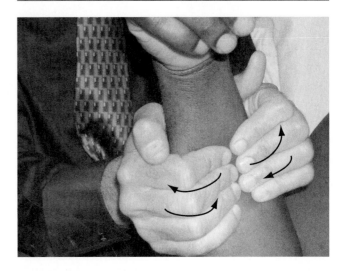

Figure 14-29 Inward and outward roll. Patient position: supine or sitting. Contacts: grasp the distal aspects of the radius and ulna, with pads of fingers contacting volar surface and thenar eminences contacting dorsal surfaces. Direction of movement: roll the radius and ulna inward and outward on one another.

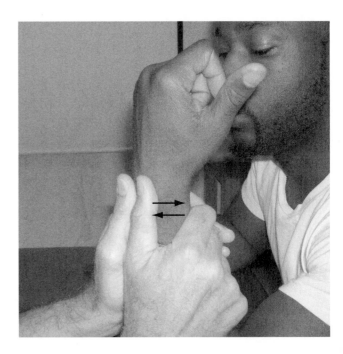

Figure 14-30 Anteroposterior glide. Patient position: sitting or supine, elbow flexed. Contacts: stabilize the ulna with thenar grasp; the other hand grasps the radius with the thumb and forefinger. Direction of movement: glide the radius anteriorly and posteriorly.

Radiocarpal Joints

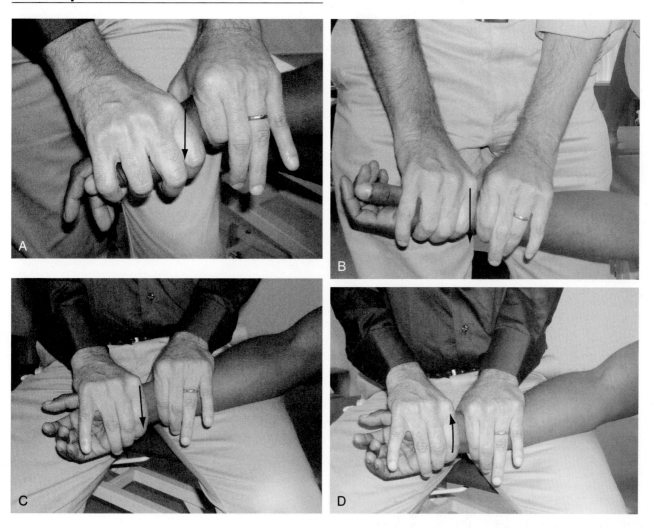

Figure 14-31 Radiocarpal (RC) glides. Patient position: supine or sitting. Contacts: with the thumb, index finger, and first web space, stabilize the radius and ulna dorsally; the other hand grasps the proximal row of carpal bones. Direction of movement: glide the carpal bones **(A)** volar direction (in pronation), **(B)** dorsal direction (in supination), **(C)** ulnar direction, and **(D)** radial direction.

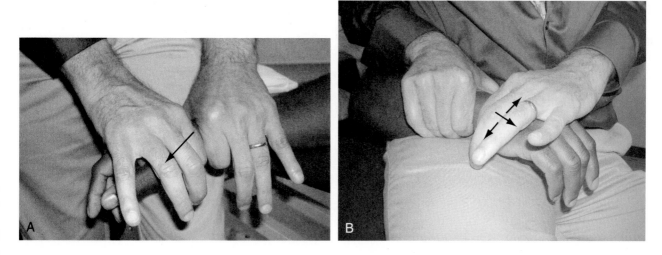

Figure 14-32 Distraction. Patient position: supine or sitting. Contacts: same as in Figure 14-31. Direction of movement: **A,** distract the carpal bones distally; **B,** distract with volar and dorsal glides.

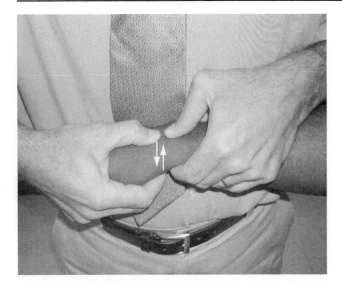

Figure 14-33 Scaphoid on radius. Patient position: supine or sitting. Contacts: using the thumbs and forefingers, stabilize the radius and grasp the scaphoid. Direction of movement: glide the scaphoid anteriorly and posteriorly on the radius.

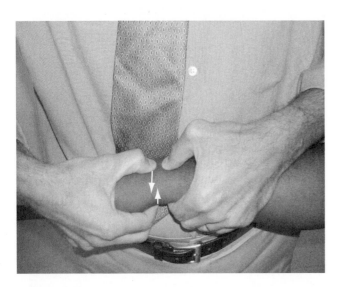

Figure 14-34 Lunate on radius. Patient position: supine or sitting. Contacts: stabilize the radius; grasp the lunate. Direction of movement: glide the lunate anteriorly and posteriorly on the radius.

Ulnomeniscotriquetral joint

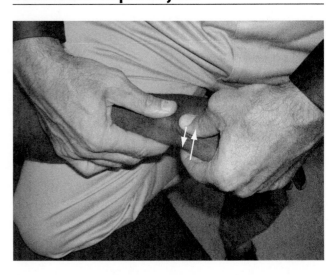

Figure 14-35 Ulnomeniscotriquetral glide. Patient position: supine or sitting. Contacts: stabilize the ulna and grasp the triquetrum. Direction of movement: glide the triquetrum anteriorly and posteriorly on the ulna.

Pisiform Joint

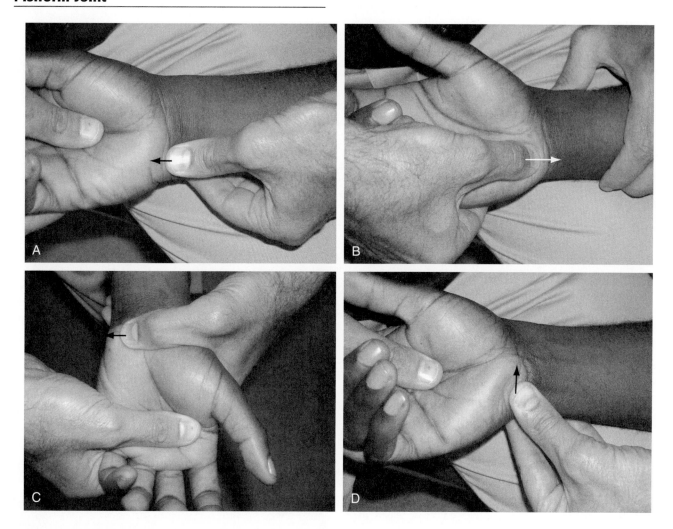

Figure 14-36 Pisiform glides. Patient position: supine or sitting. Contacts: grasp the patient's hand firmly to stabilize; contact the thumb tip against the pisiform bone. Direction of movement: glide the pisiform **(A)** cephalad, **(B)** caudally, **(C)** medially, and **(D)** laterally.

Intercarpal Joints

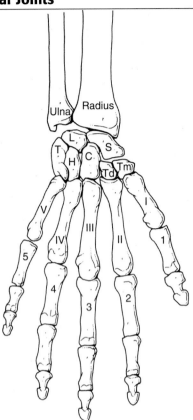

Figure 14-37 The bones of the wrist, hand, and fingers (dorsal view of the right wrist). *S,* Scaphoid; *L,* lunate; *T,* triquetrum; *Tm,* trapezium; *Td,* trapezoid; *C,* capitate; *H,* hamate; *I-V,* metatarsals; *1-5,* proximal phalanges.

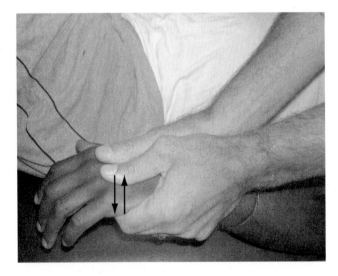

Figure 14-38 Intermetacarpal glide. Patient position: supine or sitting. Contacts: stabilize the head of the third metacarpal with the thumb and forefinger; the other hand grasps the head of the second metacarpal. Direction of movement: glide the second metacarpal anteriorly and posteriorly; repeat for the third, fourth, and fifth metacarpals.

Metacarpophalangeal Joints

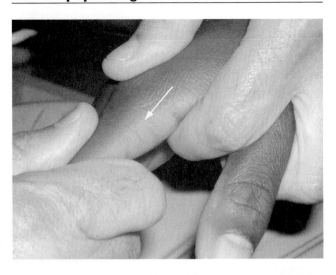

Figure 14-39 Metacarpal-phalangeal (MP) distraction. Patient position: supine or sitting. Contacts: stabilize the shaft of the second metacarpal; the other hand grasps the shaft of the proximal phalanx. Direction of movement: distract the phalanx from the metacarpal; repeat at each MP joint.

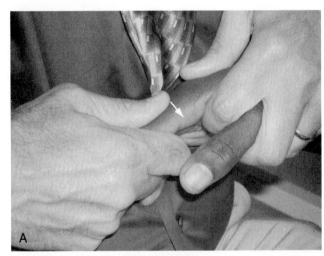

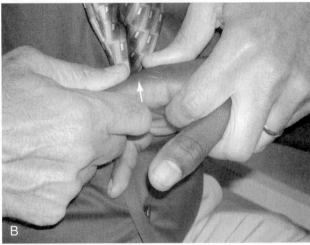

Figure 14-40 Anteroposterior glide. Patient position: supine or sitting. Contacts: same as for metacarpal-phalangeal (MP) distraction. Direction of movement: glide the proximal phalanx anteriorly **(A)** and posteriorly **(B)**; repeat at each joint.

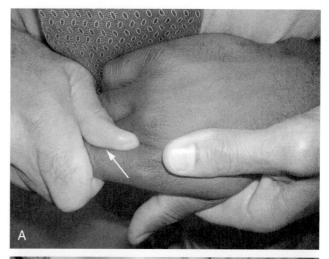

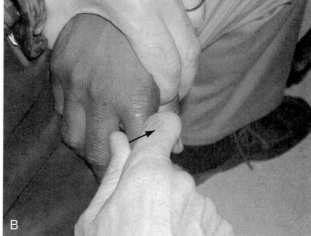

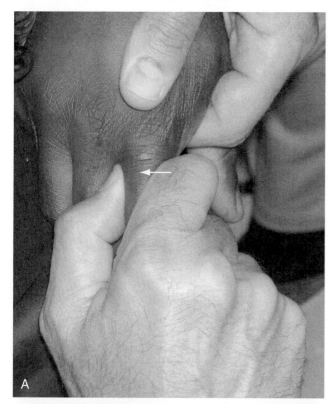

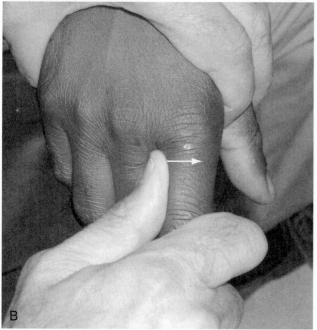

Figure 14-42 Mediolateral tilt. Patient position: supine or sitting. Contacts: stabilize the shaft of the second metacarpal; the proximal shaft is grasped the same way as for mediolateral glide. Direction of movement: tilt the phalanx medially **(A)** and laterally **(B)** by using the forefinger or thumb as a fulcrum; repeat at each metacarpal-phalangeal (MP) joint.

Figure 14-41 Mediolateral glide. Patient position: supine or sitting. Contacts: stabilize the shaft of second metacarpal as previously described; the proximal phalanx is grasped on the medial and lateral aspects of the shaft. Direction of movement: glide the phalanx medially **(A)** and laterally **(B)**; repeat at each metacarpal-phalangeal (MP) joint.

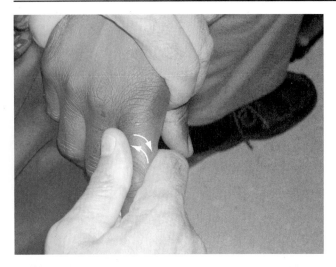

Figure 14-43 Rotation. Patient position: supine or sitting. Contacts: same as for mediolateral tilt. Direction of movement: rotate the phalanx medially and laterally; repeat at each metacarpal-phalangeal (MP) joint.

Interphalangeal joints

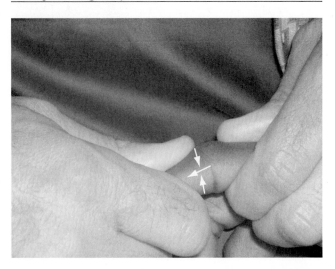

Figure 14-44 Interphalangeal (IP) distraction and anteroposterior glide. Patient position: supine or sitting. Contacts: stabilize the shaft of the proximal phalanx; the other hand grasps the anterior and posterior aspects of the middle phalanx. Direction of movement: the middle phalanx can be distracted or glided in an anterior or posterior direction; repeat for all proximal and distal IP joints.

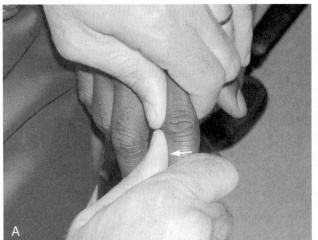

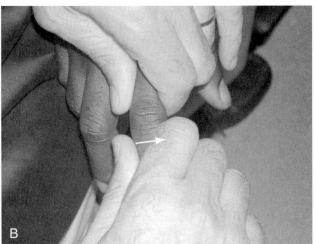

Figure 14-45 Interphalangeal (IP) mediolateral glide and tilt. Patient position: supine or sitting.
Contacts: stabilize the shaft of the proximal phalanx; the other hand grasps the medial and lateral aspects of the shaft of the middle phalanx. Direction of movement: glide or tilt the middle phalanx in a medial **(A)** or lateral **(B)** direction; repeat for all proximal and distal IP joints.

ACKNOWLEDGMENTS

The authors thank Robert E. Metzger Jr., a Doctor of Physical Therapy student at Emory University, who served as the model for the figures in this chapter.

REFERENCES

1. Clayton L, editor: Taber's cyclopedic medical dictionary, Philadelphia, 1977, FA Davis.
2. Basmajian JV, MacConail C: Arthrology. In Warwick R, Williams P, editors: Gray's anatomy, ed 35, Philadelphia, 1973, Saunders.
3. Mennell JM: Joint pain: diagnosis and treatment using manipulative techniques, Boston, 1964, Little, Brown.
4. Paris SV: Extremity dysfunction and mobilization, Atlanta, 1980, Institute Press.
5. Kaltenborn F: Manual therapy of the extremity joints, Oslo, 1973, Olaf Norlis Borkhandel.
6. McClure PW, Flowers KR: Treatment of limited shoulder motion: a case study based on biomechanical considerations, Phys Ther 72:929, 1992.
7. Poppen NK, Walker PS: Normal and abnormal motion of the shoulder, J Bone Joint Surg 58A:195, 1976.
8. Johnson AJ, Godges JJ, Zimmerman GJ, et al: The effect of anterior versus posterior glide joint mobilization on external rotation range of motion in patients with shoulder adhesive capsulitis, J Orthop Sports Phys Ther 37:88, 2007.
9. Akeson WH, Amiel D, Woo S: Immobility effects of synovial joints: the pathomechanics of joint contractures, Biorheology 17:95, 1980.
10. Woo S, Mathews JV, Akeson WH, et al: Connective tissue response to immobility: correlative study of biomechanical and biochemical measurements of normal and immobilized rabbit knees, Arthritis Rheum 18:257, 1975.
11. Akeson WH, Amiel D, LaViolette D, et al: The connective tissue response to immobility: an accelerated aging response, Exp Gerontol 3:289, 1968.
12. LaVigne A, Watkins R: Preliminary results on immobilization: induced stiffness of monkey knee joints and posterior capsules. In Proceedings of a symposium of the Biological Engineering Society, University of Strathclyde, Baltimore, 1973, University Park Press.
13. Enneking W, Horowitz M: The infra-articular effects of immobilization on the human knee, J Bone Joint Surg 54(A):973, 1972.
14. Tabary JC, Tabary C, Tardieu C, et al: Physiological and structural changes in cat soleus muscle due to immobilization at different lengths by plaster cast, J Physiol 224:231, 1972.
15. Cooper R: Alterations during immobilization and regeneration of skeletal muscle in cats, J Bone Joint Surg 54(A): 919, 1972.
16. Ham A, Cormack D: Histology, ed 8, Philadelphia, 1979, Lippincott Williams and Wilkins.
17. Akeson WH, Amiel D, Mechanic GL, et al: Collagen cross-linking alterations in joint contractures: changes in reducible cross-link's in periarticular connective tissue collagen after 9 weeks of immobilization, Connect Tissue Res 5:5, 1977.
18. Peacock E: Wound repair, ed 3, Philadelphia, 1984, Saunders.
19. Arem AJ, Madden JW: Effects of stress on healing wounds: intermittent non-cyclical tension, J Surg Res 20:93, 1976.
20. Kelly M, Madden JW: Hand surgery and wound healing. In Wolfort FG, editor: Acute hand injuries: a multidisciplinary approach, Boston, 1980, Little, Brown.
21. Evans E, Eggers G, Butler J, et al: Immobilization and remobilization of rats' knee joints, J Bone Joint Surg 42(A):737, 1960.
22. Wyke B: Articular neurology—a review, Physiotherapy 58:94, 1972.
23. Melzack R, Torgerson WS: On the language of pain, Anesthesiology 34:50, 1971.
24. Maitland G: Peripheral manipulation, ed 2, London, 1978, Butterworth-Heinemann.
25. Mulligan BR: Manual therapy: NAGS, SNAG, MWMS, etc, ed 4, Wellington, New Zealand, 1999, Plane View Services.
26. Vicenzino B, Paungmali A, Teys P: Mulligan's mobilization-with-movement, position faults and pain relief: current concepts from a critical review of literature, Man Ther 12:98, 2007.
27. Yang JI, Chang CW, Chen SY, et al: Mobilization techniques in subjects with frozen should syndrome: randomized multiple-treatment trial, Phys Ther 87:1307, 2007.
28. Paungmali A, O'Leary S, Souvlis T, et al: Hypoalgesic and sympathoexcitatory effects of mobilization with movement for lateral epicondylalgia, Phys Ther 83:374, 2003.
29. Vicenzino B, Branjerdporn M, Teys P, et al: Initial changes in posterior talar glide and dorsiflexion of the ankle after mobilization with movement in individuals with recurrent ankle sprain, J Orthop Sports Phys Ther 36:464, 2006.

SUGGESTED READINGS

Basmajian JV, MacConail C: Arthrology. In Warwick R, Williams P, editors: Gray's anatomy, ed 35, Philadelphia, 1973, Saunders.
Brooks-Scott J: Handbook of mobilization in the management of children with neurologic disorders, London, 1998, Butterworth-Heinemann.
Butler D: Mobilization of the nervous system, Melbourne, 1991, Churchill Livingstone.
Corrigan B, Maitland GD: Practical orthopaedic medicine, London, 1985, Butterworth-Heinemann.
Cyriax J: Textbook of orthopaedic medicine. I. Diagnosis of soft tissue lesions, London, 1978, Balliere Tindall.
Cyriax J, Cyriax PL: Illustrated manual of orthopaedic medicine, London, 1983, Butterworth-Heinemann.

D'Ambrogio KJ, Roth GB: Positional release therapy: assessment and treatment of musculoskeletal dysfunction, St Louis, 1997, Mosby.

Donatelli RA, editor: Physical therapy of the shoulder, ed 3, Philadelphia, 1997, Churchill Livingstone.

Glasgow EF, Twomey L, editors: Aspects of manipulative therapy, Melbourne, 1986, Churchill Livingstone.

Hoppenfeld S: Physical examination of the spine and extremities, East Norwalk, Conn, 1976, Appleton-Century-Crofts.

Konin JG, Wiksten DL, Isear JA: Special tests for orthopaedic examination, Thorofare, NJ, 1997, Slack.

Loudon J, Bell S, Johnston J: The clinical orthopedic assessment guide, Champaign, Ill, 1998, Human Kinetics.

Magee DJ: Orthopedic physical assessment, Philadelphia, 1987, Saunders.

Maitland GD: Peripheral manipulation, London, 1978, Butterworth-Heinemann.

Mennell JM: Joint pain: diagnosis and treatment using manipulative techniques, Boston, 1964, Little, Brown.

15

Robert A. Donatelli
and Kenji Carp

Evaluation and Training of the Core

Previous chapters describe the link between impairment of the trunk and hip core to injury of the spine and lower extremities.[1-3] This chapter describes available tests and measures to evaluate the core that allow the orthopaedic physical therapist to identify the underlying impairments that predispose patients to injury. These tests also help the therapist design evidence-based rehabilitation protocols and monitor therapeutic outcomes. Many tests in this chapter have been shown to have good evidence as to their clinical use. Unfortunately many commonly used orthopaedic core assessment tools still lack validation. The authors chose to describe these tests as they are still widely used in orthopaedic physical therapy practice. For these tests the authors attempted to discuss the clinical rationale behind them and allow the reader to judge their worth as clinical tools. Together these tests and measures will provide a battery of core tests useful in the assessment of nearly all orthopaedic clients regardless of specific diagnosis. In addition, the reader should gain an understanding of current approaches to core stabilization training, as well as the evidence these approaches produce.

OVERVIEW OF CORE EVALUATION

History and observation allow the therapist to form a diagnostic hypothesis and select the most appropriate tests to explore it. Motion and special screening tests help detect derangement of core tissue that could prevent successful training programs and/or rule out other significant pathologic conditions. Several methods of assessing neuromuscular control or recruitment patterns in core muscles are presented. Global tests of trunk muscle endurance and hip muscle strength are also discussed.

History

A thorough history is a crucial first component of any evaluation. The authors assume that the reader will perform a com-

prehensive systems screening to rule out conditions not appropriate for therapy as described by the American Physical Therapy Association (APTA)'s *Guide to PT Practice*.[4] Mechanism of injury can often clue the therapist into the core deficit. For example, excessive genu valgus is linked with anterior cruciate ligament (ACL), patellofemoral pain, hip abduction weakness, and/or abnormal core stabilization.[1-5] A description of core-training habits (or lack thereof) is often very helpful for evaluating chronic injuries. Changes in training programs, environment, event, or position often precede injury. As with all patients, a description of current symptoms, location, severity, and provoking factors is helpful.[5]

Observation

Muscle imbalance, joint derangement, and abnormal recruitment patterns can lead to observable changes in lumbopelvic posture. Poor core stabilization leads to altered biomechanics down the lower-extremity kinetic chain.[1-3,5] Thus observation of the lower-extremity during core evaluation will guide the therapist in selection of other core tests and measures.

Sagital Plane

Patients with normal alignment of the pelvis in the sagital plane demonstrate the anterior superior iliac spine (ASIS) at 15 degrees lower than the posterior superior iliac spine (PSIS).[6,7] Comparisons of the superior iliac spines should use this normal as reference for determining anterior or posterior pelvic tilt. Anterior tilted pelvis suggests poor recruitment of abdominal stabilizers. It may also suggest weak hamstrings, weak gluteals, and relative shortening of the rectus femoris. Increased lumbar lordosis will usually accompany anterior tilted pelvis. Posterior tilted pelvis suggests possible relative shortening of the hamstrings.[6-10] Athletes with anteriorly tilted pelvis often display hyperextended knees or genu recurvatum.[6-9]

Transverse and Frontal Planes

Visual comparison of the iliac crest heights provides a rough estimate of pelvic alignment in the frontal plane. Initial observation in normal standing posture should then be compared with feet together and apart. This allows for screening of functional leg length differences.[7,8] A lateral shift of the trunk shifting is indicative of possible lumbar discopathologic condition and warrants further testing for radicular symptoms described following.[5,11] Resting genu valgus, commonly referred to as *knock knees,* can be attributed to boney architecture but also weakness in the gluteus medius (Figure 15-1). Similarly, hip external rotator weakness can contribute to excessive femoral internal rotation in stance and with gait.[6,7,9-19]

Observation of excessive genu valgus, hip internal rotation, and/or pelvis level deviations from neutral during single-legged squatting is a commonly used screen test for hip abduction and external rotation weakness (Figure 15-2). In 2003, Zeller et al.,[19] using electromyography (EMG) and video motion analysis, demonstrated that female college athletes exhibited greater genu valgus than male subjects with single-leg squatting.[19] However, in 2005, DiMattia et al.[20] studied the single-legged squat in healthy active subjects (using unassisted clinician observation) and found poor interrater reliability and poor predictive value of hip abduction strength.

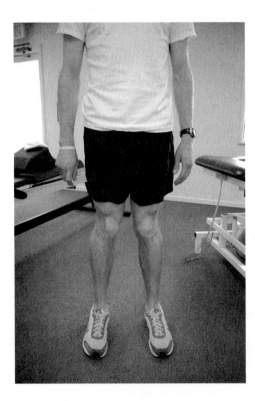

Figure 15-1 Genu valgus.

Similarly, Chmielewski et al.[21] examined the intra- and interrater reliability of single-leg squat on floor and laterally from a step using ordinal and nominal rating scales and found poor agreement among clinicians. It is possible that this was secondary to the use of complex rating systems. These findings suggest that unassisted clinical observation of single-legged squatting is a poor special test for hip abduction weakness. However, these researchers still suggested its use as a simple screening tool (i.e., graded as simply *positive* or *negative* for "excessive" genu valgus) to direct the therapist to further hip muscle testing.[19-21]

In 2005, Noyes et al.[22] studied the drop-jump screening test (Figure 15-3) using digital video analysis of frontal plane lower-extremity motion during landing. Subjects were fitted with markers of hip, knee, and ankle joint centers and videotaped while performing a depth jump from a box that was 12 inches high. This jump was immediately followed by a maximal vertical jump. They found this method to have excellent test-retest and within-test reliability in measuring relative hip, knee, and ankle motion in the frontal plane. Their findings again suggest simple visual observation of excessive genu valgus during landing should lead the clinician to further test hip strength.[22]

Gait Observation

Clients exhibiting decreased relative hip extension at terminal stance phase or "toe off" typically display relative shortening of the hip flexors and accompanying weakness of hip extensors. To compensate for the shorter stride length caused by decreased hip extension, these clients often overstride via increased relative hip flexion at initial contract or "heel strike." This overstriding increases the trunk flexion moment at initial contact by magnifying the ground reaction lever arm. As a result the therapist may be able to observe sometimes-violent muscle action of the lumbar paraspinals at initial contact. In patients with knee instability, "overstriding" contributes to hyperextension or posterior "giving way" of the knee by shifting the center of mass behind the knee axis of rotation.[13]

The classic Trendelenburg's gait pattern is seen when the stance phase hip abductors cannot resist the pull of gravity on the unsupported swing phase lower extremity. The therapist will observe the swing phase pelvis dip below level.[5,8,13] A compensated Trendelenburg's pattern is observed when the client deviates the body in the frontal plane toward the stance leg to decrease the moment arm of gravitational forces pulling on the swing side, decreasing load on the stance side abductors.[8,13] Although Dimattia et al.[20] found that alone, the Trendelenburg's position was a poor predictor of hip abduction strength, it remains a useful observational tool to clue the therapist to core impairments affecting gait (Table 15-1).

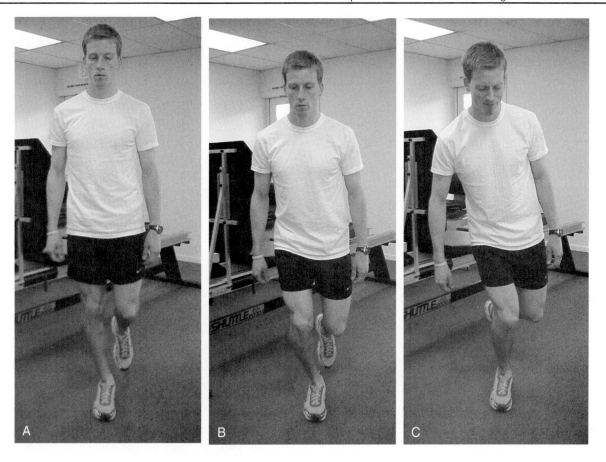

Figure 15-2 Single-leg squat screening test. **A,** Start. **B,** Normal. **C,** Positive valgus.

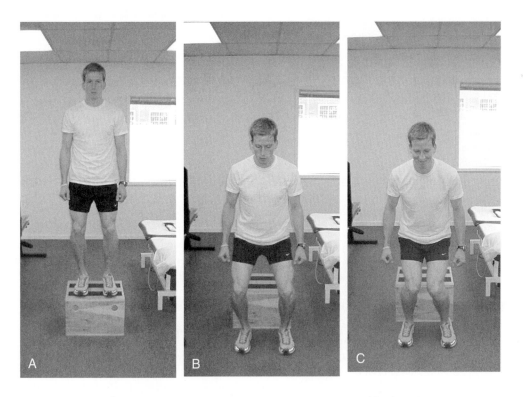

Figure 15-3 Drop-jump screening test. **A,** Start. **B,** Normal landing. **C,** Positive.

Table 15-1	Sample of Observation Section of Core Evaluation Sheet			
Observation	Date:	Date:	Date:	Date:
Anterior pelvic tilt				
Posterior pelvic tilt				
Iliac crest asymmetry				
Feet together				
Feet apart				
Genu recurvatum				
Genu valgus				
Single-legged squat				
Drop-jump screening				
Gait				

Table 15-2	Sample of Trunk Motion Section of Core Evaluation Sheet*			
Trunk Motion	Date:	Date:	Date:	Date:
Flexion				
Extension				
Right-side bending				
Left-side bending				
Knees to chest				
Prone prop				

*Note motion, peripheralization, and/or centralization.

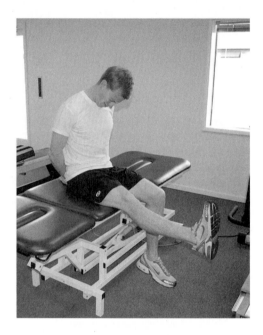

Figure 15-4 Slump test.

Tissue Derangement Screening Tests

Core stabilization is a function of the interaction of the mechanical core structures (hardware) and the neuromuscular control (software) dictating the muscle actions about the core. Thus the orthopaedic therapist needs to screen for hardware deficits or mechanical derangements of core structures. The following tests and measures screen for conditions such as lumbar disc herniation or sacroiliac dysfunction that could prevent success with core training and warrant more thorough evaluation.

Trunk Motion

Goniometry, tape measure along the spine, inclinometry, and visual estimation of motion are all commonly used clinical measures of trunk motion. Existing literature disagrees regarding the intra- and intertester reliability of all methods currently used to measure trunk motion.[23] Regardless, the therapist should attempt to quantify trunk motion with an eye toward identifying gross deficits in motion that could indicate facet, disc, and/or trunk muscle pathologic condition that would mechanically affect core stabilization. McKenzie-based assessments use knees-to-chest and prone extension on elbows to further assess trunk flexion and extension respectively (Table 15-2).[11,24] Peripheralization (report of lower-extremity symptoms moving distally) or centralization (moving proximally) with any of the trunk motions described previously are commonly associated with lumbar disc derangement.[5,11,24-27]

Slump Test

In 1991, researchers hypothesized that pathologies of the nervous system restrict the normal gliding of neural tissues around other tissues along their anatomic path.[26] The slump test is commonly used to detect "adverse neural tension" via the combined movements of the trunk and lower extremity (Figure 15-4). The client sits in combined cervical, thoracic, and lumbar flexion and then slowly extends the knee, noting any reproduction of symptoms. Next the client dorsiflexes the

ankle and again notes reproduction or worsening of symptoms. Many healthy individuals will experience pain with these tests because they stress neurologic tissues over multiple joints. Thus the slump test is considered positive only if it reproduces the patient's complaint of symptoms.[5,24,26,27] Positive slump testing can be further confirmed by manipulating the "sensitizing" aspects of the test. For example, dorsiflexing the ankle to maximally heighten neural tension sensitizes the test and should increase symptoms. Conversely, plantarflexing the ankle relieves neural tension and should decrease sypmptoms.[26] The slump test has been found to have excellent intrarater reliability and good interrater reliability for tests on the same day and between days.[24]

Straight-Leg Raise Testing

Passive straight-leg raise testing is the most commonly used test for lumbar discopathologic condition and nerve root irritation. As the name implies, the therapist raises the patient's leg while maintaining knee extension. A positive test for disc

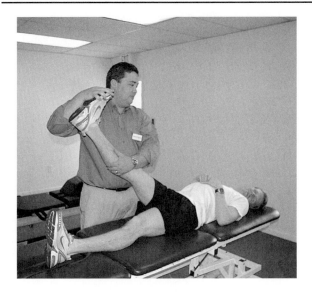

Figure 15-5 Straight-leg raise.

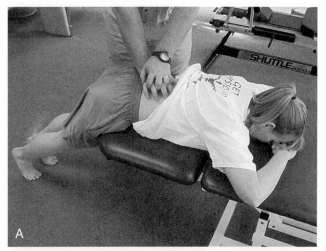

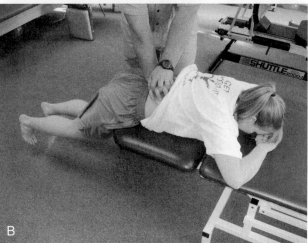

Figure 15-6 Prone instability test. **A,** Pain on first trial with anterior glide of vertebrae. **B,** Pain eliminated when patient raises legs from floor.

protrusion is reproduction of low-back pain with radiating pain to posterior thigh noted before 60 degrees of elevation. Reproduction of back pain only with motion past 70 degrees is typically associated with the sacroiliac or lumbar spine joints because this range of motion causes negligible further nerve root deformation.[5,24,26-28]

The opposite straight-leg raise or well-leg raising test uses the same technique as described previously, but a positive test is reproduction of ipsilateral radicular symptoms with raising the unaffected leg (Figure 15-5). The opposite straight-leg raise has low sensitivity but high specificity for lumbar disc herniation. Thus positive testing does not tend to rule in a significant intervertebral disc protrusion. However, a negative opposite straight-leg raise test is useful in ruling out disc protrusion.[5,24,26-28]

Prone Instability Test

To perform the prone instability test, the patient begins in prone with his or her hips at the edge of the plinth and the feet touching the floor (Figure 15-6). Then the therapist applies posterior-to-anterior pressure through the specific lumbar spinous process tested. The therapist repeats the test with the patient lifting his or her feet off the floor. Lifting the feet causes recruitment of the iliocostalis lumborum pars thoracis discussed earlier in Chapter 15, resulting in a posterior action of the vertebrae that stabilizes the segment against the therapist's anterior glide. The test is positive with reproduction of pain with the first position, which is reduced or eliminated with the feet off the floor. Unlike the posterior shear test, the prone instability test has been shown to have good reliability.[5,25]

Facet Scour

The facet scour test (also known as the *lumbar quadrant test*) is frequently used as a screening tool for lumbar facet joint patho-

logic condition and radiculopathy. The patient sits with the arms folded across the chest. The clinician passively moves the patient into coupled lumbar extension and rotation that increases compression and shear in the facet joints. Although evidence is lacking as to the sensitivity and specificity of this test, reproduction of localized low-back pain is suggestive of facet joint pathologic condition.[5,8,25] Reproduction of radiating lower-extremity symptoms is associated with neural foramen encroachment.

Sacroiliac Joint Test

The sacroiliac pain provocation tests described following have been shown to have good to excellent interrater reliability. In addition, when performed in conjunction with the McKenzie evaluation methods, provocation tests are highly valid in diagnosing sacroiliac joint pain. Specifically, in 2003, Laslett et al.[25] found three or more positive sacroiliac provocation tests with the absence of peripheralization or centralization phenomena (to rule out discopathologic condition) greatly improved the

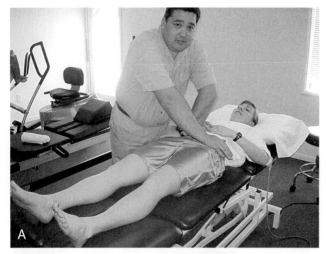

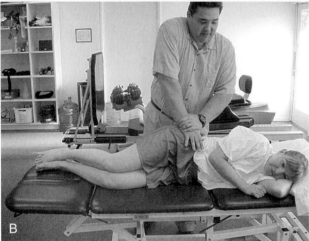

Figure 15-7 A, Sacroiliac distraction test. **B,** Sacroiliac compression test.

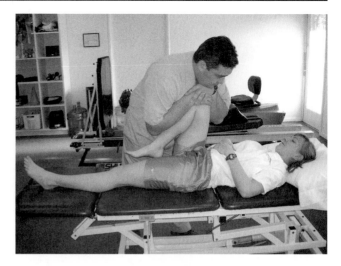

Figure 15-8 Sacroiliac thigh thrust.

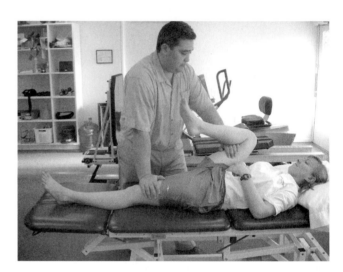

Figure 15-9 Gaenslen's test.

positive likelihood ratio for sacroiliac pain. Reproduction of the patient's complaint of pain is considered positive for all the following provocation tests. Not surprisingly, patients with sacroiliac joint pain often display poor stability of the sacroiliac joint and greater core (tests for which are described following). However, it is reasonable to expect patients with positive sacroiliac pain provocation tests will require a slightly slower course of progression of stabilization training than those without pain.

The distraction test begins with the patient in supine; the therapist then applies an anterior-to-posterior force to both ASISs (Figure 15-7, *A*). At first glance this may seem like compression to the sacroiliac joints, but the levering action of the innominates actually results in joint distraction. A sacroiliac compression test is performed with the patient in side lying; the patient flexes his or her hips and knees to 90 degrees (Figure 15-7, *B*). The examiner applies force down through the top iliac crest to compress the sacroiliac joints.

With the thigh thrust, the patient is positioned in supine, lying with one hip flexed to 90 degrees and slightly adducted (Figure 15-8). The therapist stabilizes the sacrum by cupping

his or her hand underneath the sacrum. The therapist then uses his or her other hand and body to axially load the femur, thus producing the posterior shear force on the sacroiliac joint.

For Gaenslen's test the patient lies supine with one leg hanging over the edge of the table while the therapist flexes the contralteral hip (Figure 15-9). The therapist then applies firm pressure to move the legs apart and torsion the sacroiliac joint. Performing this test immediately after the Thomas test minimizes patient position changes, which improves efficiency with testing.

To administer the sacral thrust, the therapist applies a posterior-to-anterior glide to the center of the sacrum to produce shearing of both sacroiliac joints while the patient lies in prone (Figure 15-10).

Tests of Sacroiliac Joint Dysfunction

Many orthopaedic manual therapists apply joint mobilization or manipulation to address sacroiliac joint dysfunction.

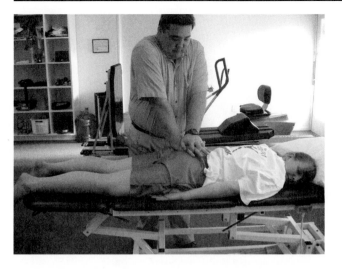

Figure 15-10 Sacral thrust.

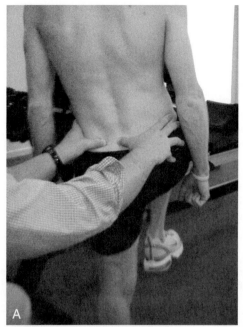

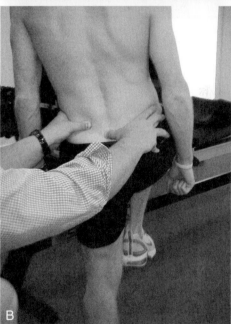

Figure 15-11 Support side stork test. **A,** Negative. **B,** Positive (stance side posterior superior iliac spine [PSIS] moves superior to sacral base).

Although operational definitions of joint dysfunction vary widely, most manual therapists describe hypomobility secondary to subtle misalignments of joint congruency. However, most studies into estimations of sacroiliac joint alignment or symmetry using visual observation, palpation, inclinometry, and calipers were shown to be unreliable.[25,28,29] Likewise, studies of commonly used manual therapy assessment for "positional diagnosis" were found to be unreliable.[29-36]

In contrast, Hungerford et al.[37] found the support side stork test to have good interrater reliability among three experienced manual therapists when using a two-point (either positive or negative) rating scale. During single-leg stance in nonpainful normal subjects, the stance side innominate should rotate posterior relative to the sacrum. The support side stork test is positive with observation and palpation of the innominate rotating anterior, and it is thought to indicate failure of the sacroiliac joint's ability to attain a closed pack, stable position (Figure 15-11). However, further research as to the validity, specificity, and sensitivity of this test is required.[37]

Somewhat paradoxically, good evidence shows the benefit of manual therapy including joint manipulation by physical therapists for low-back pain, including the sacroiliac joint.[34] Recent research has focused on identification of patients likely to respond to lumbar manipulation with the use of clinical prediction rules.[32-34] One of many implications is that assessment of sacroiliac joint dysfunction may not be necessary at all (Table 15-3). This represents a dramatic shift in the philosophy of assessment of sacroiliac (and other) joint dysfunction, and it is likely to be debated in the realm of orthopaedic manual therapy for some time.

Hip Testing

Goniometry of the lower-extremity joints has been shown to be reliable to within 5 degrees of motion.[23] In 1985, Norkin and White[23] provided a thorough description of all hip goniometry. It is important to stabilize the client's pelvis because compensation for lack of hip motion with pelvic hiking is common. Likewise, observation of compensations can provide vital additional information as to the maladaptive strategies your client is making secondary to hip core deficits. The authors also recommend testing of hip rotation in both the sitting and the prone positions to assess the effect of hip extension on hip rotation (Table 15-4). The authors most commonly observe impairments in hip extension and hip rotation range of motion.

The following tests are useful in identifying the hip structures that may be limiting hip motion. The Thomas test is useful in assessing the effect of rectus femoris restriction on hip and knee position and has been shown to have good interrater

Table 15-3	Sample of Trunk Special Tests Section of Core Evaluation Sheet			
Trunk Special Tests	Date	Date	Date	Date
Slump test				
Single-leg raise				
Prone instability				
Facet scour				
Sacroiliac joint				
Distraction				
Thigh thrust				
Gaenslen's test				
Compression				
Sacral thrust				

Table 15-4	The American Academy of Orthopaedic Surgeon's Established Mean Normal Values for Hip Range of Motion
Flexion	120 degrees
Extension	30 degrees
Abduction	45 degrees
Adduction	30 degrees
Medial rotation	45 degrees
Lateral rotation	45 degrees

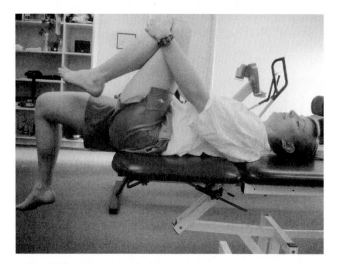

Figure 15-12 Thomas test.

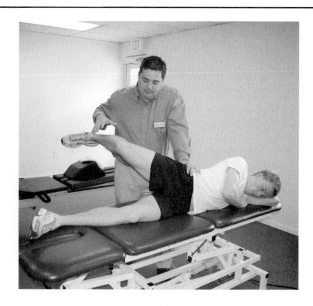

Figure 15-13 Ober's test.

tightness. Hip flexion of the free leg with knee flexion is indicative of selective restriction of the iliopsoas. The Thomas test can be further quantified with addition of goniometric measurement of hip and knee position during the test. The therapist should also observe for hip abduction of the down leg or "J-sign," which suggests iliotibial band tightness.[5,12]

Ober's test assesses tissue extensibility in the iliotibial band and tensor fasciae latae. The patient is positioned in side lying, with the down leg in hip-and-knee flexion to stabilize the patient (Figure 15-13). The therapist extends and abducts the top hip while stabilizing the pelvis to prevent a "rolling back" compensation. Knee position for the Ober's test was originally described with knee flexion, but more recent anatomic studies show that knee extension places further tension on the iliotibial band. The therapist then slowly lowers the up leg, watching for the leg to remain abducted (indicating a positive test).[5]

Craig's test is a clinical measure of femoral anteroversion or retroversion, which is the degree of femoral neck angulation in the transverse plane (Figure 15-14).[5] A handy way to remember this relationship is to point the index finger straight ahead to represent the femur and then move the thumb up and down as when striking the space bar on a keyboard. Movement of the thumb upwards is analogous to femoral anteroversion, and downwards is analogous to retroversion.

With the patient prone and knees flexed to 90 degrees, the therapist palpates the greater trochanter of the femur until it is perpendicular to the sagital plan and then measures the angle for the lower leg to vertical. Lateral to vertical is anteroversion, with the normal degree of femoral anteroversion in the adult being 8 to 15 degrees. Less than this amount of anteroversion, or when the lower leg points medially to vertical, is referred to as a *relative retroversion.*[5]

Anteroverted individuals will typically have much greater ease achieving hip internal rotation and often related decreased hip external rotation strength. Subjects with retroversion will have difficulty with hip internal rotation, which may predis-

reliability (Figure 15-12).[5-9,12] Lying in supine with hips nearly off the edge of the plinth, the patient holds the contralateral knee into the chest to prevent lumbar hyperextension, anterior pelvic tilt compensations. A negative test result is when the thigh of the free leg remains flat on the plinth with the knee flexed. If the free thigh rises from the plinth accompanied by knee extension, then the test is positive for rectus femoris

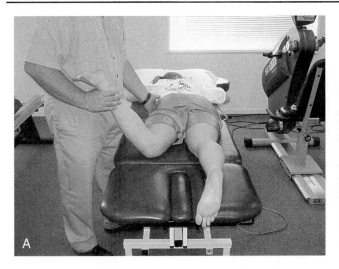
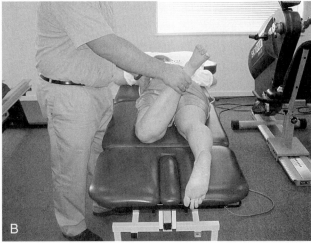

Figure 15-14 Craig's test. **A,** Anteroversion. **B,** Retroversion.

Table 15-5	Sample of Hip Motion Section of Core Evaluation Sheet							
	Date		Date		Date		Date	
	R	L	R	L	R	L	R	L
Flexion								
Extension								
Abduction								
Adduction								
Internal and external rotation sitting								
Internal and external rotation prone								
Thomas test								
Ober's test								
Craig's test								

pose the trunk core to increased reaction forces during closed chain activities because the hip arrives at closed pack position earlier (Table 15-5).

EVALUATION OF CORE STABILIZATION

Earlier models of spinal stabilization focused more on the mechanical properties of joints, ligaments, and muscles, whereas current theoretical constructs focus on neuromuscular control. In 2006, Panjabi[38] hypothesized that spinal injury begins with subclinical damage to passive stabilizing structures such as the intervertebral discs, ligaments, and facet capsules, as well to the somatosensory receptors within these tissues. This leads to corrupted sensory input to the central nervous system, resulting in abnormal neuromuscular control of the stabilizing muscles of the spine and reduced ability to dampen the shear forces produced when the larger mobilizers of the body fire. This eventually results in macrotrauma of the tissues. This neuromuscular control model of spinal stability accommodates the current principle clinical approaches of local and global core stabilization.[38] Numerous studies have docu-

mented abnormal postural control in subjects with back pain, supporting the neuromuscular control model of core stabilization.[39-44] Likewise, Cholewicki et al.[45] used EMG to study the response of core muscles in response to perturbation via surprise release of weights from the trunk and found significant delays in core muscle response.

There has been extensive recent research into the role of the transversus abdominis, lumbar multifidus, and pelvic floor or local stabilizers, in preventing and rehabilitating low-back pain, sacroiliac pain, and groin pain. Early studies into local spinal stabilization that investigated muscle recruitment using fine wire EMG followed by diagnostic or real time ultrasound (RTUS) showed these small, locally enervated muscles fire in response to perturbation, indicating a feed-forward mechanism of neuromuscular control.[45-53] However, the latency of these local stabilizers is increased as much as 200 mS in subjects with chronic episodic low-back pain.[45-53]

Measures of Local Core Stabilization

Richardson et al.[46] described a three-tiered system for assessing recruitment of local stabilizers consisting of screening tests,

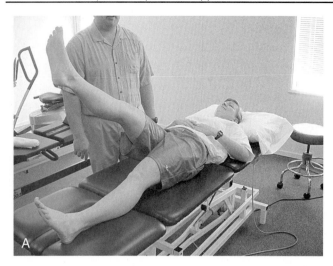
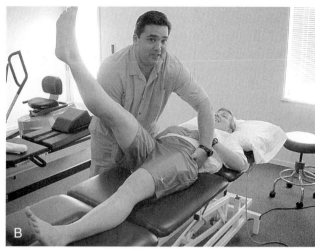

Figure 15-15 A, Positive active straight-leg raise test (posterior pain with 20 cm lift). **B,** Reduction in pain with external stabilization of pelvis suggests patient will respond well to core stabilization training.

clinical measures, and diagnostic measures. The screening test consists of an abdominal drawing in action without spinal or pelvic motion based on observation and palpation. One clinical measure, the abdominal drawing in maneuver, is essentially the same as the screening test, with the addition of the use of pressure biofeedback while the patient is prone lying with arms at sides. The patient is instructed to draw in the abdominal wall and educated in the corset-like anatomy of the transversus abdominis. The pressure biofeedback is placed under the abdomen, the distal edge of the bladder is aligned with the anterior iliac spines, and the bladder is inflated to 70 mm Hg. A correct isolated transversus abdominis contraction is reported to reduce pressure by 6 to 10 mm Hg as the abdominal wall moves away from the bladder. A drop in pressure less than 6 mm, or an increase in pressure, indicates a poor transverses abdominis contraction. Hodges et al.[49] reported "good agreement" between subjects with a poor ability to decrease pressure with the abdominal drawing in maneuver and those with delayed transversus abdominis activation in laboratory study, but they did not statistically demonstrate this relationship.

Hides et al.[51] studied the agreement between RTUS and palpation in assessing lumbar multifidus atrophy and abnormal recruitment. Clinicians agreed with RTUS assessment of atrophy in 24 of 26 cases of acute low-back pain. However, they also found fatty infiltration of the multifidus may confound the use of palpation of atrophy in patients with chronic low-back pain. To the authors' knowledge, no evidence exists supporting palpation as a reliable test of lumbar multifidus activation compared with the RTUS method used in laboratory study.

The active straight-leg raise (ASLR) is a clinical measure of local pelvic stabilization that has high test-retest and intrarater reliability. The ASLR is also a valid diagnostic test of posterior pelvic pain since pregnancy and has concurrent validity with the Quebec Back Pain Disability Score.[54-56] To perform the

ASLR, the subject lies supine with his or her arms at the sides; then the patient actively raises his or her leg 20 cm from the plinth and repeats with the other leg. It can also be applied prone with hip extension (Figure 15-15). The ASLR can be scored on a numeric scale but demonstrates high specificity and sensitivity when scored either positive (any degree of difficulty) or negative (not difficult at all and without compensatory movements of the pelvis). Some researchers endorse a second trial, with the therapist simulating the action of the transverses abdominis by pushing inwards from the lateral border of the pelvis or using a pelvic support belt.[54-56] Reduction or elimination of symptoms with the simulation of core stabilization suggests abnormal recruitment of the local stabilizers and that the patient will benefit from core stabilization training. Cowan et al.[56] supported this position when they demonstrated delayed activation of the transversus abdominis in subjects with long-standing groin pain who performed ASLR (as compared with nonpainful controls).

The third tier of local stabilization suggested by Richardson et al.[46] was initially the fine wire EMG that was replaced with RTUS to quantify the recruitment patterns in the transverses abdominis, multifidus, and pelvic floor. RTUS is becoming much more prevalent in orthopaedic practice as the cost of these devices becomes more economical and practice acts evolve. It appears RTUS provides good intra- and interrater reliability of the cross-sectional area in select lumbar and cervical spinal muscles when viewing the same image; however, it has yet to be shown reliable when rating images from different days.[57-61] In 2007, Kiesel et al.[61] found high same-day reliability with RTUS measurement of thickness (as a measure of muscle action) in the transversus abdominis and lumbar multifidus muscles. They also found significant impairment in the ability of subjects with low-back pain to change thickness in these muscles as compared with asymptomatic controls.

Measures of Global Core Stabilization

Global stabilization refers to the actions of muscles that cross more than one joint to prevent excessive motion in the trunk and hip core. In the presence of normal local stabilization, global stabilization is necessary for most functional activities. A wealth of studies shows that global stabilizers are active throughout sports motions.[62-66] The following tests are designed to test the muscle activation and endurance of these global core stabilizers in standardized positions.

Closed kinetic chain bridging test with knee extended is thought to test the muscular endurance of all stabilizers of the trunk and hip core. The patient begins in supine hook lying position and then executes the abdominal drawing in maneuver described previously to engage the local stabilization system. The patient then raises the trunk from the floor by extending the hip. During this test the quadratus lumborum and gluteus medius are active in maintaining frontal plane stability of the trunk and hip respectively. The gluteus medius in conjunction with the lessor hip rotators also stabilizes the hip in the transverse plane. The clinician measures the total time the patient can maintain the position.[7,8] For an additional challenge, one leg can be raised from the floor.

Reciprocal upper-extremity and lower-extremity raising out of the quadruped position is commonly called the *bird dog test*. Studies have correlated this motion to activation of the lumbar multifidus and iliocostalis pars thoracis.[6,9,62-66] The patient begins kneeling on all fours with a neutral spine and then raises one arm and the opposite leg until level with the trunk. The clinician measures total time that the patient can maintain the position correctly. Normal values for this test have not yet been established.

The side-lying pelvic bridge test has been shown by multiple researchers to recruit nearly all of the trunk and hip stabilizers, especially the bilateral isometric muscle action of the quadratus lumborum (Figure 15-16). Study of this test provides normal values, which explain its wide use by many researchers and common use in orthopaedic clinical assessment.[8] Normal values are displayed in the Table 15-6. The patient begins in side lying with the top leg crossed over the bottom and both feet touching the support surface. Timing begins when the patient raises the body from the floor by propping up on the down forearm and both feet.[8] The test is concluded when the patient drops or can no longer maintain the position correctly.

Abdominal bracing measures static endurance of the rectus abdominis and has fair interrater reliability. The patient begins with the feet fixed and with a 60-degree wedge placed behind the trunk as in a sit-up (Figure 15-17). Timing begins when the wedge is removed and ends when the patient can no longer hold the correct position.[8] This test also has normal values displayed in Table 15-6.

Table 15-6	Global Stabilization Test Norms		
	Male Subjects	Female Subjects	Combined Male and Female Subjects
Bridging with extended knee	Not established	Not established	Not established
Bird dog position	Not established	Not established	Not established
Right pelvic side lift	95 seconds	75 seconds	83 seconds
Left pelvic side lift	99 seconds	78 seconds	86 seconds
Abdominal bracing	136 seconds	134 seconds	134 seconds
Back extensor endurance	160 seconds	185 seconds	173 seconds

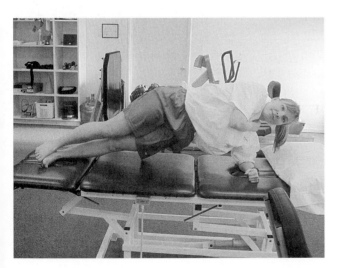

Figure 15-16 Side-lying bridge test.

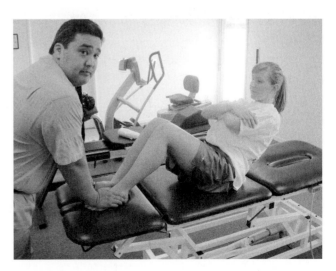

Figure 15-17 Abdominal bracing endurance test.

Multiple studies have shown poor endurance in the lumbar extensors is associated with increased risk of low-back problems. Unlike manual muscle testing (MMT), the back extensor endurance test measures the ability of the lumbar erector spinae to maintain the spine in neutral lordotic curve over time (Figure 15-18). The patient begins in prone lying, with the pelvis supported at the edge of the plinth. The therapist must apply considerable pressure to stabilize the patient's pelvis and lower extremities on the plinth, which is why strapping or other aids are commonly used for safety. The patient is timed for as long as he or she can maintain the trunk parallel to the floor (Table 15-7).[8,62-66] Normal values are displayed in Table 15-6. In 1997, Moreland et al.[64] found fair reliability for these tests. In 2007, Flanagan and Kulig[65] studied the use of the lumbar extensor endurance test in patients 4 to 6 weeks after single-level microdiscectomy and found the majority of these subjects could not tolerate the test but that this may have been secondary to fear of movement.

Balance Tests as Measures of Core Stabilization

Several researchers have used computerized posturography to establish increased postural sway in the presence of abnormal dynamic stabilization of the lower extremities.[19,39] Many researchers have found similar increases in sway in patients with back pain and core deficits.[39-44] This suggests that many of the balance tests described in Chapter 30 may also be used as measures of core stabilization. In 2005, Liemohn et al.[66] studied several commonly used clinical global stabilization tests while atop a computerized posturography platform. They found excellent reliability for the kneeling arm raise, quadruped arm raise parallel to trunk, quadruped arm raise perpendicular to trunk, and bridging after 3 days of testing, likely reflecting passage of training effect. This protocol offers excellent means for objective quantification of global stabilization testing.

Hip Mobilizer Tests

The muscles of the hip appear to function as both stabilizers and mobilizers. Many of the global tests described previously assess the hip muscles' role as stabilizers as part of a kinetic chain required to maintain the test positions. However, research clearly shows a link between hip muscle weakness or their action as mobilizers to back and lower-extremity injury.[1-3,6-8,12,14-22] Thus muscular strength is most pertinent to hip core assessment. A variety of tests and measures is available to clinically assess hip muscular strength. It appears trunk muscles function primarily as stabilizers and much less as

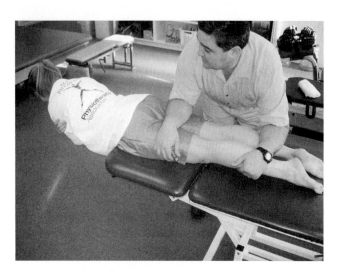

Figure 15-18 Back extensor endurance test.

Table 15-7	Sample of Trunk Stabilization Section of Core Evaluation Sheet							
	Date		Date		Date		Date	
Transverse abdominus drawing in								
Multifidus palpation								
	R	L	R	L	R	L	R	L
Active straight-leg raise (ASLR)								
Single-leg bridging								
Bird dog								
Side bridge								
Normal ranges								
Right	M = 99 sec, F = 78 sec, M/F = 86 sec							
Left	M = 95 sec, F = 75 sec, M/F = 83 sec							
Abdominal bracing								
Normal ranges	M = 136 sec, F = 134 sec, M/F = 134 sec							
Back extensor test								
Normal ranges	M =160 sec, F = 185 sec, M/F = 173 sec							

mobilizers. Likewise, trunk muscle endurance (but not strength) correlates with back injury.

Since the polio epidemic, isometric MMTs have been commonly used by physical therapists. Table 15-8 describes commonly accepted test positions used to assess hip mobilizers.[8,39]

The modified Ashworth 0 to 5 grading scale of MMT has been shown a reliable measure of isometric muscle strength.[9,67-70] Table 15-9 describes the grading system for MMT.

However, it is important to remember this unassisted MMT system was originally intended for use in subjects with acute polio or suffering from postpolio sequelae typically exhibiting obvious muscle weakness.[9,67] Although this is still commonly used in orthopaedic physical therapy, the clinician should seriously consider the fact that the 0 to 5 grading system is often not sensitive enough to detect relative weakness in the patient population. Hand-held dynamometry is a reliable and more sensitive measure of isometric strength testing that can be used with existing MMT positions.[68-70]

The standard hip abduction manual muscle test with dynamometry has been used to identify weakness in multiple studies.[14-18] The authors also advocate the hip drop test and hypothesize it is more sensitive in detecting gluteus medius weakness by preferentially recruiting the posterior muscle fibers. In addition, these authors believe it avoids common compensation for weakness with recruitment of the hip flexors and tensor fascia lata. To perform the hip drop test, the therapist takes the patient's hip passively to the end-of-range abduction and extension and then asks the patient to hold the position (Figure 15-19). At end range weak posterior fibers of the gluteus medius will cause the leg to drop 6 to 12 inches once the therapist's stabilization of the limb is removed. MMT can also be applied in this modified position, but the clinician must be mindful to perform repeat tests in the same position.

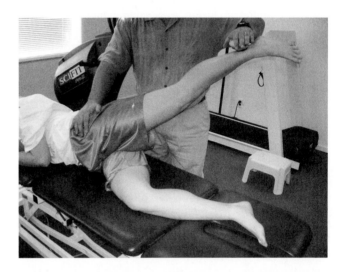

Figure 15-19 Hip drop test. To perform as a special test of gluteus medius weakness, the patient is placed in end-range hip extension and abduction. The therapist releases the leg and watches for a drop of 6 inches or more, indicating a positive special test. This also serves as an alternate position for manual muscle testing (MMT) as shown here.

Table 15-8	Manual Muscle Test Procedures
Motion Tested	**Test Procedure**
Hip abduction	The patient lies on the side with underside knee flexed. The test hip is abducted to midrange, slightly extended, and slightly externally rotated. Many patients will rotate the pelvis backwards to compensate for weak posterior gluteus medius with the tensor fascia latae.
Hip adduction	The patient is positioned in a side-lying position, with the leg to be tested in the down position. The therapist supports with top leg while resisting hip adduction on the medial distal femur of the down leg.
Hip extension	The patient is positioned prone, with the knee flexed to 90 degrees. The therapist extends the hip by lifting the thigh from the plinth and applies downward pressure against the distal posterior thigh while stabilizing the pelvis with the other hand.
Hip flexion	The patient is seated on the edge of the plinth, with the knees flexed to 90 degrees. The patient flexes the hip to midrange. The therapist applies resistance against the distal anterior thigh while stabilizing the trunk with one hand on the anterior shoulder.
Hip internal rotation	The patient is seated on the edge of the plinth, with knees flexed to 90 degrees. The therapist rotates the femur medially by moving the lower leg laterally to midrange; then the therapist applies pressure in a medial direction against the lateral lower leg while stabilizing the hip and pelvis with a hand on the thigh.
Hip external rotation	The patient is positioned as with internal rotation. The therapist moves the test leg into midrange of external hip rotation by moving the lower leg medially. Resistance is now applied laterally against the medial distal lower leg.

Table 15-9	Grading System for Manual Muscle Testing	
Grade	**Value**	**Criteria**
5	Normal	Complete range of motion against gravity with maximal resistance
4	Good	Complete range of motion against gravity with moderate resistance
3	Fair	Complete range of motion against gravity
2	Poor	Complete range of motion with gravity eliminated position
1	Trace	Evidence of slight contraction but no observable joint motion
0	Zero	No contraction palpated

Modified from Magee DJ: Orthopedic physical assessment, St Louis, 2008, Saunders.

Table 15-10	Hip Abductor to Adductor Isokinetic Muscle Force	
Male Subjects	Female Subjects	Combined Male and Female Subjects
1 : 2.09	1 : 2.46	1 : 2.46

Table 15-11	Ratios for Calculation of One Repetition Maximum
Number of Repetitions Lifted	Conversion Factor (CF) (Weight lifted × CF = 1 rep max)
1	1.00
2	1.03
3	1.06
4	1.09
5	1.13
6	1.16
7	1.20
8	1.24
9	1.29
10	1.33

Once extremely popular, isokinetic devices have more recently been alleged as *nonfunctional* because they test strength in open kinetic chain movement and are expensive. In addition, isokinetic testing tests strength at a constant joint speed, which critics are quick to point out does not occur with normal motion. However, research has clearly documented a link between hip abduction weakness and muscle imbalance to functional limitation in lower-extremity injury. Despite its limitations, isokinetic testing remains a reliable method of strength testing and inferring agonist and antagonist imbalance. Thus it begs the question: How is a reliable measure of the same variable not a functional test?

Researchers established normal hip abductor-to-adductor ratios for adults, which are displayed in Table 15-10.[71,72]

Most patients who lift weights typically know exactly what their one-repetition maximum of bench press is. This is because single-repetition isotonic maximum lifts are still considered the gold standard for measuring muscular strength.[73-75] Most nonrehabilitation strength-training programs use one-repetition maximum as the preferred baseline and outcomes measure of strength. Likewise, most strengthening programs specify intensity or load as a percentage of one-repetition maximum. However, many orthopaedic physical therapists do not use one-repetition maximum to assess strength because they fear further injuring the patient with a maximal production of force. Safety with testing is understandable but not at the cost of preventing accurate assessment of strength and thus imprecise strength training.

One alternative method recommended by the American College of Sports Medicine is 8 to 12 repetition maximum, which establishes a baseline for criterion reference but avoids maximal force production.[75,76] The subject performs the desired motion on cable machines, hydraulic machines, free weights, or any other from of isotonic resistance. With each successful completion of 8 or 12 repetitions, resistance is increased until the patient is unable to maintain correct form or fails to achieve the desired number of repetitions. The resistance level of the last successfully completed full set of the desired number of repetitions is used for the maximum.

Brzycki[77] developed a mathematic formula for calculating single-repetition maximum from multiple repetitions performed with submaximal (and thus safer) resistance. Table 15-11 reflects the conversion factors for calculating single-repetition maximum. For example, for a patient who can correctly perform hip abduction for eight repetitions at 5 lb, the clinician multiplies the 5 lb by a conversion factor of 1.24 and derives a calculated single-repetition maximum of 6.2 lb. The advantage of this method is that it will provide the therapist with the measure of muscular strength most commonly used in researched strength-training protocols but without the risks associated with actual single-repetition maximum testing.

Regardless of what number repetition maximum (single or 8 to 12) is to be tested, begin with a warm-up of 5 to 10 repetitions at approximately 50%, 70%, and 90% of an estimated repetition maximum before the actual test (Table 15-12). To prevent confounds from fatigue, a 2- to 3-minute rest period should be allowed between each set of repetitions. The last successfully completed set before failure or inability to complete the repetitions with correct form is the repetition maximum.[73-75]

Power

Power is defined as the amount of work (force × distance) produced in a given period of time.[75,78] Measures of whole-body power that require movement of body weight with direction changes are affected by core deficits of one to three. This is thought to reflect the stabilizing action of the core muscles, which provide a base for the larger torque-producing lower-extremity muscles to act against and thus transmit maximal forces down the kinetic chain to the floor. The T-test is a highly reliable measure of power.[78] The athlete sprints around a *T*-shaped course laid out measuring 10 m long by 10 m wide on the gym floor (Figure 15-20). In 2002, Nadler et al.[1] studied previously injured and uninjured NCAA Division I freshman athletes using the shuttle run. The athlete runs a course between two lines placed 6.7 m (22 feet) apart. The time to run the line three times (begin at line A, run to touch line B, return to touch line A, and finally run to line B) is recorded. The data for uninjured freshman college athletes are displayed in Table 15-13.

The countermovement vertical jump is a widely used a measure of lower-extremity power. The clinician obtains a

| Table 15-12 | **Sample Of Hip Mobilizer Section of Core Evaluation Sheet** |

Leg Drop Test (Abduction and Extension)

	Date		Date		Date		Date	
	R	L	R	L	R	L	R	L
Unable to hold								
Unable to resist								

Manual Muscle Tests (MMTs)

	Date		Date		Date		Date	
	R	L	R	L	R	L	R	L
Abduction								
Adduction								
Extension								
Flexion								
Internal rotation sitting								
External rotation sitting								

Table 15-13	**Shuttle Run Times For Uninjured NCAA Division I Freshman Athletes**
Male subjects	5.7 seconds
Female subjects	6.4 seconds

Table 15-14	**Average Values for Jump Height, Body Mass Index, and Power***			
Gender	Age Range	Number	Jump (Inches)	Power (W)
Female subjects	21-30	224	14.1	834
	21-25	182	14.1	833
	26-30	42	14.0	837
Male subjects	21-30	500	22.1	1332
	21-25	312	22.2	1309
	26-30	188	21.9	1370

*Power calculated via Lewis Power Equation: Power = $2.21 \times$ wt (kg) $\times \sqrt{\text{jump}}$ (m).

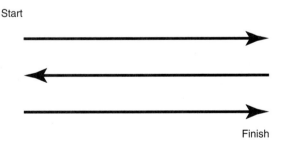

6.7 Meters (22 feet)

Start

Finish

Figure 15-20 Shuttle run diagram.

baseline standing-reaching height by marking a spot on a wall where the patient is asked to reach (as high as possible) while standing with the feet flat on the floor. The patient then jumps and reaches as high as possible, making a mark at the apex of the jump. The patient is allowed to gather the lower extremities without taking any steps and also pump the upper extremities. The therapist calculates vertical jump from highest point reached during jump minus baseline reach. Automated systems such as the Vertec and Just Jump automatically calculate vertical jump for the clinician and ease standardization of measurement.[79] Studies into normal values for vertical jump in athletes vary widely, most likely because of variance in methodology. Patterson and Peterson,[80] established vertical jump normal values for college students aged 21 to 24 years (Table 15-14).

Numerous researchers have studied single-leg hop tests as a means to evaluate lower-extremity neuromuscular function and power. Initially they were used as functional outcomes measures after ACL and ankle injury and were found to be reliable and valid predictors of return to sports.[81-91] Their relative simplicity and little to no cost make them an easy choice for indirect measures of power for most orthopaedic patients.

Clinical Tip

Limb symmetry index (LSI) for any single-leg hop test is defined as the value of the affected limb score divided by the unaffected. In post-ACL or ankle injury patients, an LSI of <85% with any of the single-leg hop tests indicates abnormal test and the need for a core, plyometric, and neuromuscular training program before return to full sports participation.[83-95] The authors still advocate the use of single-leg hop tests as a measure of core stability in patients without lower-extremity injury. In this case LSI is determined using the side with hip muscle weakness in place of the affected limb.

Table 15-15 describes the four most commonly used single-leg hop tests. Some difference exists between the methodologies of different researchers of single-leg hops. As such, the authors have attempted to provide easy to understand descriptions of the single-leg hop tests following.

Throwing tests of power reflect the core's ability to stiffen the trunk and efficiently transmit force from the lower extremities up the kinetic chain (Table 15-16). In 2003, Stockbrugger and Haennel,[91] demonstrated the backward overhead medicine ball toss to be a reliable measure of total body power. To perform this test the clinician needs a large area such as a baseball outfield in which the athlete can throw the medicine ball safely. The patient stands with the back to the scratch line and uses the entire body to throw the ball as far as possible backward overhead. Horizontal distance is measured from the scratch line to the landing point of the ball.[91] In 2004, Ellenbecker and Roetert[96] demonstrated significant correlation between the stationary rotational medicine ball toss and isokinetic trunk rotation peak torque. The patient stands with feet planted and uses a two-handed tennis forehand or backhand method to throw a 6 lb medicine ball. The therapist keeps the longest of three trials as the maximal rotational power per respective side. Szymanski et al.[93] found that maximal distance with a 1 kg medicine ball using a baseball swing motion was also reliable and had concurrent validity to isokinetic rotational power.

Overview of Core Stabilization Training

Perhaps because of the fundamental disagreement between leading researchers about the theoretical constructs of core stability, the optimal exercise prescription for core stabilization

Table 15-15	Single-Leg Hop Tests	
Time	Lines or cones placed 6 m apart	Hop from one line to other with only one leg while therapist measures time.
Distance	Starting line and open space forward of line to jump into	Patient begins with toes behind line. Must take off and land on the test limb. Distance from start line to front of toe is measured.
Triple hop for distance	Starting line with longer open space forward of line	As described previously, must take off and land on only the test leg but is allowed three consecutive hops. Test can be measured for time to complete set distance or distance covered in three maximal jumps.
Triple-crossover hop for distance	As described previously with addition of longitudinal line for athlete to jump over	Patient starts on a single limb and jumps at a diagonal across the body, lands on the opposite limb with the foot pointing straight ahead and immediately jumps in the opposite diagonal direction.

Table 15-16	Sample of Power and Agility Testing Section of Core Evaluation Sheet							
	Date		Date		Date		Date	
T-test								
Shuttle run								
Backward overhead toss								
	R	L	R	L	R	L	R	L
Vertical jump								
Six-pound rotational throw								
One-kilogram baseball swing throw								
Six-meter hop for time								
Single-leg hop test for distance								
Triple hop for distance								
Triple-crossover hop								

is a widely debated topic in orthopaedic physical therapy. However, the authors of this chapter caution clinicians to avoid polarization. It is safe to say that evidence exists for a feed-forward mechanism of neuromuscular control that activates the small local muscles in anticipation of motion or response to perturbation. Some compelling evidence suggests new technologies provide means of feedback training, which appear to recruit these local muscles and produce favorable outcomes in rehabilitation. It is also hard to deny the strong research regarding the protective action of endurance training of global core muscles. Many studies also suggest that perturbation protocols similar to those used in stabilizing the extremities have a similar effect in training feed-forward stabilization of the core.

By now it is obvious a wealth of research demonstrates delayed action of the local stabilizers in patients with back pain. Studies have identified several exercises, which preferentially recruit the local stabilizers and appear to produce favorable outcomes. Studies using pressure-sensing devices and more recently RTUS biofeedback devices have shown to enhance volitional recruitment of these muscles.[94-96] In a randomized controlled trial using healthy subjects, Van et al.[97] demonstrated that subjects improved volitional muscle action of the multifidus in the acquisition phase of motor learning, both with and without the use of RTUS biofeedback (but RTUS provided better gains). RTUS also appeared to provide superior skill retention over a 1-week period. Hides et al.[98] conducted a single blind pre- and posttest assessment study of the effect of RTUS feedback training in elite cricket players with low-back pain. They found that subjects who performed volitional local stabilization exercises with RTUS feedback improved fifth lumbar vertebral level multifidus crosssectional area comparable to controls without low-back pain with a concomitant decrease in pain.

However, these remain forms of feedback neuromuscular training, which is somewhat curious because the initial basic research into local stabilization attributed the increased latency of local stabilizer muscles to impairment in a feed-forward mechanism of neuromuscular control. It is fairly established that clinical and subclinical instability of extremity joints correlates with increased latency of stabilizers and that neuromuscular training programs focusing on perturbation result in decreased latencies and improved stabilization.[14-22] Then why would therapists use only feedback methods of core stabilization?

Several researchers have documented abnormal postural sway and balance in patients with low-back pain and hypothesized a similar abnormality in somatosensory perception and neuromuscular control as the cause.[81-91] Several studies show increased activation of global core stabilizers while performing standing balance drills or global stabilization drills on unstable surfaces.[99-105] Butcher et al.[103] included single-leg stance with eyes closed in a global stabilization program and found improved vertical jump. Figure 15-21 depicts several exercises using unstable surfaces to provide perturbation to drive feed-forward neuromuscular training of core stabilization. O'Sullivan et al.[104] compared postural sway and lumbar motion in subjects

sitting on stable and compliant surfaces and found no significant differences. It may be that the air-filled disc used did not provide sufficient perturbation in sitting to provoke the error signal required to force neuromuscular adaptation.[100] These studies have not examined the activity of the local stabilizers in response to perturbation-based exercise protocols. This may be because of methodological problems with the use of fine wire EMG and RTUS in subjects during exercise.

In addition, good evidence exists for global stabilization programs focusing on static holding or continuous movement in selected positions. In 2005, Koumantakis et al.[105] conducted a randomized control trial of 8 weeks of local stabilization training without feedback versus global stabilization training for patients with subacute or chronic nonspecific low-back pain without evidence of clinical instability. They found similar positive outcomes of decreased pain, increased mobility, and with functional outcomes measures. Global programs typically encompass a wider range of exercises designed to preferentially recruit core muscles. In 2007, Eckstrom et al.[106] used EMG to validate nine commonly used core stabilization exercises. They found bridging, unilateral bridging, side bridging, and quadruped alternate upper- and lower-extremity lifting produced sufficient recruitment of abdominal and lumbar extensor muscles to preferentially train endurance in the core. The prone bridging exercise appears redundant because superior recruitment of core muscles was observed with side bridging. Butcher et al.[103] found similar exercises with the addition of single-leg stance progressing from eyes open to closed (resulting in relative instability and perturbation) produced similar improvement in vertical jump to lower-extremity strengthening. In 2004, Sherry and Best[10] found global stabilization programs were more effective in addressing recurrent hamstring strains than traditional protocols focusing on direct hamstring stretching and strengthening. Because research clearly shows that lack of endurance in global stabilizers correlates with injury, global stabilization programs should focus on steady increases of time holding or continuously moving.

Research strongly correlates gluteus medius weakness to lower-extremity injury. Several studies have identified exercises that preferentially recruit the gluteus medius. Side-lying open chain hip abduction has been shown a valid exercise for isolating the gluteus medius.[106,107] In 2007, Bolgia and Uhl[107] showed commonly used closed chain strengthening exercises produced sufficient EMG of the stance leg gluteus medius for strengthening (Figure 15-22). The pelvic drop (single-leg stance with concentric and eccentric lowering of the pelvis) and single-leg standing and single-leg standing in 20 degrees of hip and knee flexion with the nonweight-bearing hip abducting were validated as effective strengthening exercises. Of course, application of progressive overload with relatively higher weight and lower repetitions is still required to produce the neuromuscular and muscle hypertrophy benefits of strength training.

SUMMARY

The tests and measures of the trunk and hip core described in this chapter allow the clinician to systematically identify core

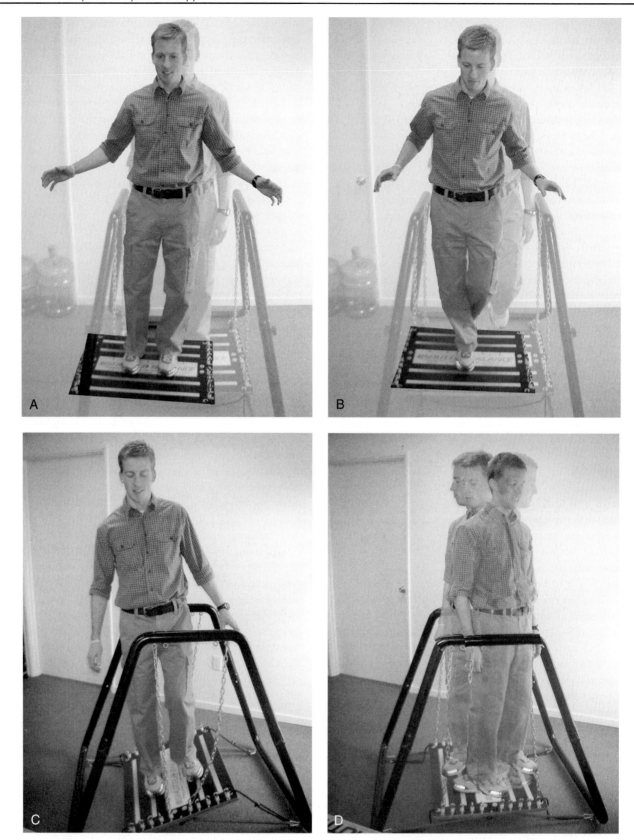

Figure 15-21 Feed-forward neuromuscular training of core stability on shuttle balance. **A,** Double-leg translation perturbation. **B,** Single-leg translation perturbation. **C,** Tilt perturbation. **D,** A 360-degree turn.

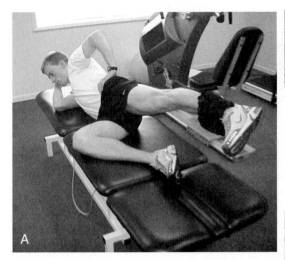
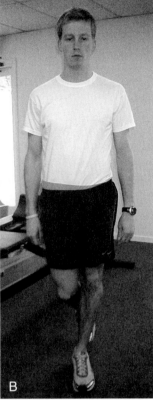
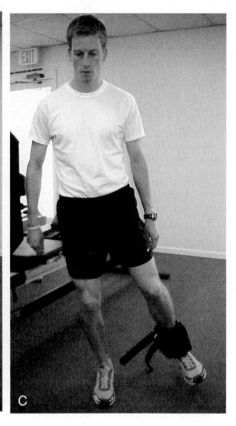

Figure 15-22 Gluteus medius strengthening exercises. **A,** Side-lying abduction and extension. **B,** Closed chain pelvic hiking. **C,** Standing hip abduction.

impairments shown to correlate with spinal and lower-extremity injury. Using this assessment format, the authors and other researchers have found the following cluster of signs extremely common in orthopaedic patients regardless of the anatomic area of diagnosis:

- Abnormal trunk and hip biomechanical alignments
- Hip muscle imbalance
- Decreased hip rotation
- Abnormal gait patterns
- Abnormal muscle activation patterns in trunk stabilizers
- Decreased endurance in the trunk stabilizers
- Decreased hip mobilizer strength (particularly in posterior fibers of gluteus medius)
- Insufficient core power
- Impaired neuromuscular control of posture and balance

Identifying core impairments allows the clinician to design optimal core stabilization and hip-strengthening programs. Debate regarding which core muscles are the best stabilizers of the spine continues. However, adoption of a neuromuscular model of core stabilization allows for integration of evidence from both the local and the global stabilization into exercise prescription for core stabilization. It appears that local stabilization programs focusing on the use of RTUS provide feedback neuromuscular training, over time hypertrophies the local core muscles, and produce favorable clinical outcomes for patients

with low-back pain. Likewise, research shows that global stabilization programs training larger, less specifically innervated core muscles are also effective for patients with back pain, lower-extremity injury, and in sports performance enhancement. Studies show abnormal neuromuscular control of posture and related deficits in standing balance in patients with back pain. This suggests many of the balance tests described in Chapter 30 may be used as measures of core stability. Some studies suggest neuromuscular training exercises focusing on perturbation also provide global stabilization and positive outcomes.

REFERENCES

1. Nadler SF, Malanga GA, Feinberg JH, et al: Functional performance deficits in athletes with previous lower extremity injury, Clin J Sport Med 12(2):73-78, 2002.
2. Nadler SF, Malanga GA, Bartoli JH, et al: Hip muscle imbalance and low back pain in athletes: influences of core strengthening, Med Sci Sports Exerc 34(1):9-16, 2002.
3. Nadler SF, Malanga GA, DePrince M, et al: The relationship between lower extremity injury low back pain and hip muscle strength in male and female collegiate athletes, Clin J Sport Med 10(2):89-97, 2000.

4. American Physical Therapy Association (APTA): Guide to physical therapist practice, ed 2, Alexandria, Va, 2001, The Association.

5. Magee DJ: Orthopedic physical assessment, ed 3, Philadelphia, 1997, Saunders.

6. Lee D: The pelvic girdle, ed 3, London, 2004, Churchill Livingstone.

7. Sahrmann S: Diagnosis and treatment of movement impairment syndromes, St Louis, 2002, Mosby.

8. McGill S: Low back disorders: evidence based prevention and rehabilitation, Champaign, Ill, 2002, Human Kinetics.

9. Kendall FP, McCreary EK, Provance PG: Muscles testing and function, ed 4, Baltimore, 1993, Williams & Wilkins.

10. Sherry MA, Best TM: A comparison of two rehabilitation programs in the treatment of acute hamstrings strains, J Orthop Sports Phys Ther 34(3):116-125, 2004.

11. Razmjou H, Kramer JF, Yamada R: Intertester reliability of the McKenzie evaluation in assessing patients with mechanical low-back pain, J Orthop Sports Phys Ther 30(7):368-389, 2000.

12. Van Dillen LR, McDonnel MK, Flemming DA, et al: Effect of knee and hip position on hip extension range of motion in individuals with and without low back pain, J Orthop Sports Phys Ther 30(6):307-316, 2000.

13. Perry J: Gait analysis normal and pathological function, Thorofare, NJ, 1992, SLACK Inc.

14. Ireland ML, Wilson JD, Ballantyne BT, et al: Hip strength in females with and without patellofemoral pain, J Orthop Sports Phys Ther 33(11):671-676, 2003.

15. Leetun DT, Lloyd, Ireland ML, et al: Core stability measures as risk factors for lower extremity in athletes, Med Sci Sports Exerc 36(6):926-934, 2004.

16. Ballantyne BT, Leetun DT, Ireland ML, et al: Differences in core stability between male and female collegiate basketball athletes as measured by trunk and hip muscle performance, Med Sci Sports Exec 33(5):S331, 2001.

17. Piva SR, Goodnite EA, Childs JD: Strength around the hip and flexibility of soft tissues in individuals with and without patellofemoral pain syndrome, J Orthop Sports Phys Ther 35:793-801, 2005.

18. Robinson RL, Nee RJ: Analysis of hip strength in females seeking physical therapy treatment for unilateral patellofemoral pain syndrome, J Orthop Sports Phys Ther 37(5):232-238, 2007.

19. Zeller B, McCrory J, Kibler B, et al: Differences in kinematics and electromyographic activity between men and women during the single-legged squat, Am J Sports Med 31(3):449-456, 2003.

20. DiMattia MA, Livengood AL, Uhl TL, et al: What are the validity of the single-leg-squat test and its relationship to hip-abduction strength? J Sport Rehabil 121:108-123, 2005.

21. Chmielewski TL, Hodges MJ, Horodyski M, et al: Investigation of clinician agreement in evaluating movement quality during unilateral lower extremity functional tasks: a comparison of two rating methods, J Orthop Sports Phys Ther 37(3):122-129, 2007.

22. Noyes FR, Barber-Westin S, Fleckenstein C, et al: The drop-jump screening test: difference in lower limb control by gender and effect of neuromuscular training in female athletes, Am J Sports Med 33(2):197-207, 2005.

23. Norkin CC, White DJ: Measurement off joint motion: a guide to goniometry, ed 2, Philadelphia, 1985, FA Davis.

24. Tucker N, Reid D, McNair P: Reliability and measurement error of active knee extension range of motion in a modified slump test position: a pilot study, J Man Manip Ther 15(4):E85-E91, 2007.

25. Laslett M, Young SB, Aprill CN, et al: Diagnosing painful sacroiliac joints: a validity study of McKenzie evaluation and sacroiliac provocation tests, Aust J Physiother 49:89-97, 2003.

26. Butler DA: Mobilization of the nervous system, Melbourne, 1991, Churchill Livingstone.

27. Scham SM, Taylor T: Tensions signs in lumbar disc prolapse, Clin Orthop Relat Res 75:195-204, 1971.

28. Cibulka MT, Aslin K: How to use evidence-based practice to distinguish between three different patients with low back pain, J Orthop Sports Phys Ther 31(12):678-695, 2001.

29. Hicks GE, Fritz JM, Delitto A, et al: Interrater reliability of clinical examination measures for identification of lumbar segmental instability, Ach Phys Med Rehabil 84:1858-1864, 2003.

30. Levangie PK: Four clinical tests results with innominate torsion among patients with and without low back pain, Phys Ther 79:1043-1057, 1999.

31. Freburger JK, Riddle DL: Measurement of sacroiliac joint dysfunction: a multicenter intertester reliability study, Phys Ther 79(12):1134-1141, 1999.

32. Freburger JK, Riddle DL: Using published evidence to guide the examination of the sacroiliac joint region, Phys Ther 81(5):1135-1143, 2001.

33. Flynn T, Fritz J, Whitman J, et al: A clinical prediction rule for classifying patients with low back pain who demonstrate short-term improvement with spinal manipulation, Spine 27(24):2835-2843, 2002.

34. Chiradejnant A, Maher CG, Latimer J, et al: Efficacy of "therapist-selected" versus "randomly-selected" mobilization techniques for the treatment of low back pain: a randomized controlled trial, Aust J Physiother 49:233-241, 2003.

35. Childs JD, Fritz JM, Piva SR, et al: Clinical decision making in the identification of patients likely to benefit from spinal manipulation: a traditional versus an evidenced-based approach, J Orthop Sports Phys Ther 33(5):259-271, 2003.

36. Cleland JA, Fritz JM, Whitman JM, et al: The use of a lumbar spine manipulation technique by physical therapists in patients who satisfy a clinical prediction rule: a

case series, J Orthop Sports Phys Ther 36:209-214, 2006.

37. Hungerford BA, Gilleard W, Moran M, et al: Evaluation of the ability of physical therapists to palpate intrapelvic motion with the stork test on support side, Phys Ther 87:879-887, 2007.

38. Panjabi MM: A hypothesis of chronic back pain: ligament subfailure injuries lead to muscle control dysfunction, Eur Spine J 15:668-676, 2006.

39. Shumway-Cook A, Woolacoot M: Motor control theory and practical applications, Baltimore, Md, 1995, Lippincott Williams & Wilkins.

40. Flanagan SP, Kulig K: Assessing musculoskeletal performance of the back extensors following a single-level microdiscectomy, J Orthop Sports Phys Ther 37(7):356-363, 2007.

41. Kuukkanen TM, Malkia EA: An experimental controlled study on postural sway and therapeutic exercise in subjects with low back pain, Clin Rehabil 14:192-202, 2000.

42. Bouche K, Stevens V, Cambier D, et al: Comparison of postural control in unilateral stance between health controls and lumbar discectomy patients with and without pain, Eur Spine J 15:423-432, 2006.

43. Popa T, Bonifazi M, Della Volpe R, et al: Adaptive changes in postural strategy selection in chronic low back pain, Exp Brain Res 178:411-418, 2007.

44. Smith M, Coppieters MW, Hodges PW: Effect of experimentally induced low back pain on postural sway with breathing, Exp Brain Res 166:109-117, 2005.

45. Cholewicki J, Greeen HS, Polzhofer GK, et al: Neuromuscular function in athletes following recovery from a recent acute low back injury, J Orthop Sports Phys Ther 32:568-575, 2002.

46. Richardson CA, Jull G, Hodges P, et al: Therapeutic exercise for spinal segmental stabilization in low back pain: scientific basis and clinical approach, Philadelphia, 1999, Churchill Livingstone.

47. Richardson CA, Jull GA, Richardson BA: A dysfunction of the deep abdominal muscles exists in low back pain patients. In Proceedings of the World Confederation of Physical Therapists, Washington, DC, 1995, The World Confederation, p 932.

48. Richardson CA, Snijders CJ, Hides JA, et al: The relationship between the transversus abdominis muscles, sacroiliac joint mechanics, and low back pain, Spine 27(4):399-405, 2002.

49. Hodges PW, Richardson CA: Inefficient muscular stabilization of the lumbar spine associated with low back pain: a motor control evaluation of transverses abdominis, Spine 21(22):2640-2650, 1996.

50. Hodges PW, Richardson CA, Jull GA: Evaluation of the relationship between the findings of a laboratory and clinical test of transverses abdominis function, Physiother Res Int 1:30-40, 1996.

51. Hides JA, Stokes MJ, Saide M, et al: Evidence of lumbar multifidus muscles wasting in ipsilateral to symptoms

52. Hides J, Richardson C, Jull G: Multifidus muscle recovery is not automatic following resolution of acute first episode low back pain, Spine 21:2763-2769, 1996.

53. Hodges PW, Richardson CA: Inefficient muscular stabilization of the lumbar spine associated with low back pain. A motor control evaluation of transversus abdominis, Spine 21(22):2640-2650, 1996.

54. Mens JMA, Vleeming A, Snijders CJ et al: The active straight leg raising test and mobility of the pelvic joints, Eur Spine J 8:468-473, 1999.

55. Mens JMA, Vleeming A, Snijders CJ et al: Validity and reliability of the active straight leg raise test in posterior pelvic pain since pregnancy, Spine 26(10):1167-1171, 2001.

56. Cowan S, Schache A, Brukner P et al: Delayed onset of transverses abdominis in long-standing groin pain, Med Sci Sports Exerc 36(12):2040-2045, 2004.

57. Hodges PW, Pengel LHM, Herbert RD et al: Measurement of muscle contraction with ultrasound imaging, Muscle Nerve 27:682-692, 2003.

58. Wallwork TL, Hide JA, Stanton WR: Intrarater and interrater reliability of assessment of lumbar multifidus muscle thickness using rehabilitative ultrasound imaging, J Orthop Sports Phys Ther 37:608-612, 2007.

59. Hides JA, Miokovic T, Belavy DL et al: Ultrasound imaging assessment of abdominal muscle function during drawing-in of the abdominal wall: an intrarater reliability study, J Orthop Sports Phys Ther 37(8):480-486, 2007.

60. Stokes M, Hides J, Elliot J et al: Rehabilitative ultrasound imaging of the posterior paraspinal muscles, J Orthop Sports Phys Ther 37(10):581-595, 2007.

61. Kiesel KB, Underwood FB, Mattacola CG et al: A comparison of select trunk muscle thickness change between subjects with low back pain classified in the treatment-based classification system with asymptomatic controls, J Orthop Sports Phys Ther 37(10):596-607, 2007.

62. Biering-Sorensen F: Physical measurements as risk indicators for low back trouble over a one-year period, Spine 9:106-119, 1984.

63. Nourbakhsh MR, Arab AM: Relationship between mechanical factors and incidence of low back pain, J Orthop Sports Phys Ther 32:447-460, 2002.

64. Moreland J, Finch E, Stratford P et al: Interrater reliability of six tests of trunk muscle function and endurance, J Orthop Sports Phys Ther 26(4):200-209, 1997.

65. Flanagan SP, Kulig K: Assessing musculoskeletal performance of the back extensors following a single-level microdiscectomy, J Orthop Sports Phys Ther 37(7):356-363, 2007.

66. Liemohn WP, Baumgartner TA, Gagnon LH: Measuring core stability, J Strength Cond Res 19(3):583-586, 2005.

67. Hislop HJ, Montgomery J: Daniels and Worthinghams' muscle testing: techniques of manual examination, ed 6, Philadelphia, 1995, WB Saunders.

68. Bohanan RW, Andrews AW: Interrater reliability of hand-held dynamometry, Phys Ther 67:931-933, 1987.

69. Wadsworth CT, Krishnan R, Sear M, et al: Intrarater reliability of manual muscle testing and hand-held dynametric muscle testing, Phys Ther 67(9):1342-1347, 1987.

70. Dunn JC, Iversen MD: Interrater reliability of knee muscle forces obtained by hand-held dynamometer from elderly subjects with degenerative back pain, J Geriatr Phys Ther 26(3):23-29, 2003.

71. Mont MA, Cohen DB, Campbell KR, et al: Isokinetic concentric versus eccentric training of shoulder rotators with functional evaluation of performance enhancement in elite tennis players, Am J Sports Med 22(4):513-517, 1994.

72. Donatelli R, Catlin PA, Backer GS, et al: Isokinetic hip abductor to adductor torque ratio in normals, Isokinet Exerc Sci 1(2):103-111, 1991.

73. Kraemer WJ, Fry AC: Strength testing: development and evaluation of methodology. In Maud P, Nieman C: Fitness and sports medicine: a health-related approach, ed 3, Palo Alto, Calif, 1995, Bull Publishing.

74. Fleck S, Kraemer W: Periodization breakthrough, Ronkonkoma, NY, 1996, Advanced Research Press.

75. American College of Sports Medicine: Principles of exercise prescription, Baltimore, 1995, Lippincott William & Wilkins.

76. American College of Sports Medicine: American College of Sports Medicine position stand on progression models in resistance training for healthy adults, Med Sci Sports Exerc 34(2):364-380, 2002.

77. Brzycki M: Strength testing: predicting a one-rep max from a reps-to-fatigue, J Phys Ed Rec Dance 64(1):88-90, 1993.

78. Pauole K, Madole K, Garhammer J et al: Reliability and validity of the T-test as a measure of agility leg power, and leg speed in college-aged men and women, J Strength Cond Res 14(4):443-450, 2003.

79. Isaacs LD: Comparison of the Vertec and Just Jump system for measuring height of vertical jump for young children, Percept Mot Skills 86:659-663, 1998.

80. Patterson D, Peterson D: Vertical jump and leg power norms for young adults, Measurement in Physical Education and Exercise Science 8(1):33-41, 2004.

81. Fitzgerald KG, Lephart SM, Hwang JH, et al: Hop tests as predictors of dynamic knee stability, J Orthop Sports Phys Ther 31(10):588-597, 2001.

82. Myer GD, Ford KR, Palumbo JP, et al: Neuoromuscular training improves performance and lower-extremity biomechanics in female athletes, J Strength Cond Res 19(1):51-60, 2005.

83. Rudolph KS, Axe MJ, Synder-Mackler L: Dynamic stability after ACL injury: who can hop? Knee Surg Sports Traumatol Arthosc 8:262-269, 2000.

84. Cerrulli G, Benoit DL, Caraffa A, et al: Proprioceptive training and prevention of anterior cruciate ligament injuries in soccer, J Orthop Sports Phys Ther 31(11):655-660, 2001.

85. Hiemstra LA, Lo KY, Fowler PJ: Effect of fatigue on knee proprioception: implications for dynamic stabilization, J Orthop Sports Phys Ther 31(10):598-605, 2001.

86. Risberg MA, Mork M, Jenssen HK, et al: Design and implementation of a neuromuscular training program following anterior cruciate ligament reconstruction, J Orthop Sports Phys Ther 31(11):620-631, 2001.

87. Williams GN, Chmielewski T, Rudolph KS, et al: Dynamic knee stability: current theory and implications for clinicians and scientists, J Orthop Sports Phys Ther 31(10):546-566, 2001.

88. Holm I, Fosdahol MA, Friis A, et al: Effect of neuromuscular training on proprioception, balance, muscle strength, and lower limb function in female team handball players, Clin J Sport Med 14(2):88-94, 2004.

89. Lephart SM, Abt JP, Ferris CM: Neuromuscular contributions to anterior cruciate ligament injuries in females, Curr Opin Rheumatol 14(2):168-173, 2002.

90. Ross MD, Langford B, Whelan PJ: Test-retest reliability of four single-leg horizontal hop tests, J Strength Cond Res 16(4):617-622, 2002.

91. Stockbrugger B, Haennel R: Validity and reliability of medicine ball explosive power test, J Strength Cond Res 15(4):431-438, 2003.

92. Ellenbecker T, Roertert E: An isokinetic profile of trunk rotation strength in elite tennis players, Med Sci Sports Exerc 1959-1963, 2004.

93. Szymanski DJ, Szymanski JM, Bradford TJ, et al: Effect of twelve weeks of medicine ball training on high school baseball players, J Strength Cond Res 21(3):894-901, 2007.

94. Hides JA, Jull GA, Richardson CA: Long-term effects of specific stabilizing exercises for first-episode low back pain, Spine 26:E243-E248, 2001.

95. Ferreira PH, Ferreira ML, Maher CG, et al: Specific stabilization exercise for spinal and pelvic pain: a systematic review, Aust J Physiother 52:79-88, 2006.

96. Hides JA, Richardson CA, Jull G: Use of real-time ultrasound imaging for feedback in rehabilitation, Man Ther 3:125-131, 1998.

97. Van K, Hides JA, Richardson CA: The use of real-time ultrasound imaging for biofeedback of lumbar multifidus muscle contraction in healthy subjects, J Orthop Sports Phys Ther 36(12):920-925, 2006.

98. Hides J, Stanton W, McMahon S, et al: Effect of stabilization training on multifidus muscle cross-sectional area among your elite cricketers with low back pain, J Orthop Phys Ther 38(3):101-108, 2008.

99. Vera-Garcia FJ, Grenier SG, McGill SM: Abdominal muscle response during curl-ups on both stable and labile surfaces, Phys Ther 80(6):564-569, 2000.

100. Willardson JM: Core stability training: applications to sports conditioning programs, J Strength Cond Res 21(3):979-985, 2007.

101. Faries MD, Greenwood M: Core training: stabilizing the confusion, J Strength Cond Res 29(2):10-25, 2007.

102. Marshal PW, Murphy BA: Increased deltoid and abdominal muscle activity during Swiss ball bench press, J Strength Cond Res 20(4):745-750, 2006.

103. Butcher SJ, Craven BR, Chilibeck PD, et al: The effect of trunk stability training on vertical takeoff velocity, J Orthop Sports Phys Ther 37(5):223-231, 2007.

104. O'Sullivan PO, Dankaerts W, Burnett A, et al: Lumbo-pelvic kinematics and trunk muscle activity during sitting on stable and unstable surfaces, J Orthop Sports Phys Ther 36:19-25, 2006.

105. Koumantakis GA, Watson PJ, Oldham JA: Trunk muscle stabilization training plus general exercise versus general exercise only: randomized controlled trial of patients with recurrent low back pain, Phys Ther 85:209-225, 2005.

106. Ekstrom RA, Donatelli RA, Carp KC: Electromyographic analysis of core trunk, hip, and thigh muscles during nine rehabilitation exercises, J Orthop Sports Phys Ther 37(12):754-762, 2007.

107. Bolgia LA, Malone TR, Umberger BR, et al: Electromyographic analysis of hip rehabilitation exercises in a group of healthy subjects, J Orthop Sports Phys Ther 35:487-494, 2005.

Trunk and Hip Core Evaluation Sheet

History/Pain Provocation:

Observation

	Date:	Date:	Date:	Date:

Anterior pelvic tilt
Posterior pelvic tilt
Iliac crest asymmetry
Feet together
Feet apart
Genu recurvatum
Genu valgus
Single-leg squat
Drop-jump screening
Gait

Trunk Motion (Note motion, peripheralization and/or centralization)

	Date:	Date:	Date:	Date:

Flexion
Extension
Right-side bending
Left-side bending
Knees to chest
Prone prop extension

Trunk Special Tests

	Date:	Date:	Date:	Date:

Slump test
Single-leg raise
Prone instability
Facet scour
Sacroiliac joint
Distraction
Thigh thrust
Gaenslen's test
Compression
Sacral thrust

History/Pain Provocation:—cont'd

Hip Motion

	Date:		Date:		Date:		Date:	
	R	L	R	L	R	L	R	L
Flexion								
Extension								
Abduction								
Adduction								
Internal and external rotation sitting								
Internal and external rotation prone								
Thomas test								
Ober's test								
Craig's test								

Trunk Stabilization

	Date:		Date:		Date:		Date:	
Transverse abdominus drawing in								
Multifidus palpation								
	R	L	R	L	R	L	R	L
Active single-leg raise								
Leg-loading test								
Bird dog								
Side bridge								

Normal Ranges
Right   M = 95 sec, F= 75 sec, M/F = 83 sec
Left   M = 99 sec, F = 78 sec, M/F = 86 sec

Abdominal bracing
Normal Ranges   M = 136 sec, F = 134 sec, M/F = 134 sec

Back extensor test
Normal Ranges   M = 160 sec, F = 185 sec, M/F = 173 sec

HIP Mobilizer Testing

Leg Drop Test (Abduction and extension for posterior fibers of gluteus medius)

	Date:		Date:		Date:		Date:	
	R	L	R	L	R	L	R	L
Unable to hold								
Unable to resist								

Manual Muscle Testing (MMT)

	Date:		Date:		Date:		Date:	
	R	L	R	L	R	L	R	L
Abduction								
Adduction								
Extension								
Flexion								
Internal rotation sitting								
External rotation sitting								

History/Pain Provocation:—cont'd

Power and Agility Testing

	Date:		Date:		Date:		Date:	
T-test								
Shuttle run								
Backward overhead toss								
	R	L	R	L	R	L	R	L
Vertical jump								
Six-pound rotational throw								
Six-meter hop for time								
Single-leg hop test for distance								
Triple hop for distance								
Triple-crossover hop								

CHAPTER

16

Wendy J. Hurd and
Lynn Snyder-Mackler

Neuromuscular Training*

This chapter will begin by discussing the importance of proprioception in the lower limb and upper limb, then the components of the sensorimotor system, and the role of the sensorimotor system in neuromuscular control. It will define postural control and describe how postural control is achieved in stance and gait and identify techniques used for assessment of neuromuscular function. It will then discuss the various effects an injury may have on neuromuscular function and summarize the purpose(s) and components of a neuromuscular training program.

Neuromuscular control involves the subconscious integration of sensory information that is processed by the central nervous system (CNS), resulting in controlled movement through coordinated muscle activity.[1] Dynamic joint stability and postural control are the result of coordinated muscle activity achieved through neuromuscular control. Any injury that disrupts the mechanoreceptors, alters normal sensory input, or interferes with the processing of sensory information may result in altered (also referred to as *decreased* or *dysfunctional*) neuromuscular control. Consequently, impairments of the neuromuscular system often result in dysfunctional dynamic joint stability and postural control. Neuromuscular control impairments can also change movement patterns and increase the risk for musculoskeletal injury. Conversely, musculoskeletal injury, by disrupting the interactions within the neuromuscular system, can be a cause of altered neuromuscular control. The authors believe an understanding of the neuromuscular control system and the functional manifestations of neuromuscular control are fundamental to designing effective treatment programs and meaningful research studies related to dynamic joint stability.

---

*This chapter is reprinted from Hurd WJ, Snyder-Mackler L: Neuromuscular training. In Donatelli R: Sports-specific rehabilitation, St Louis, 2007, Churchill Livingstone.

PROPRIOCEPTION

Why can one baseball pitcher exhibit excessive glenohumeral motion yet never experience injury, whereas another pitcher with the same glenohumeral motion require surgery to throw effectively without pain? Why does one athlete experience a single-episode lateral ankle sprain but the next athlete develop chronic ankle instability? The answer to both questions is most commonly *proprioception*. For the healthy athlete, high levels of proprioception can contribute to enhanced neuromuscular control and functional joint stability, thus decreasing the risk for injury. For the injured athlete, restoration of proprioception is critical to ward off repetitive injury (Figure 16-1). Therefore proprioceptive training plays a key role for the athlete in both injury prevention and rehabilitation.

Proprioception may be inferred from Sherrington's 1906 description of the "proprioceptive-system" as the afferent information from proprioceptors (e.g., mechanoreceptors) located in the proprioceptive field that contributes to conscious sensations, total posture, and segmental posture.[2,3] Proprioception is a product of sensory information gathered by mechanoreceptors.[2] This definition views proprioception primarily as a sensory activity. More recently, authors have expanded the definition of the proprioceptive system to include the complex interaction between the sensory pathways and the motor pathway (efferent system).[4] One assumption underlying both definitions of proprioception is that incoming sensory information processed by the CNS has not been compromised. In the presence of an injury that disrupts mechanoreceptor input, proprioceptive function will be compromised and may lead to movement dysfunction.

Over the years many terms have been used either synonymously with proprioception or to describe proprioception including *kinesthesia, joint position sense, joint stability,* and *postural control.* Kinesthesia and joint position sense may both

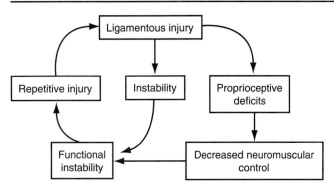

Figure 16-1 Functional stability paradigm depicting the progression of functional instability because of the interaction between mechanical stability and decreased neuromuscular control. (From Lephart S, Reimann B, Fu F: Proprioception and neuromuscular control in joint stability, Champaign, Ill, 2000, Human Kinetics.)

be viewed as submodalities of proprioception.[3] Kinesthesia refers to the sensation of joint movement (both active and passive), whereas joint position sense refers to the sensation of joint position.[3] Joint stability is accomplished through both passive (osseous congruity and ligamentous restraints) and dynamic (coordinated muscle contractions) mechanisms. Dynamic joint stability is the result of neuromuscular control and proprioception, whereas postural control is the result of integrated visual, vestibular, and proprioceptive inputs.[5,6] Consequently, any disruption in mechanoreceptor input that affects proprioception will negatively affect dynamic joint stability and posture.

SENSORIMOTOR SYSTEM

The sensory organs in the neuromuscular system are referred to as *mechanoreceptors*. Sensitive to various forms of mechanical deformation including tension, compression, and loading rate, these small sensors are located in various connective tissues throughout the body. The three classifications of mechanoreceptors are based on tissue location: joint receptors, cutaneous (skin) receptors, and muscle receptors.

Joint Receptors

Ruffini's receptor endings are described as slowly adapting mechanoreceptors because they continue their discharge in response to a continuous stimulus.[7] These receptors have a low activation threshold and are active during both static and dynamic joint conditions. Consequently, Ruffini's endings may signal static joint position, intraarticular pressure, and amplitude and velocity of joint rotations.[7-10]

Golgi tendon organ (GTO)-like receptors are the largest of the articular mechanoreceptors. They are also slow to adapt to stimuli, have a high activation threshold, and are active only during dynamic joint states. Some researchers have suggested that the high threshold of the GTO-like ending makes this

receptor ideally suited for sensing the extremes of the joint's normal movement range.[11] The Golgi and Ruffini's endings belong to a group called *spray endings*. Collectively, these mechanoreceptors represent a virtually continuous morphological spectrum of receptors.[12] Whether the spray endings should be divided into distinct receptor types has not been resolved.

Pacini's corpuscles are the only rapidly adapting joint receptor. Sensitive to low levels of mechanical stress, the pacinian corpuscle is active only during dynamic joint states. Therefore this receptor is silent during static conditions and constant velocity situations but is sensitive to joint acceleration and deceleration.[13]

Free nerve endings constitute the fourth type of joint receptor. Free nerve endings are widely distributed throughout most joint structures. These receptors are typically inactive during normal activities, but when activated by high levels of noxious stimuli they are slow to adapt during both static and dynamic states.

Cutaneous Receptors

The CNS processes sensory information from cutaneous (skin) receptors in conjunction with joint and muscle receptors. The role of cutaneous receptors in initiating reflexive responses, such as the flexion withdrawal reflex in response to potentially harmful stimuli, is well established.[15] Cutaneous receptors may also signal information regarding joint position and kinesthesia when the skin is stretched.[15,16] However, no evidence indicates that these receptors contribute significantly to these sensations[17] or that cutaneous receptors contribute to joint stability.[18]

Muscle Receptors

The muscle spindle and the GTO are the two primary types of muscle receptors.[15] The muscle spindle lies in parallel with extrafusal muscle fibers and has three main components: (1) intrafusal muscle fibers, (2) sensory axons that wrap around the intrafusal fibers and project afferent information to the CNS when stimulated, and (3) motor axons that innervate the intrafusal fibers and regulate the sensitivity of the muscle spindle (Figure 16-2).[1,15,19,20] The primary sensory axons from the spindle make monosynaptic connections with alpha motor neurons in the ventral roots of the spinal cord that, in turn, innervate the muscle where the muscle spindle is located.[1] Collectively, this feedback loop is called the *muscle stretch reflex*.[15] Although extrafusal muscle fibers comprise the bulk of the muscle responsible for generating force and are innervated by alpha motor neurons, intrafusal fibers are composed of a small bundle of modified muscle fibers that function to provide feedback to the CNS and are innervated by gamma motoneurons.[21] Sensitivity of the muscle spindle is continually modulated by the gamma motor system. This allows the spindle to be functional at all times during a contraction[21] and modulate muscle length.[15,22-24] Sensory output from the muscle spindle is triggered at low thresholds, is slowly adapting, and senses joint position throughout the range of motion.[15,20]

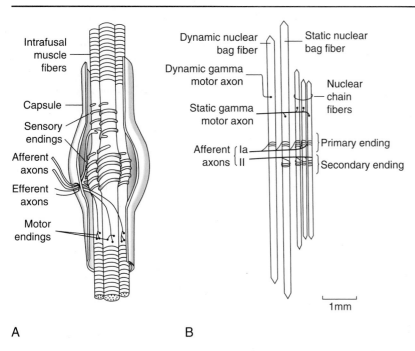

Intrafusal muscle fibers

Capsule

Sensory endings

Afferent axons

Efferent axons

Motor endings

Dynamic nuclear bag fiber

Dynamic gamma motor axon

Static gamma motor axon

Afferent { Ia
axons { II

Static nuclear bag fiber

Nuclear chain fibers

} Primary ending

} Secondary ending

1mm

A   B

Figure 16-2 A, Gross structure. **B,** Structure and innervation of the intrafusal fibers of the muscle spindle. (From Williams GN, Chmielewski TL, Rudolph KS, et al: Dynamic knee stability: current theory and implications for clinicians and scientists, J Orthop Sports Phys Ther 31(10):546-566, 2001.)

The GTO is located at the musculotendinous junction and is positioned in series with extrafusal muscle fibers and tendon. A single axon enters the GTO and then branches into many unmyelinated endings that are woven in and between the collagen fibers at the musculotendinous junction. Thus during a muscle contraction the tendon is stretched, straightening the collagen fibers and distorting the receptor endings of the GTO afferent neurons.[25] Increased activity of the GTO afferents results in inhibition of the motor neurons innervating the muscles that were stretched while exciting the motor nerves of the antagonistic muscles. This feedback loop is often referred to as the *inverse myotatic reflex.* Because each organ is connected to a small number of muscle fibers and can respond to low levels of force (as little as 0.1 g),[22] the GTO can provide the CNS with specific force feedback.[22-24]

Motor Response Pathways

Sensory information gathered by mechanoreceptors is sent to the spinal cord via afferent pathways for processing and ultimately results in a regulation of reflexes and muscle activity. In addition to being influenced by incoming afferent information, the resulting motor response also depends on the level of processing of afferent inputs within the CNS. The processing can occur at three different levels: the spinal cord, the brainstem and cerebellum, and the cerebral cortex (Table 16-1).

Spinal reflexes represent the shortest neuronal pathways and consequently the most rapid responses to afferent stimuli. These responses are typically uniform in nature and modified by the intensity of the afferent signals.[15] Spinal reflexes range from simple monosynaptic reflexes to complex multisynaptic circuits resulting in coordinated activity of groups of muscles.[13,15,26] The speed of spinal reflexes is faster than liga-

Table 16-1	Motor Response Intervals	
Motor Response Type	Level of Mediation	Able to be Modified
Spinal reflexes	Segmental level of spinal cord	No
Long-loop reflexes	Brainstem and cerebellum	No
Triggered reactions	Cortical centers	Yes
Voluntary reactions	Cortical centers	Yes

From Hurd WJ, Snyder-Mackler L: Neuromuscular training. In Donatelli R: Sports-specific rehabilitation, St Louis, 2007, Churchill Livingstone.

mentous failure, yet is not considered modifiable through training to aid in dynamic joint stability.[27,28]

Sensory information mediated at the brainstem and cerebellum is typically referred to as a *long-loop reflex.*[27-29] Because sensory information travels a greater distance before being processed, these responses are typically longer than spinal reflexes. However, because these pathways are multisynaptic with potentially more sources of sensory input, long-loop reflexes are flexible and may adapt when feed-forward information is provided to the system.[27,28,30] As a result of both the adaptability and the relative quickness with which they occur, these pathways are thought to be important in the maintenance of dynamic joint stability.[1,31]

Both voluntary reactions and triggered reactions are processed at the cortical level of the brain and represent the longest motor response times. Voluntary reactions involve the processing of multiple variables and are highly flexible.[27,28,32] In contrast, "triggered" reactions represent preprogrammed, coordinated reactions that occur in response to afferent stimuli that trigger them into action.[1,28] One example of a triggered reaction has been termed the *wine glass effect*[28]: When one holds an expensive wine glass, one instinctively tightens the grip on it if the glass begins to slip. The cutaneous message that the object is slipping comes from the fingertips, but the muscle response to increase grip pressure comes from the forearm.

In this case the reaction occurs quickly, is probably not conscious in nature, and appears to have the overall purpose of reorganizing the system slightly to complete an action successfully. Because of their preprogrammed nature, triggered reactions occur slightly more quickly than voluntary reactions but may be unable to accommodate to circumstances in atypical situations.[1]

POSTURAL CONTROL

Postural control involves controlling the body's position in space for the dual purposes of stability (balance) and orientation (maintaining an appropriate relationship between the body segments and between the body and the environment for a task).[6,33] The postural control system uses complex processes involving both sensory and motor components and results from the combined integration of visual, vestibular, and proprioceptive afferent inputs.[5,6] The combined effort of these sensory modalities lays the framework for dynamic balance (stability). If feedback from any one of these modalities is impaired, then postural stability suffers.[1]

Investigators have identified several postural control strategies that result from different types of perturbations applied during stance. Typically, if forward sway is induced as a result of a posterior horizontal perturbation, then muscles on the posterior aspect of the body are recruited.[34] Conversely, if backward sway is induced from an anterior horizontal perturbation, then muscles on the anterior aspect of the body are recruited.[34] Additionally, small perturbations applied during standing result in sway at the ankle joint; this is called an *ankle strategy*.[35] On the other hand, large perturbations result in large movements at the hip; this is called a *hip strategy*.[35] The hip strategy is also implemented when the individual cannot generate enough force with the ankle strategy. A third strategy, called the *stepping strategy*, is implemented when the perturbation displaces the center of mass outside the individual's base of support.[6] Postural control strategies can be modified and are adaptive to the circumstances of the moment; however, in the absence of other instructions, they are predictable.[6] Evidence suggests that a person's expectations of impending perturbations and training can have a significant effect on the magnitude and variability of the responses.[6] These postural control strategies provide stability in stance and therefore are applicable to the maintenance of joint stability in the lower extremity during stance.[1]

The motor skills that people perform daily, including walking, pose a complicated problem for the neuromuscular system because many muscles crossing multiple joints must be coordinated to produce a given outcome. Bernstein[36] called this the *degrees of freedom problem*. One theory for controlling the degrees of freedom problem is based on the concept of motor programs (a set of commands that are prestructured at higher brain centers and define the essential details of a skilled action). The most recent update to this theory, put forth by Schmidt and Lee,[28] contends that features that do not vary among different skills—the relative timing, force, or sequence of components—are stored in memory as motor programs, whereas the parameters that do vary (e.g., speed, duration) are specified according to the task at hand. These programs are under central control and are generally not dependent on feedback from the periphery.[28] Feedback is, however, used to select the appropriate motor program, monitor whether the movement is in keeping with the program, and reflexively modulate the movement when necessary.[27,28]

The idea of a central pattern generator is similar in concept to a motor program. These control mechanisms located in the spinal cord produce mainly genetically defined, repetitive actions, such as gait.[37] The concept of the central pattern generator is supported by animal studies including spinalized models, which have shown that the rhythmic pattern of gait can continue in the absence of feedback from the limbs or descending control from the brain.[38-40] Central pattern generators may be turned on or off by a variety of stimuli, although they are primarily stimulated or inhibited by signals originating in the brainstem.[39-41] Although gait is centrally controlled at the lower brain and spinal cord level, descending influences from higher brain centers including the cerebellum, visual cortex, hippocampus, and frontal cortex, along with peripheral sensory input, permit effective gait even when unexpected changes in the environment are encountered.[6,27,28] Thus gait is controlled through the complex interaction of central pattern generators, descending input from higher brain centers, and feedback from peripheral sensory receptors. Through this complex interaction and similar processes that occur with other motor programs, the neuromuscular system acts to maintain joint stability during dynamic situations.[1]

ASSESSMENT OF NEUROMUSCULAR FUNCTION

After injury, assessment of neuromuscular function is necessary to determine if impairments are present, aid in the development of an appropriate treatment intervention, and assess the effectiveness of the intervention.[1] Various analysis techniques are available for testing neurosensory components (e.g., kinesthesia) and neuromuscular performance (e.g., biomechanical gait analysis). Readily available clinical assessment techniques include joint position testing; observational analysis; functional testing, such as hop testing; and threshold to detection of passive motion (TTDPM) testing. Stabilometry and strength testing are common clinical assessment techniques that are performed with the aid of commercially available equipment.

Other techniques for identifying neuromuscular control deficits include kinetic and kinematic evaluation with motion analysis, force plates, and electromyography. These measures are more commonly used in the laboratory versus the clinical setting. An advantage to these laboratory-testing techniques includes a high level of precision and sensitivity, allowing the investigator to identify complex yet often subtle neuromuscular dysfunction. Because of the variety of testing methods and strategies available, it is important that clinicians and scientists carefully consider the question they are trying to answer when selecting neuromuscular assessment methods.[1]

EFFECT OF INJURY ON NEUROMUSCULAR FUNCTION

The effects of injury on the neuromuscular system have been assessed in many studies. Receiving the most attention in the literature is what neuromuscular adaptations occur to maintain dynamic joint stability after ligament injury. Injury to the anterior cruciate ligament (ACL) is a common ligament injury and typically requires surgical reconstruction and prolonged rehabilitation for a return to preinjury activity levels. This section focuses on specific neuromuscular adaptations that occur after ACL injury. The subsequent section addresses the design and implementation of a training program to improve neuromuscular function after ACL injury.

Some individuals can stabilize their knees after ACL rupture, even during activities involving cutting and pivoting, although most experience instability with daily activities.[42] Because there can be vast differences in functional outcome after ACL injury, a classification scheme was developed at the University of Delaware to improve studies of knee stabilization strategies in patients after ACL rupture. Those patients with ACL rupture who returned to activities involving cutting, jumping, or pivoting for a minimum of 1 year and had not experienced knee instability were classified as *copers*, and those who experienced episodes of giving way were classified as *noncopers*.[42] Potential copers are individuals identified early after injury through a screening process (Box 16-1) who have the potential to develop dynamic knee stability.[43] Once a potential coper returns to preinjury, high-level activities for a minimum of 1 year without experiencing episodes of giving way, the potential coper is classified as a *coper.*

The authors have conducted research to delineate knee stabilization strategies of copers, potential copers, and noncopers. Copers use strategies involving more coordinated muscle activation that stabilize the knee without compromising knee motion.[44,45] An analysis of movement patterns during walking

and jogging shows that copers have sagittal plane knee motions and moments during weight acceptance that are similar to uninjured individuals (Figure 16-3).[44,45] Copers do have differences in onset timing and magnitude of muscle activity when compared with uninjured subjects. These alterations in muscle activity allow copers to stabilize their knees while maintaining normal movement patterns.[45] However, no single pattern has been adopted by the copers; individuals adopt idiosyncratic compensation patterns that are related to rate of muscle activation and unrelated to quadriceps strength[42,44] or knee laxity.[42]

Conversely, noncopers adopt a remarkably limited strategy to stabilize their knees across activities with widely differing demands on the knee.[44-46] The pattern is a robust stiffening strategy that includes reduced knee motion, reduced internal knee extension moment, distribution of support moment away from the knee, slower muscle activation, and generalized cocontraction of the muscles that cross the knee. This pattern is present in activities ranging from walking to jumping.[45-47] Rudolph hypothesized that this reduced knee motion and internal knee extensor moment during weight acceptance, which has been observed by other researchers,[48] is the hallmark of a noncoper. The joint stiffening strategy seen in the noncopers may reflect the early stages of motor skill acquisition. Vereijkin et al.[49] demonstrated that individuals often freeze the degrees of freedom of a task via massive cocontraction of muscles. As the skill level improves, joint stiffening gives way to a larger variety of movements and more selective motor responses during the activity. The muscle cocontraction strategy seen in the noncopers reflects an unsophisticated adaptation to the ACL rupture for which appropriate muscle activation strategies to dynamically stabilize the injured knee have not yet developed. The authors speculate that the noncopers' stiffening strategy bodes poorly for long-term joint integrity and that it could contribute to the high incidence of early-onset knee osteoarthritis in individuals after ACL rupture.

Recent research at the University of Delaware has illuminated a short-term differential response to acute ACL injuries, which the authors believe is based on the potential for the neuromuscular system to reorganize appropriate responses soon after injury to better stabilize the knee. Potential copers are identified through a screening process to determine which patients are appropriate candidates for nonoperative rehabilitation.[43] The screening tool was validated on 93 consecutive patients with acute ACL rupture.[50] Thirty-nine subjects (42%) met the criteria for classification as appropriate rehabilitation candidates, and 28 of these elected to pursue nonoperative management. Of those subjects participating in nonoperative rehabilitation, 79% were successful in returning to preinjury activity levels for a short time. Success was defined as the absence of giving way on return to activity. The results demonstrate that the high success rate of nonoperative management appears to be contingent on appropriate rehabilitation candidates.

Subsequent studies have since identified characteristics of the potential coper before and after specialized rehabilitation to determine which neuromuscular adaptations are occurring to aid in the development of dynamic joint stability. If the

---

BOX 16-1   Screening Tool Selection Criteria for Rehabilitation Candidate Classification

- Episodes of giving way since initial injury ≤1
- Timed hop test score ≥80%
- KOS-ADL score ≥80%
- Global rating score ≥60%

KOS-ADL, Knee Outcome Survey-Activities of Daily Living.

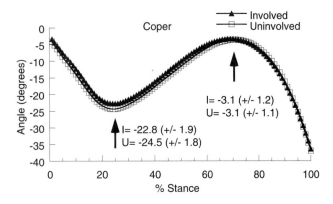

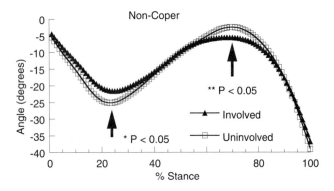

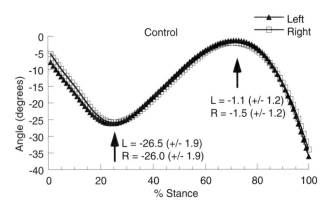

Figure 16-3 Sagittal plane knee angles during the stance phase of walking in copers *(top)*, noncopers *(middle)*, and uninjured *(bottom)* subjects. The noncopers demonstrate a reduced knee angle, although the copers maintain knee angles that are similar to both the uninvolved side and the knee angles of the uninjured subjects. *I,* Involved; *U,* uninvolved. *Significant differences at peak knee flexion. **Differences in peak knee extension on the injured versus the uninjured limb. (Modified from Rudolph KS, Eastlack ME, Axe MJ, et al: Movement patterns after anterior cruciate ligament injury: a comparison of patients who compensate well for the injury and those who require operative stabilization (1998 Basmajian Student Award paper, J Electromyogr Kinesiol 8(6):349-362, 1998.)

hallmark of the noncoper is reduced knee motion and reduced internal knee extension moment during weight acceptance, then the potential copers appear to be intermediate to noncopers and uninjured subjects.[51] Before training, potential copers stiffen their knees with significantly higher muscle cocontraction and slightly lower peak knee flexion angles. These altered movement patterns indicate an undeveloped knee stabilization strategy. After perturbation training, potential copers can increase knee flexion during weight acceptance and reduce the level of muscle cocontraction; they became more similar to uninjured subjects.[51] An increase in knee flexion after training in conjunction with a decrease in rigid muscle cocontraction indicates the adoption of a movement pattern that is consistent with clinical findings of improved dynamic knee stability.

NEUROMUSCULAR TRAINING PROGRAMS

Like the injury research, studies assessing the effectiveness of neuromuscular training programs have predominantly investigated individuals with ACL injuries as their subjects.[50,52-55] The purpose of the training program may be to prevent injury or to return the injured patient to preinjury activities either nonoperatively or postoperatively. Several training techniques have been used including balance training, functional training (jump and agility drills), technique instruction, and perturbation training.[50,52,54,56,57]

Injury Prevention Training Programs

Multiple training programs have been shown to be effective in reducing injury rates.[56-60] Retrospective analysis has suggested that body positioning during noncontact ACL injury includes external rotation of the tibia, the knee in close-to-full extension, the foot planted, and limb deceleration followed by a valgus collapse.[61] Hewett et al.[62] have termed this *collective positioning* of the lower extremity dynamic valgus. Both male and female athletes commonly adopt similar dynamic valgus body alignment during competitive play,[63] and with sufficient neuromuscular control, knee stability can be maintained without ACL injury.[64] Female athletes often demonstrate insufficient neuromuscular control during performance of high-risk maneuvers, which may result in valgus collapse (Figure 16-4) and ACL rupture.[61,63,65] Neuromuscular imbalances that women may demonstrate include ligament dominance, quadriceps dominance, and leg dominance.[62] Evidence that neuromuscular training is effective in reducing neuromuscular imbalances and preventing ACL injuries is increasing.

Secondary to the high rate of noncontact ACL injuries among physically mature female athletes, many injury prevention studies have focused on decreasing injury rates within this highly select population.[66] Henning identified potentially dangerous maneuvers in sports and recommended modifications of these potentially dangerous athletic maneuvers that may contribute to ACL injury.[67] These recommendations included landing from a jump in a more bent-knee position and decelerating before a cutting maneuver. Early results

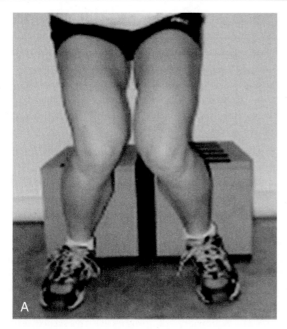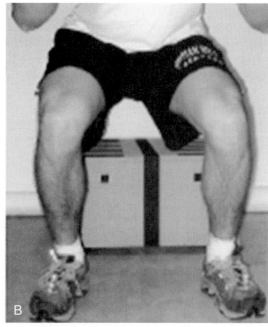

Figure 16-4 A, Valgus collapse position for a female athlete on jump landing secondary to poor neuromuscular control compared with **(B)** good lower extremity limb positioning when landing from a jump for a male athlete. (From Hewett TE, Paterno MV, Myer GD: Strategies for enhancing proprioception and neuromuscular control of the knee, Clin Orthop Relat Res 402:76-94, 2002.)

have suggested that technique modifications are successful in decreasing injury rates among trained subjects. Hewett et al.[57] later developed a training program that was based on a thorough review of the literature and prior athletic experience. Hewett's training program included an initial phase devoted to correcting jump and landing techniques in female athletes. Four basic techniques were stressed: (1) correct posture throughout the jump, (2) jumping straight up with no excessive side-to-side movement, (3) soft landings including toe-to-heel rocking and bent knees, and (4) instant recoil preparation for the next jump. Hewett's program was successful in reducing noncontact ACL injuries among trained women. The studies by both Henning[67] and Hewett[57] demonstrate the importance of incorporating dynamic, biomechanically correct movements into training protocols aimed at injury prevention.[62]

In a prospective study of 300 semiprofessional male soccer players, Caraffa et al.[56] demonstrated a significant reduction of ACL injury rates after participation in a balance-board program. The training consisted of 20 minutes of balance-board exercises divided into five phases. Athletes who participated in proprioception training before their competitive season had a significantly decreased rate of knee injuries. In an attempt to validate Caraffa's injury prevention program among a comparable cohort of female athletes, Soderman et al.[68] implemented Caraffa's wobble board balance program with 221 female soccer players. In contrast to Caraffa's results, Soderman found no difference between the control and intervention groups with respect to the number, incidence, or type of traumatic injuries of the lower extremities. Subsequently, Myklebust et al.[59]

examined the effects of a more comprehensive and dynamic neuromuscular training program on female athletes. Their program incorporated the wobble board protocol of Caraffa et al.[56] and the techniques of Hewett[57] by adding a focus to improve awareness and knee control during standing, cutting, jumping, and landing. Myklebust was able to reduce the incidence of ACL injury in women's elite handball players over two consecutive seasons. These studies demonstrate the ability of a neuromuscular-balance component to reduce knee injury risk for athletes when incorporated into an injury prevention protocol.[62]

NONOPERATIVE AND POSTOPERATIVE TRAINING PROGRAMS

Training objectives for the ACL-injured patient include improving the nervous system's ability to generate fast and optimal muscle firing patterns, to increase dynamic joint stability, to decrease joint forces, and relearn movement patterns and skills.[69] Limited work has been done to evaluate the effectiveness of neuromuscular training in achieving these objectives among ACL-injured or reconstructed patients. Risberg et al.[69] developed a neuromuscular training program for the ACL-reconstructed patient. The main areas considered when developing this program were ACL graft healing and ACL strain values during exercises, proprioception and neuromuscular control, and clinical studies on the effect of neuromuscular training programs. The program consists of balance exercises, plyometric exercises, agility drills, and sport-specific exercises. The program is divided into six phases, each 3 to 5 weeks in length. Progression through the program is criteria based and includes no increase in pain or swelling and the ability to maintain postural control of the position before movements are superimposed on the position. The scientific rationale underlying the program design, as well as the clinical assessment of patient performance and progression, are key components to the Risberg program. The effectiveness of this rehabilitation program is not known at this time; however, ongoing work is evaluating the effect of training on proprioception, balance, muscle activity patterns, muscle strength, and knee joint laxity.

Ihara and Nakayama[70] were the first to assess a neuromuscular training program consisting of balance and perturbation exercises among an ACL-deficient group. The experimental group consisted of four ACL-deficient female athletes who had suffered the sensation of "giving way" during sports activity. Training for the experimental group consisted of four training sessions per week for 3 months. Patients were compared with a control group of five subjects who did not participate in a training program. After training, the experimental group demonstrated significant improvement in peak torque time and rising torque value of the hamstrings compared with the control group. The authors concluded that simple muscle training does not increase the speed of muscular reaction, but dynamic joint control training has the potential to shorten the time lag of muscular reaction.

Beard et al.[54] also studied the effects of neuromuscular training among ACL-deficient subjects. In this study, 50 ACL-deficient patients were randomly assigned to either a neuromuscular and weight-training program or a weight training–only program. Neuromuscular training consisted of balance, dynamic stability, and perturbation training all performed in a weight-bearing position; the program was 1 hour in length and performed twice a week for 12 weeks. Results for the neuromuscular training group included significant improvement in Lysholm scoring and mean hamstring contraction latency compared with the weight training–only group.

The studies by Ihara and Nakayama[70] and Beard et al.[54] underscore the importance of neuromuscular training in promoting components of dynamic joint stability. Neither study, however, assessed the effectiveness of neuromuscular training in returning patients to preinjury activities. Fitzgerald et al.[50] used return to sport as the primary outcome measure after a select group of ACL-deficient patients (potential copers identified through a screening process) had participated in either a traditional or perturbation-enhanced training program. The traditional training performed by both groups included lower-extremity resistance training and agility drills performed while in a brace. Perturbation training consisted of a series of progressively challenging drills performed on unstable support surfaces. The researchers found that 93% of the subjects who received the additional perturbation training could return to sports for at least 6 months without episodes of giving way. Only 50% of those who participated

in traditional training alone returned to sporting activities. The results of this study indicate that the subjects receiving perturbation training were able to improve their dynamic knee stability, which manifested in improved functional levels.

At the University of Delaware, the authors use the perturbation training program developed by Fitzgerald et al.[71] as their primary treatment intervention for ACL-deficient patients. Nonoperative rehabilitation candidates at this time consist of high-level athletes who are identified as good nonoperative candidates after successfully completing the screening process.[43] Ongoing work is being conducted to determine the efficacy of perturbation training among patients who have lower functional activity levels, as well as those who do not pass the screening process.

The perturbation training protocol developed by Fitzgerald et al.[71] is a multifaceted, 10-session neuromuscular training program that incorporates strength training, agility drills, and three perturbation tasks (Figure 16-5) (Table 16-2). A variety of progressive resistance exercises are implemented and systematically advanced to address lower-extremity muscle weakness. Agility and perturbation drills are also included and progressed based on the successful completion of each task. Verbal cues, such as "keep your knees soft," "keep your trunk still," and "relax between perturbations" are provided during perturbation training early in the program to provide patients with a framework for successful task completion. The focus of training is not on developing specific muscle activation patterns. Instead, patients are allowed to develop individualized patterns as long as the task is successfully completed (i.e., maintain balance and dynamic joint stability without rigid muscle cocontraction). During the first five sessions, perturbations are initiated in a block manner in anterior-posterior, medial-lateral, or rotational planes, and verbal cues are gradually decreased as the patient becomes more proficient with the task. During the last five treatments, the perturbation directions are applied randomly while the patient performs a sport-specific task (e.g., kicking a ball). Intensity, speed, and force of perturbations are advanced throughout the program.

Patients can usually begin a partial return to sport by the eighth perturbation training session. Patients are generally discharged to competition after the tenth session as long as they successfully pass a posttreatment ACL screening by scoring greater than or equal to 90% on the screening criteria (timed hop test, Knee Outcome Survey-Activities of Daily Living Scale, global rating) and demonstrate greater than or equal to 90% contralateral quadriceps maximum voluntary isometric contraction strength.

SUMMARY

Neuromuscular control represents the complex interaction among sensory input, central processing, and efferent output. Dysfunction at any level can result in altered neuromuscular control and consequently lead to injury or reduced functional levels. An appreciation of how injury influences the sensorimotor system, as well as proprioception, dynamic joint stability,

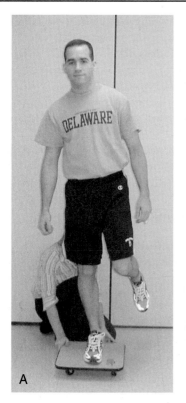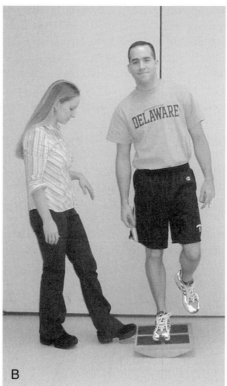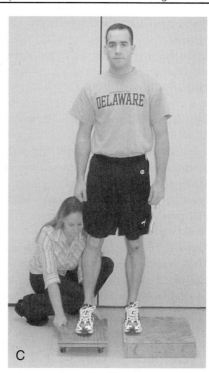

Figure 16-5 Perturbation training involves maintaining balance on three unstable support surfaces. **A,** Rollerboard. **B,** Rockerboard, **C,** Rollerboard with block.

Table 16-2	**Perturbation Training Protocol**		
Rockerboard	2-3 sets 1 min each	A/P, M/L	Begin in bilateral stance for first session. Perform in single-leg stance for remaining sessions.
Rollerboard/ platform	2-3 sets 1 min each Perform bilaterally	Initial: A/P, M/L Progression: Diagonal, rotation	Subject force is counter-resistance opposite of rollerboard, matching intensity and speed of application so that rollerboard movement is minimal. Leg muscles should not be contracted in anticipation of perturbation, and response should not be rigid cocontraction.
Rollerboard	2-3 sets 30 sec to 1 min each	Initial: A/P, M/L Progression: Diagonal, rotation	Begin in bilateral stance for first session. Perform in single-leg stance for remaining sessions. Perturbation distances are 1-2 inches.
Early phase (sessions 1-4)	Treatment goals: Expose athlete to perturbations in all directions. Elicit an appropriate muscular response to applied perturbations (no rigid cocontraction). Minimize verbal cues.		
Middle phase (sessions 5-7)	Treatment goals: Add light sport-specific activity during perturbation techniques. Improve athlete accuracy in matching muscle responses to perturbation intensity, direction, and speed.		
Late phase (sessions 8-10)	Treatment goals: Increase difficulty of perturbations by using sport-specific stances. Obtain accurate, selective muscular responses to perturbations in any direction and of any intensity, magnitude, or speed.		

A/P, Anterior/posterior plane; *M/L,* medial/lateral plane.

and postural control will aid in the identification of altered neuromuscular control. Once specific alterations in neuromuscular control are identified, implementation of appropriate treatment strategies will assist in returning the athlete to competition.

REFERENCES

1. Williams GN, Chmielewski T, Rudolph K, et al: Dynamic knee stability: current theory and implications for clinicians and scientists, J Orthop Sports Phys Ther 31:546-566, 2001.

2. Sherrington CS: The integrative action of the nervous system, New Haven, Conn, 1906, Yale University Press.

3. Lephart S, Reimann B, Fu F: Proprioception and neuromuscular control in joint stability, Champaign, Ill., 2000, Human Kinetics.

4. Hewett TE, Paterno MV, Myer GD: Strategies for enhancing proprioception and neuromuscular control of the knee, Clin Orthop 492:76-94, 2002.

5. Ghez C: Posture. In Kandel E, Schwartz J, Jessell T, editors: Principles of neural science, ed 4, New York, 2000, McGraw-Hill Medical.

6. Shumway-Cook A, Woollacott M: Motor control: theory and practical applications, Baltimore, 1995, Williams & Wilkins.

7. Grigg P, Hoffman AH: Ruffini mechanoreceptors in isolated joint capsule: responses correlated with strain energy density, Somatosens Res 2:159-162, 1984.

8. Eklund G, Skoglund S: On the specificity of the Ruffini-like joint receptors, Acta Physiol Scand 49:184-191, 1960.

9. Grigg P: Peripheral neural mechanisms in proprioception, J Sport Rehabil 3:1-17, 1994.

10. Ferrell WR: The effect of acute joint distension on mechanoreceptor discharge in the knee of the cat, Q J Exp Physiol 72:493-499, 1987.

11. Zimny ML: Mechanoreceptors in articular tissues, Am J Anat 182:16-32, 1988.

12. Stilwell DL Jr: The innervation of deep structures of the hand, Am J Anat 101:75-99, 1957.

13. Boyd IA: The histological structure of the receptors in the knee-joint of the cat correlated with their physiological response, J Physiol 124:476-488, 1954.

14. Gordon J, Ghez C: Muscle receptors and spinal reflexes: the stretch reflex. In Kandel ER, Schwartz JH, Jessell TM, editors: Principles of neural science, ed 4, New York, 2000, McGraw-Hill Medical.

15. Hulliger M, Nordh E, Thelin AE, et al: The responses of afferent fibers from the glabrous skin of the hand during voluntary finger movements in man, J Physiol 291:233-249, 1979.

16. Edin BB, Johansson N: Skin strain patterns provide kinaesthetic information to the human central nervous system, J Physiol 487:243-251, 1995.

17. Prete ZD, Grigg P: Responses of rapidly adapting afferent neurons to dynamic stretch of rat hairy skin, J Neurophysiol 80:745-754, 1995.

18. Burgess PR, Wei JY, Clark FJ, et al: Signaling of kinesthetic information by peripheral sensory receptors, Annu Rev Neurosci 5:171-187, 1982.

19. Matthews PB: Recent advances in the understanding of the muscle spindle, Sci Basis Med Annu Rev 99-128, 1971.

20. Matthews PB: Evolving views on the internal operation and functional role of the muscle spindle, J Physiol 320:1-3, 1981.

21. Lephart SM, Pincivero DM, Giraldo JL, et al: The role of proprioception in the management and rehabilitation of athletic injuries, Am J Sports Med 25:130-137, 1997.

22. Houk J, Henneman E: Responses of Golgi tendon organs to active contractions of the soleus muscle of the cat, J Neurophysiol 30:466-481, 1967.

23. Houk JC: Regulation of stiffness by skeletomotor reflexes, Annu Rev Physiol 41:99-115, 1979.

24. Nichols TR, Houk JC: Improvement in linearity and regulation of stiffness that results from actions of stretch reflex, J Neurophysiol 39:119-142, 1976.

25. Schauf CL, Moffett DF, Moffett SB, editors: Human physiology: foundations and frontiers. New York, 1993, William C. Brown.

26. Nichols TR, Cope TC, Abelew TA: Rapid spinal mechanisms of motor coordination, Exerc Sport Sci Rev 27:255-284, 1999.

27. Brooks VB: The neural basis of motor control, New York, 1986, Oxford University Press.

28. Schmidt R, Lee T: Motor control and learning: a behavioral emphasis, ed 4, Champaign, Ill., 2006, Human Kinetics.

29. Lee R, Tatton W: Clinical applications. In Desmedt JE, editor: Cerebral motor control in man: long loop mechanisms. Progress in clinical neurophysiology, vol 4, Basel, Switzerland, 1978, S Karger Publishers, pp 320-333.

30. Evarts EV: Motor cortex reflexes associated with learned movement, Science 179:501-503, 1973.

31. Di Fabio RP, Graf B, Badke MB, et al: Effect of knee joint laxity on long-loop postural reflexes: evidence for a human capsular-hamstring reflex, Exp Brain Res 90:189-200, 1992.

32. Ghez C: Voluntary movement. In Kandel ER, Schwartz JH, Jessell TM, editors: Principles of neural science, ed 4, New York, 2000, McGraw-Hill Medical.

33. Horak F, Macpherson J: Postural orientation and equilibrium. In Rowell LB, Shepard JT, editors: Handbook of physiology, New York, 1997, American Physiological Society, pp 255-292.

34. Nashner LM: Fixed patterns of rapid postural responses among leg muscles during stance, Exp Brain Res 30:13-24, 1977.

35. Horak FB, Nashner LM: Central programming of postural movements: adaptation to altered support-surface configurations, J Neurophysiol 55:1369-1381, 1986.

36. Bernstein NA: The coordination and regulation of movements, London, 1967, Pergamon Press.

37. Schmidt RA, Wrisberg CA, editors: Motor learning and performance: a situation-based learning approach, ed 4, Champaign, Ill, 2008, Human Kinetics.

38. Duysens J, Van de Crommert HW: Neural control of locomotion; the central pattern generator from cats to humans, Gait Posture 7:131-151, 1998.

39. Grillner S: Locomotion in vertebrates: central mechanisms and reflex interaction, Physiol Rev 55:247-304, 1975.

40. Grillner S, Wallen P: Central pattern generators for locomotion, with special reference to vertebrates, Annu Rev Neurosci 8:233-261, 1985.

41. Van de Crommert HW, Mulder T, Duysens J: Neural control of locomotion: sensory control of the central

pattern generator and its relation to treadmill training, Gait Posture 7:251-263, 1998.

42. Eastlack ME, Axe MJ, Snyder-Mackler L: Laxity, instability, and functional outcome after ACL injury: copers versus noncopers, Med Sci Sports Exerc 31:210-215, 1999.

43. Fitzgerald GK, Axe MJ, Snyder-Mackler L: A decision-making scheme for returning patients to high-level activity with nonoperative treatment after anterior cruciate ligament rupture, Knee Surg Sports Traumatol Arthrosc 8:76-82, 2000.

44. Rudolph KS, Axe MJ, Buchanan TS, et al: Dynamic stability in the anterior cruciate ligament deficient knee, Knee Surg Sports Traumatol Arthrosc 9:62-71, 2001.

45. Rudolph KS, Eastlack ME, Axe MJ, et al: Movement patterns after anterior cruciate ligament injury: a comparison of patients who compensate well for the injury and those who require operative stabilization (1998 Basmajian Student Award paper), J Electromyogr Kinesiol 8(6):349-362, 1998.

46. Rudolph KS, Axe MJ, Snyder-Mackler L: Dynamic stability after ACL injury: who can hop? Knee Surg Sports Traumatol Arthrosc 8:262-269, 2000.

47. Ramsey DK, Lamontagne M, Wretenberg PF, et al: Assessment of functional knee bracing: an in vivo three-dimensional kinematic analysis of the anterior cruciate deficient knee, Clin Biomech (Bristol, Avon) 16:61-70, 2001.

48. Berchuck M, Andriacchi TP, Bach BR, et al: Gait adaptations by patients who have a deficient anterior cruciate ligament, J Bone Joint Surg Am 72:871-877, 1990.

49. Vereijkin B, van Emmerik REA, Whiting HTA, et al: Freezing degrees of freedom in skill acquisition, J Mot Behav 24:133-152, 1992.

50. Fitzgerald GK, Axe MJ, Snyder-Mackler L: The efficacy of perturbation training in nonoperative anterior cruciate ligament rehabilitation programs for physical active individuals, Phys Ther 80:128-140, 2000.

51. Chmielewski T, Hurd W, Rudolph K, et al: Perturbation training decreases knee stiffness and muscle co-contraction in the ACL injured knee, Phys Ther 85:740-749, 2005.

52. Zatterstrom R, Friden T, Lindstrand A, et al: The effect of physiotherapy on standing balance in chronic anterior cruciate ligament insufficiency, Am J Sports Med 22:531-536, 1994.

53. Barrett DS: Proprioception and function after anterior cruciate reconstruction, J Bone Joint Surg Br 73:833-837, 1991.

54. Beard DJ, Dodd CA, Trundle HR, et al: Proprioception enhancement for anterior cruciate ligament deficiency: a prospective randomized trial of two physiotherapy regimens, J Bone Joint Surg Br 76:654-659, 1994.

55. Carter ND, Jenkinson TR, Wilson D, et al: Joint position sense and rehabilitation in the anterior cruciate ligament deficient knee, Br J Sports Med 31:209-212, 1997.

56. Caraffa A, Cerulli G, Projetti M, et al: Prevention of anterior cruciate ligament injuries in soccer: a prospective controlled study of proprioceptive training, Knee Surg Sports Traumatol Arthrosc 4:19-21, 1996.

57. Hewett TE, Lindenfeld TN, Riccobene JV, et al: The effect of neuromuscular training on the incidence of knee injury in female athletes: a prospective study, Am J Sports Med 27:699-706, 1999.

58. Heidt RS Jr, Sweeterman LM, Carlonas RL, et al: Avoidance of soccer injuries with preseason conditioning, Am J Sports Med 28:659-662, 2000.

59. Myklebust G, Engebretsen L, Braekken IH et al: Prevention of anterior cruciate ligament injuries in female team handball players: a prospective intervention study over three seasons, Clin J Sport Med 13:71-78, 2003.

60. Wedderkopp N, Kaltoft M, Lundgaard B, et al: Prevention of injuries in young female players in European team handball: a prospective intervention study, Scand J Med Sci Sports 9:41-47, 1999.

61. Boden BP, Dean GS, Feagin JA Jr, et al: Mechanisms of anterior cruciate ligament injury, Orthopedics 23:573-578, 2000.

62. Myer GD, Ford KR, Hewett TE: Rationale and clinical techniques for anterior cruciate ligament injury prevention among female athletes, J Athl Train 39:352-364, 2004.

63. Teitz CC: Video analysis of ACL injuries. In Griffin LY, editor: Prevention of non-contact ACL injuries, Rosemont, Ill., 2001, American Academy of Orthopaedic Surgeons, pp 93-96.

64. Myer GD, Ford KR, Hewett TE: The effects of gender on quadriceps muscle activation strategies during a maneuver that mimics a high ACL injury risk position, J Electromyogr Kinesiol 15:181-189, 2005.

65. Ford KR, Myer GD, Hewett TE: Valgus knee motion during landing in high school female and male basketball players, Med Sci Sports Exerc 35:1745-1750, 2003.

66. Hewett TE, Myer GD, Ford KR: Decrease in neuromuscular control about the knee with maturation in female athletes, J Bone Joint Surg Am 86-A:1601-1608, 2004.

67. Griffin LY: The Henning Program. In Griffin LY: Prevention of noncontact ACL injuries, Rosemont, Ill, 2001, American Academy of Orthopaedic Surgeons.

68. Soderman K, Werner S, Pietila T, et al: Balance board training: prevention of traumatic injuries of the lower extremities in female soccer players? A prospective randomized intervention study, Knee Surg Sports Traumatol Arthrosc 8:356-363, 2000.

69. Risberg MA, Mork M, Jenssen HK, et al: Design and implementation of a neuromuscular training program following anterior cruciate ligament reconstruction, J Orthop Sports Phys Ther 31:620-631, 2001.

70. Ihara H, Nakayama A: Dynamic joint control training for knee ligament injuries, Am J Sports Med 15:309-315, 1986.

71. Fitzgerald GK, Axe MJ, Snyder-Mackler L: Proposed practice guidelines for nonoperative anterior cruciate ligament rehabilitation of physically active individuals, J Orthop Sports Phys Ther 30:194-203, 2000.

17

Victor Katch*

The Lumbopelvic System
Anatomy, Physiology, Motor Control, Instability, and Description of a Unique Treatment Modality

This chapter discusses anatomy, physiologic condition, and motor control of the lumbopelvic region. Recent research on defining the cause of low-back pain (LBP) is introduced, including a new evaluation and treatment option. The physical therapist's role in treating LBP centers on three principles: reducing pain, enhancing healing, and promoting optimum function. Most therapists who treat LBP rely on the premise that the cause of LBP represents a gradual breakdown of the joint structures and soft tissues over a relatively long time. This "wear-and-tear" hypothesis, however, has received little confirmation in the research literature. Most treatments for LBP, including progressive resistance rehabilitation exercises, are based on assumptions with little outcome research to indicate success. In contrast to traditional resistance exercise therapy, this chapter presents a new LBP treatment modality based on closed-kinetic chain, suspension exercise movements that use slings, ropes, and bungee cords.

Typically, LBP treatment has been related to a diagnostic label, generally guided by the history of signs and symptoms of the low-back disorder and clinical knowledge related to the diagnosis. Two broad treatment categories exist: those that are pathologic-condition focused and those that focus on patients' "signs and symptoms." Before Hippocrates, the Cnidian School of Medicine taught that *one specific cause* and *one specific treatment* existed for every illness.[1] This approach has become known as *pathology-focused treatment*; the therapy professional focuses on the patient's diagnosis and then offers "standard" treatment. Unfortunately, this approach fails to appreciate the broader picture of interactions between different systems, such as neural-spinal and physical-mental faculties that produce perceptions and responses, both independent of pathologic condition. The other approach, traced to Hippocrates, represents *a patient-focused treatment* model. It looks at the patient's total wellness and focuses on how to strengthen the body's defenses against illness or injury.

LUMBOPELVIC STRUCTURE AND MOVEMENTS

The spinal column represents a segmented, multiarticular pillar with the following six functions:
1. Support
2. Force (shock) absorption
3. Protection
4. Leverage
5. Metabolic (bone marrow production)
6. "Physical" expression of posture

The fundamental design of the structures within the seven cervical, twelve thoracic, and five lumbar spinal sections reflects a unified purpose (except C1 and C2) (Figure 17-1). The unified purpose of the spinal column is to provide movement in all three planes (Figure 17-2): flexion and extension, lateral flexion (side bending), and rotation.

An Expanded View of the Lumbopelvic System: The Concept of the "Functional Core"

Academic reference to *the core* dates back at least 50 years to the popular college text *Kinesiology* by Logan and McKinney.[2] They referred to the *serape effect* of the hip-to-shoulder muscle link that includes the rhomboids, serratus anterior, and external and internal oblique muscles connected to deeper core muscles to control distal segmental movement. They attempted to explain the role of the core (spine + dependent muscles) as a connector and anchor that determines diagonal rotational movement patterns of the hip and shoulders during movement (Figure 17-3).

The serape effect explained, in a common-sense way, what was already known by top mountain climbers, off-road cyclists,

*Appreciation is expressed to Oyvind Pedersen, Redcord AS., and the Redcord Clinic, Santa Barbara, California; Art Weltman and Kate Jackson from the University of Virginia, and Frank Katch, University of Massachusetts (retired) for editorial assistance and help.

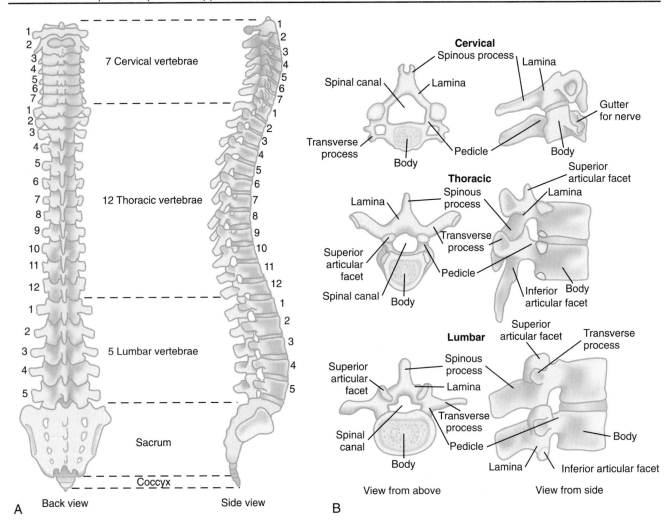

Figure 17-1 Structural features of vertebrae. **A,** Seven cervical, twelve thoracic and five lumbar vertebrae exist, each with a similar structure that reflects common functions, except for the highly specialized C1 and C2 structures. **B,** Vertebrae specifics. (From Marx JA: Rosen's emergency medicine: concepts and clinical practice, ed 6, Philadelphia, 2006, Mosby.)

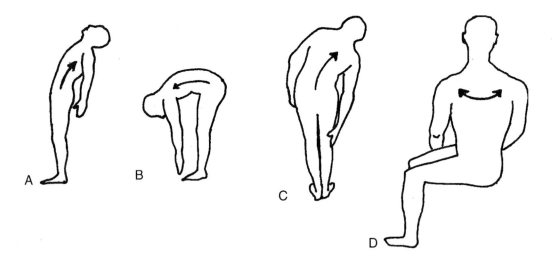

Figure 17-2 Spinal movements. **A,** Extension. Mainly cervical and lumbar regions because of orientation of apophyseal facet joints. **B,** Flexion. Possible in all regions because of orientation of apophyseal facet joints. **C,** Side bending (lateral flexion). Possible in all regions but somewhat restricted in thoracic region because of the ribs. **D,** Rotation. Mainly cervical and thoracic regions because of orientation of apophyseal facet joints. (From Kingston B: Understanding muscles: a practical guide to muscle function, ed 2, Philadelphia, 2005, Nelson Thornes.)

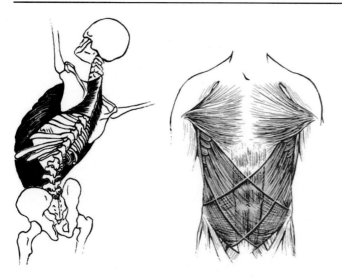

Figure 17-3 Serape effect of the core muscles. (From Logan G, McKinney W: Kinesiology, New York, 1970, McGraw-Hill.)

tight-rope walkers, various circus performers, surfers, and many other elite athletes: that performance, injury prevention, and overall success starts with a strong, stable, neuromuscularly coordinated, and healthy "athletic core." They knew intuitively that simple muscular development without corresponding muscular coordination and balance was not sufficient to enhance performance, decrease injury potential, or optimize movement.

Developing a functional serape effect places emphasis on what is now termed *core training*. This term has taken on its own lexicon in different fields and often is referred to as the following:
1. *Lumbar stabilization*
2. *Core strengthening*
3. *Dynamic stabilization*
4. *Neutral spine control*
5. *Trunk stabilization*
6. *Abdominal strength*
7. *Core "pillar" strength*
8. *Functional strength*

Describing the Functional Core

The core has been described many different ways, most often as the musculature that crosses the body's midsection. This is an oversimplification, negating an understanding that the core represents more than just a static component. Instead, the core (and its stability) needs to be viewed as a dynamic system to maintain spinal positioning and allow for controlled trunk movement.[3-5]

It can be helpful to view the core as a muscular frame with abdominal muscles located in front, paraspinals and gluteals in back, the diaphragm at the top, and the pelvic floor and hip girdle musculature at the bottom. This frame contains 29 pairs of muscles that balance and stabilize the bony structures of the spine, pelvis, and lower extremities during movement. The spine-frame would become mechanically unstable without involvement of the core musculature, and it most surely would collapse under the weight of the upper body.[6]

Successful neuromotor control and efficient, pain-free movement requires appropriate distribution of forces, optimal control and efficiency of movement, adequate absorption of ground reaction forces, and absence of excessive compressive, translation, or shearing forces on the joints of the kinetic chain. In this context, the development of a strong and stable core is critical.

Muscle Systems of the Core: Static View

Spinal muscles attach principally to the bony levers formed by the transverse and spinous processes of individual vertebrae. The flexor muscles attach anteriorly and the extensor muscles posteriorly.

Five anterior spinal muscles perform head and cervical spine flexion:
1. Longus colli
2. Longus capitis
3. Sternocleidomastoid
4. Rectus capitis anterior
5. Scalenes

Nine posterior vertebral muscles control head and neck extension:
1. Trapezius (upper fibers)
2. Splenius capitis
3. Splenius cervicis
4. Longissimus capitis and cervicis
5. Spinalis and semispinalis capitis
6. Spinalis cervicis
7. Iliocostalis cervicis
8. Semispinalis
9. Suboccipital muscles

Superficial Muscle Layer

The superficial muscles of the spine (or those attached to the spine) give shape and form to the back and are palpable. Figure 17-4 presents the visible and palpable spinal muscles.

Intermediate Muscle Layer

The intermediate muscles are located immediately below the superficial layer (Figure 17-5).

Deep Muscle Layer

The erector spinae (sacrospinalis) muscles are located under the intermediate muscles in three medial-to-lateral bands according to their attachment location (Table 17-1). Their primary functions include extension, rotation, and lateral flexion.

Muscle Systems of the Core: Functional View

The muscles of the core represent an active subsystem; they modulate the stability of the spine and interact with the central

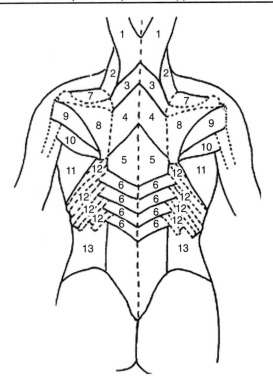

Figure 17-4 Superficial (visible and palpable) spinal muscles. (From Kingston B: Understanding muscles: a practical guide to muscle function, ed 2, Philadelphia, 2005, Nelson Thornes.)

Table 17-1	Distribution of the Erector Spinae Muscles According to Their Attachment Location			
Superior to Inferior	Attachment Region	Spinalis	Longissimus	Iliocostalis
	Head	X	X	
	Cervical	X	X	X
	Thoracic	X	X	X
	Lumbar			X
	‹– – – – – Medial to Lateral – – – – – –›			

nervous system (CNS). Considering the complexity of spinal stability, it is difficult to designate the most important core muscle, but it is not necessary to do so. Rather, the differential motor control that governs all of the muscle groups under different conditions supersedes any one muscle's contribution to stability and function.[7-10]

Two major structural, anatomic, and functional muscle classification systems describe elements of the core musculature. These divisions are (1) central-lateral and (2) local-global.

The central-lateral view was first mentioned by Leonardo da Vinci, who originally represented the vertebral neck muscles as ropes, with the deeper underlying central muscles serving as stabilizers (Figure 17-6). Da Vinci hypothesized that the muscles of the cervical spine stabilized the neck analogous to

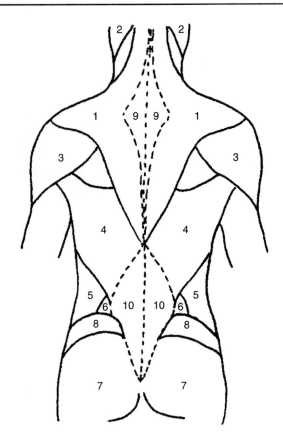

Figure 17-5 The intermediate muscle layer of the back. 1, Trapezius; 2, sternocleidomastoid; 3, deltoid; 4, latissimus dorsi; 5, oblique externus abdominus; 6, oblique internus abdominus; 7, gluteus maximus; 8, gluteus medius; 9, fascia; 10, thoracolumbar fascia. (From Kingston B: Understanding muscles: a practical guide to muscle function, ed 2, Philadelphia, 2005, Nelson Thornes.)

guy ropes of a ship's mast; whereas the more lateral muscles bend the neck.[11]

A second but more sophisticated and accepted model of muscle division for the purpose of explaining spinal stability (of the trunk) categorizes muscles into local and global muscles, based on their architectural properties.[12]

Box 17-1 lists the major global (dynamic, phasic, torque producing) and local (postural, tonic, segmental stabilizer) core muscles. In this model the local muscle system includes the deep muscles and deeper portions of other muscles that have origins or insertions on lumbar vertebrae. These muscles control stiffness and the intervertebral relationship of spinal segments and the posture of lumbar segments. These deeper muscles are essential (but by themselves not sufficient) to establish lumbar stability. The lumbar multifidi muscles (with vertebrae-to-vertebrae attachments) represent a prime example of local muscles of the lumbar spine (Figure 17-7). Other examples include the smaller intersegmental, intertransversarii, and interspinales muscles. In the abdominal region, the posterior fibers of the internal obliques are part of the local muscle systems, as are the deep transverse abdominis, with its direct attachment to the lumbar vertebrae through the thoracolumbar region.

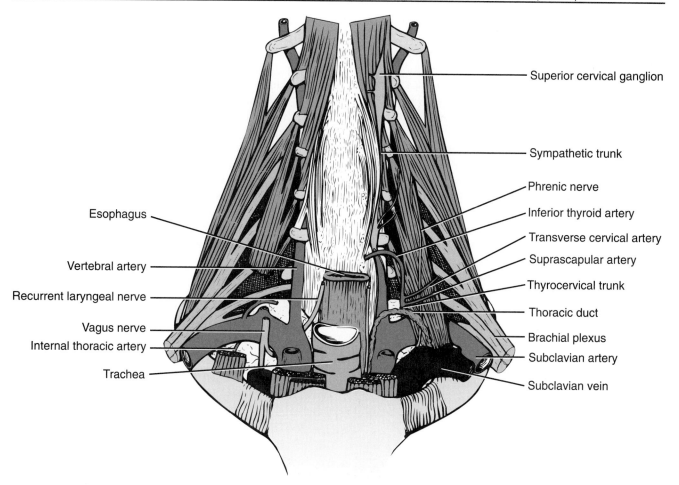

Superior cervical ganglion

Sympathetic trunk

Phrenic nerve

Inferior thyroid artery

Transverse cervical artery

Suprascapular artery

Thyrocervical trunk

Thoracic duct

Brachial plexus

Subclavian artery

Subclavian vein

Esophagus

Vertebral artery

Recurrent laryngeal nerve

Vagus nerve

Internal thoracic artery

Trachea

Figure 17-6 Muscles of the neck. Sketches by Leonardo da Vinci show "lateral" muscles of the neck and his illustrated analogy between the stability provided by the guy ropes of a ship's mast and the stability provided by the spinal muscles. Da Vinci hypothesized that the more central muscles stabilized the spine and the lateral muscles moved the neck (spine). (From Liebgott B: The anatomical basis of dentistry, ed 2, St. Louis, 2002, Mosby.)

BOX 17-1	**Most Important Global and Local Muscles of the Lumbar Region**

Global Muscles

- Rectus abdominis
- External oblique
- Internal oblique (anterior fibers)
- Iliocostalis (thoracic fibers)
- Quadratus lumborum
- Erector spinae

Local Muscles

- Multifidi (medial fibers)
- Psoas major (posterior fibers)
- Transverse abdominis
- Quadratus lumborum (medial fibers)
- Diaphragm
- Internal oblique (posterior fibers)
- Iliocostalis and longissimus (lumbar fibers)

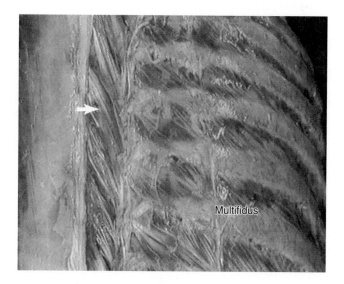

Multifidus

Figure 17-7 Multifidus muscle *(arrow)* consists of a number of fleshy and tendinous fasciculi that fill up the groove on either side of the spinous processes of the vertebrae, from the sacrum to the axis.

The global muscles encompass the large, superficial muscles of the trunk with no direct attachment to vertebrae; they cross multiple segments and generate torque for spinal motion. These muscles act similar to guy ropes (see Figure 17-6) to control segment orientation, balance the external loads applied to the trunk, and transfer loads from the thorax to the pelvis.[13] Other global muscles include the abdominal internal and external obliques, the rectus abdominis, and lateral fibers of the quadratus lumborum and portions of the erector spinae.

Hodges et al.[4] eloquently described the relationship between local and global muscles as follows: "Consider the spine as an orchestra... at one extreme we have load instruments that give volume with ease, such as a tuba. This is akin to the superficial muscles, which efficiently provide control of buckling forces and stiffen the spine. At the other extreme, we have the instruments that contribute to the finer elements of melody, such as a violin or flute. This is similar to the contribution of the deep segmental muscles, which provide minimal contribution to the control of buckling forces but provide an efficient mechanism to fine-tune the control of intervertebral motion and the segments of the pelvis. Neither system alone can provide optimal spinal control, and both elements must be coordinated to meet the demands for spinal health."

Muscle Fiber Types

Two general fibers types comprise the core muscles: slow-twitch and fast-twitch fibers (Table 17-2).[14] The local muscle system (the deep muscle layer) consists primarily of slow-twitch fibers. These muscles are shorter in length, have high oxidative properties that contribute to fatigue resistance, are well suited for intersegmental motion control, and they respond well to changes in posture and extrinsic loads. The five key local muscles are as follows:

1. Transverses abdominis
2. Multifidi
3. Internal oblique
4. Deep transversospinalis
5. Pelvic floor muscles

These local muscles control the stiffness and intervertebral relationship of the spinal segments including posture of the lumbar segments. These muscles play a substantial role in proprioception.[4,15]

The global muscle's superficial layer consists of fast-twitch fibers. These muscles tend to be long and possess long lever arms, have high glycolytic capabilities, and are able to produce large torque outputs. They also act to control spinal orientation, balance the external loads applied to the trunk, and transfer loads from thorax to pelvis.[13] Related biomechanical data indicate that the large muscles linking the pelvis to the rib cage also provide a significant amount of stiffness to the spinal column and provide stability to spinal segments.[16] Four key global muscles are the erector spinae, external oblique, rectus abdominis, and quadratus lumborum.

Lumbar Aging

The normal spine ages over time with respect to shape, orientation, and range of motion.[17-19] It is difficult to define a normal aging spine because of inter and intraindividual variability that coincides with aging. Although fairly uniform changes occur in the lumbar spine with aging, most of these changes may not associate with symptoms of dysfunction and may not be pathologic.[20] Fundamental lumbar spine age changes occur at the biochemical level; they affect biomechanical properties and ultimately morphologic conditions, and subsequent patterns of movement.

Age Changes: A Continuous Process

With increasing age, continuous biochemical changes occur in lumbar spine nuclei, represented by an increase in the nucleus' collagen content and collagen-proteoglycan binding.[20] The collagen of the intervertebral disc increases in both quantity and diameter. However, a decrease in the annulus elastic fibers occurs from about 13% at age 26 to about 8% at age 62. The nucleus pulposus dries out and becomes more fibrous and less able to exert fluid pressures. This makes the nucleus less able

Table 17-2	**Classification Schemes of Skeletal Muscle Fiber Types**		
	Fiber Type		
	Fast-Twitch, Type II		
Characteristic	Fast-Twitch Type IIB	Fast-Twitch Type IIA	Slow-Twitch Type I
Electrical Activity Patterns	Phasic: High Frequency		Tonic: Low Frequency
Color	White	White/red	Red
Fiber diameter	Large	Intermediate	Small
Speed of contraction	Fast	Fast	Slow
Speed of fatigue	Fast	Fast	Slow
Speed of relaxation	Fast	Fast	Slow
Fatigue resistance	Low	Moderate/high	High
Force capacity	High	Intermediate	Low

to transmit forces directly; consequently, the spine is subject to greater stress and strain.

Narrowing of the intervertebral discs has been considered a pathologic condition of aging, but more recent postmortem studies refute this common belief.[21] In fact, lumbar intervertebral disc dimensions increase with age. Between ages 20 and 70, the lumbar disc increases by 10% in female subjects and 2% in male subjects. This coincides with about a 10% increase in disc height and an increase in disc convexity.[22-24]

Eight additional changes in the vertebral bodies occur with aging:[17,18,25]

1. Overall decrease in bone density
2. Decrease in strength
3. Loss of horizontal trabeculae in the central portion of the vertebral body
4. Lumbar intervertebral discs become drier
5. Increase in collagen
6. Loss of elastin
7. Reduction in the mobility and range of motion
8. Increased joint stiffness

Often a change in the spine with aging, when viewed relative to a "normal" spine (i.e., in youth and young adults), usually presents as a disease like spondylosis, osteoarthritis, or degenerative joint disease. It is equally possible, however, that these changes reflect aging and accumulated stresses applied to the spine. This raises the issue confronting the therapist: Does the patient with LBP have a treatable disease, or does pain resolution require the attention of other factors to resolve pain?

LUMBOPELVIC INSTABILITY AND PAIN

LBP represents one of the most common medical problems and a major cause of worker's disability compensation. Research suggests a 50% to 70% chance of any one adult suffering LBP during their lifetime,[14] with a prevalence of about 18% to 20%.[26] LBP is expensive; costing an estimated $20 to $55 billion annually in the United States alone.[27,28] Specific origins of LBP are poorly understood and controversial without a specific cause (i.e., nonspecific LBP). A significant proportion of LBP is of mechanical origin and related to clinical spinal instability.[29] Often it is identified clinically without regard to available biomechanical or motor control issues and diagnostic techniques. In many instances, instability itself has become a diagnostic entity.

Low-Back Pain

The causes of LBP are poorly understood, diagnosed, and treated. Many traditional treatments have proven unsatisfactory, and new treatments are often implemented without clinical evidence.

Definitions

The International Association for the Study of Pain (IASP) taxonomy defines pain in clinical terms and sets criteria for the diagnosis of specific entities.[30] The taxonomy defines pain topographically as *lumbar spinal pain* and *sacral spinal pain*. Descriptions of pain do not indicate cause or imply that its source actually generates in the lumbar spine or sacrum. Instead, it simply defines the area identified by the sufferer when asked to specify the location of the pain.

Lumbar pain is often defined as pain perceived within a region bounded laterally by the borders of the erector spinae, superiorly by an imaginary transverse line through the T12 spinous processes, and inferiorly by a line through the S1 spinous process. Sacral spinal pain refers to pain perceived within a region overlying the sacrum, bounded laterally by imaginary vertical lines through the posterior superior and posterior inferior iliac spines, superiorly by a transverse line through the S1 spinous process, and inferiorly by a transverse line through the posterior sacrococcygeal joints.[30]

Types of Pain

Somatic Pain

Somatic pain results from harmful stimulation of one or more musculoskeletal components of the body, particularly nerve endings in a bone, ligament, joint, or muscle. Visceral pain, in contrast, represents noxious stimulus that occurs in a body organ. Neurogenic pain originates as irritation or damage to a peripheral nerve's axons or cell bodies.

Referred Pain

Referred pain is perceived in a body area innervated by nerves other than those innervating the actual source of pain. Referred pain is often remote from its actual source. An example would be back pain associated with hip girdle dysfunction. The physiologic basis for referred pain is convergence.[10] This occurs when converging neurons innervate different peripheral sites that relay signals to higher brain centers. Without additional sensory information, the brain does not determine whether other peripheral inputs initiate activity in the common-convergent neurons. Referred pain occurs from misperception of the origin of the signal from the common-convergent sensory pathway to the brain.

Radicular Pain

Radicular pain arises from irritation of a spinal nerve or its roots and often associates with radiculopathy. The pain does not associate with compression of nerve roots because nerve root compression does not evoke nociceptive activity. Radicular pain often presents as shooting pain, whereas somatic referred pain is constant in position but poorly localized and diffuse. It is perceived as an aching sensation in a lower limb (not the back).

Radiculopathy refers to a neurologic condition in which conduction blocks in the axons of spinal nerves or roots produce numbness in the sensory axons and/or weakness in the motor axons. Radiculopathy can be caused by compression or ischemia of affected axons.[21]

Sources of Low-Back Pain

Skeletal, muscular, and neurologic sources help explain the causes of LBP (Table 17-3). Some have a sound theoretical basis, whereas others do not. Each of the proposed sources (or causes) of pain include only those that meet one or all of the following four criteria[4]:

1. The structure requires a nerve supply (without nerve innervations there would be no pain).
2. The structure needs to cause pain similar to what is seen clinically. This should be demonstrated in normal volunteers (clinical studies introduce observer bias or poor patient reliability).
3. The structure should be susceptible to disease or injuries that are known to be painful (certain conditions may not be detectable because of poor techniques).
4. The structure needs be a source of pain in patients and should be evaluated using diagnostic techniques with known reliability and validity (large intraindividual variability sometimes inhibits estimates of true prevalence).

Attractive explanations and/or sources of LBP in terms of treatment (regardless of actual cause) include sprains, spasms, imbalances, and trigger points.

Strains

Data confirming that strained back muscles commonly cause LBP are suspect and not impressive.[31] Little evidence shows that sustained exertion or sudden stretching produces a "strained" muscle. When animal muscle is forcibly stretched against contraction, they characteristically fail at the myotendinous junction.[32] This presumably could be a cause of LBP after lateral flexion or combined flexion-rotation injuries; it can be associated with tenderness near the myotendinous junctions of the affected muscles, but confirming data with magnetic resonance imaging (MRI) have not been published.

Spasm

The muscle spasm notion of pain implies that some postural or movement abnormality (or malalignment) makes muscle more chronically active and therefore painful. The exact physiologic condition of spasm, particularly in the lumbar region, is difficult to duplicate reliably with or without tonic contractions, ischemia, or hyperflexion.

Imbalance

The clinical detection of muscle imbalance with resulting pain comes from observations of an imbalance between postural and phasic muscles, between trunk extensors and psoas major, or between trunk flexors and hip extensors. Surprisingly, such observations have not been validated, and normative data have not been established. No studies have established how an imbalance triggers pain, or identified any structures involved. However, it has been suggested that weak back muscles are compensated by tight chest muscles, resulting in increased risk of nerve impingement.

Table 17-3	Various Proposed Sources and Causes of Back Pain					
Structure or Cause	Innervated	Pain in Normal Volunteers	Pathologic Condition Known	Identified in Patients	Prevalence	
					Acute LBP	Chronic LBP
Vertebral bodies	Yes	No	Yes	Yes	Rare	Rare
Kissing spines	Yes	No	Presumed	Yes	Unknown	Unknown
Lamina impaction	Yes	No	Presumed	No	Unknown	Unknown
Spondylolysis	Yes	No	Yes	Yes	<6%	<6%
Muscle sprain	Yes	Yes	Yes	Anecdotal	Unknown	Unknown
Muscle spasm	Yes	Yes	No	No	Unknown	Unknown
Muscle imbalance	Yes	No	No	Uncontrolled	Unknown	Unknown
Trigger points	Yes	Yes	No	Unreliable	Unknown	Unknown
Iliac crest syndrome	Yes	Yes	No	Yes	Unknown	30%-50%
Compartment syndrome	Yes	No	No	Yes	Unknown	Unknown
Fat herniation	Yes	No	Yes	Yes	Unknown	Unknown
Dural pain	Yes	Yes	Presumed	Yes	Unknown	Unknown
Epidural plexus	Yes	No	No	No	Unknown	Unknown
Interspinous ligament	Yes	Yes	Presumed	Uncontrolled	Unknown	<10%
Iliolumbar ligament	Probably	No	No	No	Unknown	Unknown
Sacroiliac joint pain	Yes	Yes	No	Controlled studies	Unknown	13% (+/- 7%)
Zygapophysial joint pain	Yes	Yes	No	Controlled studies	Unknown	<10% (31% older adults)
Internal disc disruption	Yes	No	Yes	Controlled studies	Unknown	39% (+/- 10%)

Modified from Richardson C, Hodges P, Hides J: Therapeutic exercise for lumbopelvic stabilization, Edinburgh, 1999, Churchill Livingstone.
LBP, Lower-back pain.

Trigger Points

Trigger points represent tender areas located within a palpable band of fibers that, with applied pressure, produces referred pain.[33] Trigger points probably originate from acute or chronic overload, or perhaps from underlying joint disease. Another possible cause involves hypercontracted muscle cells that deplete local energy stores and impair local calcium pumps, or they originate from obstruction of local blood flow and accumulation of algogenic metabolites (perhaps bradykinin). Specific stretching techniques, ultrasonography, manipulative and manual therapy, and injections are used to treat trigger points. However, no consensus exists regarding the cause of trigger points or the success of any one treatment.

Causes of Low-Back Pain

Many researchers have used a simple biomechanical model to suggest that stimulation of one or several peripheral nociceptors serves as the primary agent (or agents) for pain. A more contemporary and comprehensive view posits that the interaction between biologic, psychologic, and social elements interact in pain generation and modulation.[5] A multivariate view of the pain experience directly links one or several biomechanical or physiologic causes to the variety of LBP conditions.

It is not clear which comes first—pain or changes in biomechanics and motor control of movement. Is pain the cause or the response? It has been shown, for example, that induced pain can cause motor control dysfunction similar to clinically reported LBP.[34] In contrast, others have shown that deficits in motor control can lead to poor control of joint movement, repeated microtrauma, and pain.[7]

Figure 17-8 presents a contemporary view of different mechanisms to explain the effect of pain on motor control of the lumbopelvic segment. The model also can explain possible mechanisms in the pain response.[34]

Lumbopelvic Instability

For many years, lumbopelvic instability has served as a diagnostic criterion to identify LPB. One of the first studies in 1944 used functional radiographs to relate LBP to retrodisplacement of vertebrae during trunk flexion.[35] Other studies followed, but the cumulative results are unclear, and no consensus emerged. Some researchers find increased motion in association with back or neck pain,[15,36,37] whereas other researchers report decreased motion.[18,38,39]

The lack of a causal relationship between LBP and instability are most likely because of (1) variability in the voluntary efforts of patients to produce spinal motion (in the presence of pain), (2) the presence of muscle spasm and pain during the radiographic examination, (3) lack of appropriate controls matched for age and gender, and (4) the limited accuracy of in vivo methods to measure motion. The instability–pain hypothesis implies that a person with LBP has a biomechanical dysfunction in their lumbopelvic region, which somehow links to their pain symptoms.[8,40-42]

The two major definitions of instability include mechanical and clinical instability, with the assumption that these two states are causally linked.

White and Panjabi[43] define spinal clinical instability as "the loss of the spine's ability to maintain its patterns of displacement under physiologic loads, so there is no initial or additional neurologic deficit, no major deformity, and no incapacitating pain."

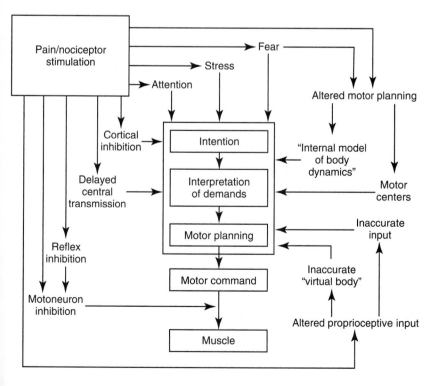

Figure 17-8 Comprehensive mechanistic view of the factors (biologic, biomechanical, and social) involved in the lumbopelvic pain response. (Modified from Hodges PW, Moseley GL: Pain and motor control of the lumbopelvic region: effect and possible mechanisms, J Electromyogr Kinesiol 13(4):361-370, 2003.)

Table 17-4	Checklist for the Diagnosis of Clinical Instability in the Lumbar Spine*

Element	Point Value
Anterior elements destroyed or unable to function	2
Posterior elements destroyed or unable to function	2
Radiographic criteria	4
Flexion-extension radiographs	
Sagittal plane translation >4.5 mm or 15%	2
Sagittal plane rotation	
15 degrees at L1-2, L2-3, and L3-4	
20 degrees at L4-5	2
25 degrees at L5-S1	2
Resting radiographs	
Sagittal plane displacement >4.5 mm or 15%	2
Relative sagittal plane annulation >22 degrees	2
Cauda equina damage	3
Dangerous loading anticipated	1

Modified from White AA, Panjabi MM, editors: Clinical biomechanics of the spine, ed 2, Philadelphia, 1990, JB Lippincott.
*A point value total of 5 or more indicates clinical instability.

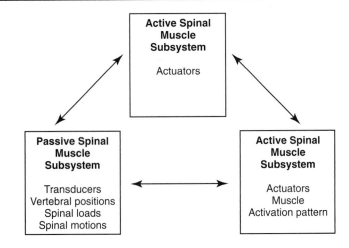

Figure 17-9 Panjabi spinal stabilizing system of the spine consists of three major subsystems: spinal column providing intrinsic stability, spinal muscles surrounding the spinal column providing dynamic stability, and neural control unit evaluating and determining the requirements for stability and coordinating the muscle response. (Modified from Panjabi MM: Clinical spinal instability and low back pain, J Electromyogr Kinesiol 13:371-379, 2003.)

Mechanical instability usually refers to a condition in which application of a small load causes an inordinately large (and harmful) spinal displacement and somehow links causally to clinical symptoms.[13]

Lumbopelvic instability is difficult to define because of its diverse nature and large inter- and intravariability of symptoms. White and Panjabi[43] produced a checklist to document clinical instability that included biomechanical parameters, neurologic damage, and anticipated spinal loading (Table 17-4). Each item on the checklist associates with a point value, and a total score of 5 or higher indicates presence of clinical lumbar spine instability.

A model of the spinal stabilizing system shown in Figure 17-9 consists of three subsystems:[7]

1. Spinal column that provides intrinsic (passive) stability
2. Spinal muscles, surrounding the spinal column, that provide dynamic (active) stability
3. Neural control unit that evaluates and determines the requirements for stability while simultaneously coordinating the active, muscular response

Under normal conditions, the three subsystems work in harmony. The passive structures of the spine and pelvis (i.e., the core) contribute to control of all elements of spinal stability. The passive subsystem incorporates bones, joint structures, and spinal ligaments that control movement and stability, particularly toward the end of the range of motion. The active subsystem refers to the force and tension–generating capacity of muscles that provide mechanical ability to stabilize the spine in the upright posture. Various components of the spinal column generate input information about the spinal position,

load, and displacement in a dynamic, real-time fashion. The neural control unit computes needed stability requirements and generates an appropriate efferent neuromuscular response, providing information to control patterns and amounts of required muscle activation to maintain stability.

This model suggests the three subsystems are interdependent components, with one capable of compensating (within limits) for deficits in another to maintain spinal stability. Moreover, the coordinating center must be able to recognize input (from mechanoreceptors) in advance of predictable challenges to stability (planned bodily movements) and coordinate responses to afferent feedback from unpredictable challenges (unforeseen body perturbations [i.e., misstep, awkward movement]).

Under this system, the neural subsystem must be able to activate muscles with the correct timing, amplitude, and sequencing to maintain successful core stability in static and dynamic situations. A sufficient deficit or system failure in any of the subsystems would cause the whole system to malfunction, resulting in overcompensation, underperformance or dysfunction, and pain.

Because the active muscle subsystem modulates spine stability, this system is most susceptible to dysfunction. Muscles provide mechanical stability in the same manner as the load-carrying capacity of upright, slender columns, first described by Swiss mathematician Leonhard Euler in 1744.[44] The greatest mathematician of the eighteenth century, Euler calculated the critical load a column could sustain, defining it as the minimum weight placed on the top of the column that would cause buckling. In other words, the critical load of a column directly relates to the column's stiffness. The thickest (or stiffer) column has the greater critical minimum load and is a more stable column; the thinnest column (with lower stiffness) experiences more column buckles at the same critical load.

The critical load for the lumbar spine column is about 90 N (newtons) (<20 lb),[6] that is smaller than measured in vivo spinal loads of 1500 N or greater.[29] The ability for the spinal column to not buckle (based on the differences between the in vitro and in vivo loads) can only be explained if the spinal muscles act as guy wires (see Figure 17-6) to stiffen the spine and thereby increase its critical load potential.

The previous model was validated by Cholewicki and McGill with young, healthy subjects performing tasks that involved trunk flexion, extension, lateral bending, and twisting.[45] The researchers demonstrated that spinal stability produced mostly by the muscles was proportional to the demands placed on the spine. Thus if the spinal system was challenged by a sudden increase in dynamic loading (e.g., misstep; awkward movement; sudden hip flexion, extension, or rotation), then the spine would be at greater risk for injury even while minimally loaded. Any sudden loading challenges to the spinal stability muscles could produce suboptimal neuromuscular activation via feedback from the neural subcenter to redirect signaling to global muscles to maintain spinal stability. Any redirection of neuromotor signal control could result in sensorimotor dysfunction and subsequent pain. Altered signal streaming would occur within certain regions of movement (beyond a pain-free zone) when muscle signal interruption occurs. Evidence of sensorimotor dysfunction is evident in reduced lumbar stability measurements on movement.[9] Stated somewhat differently, the spinal-stabilizing system responds to injury by decreasing the range of motion when any movement provokes pain. Further stabilizer muscle deactivation

from disuse also could produce pain, as could increased adaptive stiffening of the spinal column over time that forms osteophytes.

Redcord: Applications of Suspension Exercise to Core Strengthening and Lumbopelvic Dysfunction

Developed in Norway in 1991, the Redcord apparatus provides for suspension exercises that introduce high levels of neuromuscular input to optimize muscle activation of both local and global muscle systems. In both clinical and research applications for the lumbopelvic region, use of this technique shows promise in therapy, rehabilitation, and functional training applications.[19,46-50]

Figure 17-10 shows the Redcord apparatus. This device—along with the use of straps, elastic expanders (bungee cords), and ropes—provides for open and closed chain movements incorporating controlled instability to challenge the neuromuscular system to restore coordinated muscle activation. Clinical experience with this modality has shown enhanced muscle activation and improved joint stabilization and substantial reduction (or elimination) of LBP.

The Redcord approach is typically used in four crossover applications that include evaluation using weak-link assessments, therapeutic exercise, preventive exercise, and functional exercise training for fitness and sport.

Following are six principle applications of Redcord for lumbopelvic muscle activation:
1. Reestablish the simultaneous activation of the deep lumbopelvic muscle complex (transverse abdominis, deep multifi-

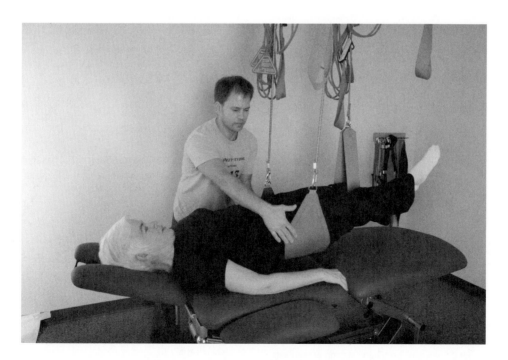

Figure 17-10 The Redcord Trainer. Patient performing supine bridge, illustrating use of slings, straps, and cords to modulate body weight unloading, as determined by the therapist. (Courtesy Redcord AS, Staubo, Norway.)

dus, pelvic floor, and diaphragm) independently of global muscle interaction (weight-bearing and nonweight-bearing muscles).

2. Precisely grade the overload (i.e., control the intensity) to permit concentration on quality of movement coordination.

3. Master muscular control and restore kinesthetic awareness of lumbopelvic position sense (posture with body weight loading).

4. Activate local (stabilizing) muscles with controlled incremental body weight loading and controlled instability (control the antigravity muscle support system). The body weight loading can be incremented as needed (Figure 17-11).

5. Enhance range of motion with graded overload.

6. Establish pain-free movement in all planes.

An important feature of Redcord's application of body weight loading is the ability to grade overload and use the response as a simple assessment tool, termed a *weak-link test* (see following).

Figure 17-12 shows an example of a standard Redcord supine pelvic lift, a typical body weight–bearing movement, performed on the therapy table. (Note: These kinds of movements, in which the end segment bears the body weight, are often referred to as *closed kinetic chain movements*.) Different starting positions (Figure 17-12, *B* to *D*) dictate how much unloading and/or assistance the patient requires to correctly perform the movement. In the pelvic lift example, the progression ladder shown in Figure 17-13 is used to make the movement more challenging and consists of the following sequence:

1. Gradually lower the elastic cords to reduce the body weight.

2. Rotate the pelvis with the arms parallel to the body. The pelvis is rotated around the longitudinal axis on the supporting leg to judge how well the individual performs rotation in the full range of motion.

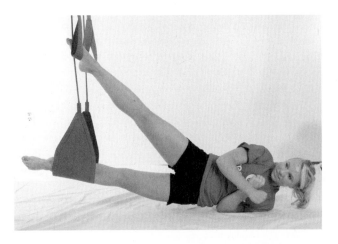

Figure 17-11 Example of Redcord body weight–bearing exercise (distal segment bearing the body weight load or part of the body weight). These exercises tend to involve both agonists and antagonists about a joint and other muscle groups in the kinematic chain. (Courtesy ActivCore Inc., Ann Arbor, Michigan.)

3. Rotate the pelvis with arms folded across the chest. The pelvis is rotated around the longitudinal axis on the supporting leg to judge how well the individual performs rotation in the full range of motion.

4. Abduct the hip of the free leg with the arms parallel to the body with the pelvis a horizontal level and the free leg abducted.

5. Combine maximum free leg abduction and pelvic rotation with the arms parallel to the body.

6. Increase the difficulty of the movements by placing a balance cushion between the scapulae in all progressions.

Weak-Link Assessment

Redcord's weak-link assessment represents a useful tool to identify a deficit within the biomechanical and kinetic chain that often associates with pain. The deficit often produces dysfunction and usually associates with pain provocation. This deficit appears as a decrease in the range of motion, reduced neuromuscular control, impaired joint stability and/or balance, impaired (reduced) muscle force, or pain avoidance. After typical functional testing (Trendelenburg's test) and active movements (walking, running, one- and two-legged balancing), bilateral weak-link testing is initiated (for the appropriate muscle group [e.g., supine pelvic lift, side-lying hip abduction]). This is done at the lowest body weight (using appropriate off-loading with bungee cord support) overload level at which the test can be performed correctly without provoking pain or uncoordinated movement patterns. Overload, achieved by manipulating either lever arm position, suspension point, and/or movement plane, can be gradually increased until one of the following three events occurs:

1. The patient cannot perform the test correctly.

2. Pain occurs.

3. An imbalance occurs on either the left or right side of the body (where the movement occurs).

Figure 17-14 shows an example of the supine pelvic lift weak-link test. No weak link is present when the person can lift the pelvis and free leg to the level of the leg already in the sling, with the arms crossed on the chest (or resting by the side), and can also do the following:

1. Hold the position horizontally for 3 to 5 seconds.

2. Maintain normal lordosis in the lumbar spine.

3. Maintain a neutral body position without rotating or side bending.

4. Perform the test pain free.

Clinical experience shows that most patients with LBP cannot successfully complete this movement with body weight loading without provoking pain. To determine the level of performance (without pain), and to set the level for the initiation of Neurac treatment (see following), the therapist can do the following:

1. Increase the base of support by putting the arms parallel to the body.

2. Activate the latissimus dorsi on the opposite side of the supporting leg by grabbing a support above the head and

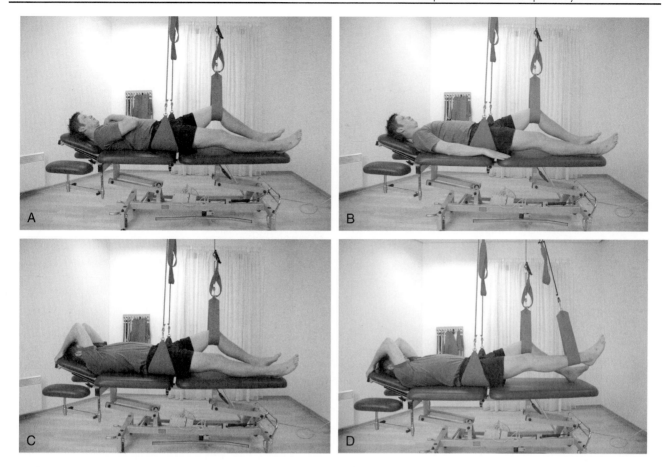

Figure 17-12 Redcord supine pelvic lift, closed kinetic chain movement. **A,** Basic starting position: Patient supine; arms on chest; strap or narrow sling under one knee, with knee flexed; vertical rope with sling about 30 cm above surface; wide sling attached with elastic cords under the pelvis. The patient extends the knee in the sling, brings the free leg up and parallel to the other, and lifts the pelvis up to a straight body position. **B-D,** Alternative starting positions, making it progressively easier to perform the pelvic lift. (Courtesy Redcord AS, Staubo, Norway.)

pulling downwards (grabbing a person's lower leg works well).

3. Activate the latissimus dorsi on both sides by grabbing a support above the head and pulling downwards (grabbing a person's lower leg as described in step 2).

4. Unload the weight of the free leg by placing it in a narrow sling attached with an elastic cord.

5. Activate the transverse abdominis.

6. Use a combination of steps 1 to 5.

Neuromuscular Activation Treatment (Neurac)

The application of the body weight–bearing neuromuscular activation technique termed *Neurac* focuses on restoring tonic function of the local and weight-bearing muscles typically impaired with LPB. The unique aspect of this technique is the introduction of high levels of neuromuscular overload, as well as the introduction of controlled instability and vibration to both local and weight-bearing muscles, to restore functional movement patterns. The ability to unload (unweight) with slow, controlled movements in pain-free positions enhances muscle activation of the weight-bearing muscles.

The hallmark of Neurac is the ability to carefully increase body weight loading, with the introduction of controlled vibration, during movement (often to the point of muscle fatigue) without pain provocation. This represents a major difference with typical strength-training techniques, where increased loading with fast or jerky and uncontrolled movement patterns, with pain-induced fatigue, often leads to poor joint control and pain exacerbation.

The support slings and ropes make it possible to suspend the patient in a pain-free position and passively move the pelvis (decrease lordosis) by activating the lumbopelvic stability muscles (Figure 17-15). Patients with LPB often cannot maintain this position with the desired quality because of muscle disactivation. By placing the patient in a pain-free position, this prone lumbar setting stimulates these disactivated (dormant) muscles and often dramatically restores pain-free lumbar movements.

Although the mechanism underlying the success of Neurac is not well understood, nor documented, the technique represents a promising new methodology. Current basic research and random controlled trials are underway in Europe and the United States to facilitate this novel approach to pain modulation.

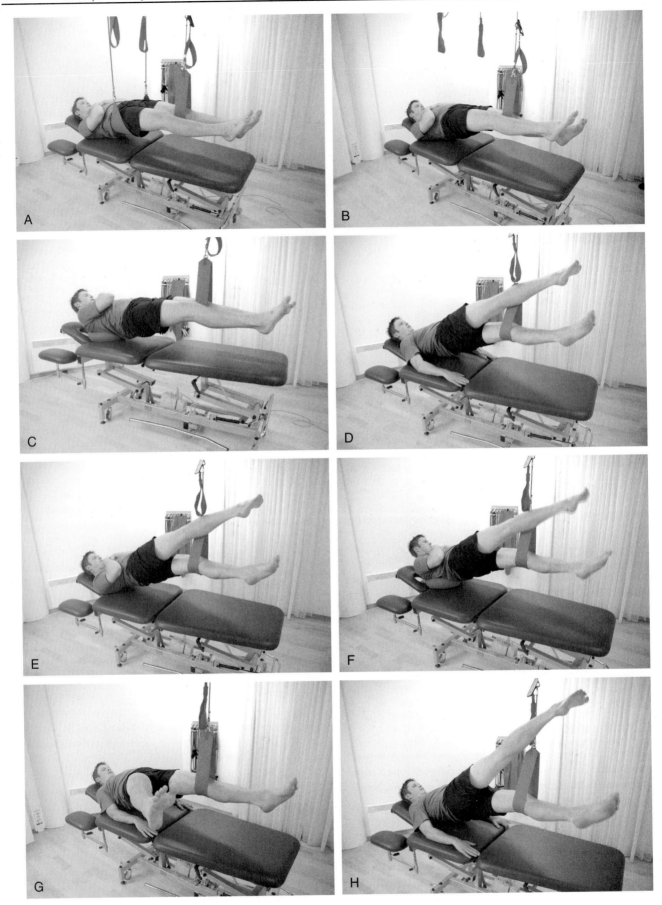

Figure 17-13 Supine pelvic lift progression. (Courtesy Redcord AS, Staubo, Norway.)

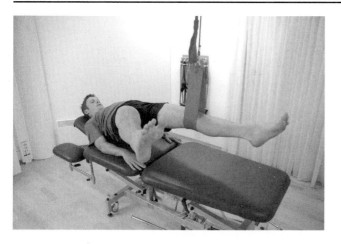

Figure 17-14 Supine pelvic lift with abduction of free leg used as a weak-link test of lumbopelvic stability performed without elastic support. The patient lifts the pelvis and free leg to the level of leg in the sling and performs hip abduction with the arms crossed on the chest. The therapist judges that the pelvis can be held horizontally, that the lumbar spine can be maintained in normal lordosis, and that no rotation or side bending of the body occurs. If these conditions are attained, then the therapist can record the degree of hip abduction at the level of failure (defined as the point where the hip drops below horizontal). The degree of hip abduction can be used as an objective measure of change after appropriate intervention. (Courtesy Redcord AS, Staubo, Norway.)

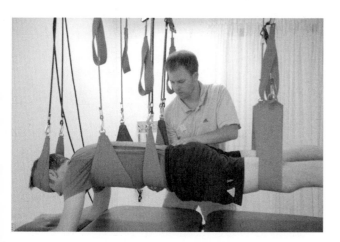

Figure 17-15 Redcord prone lumbar setting. This procedure is used both to assess and activate the deep stabilizing muscles of the lumbopelvic region when the patient exhibits decreased range of motion, stiffness, discomfort, or pain and reduced neuromuscular control of the low back. The therapist places one hand on the sacrum and one hand under the abdomen. Next the therapist gently squeezes the hands together to slightly induce lumbar flexion by reducing lumbar lordosis about 2 mm. The therapist slowly removes the hands and tells the patient to maintain the corrected position with minimal effort for 120 seconds (and to do so without pain or fatigue). (Courtesy Redcord AS, Staubo, Norway.)

REFERENCES

1. Arey BL, Burrows W, Greenhill JP, et al, editors: Dorland's illustrated medical dictionary, ed 23, Philadelphia, 1959, WB Saunders.
2. McArdle WD, Katch FI, Katch VL: Exercise physiology: energy, nutrition, and human performance, ed 6, Philadelphia, 2007, Lippincott Williams & Wilkins.
3. Bogkuk N, Amevo B, Pearcy M: A biological basis for instantaneous centers of rotation of the vertebral column, Proceeding of the Institute of Mechanical Engineering (H) 209:177-183, 1995.
4. Hodges PW, Moseley GL, Gabrielsson A, et al: Experimental muscle pain changes feed-forward postural responses of the trunk muscles, Exp Brain Res 151(2):262-271, 2003.
5. Seiler S, Skaanes PT, Kirkesola G: Effects of sling exercise training on maximal club head velocity in junior golfers, Med Sci Sports Exerc 38(5):S286, 2006.
6. Crisco JJ, Panjabi MM, Yamamoto I, et al: Stability of the human ligamentous lumbar spine. II. Experiment, Clin Biomech 7:27-32, 1992.
7. Panjabi MM: Clinical spinal instability and low back pain, J Electromyogr Kinesiol 13:371-379, 2003.
8. Panjabi MM: The stabilizing system of the spine. I. Function, dysfunction, adaptation, and enhancement, J Spinal Disord 5:389-390, 1992.
9. Panjabi MM: The stabilizing system of the spine. II. Neutral zone and instability hypothesis, J Spinal Disord 5:390-397, 1992.
10. Pope MH, Frymoyer JW, Krag MH: Diagnosing instability, Clin Orthop 279:60-67, 1992.
11. Kirkaldy-Willis WH: Presidential symposium on instability of the lumbar spine: introduction, Spine 10:290-291, 1985.
12. Bergmark A: Stability of the lumbar spine: a study in mechanical engineering, Acta Orthop Scand 20(suppl):20-24, 1989.
13. Bernick S, Walker JM, Paule WJ: Age changes to the annulus fibrous in human intervertebral disc, Spine 16:520-524, 1991.
14. Mearcy M, Portek I, Shepherd J: The effect of low-back pain on lumbar spinal movements measured by three-dimensional x-ray analysis, Spine 10:150-153, 1985.
15. Dvorak J, Panjabi MM, Grob D, et al: Clinical validation of functional flexion/extension radiographs of the cervical spine, Spine 18:120-127, 1993.
16. Cholewicki J, McGill SM: Mechanical stability of the in vivo lumbar spine: implications for injury and chronic low back pain, Clin Biomech (Bristol, Avon) II:1-15, 1996.
17. Buckwalter JA: Spine update: aging and degeneration of the human intervertebral disc, Spine 20:1307-1314, 1995.
18. Ericksen MF: Aging changes in the shape of the human lumbar vertebrae, Am J Phys Anthropol 41:477, 1974.
19. White AA, Panjabi MM, editors: Clinical biomechanics of the spine, ed 2, Philadelphia, 1990, Lippincott Williams & Wilkins.

20. Cholewicki J, et al: Stabilizing function of trunk flexor-extensor muscles around a neutral spine posture, Spine 22:2207-2212, 1997.

21. Vikne J, Oedegaard A, Lærum E, et al: Randomized study of new sling exercise treatment vs. traditional physiotherapy for patients with chronic whiplash-associated disorders with unsettled compensation claims, J Rehab Med (3):252-259, 2007.

22. Ericksen MF: Some aspects of aging in the lumbar spine, Am J Phys Anthropol 45:578-580, 1975.

23. Friberg O: Lumbar instability: a dynamic approach by traction-compression radiography, Spine 12:119-129, 1987.

24. Logan G, McKinney W: Kinesiology, New York, 1970, McGraw-Hill.

25. Dvorak J, Antinnes JA, Panjabi MM, et al: Age and gender related normal motion of the cervical spine, Spine 17(suppl 10):S393-S398, 1992.

26. Panjabi MM: A hypothesis of chronic back pain: ligament subfailure injuries lead to muscle control dysfunction, Eur Spine J 15(5):668-676, 2006.

27. Hides JA, Stanton WR, McMahon S, et al: Effect of stabilization training on multifidus muscle cross-sectional area among young elite cricketers with low back pain, J Orthop Sports Phys Ther 38(3):101-108, 2008.

28. Stray Pedersen JI, Magnussen R, Kuffel E, et al: Sling exercise training improves balance, kicking velocity and torso stabilization strength in elite soccer players, Med Sci Sports Exerc 38(5):S243, 2006.

29. Nachemson AL: Instability of the lumbar spine: pathology, treatment, and clinical evaluation, Neurosurg Clin N Am 2:785-790, 1991.

30. Nachemson AL, Morris JM: In vivo measurements of intradiscal pressure: discovery, a method for the determination of pressure in the lower lumbar discs, J Bone Joint Surg 46A:1007-1092, 1964.

31. Grenier SG, McGill SM: Quantification of lumbar stability by using two different abdominal activation strategies, Arch Phys Med Rehabil 88:54-62, 2007.

32. Hodges P: Lumbopelvic stability: a functional model of the biomechanics and motor control. In Richardson C, Hodges P, Hides J: Therapeutic exercise for lumbopelvic stabilization, Edinburgh, 2004, Churchill Livingstone.

33. Spengler DM, Bigos SJ, Martin NA, et al: Back injuries in industry: a retrospective study. I. Overview and cost analysis, Spine 11:241-245, 1986.

34. Keele KD: Leonardo da Vinci's elements of the science of man, New York, 1983, Academic Press, pp 86-287.

35. Lawrence JS: Disc degeneration, its frequency and relationship to symptoms, Ann Rheum Dis 28:121-138, 1969.

36. Dvorak J, Dvorak V: Manual medicine: diagnostics, New York, 1984, Thieme-Stratton.

37. Garrett W, Bradley W, Bryd S, et al: Muscle basic science perspectives. In Frymoyer JW, Gordon SL, et al: New perspectives on low back pain, Park Ridge, Ill, 1989, American Academy of Orthopedic Surgeons, pp 335-372.

38. Knutsson F: The instability associated with disk degeneration in the lumbar spine, Acta Radiol 25:593-609, 1944.

39. Merskey H, Bogduk N, editors: Classification of chronic pain: descriptions of chronic pain syndromes and definitions of pain terms, ed 2, Seattle, 1994, IASP Press.

40. Klein GN, Mannion AF, Panjabi MM, et al: Trapped in the neutral zone: another symptom of whiplash-associated disorders? Eur Spine J 10(2):141-148, 1997.

41. Nagi SZ, Riley LE, Newby LG: A social epidemiology of back pain in a general population, J Chronic Dis 26:769-779, 1973.

42. Resnick D: Common disorder of the aging lumbar spine: radiographic-pathologic correlation. In Genanat HK, editor: Spine update 1984, San Francisco, 1983, Radiology Research and Education Foundation.

43. White AA, Panjabi MM, editors: Clinical biomechanics of the spine, Philadelphia, 1978, Lippincott Williams & Wilkins.

44. Tsauo JY, Cheng PF, Yang RS: The effects of sensorimotor training on knee proprioception and function for patients with knee osteoarthritis: a preliminary-report, Clin Rehabil 22:448, 2008.

45. Crisco JJ: The biomechanical stability of the human spine: experimental and theoretical investigations, dissertation, New Haven, CT, 1989, Yale University.

46. Simmons EH, Segil CM: An evaluation of discography in the localization of symptomatic levels in disease of the spine, Clin Orthop Relat Res 108:57, 1975.

47. Stuge B, Lærum E, Kirkesola G, et al: The efficacy of a treatment program focusing on specific stabilizing exercises for pelvic girdle pain after pregnancy: a randomized controlled trial, Spine 29(4):351-359, 2004.

48. Stuge B, Veierød MB, Lærum E, et al: The efficacy of a treatment program focusing on specific stabilizing exercises for pelvic girdle pain after pregnancy: a two-year follow-up of a randomized clinical trial, Spine 29(10):E197-E203, 2004.

49. Timoshenko SP, Gere JM, editors: Mechanics of materials, Reinhold, NY, 1972, Van Nostrand.

50. Vernon-Roberts B, Pirie CJ: Degenerative changes in the intervertebral discs of the lumbar spine and their sequelae, Rheumatol Rehabil 16:13-21, 1977.

ADDITIONAL READINGS

Akuthota V, Nadler SF: Core strengthening, Arch Phys Med Rehabil 85:86-92, 2004.

Arokoski JP, Valta T, Kankaanpaa M, et al: Activation of lumbar paraspinal and abdominal muscles during therapeutic exercises in chronic low back pain patients, Arch Phys Med Rehabil 85:823-832, 2004.

Biering-Sorensen G: Low back trouble in a general population of 30-, 40-, 50-, and 60-year-old men and women: study design, representativeness, and basic results, Dan Med Bull 29:289-299, 1982.

Cairns MC, Foster NE, Wright C: Randomized controlled trial of specific spinal stabilization exercises and conventional physiotherapy for recurrent low back pain, Spine 31:E670-E681, 2006.

Delitto A, Erhard RE, Bowling RW: A treatment-based classification approach to low back syndrome: identifying and staging patients for conservative treatment, Phys Ther 75:470-485, 1995.

Fahrni WH: Backache: assessment and treatment, Vancouver, 1978, Evergreen Press.

Falla D: An endurance-strength training regime is effective in reducing myoelectric manifestations of cervical flexor muscle fatigue in females with chronic neck pain, Clin Neurophy 117:828-837, 2006.

Falla D, Jull G, Hodges PW: Feed-forward activity of the cervical flexor muscles during voluntary arm movements is delayed in chronic neck pain, Exp Brain Res 157(1):43-48, 2004.

Falla D, Jull G, Russell T, et al: Effect of neck exercise on sitting posture in patients with chronic neck pain, Phys Ther 87(4):408-417, 2007.

Foster NE, Konstantinou K, Lewis M, et al: A randomized controlled trial investigating the efficacy of musculoskeletal physiotherapy on chronic low back disorder (comment), Spine 31:2405-2406, 2006.

Fredericson M, Moore T: Muscular balance, core stability, and injury prevention for middle- and long-distance runners, Phys Med Rehabil Clin N Am 16:669-689, 2005.

Fritz JM, Cleland JA, Childs JD: Subgrouping patients with low back pain: evolution of a classification approach to physical therapy, J Orthop Sports Phys Ther 37:290-302, 2007.

Frymoyer JW, Pope MH, Clements JH, et al: Risk factors in low-back pain: an epidemiological survey, J Bone Joint Surg 65A:213-218, 1983.

Hicks G, Fritz JM, Delitto A: Preliminary development of a clinical prediction rule for determining which patients with low back pain will respond to a stabilization exercise program, Arch Phys Med Rehabil 86:1753-1762, 2005.

Hicks GE, Fritz JM, Delitto A, et al: Inter-rater reliability of clinical examination measures for identification of lumbar segmental instability, Arch Phys Med Rehabil 84:1858-1864, 2003.

Hides J, et al: An MRI investigation into the function of the transversus abdominis muscle during "drawing-in" of the abdominal wall, Spine 31(6):E175-E178, 2006.

Hides JA, Belavy DL, Stanton W, et al: Magnetic resonance imaging assessment of trunk muscles during prolonged bed rest, Spine 32(15):1687-1692, 2007.

Hides JA, Jull GA, Richardson CA: Long-term effects of specific stabilizing exercises for first-episode low back pain, Spine 26:E243-E248, 2001.

Hides JA, Richardson CA, Jull GA: Multifidus muscle recovery is not automatic after resolution of acute, first-episode low back pain, Spine 21:2763-2769, 1996.

Hodges PW: Core stability exercise in chronic low back pain, Orthop Clin North Am 34:245-254, 2003.

Hodges PW, Richardson CA: Altered trunk muscle recruitment in people with low back pain with upper limb movement at different speeds, Arch Phys Med Rehabil 80:1005-1012, 1999.

Hodges PW, Richardson CA: Inefficient muscular stabilization of the lumbar spine associated with low back pain: a motor control evaluation of transversus abdominis, Spine 21:2640-2650, 1996.

Kibler WB, Press J, Sciascia A: The role of core stability in athletic function, Sports Med 36:189-198, 2006.

Koumantakis GA, Watson PJ, Oldham JA: Trunk muscle stabilization training plus general exercise versus general exercise only: randomized controlled trial of patients with recurrent low back pain, Phys Ther 85:209-225, 2005.

Liddle SD, Baxter GD, Gracey JH: Exercise and low back pain: what works? Pain 107:176-190, 2004.

MacDonald D, Moseley L, Hodges PW: The lumbar multifidus: does the evidence support clinical beliefs? Man Ther 11(4):254-263, 2006.

Morris A: Identifying workers at risk to back injury is not guesswork, Occup Health Saf 54:16-20, 1985.

Nachemison AL: Advances in low-back pain, Clin Orthop Relat Res 200:266-278, 1985.

Newcomer KL, Jacobson TD, Gabriel DA, et al: Muscle activation patterns in subjects with and without low back pain, Arch Phys Med Rehabil 83:816-821, 2002.

O'Sullivan PB, Phyty GD, Twomey LT, et al: Evaluation of specific stabilizing exercise in the treatment of chronic low back pain with radiologic diagnosis of spondylosis or spondylosis-thesis, Spine 22:2959-2967, 1997.

Shaughnessy M, Caulfield B: A pilot study to investigate the effect of lumbar stabilization exercise training on functional ability and quality of life in patients with chronic low back pain, Int J Rehabil Res 27:297-301, 2004.

Willardson JM: Core stability training: applications to sports conditioning programs, J Strength Cond Res 21(3):979-985, 2007.

Willson JD, Dougherty CP, Ireland ML, et al: Core stability and its relationship to lower extremity function and injury, J Am Acad Orthop Surg 13:316-325, 2005.

Advances in Lumbar Spine Surgery

Over the past several decades, some exciting advances have occurred in the field of spinal surgery. Many of the core principles surrounding operative intervention remain the same; however, as our understanding in the fields of spinal biomechanics, bone biology, and degenerative disease improves, newer technologies and techniques have been developed, allowing for better care of the spine patient.

Much emphasis has been placed on evidence-based medicine to help define standards of care and to measure outcomes of surgical procedures, thus identifying effectiveness and defining limitations of surgical interventions. For the majority of spine patients, surgery is only considered an option after the patient has exhausted an appropriate course of conservative treatment. New technologies have not altered this view.

Proper patient selection remains one of the most important factors in obtaining successful outcomes. As more technologies become available to the spinal patient and surgeon, one must balance novel methods against the historical "gold standards." Furthermore, with the escalating cost of health care, financial issues cannot be ignored.

This chapter reviews the operative treatment of disorders of the lumbar spine. It begins by looking at the key role that the lumbar intervertebral disc is thought to play in the development of spinal disease, with a focus on the indications and methods of operative management. New technologies and techniques are discussed. Some of these advances have not been established as the standard of care and as such must still be considered experimental. Outcome studies and prospective clinical data are required to help define the roles that these technologies will play in the future treatment of the spine patient.

INTERVERTEBRAL DISC AND THE DEGENERATIVE LUMBAR SPINE

The intervertebral disc is a fibrocartilaginous structure linking two adjacent lumbar vertebrae. Its viscoelastic properties play a vital role in the normal functions of the lumbar spine, such as stress absorption and load distribution. Furthermore, the disc is considered to be a principal stabilizer in the vertebral column.[1] Intervertebral discs naturally undergo an age-related process of degeneration, which implies a deterioration of their anatomic, biochemical, and biomechanical properties. The physical and chemical deterioration of discs is typically asymptomatic. Several imaging studies have described MRI evidence of disc degeneration in approximately one third of young patients and in greater than 50% of older individuals, none of who were symptomatic.[2,3]

The exact sequence and cause of age-related changes in the lumbar spine remains poorly defined, as does the process by which disc failure leads to symptomatic disorders. Repetitive loading of a degenerating disc may lead to fatigue failure at the microscopic level, resulting clinically in low-back pain, mechanical instability, disc herniation, and/or nerve compression.[4] The treatment of these pathologic conditions is further discussed following.

GENERAL INDICATIONS FOR SURGICAL TREATMENT OF THE LUMBAR SPINE

Lumbar Disc Herniation

The excision of herniated lumbar disc material remains the most common surgical intervention for spinal disorders. With proper patient selection, this procedure has been one of the most successful.[5] Herniation of a lumbar disc occurs when material within the center of the disc (known as the *nucleus pulposus*) pushes through fissures or tears in the outer portion of the disc (the annulus). Degeneration of the disc typically begins as an asymptomatic process, as mentioned previously. When fragmentation or fissuring of the disc spreads to the densely innervated outer fibers of the annulus, patients may have the sudden onset of back pain.[6] As material herniates through the annular tear, spinal nerve roots may become compressed, resulting in radiating pain into the lower extremity, often referred to as *sciatica*.

The leg pain associated with lumbar disc herniations may present insidiously, or it may be associated with a traumatic event. Any activity that tends to increase intraspinal or intra-discal pressure, such as lifting, sneezing, or bearing down, can exacerbate the pain.[6] Disc material typically herniates in a posterolateral direction, where the annulus is no longer rein-forced by the fibers of the posterior longitudinal ligament (PLL). It then compresses the traversing or exiting nerve root. When the nuclear material remains within the annular or PLL fibers, it is considered to be a contained herniation; whereas disc material that has violated these fibers and enters the spinal canal as a free fragment, creates what is known as an *extruded disc herniation* (Figure 18-1). This must be distinguished from the disc bulge or prolapse, which is a typical radiographic finding in the asymptomatic degenerative lumbar spine.[5] Disc prolapse occurs when the degenerative disc becomes dehy-drated and compresses under load, causing the annular ring to bulge outward.

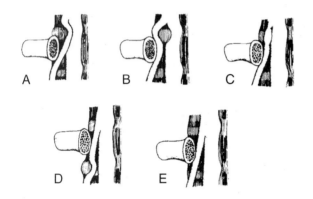

Figure 18-1 Disc herniation may occur in one of several positions. The physician should always identify the nerve root before incising the presumed herniation. (From Kirkaldy-Willis WH, editor: Managing low back pain, ed 2, New York, 1988, Churchill Livingstone.)

Patients with lumbar disc herniations may have back pain and/or leg pain, a positive straight-leg raise, limitation in bending, decreased sensation in a dermatomal distribution, a decreased patellar or Achilles reflex, and possibly a neurologic deficit such as motor weakness (commonly in the ankle or foot). A progressive motor deficit and/or intractable leg pain are strong indications for surgical intervention. In rare circum-stances, a large disc herniation or one superimposed on a very tight spinal canal, may cause cauda equina syndrome; whereby the terminal nerve roots become acutely and severely com-pressed. Patients may have loss of bowel and/or bladder control, and possibly profound functional impairment. This is consid-ered a surgical emergency.

The diagnosis of lumbar disc herniation is confirmed using advanced diagnostic imaging (Figure 18-2). The gold standard is a magnetic resonance imaging (MRI) scan. Clinical correla-tion of MRI findings is imperative, given the high rate of asymptomatic disc degeneration. In certain clinical situations, a computed tomography (CT) scan or a CT myelogram may be used to make the diagnosis.

The natural history and success of nonoperative treatment for lumbar radiculopathy is quite favorable.[6] Up to 90% of patients will have a gradual improvement in symptoms over the course of 3 months, obviating the need for surgical inter-vention.[6] Most physicians recommend a 6-week minimum of conservative therapies, such as a short period of bed rest, oral antiinflammatory medication, and activity modification. Physi-cal therapy remains a mainstay of treatment and involves core and paraspinal strengthening and general aerobic conditioning. A paucity of high-quality long-term data exist concerning spinal manipulation for the treatment of lumbar disc hernia-tions, and as such, its role for this diagnosis remains poorly defined.

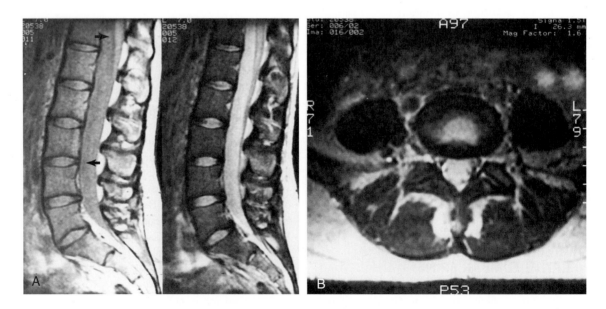

Figure 18-2 Lumbar spine magnetic resonance imaging (MRI) scan. **A,** Sagittal view showing disc protrusion at L4-L5. **B,** Image through the L4-L5 intervertebral disc showing a normal posterior disc margin. (From Kirkaldy-Willis WH, Bernard TH: Managing low back pain, ed 4, Philadelphia, 1999, Churchill Livingstone.)

Inflammation of compressed nerve roots plays a significant role in the symptomatic disc herniation. Epidural injections of steroid medication can decrease the inflammation and pain from irritated nerve roots. Complications from epidural steroids are extremely rare but can be quite serious. When patients fail an appropriate course of conservative treatment, or have progressive motor weakness or intolerable pain, they are candidates for surgical treatment.

The standard of surgical care for the herniated lumbar disc is a microdiscectomy. This procedure involves an open limited laminotomy and excision of herniated disc material. A natural space exists between two adjacent lamina that is covered on its undersurface by the ligamentum flavum. A laminotomy takes advantage of this natural window, making it larger by the partial removal of the cephalad and caudal lamina. The ligament is removed, allowing access to the neural elements below. The dural sac is carefully retracted, allowing the herniated disc fragments to be removed. Often an annulotomy (a partial removal of the annular and/or PLL fibers) is required to fully decompress the nerves.

Arthroscopic techniques have been developed that theoretically allow the surgeon to perform this procedure with less tissue dissection. However, the amount of disc and laminar bone removed are the same. The proposed advantage of less dissection and quicker recovery time may be counterbalanced by the concern of higher rates of retained disc material.[6]

Outcome studies have recently been published comparing surgical and nonoperative treatment of lumbar disc herniations.[7] This expansive study randomized approximately 500 patients to one of two groups: those receiving microdiscectomy versus those with an individualized nonoperative treatment plan. The authors observed better outcomes in the surgically treated group at all follow-up intervals up to 2 years. Nevertheless, the results were small and not statistically significant. The study methodology has been criticized because of a high crossover of patients between the two groups that may obscure the data (i.e., 50% of the patients assigned to the surgery group did not receive surgery by 3 months, whereas, 30% of nonoperative patients elected to undergo surgery).

Lumbar Spondylolisthesis

Lumbar spondylolisthesis refers to the forward slippage of one vertebra on its caudal level. Different types of lumbar spondylolisthesis exist. In 1976, Wiltse et al.[8] described these types in a classic article. The two most common forms of spondylolisthesis are isthmic and degenerative spondylolisthesis.

Degenerative spondylolisthesis refers to the anterior slippage of a vertebra related to the collapse of a failing disc, causing hypermobility between two adjacent vertebrae. In this situation, the degenerated disc presumably undergoes an extensive decline in its biomechanical properties, allowing for the instability. Isthmic spondylolisthesis occurs as the result of a defect in a portion of the bone known as the *pars interarticularis*. The deficient bone is known as a *spondylolytic defect*. It may occur at any level in the lumbar spine but is most common at L5-S1. The spondylolytic defect is generally present by the age of 5

or 6 years and is commonly the result of repetitive hyperextension (as seen in young gymnasts). Subsequently, the slip or spondylolisthesis typically occurs during adolescence. The majority of isthmic spondylolistheses that become symptomatic do so during the adult years, generally in the fourth and fifth decades. A minority of isthmic spondylolistheses become symptomatic during the teenage years and very occasionally require surgical treatment during this period. It is fairly common for an isthmic spondylolisthesis to become symptomatic in adults after an injury, when no symptoms existed previously.

The typical symptoms associated with isthmic spondylolisthesis are radicular leg pain and/or back pain. At L5-S1 the spondylolysis involves the L5 pars interarticularis and may ultimately lead to compression of the L5 nerve root. An L4-L5 isthmic spondylolisthesis most commonly involves the L4 nerve root and causes dermatomal pain in the leg after the L4 distribution. In adolescence, isthmic spondylolisthesis may present primarily as back pain. In adults, a combination of back and leg pain may be reported. Whether axial back pain without leg pain in an adult with spondylolisthesis is entirely attributable to the slip has not been determined.

Treatment of symptomatic spondylolisthesis begins in much the same way as treatment of the herniated lumbar disc. An initial period of activity modification, physical therapy, and oral antiinflammatory medication is the first level of treatment. Epidural steroid injections can be helpful in treating the radicular leg pain (Figure 18-3).[9] After appropriate conservative treatment, if the patient continues to have symptomatic leg or back pain, then surgical intervention may be considered. The most widely accepted surgical treatment for isthmic spondylolisthesis at this time is laminectomy and decompression of the

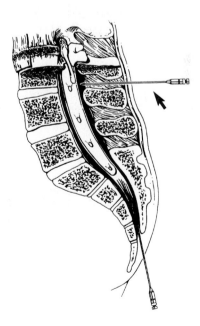

Figure 18-3 Epidural injection may be performed through the sacral hiatus or by the interlaminar technique. (From Kirkaldy-Willis WH, Bernard TH: Managing low back pain, ed 4, Philadelphia, 1999, Churchill Livingstone.)

effected nerve roots (Gill's procedure) along with posterolateral fusion. The decompression portion of the procedure involves the removal of bone and ligament that cause nerve compression. When the spinal elements are unstable, as with a spondylolisthesis, the removal of tissue may further destabilize the spine, thus necessitating a concomitant fusion procedure.

Lumbar Spinal Stenosis

The word *stenosis* generally refers to the narrowing of a space. In lumbar spinal stenosis, the spinal canal (the space where the dural sac passes through the spine) is the structure that is at risk for becoming narrowed. Spinal stenosis is generally an end-stage process whereby the arthritic involvement of facet joints, the progressive degenerative collapse of the lumbar disc, and the thickening of the ligamentum flavum concentrically narrow the dimensions of the spinal canal.[4] One theory suggests that disc failure leads to increased stress on the facet joints, which then become arthritic and develop bone spurs. In contrast to a disc herniation, which is an acute nerve compression, lumbar spinal stenosis is a gradual compression of the lumbar nerve roots and/or the cauda equina (the terminal extension of nerve roots below the conus).

The classic symptoms associated with lumbar spinal stenosis are leg pain, frequently involving both legs and almost always becoming more severe with ambulation. The term *neurogenic claudication* has been applied to the progressive radicular pain in the legs that can occur with ambulating distances of less than 100 to 200 feet. Over time, patients will commonly describe a decreasing distance that is required to provoke symptoms. The patient frequently walks with a forward-bent posture and must sit or bend forward to relieve the leg pain.

Physical findings may be very sparse, and in most instances no pain occurs with lumbosacral bending and no neurologic findings in the legs. A consistent observation in spinal stenosis is the absence of a straight-leg raise or nerve tension sign. In rare cases a motor or sensory deficit is noted. Many older adult patients are areflexic, so the absence of a reflex is very seldom helpful in the diagnosis.

Radiographs may show diffuse arthritic and degenerative disc changes throughout the lumbar spine (Figure 18-4). Associated spondylolisthesis is fairly common in spinal stenosis and often contributes to the canal compromise at the level of the slip. The diagnosis is typically made by its classic history and is confirmed by imaging studies such as an MRI scan. In spinal stenosis, lumbar myelography can still be helpful in certain clinical situations, but its use has essentially been supplanted by MRI secondary to its efficacy and noninvasive nature.

The treatment of lumbar spinal stenosis follows the same stages as the previously mentioned lumbar conditions, with oral antiinflammatory medications, activity modification, and physical therapy being instituted initially, followed by epidural steroid injections. A surgical decompression or laminectomy is frequently the appropriate treatment for spinal stenosis with progressive symptoms and/or a neurologic deficit. Care must be taken to ascertain whether the patient has any evidence of instability. In the presence of instability, the laminectomy

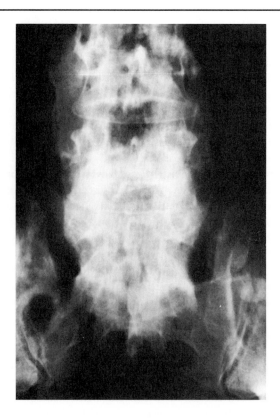

Figure 18-4 Severe degenerative arthritis of L5 with spinal canal stenosis. The actual canal stenosis is imaged with computed tomography (CT) or magnetic resonance imaging (MRI).

procedure must often be accompanied by a spinal fusion to prevent any further destabilization of the spine.

Lumbar Fracture

Fractures of the lumbar spine may occur in response to multiple forms of trauma. The thoracolumbar spine is frequently involved when a high-velocity or high-impact trauma occurs. This region is likely at risk for injury secondary to a differential in biomechanical stiffness between the thoracic and lumbar spines. Fractures of the lumbar spine can compromise the stability of the spine and/or lead to nerve compression. The majority of lumbar fractures are treated nonoperatively. However, if the spine is determined to be unstable despite appropriate bracing, or if a patient has a progressive neurologic deficit, then a surgical decompression and stabilization procedure may be required. These procedures may be performed from an anterior or posterior approach, depending on the pathologic condition and the resources available to the surgeon.

A vertebral body may additionally become weakened secondary to osteoporosis or a malignant process (either a primary bone tumor or a metastasis). A compression fracture may then result, even in the absence of significant trauma. An osteoporotic compression fracture is typically painful and can cause a progressive kyphotic deformity (dowager's hump) that may predispose the patient to additional fractures. Older adult patients, thus afflicted, may then experience a significant decline in their quality of life secondary to pain and deformity.

Traditionally, these fractures are treated nonoperatively with a brace to prevent progressive vertebral collapse. Two procedures have been developed that are designed to provide immediate surgical stabilization of these fractures, through a minimally invasive technique.

A vertebroplasty is a procedure that involves injecting polymethylmethacrylate or "bone cement" into a vertebral body through a cannula. The cannulae are percutaneously placed into the vertebrae through the pedicle. Fluoroscopy is required for safe placement of the instrumentation and cement. Polymethylmethacrylate is a polymer that is created in a liquid state. Over several minutes the polymer anneals or cures, becoming solidified. This can provide immediate stabilization of a fractured vertebral body and, consequently, excellent pain relief. One concern is that the cement, when injected, is in a state of low viscosity, allowing it to infiltrate the trabecular bone. Before curing, the liquid cement is hard to control and may infiltrate unintended areas of the spine (e.g., the spinal canal), causing neurologic compression and injury.

Kyphoplasty also uses cement to stabilize the fractured vertebral body. However, before the injection of cement, a cavity is created within the bone using an inflatable tamp. The cement can then be injected in a state of higher viscosity, theoretically making the placement of cement easier to control. Creating a cavity in the bone has the added benefit of attempting to reverse the compression (or kyphosis) of the fractured spine.

These procedures may be considered in patients who have failed conservative bracing for their fractures. Additionally, it may be appropriate in situations in which a high concern exists that a malignant process, as opposed to osteoporosis, weakened the vertebral body. A bone biopsy can be performed concomitantly during a vertebroplasty or kyphoplasty, allowing for direct pathologic analysis of the vertebral bone.

Lumbar Scoliosis

Scoliosis is defined as a spinal curve measuring 10 degrees or greater. It can occur in adolescents and adults. The majority of young patients who have a spinal curvature do not have a definable cause for scoliosis and are classified as *idiopathic*. Many other types of scoliosis must be considered in the differential diagnosis. Some examples are curves associated with a congenitally deformed vertebrae; those associated with a neuromuscular disease or connective tissue disorder; or curves associated with tumor, trauma, or infection.[10]

Typically, scoliosis will involve both the thoracic and the lumbar spine; only rarely is the lumbar spine solely affected. The natural history of idiopathic scoliosis depends on many factors, such as curve pattern, location, magnitude, and degree of skeletal maturity.[10] Curves with apexes within the thoracic spine are at higher risk of progression than those within the lumbar spine. Thoracic curves greater than 50 degrees and lumbar curves greater than 30 degrees are also at high risk. After patients reach skeletal maturity, curve progression proceeds at an average rate of 1 degree per year.[10]

Bracing has been shown to be an effective method of nonsurgical treatment in the growing patient. The goal of bracing is to prevent curve progression until the patient reaches maturity, when the rate of progression is expected to slow down.[10] Surgery may be necessary in patients with large curves or in curves that create significant imbalance. Surgical techniques have evolved over the years; however, the goals of balance and deformity correction remain the same. An instrumented fusion is performed with hooks and rods, or it is performed with the judicious placement of pedicle screws. Anterior techniques have also been developed that have the advantage of avoiding disruption of the posterior musculature and potentially minimizing the number of levels fused.

Adult scoliosis is commonly the result of prior idiopathic scoliosis or de novo degenerative scoliosis that occurs secondary to asymmetric collapse of failing discs.[11] Adults are more likely than adolescents to have pain associated with their deformities. Additionally, their disease process may be complicated by other sequelae of degenerative disc disease, such as symptomatic spinal stenosis.[11] Nonsurgical treatment in adults consists of physical therapy, nonsteroidal antiinflammatory drugs (NSAIDs), and activity modification. The goal is to decrease symptoms and improve function; bracing is contraindicated, and curve correction is not anticipated without surgery.[11] As with younger patients, a variety of surgical options are available, including anterior-only, posterior-only, or combined anterior and posterior surgery.[11] A decompressive laminectomy may be required when significant stenosis is present.

DISCOGENIC LOW-BACK PAIN AND DEGENERATIVE DISC DISEASE

As mentioned previously, the majority of individuals undergo disc degeneration as part of the normal aging process. For poorly defined reasons, some patients may experience varying degrees of disc-related pain. The primary symptom associated with degenerative disc disease is lower-back pain. This generally occurs as an episodic recurrence of lower-back pain that can be accompanied by trunk listing and muscle spasm. Although the pathophysiologic condition of discogenic pain is not fully understood, it has been suggested that mechanical loading of a disc with annular fibers that have become disrupted can sensitize nociceptors and stimulate an inflammatory response.[4] These annular tears can be visualized with MRI scanning, and they show up as a bright signal (or high-intensity zone) at the posterior aspect of the disc. The practitioner must keep in mind that asymptomatic degenerative change will also be visualized on MRI and further diagnostic testing may be required to attribute back pain to a specific disc.

Lumbar discography is a pain provocation test designed to identify symptomatic disc disease. Over the years, considerable controversy has surrounded the indications and usefulness of discography as a diagnostic tool. Currently, discography is a generally accepted method used to identify patients with clinically relevant discogenic back pain. A positive result involves the reproduction of a patient's subjective pain complaint, when a particular disc is injected with contrast solution.

The physical findings suggestive of discogenic back pain include muscle spasm, trunk listing, and pain with bending. The neurologic examination is typically normal. Patients may have referred pain into the lower extremities; however, it does not follow a typical dermatomal or radicular pattern.[4] Disc-related low-back pain is self-limiting in the majority of circumstances. Symptomatic relief may be accelerated with an appropriately designed conservative management program. Surgical treatment is rarely indicated, but it may be considered in the patient with recurrent, episodic low-back pain or chronic pain that lasts longer than 6 months and produces symptoms that can be clearly attributed to a specific disc level with a positive discography.

Once again, a wide variety of surgical options exist; however, the primary objective is to achieve a solid fusion at the painful disc level. This may be performed with a classic posterolateral fusion with instrumentation. Many surgeons prefer to address the pathologic condition directly by performing a subtotal discectomy followed by an interbody fusion. This technique may be achieved through an anterior or posterior approach.

Infection

Infections in the spine are rare, but their incidence can be associated with significant morbidity, neurologic complications, and even death.[12] The lumbar spine is most commonly involved. Most cases are believed to result from hematogenous spread of bacteria. In young patients, infection is thought to begin as a discitis secondary to the vasculature of the disc, whereas in adults the vertebra is thought to be primarily involved.[13] The most common presenting complaint is back pain that is worsened by activity and spinal motion. The pain is typically gradual in onset, and constitutional symptoms are infrequent. If the infection causes a psoas abscess, then patients may have flexion of the hip to alleviate psoas tension.[13] Leg pain is also uncommon but may occur with the neural compression from an epidural abscess.

The diagnosis is often based on clinical suspicion. An elevation of leukocytes is rarely seen; however, inflammatory markers (erythrocyte sedimentation rate [ESR] and C-reactive protein [CRP]) are usually elevated. With progressive infection, radiographic changes become apparent. MRI is significantly more sensitive at identifying the early stages of infection. Blood cultures are routinely performed; however, they are not commonly successful in isolating an organism.[12] When necessary, a CT-guided biopsy of the involved levels may provide a definitive diagnosis.

Management of spinal infections usually begins with a trial of high-dose parenteral antibiotic agents and bracing for symptomatic relief. Failure of conservative treatment warrants surgical intervention, including débridement of the infected disc and bone, decompression of abscesses, and reconstruction-fusion of the spine.

Pseudoarthrosis of a Previous Fusion

An uncommon cause of low-back pain may result from a previous surgical fusion attempt that does not heal, causing a non-union. Great care must be used to distinguish a painful pseudoarthrosis from other sources of back pain. The treating surgeon must always be vigilant that the original indications for surgery were appropriate before considering further surgery to create a successful fusion.

A symptomatic pseudoarthrosis patient typically has a history of temporary pain relief after a spinal fusion followed by recurrent back pain that is often activity related. A CT scan with sagittal and coronal reconstructions may be helpful in establishing the diagnosis of pseudoarthrosis. Plain radiography may demonstrate loosening or hardware failure. Steroid injections placed in the region of the nonunion, which provide temporary relief, may lend support to the diagnosis of a symptomatic pseudoarthrosis.

If a high clinical suspicion exists that a patient's symptoms are attributable to a nonunion, then revision fusion may be warranted. Typically, the original hardware is removed and the fusion mass is explored. If a nonunion is observed, then the fusion mass is decorticated and new bone graft is placed. The graft material may be augmented with new instrumentation and possibly biologic material known as *bone morphogenic protein* (to be discussed following).

Standard Techniques for Surgical Treatment

Laminotomy and Microdiscectomy

The standard technique for lumbar disc excision is to create a laminotomy at the herniated disc level and perform a procedure known as a *microdiscectomy*. The procedure involves a limited exposure of the hemilamina on the right or left side, depending on the location of the herniation. A small amount of hemilamina on the cephalad and caudal sides of the disc level is removed, along with the ligamentum flavum (Figure 18-5). A small portion of the medial aspect of the facet joint is also removed. The underlying nerve root is identified and retracted toward midline with a small retractor, and the herniated disc material is removed (Figure 18-6). An annulotomy is often created that involves the removal of a small portion of the

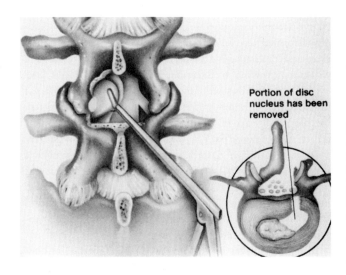

Portion of disc nucleus has been removed

Figure 18-5 Laminotomy and discectomy.

Figure 18-6 Disc removal. The physician avoids damaging the nerve by inserting the pituitary forceps with its jaws closed. Damage to the great vessels is avoided by referring to the depth mark scored on the forceps. (From Kirkaldy-Willis WH, editor: Managing low back pain, ed 2, New York, 1988, Churchill Livingstone.)

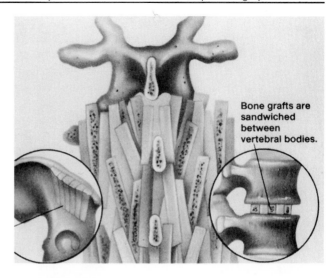

Figure 18-7 Lumbar spine fusion. Bone is rarely placed in the midline in a posterolateral fusion, as depicted here. The majority of the bone is placed in the posterolateral position between the transverse processes and in the area of the facets.

posterior annular fibers, allowing access to the disc fragments.

The technique may involve division of the lumbodorsal fascia at the tips of the spinous processes with lateral retraction of the unilateral paraspinal muscles, or it may involve splitting the muscle more laterally, with less muscular retraction, allowing for the treatment of a more lateral disc herniation. Some type of magnification is typically used, depending on surgeon preference. Loupe magnification is a unique set of eyeglasses worn by the operating surgeon that can provide ×2.5 to ×3.5 magnification. Some surgeons prefer the use of an operating microscope, which has the advantage of providing a better field of view for the assistant. An accessory headlight is often used to illuminate the small exposure.

The advantages of this procedure involve minimal disruption of important stabilizing structures. The interspinous ligaments are left intact, and the facet joint and capsule are largely undisturbed. Essentially no destabilizing effect occurs from removal of small portions of the lamina and ligamentum flavum. This technique may be performed at one or more levels, or it may be performed bilaterally at the same level, depending on the needs of the individual patient.

Laminectomy

A laminectomy procedure is performed to decompress the neural elements. It involves the removal of the posterior laminar bone, the spinous process, and hypertrophied ligamentum flavum that may play a significant role in the compression of spinal nerves. The procedure requires the subperiosteal exposure of the lamina while maintaining the integrity of the facet capsules bilaterally. The pars interarticularis is identified and provides a reference for the limit of bone removal; the pars bone is typically left intact to allow for postoperative stability.

Once the lamina is removed, the spinal canal and dura are exposed. Partial facetectomies and bilateral foraminotomies are performed to fully decompress the nerve roots. In spinal stenosis, it is common to perform a laminectomy at multiple levels. An adequate decompression can typically be performed without creating a destabilizing effect on the spine. Postlaminectomy instability is a well-described complication of surgery; however, it is uncommon unless the spine is unstable before the laminectomy. If the preoperative workup demonstrates evidence of spinal instability in the sagittal or coronal planes, then consideration should be give to performing a concomitant fusion. When a laminectomy is performed for the decompression of a spondylolisthesis, it is often referred to as a *Gill's procedure*. In this situation the pars bone is not intact, thus necessitating a lumbar fusion.

Fusion

The standard technique for lumbar spinal fusion is a posterolateral fusion. This is also called an *intertransverse process fusion* (Figure 18-7). The original fusion technique involves the harvesting of iliac crest bone graft, which is either performed through the same midline incision or through a separate incision. The outer table of the iliac wing is exposed, then harvested with the corticocancellous bone between the inner and outer tables. The bone graft is then placed on top of the transverse processes at the fusion levels. The transverse processes are decorticated using an osteotome or a burr, allowing for the egress of autologous blood products that play a vital role in the formation of a fusion. Generally, the facet joint that is involved in the area to be fused is denuded of its capsule, then decorticated with a high-speed burr.

Posterolateral fusions may be performed with or without the use of spinal instrumentation (Figure 18-8). Before the development of pedicle screws, lumbar fusions were commonly

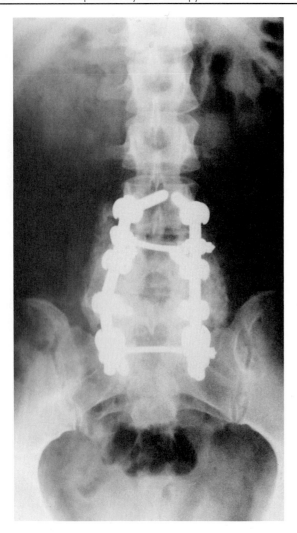

Figure 18-8 Lumbar spinal fusion with internal fixation by pedicle screws.

attempted with bone graft alone. With the advent of pedicle screw fixation, fusion constructs have achieved significantly higher levels of stiffness. This has led to higher rates of successful bony union. Nevertheless, it remains controversial as to whether a successful union results in better clinical outcomes.

New Techniques in Lumbar Surgery

Microendoscopic Surgery

Microendoscopic discectomy is a newer technique for microdiscectomy that is performed through a tubular structure known as a *cannula*. The lumbar paraspinal muscle is split, and a cannula is placed at the intralaminar level of pathology. Small portions of the lamina are removed, along with a portion of the ligamentum flavum. The technique involves the use of an endoscope or camera, which projects the operative field onto a screen in much the same way as arthroscopic surgery of the knee or shoulder (Figure 18-9).[14]

This technique may be performed under local or spinal anesthetic agent, but it is most commonly performed under general anesthetic agent because it may require more time than a standard microdiscectomy. The size of the skin incision and the amount of bone removal are essentially the same with both procedures. The proposed advantage of the endoscopic technique is less muscle dissection and consequently a quicker postoperative recovery. One criticism of the procedure is a potentially higher rate of retained disc fragments. The goals of less invasive surgery, such as quicker recovery time and postoperative rehabilitation, must be weighed against the gold standards of well-established techniques, such as a microdiscectomy. Microendoscopic surgery may play an important role in more expansive procedures, such as minimally invasive fusions. Its role in the future of spine surgery remains to be established.

Biologics

One of the most exciting and intense area of research in orthopaedics has been in the area of bone morphogenetic proteins (BMPs). Some years ago, it was discovered that demineralized bone matrix induced bone formation. A group of proteins, BMPs, were isolated and cloned from demineralized bone matrix. Initial studies of BMP involved its use in fracture repair, but this was soon expanded to evaluate its use as a potential bone graft substitute in fusions. Pilot studies have been performed using BMP for anterior spinal fusions, resulting in recent Food and Drug Administration (FDA) approval. It has also been used experimentally in posterolateral fusion and has shown significant promise as a bone graft alternative.

Interbody Fusion

Interbody fusion is a technique in which a subtotal discectomy is performed, and bone graft is placed into the disc space to create a fusion within the anterior column of the spine. This procedure may be performed from an anterior approach across the abdomen, called an *anterior lumbar interbody fusion* (ALIF). It may also be performed through a posterior approach, referred to as *posterior lumbar interbody fusion* (PLIF). These interbody techniques have traditionally used structural autograft or allograft bone to create a fusion.

Fusing the anterior column of the spine has many proposed advantages. The majority of stress within the lumbar spine is supported through the anterior two thirds of the spine. Bone graft within the disc space is therefore under compressive load, which is more conducive to a successful fusion, as opposed to a posterolateral fusion that is in a tension environment. Additionally, in the case of discogenic back pain, the removal of disc material may directly address the patient's pain generator. Some researchers have demonstrated that a successful posterior fusion does not eliminate motion across the disc space, and they have surmised that this may be a source of persistent pain.[15] Reconstructing the anterior column of the spine with the placement of a structural graft may also help to restore the

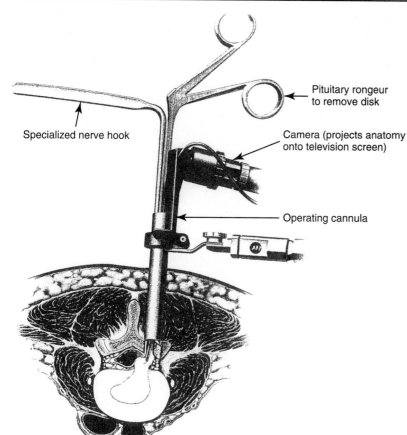

Specialized nerve hook

Pituitary rongeur
to remove disk

Camera (projects anatomy
onto television screen)

Operating cannula

Figure 18-9 Lumbar discectomy by the microendoscopic technique. (From MED surgical technique
booklet, Memphis, Tenn, 1997, Medtronic Sofamor
Danek.)

natural lordotic curvature of the lumbar spine, reestablishing
the sagittal and/or coronal balance of the spine.

An interbody fusion may be preferred instead of (or in addition to) a posterolateral fusion when treating discogenic back
pain, as well as when angular instability is seen in the sagittal
or coronal plane. It is also useful when treating patients with
a failed posterolateral fusion.[15] Over the past decade, synthetic
devices, known as *cages* (i.e., the BAK cage and Ray cage), have
been popularized for use in anterior interbody fusions. These
devices decrease the risk of graft subsidence and collapse, and
they can prevent the pain associated with harvesting large
structural grafts from donor sites. Threaded cylindrical cages
filled with morselized bone graft can be "screwed" into the disc
space after removal of disc material, providing excellent stability and high fusion rates, while restoring alignment.[16]

In recent years, laparoscopy has been used as an aid in performing an ALIF. A general surgeon, working with a spinal
surgeon, performs the laparoscopic portion of the procedure,
and the interbody fusion is performed entirely through a
cannula rather than through an open abdominal or retroperitoneal procedure. At this time, laparoscopic techniques are
being used primarily for L5-S1 interbody fusions and occasionally for L4-5 interbody fusions. The location of the great vessels
has limited the use of this technique above the L4-5 level,
although some retroperitoneal techniques are being developed
for laparoscopic interbody fusion above L4-5.

Cages made out of titanium, carbon fiber, or polyethyleth-
ylketone (PEEK) have also been developed for use as interbody

devices that can be inserted through a posterior approach
(Figure 18-10). A large laminotomy and partial facetectomy is
required for this procedure to be performed safely. Alternatively, the entire facet may be removed, allowing access to the
disc space through a transforaminal approach (transforaminal
lumbar interbody fusion [TLIF]). This technique has the
advantage of requiring minimal nerve retraction for disc space
exposure; it does, however, significantly destabilize the spine
and typically requires additional fixation such as pedicle screws
and a posterolateral fusion.

Intradiscal Electrothermography

A pilot study by Saal et al.[17] proposed that an electrothermal
coil may be used to treat degenerative disc pain. This technique was adapted from electrothermal treatment for disorders
of the shoulder capsule. Electrothermal treatment of the
anterior capsule of the shoulder causes a capsular contraction,
presumably creating greater shoulder stability. The theory
of electrothermal treatment of degenerative disc disease is that
heat can be used to coagulate the internal portions of the
annulus fibrosis where innervation is supplied by the sinuvertebral nerve. Theoretically, thermal destruction of this
nerve could eliminate the pain associated with annular
tears and internal disc disorders. Additionally, it has been suggested that thermal breakdown of fibrocartilage could repair
annular tears as the heated fibers reorganize during the healing
process.

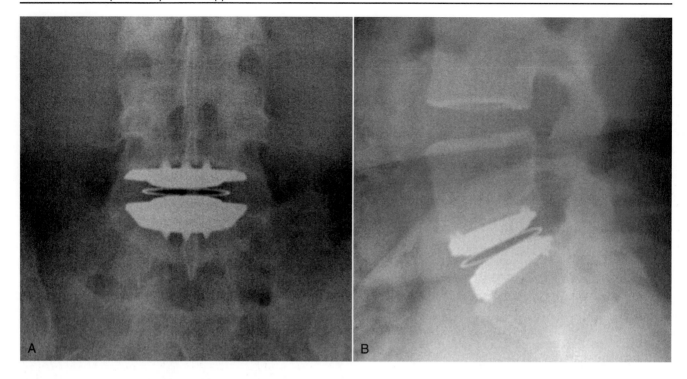

Figure 18-10 Anteroposterior **(A)** and lateral **(B)** views of patient with internal disc derangement treated with Charité total disc replacement. (From Canale ST, Beaty JH: Campbell's operative orthopedics, St Louis, 2008, Mosby.)

Intradiscal electrothermography (IDET) received FDA approval in 1999. It is performed through a minimally invasive approach. One advantage of this procedure is the paucity of successful alternative treatments for the painful degenerative disc. Additionally, the IDET procedure has a significant financial advantage over attempted spinal fusion surgery. If IDET is unsuccessful, then a patient may still remain a candidate for a fusion procedure, if deemed appropriate.

Preliminary studies suggest that IDET may be an effective treatment for discogenic low-back pain. However, the initial successful results have been difficult to reproduce. A recent cadaveric study indicated that the heat produced by the thermal coil was insufficient to cause nerve ablation (one of the proposed mechanisms by which IDET relieves pain).[18] Additionally, follow-up clinical studies have not consistently demonstrated successful results.[19] A considerable amount of research will be necessary to determine whether this treatment is truly effective for degenerative disc–related pain in the lumbar spine.

Motion-Sparing Technology

Over the past several decades, surgical technologies have been developed that were designed to preserve spinal motion, while simultaneously addressing pathologic condition. The greatest interest has focused on the creation of a total disc arthroplasty, although efforts have also addressed other areas of the spinal

motion segment. Historically, the treatment of various spinal disorders has involved a fusion procedure to address the instability of the degenerated spine and/or the instability created by operative decompression. Fusion of one or more lumbar motion segments is thought to alter the natural biomechanics of the spine, transferring stress to adjacent unfused levels.

Biomechanical studies have found increased intradiscal pressure and motion at adjacent levels, which is amplified with an increasing number of fused levels.[20] The concern is that increased stress at these unfused motion segments will lead to an acceleration of symptomatic disc failure, leading to disc herniation, instability, or stenosis (a theoretical cause of long-term failure).[20] It is currently unclear, however, whether observed degeneration at an adjacent disc level is a function of a neighboring fusion and the transfer of stresses, or if it is simply the natural history of degenerative disc disease being manifested.

The concept of disc arthroplasty and motion preservation dates back to the 1950s, when the earliest attempts consisted of the implantation of ball bearings. The first prosthesis to gain FDA approval (in 2004) is the Charité prosthesis (DePuy Spine). This device uses a metal-on-polyethylene bearing in an attempt to recreate the complex mechanical behavior of a natural disc. Many other prostheses are in various stages of development, and they use a variety of bearing surfaces and kinematic designs.

Some theoretical concerns with disc arthroplasty involve the long-term survivorship of the device and the consequences of mechanical failure. From the total joint literature, it is clear that artificial debris and foreign bodies can have a deleterious effect on surrounding bone and soft tissue in the long term. Apart from longevity, other areas of concern are the relative safety of insertion (and particularly removal), their efficacy, the proper indications and contraindications for use, the compatibility of biomaterials, and the learning curve required for proper implantation. Clinical trials should demonstrate safety and have proper outcome measures to validate their effectiveness.[21] Comparison must be made to existing standards of care, and long-term studies are necessary to establish the role that motion-sparing devices will play in the future of spinal surgery.

Postoperative Rehabilitation

It is difficult to fashion a single rehabilitation program for any given postoperative setting after lumbar spine surgery. The following are general guidelines for postoperative rehabilitation after lumbar decompressive surgery with and without fusion.

In a patient who has undergone a microdiscectomy or laminectomy procedure, rehabilitation may begin shortly after surgery. During the first 6 weeks, therapy is focused on gentle stretching and nerve glide exercises on the lower extremities. Some surgeons prefer to place their patients in a lumbar corset brace for support and comfort. Walking to tolerance is generally encouraged, increasing the pace and distance as symptoms allow. The wound is checked 1 to 2 weeks postoperatively. Forward-bending and twisting activities are often restricted during this time, and heavy lifting is to be avoided. Between 4 to 6 weeks after surgery, once the operative site has had a chance to heal, physical therapy begins in earnest. Lumbar and core-strengthening exercises are initiated and increased gradually, depending on the individual patient. Range-of-motion and return-to-flexion exercises begin as the supporting musculature allows. Low-impact aerobic conditioning such as the stationary bicycle or pool therapy may commence during these initial stages of rehabilitation, with the expectation that exercise intensity will slowly increase over the course of a 6-week program. Return to higher-impact athletics typically occurs after 3 months postoperatively.

Postoperative rehabilitation in fusion patients is typically delayed to allow the fusion mass to heal. This process typically takes a minimum of 12 weeks. During this time, patients usually wear a structurally supportive brace (e.g., lumbar sacral orthosis [LSO], thoracic lumbar sacral orthosis [TLSO]). Ambulation and nerve glide exercises are encouraged early on; however, trunk strengthening is deferred until the tenth or twelfth postoperative week. An unfortunate consequence of minimizing trunk and lumbar mobility is the unavoidable deconditioning that will occur in the core and paraspinal musculature. Once radiographs demonstrate signs of bone healing and the brace is discontinued, a strengthening and mobilization program may begin. Aerobic conditioning is introduced gradually, as the patient's symptoms allow.

REFERENCES

1. Rolander SD: Motion of the lumbar spine with special reference to the stabilizing effect of posterior fusion, Acta Orthop Scand Suppl 90:1-144, 1966.
2. Boden SD, McCowin PR, Davis DO, et al: Abnormal magnetic resonance scans of the lumbar spine in asymptomatic subject, J Bone Joint Surg Am 72:403-408, 1990.
3. Powell MC, Szypryt P, Wilson K, et al: Prevalence of lumbar disc degeneration observed by MRI in symptomless women, Lancet 2:1366-1367, 1986.
4. St John T, et al: The aging lumbar spine: the pain generator. In Vaccaro AR, Betz RR, Zeidman SM, editors: Principles and practice of spine surgery, Philadelphia, 2003, Mosby, pp 83-96.
5. Greenough CG: Operative treatment of disc herniation: natural history and indications for surgery. In Herkowitz HN, Dvorak J, Bell GR et al, editors: The lumbar spine, ed 3, Philadelphia, 2005, Lippincott Williams & Wilkins, pp 437-442.
6. Bendo JA, Awad JN: Lumbar disk herniation. In Spivak JM, Connolly PJ, editors: Orthopaedic knowledge update: spine, ed 3, Rosemont, Ill, 2006, American Academy of Orthopaedic Surgeons, pp 289-298.
7. Weinstein JN, Lurie JS, Tosteson TD, et al: Surgical vs. nonoperative treatment for lumbar disc herniation: the spine patient outcomes research trial (SPORT), JAMA 20:296, 2006.
8. Wiltse LL, Newman PH, McNab I: Classification of spondylolysis and spondylolisthesis, Clin Orthop Relat Res 117:23-24, 1976.
9. Bernard TN Jr: Diagnostic and therapeutic techniques. In Kirkaldy-Willis WH, Burton CV, editors: Managing low back pain, ed 3, New York, 1992, Churchill Livingstone.
10. Akbarnia BA, Segal LS: Infantile, juvenile, and adolescent idiopathic scoliosis. In Spivak JM, Connolly PJ, editors: Orthopaedic knowledge update: spine, ed 3, Rosemont, Ill, 2006, American Academy of Orthopaedic Surgeons, pp 289-298.
11. Anderson DG, Albert T, Tannoury C: Adult scoliosis. In Spivak JM, Connolly PJ, editors: Orthopaedic knowledge update: spine, ed 3, Rosemont, Ill, 2006, American Academy of Orthopaedic Surgeons, pp. 289-298.
12. Weinstein MA, et al: Evaluation of the patient with spinal infection. In Wiesel SW, Boden SD, Garfin SR, editors: Seminars in spine surgery: infections of the spine, Semin Spine Surg 12(4):160-175, 2000.
13. Vaccaro AR, Harris BM: Presentation and treatment of pyogenic vertebral osteomyelitis. In Wiesel SW, Boden SD, Garfin SR, editors: Seminars in spine surgery: infections of the spine, Semin Spine Surg 12(4):183-191, 2000.
14. MED surgical technique booklet, Memphis, Tenn, 1997, Medtronic Sofamor Danek.
15. Lee CK, Kopacz KJ: Posterior lumbar interbody fusion. In Herkowitz HN, et al, editors: The lumbar spine, Philadelphia, 2004, Lippincott, pp 324-330.

16. Hannani K, Delamarter R: Operative treatment of anterior procedures. In Herkowitz HN et al, editors: The lumbar spine, Philadelphia, 2004, Lippincott, pp 331-337.

17. Saal JA, Saal JS: Intradiscal electrothermal treatment (IDET) for chronic discogenic low back pain: a prospective outcome study with minimum two year follow up. Paper presented at the North American Spine Society meeting, New Orleans, LA, October 2000.

18. Kleinstuek FS, Diederich CJ, Nam WH, et al: Temperature and thermal dose distributions during intradiscal electrothermal therapy in the cadaver spine, Spine 28:1700-1708, 2003.

19. Freeman BJ, IDET: a critical appraisal of the evidence, Eur Spine J 15(suppl 3):S448-S457, 2006.

20. Yang JY, Lee JK, Song HS, et al: The impact of adjacent segment degeneration of the clinical outcome after lumbar spinal fusion, Spine 33(5):503-507, 2008.

21. Hilibrand AS, Kirkpatrick JS: Motion-sparing technologies. In Spivak JM, Connolly PJ, editors: Orthopaedic knowledge update, spine, ed 3, Rosemont, Calif, 2006, AAOS, pp 495-502.

SUGGESTED READING

An HS: Principles and techniques of spine surgery, Baltimore, 1998, Lippincott Williams & Wilkins.

Bolender NF: The role of computed tomography and myelography and the diagnosis of central spine stenosis, J Bone Joint Surg 67(A):240, 1985.

Bostrom MP, Camacho NP: Potential role of bone morphogenetic proteins in fracture healing, Clin Orthop Relat Res 255(suppl):S274-S282, 1990.

Bradford DS, Lonstein JE, Moe JH, et al: Moe's textbook of scoliosis and other spinal deformities, ed 2, Philadelphia, 1987, Saunders.

Brown CA, Eismont FJ: Complications in spinal fusion, Orthop Clin North Am 29(4):679-699, 1998.

Eismont FJ: Lumbosacral spine, Maine Orthop Rev 151:101,1985.

Frymoyer JW, editor: The adult spine: principles and practice, New York, 1991, Raven Press.

Herkowitz HN, et al: The lumbar spine, ed 3, Philadelphia, 2004, Lippincott Williams & Wilkins.

Karahalios DG, Apostolides PJ, Sonntag VK: Degenerative lumbar spinal instability: technical aspects of operative treatment, Clin Neurosurg 44:109-135, 1997.

MacNab I: Backache, Baltimore, 1977, Lippincott Williams & Wilkins.

Niggemeyer O, Strauss JM, Schultz KP: Comparison of surgical procedures for degenerative lumbar spinal stenosis: a metaanalysis of the literature from 1975 to 1995, Eur Spine J 6(6):423-429, 1997.

Reddi AH: Initiation of fracture repair by bone morphogenetic proteins, Clin Orthop Relat Res 355(suppl):S66-S72, 1998.

Rosen C, Kahanovita N, Viola K: A retrospective analysis of the efficacy of epidural steroid injections, Clin Orthop Relat Res 228:270, 1988.

Sakou T: Bone morphogenetic proteins: from basic studies to clinical approaches, Bone 22(6):591-603, 1998.

Schneiderman G, Flannigan B, Kingston S: Magnetic resonance imaging in the diagnosis of disc degeneration: correlation with discography, Spine 12:276, 1987.

Waddell G: A new clinical model for the treatment of low back pain, Spine 12:632, 1987.

Watkins RG, Collis JS: Lumbar discectomy and laminectomy, Rockville, Md, 1987, Aspen.

Weinstein JN, Wiesel SW, editors: The lumbar spine, Philadelphia, 1990, Saunders.

White AA, Punjabi MM: Clinical biomechanics of the spine, ed 2, Philadelphia, 1990, Lippincott Williams & Wilkins.

White AA, Rothman RH, Rey CD, editors: Lumbar spine surgery: techniques and complications, St Louis, 1987, Mosby.

Williams RW, McCullouch JA, Young PH: Microsurgery of the lumbar spine: principles and techniques in spine surgery, Rockville, Md, 1990, Aspen.

Young Hing K: Surgical techniques. In Kirkaldy-Willis WH, editor: Managing low back pain, ed 2, New York, 1988, Churchill Livingstone, p 315.

Evaluation, Diagnosis, and Treatment of the Lumbar-Pelvic-Hip Complex

Musculoskeletal experts continue to debate how the low back, pelvic girdle, and lower-extremity function in synchrony. The literature contains information on a plethora of diagnostic tests, some with good psychometric properties. However, little consistency is seen in the tests used by different clinicians. Exercise and manual treatments selected by clinicians also vary greatly, depending on their experience, education, and exposure to continuing education. Few diagnostic tests used by the physical therapist in the pelvic-hip complex should be used in isolation; instead the clinician must use selected special tests and combine all information gleaned from the examination to form a diagnosis. When evaluating the pelvic-hip complex, it is essential to consider the anatomy, biomechanical state, and neurologic condition of this region, as well as the subjective history and emotional state of the patient.

FUNCTIONAL ANATOMY AND MECHANICS OF THE HIP

Osteology of the Hip

The hip, or coxofemoral joint (CFJ) is formed by the articulation of the head of the femur with the acetabulum of the pelvis (Figure 19-1, A). This joint is a classic example of a ball-and-socket joint and has three degrees of freedom in motion. The primary functions of the hip joint are to increase stability and to provide support for the transmission of forces between the pelvis and lower extremities with dynamic activities such as running, jumping, and walking. Stability is produced in three ways: (1) bony congruency, (2) capsular reinforcement, and (3) the neuromuscular system. In addition, the hip joint allows significant mobility for those activities and supports the weight of the upper body during static erect posture. The hip joint must be able to resist loads, both tensile and compressive, much more than body weight.

The femur is the longest and strongest bone in the body. The proximal end of the femur includes the head, neck, and trochanters. The head of the femur is ellipsoid in shape, forming roughly two thirds of a sphere approximately 4 to 5 cm in

diameter. It is covered with hyaline cartilage, which is thicker centrally[1] and thinner at the periphery. Just below the center of the head lies the fovea centralis (capitis), which is where the "teres" ligament inserts. The ligamentum teres, comprised of three bundles, is a flattened fibrous band 3 to 3.5 cm long that arises from the acetabular notch and inserts into the fovea capitis (Figure 19-1, B). It lies in the floor of the acetabulum and has minimal, if any, mechanical function in the hip joint, because it comes under tension only in adduction. Its primary function is to protect the delicate posterior branch of the obturator artery, which supplies the head of the femur. In infants and children, this artery is a significant source of blood to the femoral head.[2] Avascular necrosis (AVN) of the femoral head has been linked to interruption of this artery.

The femoral neck projects laterally from the head and fans out; this projection is usually between 120 and 125 degrees in adults and is known as the *angle of inclination* (Figure 19-2, A). At birth this angle is 135 degrees; by the end of the second year of life, this head-to-neck angle can be as great as 150 degrees. The decrease in this angle from infancy to adulthood is the result of compression and bending forces acting on the head during weight bearing. *Coxa vara* is an angle less than 120 degrees, and *coxa valga* is an angle larger than 135 degrees.[3]

Coxa vara is a deformity that causes a decreased joint load because of more balanced force distribution. The femoral neck tends to be shorter. The head maintains a more central position in the acetabulum because of the greater leverage associated with the adductors. This deformity, however, causes more shearing forces that can lead to a pseudoarthrosis of the femoral neck.[4]

Coxa valga is considered to be one of the most unfavorable structural configurations of the hip because it causes increased joint compression.[4] The femoral neck tends to be longer. This position of the hip leads to a loss of hip abduction moment, which causes a force imbalance and a prearthritic state, not the deformity itself. Eccentric control of the hip adduction is diminished during landing (through the pelvis), leading to increased forces borne through the joint. The acetabular weight-bearing surface may become more oblique so that the

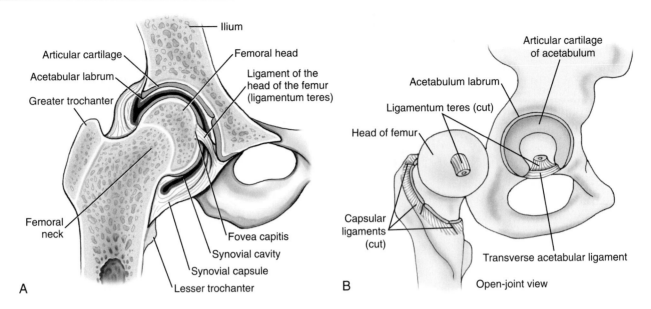

Figure 19-1 A, Coxofemoral joint (hip joint). **B,** Ligamentum teres. (**A** from Kelley L: Sectional anatomy for imaging professionals, ed 2, St Louis, 2007, Mosby. **B** from Muscolino JE: Kinesiology: the skeletal system and muscle function, St Louis, 2006, Mosby.)

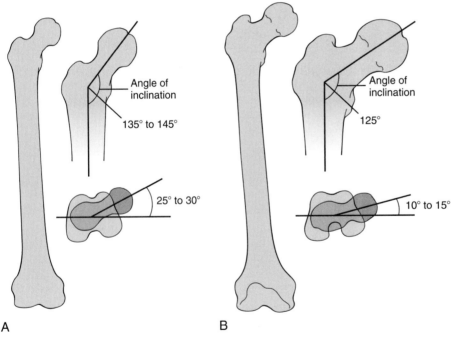

Figure 19-2 Comparison of the newborn (**A**) and adult (**B**) femoral angle of inclination (*top*) and femoral angle of torsion (*bottom*). The enlarged views of the femoral angle or torsion show a superior perspective, looking down from the head and neck of the femur to the femoral condyles. (From Cech D: Functional movement development across the life span, ed 2, Philadelphia, 2003, Saunders.)

femoral head no longer sits in the center. The outer aspect of the acetabulum must then absorb more force from the femoral head, increasing the load on the labrum.[5]

Two basic functional adaptations have been identified in the structure of the femoral head (Figure 19-3). In the first (type I), the femoral head is greater than two thirds of a sphere with maximal angles. Its shaft is slender, and the associated pelvis is small and high slung. This adaptation is suited for speed and movement. The type II adaptation has a femoral head that is nearly a full hemisphere and has minimal angles. Its shaft is thick, and its associated pelvis is broad. This adaptation is for power and strength.

The trabecular bone in the femoral head and neck is designed to withstand high loads (see Figure 19-1, *A*). The design includes both primary and secondary tensile and compressive patterns. The Ward triangle is a site of weakness; this weakness increases with age and this site often sustains osteoporotic fractures. A 5- to 7-degree angle exists in the shaft of the femur with respect to the vertical plane, thus causing an anteroposterior bend. This bend produces strength to withstand ground reaction forces.

The femoral head and neck project anteriorly in relation to the femoral condyles. This angle is known as the *angle of declination* or *femoral torsion angle* (Figure 19-2, *B*), which changes

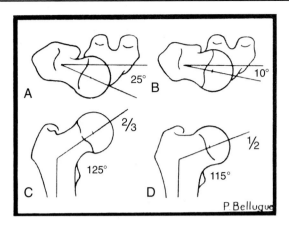

Figure 19-3 Functional adaptations of the femoral head and neck. Type I (**A** and **C**) has a head equal to two thirds of a sphere and maximal angles; type II (**B** and **D**) has a head greater than half of a hemisphere and minimal angles. The angle of inclination is shown in parts **C** and **D**, and the angle of declination is shown in parts **A** and **B**. (From Kapandji IA: The physiology of the joints. II. The lower limb, ed 2, Edinburgh, 1970, Churchill Livingstone.)

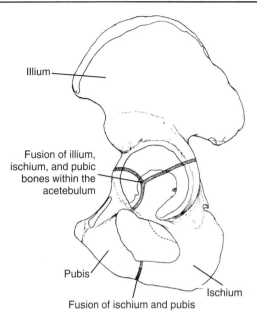

Figure 19-4 The innominate, acetabulum, and labrum. Left innominate, lateral view. Reader should note the junction of the ischium, ilium, and pubic bones in the fossa of the acetabulum.

from birth to adulthood. This angle is approximately 25 to 30 degrees at birth and 10 to 15 degrees in the adult. If this angle is significantly increased, then the condition known as *anteversion* can result in a greater amount of internal rotation (toe in). The hip internal rotation will be increased, and hip external rotation will be decreased; this condition is usually seen in children. Anteversion may also induce genu valgus and or ankle-foot eversion, because the femoral head points back toward the acetabulum. If the angle of declination is significantly decreased, then retroversion results in a greater amount of external rotation (toe out), whether the hip is positioned in 0 or 90 degrees of hip flexion. Anteversion and retroversion affect both the pattern and the range of motion available at the hip joint.[6]

The acetabulum (or socket portion) of the hip joint is comprised of the ilium, ischium, and pubic bones, which fuse to form the innominate (Figure 19-4). It is ellipsoidal shape, not quite hemispheric. Its orientation is directed anterolateral and inferiorly about 30 degrees in the transverse plane (from the sagittal plane); this angle is known as the *anteversion angle*. A fibrocartilaginous ring called the *labrum* inserts into the acetabular rim (see Figure 19-1, *B*). The labrum is triangular in cross section and serves to deepen the acetabulum, increasing contact with the femoral head by about 30%.[7] Tightly packed type I collagen bundles make up the labrum and run parallel to the edge of the acetabulum; some dispersed fibers run obliquely as well.[8] The labrum bridges the acetabular notch along with the transverse acetabular ligament in the ventrocaudal labrum. Within the acetabulum is a horseshoe-shaped (or an inverted *U*) feature with hyaline cartilage lining, which is thicker and broader at the roof and thinner and narrower at the floor. The outer portion of the labrum is vascularized, and the middle portion is sometimes vascularized; however, the inner portion of the labrum is never vascularized.[9] The fovea capitis is the area in the central cartilage occupied by the liga-

mentum teres and the obturator artery where no collagen exists (see Figure 19-1, *B*). A fat pad covers the acetabular floor at this point because no compression or contact by the head occurs there. The labrum of a healthy hip appears to have three functions: as (1) a shock absorber, (2) a closure ring, and (3) a force transmitter.[1]

The Wiberg angle, also called the *center-edge* (CE) angle, is another architectural angle to consider (Figure 19-5). This angle indicates how much the acetabulum overlaps the head. To determine the angle, first connect both centers for a baseline. Then from the center of the head, draw one line perpendicular and a second line connecting with the edge of the acetabular roof. According to Dihlmann,[10] the CE angle is represented by the angle between these lines. Angles between 30 and 35 degrees are considered within normal range for adults.[11] Within the first 2 years of age, values under 10 degrees are considered pathologic conditions. The angle should be at least 15 degrees from age 3 to the early teenage years. By the age of 14, the angle should reach 20 degrees. Murphy et al.[12] demonstrated that a CE angle of less than 16 degrees in adults near the age of 65 or who are suffering from hip dysplasia was associated with severe arthritic changes of the hip.

The osteology of the pelvis is described in greater detail in the discussion of the sacroiliac joints (SIJs). For now, the pelvis can be described as a closed ring composed of the two innominate bones, which are joined anteriorly by the pubic symphysis and posteriorly by the interposed sacrum and the resulting two SIJs. The pelvis functions to transmit vertical forces from the vertebral column to the hips via the SIJs and to transmit ground reaction forces from the legs and hips to the vertebral column (and also via the SIJs). These force transmissions and

"Center-edge" angle

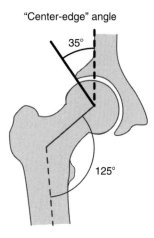

Figure 19-5 The center-edge (CE) angle indicates the relative coverage provided by the acetabulum over the femoral head within the frontal plane. This angle (the Wiberg angle) is formed by the intersection of a vertical reference line (*stippled*) and a line that connects the upper edge of the acetabulum to the center of the femoral head. The normal 125-degree angle of inclination of the proximal femur is also indicated. (From Neumann DA: Kinesiology of the musculoskeletal system: foundations for physical rehabilitation, St Louis, 2002, Mosby.)

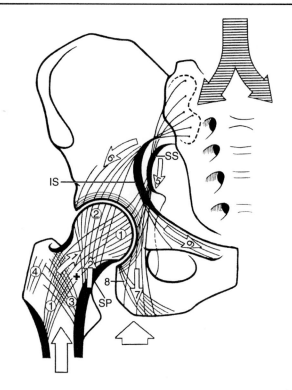

Figure 19-6 Trabecular systems of the hip and pelvis. Main system: (*1*) arcuate and (*2*) supporting bundles. Accessory system: *3* and *4*. The intersections of *1* with *3* and *1* with *2* form the main gothic arches of the hip. A third arch, of less importance, is formed by the intersection of *3* and *4*. Sacroacetabular trabeculae (*5* and *6*) reduce the stress on the sacroiliac joint (SIJ). Set *5* converges with set *1* from the femur; set *6* converges with set *2*. Sacroischial trabeculae (*7* and *8*) intersect to bear the body weight in sitting. (From Kapandji IA: The physiology of the joints, ed 2, vol 3, Edinburgh, 1974, Churchill Livingstone.)

dissipations are accomplished through two trabecular systems: (1) the sacroacetabular system and (2) the sacroischial system (Figure 19-6). The sacroacetabular system resists the forces of compression and traction through the kinetic chain, whereas the sacroischial system resists the forces of compression applied to the pelvis. The sacroischial system bears the weight of the trunk, particularly when the individual is seated.

Arthrology of the Hip

Maximal joint congruence (about 50%) of the hip is achieved in 30 to 60 degrees of flexion, 15 to 30 degrees of abduction, and about 15 degrees of external rotation.[13] This position is termed the *maximally loose-packed position* (MLPP). The ligamentous maximally close-packed position (MCPP) is found instead in maximal extension, adduction, and internal rotation, as well as in maximal extension, abduction, and external rotation.[13] The MCPP provides the greatest joint stability because of the combination of ligamentous tightness and joint congruity. The bony close-packed position is in maximal flexion, abduction, and external rotation.[13] Note that in the erect posture, the femoral head is not completely covered by the acetabulum but is exposed superiorly and anteriorly.

The capsular pattern of motion restriction has the greatest limitation of internal rotation; flexion, extension, and abduction have about equal limitations of motion; external rotation and adduction are least limited. The internal rotation is limited in 0 and 90 degrees of hip flexion.[14]

The fibrous membrane of the hip joint capsule is cylindrical and runs caudolaterally from the acetabular rim to the base of the femoral neck (Figure 19-7). The fibrous membrane is comprised of a superficial layer of longitudinal bands and a deep layer of circular fibers.[15,16] The capsule inserts into the base of

the acetabular labrum, the edge of the acetabulum, and the outer edge of the transverse acetabular ligament. Distally, the posterior capsule attaches just proximal to the intertrochanteric crest. The lateral capsule inserts into the anterior femur along the trochanteric line. The capsule has synovial folds (at the femoral neck) that are located anterior, medial (also called *frenulum of Amantini* or *pectineofoveal fold and/or plica*), and lateral.[3] Blood vessels run within the capsule and reach the femoral head through these folds.

The extraarticular ligaments, including the iliofemoral ligament, pubofemoral ligament, ischiofemoral ligament, and the femoral arcuate ligament, blend with and support the capsule. The two intraarticular ligaments are (1) the transverse acetabular ligament and (2) the ligamentum teres (see Figure 19-7). The anterior ligaments of the hip are arranged in a *Z* shape and are analogous to the glenohumeral ligaments of the shoulder. The iliofemoral ligament (the *Y*-shaped Bertini's ligament or Bigelow's ligament) is considered the strongest ligament of the body and is comprised of two bands: (1) the iliotrochanteric (superior/lateral) band and (2) the inferomedial band. The superior band is stronger and is 8 to 10 mm thick. The inferior band inserts into the lower trochanteric line. Together, these two bands restrict hip extension. This ligament is able to resist

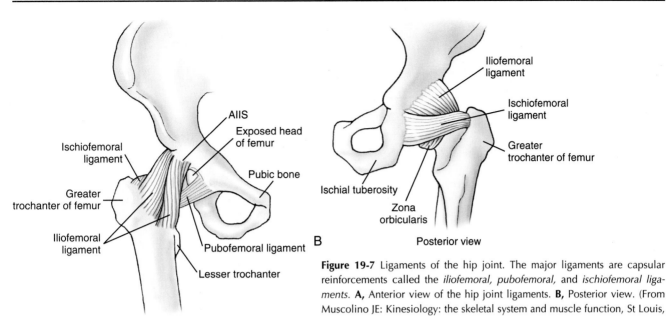

Figure 19-7 Ligaments of the hip joint. The major ligaments are capsular reinforcements called the *iliofemoral, pubofemoral,* and *ischiofemoral ligaments.* **A,** Anterior view of the hip joint ligaments. **B,** Posterior view. (From Muscolino JE: Kinesiology: the skeletal system and muscle function, St Louis, 2006, Mosby.)

much greater tensile forces than the posterior ligaments.[16,17] The great strength of this ligament may explain why only 10% to 15% of hip dislocations and subluxations occur anteriorly.[18] The second anterior ligament, the pubofemoral ligament, attaches on the superior ramus of the pubic bone, blends medially with the pectineus muscle and the inferior band of the iliofemoral ligament, and attaches anteriorly to the intertrochanteric line. Tschauner[1] describes this ligament as the weakest structural link of the hip capsule. This ligament is located between the arms of the *Z,* where the capsule is thinner. The iliofemoral bursa lies here as well, between the iliopsoas tendon and the capsule.

The posterior ligament of the hip, the ischiofemoral ligament (Figure 19-7, *B*), arises from the posterior acetabular rim and the labrum and attaches to the trochanteric line, deep to the iliofemoral ligament. The capsule is strengthened by the ischiofemoral ligament as it winds posteriorly around the femur to attach anteriorly. The femoral arcuate ligament, formerly called the *zona orbicularis,*[16] has some fibers that run transversely to blend with the ischiofemoral ligament. The femoral arcuate ligament originates on the greater trochanter and inserts onto the lesser trochanter. Although it does not cross the hip joint, it creates tension in the capsule at the end ranges flexion and extension. In tension studies, this ligament achieved the least amount of stiffness and failed at the lowest forces when compared with the other hip ligaments. The ligamentum teres (see Figure 19-1, *B*) attaches to the fovea of the femoral head and has three bands that extend to the pubic portion of the lunate surface of the acetabulum, to the upper border of the transverse acetabular ligament, and to the ischial side of the lunate fossa. When ruptured by trauma, the teres ligament has been identified as a pain generator.[19] The tension in this ligament increases with maximal adduction.

In bipedal stance, both the anterior and the posterior ligaments coil in the same direction around the hip. In the erect posture, all ligaments are under modest tension. In extension, all ligaments tighten, especially the inferior band of the iliofemoral ligament, which blends with the iliopsoas muscle and checks posterior tilting of the pelvis. In flexion, all ligaments relax. In external rotation, all anterior ligaments tighten and the posterior relax; the reverse occurs with internal rotation. With adduction, the iliotrochanteric band tightens, the pubofemoral ligament slackens, and the ischiofemoral ligament relaxes. In abduction, the pubofemoral ligament tightens, the iliotrochanteric band slackens, and the ischiofemoral band tightens (Table 19-1).

Neurovascular Supply of the Hip

The innervation of the hip joint and capsule is primarily derived from the L3 segment with spinal cord connections from L2 to S1.[20] The nerve supply is derived directly from the femoral nerve through its muscular branches: the obturator nerve, the accessory obturator nerve, the nerve to the quadratus femoris, and the superior gluteal nerve (Figure 19-8, *A*). The great overlap of the nerves in this region creates the potential for a variety of pain referral patterns; therefore the clinician must check the lumbar spine, the SIJ, and CFJ in patients with complaints in this region.

The blood supply is derived from the obturator, the medial and lateral circumflex femoral arteries and veins, and the superior and inferior gluteal arteries and veins (Figure 19-8, *B*).[21] The acetabular fossa and head of the femur receive blood supply from the acetabular branch of the obturator and medial femoral circumflex vessels, which run through the ligamentum teres. Necrosis of the femoral head typically begins at the anterior aspect, because of closure of the lateral circumflex network. Early traumatic dislocation can predispose one to later AVN.

Lymphatic drainage is accomplished primarily by the deep inguinal lymphatic chain, particularly the upper and middle

Table 19-1	Overview of the Ligaments and Their Restraining Function of Anatomic Motions

Ligament	Restraining Function
Iliofemoral, medial part	Extension (end range) of the hip or posterior tilt of the pelvis
	External rotation
	Internal rotation (to some extent)
Iliofemoral magnum	Extension of the hip or posterior tilt of the pelvis
Iliofemoral, lateral part	Extension (end range) of the hip or posterior tilt of the pelvis
	Adduction
	External rotation
Pubofemoral	Extension
	Adduction
	External rotation
Ischiofemoral (Tillman, 1998)	Internal rotation
	Extension
	Adduction
Ischiofemoral, superior part (Fuss, 1991)	Internal rotation
	Extension
	Adduction
Ischiofemoral, lateral inferior part (Fuss, 1991)	Flexion, from an extreme adducted or from a middle position
Ischiofemoral, medial inferior part (Fuss, 1991)	Flexion
Arcuate femoral	Flexion (end range)
	Extension (end range)

From Sizer PS, Phelps V, Brismeé et al: Diagnosis-specific orthopedic management of the hip, Minneapolis, 2008, Orthopedic Physical Therapy Products.

	Muscle	Innervation
Posterior	Gluteus maximus	Inferior gluteal nerve, L5 to S2
	Gluteus medius	Superior gluteal nerve, L5 and S1
	Gluteus minimus	Superior gluteal nerve, L5 and S1
	Piriformis	L5 to S2
	Superior and inferior gemelli	L5 and S1
	Obturator externus	Posterior obturator nerve, L3 L4
	Obturator internus	L5 and S1
	Quadratus femoris	L5 and S1
	Semitendinous membranous	Sciatic nerve tibial portion L5-S2
	Biceps femoris	Sciatic nerve long head tibial portion short head common peroneal L5 to S2
Medial	Adductor longus	Anterior obturator nerve, L2 L4
	Adductor magnus	Obturator nerve
		Tibial division of the sciatic nerve, L2 L4
	Adductor brevis	Obturator nerve, L2 IA
	Pectineus	Accessory obturator nerve, L2 L3
		Femoral nerve, L2 L3
	Gracilis	Obturator nerve, L2 L3
Anterior	Iliopsoas	Femoral nerve, L2 L3
		Lumbar nerves, L1 L3
	Rectus femoris	Femoral nerve, L2 L4
	Sartorius	Femoral nerve, L2, L3, and L4
Lateral	Tensor fasciae latae	Superior gluteal nerve, L4 L5

nodes (which lie in the femoral canal and the lateral part of the femoral ring) and the extrailiac lymph nodes.

Myology of the Hip

The muscles that run parallel to the femoral neck—the gluteals, piriformis, obturator externus, and quadratus femoris—are considered the rotator cuff of the hip.[22] These muscles work together to improve functional mobility. The flexors and extensors include the gluteus maximus, all hamstring muscles, iliopsoas, rectus femoris, tensor fasciae latae (TFL), and sartorius. These muscles provide pelvic stability in the sagittal plane. The deep muscles include the gemelli, obturators, and piriformis. These muscles are rarely implicated as the primary cause of buttock pain, unless resisted abduction and external rotation causes pain (from a position of hip flexion with internal rotation), which indicates involvement of the piriformis. The abductors and adductors increase pelvic stabilization in a closed kinetic chain.[23]

The muscles of the hip divided into four compartments: (1) posterior, (2) medical, (3) anterior, and (4) lateral (Figures 19-8 and 19-9).

For a discussion of the influence of many of these muscles on the pelvis, refer to "Myology of the Pelvis."

POSTERIOR MUSCULATURE

Gluteus Maximus

The gluteus maximus is innervated by the inferior gluteal nerve, L5 to S2. This muscle is primarily an extensor of the hip from 0 to 90 degrees of flexion, an external rotator of the hip at 0 degrees, and an internal rotator and abductor the hip at 90 degrees of flexion. The gluteus maximus also assists in pelvic stability at heel-strike during the gait cycle. It is a phasic muscle and tends to weaken with dysfunction.

Gluteus Medius

The gluteus medius is innervated by the superior gluteal nerve, L5 and S1. It is primarily an abductor at 0 degrees, but its anterior fibers can flex, abduct, and internally rotate the hip in

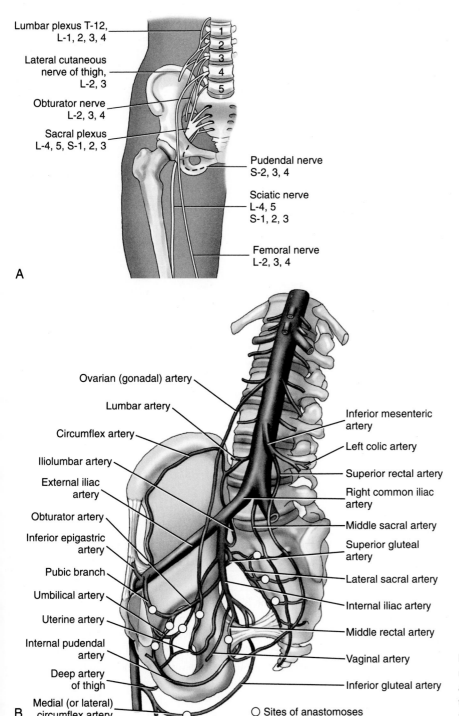

Figure 19-8 A, Anterior and posterior views of right leg with nerves. **B,** Anterior view of iliac arteries. (From Kelley LL, Petersen CM: Sectional anatomy for imaging professionals, ed 2, St Louis, 2007, Mosby.)

90 degrees of flexion while the posterior fibers extend and externally rotate the hip. It serves as the main lateral stabilizer of the hip and pelvis. The gluteus medius also decelerates hip adduction. Its fibers run parallel to the femoral shaft, with the anterior part coursing slightly backward and the posterior part running slightly forward. It is not a very strong muscle until the femur is abducted 30 degrees or more, which brings its fibers more perpendicular to the shaft. Only the anterior part of this muscle can be palpated (directly behind the TFL)

because the posterior third is covered by the gluteus maximus. It is a phasic muscle and tends to weaken with dysfunction, producing the Trendelenburg's gait pattern.

Gluteus Minimus

The gluteus minimus is completely covered by other muscles; it lies deep to the medius and is likewise innervated by the superior gluteal nerve, L5 and S1. It functions as a medial

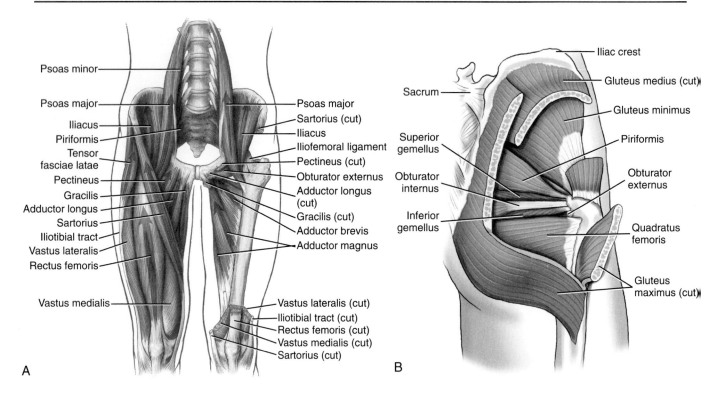

Figure 19-9 A, Muscles of the anterior hip region. The right side shows the primary flexors and adductor muscles of the hip. Many muscles on the left side are cut to expose the adductor brevis and adductor magnus. **B,** Posterior view of deep muscles of right hip and thigh. (**A** from Neumann DA: Kinesiology of the musculoskeletal system: foundations for physical rehabilitation, St Louis, 2002, Mosby. **B** from Kelley LL, Petersen CM: Sectional anatomy for imaging professionals, ed 2, St Louis, 2007, Mosby.)

lateral stabilizer of the hip, as well as an internal rotator and abductor of the femur.[24]

Piriformis

The piriformis muscle arises on the anterior surface of the sacrum (S2 to S4), the sacroiliac ventral capsule, and the anterior part of the posterior inferior iliac spine (PIIS) of the ilium (and often the upper part of the sacrotuberous ligament). Its tendon passes through the greater sciatic foramen to the greater trochanter of the femur. The piriformis muscle is the most superficial external rotator of the hip. It is a two-joint muscle, acting on both the sacrum and the femur. The function of this muscle changes depending on the position of the hip joint. The piriformis muscle externally rotates, abducts and extends the thigh in 0 degrees (neutral position), up to 60 degrees of hip flexion. However, in 90 degrees of hip flexion, the piriformis internally rotates and abducts.[25] To stretch this muscle in maximal hip flexion, the hip must be flexed, adducted, and externally rotated. The piriformis derives its innervation from the L5 to S2 nerve roots. The nerves of the sciatic plexus and the inferior gluteal vessels run intimately together. In 90% of individuals, these nerves and vessels pass under the piriformis. In 10% of the population, the nerves and vessels pierce the body of the muscle, passing through it. Thus dysfunction of the piriformis can compress the sciatic nerve against the foramen. The piriformis is a postural muscle and tends to tighten with dysfunction, producing external rotation of the

femur and restriction of internal rotation. Dysfunction of the piriformis can thus cause problems with both the SIJ and the hip.

Superior and Inferior Gemelli, Obturator Externus and Internus, Quadratus Femoris

All these muscles are external rotators of the hip and function best when the hip is in extension, although they also abduct the hip when it is flexed.[26] The obturator externus and quadratus femoris externally rotate and adduct the thigh (see Figure 19-9). They run close to the capsule and help reinforce it. The obturator externus is innervated by the posterior obturator nerve, L3 L4, and the obturator internus is innervated by the nerve to the obturator internus, L5 and S1. All the others are innervated by nerve roots L5 and S1.

Hamstrings

The hamstrings are two-joint muscles acting at both the knee and the hip. They have a common origin on the lateral border of the ischial tuberosity, with the exception of the short head of the biceps femoris muscle, which attaches on the linea aspera on the posterior aspect of the femur. Bilateral tightness or contracture produces a posterior pelvic tilt. The semimembranosus and semitendinosus both extend the hip, flex the knee, and internally rotate the tibia.[27] The long head of the biceps femoris acts on the hip, whereas the short head acts on the knee.

The long head is active during less forceful activities, such as decelerating the leg at the end of the swing phase, and during forceful hip extension.[28] It extends the hip, flexes the knee, and externally rotates the tibia. The biceps femoris usually has an interrelationship with the sacrotuberous ligament; therefore its function is related to SIJ function.[29,30] As the sciatic nerve loops through a groove around the ischial tuberosity, the hamstring tendon sends a fascial envelope around the sciatic nerve, which can potentially entrap it (a condition known as *hamstring syndrome*). A strong relationship exists between a history of severe biceps femoris strain and latent onset of this condition.[23] The semitendinosus and semimembranosus are innervated by the tibial division of the sciatic nerve, L5 to S2. The biceps femoris long head innervated by the tibial division of the sciatic nerve, L5 to S2, whereas the short head is innervated by the peroneal division.

MEDIAL MUSCULATURE

The medial muscles as a group arise from the pubis and insert on the posterior and posteromedial aspects of the femur. They are postural muscles and tend to tighten with dysfunction. Tightness unilaterally produces a lateral pelvic tilt high to the involved side, creating the appearance of a long leg.

Adductors

With resisted adduction, the adductor longus is the most visible and palpable of the adductors. This muscle originates on the pubic tubercle and inserts on the middle third of the linea aspera of the femur. In extension, this muscle also assists with external rotation, and when the hip is in other positions it aides in internal rotation. Sports that exert excessive force to the adductors (e.g., soccer, swimming, long-distance running) can cause chronic tendonitis in the adductor longus. The adductor magnus is the most powerful (and the least often injured) adductor. This muscle also originates on the pubis to inserts on the linea aspera and adductor tubercle of the femur. The primary function of the magnus is to adduct the femur, with anterior fibers that simultaneously flex the femur and posterior fibers that extend the femur. The adductor brevis arises from the body and inferior ramus of the pubis and inserts on the line from the greater trochanter of the linea aspera of the femur. This muscle adducts, flexes, and medial rotates the femur. The adductor longus is innervated by the anterior obturator nerve, L2 to L4; the adductor magnus is innervated by the obturator nerve and the tibial division of the sciatic nerve, L2 to L4; the adductor brevis is innervated by the obturator nerve, L2 Ia.

Pectineus

The pectineus muscle—along with the iliopsoas and the adductor longus—form the floor of the femoral triangle. The pectineus originates on the superior ramus of the pubis, and inserts on the femur, just below the lesser trochanter. It flexes, adducts and internally rotates the femur. It is innervated by the accessory obturator nerve, L2 and L3, and the femoral nerve, L2 and L3. The pectineus, gracilis and adductor longus are the three most common muscles involved in pubalgia.

Gracilis

The gracilis is the only two joint adductor and is innervated by the obturator nerve, L2 and L3. It is the longest, most superficial and medial of the hip adductors. This muscle originates on the inferior pubic ramus and inserts on the medial surface of the proximal tibia at the pes anserinus, where it also inserts with the sartorius and semitendinosus muscles. The functions of the gracilis are to adduct, flex, and internally rotate the femur, as well as to aid in knee flexion.

ANTERIOR MUSCULATURE

Iliopsoas

The iliopsoas forms at the junction of the iliacus—from the iliac fossa—with the psoas major, which arises from the transverse processes of L1 to L5. Their common tendon inserts into the lesser trochanter of the femur. The iliopsoas is a two-joint muscle and the most powerful hip flexor. When the spine is stable, it flexes the hip (and adducts and externally rotates it to some degree); when the femur is stable, it extends the lumbosacral spine. Unilateral contraction side bends the spine ipsilaterally and rotates the spine contralaterally. The iliopsoas acts as a primary stabilizer of the hip in erect posture. Because it is a postural muscle, it tightens with dysfunction, producing hip flexion and increased lumbar lordosis. The iliopsoas is innervated by the femoral nerve, L2 to L3, and the lumbar nerves, L1 to L3.

Rectus Femoris

The rectus femoris is a two-joint muscle comprised of two heads. The straight head arises from the anterior inferior iliac spine (AIIS); the reflected head arises from the margins of the hip joint capsule along the groove above the acetabulum. The rectus femoris inserts into the common quadriceps tendon on the upper border of the patella and into the tibial tuberosity. It is a hip flexor and a knee extender and is innervated by the femoral nerve, L2 to L4.

Sartorius

The sartorius cuts across the thigh obliquely from the ASIS and runs posteriorly to the medial femoral condyle before reaching the superomedial tibia. Along with the gracilis and semitendinosus, the sartorius forms the pes anserinus, which inserts just medial to the tibial tuberosity. It is the longest muscle in the body and crosses two joints. It flexes, externally rotates, and abducts the hip, as well as flexes the knee. It forms the lateral border of the femoral triangle (the superior border is the inguinal ligament, and the medial border is the adductor longus). It is innervated by the femoral nerve, L2, L3, and L4.

LATERAL MUSCULATURE

Tensor Fasciae Latae

The TFL arises from the anterior part of the outer lip of the iliac crest and from the lateral surface of the ASIS, and it inserts into the iliotibial band, which continues distally to the tibial tuberosity (see Figure 19-9). It should be noted that the biceps femoris tendon and the lateral collateral ligament insert more posteriorly and attach on the fibula, not to be mistaken for the iliotibial tract on the tibia. The TFL, along with the superior fibers of the gluteus maximus, form the deltoid of the hip. It is primarily an abductor, but it can also flex and internally rotate the hip. The TFL has a very long lever arm where the iliotibial band crosses the knee. It tends to tighten with dysfunction. Unilateral tightness produces a lateral pelvic tilt low ipsilaterally. Bilateral tightness produces an anterior pelvic tilt. The trochanteric bursae lie deep to this muscle where it passes over the greater trochanter. The TFL is innervated by the superior gluteal nerve, L4 and L5.

ENTRAPMENT SYNDROMES OF THE HIP AND PELVIS

Several peripheral nerve entrapment syndromes that can occur in and around the hip and pelvis are briefly mentioned here, not only to alert the clinician to the possibility of neurogenic pain in this region but also to emphasize the anatomic considerations of such entrapment. The nerves of the muscles that cross the hip that can be entrapped include the femoral, obturator, and superior gluteal nerves, as well as the nerve to the quadratus femoris and the sacral plexus. The previously mentioned nerves are important because they also supply the joint and the joint capsule. Therefore the hip joint can refer pain anywhere in the hip, buttock, groin, thigh, leg, or foot.

Femoral Nerve

The femoral nerve, L2 to L4, descends through the psoas and traverses over the iliacus (see Figure 19-8, *A*). It exits the pelvis behind the inguinal ligament and passes through the lacuna musculorum, which sits lateral to the femoral artery. The femoral nerve lies close to the femoral head, separated by only a thin layer of muscle and capsule. Trauma or hematoma here may cause entrapment, producing pain and muscle weakness in the iliopsoas, sartorius, pectineus, and quadriceps muscles. The main complaint is generally pain that starts below the inguinal ligament and can encompass the anteromedial surface of the thigh, as well as the medial surface of the leg all the way down to the medial surface of the foot. Local tenderness in the groin is almost always present. Muscle stretch reflexes of the knee will be diminished. Femoral nerve palsy has also been reported after cardiac catheterization, anterior lumbar spine fusion, acetabular fracture, total hip arthroscopy, and spontaneously in hemophilia.[31-33]

Sciatic Nerve

The sciatic nerve, L4 to S2, usually exits the sciatic notch along the inferior edge of the piriformis muscle (see Figure 19-8, *A*). From there it runs inferiorly along the lateral border of the ischial tuberosity. Occasionally, the lateral division of this nerve pierces the piriformis, which can compress the sciatic nerve with contraction.[34] The lateral division forms the peroneal trunk. Piriformis syndrome is an umbrella term that describes many causes of buttock pain and symptoms. Such symptoms may stem from compression of the sciatic nerve or issues external to the nerve such as disc herniation, irritation from inflammation caused by a bulged disc, or other conditions.[35-37] Piriformis syndrome may also be caused by cumulative trauma from repetitive activities such as running that create tension in the sciatic nerve.[38] Straight-leg raise (SLR) and slump testing will be painful, and the most painful test will be resisted hip external rotation from full internal rotation with the patient reclined at 45 degrees of trunk flexion.[35] A true neuropathic condition produces a flail leg and foot, although neuropathic condition secondary to direct external trauma at the sciatic notch is rare. Another condition resulting from sciatic nerve entrapment is hamstring syndrome. This condition is characterized by epineural irritation as the nerve runs around the ischial tuberosity and goes through a fibrous band from the insertion of the biceps femoris at the tuberosity.[39] The common triad seen in this syndrome will be pain at the ischial tuberosity with sitting, pain with resisted knee flexion with the leg in a SLR position (although resisted knee flexion prone can be painless), and pain with neural testing (e.g., SLR, slump test). Palpation will be tender over the sciatic nerve just lateral to the ischial tuberosity.[38] Previous hamstring injury, low-back pain, or surgery that could predispose the sciatic nerve to more risk of injury often precede this condition. This syndrome is often seen in jumping athletes, power sprinters, and distance runners.[40] The sciatic nerve innervates the hamstrings, the adductor magnus, and all the muscles of the leg and foot. It provides sensory innervation to the posterolateral leg and the plantar and dorsal aspects of the foot (see the section on the piriformis under "Myology of the Hip").

Obturator Nerve

The two most common causes of obturator nerve (L2 to L4) entrapment are obturator hernias and osteitis pubis (see Figure 19-8, *A*). Both conditions entrap the nerve in the obturator foramen. Obturator nerve entrapment is characterized by groin pain to the inner thigh, which is exacerbated with the Valsalva maneuver and is not relieved with rest. The fascia over this nerve may contribute to the compression of the nerve, or it may trigger development of a compartment syndrome.[41] True neuropathy will cause pain and weakness in the muscles it supplies including the adductors, the gracilis, the obturator externus, and occasionally the pectineus. Pain from this nerve refers from the medial thigh to the groin. Hip motion will cause pain, and crossing the legs (external rotation and adduction) may be difficult. Patients may exhibit a waddling gait secondary to pain and adductor weakness and in an attempt to restrict hip motion.

Ilioinguinal Nerve

The ilioinguinal nerve, L1 and L2, is vulnerable to entrapment in the region of the ASIS. This nerve follows the pattern of an intercostal nerve and emerges from the lateral border of the psoas major, arriving in the region of the ASIS. Here it turns medially and traverses the abdominal muscles, piercing the transversus abdominis and internal oblique (which it supplies) to reach the spermatic cord or mons pubis and labia majora, under the external oblique muscle. Entrapment of this nerve causes pain into the groin with some radiation to the proximal inner surface of the thigh. Pain is aggravated by increasing tension in the abdominal wall on standing erect and by hip motion, particularly extension. Pressure over a point medial to the ASIS will cause pain to radiate into the area of innervation. A high incidence of lower-back difficulties is associated with ilioinguinal nerve entrapment.

Lateral Femoral Cutaneous Nerve

The lateral femoral cutaneous nerve is a sensory nerve, L2 and L3, and is vulnerable to entrapment in the region of the proximal crest of the ASIS, where it passes through the lateral end of the inguinal ligament. The exact site where the nerve exits the pelvis varies (see Figure 19-8, A).[42] The condition, known as *meralgia paresthetica*, is characterized by a burning pain in the anterior and lateral portions of the thigh. Pressure over the ASIS usually aggravates the pain. The mechanism of onset may be traumatic, but very often the condition is idiopathic. Pelvic tilt or a short leg resulting in postural alterations may be associated with meralgia paresthetica.

FUNCTIONAL ANATOMY AND MECHANICS OF THE PELVIS

Bernhard Siegfried Albinus (1697-1770) and William Hunter were the first anatomists to demonstrate that the SIJ was a true synovial joint. Meckel (in 1816) and Von Luschka (in 1854), who first classified the joint as *diarthrodial,* later confirmed these studies. Albee (in 1909) and Brooke (in 1924) confirmed a synovial membrane and articular cartilage within the joint.[43] Solonen[44] conducted a comprehensive study in 1957 on the osteology and arthrology of the pelvic girdle.

Orientation Planes of the Pelvis

To understand the relationships of the structure and movements of the sacrum, lumbar spine, and lower extremities, one must understand and be able to relate them to the reference planes of the pelvis and the cardinal planes of the body. By understanding these planes, one is able to describe the direction and degree of motion of any given pelvic landmark in relation to any other specified landmark.

The three cardinal planes of the body are (1) the transverse plane, which bisects the body through the center of gravity into upper and lower halves; (2) the sagittal plane, which bisects the body in the midline through the center of gravity into right and left halves; and (3) the frontal plane, which bisects the body through the shoulders anteroposteriorly into ventral and dorsal halves.

The pelvic region is made up of three bony parts: (1) the right ilium, (2) the left ilium, and (3) the sacrum. The sacrum is connected to both ilia through the SIJs. The pubic symphysis connects the two ilia. The upper body averages about 65% of the total body weight and is transferred to both SIJs through the sacrum. According to Vleeming et al.[45] and Snijders et al.,[46] small amounts of motion occur at the SIJ, but this movement cannot be detected manually because the joint is too deep. Impaired load transfer through the SIJs causes sacroiliac dysfunction. There has been much debate between different practitioners regarding the biomechanics of the pelvis. Bilateral hip flexion (nutation) produces the most consistent three-dimensional (3-D) pattern.[47] In nonweight-bearing positions, the innominate external rotation (outflare) is a part of all SIJ motion that results from hip movement. Therefore the rotary axis of the SIJ must be outside the sacrum but through the pubis. All SIJ motions (rotary and translatory) are 3-D, as a result of maximal hip motions in nonweight bearing.[48,49]

The lumbar spine moves primarily in the sagittal plane (flexion and extension), whereas the hip moves in three planes including rotation (which the lumbar spine does not like). Therefore the pelvis must work together with both sides to accommodate the hip rotation while still allowing movement within the pelvis during gait. Much of the movement in the SIJ is due to deformation of cartilage on the surfaces of the innominate facets, primarily with weight bearing. The reciprocal movement that occurs is due to the pubic symphysis.

The SIJ axis of rotation direction and location depends on three factors: (1) the pelvic load and support, (2) the joint surface geometry, and (3) the physical properties of the connections between both joints. These three factors make understanding the axis of the rotation of the SIJ very complex. What is essential to understand in the clinic is what influences the mobility of the SIJ and how the different factors are related.[50]

Pelvic Anatomy

The SIJ, along with other transitional areas of the spine, are important in understanding vertebral joint problems.[21] A functional unit is formed by the lumbar spine, the sacrum, the innominates, and the hip joints. Almost every movement of the lumbar spine influences the pelvic ring (SIJs and pubic symphysis). Forces are transmitted either up or down from the lower extremities to the spine through the pelvic ring. The lumbosacral junction is the weakest link in this kinetic chain. Many strong collagenous connections exist between the sacrum and surrounding bones, as well as the iliolumbar ligaments, which connect L4 and L5 to the ilium without being directly connected to the sacrum (Figure 19-10).

The SIJ is a "mobile stabilizer" and relies on form closure and force closure. The roles of the SIJ include force transduction, shock absorption, and motion control. A multitude of treatment techniques are aimed at correcting pelvic dysfunction. The pelvic joints not only produce pain but also may refer pain. Many practitioners are mistakenly taught that the articulations of the pelvis (the pubic symphysis and the SIJs) have no functional movements except in childbirth and therefore do not contribute to complaints of pain or dysfunction except in rare instances such as disease and trauma. However, the pelvic joints do indeed move[29,30,44,51] and can be involved directly or indirectly in mechanical low-back problems. Sturesson et al.[52] found the SIJ to translate less than 1 mm, whereas Smidt et al.[47] found it to move less than 3 mm.

The pelvic girdle is considered to be a closed osteoarticular ring composed of five functional pieces: the two pelvic halves/ilium (innominates), the sacrum (which could be one or two bones that together form the coccyx), and the two hip joints. The two innominates are conjoined anteriorly by the pubic symphysis and posteriorly by the sacrum and the resulting two SIJs. The pelvic girdle supports the organs of the lower pelvis and abdomen and provides a dynamic link between the spine and the lower limbs, transmitting vertical forces between them as part of the global sling system.[54]

Pelvic Types

Four types of pelves are described in *Gray's Anatomy*: (1) anthropoid, (2) android, (3) gynaecoid, and (4) platypelloid.[55] These pelvic types differ in the dimensions of the superior and inferior apertures, the greater sciatic notch, and the subpubic arches. In addition, proportional differences exist between the fore and hind pelvis, as well as between the anterior and posterior transverse diameters of the inlets. The differences among the four types depend mainly on the gender of the individual.

Gender differences between male and female pelves have to do with function. Although the primary function of both pelves is locomotion, the female pelvis must also accommodate childbirth. The male pelvis is designed more for power and strength; it is more heavily built, and the general architecture is more angular in orientation. The female pelvis is broader and deeper, with its iliac wings more vertically set but shallower than in the male pelvis.

The pelvis functions to transmit vertical forces from the vertebral column to the hips via the SIJs or to transmit ground reaction forces from the legs and hips to the vertebral column via the SIJs. These force transmissions and dissipations are accomplished through two trabecular systems previously

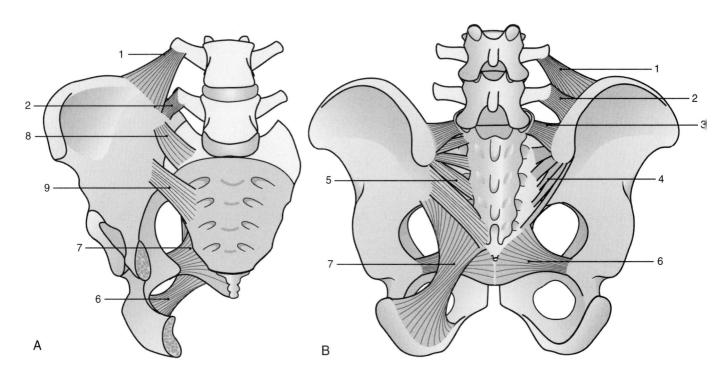

Figure 19-10 The sacral joint capsule and ligaments. **A,** Anterior view, **B,** Posterior view. *1,* Superior bundle of the iliolumbar ligament. *2,* Inferior bundle of the iliolumbar ligament. *3,* Intermediate plane ligament from the iliac crest to the transverse process of S1. *4,* Posterior sacroiliac ligaments. *5,* Anterior plane of the sacroiliac ligaments (deep fibers of the interosseous ligaments). *6,* Sacrospinous ligament. *7,* Sacrotuberous ligament. *8,* Anteroposterior bundle of the anterior sacroiliac ligaments. *9,* Anteroinferior bundle of the anterior sacroiliac ligaments. (From Kapandji IA: The physiology of the joints, ed 6, vol 3, Edinburgh, 2008, Churchill Livingstone.)

mentioned: (1) the sacroacetabular system and (2) the sacroischial system (see "Osteology of the Hip").

Osteology of the Pelvis

Innominate Bones

Each of the innominate bones is comprised of three bones—(1) the ilium, (2) ischium, and (3) pubis—that are fused in adults at the acetabulum. Because no functional movement occurs between these fused bones, each innominate is a functional unit (Figure 19-11).

Ilium

The fan-shaped ilium makes up the superior portion of the acetabulum. The anterior superior iliac spine (ASIS) and the posterior superior iliac spine (PSIS) are on the front and back, respectively, of the iliac crest. The ilium has an irregular curve inferior to the PSIS, which ends at the PIIS.

The articular surface for the SIJ is on the posterosuperior aspect of the ilium and faces medially to articulate with the sacrum. The articular surface is L shaped, like the sacrum, with the short arm axis in the craniocaudal plane and the long arm axis in the anteroposterior plane. The iliac surface is a thin (0.5 mm), rough fibrocartilage, whereas the sacral surface consists of thicker (3 mm), smooth hyaline cartilage. The different cartilage between the two surfaces creates friction and stability. According to Salsibali et al.,[56] the sacral cartilage is thicker in female subjects than in male subjects. In adults, many ridges and depressions develop with age (by the fourth decade of life) on the articular surface. The strong interosseous sacroiliac ligaments attach to this rough surface on the medial aspect of the

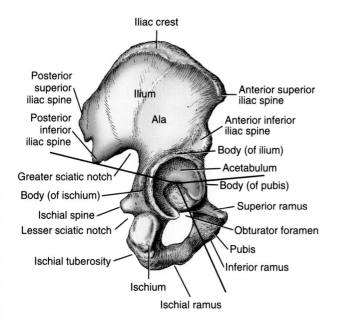

Figure 19-11 Lateral aspect of right os coxae with divisions. (From Frank ED, Long BW, Smith BJ: Merrill's atlas of radiographic positions and radiologic procedures, ed 11, St Louis, 2007, Mosby.)

ilium, superior to the articular surface. The SIJ is too deep to be palpated.

Ischium

The ischium is formed by the inferolateral third of the innominate. The upper part includes the body and forms the posterior two-fifths of the acetabulum. The ischial tuberosity is formed by the inferior aspect of the ischial body and the ramus. This tuberosity is an important landmark and serves as the attachment site for strong muscles and ligaments, including the hamstrings and the sacrotuberous ligament.

Pubis

The pubic bone of each of the innominates is joined anteriorly in the midline (to close the anterior ring) by an amphiarthrosis at the pubic symphysis (Figure 19-12). This joint is classified as a *symphysis* because it lacks synovial tissue or fluid, and a fibrocartilaginous disc sits in the lower half of the symphysis. The surface of the bones is covered by a thin layer of hyaline cartilage, separated by the disc. A cavity (nonsynovial) may often be found in the posterosuperior part of the disc, but this cavity is not present before 10 years of age.[55] The ligaments that support the pubic symphysis include the superior pubic ligament, the inferior arcuate pubic ligament, the posterior pubic ligament, and the anterior pubic ligament, which is thick and contains both transverse and oblique fibers. The anterior public ligament also receives fibers from the abdominal aponeurosis and the adductor longus (see Figure 19-12, *D*). The superior pubic ligament runs transversely between the pubic tubercles as a thick fibrous band, and the inferior arcuate ligament blends with the articular disc and attaches to the inferior pubic rami bilaterally. The arcuate ligament has diagonal ligamentous fibers running from cranial to caudal on opposite sides. These fibers serve to transfer loads cranial from the rectus abdominis and contralateral adductors (i.e., Vleeming's sling system). Symphyseal instability may irritate the arcuate ligament. The posterior pubic ligament is a membranous structure that blends with the adjacent periosteum. The pubic symphysis receives muscle attachments superiorly from the rectus abdominis and external oblique muscles and inferiorly from the adductor longus muscles.

The pubic tubercle lies on the lateral aspect of the pubic crest, just lateral to the midsymphyseal line. Chronic pubalgia may affect the rectus abdominis insertion on the cranial part of the ramus. Other soft tissues associated with this area include the inguinal ligament (located more laterally) and the adductor longus, which inserts on the caudal tubercle. The spermatic cord also runs anterior to the pubic tubercle in male subjects.

The superior pubic ramus serves as the origin of the pectineus muscle at the pectin pubis (cranial to the obturator ridge) (see Figure 19-11). This is a possible site of stress fracture at the ridge. The inferior pubic ramus is where the gracilis originates.

The anterior symphysis receives innervation from the femoral nerve (L2 to L4), which can produce groin pain. The

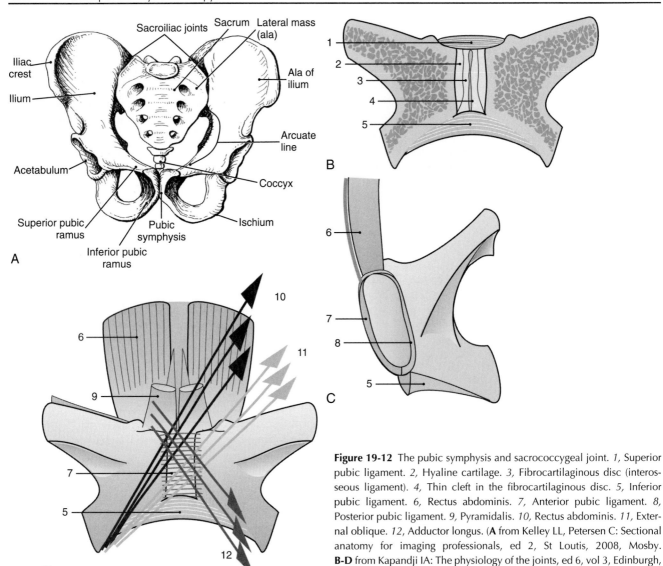

Figure 19-12 The pubic symphysis and sacrococcygeal joint. *1,* Superior pubic ligament. *2,* Hyaline cartilage. *3,* Fibrocartilaginous disc (interosseous ligament). *4,* Thin cleft in the fibrocartilaginous disc. *5,* Inferior pubic ligament. *6,* Rectus abdominis. *7,* Anterior pubic ligament. *8,* Posterior pubic ligament. *9,* Pyramidalis. *10,* Rectus abdominis. *11,* External oblique. *12,* Adductor longus. (**A** from Kelley LL, Petersen C: Sectional anatomy for imaging professionals, ed 2, St Loutis, 2008, Mosby. **B-D** from Kapandji IA: The physiology of the joints, ed 6, vol 3, Edinburgh, 2008, Churchill Livingstone.)

posterior symphysis is innervated by the pudendal nerve (S2 to S4), and can produce scrotal and/or labial pain.

Sacrum

The sacrum provides stability between the innominates and transmits the body weight from the mobile spine to the pelvic girdle. The iliac portions of the posterior innominate bones articulate with the sacrum to produce the SIJs. The sacrum is a strong triangular bone formed by the fusion of the five sacral vertebrae, and it sits as a wedge between the innominates (see Figure 19-11). The sacrum is generally asymmetrical from side to side, and its shape also varies between individuals. The base of the sacrum (S1) is wide; together with the fifth lumbar vertebra, it forms the lumbosacral junction. Its anterior projecting edge is known as the *sacral promontory.* The sacral apex (S5) articulates with the coccyx. The sacral hiatus includes the posterior aspect of the S5 vertebral body and the sacral cornua, which are bilateral downward projections that are the inferior articular processes of S5. About 2 cm from either side

of the hiatus, on the inferolateral borders, are the inferior lateral angles (ILA) (Figure 19-13). The lateral sacral crest has three deep depressions at S1, S2, and S3. The interosseous sacroiliac ligament has strong attachments to these depressions. The sacrum is curved ventrally, increasing the capacity of the true pelvis for visceral contents and childbearing. Posteriorly, the sacrum encases the spinal canal and the end of the cauda equina.

Sacroiliac Joints

The SIJs are synovial articulations or a diarthrosis.[57] The adult male auricle is *C*-form in shape and extends from S1 to S3. In the adult female subject, the joint has an inverted *L*-shaped auricular surface, because women need more translation from S1 to S2, and it is characterized by irregularities (elevations and depressions) in the joint surfaces (see Figure 19-10). The contours of the articular surface are quite variable and depend on the age and gender of the individual. The continued debate on the mechanics, testing (close to 60 tests exist for the SIJ),

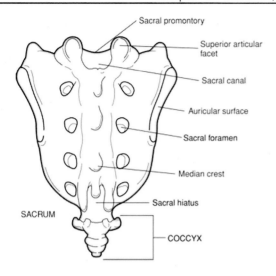

Figure 19-13 The sacrum and the coccyx. (From Applegate EJ: The sectional anatomy learning system, ed 3, St Louis, 2010, Saunders.)

and pathologic condition of the SIJ may stem from the fact that every SIJ is different, both within and among individuals.[48] These differences are likely normal physiologic adaptions, not stemming from degenerative changes or pathologic conditions.[6,29] These irregularities usually fit reciprocally with one another—lending strength to the SIJ—but also tend to restrict its movements. The SIJ adapts toward stiffness over time, especially in male subjects.[58] A healthy SIJ is one that does not cause problems.[48]

Sacroiliac Ligaments

The ligaments surrounding the SIJ are the strongest in the body and serve as attachments for some of the strongest muscles in the body. The ligaments are never completely slack. Even in supine (counternutation), the long dorsal sacroiliac ligament is tight. In nutation, all the other sacroiliac ligaments are tight. The two primary roles of these ligaments are to enhance the stability by increasing friction in the SIJ, also known as a *self-tightening mechanism*.[59] The other role is to provide proprioceptive feedback, supplied by a large number of articular receptors, because the ligaments are intimately connected to the joint capsule. The strength of these ligaments has led some authorities to believe that the SIJ is relatively immobile and thus rarely the source of pain or pathologic condition, or that the sacrum moves only as a unit with the innominates. However, in recent years the fact that the SIJs are mobile has been convincingly proved as experimental methods have improved.[49] Sturesson et al.[52] conducted a tantalum ball study in which these balls were placed in the SIJs to detect movement. During walking, the maximum nutation was found to be 3 to 5 degrees, with 1 degree around the y-axis and 1 degree around the x-axis. The maximum translation was 0.3 to 0.8 mm, attributed primarily to cartilage deformation. Sturesson et al. also found that, with hip adduction, the SIJ counternutates and, with asymmetrical movement, the SIJ is controlled more

from the pubic symphysis. Vleeming et al.[60] found that even in older age (51 to 70 years) the SIJ can still make small movements, more in women than men. Hormone levels in women may also contribute to the continued mobility of the SIJ.

For simplicity, the sacroiliac ligaments are presented here in two groups: (1) intrinsic and (2) extrinsic (see Figure 19-10).

Intrinsic ligaments	Extrinsic ligaments
Ventral sacroiliac	Sacrotuberous
Interosseous	Sacrospinous
Dorsal	Iliolumbar

Intrinsic Ligaments

The ventral sacroiliac (capsular) ligament is a thickening of the capsule[55] and is relatively weak. In addition, it is thinner than other supporting structures (and is therefore known as the *Kleenex ligament* [average thickness, 2 mm]). This ligament acts as a shock absorber for the capsule, but also allows for increased motion during pregnancy. It surrounds the joint surfaces completely and is continuous with the periosteum caudally,[61] where it is about 1 mm thick, becoming better developed at the level of the arcuate line (see Figure 19-10). This ligament can be torn,[62] and fluid can leak out to the sacral plexus and cause an irritation (severe sacroiliitis). If this ligament is stretched (with arthritis), then the patient will have pain. Because of the different innervation patterns, the location of pain will vary. Most often the ligament is innervated by L3 to S1, but it can also range from L1 to S2.[56] It can be stressed with pain provocation tests of posterior compression and anterior distraction. The psoas major lies just anterior to the ventral sacroiliac ligament and SIJ. The cranial insertions of the internal obturator muscle and obturator nerve are also located here.

The deep interosseous ligaments are massive and form the chief bond between the SIJ surfaces. This structure limits direct palpation of the SIJ and creates difficulty for intraarticular injections. They tighten when the sacrum moves anteriorly (nutation) and prevent posterior rotation of the ilium on the sacrum. The deep cranial and caudal bands blend with a more superficial sheet, which also has cranial and caudal portions that together form the short and long posterior sacroiliac ligaments (see Figure 19-10). The short posterior sacroiliac ligament refers pain from the posterior thigh to the knee. The long ligament refers pain to the lateral foot and lateral calf.

The dorsal ligaments overlie the interosseous ligaments. Their lower fibers may form a separate fasciculus known as the *long dorsal sacroiliac ligament* (LDSIL), also referred to as the *longissimus ligament*. It runs from the PSIS to the lateral sacral crest of S3 and S4, and sometimes to S5.[63] It can be palpated just caudal to the PSIS as a thick band, and can be tender with pregnancy. The skin covering this ligament is a frequent source of pain in patients with pelvic girdle and lumbosacral dysfunction.[64,65] The LDSIL has fibers that attach to the thoracolumbar fascia and the erector spinae aponeurosis.[63] Willard[66] found deeper connections between the LDSIL and the multifidus muscle. The gluteus maximus has strong connections with the deepest dorsal ligaments, as well as the dorsal and interosseous sacroiliac ligaments, and it also dynamizes the posterior ligaments. Because of these connections and because the gluteus maximus is the only contractile structure bridging the SIJ, this muscle is important in treating SIJ instability.[50]

The LDSIL blends with the extrinsic sacrotuberous ligament and connects the cranial and caudal insertions. It has three large fibrous bands[66] with a broad base attached to the PSIS, the lateral sacrum, and the LDSIL. The superior fibers connect the PSIS and the coccyx. The lateral fibers connect the PIIS and ischial tuberosity, and they receive fibers from the piriformis muscle and gluteus maximus. The medial fibers (inferior arcuate band) run anteroinferior and lateral, and attach to the transverse tubercles of S3, S4, and S5, as well as to the lateral part of the lower sacrum and coccyx. The fibers of this band have a spiral configuration so that the lateral fibers insert on the caudal sacrum and the medial fibers attach to the cranial sacrum and PSIS.[63] Because they are more distant from the axis of nutation than the medial fibers, the lateral fibers better control this motion. This spiral configuration also aids in elastic loading during the loading response of gait.[67,68] When the hip is flexed, the fibers tighten, causing the ilium to rotate posteriorly. The sacrotuberous ligament works together with the sacrospinous ligament to stabilize the pubic symphysis. With counternutation (the cranial sacrum moves posteriorly), the LDSIL is the only ligament that maximally tightens.[63] According to Smidt et al.,[53] nutation is controlled by ligaments and counternutation is more controlled by bony approximation.

Extrinsic Ligaments

The sacrotuberous and sacrospinous ligaments bind the sacrum to the ischium and stabilize the pubic symphysis (see Figure 19-10). The lower fibers of the sacrotuberous ligament blend with the gluteus maximus and the biceps femoris. This ligament resists upward tilting of the lower sacrum (nutation) under the downward thrust of the weight of the trunk imparted to the sacral base from above. The biceps femoris tendon may also insert onto the inferior aspect of the sacrotuberous ligament, even without a direct connection to the ischial tuberosity. Therefore the gluteus maximus and/or the biceps femoris can tighten this ligament.[29,30,54,67,68] It is important to be aware of this connection when conducting the SLR test: stretching of the biceps femoris explains why the SLR test can be positive with sacroiliac disorders (particularly sacroiliitis).[50] The deep multifidus tendons can also blend into the superior surface of the sacrotuberous ligament.[66] The sacrospinous ligament is thinner and triangular-shaped, and it connects the spine of the ischium to the lower lateral margins of the sacrum and coccyx. This ligament blends with the sacrotuberous ligament, runs deep (anterior) to it, and attaches to the SIJ capsule.[66]

The strong iliolumbar ligaments are comprised of five bands,[70] although according to Willard[66] these bands are quite variable in number and form. Regardless, these bands all arise at the L4 (occasionally) and L5 (always) transverse processes, blend with the SIJ ligaments inferiorly, as well as with the ventral iliac tuberosity, the deep thoracolumbosacral (TLS)

fascia, the ventrolateral sacral base, the sacral ala, and the interosseus ligaments, and move lateral to the iliac crest.[69] It is believed that these ligaments are important for maintaining stability of the lumbosacral junction.[66,70] The superior band arises at the tip of the L5 transverse process, divides on either side of the quadratus lumborum, and inserts onto the iliac crest. The anterior band connects the anteroinferior part of the entire transverse process of L5. It runs anterior to the quadratus lumborum and blends with the superior band to insert on the anterior iliac crest. The posterior band also starts on the tip of the L5 transverse process and runs posteroinferior to the superior band to insert on the iliac tuberosity. The inferior band arises on both the inferior border of the transverse process and the body of L5, and it connects to the iliac fossa. Sometimes the inferior band displays two distinct divisions: (1) a strictly iliac portion and (2) a portion that is exclusively sacral. The vertical band starts on the anteroinferior border of the L5 transverse process and runs vertical to insert on the posterior part of the arcuate line.

The influence of the iliolumbar ligaments on lumbosacral motion is discussed later.

Innervation

The innervation of the SIJ is not always symmetrical.[44,71] The joint is most consistently found to be innervated by segments S1 and S2 dorsally and ventrally by the dorsal rami of segments L2 to S2.[70] SIJ issues may cause pain in any of these dermatomes. Participation of the obturator nerve in the innervation of the SIJ has not been confirmed.[44]

MYOLOGY OF THE PELVIS

Solonen[44] noted that the SIJ is normally in a state of stable equilibrium and that much force is required to disturb this equilibrium. He further pointed out that the strongest muscles in the body surround the SIJ but that none have the primary function of moving it. Thus he concluded that no voluntary movements of the SIJ occur; movements that do occur are influenced by other regions of the body, particularly weight changes and posture.

The main two movements that occur at the SIJ are (1) nutation and (2) counternutation (Figure 19-14). With nutation, the cranial part of the sacrum moves ventral relative to the ilium, or the ilium moves dorsal relative to the sacrum. This motion occurs when one moves from bilateral stance to unilateral stance. With counternutation, the opposite occurs; the cranial sacrum moves dorsal relative to the ilium. Stepwise creep deformation of cartillage[29,30] accounts for some of the movement in the SIJ. Pain associated with deformation can take more than 1 minute to appear during a provocation test, which is why clinicians should hold the test for anywhere from 1 to 3 minutes (see "Provocation Tests").

The muscles around the pelvis most likely provide stability to the SIJ, either directly or indirectly. Some believe that the following muscle or muscle groups can indirectly impart force

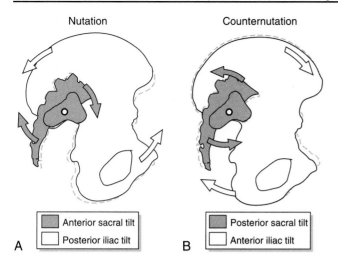

Nutation   Counternutation

A ▨ Anterior sacral tilt   B ▨ Posterior sacral tilt
   ☐ Posterior iliac tilt   ☐ Anterior iliac tilt

Figure 19-14 Kinematics of the sacroiliac joint (SIJ). **A,** Nutation. **B,** Counternutation. (From Neumann DA: Kinesiology of the musculo-skeletal system: foundations for physical rehabilitation, St Louis, 2002, Mosby.)

Box 19-1	Muscles That Attach to the Sacrum and/or Ilium

- Latissimus dorsi
- Erector spinae
- Semimembranosus
- Semitendinosus
- Biceps femoris
- Sartorius
- Inferior gemellus
- Multifidus
- Obturator internus
- Obturator externus
- Piriformis
- Tensor fascia lata
- External oblique
- Internal oblique
- Transverse abdominis (TA)
- Rectus abdominis
- Pyramidalis
- Gluteus minimus
- Gluteus medius
- Gluteus maximus
- Quadratus femoris
- Superior gemellus
- Gracilis
- Iliacus
- Adductor magnus
- Rectus femoris
- Quadratus lumborum
- Pectineus
- Psoas minor
- Adductor brevis
- Adductor longus
- Levator ani
- Sphincter urethrae
- Superficial transverse perineal ischiocavernous
- Coccygeus

From Dutton M: Orthopaedic examination, evaluation, and intervention, ed 2, New York, 2008, McGraw-Hill.

on the SIJ, either through their primary actions or by their reverse actions, depending on the points of fixation:

- Iliopsoas
- Rectus femoris
- Hip abductors and adductors
- Sartorius
- External rotators and piriformis
- Gluteus maximus
- Hamstrings
- Abdominals
- Quadratus lumborum
- Multifidi
- TFL

At least 35 muscles attach to the sacrum, innominate, or both (Box 19-1). Rather than give a detailed synopsis of each muscle in terms of its morphologic condition, some of the muscles or groups are presented according to their actions.

Iliopsoas

The iliacus arises at the iliac fossa, the iliac crest, the anterior sacroiliac ligament, the inferior part of the iliolumbar ligament,[70] and the lateral part of the sacrum. More distally, its fibers connect with the lateral part of the psoas major tendon to form the iliopsoas. This muscle travels down to insert onto the lesser trochanter of the femur. With the femur and pelvis fixed, the iliopsoas produces powerful ipsilateral flexion of the lumbar spine with contralateral rotation. It flexes the lumbar spine relative to the pelvis, increasing lordosis. When the lumbar spine and pelvis are fixed, the iliopsoas produces flexion of the hip, as well as some lateral rotation of the hip, and it may have some adduction function. Some fibers—especially from the iliacus—blend with the anterior sacroiliac ligament and joint capsule. Bilateral contraction of the iliopsoas produces an anterior force on the pelvis, causing anterior motion

of the innominate, as well as an anterior force on the sacrum because of its attachment on the sacral ala. Unilateral contraction may cause an anterior force ipsilaterally, resulting in anterior rotation of the innominate, potentially producing anterior movement of the sacrum on that side. It can also side bend the spine ipsilaterally.[72] The ventral rami of L1 and L2 innervate this muscle.

Rectus Femoris

Because it crosses the hip and knee joints, the rectus femoris can simultaneously flex the hip and extend the knee. When the pelvis is fixed, it will flex the thigh on the pelvis. If the thigh is fixed, then it will flex the pelvis on the thigh. When the thigh and the lumbar spine are both fixed and the pelvis is free to move, the rectus femoris has the potential to anteriorly rotate the innominate. It originates from the AIIS and is easiest to palpate in the lateral femoral triangle (approximately 5 cm distal from the ASIS, between the TFL and the sartorius). Because it attaches to the hip capsule, an injury to the proximal region of the rectus femoris could cause a capsular adhesion. This muscle inserts on the superior patella and is innervated by the femoral nerve; L2, L3, and L4 innervate this muscle.

Hip Abductors and Adductors

The hip abductors indirectly influence the SIJs through the pubic symphysis. (Refer to the sections on "Myology of the Hip," "Evaluation," and "Treatment.") The hip adductors exert indirect action on the SIJs through the pubis (see "Evaluation," "Treatment," and "Myology of the Hip"). Tightness or weakness of the adductors may influence the position of the hip, which in turn influences the SIJs.

Sartorius

The sartorius can simultaneously flex the knee and the hip. It assists with hip abduction and external rotation. It may exert an anterior influence on the innominate when the knee is fixed in slight flexion and the hip is extended. It is the longest muscle in the body. This muscle originates at the ASIS and the notch below, and it inserts on the medial surface of the proximal tibia, anterior to the gracilis. It is also innervated by the femoral nerve; L2, L3, and L4 innervate this muscle.

External Rotators and Piriformis

Bilateral contraction of the piriformis produces an anterior force on the sacrum and causes it to flex forward. Unilateral contraction may produce an anterior force ipsilaterally, causing rotation to occur toward the opposite side. Tightness or spasm of the piriformis may influence the SIJ (see the sections on "Myology of the Hip," "Gait and Body Position," "Evaluation," and "Treatment"). The piriformis originates from the anterior sacrum and SIJ capsule, the anterior part of the AIIS of the ilium, and the sacrotuberous ligament. It exits the pelvis through the greater sciatic foramen and attaches to the upper part of the femoral greater trochanter. It is innervated by the ventral rami of L5 and S1.

Gluteus Maximus

The gluteus maximus extends a flexed thigh and, in the gait cycle, prevents the forward momentum of the trunk from causing flexion of the hip. It is not active in standing but powerfully rotates the pelvis backward when one is returning from a forward bend. It can be a strong lateral rotator of the thigh and abductor as it exerts influence on the iliotibial tract. Bilateral contraction may assist in trunk extension when the femur is fixed. Bilateral contraction produces posterior movement of the innominates through the sacrotuberous and posterior sacroiliac ligaments. Unilateral contraction produces a posterior force on the innominate ipsilaterally, causing posterior rotation. This muscle originates on the posterior gluteal line of the ilium, iliac crest, the erector spinae aponeurosis, the inferior part of the dorsal sacrum, lateral side of the coccyx, the sacrotuberous ligament, and intermuscular fascia. This muscle has both deep and superficial parts. The deep part inserts on the femoral gluteal tuberosity; the larger, superficial part inserts on the TFL iliotibial tract. The inferior gluteal nerve, which is located in the deep part, innervates it.

Hamstrings

The hamstrings as a group are the primary knee flexors, but they can also extend the hip when the hip is flexed and the knee is in extension. (Refer to the section "Myology of the Hip.") They work to convert the posterior ligaments—especially the sacrotuberous ligament—into dynamic movers of the hip. Tightness or weakness of the hamstrings can cause either an anterior or a posterior rotation of the pelvis on the hip (see "Lumbofemoral Rhythm").

Abdominals

The abdominals are essential to support the lumbar spine and the pelvis during lifting. By contracting and exerting pressure internally (Valsalva maneuver), they significantly reduce axial compressive forces. The abdominals resist the shear forces produced by the multifidus and the psoas on the lumbar facets. A bilateral contraction, particularly of the rectus abdominis, produces a posterior rotation of the pelvis when the vertebral column and the sternum are fixed. Lack of abdominal tone results in increased lumbar lordosis and an increased sacral flexion. The transverse abdominis (TA) serves as the most important abdominal group in lumbar spinal stability.[73] The TA also contributes to stiffness in the SIJ.[74] Hodges and Richardson[75-78] found that in patients with low-back pain there was a timing delay or absence of the TA anticipation of upper- or lower-extremity movement, which would decrease stiffness and stability of the spine and SIJ. The pelvic floor muscles also play an important role in stabilizing the pelvic girdle. Research by Sapsford et al.[79,80] looked at the relationship of the coactivation pattern of the abdominals and the pelvic floor, using electromyography (EMG). They found the abdominals contract in response to a pelvic floor contraction and vice versa.[43]

Quadratus Lumborum

The quadratus lumborum fixes the twelfth rib to help the diaphragm and can be an accessory muscle of inspiration. Bilateral contraction results in stabilization of the lumbar spine, preventing deviation from the midline. Unilateral contraction produces ipsilateral side bending when the pelvis is fixed; it also helps with eccentric control of contralateral side bending. Some elevation and rotation anteriorly also occur with unilateral contraction. Bilateral contraction may produce an anterior flexion of the sacrum through (the quadratus lumborum) attachments onto the base and ala. This muscle is also active with sustained postures and when a weight is lifted in the opposite hand.[81] This muscle attaches to the ventral, inferior surface of the twelfth rib, the ventral surface of the upper four transverse processes, the anterior band of the iliolumbar ligament, and lateral to it on the iliac crest. It is innervated by the ventral rami of T12 to L2.[82]

Multifidus

The deep multifidus fibers have been shown to be recruited before movement of the upper- or lower-extremity starts and are anticipatory to stabilize the lumbosacral region.[83] The superficial and lateral fibers are direction dependent.[43] Richardson et al.[74] found increased stiffness of the SIJ with cocontraction of the TA and multifidi.

Along with the rotators (transversospinalis group), the multifidus is primarily a postural muscle and stabilizes the lumbar spinal joints. Bilateral contraction extends the vertebral column from the prone or the forward-bent position and, conversely, performs in controlled forward bending (eccentric contraction). Bilateral contraction may also produce a posterior force on the pelvis through the muscle's attachments with the erector spinae, the PSIS, and the posterior sacroiliac ligaments. The pelvic part of the multifidus lies between the posterior sacrum and the deep layers of the thoracolumbar fascia. The lumbar multifidus is segmentally innervated by the medial branch of the dorsal ramus of the same level or the level below where it originates.[84]

Tensor Fasciae Latae

Refer to the section "Myology of the Hip."

GLOBAL MUSCLE SYSTEM

The global muscle system is made up of several muscles that produce forces and act as "integrated sling systems" as described by Vleeming et al.[54] Four separate sling systems stabilize the pelvis (between the thorax and lower extremities). The posterior oblique sling (Figure 19-15, *A*) connects the latissimus dorsi through the thoracolumbar fascia to the contralateral gluteus maximus. This sling operates during loading response, the ipsilateral gluteus maximus fires, the contralateral latissimus fires, and dynamic stabilization occurs with tightening of the ipsilateral SIJ. Thus in rehabilitation, a brisk walk with increased arm swing and 2 lb hand weights may be prescribed to promote training of the latissimi dorsi and increased SIJ stability. Activation of the gluteus maximus will also increase SIJ stability.[48] The anterior oblique sling (Figure 19-15, *B*) connects the external oblique, the anterior abdominal fascia, the contralateral internal oblique, and the thigh adductors. The longitudinal sling connects the peroneals, the biceps femoris, the sacrotuberous ligament, the deep lamina of the thoracolumbar fascia, and the erector spinae. Finally, the lateral sling connects the gluteus medius and minimus, TFL, and the thoracopelvic lateral stabilizers; these are the main stabilizers of the hip joint. The concept of the sling systems provides an

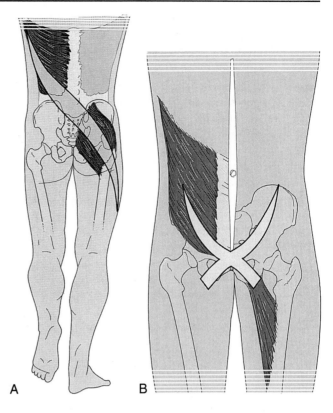

Figure 19-15 A, The posterior oblique sling of the global system includes the latissimus dorsi, gluteus maximus, and the intervening thoracodorsal fascia. **B,** The anterior oblique sling of the global system includes the external oblique, the contralateral internal oblique, the adductors of the thigh, and the intervening anterior abdominal fascia. (From Lee D: The pelvic girdle, ed 3, New York, 2004, Churchill Livingstone.)

understanding of how these muscles and tissues connect and function together to transfer loads and forces, as well as stabilize the SIJ.[85]

It is important that clinicians identify a specific muscle dysfunction (e.g., weakness, tightness, poor recruitment) to help with restoring both mobility and global stabilization between the thorax, pelvis, and lower extremities. Clinicians must also understand why part of the sling may be too flexible or too tight.[43]

Local Muscle System

The role of the lumbopelvic local muscle system is to prepare the spine and pelvic girdle for additional external loads by stabilizing these joints. Local muscle systems accomplish this in one or more of the following ways:
- Increase the intraabdominal pressure.[86-88]
- Increase the tension of the thoracodorsal fascia.[54,86,88]
- Increase the articular stiffness.[74,89]

These muscles should always work at low levels and are activated and recruited before any extra loading or motion occurs.[43]

ANATOMIC CONSIDERATIONS FOR SACROILIAC DYSFUNCTION

According to Cyriax,[14] SIJ problems are more common in female subjects than in male subjects. The following anatomic factors may explain why the occurrence of sacroiliac dysfunctions in the general population is six times greater in female subjects than in male subjects. (Refer also to "Functional Anatomy and Mechanics of the Pelvis.")

- The lateral dimension of the pelvic foramen is greater in female subjects than in male subjects.
- The bone density of the male pelvis is greater.
- The SIJ surfaces are smaller in female subjects.
- The SIJ surfaces are flatter in female subjects.
- The SIJs are located farther from the hips in female subjects than in male subjects.
- The iliac crests are set farther apart in the female pelvis than in the male pelvis.
- The vertical dimension of the pelvis is greater in the male pelvis.
- The more rectangular the shape of the sacrum (as in male subjects), the more stable it is within the innominates.
- The more vertical the orientation of the sacrum within the innominates, the flatter or less lordotic is the lumbar spine; this position increases compressive forces on the lumbar spine.
- The more horizontal the orientation of the sacrum within the innominates, the greater will be the lumbar lordosis; this increases the shear forces across the lumbosacral angle.
- Three types of sacral articular surfaces have been classified according to shape:
  - Average or normal auricular surface
  - Smooth and convex anteroposteriorly (This is the type of articular surface in which the rare inflare and outflare dysfunctional lesions of the innominates occur.)
  - Extremely irregular and concave auricular surfaces (These are very stable and usually uniform bilaterally but occasionally may be asymmetric in shape.)
- As the SIJ changes with age (>50 years old), ankylosis (bony bridging at L5 to S1 can cause L4 and L5 and the SIJ to move more) occurs, which likely decreases movement where the ankylosis is located; these changes are more marked in male subjects than female subjects.[67,68,91]

INTEGRATED MODEL OF FUNCTION

The transmission of vertical forces from the spine to the lower members, and of ground reaction forces from the lower limbs to the spine (Figure 19-16), occurs through trabecular lines (see "Osteology of the Hip"). The SIJ is a force transducer, shock absorber, and part of three different chains:[53,91,92]

1. The lower-extremity kinematic chain: sacrum-innominate-lower extremity (LE)
2. The spine kinematic chain: L4-L5-sacrum
3. The closed chain: innominate-sacrum-innominate[48]

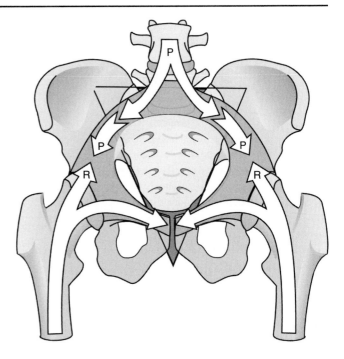

Figure 19-16 Transmission of ground reaction forces and vertical compression forces from the upper body through the sacroiliac joints (SIJs) and pubic rami. *P,* Compression forces; *R,* ground reaction forces. (From Kapandji IA: *The physiology of the joints,* ed 6, vol 3, Edinburgh, 2008, Churchill Livingstone.)

SIJ locking correlates with symphyseal irritation. The SIJ also relates to the lower lumbar spine as a compensatory movement, usually at L4 and L5, as well as L5 to S1. In individuals with ankylosis of SIJ, Brook found that 81% had hypermobility at L5 to S1, and 19% had ankylosis of L5 to S1 with hypermobility at L4 and L5. In asymmetrical ankylosis, bilateral hypermobility was noted at L5 to S1.

Because the hip must sustain pressures greater than body weight, it must use the bone, articular, and myofascial systems for stability. Each hip joint supports about 50% of body weight during normal standing.[93,94] When the passive, active, and control systems work together, proper load transfer and stability is achieved.[95] The manner in which these forces are transmitted and dispersed (i.e., from the top down versus from the bottom up) helps explain why certain dysfunctional lesions of the pelvis occur regularly with certain actions or activities. Vleeming et al.[29,30] and Snijders et al.[96] described lumbar-pelvic-hip region motion as involving *intrinsic* and *extrinsic* stability of the pelvic girdle along with the self-locking mechanism. These authors coined the terms *form closure* and *force closure* to describe the active and passive forces that help stabilize the SIJ and pelvis.

Four components make up the integrated model of function:

1. Form closure, which is structural
2. Force closure, which are forces from myofascial action
3. Motor control, which has to do with the timing of muscle contraction and inaction with loading
4. Emotions, which are psychological

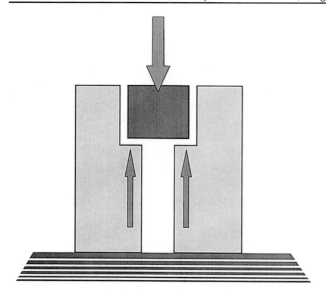

Figure 19-17 Schematic representation of form closure. (From Lee D: The pelvic girdle, ed 3, New York, 2004, Churchill Livingstone.)

Because joint mechanics are influenced by emotional, neuromuscular, and/or articular components, the clinician must address each of these factors.[43]

Form closure (Figure 19-17) describes how the joint's structure, shape, and orientation increase the stability and possible mobility of the joint. Because all joints are asymmetrical, each individual's anatomy will influence how much force closure is required for stability with increased loads. The structure of the SIJ helps to stabilize the pelvic girdle in three ways. First of all, the wedge shape of the sacrum is stabilized by the innominates. Secondly, the ridges and furrows in both the cartilage and the subchondral bone of the articular surface provide stability.[29,30] Third, the articular cartilage is irregular (not smooth), especially on the ilium. When force closure (compression) is applied to the pelvis, these factors help with stabilize the SIJ.

The elements involved in form closure include the orientation of the trabeculae, the design of the anatomy of the joint, and the capsule and ligament system. Because the hip must sustain pressures greater than body weight, it must use the bone, articular, and myofascial systems for stability. Each hip joint supports about 50% of body weight during normal standing.[78,79]

Force closure occurs with loading when increased compression, both intrinsic and extrinsic, takes place across a joint surface. The soft tissues that create force closure are the muscles, ligaments, and fascia. Both the myofascial and the neurologic systems make up these dynamic forces, producing a self-locking mechanism for the SIJ. The amount of force closure needed is dictated by the amount of load and the form closure.[43] Both form closure (articular) and force closure (myofascial) are necessary to balance a heavy load.

The joint position with the most stability, where a maximum congruence of the joint surfaces occurs along the ligaments, placing the most tension on them, is called a *closed-packed position*. Here the joint can resist shear forces better.[30,96,97] For the

SIJ, the closed-packed position involves full nutation of the sacrum or posterior rotation of the innominate.[67,68] For the hip it involves full extension along with maximum adduction and internal rotation or full extension with abduction and external rotation.[38] Positions that involve nutation include bilateral hip flexion, standing or landing, sitting with passive lordosis, and trunk flexion.[58] Sacral nutation winds up most of the SIJ ligaments, particularly the sacrotuberous, sacrospinous, and interosseous ligaments.[45,46,98] Often fractures and dislocations occur when a joint is in its close-packed position and an external force is applied.

When the joint is out of the close-packed position, it is considered an open-packed (or loose-packed) position. In these positions the joint has minimal stability, minimal joint surface contact or congruency, and the ligaments are on slack. Loose-packed position for the SIJ is counternutation of the sacrum or anterior rotation of the innominate. For the hip it is from 30 to 60 degrees of flexion, 15 degrees to 30 degrees of abduction, and about 15 degrees of external rotation.[38] Positions that involve counternutation of the SIJ include trunk extension, lying supine, and hip hyperextension; the long dorsal ligament tightens with counternutation. The counternutation position is also important for childbirth. In the third trimester, the low back moves into a lordotic position and slight nutation. The position the baby is in at that time pulls the pelvic ring forward, which creates a relative counternutation.[48] In loose-packed positions, the joint capsule and/or ligaments must sustain outside forces; therefore the injuries sustained in these positions are often ligament or capsule sprains. Joint mobilization techniques are often performed in the open-packed positions.

According to Shumway-Cook and Wollacott,[99] motor control is the ability to regulate or direct the mechanisms essential to movement, including proper muscle activation patterns.[69] It involves the timing of specific muscle action and relaxation, and such coordinated muscle action provides stability with mobility.[88] The coordination between the local and global systems creates stability without rigid posture or collapse of the lumbopelvic region. Exercises that focus on balancing tension and decreasing compression using the sling system, as well as with mental imagery for the patient, help improve motor control.[43]

PATIENT EMOTIONAL STATE AND DYSFUNCTION

The emotions play an important role in function of the neuromusculoskeletal system. Often chronic pain patients who have functional complaints have also had traumatic life experiences. Many of these patients will use motor control patterns with defensive posturing. In addition, a negative emotional state induces increased stress. Such stress is a normal response required to stimulate flight or fight reactions. However, if this response continues for an extended period of time, then high levels of epinephrine (adrenaline) and cortisol circulate in the system[100] and may exert negative effects.

These emotional states of fight or flight (or freeze reactions) are demonstrated through muscle action; over time they will influence muscle tone and patterns.[100] The SIJ compression will increase if the pelvic muscles become hypertonic.[85,74] Therefore it is important to consider and influence the patient's emotional state to change any poor motor patterns. The best strategy is for the clinician to validate the patient's feelings and to increase his or her awareness of the mechanical problem with education. Such intervention increases hope in the patient and leads them toward the road to recovery. In more severe cases, the patient may need professional cognitive-behavioral therapy to help retrain and restore more positive thought patterns. It is essential to teach patients about the effect that physical and emotional stress may have on the body so that they may try to relax and decrease muscle tone in periods of stress.[101]

LUMBOFEMORAL RHYTHM

The concept of normal functional integration among the lumbar spine, pelvis, and hip joints is fundamental to the understanding of dysfunction in this region. In the total forward bending of the spine, synchronous movement occurs in a rhythmic pattern of the lumbar spine to that of pelvic rotation about the hips (Table 19-2). Cailliet[102] describes this relationship between the hip, pelvis, and lumbar spine as *lumbofemoral rhythm*.

As one bends forward, the lumbar lordosis progresses from concave to flat to convex. At the same time, a proportionate amount of pelvic rotation occurs about the hips. The pelvic girdle tilts anteriorly on the femoral heads, causing hip flexion. The amount of movement between each lumbar level will vary, with the most movement occurring at L5 and S1 and lesser amounts at successively higher levels. Thus to achieve full forward bending, the lumbar spine must fully reverse itself, and the pelvis must rotate to its fullest extent. Nonetheless, the rhythm between levels should be smooth and precise, creating a balance between lumbar movement and pelvic rotation (Figure 19-18).

Many muscles are involved in controlling this motion, including the low-back local and global muscles, most of the

Table 19-2	Sacroiliac Joint Responses to Movements or Positions
Movement/Position	**Response**
Standing	Nutation
Unilateral standing	Nutation on weight-bearing side
	Counternutation on nonweight-bearing side
Supine	Counternutation
Standing with active lordosis	Variable
Standing or supine with passive lordosis	Nutation (always)
Sitting	Counternutation

hip muscles, and the lower abdominals. Other factors that can influence this rhythm include facet restriction, degenerative joint disease, and tight hamstring muscles. Tully et al.[103] found that in adults for every 3 degrees of hip flexion, there will be 1 degree of lumbar flexion. It appeared that the first 3 to 5 degrees of movement started at the hip. The authors found that the lumbar spine made up approximately 26% of the total flexion and 24% of total extension. During these movements, the sacrum is also moving within the ilia. Initially, the sacrum nutates (flexes relative to the innominates) and remains in this position until the individual returns to an upright posture, where it slightly counternutates (extends, but stays relatively nutated) within the ilia. The sacrum nutates in standing and counternutates in supine.[104]

Comments for sitting are as follows:
- Ground reaction forces induce anterior rotation of the innominate.
- Sitting forward-flexion test begins in counternutation.
- A lumbar roll may help patients with instability because increased nutation will give increased stability.[48]

Backward bending of the trunk (spinal extension) involves anterior displacement of the pelvic girdle. The sacrum remains nutated, and the pelvic girdle tilts posteriorly on the femoral heads, causing hip extension; L5 extends on the sacrum. If L5 and S1 move first, then counternutation occurs.

Side bending to the right displaces the upper legs to the left and tilts the pelvic girdle laterally to the right; the right femur abducts, and the left femur adducts. The right innominate rotates anteriorly while the sacrum side bends to the right. L5 appears to side bend and rotate with the sacrum.

Axial trunk rotation to the left causes both femurs to rotate to the left, which leads the right proximal femur to displace anteromedially and the left proximal femur to displace posteromedially. At the same time the pelvic girdle rotates left, the right innominate rotates anteriorly relative to the left innominate, and the sacrum counternutates at the right SIJ and nutates at the left SIJ (i.e., rotates left). L5 seems to side bend and rotate with the sacrum.

Sacral Motion

Vleeming et al.[45] proposed that when the sacrum nutates relative to the innominates, the sacrum makes a small inferior glide down the short arm of the joint surface (at S1) and posteriorly down the long arm (at S2, S3, and S4) of the joint surface (see Figure 19-14). The wedge of the sacrum; the ridges and furrows of the joint surfaces (and joint surface friction); and the sacrotuberous, dorsal, and interosseous ligaments (as well as the muscles that attach to these ligaments) resist this movement.

With sacral counternutation (extension), it is proposed that the sacrum glides anteriorly along the long arm and superiorly up the short arm. The LDSIL resists this motion,[63] which is supported by the multifidus contraction and helps to nutate the sacrum.

At the same time as these movements are occurring in the sagittal plane, a backward translation of the pelvis and the hips occurs in the horizontal plane. This represents a shift in the

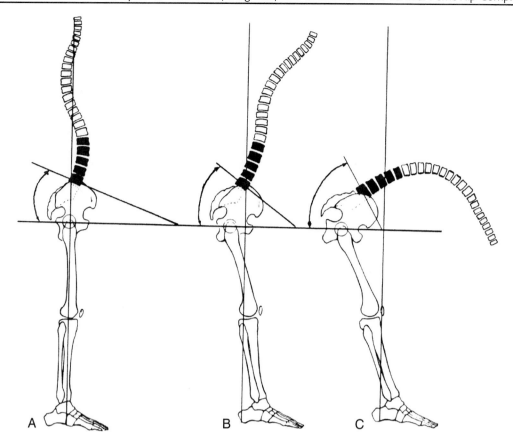

Figure 19-18 Lumbopelvic rhythm. **A,** Normal standing posture with lumbar concavity; body weight superimposed directly over the hip joints; normal pelvic inclination with respect to horizontal. **B,** Flattening of the lumbar spine. The pelvis begins to rotate anteriorly around the hips; the hips and pelvis move posteriorly in the horizontal plane. **C,** Reversal of the lumbar spine into lumbar convexity. The pelvis rotates anteriorly to the fullest extent; the hips and pelvis are posteriorly displaced in the horizontal plane. (From Saunders HD: Evaluation, treatment, and prevention of musculoskeletal disorders, ed 2, Minneapolis, 1985, H Duane Saunders.)

pelvic fulcrum so that the center of gravity is maintained over the feet. If such a shift did not occur, then the person would fall forward.

As the person returns to the standing position, the reverse process should occur in an equally smooth manner. It is a fallacy to think that just because a person can bend forward and touch the toes, he or she has full range of motion of the lumbosacral spine. Such an individual may have loose hamstrings, which never engage the pelvis to tether it (Box 19-2). Thus the lumbar spine could remain relatively concave or flat and the sacrum in relative nutation. Conversely, the hamstrings may be tight and can markedly restrict pelvic rotation about the hips. Should this person try to force flexion of the trunk (as in lifting), a strain may occur in the lumbosacral area. Thus the clinician must assess closely the integration of motion between the lumbar spine and pelvic components.

The iliolumbar ligaments directly influence the integration of movement between the lumbar and pelvic components of the complex. The superior and inferior bands are selectively stretched during different movements and greatly limit motion and stabilize the lumbosacral junction. In side bending, the iliolumbar ligaments become taut contralaterally and relax ipsilaterally. They allow only 8 degrees of movement of L4

Box 19-2	**Factors Affecting Nutation and Counternutation**
Factors That Can Limit Nutation and Facilitate Counternutation	**Factors That Can Limit Counternutation and Facilitate Nutation**
• Shortening/increased tone of the hip flexors (e.g., tensor fascia latae [TFL], iliacus, rectus femoris, adductor longus) • Capsular hip extension limitation • Rotation left at L5 and S1 (causing limited nutation on the right side) • Short leg ipsilaterally	• Shortening/increased tone of the hip extensors (i.e., gluteals, hamstrings) • Capsular hip flexion limitation • Rotation right at L5 and S1 (counternutation will be limited on right side) • Long leg ipsilateral • Weak sacrospinous and sacrotuberous ligaments

Data from Gerlach, UJ, Lierse W: Functional construction of the sacroiliac ligamentous apparatus, Acta Anatomica 144:97-102, 1992.

Table 19-3	Hip Motion and Innominate Motions
Hip Motion	Motion of Ipsilateral Innominate
Flexion	Posterior rotation
Extension	Anterior rotation
Internal rotation	Internal rotation (inflare)
External rotation	External rotation (outflare)
Abduction	Superior glide
Adduction	Inferior glide

From Dutton M: Orthopaedic examination, evaluation, and intervention, ed 2, New York, 2008, McGraw-Hill.

Table 19-4	Lumbar Motions and Sacroiliac Motions	
Lumbar Motion	Innominate Motion	Sacrum Motion
Flexion	Anterior rotation	Nutation, then counternutation
Extension	Slight posterior rotation	Nutation
Rotation	Ipsilateral: posterior rotation	Nutates ipsilaterally
	Contralateral: anterior rotation	Nutates ipsilaterally
Side bending	Ipsilateral: anterior rotation	Ipsilateral: side bends ipsilaterally
	Contralateral: posterior rotation	Contralateral: side bends contralaterally

From Dutton M: Orthopaedic examination, evaluation, and intervention, ed 2, New York, 2008, McGraw-Hill.

relative to the sacrum. In flexion, the inferior band is relaxed and the superior band tightens. In extension, the inferior band tightens and the superior band relaxes. These ligaments monitor both lumbosacral and SIJ movement.

Innominate Motion

The motion of the innominate relative to the sacrum occurs through the interosseous ligament of the SIJ. Movement of the innominate can be induced by hip or trunk motion. Posterior rotation (relative to the sacrum) occurs on the nonweight-bearing side when the ipsilateral hip is flexed; the weight-bearing side either posteriorly rotates or remains posterior relative to the sacrum. Therefore the sacrum is relatively nutated and ready for load transfer in a close-packed position (Tables 19-3 and 19-4).[104,105]

FUNCTIONAL BIOMECHANICS

The following describes a functional biomechanical model for SIJ movement as taught by Vleeming et al.[45] and Snijders et al.[46] According to this model, the SIJ moves very little and

Box 19-3	Dysfunctions of the Posterior and Anterior Innominate
Posterior Innominate Dysfunctions Occur Most Frequently in the Following Situations:	**Anterior Innominate Dysfunctions Occur Most Frequently in the Following Situations:**
• Repeated unilateral standing • A fall onto an ischial tuberosity • A vertical thrust onto an extended leg • Lifting in a forward-bent position with the knees locked • Intercourse positions in female subjects (hyperflexion and abduction of the hips)	• Golf or baseball swing • Horizontal thrust of the knee (dashboard injury) • Any forceful movement on a diagonal (ventral proprioceptive neuromuscular facilitation [PNF] pattern)

dysfunction is a result of improper load transfer through the joints. The clinician must remember that very few if any motions in the human body occur in a single plane about a single axis; so it is in the SIJ. It is also important to remember that pelvic asymmetry is often seen on radiologic examination, even without symptoms. The models by Vleeming et al. and Snijders et al. described present concepts of motion and form a basis for examination and a rationale for treatment. The less common models will be briefly mentioned (see "Signs of Sacroiliac Problems").

Innominate Rotation

Two principal rotatory movements of the innominates occur: (1) anterior (forward) and (2) posterior (backward), both relative to the sacrum. Anterior rotation usually occurs during nonweight-bearing extension of the leg. The innominate glides inferiorly down the short arm of the joint surface and posteriorly down the long arm of the joint surface—the same way the sacrum moves into counternutation. Posterior rotation occurs with the same glide as nutation of the sacrum; it glides anteriorly along the long arm and superiorly up the short arm. Posterior rotation can occur with forward bending at the waist. According to Hungerford et al.,[106] an arthrokinematic glide between the sacrum and innominate in nonweight-bearing is a physiologic motion, with posterior rotation of the innominate. In weight-bearing, however, the SIJ assumes the close-packed position, thus preventing this physiologic glide. The clinician should keep in mind that asymmetrical movements of the innominates are variable because of the influence of the symphysis pubis (Box 19-3).[91]

Pubic Shear Lesions

As the name implies, pubic shears involve the sliding of one joint surface in relation to the other, either vertically or horizontally. The pubic symphysis relies on the myofascial and the passive structures for stability. Because the joint surfaces are more flat, this joint does not have form closure as described for the SIJ. A fibrocartilaginous disc sits between the joint surfaces, supported by four ligaments: anterior, posterior, superior, and inferior.

Pubic shears are likely the most often overlooked pelvic dysfunction. Their recognition and proper treatment, however, are mandatory for success in treating pelvic dysfunctions. These shears are usually traumatic and result from a fall onto an ischial tuberosity or from an unexpected vertical thrust onto an extended leg. Pubic shears very frequently occur with innominate rotations and upslips and are often the cause of groin pain as a presenting symptom (see "Evaluation").

CAUSE OF SACROILIAC JOINT DYSFUNCTION

Four classifications of SIJ pathologic condition exist:
1. Inflammatory disorders
2. Instability
3. Intraarticular derangement (locking)
4. Other mechanical disturbances

Problems that occur as a result of dysfunction in other joints of the pelvic girdle are termed *other mechanical disturbances.* Often this has to do with lumbar spine disease or hip problems.

Inflammatory disorders may include rheumatoid-related illnesses or infectious sacroiliitis, neither of which is very common. An acute sacroiliitis is usually unilateral and caused by an infection, sometimes from gout. Bacteria can enter the SIJ directly from the surrounding tissues or through hematogenic or lymphatic pathways. Antibiotic agents are the preferred treatment for infectious sacroiliitis. In the examination, every movement that involved the SIJ is painful, including sacroiliac provocation tests, lumbar spine movements, and passive hip movements. The patient experiences pain with coughing, sneezing, and walking and may complain of pain at the affected joint; in other patients the pain may radiate down into the buttock and/or posterior thigh.

Chronic sacroiliitis may be seen in patients with ankylosing spondylitis and is more often symmetrical, although initially it may present unilaterally. A chronic unilateral sacroiliitis could be a tuberculosis. Bilateral (sometimes unilateral) sacroiliitis often stems from rheumatoid-related disorders including Reiter's disease, psoriasis, Crohn's disease, juvenile chronic arthritis, ulcerating colitis, reactive arthritis (particularly after infections in the intestines), and Behçet's disease.[50]

With instability, movement of the ilium in relation to the sacrum is easy to feel. When a dysfunction is found, it is not always clear as to which of the SIJs is the cause. As proposed by Chamberlain,[107] sometimes mobility can be seen objectively with three pelvic radiographic anteroposterior views:
1. In left unipodal position
2. In right unipodal position
3. With equal weight on both legs

The mobility of one innominate versus the other can be seen very well at the symphysis.

Sacroiliac instability often contributes to irritation of one or more ligaments, or even arthritis of the SIJ. Instability usually increases between the ages of 18 to 35 years (in female subjects more than male subjects). Then instability usually decreases after the age of 35 years in men and 45 years in women, unless they are taking hormones or birth control pills.[48] In the first few months of pregnancy and after childbirth, women may experience SIJ hypermobility and pain.[108] The width of the pubic symphysis increases an average of 5 mm. The hormone relaxin causes the pelvic ligaments to loosen and relax.[109] Some female subjects may notice cyclic symptoms because of monthly hormone changes. The patient may have tenderness over the SIJ and/or pubic symphysis because of loss of force closure. Such a patient may benefit from a SIJ belt designed for pregnant women.

Internal derangement or locking is a pathologic form of decreased mobility that is different from a capsular pattern limitation. With a capsular pattern the entire capsule would be equally involved. Internal derangements can have an intra- or extraarticular involvement, or both. Intraarticular problems include meniscal lesions, loose bodies, intraarticular adhesions, and subluxations. In general, space-occupying lesions (e.g., shortened and hypertonic muscles, inflammation, infection, tumor) cause extraarticular locking.[50]

To confirm a diagnosis of SIJ instability and/or locking, the clinician must have a corresponding subjective history and more than two positive provocation tests (see "Provocation Tests"). Other pathologic conditions that can stem from SIJ instability are trochanteric bursitis and piriformis syndrome.

Sacroiliac joint dysfunctions—whether mechanical or disease related—are often characterized by localized pain in and around the sulcus. In the general population, acute strains with joint involvement are rare, excluding certain special populations such as athletes and the military.

SIGNS OF SACROILIAC PROBLEMS

Pain that occurs with sacroiliac dysfunction may be acute or chronic, sharp or dull, and aching or tingling. The two sources of pain are intraarticular and periarticular, including the ligaments (anterior and osseous).

Following are some of the most common signs of pain from the SIJ:
- The pain is never midline and is always caudal to the PSIS.[110]
- Pain has a high correlation with the SIJ if the patient points to the PSIS.[71]
- The pain is most often unilateral (chronic SIJ problems may be bilateral or unilateral) and local to the joint (sulcus) itself.
- Typically the pain is present in the upper, inner buttock region (S1, S2 dermatomes)

- The pain may refer down the leg (usually posterolaterally along the sciatic distribution and not often below the knee) because of innervation from the L2 to S2 segments.
- Pain may also be referred to the anterolateral pelvis and even the groin or abdominal region.[111] The possibility of referred pain exists because of a systemic pathologic condition (including from the anterior SIJ with different types of arthritis).
- The clinician should consider involvement of the symphysis pubis if groin pain occurs with provocation tests (and recheck it with a sacroiliac belt). A positive test for symphysis pubis includes lower abdominal or genital pain with resisted adduction at 45 degrees of hip flexion (in supine). This test is negative with the patient wearing the sacroiliac belt.
- No neurologic symptoms are associated with sacroiliac dysfunction.
- A SLR test may be positive but only for pain and usually in the higher arc above 60 degrees. The SLR test should also be retested with the sacroiliac belt on to check for instability.
- The pain is usually worse with weight bearing,[100] walking and stair climbing, and the patient usually limps (with a Trendelenburg's or similar gait pattern).
- The intensity of pain usually does not increase with prolonged sitting; when the condition is acute, however, the patient may sit shifted onto one ischium.
- The patient often maintains lumbar lordosis in forward bending, recruiting motion around the acetabuli (see "Lumbofemoral Rhythm"), and may also complain of lumbar pain.
- The clinician may note ipsilateral tension over the erector spinae muscles and a slight swelling over the dorsal aspect of the sacrum.
- Pain may often arise from the nonblocked side (i.e., the dysfunctional side may be nonpainful, but it causes the opposite side to become hypermobile and painful).
- Sacroiliac pain is more common in female subjects (see "Anatomic Considerations for Sacroiliac Dysfunction").
- No findings of weakness, paresthesia, or numbness.
- The diagnosis is made based on three things: (1) a positive history, (2) a negative result on a basic functional examination of the lumbar spine, and (3) three or more positive SIJ provocation tests.[48]

GAIT AND BODY POSITION

A patient with SIJ dysfunction often complains of pain during walking or climbing stairs. An understanding of the relative positions and movements of the sacrum, innominates, and other body parts helps to account for the pain produced during locomotion. The lumbo-pelvic-hip complex must work together for optimal gait. The movement of the pelvis in walking is described in sequence as though the patient were starting to walk by advancing the right foot first:

1. Trunk rotation in the thoracic region occurs to the left, accompanied by left side bending of the lumbar spine, forming a convexity to the right.
   - The pelvic girdle rotates counterclockwise, translates anteriorly, and adducts on the femoral head. The right innominate rotates posteriorly, whereas the left rotates anteriorly. The left innominate rotates anteriorly and pulls the sacrum into right rotation.
   - At this time the lower lumbar vertebrae flex and side bend contralaterally in the same direction of the rotating sacrum,[112] and the iliolumbar ligament then controls the movement of the L5 to S1 segment.[113] The side bending and lumbar rotation appear to occur in an isolated manner.
   - Before the right foot makes contact and the left foot starts the swing phase, tension is increased in the right sacrotuberous ligament, biceps femoris, and interosseous ligament. At heel-strike, the right innominate rotates posteriorly, tightening the sacrotuberous ligament. Biceps femoris contraction further tightens this ligament. This increased tension stabilizes the SIJ on the side of initial contact[43] (Figure 19-19).
2. From heel-strike to midstance, the right innominate rotates anteriorly relative to the sacrum, and the ipsilateral gluteus medius and contralateral adductors stabilize the pelvic girdle on the femoral head. When the left foot leaves the

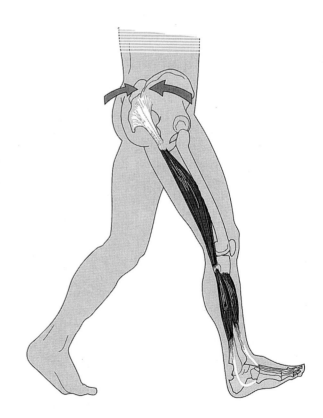

Figure 19-19 At heel-strike, posterior rotation of the right innominate increases the tension of the right sacrotuberous ligament. Contraction of the biceps femoris further increases tension in this ligament, preparing the sacroiliac joint (SIJ) for impact. (Redrawn from Lee D: The pelvic girdle, ed 3, New York, 2004, Churchill Livingstone.)

ground, the pelvis lists to the left. The right hip abductors and right lumbar side benders control this listing.

3. With single-leg stance phase on the right, the pelvic girdle translates anteriorly and adducts on the right femoral head. The right innominate starts to anteriorly rotate, whereas the left innominate posteriorly rotates both relative to the sacrum. The biceps femoris relaxes while the gluteus maximus tightens.[114] At the same time the contralateral latissimus dorsi fires.[115] The simultaneous contraction of these muscles dynamizes the thoracolumbar fascia (force closure), which helps to stabilize the SIJ according to Vleeming's "sling system."

QUALITY OF MOTION

The ease with which a patient moves through a range of motion is as significant as the total range of motion itself. With careful palpation, the clinician can assess subtle aberrations in the freedom of motion within a segment or group of segments that exhibit normal range of motion. Thus the clinician must be able to evaluate quality, as well as quantity, of motion for diagnostic and therapeutic considerations. Alternatively, segments with restricted range of motion may have normal movement or ease of motion, although this situation tends to occur symmetrically. Hypermobility is increased range and freedom (laxity) of joint motion. Hypermobile segments are frequently symptomatic, and thrust mobilizations are generally contraindicated. Hypermobile joints are most frequently the result of compensatory change caused by restricted motion (above or below the joint) or are traumatic in origin.

BARRIER CONCEPT OF MOTION RESTRICTION

A normal functional range of motion exists in or across the three planes of motion for each segment. If, for whatever reason, motion becomes restricted in one plane, motion in the other two planes is also reduced (Fryette's third law) (Table 19-5). This may be perceived as a restriction in overall movement during an analysis of spinal movement.

Table 19-5	Laws of Physiologic Spinal Motion (Fryette's Laws)
Law I	If the vertebral segments are in the neutral (or easy normal) position without locking of the facets, then rotation and side bending are in opposite directions (type I motion).
Law II	If the vertebral segments are in full flexion or extension with the facets locked or engaged, then rotation and side bending are to the same side (type II motion).
Law III	If motion is introduced into a vertebral segment in any plane, then motion in all other planes is reduced.

Somatic dysfunction has been described as impaired or altered function of related components of the somatic (body framework) system. Somatic dysfunction is characterized by impaired mobility, which may or may not occur with positional alteration. Figure 19-20 illustrates the total range of motion for any given joint. It is bounded at its extremes by its anatomic limits (barriers). A barrier is an obstruction or a restriction to movement. Anatomic barriers include the bone contours and/or soft tissues—particularly the ligaments—that serve as the final limit to motion in an articulation; beyond this limit tissue damage will occur. Physiologic barriers are the soft tissue tension accumulations that limit the voluntary motion of an articulation. Further motion toward the anatomic barrier can be induced passively.

Figure 19-21, A, illustrates the divisions of active and passive motion within the total range of motion of a given joint. Active motion is voluntary movement of a joint by the individual between the physiologic barriers. Passive motion is movement induced in an articulation by the clinician. It includes the range of active motion, as well as the movement between the physiologic and anatomic barriers permitted by soft tissue resilience that the individual cannot execute voluntarily. Soft tissue tension accumulates as the joint is passively moved from its active range, through physiologic barriers, and toward anatomic barriers. The clinician is assessing these barriers when examining a joint for end feel or joint play.

In somatic dysfunction, slight loss of motion sometimes occurs, implying that a restrictive barrier has formed within the normal active range of motion (AROM), thus limiting the ability of the joint to complete its full, pain-free range of motion. A minor motion loss is one in which the barrier does not cross the midpoint of the joint's normal range of motion. This concept is illustrated in Figure 19-21, B.

Loss of motion occurs when the motion barrier crosses the normal midpoint of the AROM of the joint. This is illustrated in Figure 19-21, C. Motion loss—whether major or minor—is

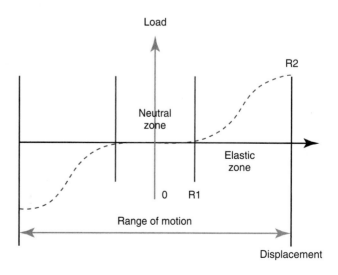

Figure 19-20 Zones of articular motion. (From Lee D: The pelvic girdle, ed 3, New York, 2004, Churchill Livingstone.)

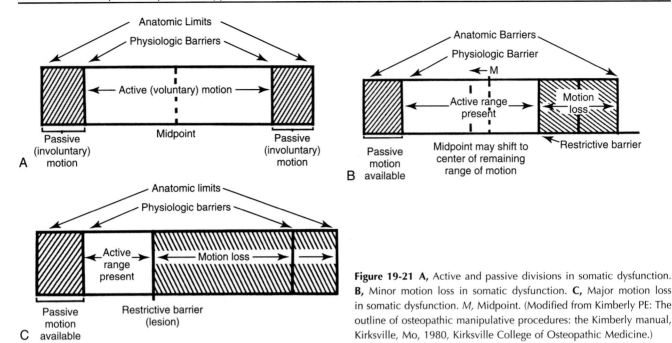

Figure 19-21 A, Active and passive divisions in somatic dysfunction. **B,** Minor motion loss in somatic dysfunction. **C,** Major motion loss in somatic dysfunction. *M,* Midpoint. (Modified from Kimberly PE: The outline of osteopathic manipulative procedures: the Kimberly manual, Kirksville, Mo, 1980, Kirksville College of Osteopathic Medicine.)

maintained until something occurs to change the barrier. Various factors influence these restrictions, including taut joint capsules, shortened ligaments and fascias, muscles shortening because of spasm or fibrosis, or a shift in the gamma gain mechanism. Long-standing lesions lead to changes in the adjacent tissues (adnexa), especially in circulatory (edema with dilation or vasoconstriction), neural (pain, tenderness, hyperesthesia, itching), and myofascial components (muscle contraction, fibrosis). These changes in turn lead to further changes in segmentally related tissues, especially circulatory (usually vasoconstriction) and neural tissues (altered efferent or afferent flow).

ADAPTATION

The lumbar spine must make certain adaptations to the position of the sacrum. It has already been noted that L5 and S1 are coupled through the iliolumbar ligaments and that the sacrum nutates and counternutates in response to lumbar flexion and extension (lumbopelvic rhythm). It has also been noted that certain spinal movements are coupled together consistently and have been defined as Fryette's laws (type I, neutral; type II, nonneutral). Neutral mechanics refers to when vertebral weight bearing is on the vertebral bodies, and the introduction of side bending results in the vertebral bodies twisting out from under the load (in the opposite direction of the side bending). Nonneutral mechanics of the spine refers to when sagittal plane motion in the vertebral facets (either through stretch or compression) is sufficient to influence motion so that the introduction of side bending results in a vertebral body twisting into the intended concavity, permitting side bending to occur. Neutral mechanics are usually grouped (three to five

segments), and nonneutral mechanics are usually single segmental.

It may be easier to think of the sacrum as behaving like a sixth lumbar vertebra when considering the functional integration of total spinal motion. Normally, if the sacrum side bends left, then L5 side bends right. In neutral (type I) spinal mechanics, if the L5 segment is side bent right, then it is coupled with rotation to the left. Thus if the sacrum is left side bent and the L5 vertebra is found to be left rotated, then one may presume—according to type I mechanics—that the spine has made a normal adaptation to the dysfunctional sacral position. When attempting to assess the presence of neutral adaptations in the lumbar spine, the clinician should start at the bottom and work up to the first segment with dysfunction. Any abnormal findings then relate to the last segment that was found to be normal.

Normal neutral adaptive lumbar spinal behavior occurs over three to five segments and produces a minimal flexion or extension restriction to overall spinal movement. The principal restriction to motion is side bending. The sacrum should always face the concavity of the lumbar spinal curve if the lumbar spine is normally adaptive.

Nonneutral or type II restrictions are coupled with side bending and rotation to the same side. Here the facets influence the motion to a greater extent, and the flexion or extension component is part of the restriction. In the L4 and L5 segments, the iliolumbar ligaments greatly influence these mechanics if flexion or extension is great enough to produce tension in them. A nonneutral restriction will restrict the segment above and below it. Thus if the sacrum is left side bent and it is found that the L5 vertebra is right rotated and right side bent, then one may presume (according to type II mechanics) that the lumbar spine has not made a normal adaptation to the sacral dysfunction. Nonadaptive lumbar responses to sacral positioning are highly significant in patients who do not get better or experience chronic recurrences. These responses must be treated before the underlying sacral lesion.

Recent research indicates that the coupled motion rules are not as predictable with flexion greater than extension of the lumbar spine.

EVALUATION

Development of the Tactile Sense

The clinician specializing in musculoskeletal disorders must refine his or her palpatory skills. Through palpation, the clinician should be able to do the following:

- Detect a tissue texture abnormality.
- Detect asymmetry of position of comparable body parts visually and tactilely.
- Detect differences in the quality and range of joint movement.
- Sense position in space (the patient's and his or her own).
- Detect changes in the palpatory findings from one examination to the next.

Development of palpatory skills involves three components within the neurophysiologic makeup of the clinician: (1) reception of information through the fingertips and eyes, (2) transmission of this information to the brain, and (3) interpretation of the information. The sensitivity or tactile discriminatory power of the fingertips is extremely fine.

The clinician's palpatory examination is usually performed last and should begin with light touch over the area of observation. This procedure allows a sort of scanning examination of the area and will reveal the presence of any great abnormalities in the superficial or deep layers of tissue, as well as increased warmth of the tissue. After the basic functional examination, the clinician can identify the structures or planes as the pressure of his or her palpation increases. The clinician may use shear movements across the tissues to discern different structures, planes, or the extent or size of a lesion. Such palpatory examination requires concentration; errors in reception often result from too much pressure (sensory discrimination actually decreases with increased pressure) and/or too much movement of the palpating fingertips.

Layer Palpation

The goal of palpatory diagnosis is to identify and define areas of somatic dysfunction. Somatic dysfunction is the impaired or altered function of related components of the somatic (body framework) system: skeletal, arthrodial, and myofascial structures and related vascular, lymphatic, and neural elements. Once such an area is identified, the goal of manual therapy is to improve function in that area (i.e., to improve the mobility of tissues [bone, joint, muscle, ligament, fascia, fluid] and to restore normal physiologic motion) as much as possible.

KEY LANDMARKS FOR PELVIC GIRDLE EVALUATION

For the experienced clinician it is important to be able to palpate accurately and consistently as part of the evaluation. For the student continued practice and anatomic review will help to improve reliability and accuracy of palpation skills. Only then will the clinician be able to assess dysfunction and accurately test, retest, and evaluate the effects of treatment. Structural asymmetry is the rule, not the exception, particularly in the lower lumbar and sacral spine. It is *normal* to see some asymmetry in the lumbopelvic region. According to Levangie, "In the absence of meaningful positive association between pelvic asymmetry and low-back pain, evaluation and treatment strategies based on this premise should be questioned."[116] In the following sections, several anatomic landmarks are discussed:

- Iliac crest
- ASIS
- Pubic tubercles
- PSIS
- Inferior lateral angle
- Sacrotuberous ligament
- Ischial tuberosity
- Medial malleolus

Iliac Crest

The iliac crests are compared with the patient in the standing and prone positions (Figure 19-22). Soft tissue must be moved

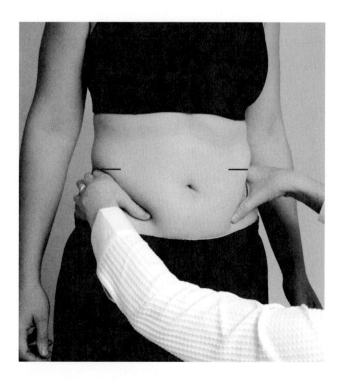

Figure 19-22 Palpation of the iliac crests. (From Magee DJ: Orthopedic physical assessment, ed 5, St Louis, 2008, Saunders.)

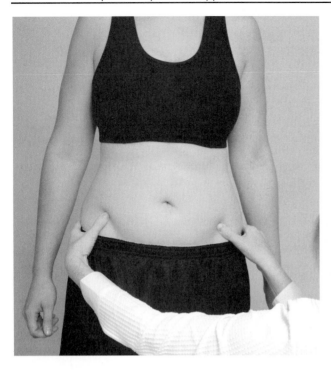

Figure 19-23 Palpation of the anterior superior iliac spine (ASIS). (From Magee DJ: Orthopedic physical assessment, ed 5, St Louis, 2008, Saunders.)

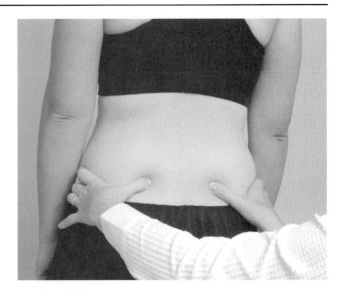

Figure 19-24 Palpation of the posterior superior iliac spine (PSIS). (From Magee DJ: Orthopedic physical assessment, ed 5, St Louis, 2008, Saunders.)

Inferior Lateral Angle

Another important landmark, the ILA, is found by palpating laterally approximately 1 to $1\frac{1}{2}$ inch from the sacral cornua. The posterior aspects can be assessed for their anteroposterior relationship, and the inferior aspects can be assessed for their superoinferior relationship.

Sacrotuberous Ligament

The sacrotuberous ligament is located between the ILA and the ischial tuberosity and must be compared for equality of tension and tenderness.

Ischial Tuberosity

The ischial tuberosities are palpated at their inferior aspects and are assessed for their relative superoinferior position and/or tenderness. The soft tissue must be moved out of the way (approached from below) to palpate the tuberosities (Figure 19-25).

Medial Malleolus

The inferior slopes of the medial malleoli can be located in both the supine and the prone positions. They are then compared for their relative superoinferior positions. The position of the malleoli gives information regarding leg length, as well as possible innominate rotation and/or pubic shear.

LOWER-QUARTER SCREENING EXAMINATION

The patient positions used in the examination of pelvic girdle dysfunction are standing, seated, supine, and prone.

out of the way by pushing it superiorly and medially above the crests. The crests are evaluated for their superoinferior relationship.

Anterior Superior Iliac Spine

The clinician should be able to locate the anterior medial aspect of the inferior slope of the ASIS, with the patient standing and in the supine position, and assess their relative positions (superoinferior and/or mediolateral) (Figure 19-23).

Pubic Tubercles

With the patient supine, the anterior aspects of the pubic tubercles are palpated for their relative anteroposterior position. Then the superior aspects of the tubercles are examined by pushing the soft tissue out of the way cranially to assess their relative craniocaudal position. The clinician should ask the patient for permission to palpate the tubercles, and have the patient show the exact location using the fingertips.

Posterior Superior Iliac Spine

The PSIS is a most important landmark and should be assessed in the standing, seated, and prone positions by locating the inferior slope of the posterior aspect of this prominence (Figure 19-24). Its relative position can be assessed as superoinferior and/or mediolateral.

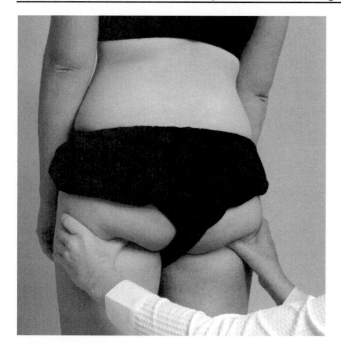

Figure 19-25 Palpation of the ischial tuberosities. (From Magee DJ: Orthopedic physical assessment, ed 5, St Louis, 2008, Saunders.)

To avoid unnecessary movement of the patient from one position to the other, which wastes time and may exacerbate the patient's condition, as many relevant tests as possible should be performed while the patient is in a particular position. The lower-quarter screening examination is included here for completeness because aspects of the screen may rule out certain diagnoses in a pelvic dysfunction examination. This examination sequence allows the clinician to rapidly evaluate the lower quarter as a whole and to avoid missing any major dysfunction (see appropriate chapters for related tests and their meanings).

The areas included in the examination are the lumbar spine screen, the SIJ, the pubic symphysis, the hip, the knee, the ankle, and the foot.

The examination begins with an inspection of the patients' facial expressions, how they move, and their posture and gait patterns, with attention to the positions of the following:
- Feet
- Knees
- Legs and leg length
- Pelvis
- Thoracolumbar spine

The clinician should note any swelling, atrophy, scar tissue (from previous surgery or injury), and/or changes in color. If palpation is performed before the functional examination, then feel only for skin temperature and swelling.

Before starting the functional examination, the clinician should ask the patient what he or she is currently feeling and where that feeling is located. The patient can also rate the pain on a scale from 0 to 10 (with 10 being the worst). Next the patient should be asked if the symptoms change with each test

and if the patient considers what he or she feels to be his or her pain. The uninvolved side should always be tested first to see what is "normal" for the patient (and compared with the involved side).

The clinician should pay attention to the range of motion with passive motions and the end feel with overpressure, as well as if the patient's symptoms are provoked. If a limitation of motion exists, then the clinician should decide if the limitation is in a capsular or noncapsular pattern. The capsular pattern of the hip is variable but usually involves a limitation primarily of internal rotation, followed by equal amounts of limited flexion, extension, and abduction. Internal rotation is limited in both 0 degrees of hip flexion and 90 degrees of hip flexion.[14,38] Adduction and external rotation are the least limited.

Resisted tests assess the contractile tissues for strength and pain associated with contraction and muscle recruitment. When pain with maintained strength occurs, it usually indicates a small muscle tendon lesion. When loss of strength and no pain occurs, it usually indicates a large muscle tendon lesion, total rupture, or a neurologic problem.

Another source of pain around the hip joint can be the bursae. Several bursae are located around the hip joint that can become compressed and painful with isometric contraction of muscles around the hip.[38]

The functional tests in Table 19-6 are then performed.

It should be remembered that the screening examination only indicates the area or areas where any lesions lie. A detailed examination should be performed of any area where a problem is detected. The clinician should not persist in the examination when it is apparent that the condition is being exacerbated.

After the functional examination is complete, the clinician should palpate gently again to feel for any change in temperature or swelling. At this point, more in-depth palpation can be performed to inspect the involved tissues or structures.

CLEARING TESTS FOR THE HIP

Should the clinician need to clear the hip to differentiate between hip and lumbar or sacroiliac problems, the following special procedures are recommended:
- Log roll test
- Thomas test
- Scour test
- Hip apprehension test
- Trochanteric bursitis tests
- Iliopectineal (iliopsoas) bursitis test
- FABER (flexion, abduction, and external rotation) test (Patrick's test)
- Piriformis tightness
- Femoral nerve stretch test
- Lateral femoral cutaneous nerve stretch test
- Fulcrum test
- Ober's test
- SLR for hamstring length
- Active straight-leg raise (ASLR) test

Table 19-6	Functional Examination of the Lower Quarter

Position	Tests
Standing	Active range of motion (AROM) in the lumbar spine, all planes; add full cervical flexion at end of trunk flexion
	Active clearing test for peripheral joints (full squat)
	Toe walking (S1, S2)
	Heel walking (L4, L5)
Sitting	Active and passive rotation of the thoracolumbar spine
	Knee jerk reflex (L3, L4)
	Slump test
Supine	Active and passive straight-leg raise tests (SLR)
	Sacroiliac joint (SIJ) dorsolateral provocation test
	Range of motion of the hip, all planes (check for sign of the buttock[38])
	Assess quality of motion, extent of motion/pain
	Passive hip flexion, internal and external rotation at 90 degrees of hip flexion, passive abduction with the knee flexed and extended, and passive adduction of the hip
	Resisted hip flexion in 90 degrees of hip flexion (LI, L2)
	Resisted hip abduction in neutral, bilaterally
	Resisted hip adduction bilaterally in neutral, 45 degrees of hip flexion, and 90 degrees of hip flexion
	Resisted ankle dorsiflexion (L4); assess for strength/pain
	Resisted eversion of the foot (L5, S1); assess for strength/pain
	Knee-clearing tests (full extension, varus and valgus stress)
	Trochanteric bursitis test (extra test)
	Iliopectineal (Iliopsoas) bursitis test (extra test)
	Resisted abdominals (extra tests)
Prone	Passive hip extension
	Passive internal and external rotation with knees in 90 degrees of flexion
	Resisted hip extension
	Resisted knee flexion (S1), with knee in 70 degrees of flexion
	Resisted knee extension (L3, L4), with knee in 70 degrees of flexion
	Resisted external rotation of the hip, with bilateral knees in 90 degrees of flexion
	Resisted internal rotation of the hip, with bilateral knees in 90 degrees of flexion
	Hip apprehension test[1]
	Ankle jerk (Achilles) reflex (S1)
	Observation of gluteal mass (assess for any asymmetry)
	Spring testing (thoracolumbar spine and sacrum)
	Ankle-clearing tests
Side lying (extra tests)	Femoral nerve stretch test (L3)
	Lateral femoral cutaneous nerve stretch test
	Ventromedial provocation sacroiliac joint (SIJ) test
Sitting (extra test)	Fulcrum test

- Medial femoral triangle
- Lateral femoral triangle

Illustrations and video demonstrations of some of these procedures can be found on the Evolve site that accompanies this text.

Log Roll Test

The log roll test is a joint play movement for internal and external rotation of the hip in extension. The clinician simply rolls the thigh under his or her hands to get an end feel of the joint in internal and external rotation (while patient is supine). By watching the excursion of the feet, the clinician can estimate range of motion.

Thomas Test

The Thomas test detects tightness of the long and short flexor muscles of the hip. While lying with one leg freely hanging over the edge of an examination table, the patient flexes the opposite hip toward the chest to a point where the lumbar spine flattens against the table. The freely hanging leg is then observed for its position in space. The knee should be flexed to 70 to 90 degrees, and the hip should be in 0 degrees of extension. Sufficient knee flexion with the hip also in flexion indicates tightness of the iliopsoas group. Proper extension of the hip with a lack of knee flexion indicates tightness and/or shortness of the rectus femoris. Abduction of the hip indicates tightness of the iliotibial band.

Scour Test

The scour test is performed to "feel" the acetabular rim. The clinician literally scours the femoral head around the acetabular rim from the point of maximal extension, abduction, and external rotation to the point of maximal flexion, adduction, and internal rotation. The second part of this test is to return to the starting position in the opposite direction. Throughout this test, axial compression is applied to the hip through the knee. The clinician thus "palpates" for any resistance, joint crepitation and for "bumps" in the smoothness of the range of motion that may indicate capsular tightness, an adhesion, or loss of joint congruity. In addition, the clinician should pay attention to any tenderness as the femur moves into flexion and internal rotation. If a click, followed by pain occurs, this test is considered positive for a labral lesion.

Hip Apprehension Test

As the patient lies prone, the clinician brings the hip into hyperextension and external rotation. The examiner applies overpressure at the end of the motion by pushing anteriorly on the posterior proximal femur. At the same time, the examiner pulls the anterior distal thigh into further hyperextension and external rotation. When a painful snap occurs, this test is positive for a labral defect and indicates a slight anterior subluxation.[38]

Trochanteric Bursitis Tests

With the patient lying supine, the examiner stands on the side to be tested. The patient's hip is put into maximal flexion and adduction. The examiner rotates the hip into maximal internal rotation, while holding the knee and ankle. If no pain occurs, then the hip is rotated into maximal external rotation. The test is positive for trochanteric bursitis if the patient feels pain posterior to the greater trochanter.[38]

Iliopectineal (Iliopsoas) Bursitis Test

The patient is lying supine, and the examiner stands on the side to be tested. The patient's hip is put into maximal flexion and slight adduction. The examiner holds the knee and ankle and applies axial pressure through the femur while bringing the hip into external rotation. The test is positive if the patient experiences anterior hip pain.

FABER (Patrick's) Test

See "Objective Examination of the Sacroiliac Joint."

Piriformis Tightness

See "Objective Examination of the Sacroiliac Joint."

Femoral Nerve Stretch Test

The patient lies on the nonsymptomatic side while the examiner stands behind. The patient moves into maximal flexion of the entire neck and spine. The bottom leg and hip are brought into maximal flexion, with the patient holding the leg inward. The examiner then puts the top leg and hip into maximal extension and slight abduction. To induce tension in the femoral nerve, the patient's knee is flexed. Lastly, the patient is asked to extend his or her neck. This test is positive for a tension sign of the lumbar plexus and/or femoral nerve pathologic condition if the patient's pain occurs with knee flexion followed by a decrease in pain with neck extension.[38]

If the femoral nerve is entrapped, this movement should produce neurologic pain in the femoral nerve distribution of the anterior thigh. This test may also be used to assess rectus femoris tightness (see "Entrapment Syndromes of the Hip and Pelvis").

Lateral Femoral Cutaneous Nerve Stretch Test

This test starts in the same position as the previous test (femoral nerve stretch test), with the spine and neck flexed and the bottom knee flexed. The examiner stabilizes the pelvis while the other hand supports the leg in slight hip adduction (so that the femur is horizontal) and knee extension. The leg is brought into maximal hip extension, which exerts tension on the lateral femoral cutaneous nerve. Then the patient is asked to extend his or her neck. The test is positive for a lateral femoral cutaneous nerve lesion if pain occurs with hip extension and is decreased with neck extension.[38]

Fulcrum Test

The patient is seated on the table with the legs bent over the edge and lower legs hanging. The examiner puts one forearm or a towel roll under the midfemur and gently presses down on the distal femur. The forearm and towel can be moved proximal to distal while applying pressure to the distal femur. The test is positive if the patient's pain is provoked. This test is used to detect stress fractures in the femoral shaft.[117]

Ober's Test

Ober's test is used to assess the length of the hip abductor muscles, particularly the gluteus medius and the TFL and iliotibial band. The patient lies on the unaffected side, facing away from the clinician. The clinician asks the patient to raise (abduct) the leg toward the ceiling, with the knee flexed to 90 degrees. Knee flexion relaxes the iliotibial tract and fascia lata. Using his or her own body weight to stabilize the pelvis (above the level of the hip joint), the clinician instructs the patient to lower the leg. Normal muscle length permits the patient's thigh to cross the midline and touch the downside leg. The reliability of Ober's test as a measure of iliotibial band tightness is controversial.[118] (For information on a modified Ober's test, see Kendall and Kendall-McCreary[119]).

Straight-Leg Raise for Hamstring Length

The patient lies supine with the legs in extension, and the examiner stands on the side to be tested. The patient's opposite ASIS is palpated, and his or her ankle is grasped on the side being tested. The patient's leg is lifted, with the knee extended until the opposite ASIS moves. The clinician measures the angle of hip flexion from the table with the opposite leg extended, and the test is repeated the test on the other side. The hamstrings are considered shortened if they cannot reach 80 degrees from the horizontal with the other leg straight.[120]

This test can also be used for neural tension (especially the sciatic nerve) by dorsiflexing the ankle before lifting the leg, while keeping the knee straight.

Active Straight-Leg Raise Test

According to Mens et al.,[121,122] the supine ASLR test measures the ability to transfer loads effectively between the lumbosacral spine and legs. If movement occurs in the pelvis (flexion, extension, side bend, or rotation) relative to the trunk or legs, then pelvic instability or poor muscle activation of the local and global systems could exist. The clinician can compress the pelvis (either manually or with an sacroiliac belt) and retest the ASLR to determine if imposed pelvic stability decreases the pain.

Medial Femoral Triangle

Palpation of the structures of the femoral triangle is important in distinguishing soft tissue problems in and around the hip. The borders of the femoral triangle are the inguinal ligament superiorly (originating at the ASIS and running medially and caudally to the pubic tubercle), the sartorius laterally (which can be palpated by active hip flexion and external rotation [figure four position]), and the adductor longus medially (which has a prominent tendon that can be palpated with slight adduction when the hip is in 45 to 60 degrees of flexion). The adductor longus originates on the pubic tubercle. The floor of the femoral triangle is formed by portions of the adductor longus, the pectineus, and the iliopsoas muscles. The femoral artery, the psoas bursa, and the hip joint may be found within the triangle. These structures are best palpated in 0 degrees of flexion. The femoral nerve is located just lateral to the artery, whereas the vein is just medial to the artery (although it is not palpable). The inguinal ligament extends from the ASIS to the pubic tubercles and should be palpated for tenderness and tightness. The FABER position is best for the examination of the femoral triangle.

Lateral Femoral Triangle

The ASIS is the apex of this triangle. The lateral border is the TFL, and the sartorius serves as the medial border. The triangle can be easily seen in active hip flexion, external rotation, slight abduction, and slight knee flexion. It serves as a good landmark for locating the rectus femoris and its insertion on the AIIS, as

well as the joint capsule, which lies approximately 5 cm infero-medial to the ASIS. When a lesion exists in the rectus femoris tendon, the patient has pain with prone resisted knee extension.

COMMON HIP SYNDROMES OR PATHOLOGIC CONDITIONS OF THE HIP

The history will provide vital information regarding the mechanism of injury and the patient's primary complaint. Positions or activities that increase or decrease symptoms must be noted, as well as how pain affects activities of daily living (ADL). The time or times of day the patient experiences pain and symptoms can also provide clues as to what structure is involved.

Sacroiliac and pubic dysfunctions often produce pain in the groin area; thus groin pain can be referred or local. Osteoarthritis (OA) of the hip can also cause pain in the groin, as well as in the anterior thigh posterior to the greater trochanter, and in the knee because of the nerves that cross the hip.[123] The clinician evaluating a patient with these complaints must be able to differentiate between complaints of hip origin and those of pelvic origin. With a functional examination, a capsular pattern of limitation of the hip is most commonly described as internal rotation being most painful and limited, with abduction, flexion, and extension less limited. The following discussion presents some of the signs and symptoms of several common hip problems that must be considered in any evaluation of this region:

- Degenerative joint disease (i.e., OA)
- Loose body
- Legg-Calvé-Perthes disease (LCPD), or Perthes disease
- Acetabular labral tear
- Iliopectineal bursitis (psoas bursitis)
- Trochanteric bursitis
- Sign of the buttock
- Hamstring syndrome
- Groin pain (pubalgia)

Degenerative Joint Disease (Osteoarthritis)

Degenerative joint disease is the most common disease process affecting the hip in adults. The degenerative tissue changes that occur with symptomatic degenerative joint disease are usually reactions to increased stress to the joint over time. Some predisposing factors include congenital hip dysplasia, osteochondrosis, SCFE, leg length discrepancy, a tight hip capsule, and shock loading.

The patient is usually middle aged or older, with an insidious onset of groin or trochanteric pain, which becomes more pronounced after use of the joint (e.g., walking, running). Typically, the pain is felt first in the groin and later in the L2 and L3 distributions (anterior thigh and knee). Later, it progresses laterally and posteriorly. The pain rarely extends below the knee. Complaints often include morning stiffness and stiffness when arising from the sitting position, with pain by the end of the day. Symptoms progress to a constant ache at night and loss of functional abilities such as tying one's shoes and climbing stairs.

The clinician should assess range of motion of the hip, noting any loss of abduction and internal rotation. The clinician should test for a capsular pattern, perform the log roll test, the scour test, the Thomas test, and the FABER test, as well as palpate the femoral triangle.

When early or even moderately advanced signs of degenerative joint disease of the hip are detected, the clinician may elect to use capsular stretch techniques and long axis distraction for pain control and improvement in function.

Loose Body

A loose body can be a piece of bone or cartilage, and may occur without previous trauma or pathology. The CFJ is more susceptible to loose bodies in advanced cases of OA. The most common symptom is a sharp, sudden pain in the groin with weight bearing followed by a feeling of giving way in the leg. The pain is usually brief, and can sometimes be felt in the thigh or knee.

A loose body causes a noncapsular pattern of limitation with a springy end feel (usually felt with passive hip extension because that is the close-packed position). Passive external rotation may be limited with the hip in 90 degrees of flexion, abduction or adduction. Imaging should be performed to rule out serious pathology such as ischemic (avascular/aseptic) necrosis of the femoral head, osteochondrosis dissecans, synovial (osteo)chondromatosis, which is rare, or pigmented villonodular synovitis. Once serious pathology is ruled out, the loose body can be treated with a rotation manipulation under traction.[38] Often the loose body will be absorbed into the synovial membrane; otherwise surgical excision may be necessary.

Legg-Calvé-Perthes Disease (Perthes Disease)

LCPD is a hip disorder typically seen in children between the ages of 3 and 10 years old, but it may occur up to age 15. This condition is characterized by necrosis of the femoral head.[124] In children, ischemic necrosis of the femoral head is usually associated with LCPD or slipped capital femoral epiphysis (SCFE). The exact cause of LCPD is unknown, but theories include poor, variable vasculature with repeated infarction episodes.[125]

This condition can lead to collapse of the femoral head and neck. Subchondral fractures may occur under the femoral head cartilage.[126] Because of the changes in the subchondral bone and ischemia, osteochondritis dissecans can develop, creating loose bodies that may require surgical removal if they interfere with hip function.[127,128] Deformation of the femoral head can occur if not diagnosed early. This disorder can occur bilaterally, but it tends to develop several months apart.[129]

Clinical presentation usually starts with limping and slight dragging of the leg. Because of the altered joint structure and decreased joint movement, the abductors are unable to function normally.[130] Muscle spasms may also occur early in the disease.

Later the pain appears in the groin, thigh, and medial knee, and the limp increases.

The examination reveals a moderate limitation in the capsular pattern. There may be some atrophy of the thigh muscles, along with a positive Trendelenburg's test (while standing on the involved leg, the pelvis tilts toward the uninvolved side). The diagnosis is confirmed with imaging. It is best visualized with an anteroposterior radiograph along with an anteroposterior view with the hip in flexion, abduction, and external rotation (Lauenstein's position).

Treatment for LCPD remains controversial but should be administered by a specialist. The treatment can be conservative or operative, depending on the stage of the disease. The primary goal is to prevent femoral head collapse and displacement by keeping the femoral head inside the acetabulum. A conservative approach to maintain this position is wearing a leg brace that keeps the legs in hip abduction and slight internal rotation. The patient can still actively flex the hip, so he or she may ride a bike and run while wearing the brace.[131]

Acetabular Labral Tear

Labral tears can be degenerative (horizontal), traumatic (vertical), dysplastic, or idiopathic.[132] The diagnosis is determined from the history and physical examination. Labral tears present in a variety of ways, with a number of clinical findings. If the history is traumatic (40%) the tear usually occurs when the hip joint is stressed in rotation (twisting or falling) or forced into adduction. The pain is usually felt in the groin, but it can also be experienced in the buttock, thigh, or trochanteric region.[133] Degenerative lesions occur 49% of the time, whereas congenital lesions occur 5% of the time.[134] The diagnosis can be confirmed with magnetic resonance arthrography, magnetic resonance imaging (MRI) with intraarticular contrast medium, or arthroscopy.[135,136] A fluoroscopic injection can differentiate extraarticular versus intraarticular symptoms.[137]

The most common tears are posterior-superior or anterior-superior on the labrum. Seldes et al.,[138] classify tears as type 1 or type 2, according to their anatomy and histology. When the labrum detaches from the articular cartilage, it is considered type 1. These tears are perpendicular to the articular surface and sometimes extend to the bone. When one or more fissures develop within the labral substance, it is considered type 2. Traumatic tears that are vertical can go to various depths in the substance of the labrum and may involve avulsion.[139] Horizontal degenerative tears can detach the labrum from the cartilage transition zone or cause separation within the labrum.[138]

The patient with a labral tear will usually complain of pain with sitting and climbing stairs. There will often be clicking, locking, catching, or giving way associated with weight bearing. With an anterior-superior tear, examination may reveal pain and possible limitation of passive internal rotation when the hip is in flexion and adduction.[133] With a posterior tear, passive hyperextension, abduction, and external rotation will elicit pain.[140] It is helpful to take the leg through a passive range of motion from hip flexion, external rotation, and full abduction, into extension, abduction, and internal rotation to test for anterior tears. The motion for posterior tears would include extension, abduction, and external rotation followed by flexion, adduction, and internal rotation.[141]

Treatment of labral lesions includes patient education focusing on pathologic condition and activities to avoid. Patients should be encouraged to decrease the stress on the labral cartilage by minimizing use of stairs and long periods of sitting with the hip flexed. The patient may require an assistive device initially. The patient may ride a stationary bike with decreased load and decreased hip flexion (with an upright bike, the seat can be raised; with a recumbent bike, the seat can be moved back).[139] The clinician may perform a rotation manipulation during traction after ruling out instability and necrotic changes. The physician may perform intraarticular injection of corticosteroid agents in chronic cases. If conservative interventions fail, then the patient may require arthroscopic excision and partial labrectomy.[38]

Iliopectineal Bursitis (Psoas Bursitis)

The iliopectineal bursa lies anterior to the hip joint between the capsule and the iliopsoas musculotendinous junction. Inflammation is fairly common and can be confused with degenerative joint disease of the hip and vice versa. In some cases a congenital communication can exist between the bursae and the hip synovial compartment.[142]

Pain from an iliopectineal bursitis is often insidious and can be acute or chronic. Acute bursitis is usually from trauma, such as a kick to the groin area. Chronic cases result from cumulative microtrauma caused by biomechanical factors (i.e., shorter leg, altered lower-extremity structure, short hip muscle). Such lesions are often missed for several years. Pain is felt in the groin, with some radiation into the L2 and L3 distributions. The pain usually occurs with activity but may also occur at rest. The clinician should check for a restriction in the capsular pattern of motion to rule out joint effusion or capsular involvement. A positive test for iliopectineal bursitis would be pain with passive hip flexion, external rotation, and extension. The pain may increase initially when adduction is added to any of the previously mentioned movements, or a painful arc may occur (whereby the pain increases during the movement and decreases as the range moves toward the end). In addition, consistent pain may be felt with full flexion combined with passive external rotation.[38] Diagnostic ultrasound or MRI are the best tests to confirm this bursitis.[143]

Treatment should include correction of any leg length discrepancy. Pulsed ultrasound directed into the bursa, coupled with the use of nonsteroidal antiinflammatory drugs (NSAIDs) may be beneficial in the treatment of iliopectineal bursitis. The bursa can be injected with a local anesthetic agent or a corticosteroid agent with fluoroscopic guidance.[144]

Trochanteric Bursitis

The onset of trochanteric bursitis is usually traumatic (acute or microtraumatic causing irritation and inflammation) but can

be insidious. Occasionally, the patient reports an incident when he or she heard a "snap" in the posterolateral region of the hip (e.g., when getting into a car). The pain is located in the lateral hip, although it may radiate into L4 or L5 distribution along the lateral thigh to the knee and lower leg. Occasionally, it may radiate proximally to the lumbar region and mimic an L5 spinal lesion. A tight TFL tendon may also produce a "snap" over the trochanter, resulting in a friction syndrome.

The pain of a trochanteric bursitis is a deep, aching sclerotogenous pain rather than the sharp dermatomal L5 pain of nerve root involvement. Sitting, stair climbing, and side lying, all of which compress the bursa, will be painful. The patient may stand in a lateral pelvic shift away from the side of involvement, which also increases valgus stress at the knee.

The clinician tests the bursa by fully flexing the patient's hip passively and then moving it into adduction and external rotation. This maneuver compresses the stretched bursa under the gluteus maximus. From this position the clinician may then resist internal rotation and would find consistent pain if positive. The patient would also consistently feel pain with passive internal or external rotation with the hip in 90 degrees of flexion. Less consistent pain may be felt with resisted hip abduction, extension, or external rotation. The clinician may also palpate the bursa, which is located posterior to the trochanter rather than directly on top of it, next to the gluteus maximus. The reader should keep in mind that several bursae are found around the greater trochanter; the largest is the trochanteric bursa.

Ultrasound and the use of a hydrocortisone-based coupling agent (phonophoresis), Iontophoresis (depending on the depth of the bursae), ice massage, and NSAIDs may prove helpful in the treatment of trochanteric bursitis. An injection would be a treatment of choice, if injected directly into the bursa. If a TFL friction syndrome is considered a possibility, then stretching exercises may be indicated for the iliotibial tract, as well as the iliopsoas muscle (including hip extension with internal rotation).[145]

Sign of the Buttock

The *sign of the buttock* is a collection of signs that indicate a serious pathologic condition with severe pain in the gluteal region and occasionally the groin. Such pathologic condition could be traumatic, including fracture of the pelvis or sacrum. Insidious onset could involve an abscess, osteomyelitis, septic bursitis, infectious sacroiliitis, rheumatic bursitis, gluteal tumor or hematoma, or a tumor in the pelvic region. A patient with a positive sign of the buttock should be referred immediately to a physician.

The patient generally experiences difficulty walking, and complains of severe pain in the gluteal region. The pain can radiate to the posterior thigh and occasionally to the foot.

The sign of the buttock is conducted with the patient supine while the clinician performs a passive SLR. A positive sign is indicated by the following:

- Extremely limited and painful SLR
- Extremely limited passive hip flexion with the knee flexed with an empty end feel
- A noncapsular pattern of the passive hip tests

To determine the cause of a positive sign of the buttock, a bone scan should be performed, along with lab tests and imaging. The treatment will depend on the cause.[38]

Hamstring Syndrome

Hamstring syndrome involves entrapment and epineural irritation of the sciatic nerve as it comes around the ischial tuberosity. At this point the nerve goes through a fibrous band where the biceps femoris attaches to the tuberosity.[39] Injuries that can predispose the sciatic nerve to this syndrome include previous history of low-back pain or surgery and hamstring strains. The most common athletes to have this syndrome include power sprinters, jumping athletes, and runners.[40]

The clinical examination reveals pain localized to the ischial tuberosity, which increases with activity and stretching. The patient will also experience pain with sitting and with resisted knee flexion while the leg is in a SLR position (yet testing in prone would be painless). Neural tension to the sciatic nerve (positive SLR or slump test) and palpation to the sciatic nerve, lateral to the ischial tuberosity (in side lying on uninvolved side, with the hips and knees in 90 degrees of flexion), also elicit pain.

Treatment should include gentle neural mobilization of the lower extremity with distal initiation at the knee or ankle and foot. Stretching should be avoided, and the patient should sit with a wedge to decrease hip flexion. A trial of iontophoresis can be performed with the electrode placed in the same places as the previously mentioned palpated areas. Severe cases may require surgical release.[38]

Groin Pain (Pubalgia)

Pubalgia is a collective term for several disorders that cause pain around the pubic tubercle and the structures that attach to it. The most common complaint is groin pain. However, the exact location of groin pain can change and be misleading. The pain can be unilateral initially and progress to bilateral in 40% of people.[146] When lower abdominal pain occurs, it is usually due to an insertion tendopathy of the abdominal muscles. The pain usually occurs during the closed-chain activity like pivoting in soccer, kicking, or sprinting.

The pain is often around the pubic symphysis and can extend into the lower abdomen and groin. The pain usually occurs after more vigorous activities than usual or if the athlete has not prepared enough for the sport or activity (as with the "weekend warrior"). The most common sports that are associated with this disorder include soccer, speed skating, track and field, swimming, and distance running.[38]

Pubalgia is most often a sports injury in which the unipodal, weight-bearing leg supports the pelvis and trunk as they rotate over the hip, while the other leg performs a movement like kicking. The abdominal and weight-bearing leg muscles

must provide a great amount of stability for the other leg to achieve an explosive movement. With this type of motion, small shearing movements take place in the pubic symphysis. One cause of shearing movements in the symphysis could be a muscle imbalance between the abdominals and adductors, with increased load on the tendon insertions and the adductor muscles. This scenario is more common in male subjects than female subjects. Occasionally, avulsion may occur at the adductor tendon insertions.[147] Which structure actually causes the pain during loading is controversial. Some believe pubalgia is due to tendopathy,[148] whereas others believe it is from a sportsman's hernia[149] or osteitis pubis.

Often the abdominal muscles can have an insertion tendopathy as well, in the rectus abdominis more than the obliques. Because this tendon combines with the arcuate ligament and adductor longus, its insertion may become tension loaded with resisted hip adduction. Cough, sneeze, and strain can be painful because the abdominal muscles pull on the irritated arcuate ligament. Pain with resisted trunk flexion in supine would confirm tendon involvement.[38]

Athletes must perform correct technique with running, swimming, or skating so that tendopathy can be avoided. If not, then the adductors are overloaded and produce microtears in the muscle belly and tendopathy at the insertion of the adductor longus. Other tendopathies that occur less often are in the adductor brevis, gracilis, and pectineus muscles. The adductors fatigue from overload, which causes increased tension and muscle shortening. This shortening and tightening results in a constant pull on the tendons and their insertion sites. An increased shearing force is seen on the symphysis, which causes the anterosuperior ligaments of the symphysis to stretch, creating instability with symphysis disc irritation.[38]

Four clinical stages of adductor tendopathy exist:[38]
- Stage 1: Short-lasting groin pain, especially after exertion
- Stage 2: Groin pain at the beginning of exertion that returns more intensely after 1 day and decreases with rest
- Stage 3: Unilateral pain in the groin and lower abdominal area during the entire exertion and lasting for several days
- Stage 4: Chronic pain that increases with exertion and only slightly decreases with rest

Examination should include the pelvis, hip, and lumbar spine. Passive hip flexion with adduction will usually be painful because the adductors get compressed at their origin. Passive hip abduction can be painful with the knee in extension or flexion. If the gracilis is involved, then the pain will decrease with the knee in flexion.
- When the most pain is with resisted hip adduction with the hips in 0 degrees of hip flexion, it indicates tendopathies of the gracilis, adductor longus, and brevis. Painful resisted knee flexion also indicates involvement of the gracilis.
- When the most pain is with resisted hip adduction with the hips in 45 degrees of hip flexion, it indicates the pubic symphysis is involved. The pain should decrease if retested with a sacroiliac belt.
- When the most pain is with resisted hip adduction with the hips in 90 degrees of flexion, it indicates pectineus involvement. Additionally, resisted abdominal testing would

produce pain if the abdominals are involved. Palpation can be performed to localize the specific tendon involved. MRI can confirm the diagnosis, along with diagnostic ultrasound.[38]

Treatment should include improving any poor techniques with the sport. For instance, track runners should alternate which direction and which edge they run around on the track. Treatment should also include correction of leg length discrepancies or muscle imbalances as needed. Athletes may continue to participate in sports if it does not increase their pain. If possible, then these athletes should receive daily treatments. If no improvement is seen after the first week, then the painful activities must be avoided; this would apply to athletes in stage 1. Those in stage 2 tendopathy should decrease their frequency, duration, and intensity by 25% until the pain starts to decrease. Stage 3 should decrease by 50%; stage 4 should stop activity until at least 50% improvement is seen, then return to the sport gradually.[38]

Conservative management can include transverse friction massage (only put pressure across one direction, rest to bring back to starting position) to the insertion of the tendon. Stretching should be performed as tolerated to the involved and surrounding myofascial tissues including the short and long adductors, the hip flexors (psoas and rectus femoris), hip internal rotators, abdominals, and gluteals. Strengthening of the adductors should be prescribed as pain allows. The abdominals should also be trained isometrically initially, progressing to concentric and eccentric, followed by isokinetic when ready. Proprioception and core stability training should also be included. If no improvement is seen, then the area may need to be injected with a corticosteroid agent.[144] Surgery may be indicated if no improvement is seen after 3 months of rest.[150] The reader should keep in mind that symphyseal instability may be treated with wearing an sacroiliac belt for 3 months, 23 hours a day. The clinician should remind the athlete to prepare correctly for his or her sport and include an effective warm-up to prevent further injury.

SUBJECTIVE EXAMINATION

Evaluation of the lumbopelvic unit begins with the subjective examination. A careful, detailed history is essential for proper diagnosis and management of these problems. The following outline by Maitland[151] provides a concise historical context and tends to focus the clinician's attention toward particular trouble spots. The outline by the International Academy of Orthopaedic Medicine includes asking five questions: *who* (age, gender, pregnancy), *what/where* (type and location of pain, referred or not), *when* (traumatic or not, what reproduces the pain, time of day), and *to what extent* (acute or chronic, bilateral or unilateral). The history should reveal the patient's main complaint; his or her occupation and sport or hobby; onset, duration, and location of complaints; any relevant past medical history; factors that influence the symptoms; and medications. These questions will help with differential diagnosis and to discern whether the pain is from mechanical, activity-related, or nonmechanical sources. This part of the examination is also essential to building trust and a healthy clinician-patient relationship.

Location of Pain

Use of a body chart is helpful. The clinician should note the length (proximal to distal), width (medial to lateral), depth (superficial to deep), type (e.g., burning, aching), and intensity (e.g., sharp, dull) of the pain. In addition, he or she should note any areas of paresthesia or anesthesia.

History and Behavior of Symptoms

The clinician should obtain a detailed account—to the best of the patient's recollection—of the first episode of similar pain. Often this is a vivid memory, and the patient will have no trouble in relating the episode. The clinician gathers information about subsequent episodes of the problem, including frequency of occurrence, how irritable the pain is, any strategies the patient uses to lessen the pain, recovery time, and any previous treatments, whether successful or not. The interview should continue through the patient's present history and behavior of symptoms (Figure 19-26).

Effect of Rest

The clinician then obtains answers to the following questions:
- How does rest affect the pain? (Note: Pain of musculoskeletal origin usually gets better with rest.)
- Does the pain ever awaken the patient during the night? (Night pain that awakens an individual from a sound sleep should be a red flag to the clinician, suggesting neoplastic activity.)
- What is the pain like in the morning? (Does the patient awaken pain free and then experience exacerbation of symptoms as the day goes on, or does the patient awaken with the same pain, which remains at a constant level throughout the day?)
- Is there any stiffness? (The clinician should consider rheumatologic or degenerative processes.)

PARTICULAR QUESTIONS CONCERNING THE PELVIC JOINTS

- Have you experienced a sudden sharp jolt to the leg, such as, after unexpectedly stepping off a curb? (This mechanism is a very common mechanism in innominate rotations and shears.)
- Have you recently experienced a fall directly onto your buttocks? (This mechanism is very common in innominate rotations and shears.)

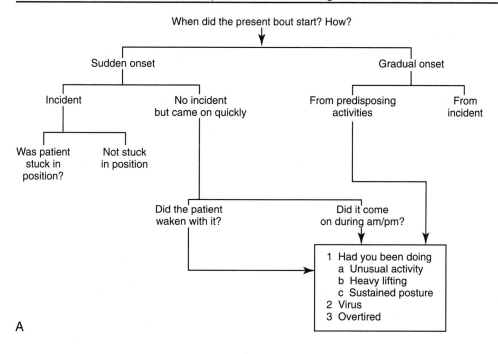

A

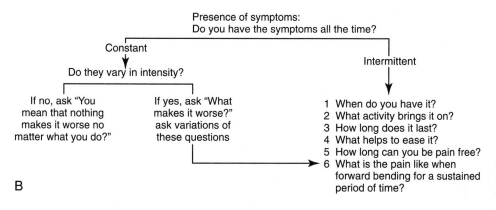

B

Figure 19-26 A, Flowchart of the patient's present history. **B,** Flowchart for determining the presence of symptoms.

- What is the effect on the pain of sitting, standing, walking, or maintaining a sustained posture? (If pain, especially radicular pain, increases with sitting, then a discogenic cause is more of a possibility; if pain increases with standing, then the SIJ may be implicated, particularly if the patient habitually tends to stand with weight borne more unilaterally; if the pain increases with walking, then the SIJ is strongly implicated.)
- Has the patient recently experienced a sudden trunk flexion with rotation? (This is a common mechanism for sacroiliac strain.)

When interpreting SIJ tests, remember that bone deformation, as well as fascial movement, can play a role.[50] Deformation of bone may occur because it contains much collagen. For example, the ilium can deform slightly with SIJ mobility tests. In addition, the sacrum can have palpable movement until around 25 years of age, because the vertebrae are not fully fused yet.

PARTICULAR QUESTIONS CONCERNING CONTRAINDICATIONS

- How is your general health? (This question is essential to glean any history of carcinoma, chronic disease, or general malaise that indicates nonmusculoskeletal origin.)
- Have you had a recent unexplained weight loss? (Recent unexplained weight loss would be a red flag to the clinician because it may indicate neoplastic activity.)
- Are you currently taking any medications? (It is helpful to know what a patient may be taking and for what reasons. The clinician should remember the potential side effects and symptoms that medications may produce in the neuromusculoskeletal system.)
- Has the patient had any recent radiographs of the spine or pelvis? (In cases of trauma, radiographs are always mandatory. In cases of chronic back pain, radiographs should probably be no more than 1 year old.)

HOW IMPORTANT IS IMAGING?

- There continues to be a considerable margin of error in the interpretation of SIJ radiographs in plain film imaging.[152]
- Computed tomography (CT) scans are limited in diagnostic value for SIJ disease because of low sensitivity (57.5%) and specificity (69%).[152,153]
- CT or MRI demonstrate poor correlation with SIJ pain invasive provocation.[154]
- Diagnostic ultrasound/color Doppler imaging that compares vibration energy between the sacrum and ilium appears to be helpful in evaluating stability and stiffness of the SIJ.[155]
- SIJ fluoroscopic blocks can be considered the gold standard in the diagnosis of SIJ pathologic conditions. The best technique appears to be a short, followed by a long-acting anesthesia.[48,156]

OBJECTIVE EXAMINATION

As with any musculoskeletal complaint, examination begins as the patient walks into the office. The clinician should observe how the patient walks, moves, and sits, especially if the patient does not know that he or she is being observed.

The following outline for planning the objective examination is based on the work of Maitland.[151]

Cause of Pain

- Name every joint and muscle that must be examined as the possible source of any part of the patient's pain:
  - Joints that lie under the painful area
  - Joints that refer pain into the area
  - Muscles that lie under the painful area
- Are you going to perform a neurologic examination?
- Identify the joints above and below that must be cleared.

Influence of Pain on the Examination

- Is the pain severe? Does it reproduce the patient's perceived pain?
- Does the subjective examination suggest an easily irritable disorder?
- Are the symptoms local or referred? Which is the dominant factor?
- Give an example of the following:
  - An activity that causes increased pain
  - The severity of the pain (so caused)
  - Duration before the pain subsides
- Does the nature of the pain indicate caution?
  - Pathologic condition (e.g., osteoporosis, rheumatoid arthritis)
  - Episodes easily caused
  - Imminent nerve root compression

Kind of Examination Indicated

- Do you think you will need to be gentle or moderately vigorous with your examination of movements?
- Do you expect a comparable sign to be easy or hard to find?
- Do you think you will be treating pain, resistance, or weakness?

Cause of the Pain (Other Factors)

- What associated factors must be examined as reasons for the present symptoms that might cause recurrence (e.g., posture, muscle imbalance, muscle power, obesity, stiffness, hypomobility, hypermobility, instability, deformity in a proximal or distal joint)?
- In planning the treatment (after the examination), what patient education measures would you include to prevent or lessen recurrences?

OBJECTIVE EXAMINATION OF THE SACROILIAC JOINT

Evaluation of the pelvic hip complex involves a common sense approach in the correlation of comparable signs. This means that a given dysfunctional lesion will reflect a fairly consistent pattern of findings, which when viewed together yield a diagnosis of the affected area in relation to adjoining areas. The clinician simply collects the raw data using his or her palpatory and observational skills together with the patient history, formulates a diagnosis, and then applies a specific technique to the affected segment based on that diagnosis. It should be kept in mind that each test viewed alone does not make a diagnosis. Only when all data are gathered and correlated can the clinician make the diagnosis. At least three or more SIJ provocation tests must be positive to make the SIJ diagnosis.[157] Table 19-7 outlines the clinical-testing procedures and their meanings according to patient position and follows a sequence that minimizes patient position changes.

Standing Position

Posture

The clinician should ensure that the feet are hip-width apart and that the knees are fully extended. Assessment needs to be made from the anterior, posterior, and lateral aspects to assess the posture of the patient (e.g., scoliosis, kyphosis, lordosis, position of the cervical spine and head, tilt of pelvis, position of the shoulder girdle, slope of waist, distances of arms from sides, obvious changes in the muscles, skin, and joints).

Gait

The patient's gait pattern should be observed. Frequently, sacroiliac lesions may produce a Trendelenburg's gait, a gluteus maximus gait, or the patient may side bend the trunk away

Table 19-7	Clinical-Testing Procedures for the Sacroiliac Joint

Position	Tests
Standing	Posture
	Gait
	Alignment and symmetry
	Iliac crest height
	Posterior superior iliac spine (PSIS)
	Anterior superior iliac spine (ASIS)
	Trochanteric levels
	Standing flexion test (forward bending of the trunk)
	Gillet test or stork test (sacral fixation test)
	Active lumbar movements
Sitting	Neurologic examination
	Sacroiliac (SIJ) examination
	Sitting flexion test (forward bending of the trunk)
Supine	Thigh thrust provocation test (also known as *Oestgaard provocation test*)
	Gaenslen's provocation test
	Modified Gaenslen's: right nutation
	Modified Gaenslen's: right counternutation
	Straight-leg raising (SLR)
	Active straight-leg raise (ASLR) test
	Long sit test (leg length test or supine to sit test)
	Distraction test (ilium dorsolateral provocation test in neutral or gapping test)
	Compression test (ilium ventromedial provocation test)
	Piriformis tightness or piriformis syndrome
	Pubic tubercles and pubic symphysis
	ASIS
Prone	Ilium cranial provocation test (shear test)
	Ilium caudal provocation test (shear test)
	Sacral thrust
	Prone knee flexion to 90 degrees

from the affected side. The patient may limp or walk with difficulty.

Alignment and Symmetry

Observations of alignment begin with the general postural assessment; then the certain features (discussed following) are checked. It should be remembered that no one is perfectly symmetrical, and positive findings can be misleading.[116] Palpation of landmarks should be used less to assess pelvic symmetry and more for bony orientation, to locate other soft tissue and bony structures, and to identify areas of tenderness. If the pelvic girdle has an altered position, then the clinician should also check for a mobility restriction of the SIJ and/or the pubic symphysis to determine if the position is of any significance.

Iliac Crest Height

Iliac crest height is best observed by using the radial borders of the index fingers and the web spaces of the hands to push the soft tissue up and medially out of the way before pushing

down on each crest with equal pressure. The clinician's eyes must be level with his or her hands to assess whether one side is more caudal or cephalad in relation to the other (see Figure 9-22). This method has been found to be quite accurate and precise in the detection of leg length discrepancies.[158] If an asymmetry is found, then a lift of appropriate dimension could be placed under the short side before any of the other motion tests in the standing position are executed. This is done to achieve symmetry of muscle tone and balance of the pelvis in space before testing motion. Placing a lift under the foot does not imply that a determination has been made as to whether the asymmetry is due to a structural or functional leg length discrepancy.

Posterior Superior Iliac Spine

In the standing position, the clinician should palpate the PSIS (see "Key Landmarks for Pelvic Girdle Evaluation"). The inferior border of the PSISs are level with the S2 spinous process. An assessment needs to be made as to the relative superoinferior and mediolateral relationships in positions. The clinician may use the ulnar borders of the thumbs or the tips of the index fingers, hooking them under the inferior aspect to the posterior spine. Again, the clinician must be at eye level with the PSISs to make an accurate assessment. If the patient has an innominate inferior relative to the opposite side, then it may indicate a rotated innominate; the iliac crests and the PSIS positions will be unlevel but in opposite directions.

Anterior Superior Iliac Spine

As with the PSIS, the superior-inferior and medial-lateral relationships of the ASIS can be assessed. This may be accomplished from the front by visual inspection and thumb palpation. If examined in the supine position and the innominate is anteriorly rotated, then the leg will be longer on the ipsilateral side. If the innominate is posteriorly rotated, then the ipsilateral leg will be shorter. Because the sartorius and TFL muscles attach to the ASIS, tenderness could occur because of an avulsion fracture, especially in young, high-level athletes.[159]

Trochanteric Levels

Greater trochanteric levels are palpated by the same method as for the iliac crests, with the radial borders of the index fingers and the web spaces resting on the tops of the greater trochanters. If the greater trochanters are palpated in prone, then the hand can be put over the widest part of the hip and passively rotate the lower leg internal and external to feel the trochanter move underneath. Levelness here and unlevelness at the iliacs could indicate pelvic dysfunction, producing an apparent leg length discrepancy. Unlevelness here indicates a structural leg length discrepancy below the level of the femoral neck.

Standing Flexion Test
(Forward Bending of the Trunk)

The standing flexion test of iliosacral motion is accomplished by localization of the PSISs, noting their relative position. The patient is asked to bend forward to midline as if to touch the toes. The head and neck should be flexed, and the arms should hang loosely from the shoulders. As the patient bends forward, the examiner should note cranial movement of the PSISs, and the relative movement of the pelvic girdle on the femoral heads. There should not be intrapelvic rotation with this test. A normal response would be symmetrical movement of the PSISs. This test may need to be repeated a few times. Many factors can affect this test including hamstring tightness, leg length discrepancy, asymmetrical weight bearing, and hypermobility versus hypomobility of the symphysis pubis. This test is primarily to screen for SIJ dysfunction because it has poor sensitivity and reliability by itself.[160]

Gillet Test or Stork Test (Sacral Fixation Test)

The Gillet test checks the osteokinematic motion of the innominate and the sacrum, as well as the lower lumbar vertebrae. The PSISs are again localized from behind. The patient is asked to stand first on one leg and then on the other while lifting the opposite knee to 90 degrees of hip flexion. The PSIS on the nonweight-bearing side will move farther inferiorly. The weight-bearing side will move very little. An alternate method of assessment uses the S2 spinous process as a fixed reference point for the relative PSIS movement as the patient alternately lifts the knees toward the waist. Hip flexion must reach at least 90 degrees. Anterior rotation of the nonweight-bearing innominate relative to the sacrum,[105,106] or if it flexes relative to the femur, indicates a positive test. These would demonstrate a load transfer through the hip and pelvis that would be less stable. This test serves only as a screen for SIJ dysfunction, because it has poor reliability and sensitivity by itself.[71,160]

Active Lumbar Movements

Because lumbar lesions often occur along with sacroiliac dysfunctions, restrictions of lumbar movement must also be assessed. Often when a sacroiliac dysfunction exists, side bending of the lumbar spine toward the affected side can cause exacerbation of pain. Pain on backward bending may also be indicative of lumbar involvement.

Sitting Position

The sitting position fixes the innominates to the chair or table and eliminates the influence of the hamstrings on the pelvis. This allows for sacroiliac movement within the innominates when testing motion. In addition, active trunk rotation can best be tested here because hip and pelvic motions are stabilized. The clinician should also note the posture of the patient in this position; the patient with sacroiliac dysfunction often tends to sit on the unaffected buttock. The sitting position also facilitates the neurologic examination, which consists of testing muscle strength, sensation, and muscle stretch reflexes, as well as the slump test.

NEUROLOGIC EXAMINATION

The examiner tests the following:
1. Muscle stretch reflexes (deep tendon reflexes)
2. Sensation
3. Resistive muscle tests
4. Slump test

SACROILIAC JOINT EXAMINATION

Sitting Flexion Test (Forward Bending of the Trunk)

The clinician must again be at eye level after having localized the inferior border of the PSISs. The patient is asked to cross the arms across the chest and pass the elbows between the knees to midline as if to touch the floor. The patient's feet should be in contact with the floor or resting on a stool if seated on the edge of an examination table. A normal response would be symmetrical movement of the PSISs. The involved PSIS will move first or farther cranially (i.e., the blocked joint moves solidly as one, while the sacrum on the unblocked side is free to move through its small range of motion with the lumbar spine). If a blockage is detected in this test and it is more positive (greater) than the restriction noted in the standing flexion test, then the test is indicative of a sacral dysfunction. If the two PSISs move symmetrically, then an innominate dysfunction is present (if the standing flexion or Gillet test was positive). If the standing flexion test and the sitting flexion test are both equally positive, then a soft tissue lesion is a possibility. This test is a screen for SIJ dysfunction, because it has poor sensitivity and reliability by itself.[160]

Supine Position

Thigh Thrust Provocation Test (Oestgaard Provocation Test)

The patient is supine with the painful hip flexed to 90 degrees, no pillow under to opposite knee. The tester can stand on the painful side and stabilize the opposite ASIS. The patient's anterior knee is grasped, and downward pressure is applied through the femur. The clinician should make sure the thigh is held in 90 degrees of flexion and neutral adduction. This test produces an innominate rotation and causes counternutation. A positive test would reproduce pain in the SIJ or posterior to the hip. If no symptoms are seen, then the clinician should apply overpressure after 1 to 3 minutes of holding the thigh with an axial load to see if pain is provoked. This test is one of the most sensitive for SIJ pathologic conditions.

A modification of this test would be to start in the same position as previously mentioned but to stand on the side opposite the pain. The tester places the hand under the sacrum, creating a "bridge" for it. Downward pressure is applied as previously mentioned. A positive test would reproduce pain on the overpressured side.

Gaenslen's Provocation Test

The patient is lying supine at the end edge of the table, and the tester assesses his or her symptoms at rest. The tester lifts the nonpainful side with the knee and hip at 90 degrees of flexion and applies a downward pressure to the lower leg (painful side) in submaximal tension first. Then the contralateral hip is repositioned in full tension, and the test is conducted again. Both sides are tested if the pain is bilateral. Each should be held for 30 to 60 seconds; if no pain is felt, then overpressure is applied.[48] A positive test reproduces SIJ pain. This test could also be positive for a pubic symphysis instability, hip pathologic condition, L4 nerve root lesion, and stress to the femoral nerve.

According to Smidt et al.,[53] the symphysis pubis influences the movement of each innominate. Putting one lower extremity into flexion and the other in extension does not necessarily reveal which way the innominate moves. This study suggests that innominate movement may not correspond to hip movement.[48]

Modified Gaenslen's: Right Nutation

The modified versions of this test are more specific to the SIJ, with less influence by the pubic symphysis. The patient is in (left) side lying with the involved (right) side up. The table should be midthigh height. To promote nutation, the patient is placed in a flexed spine position, with the lower arm behind the back. The top leg is fully flexed and wrapped around the clinician's waist and thigh for support. The clinician can put his or her knee on the table to help block the patient's upper leg. The clinician locks his or her hands and forearms around the innominate and rotates it backward into posterior rotation, then applies overpressure. A positive test reproduces SIJ pain.[48]

Modified Gaenslen's: Right Counternutation

The patient is in (left) side lying with the involved (right) side up. The table should be midthigh height. To promote counternutation, the lumbar spine is extended and rotated right. The patient's top arm is behind the back and holding the back edge of the table. The lower leg is put in flexion, with the knee stabilized on the clinician's upper thigh. The clinician locks his or her hands and forearms around the innominate (while supporting the top leg in slight extension) and pulls the innominate into anterior rotation, then overpressure.[48]

Straight-Leg Raising

The SLR test is one of the most common clinical tests used in the evaluation of low-back pain. It is perhaps one of the most commonly misinterpreted clinical tests as well. The test applies stress to the SIJ in the higher ranges of the arc and can indicate the presence of a unilateral dysfunction of the joint. The test may be positive if the biceps femoris tendon (either partially or completely) attaches to the sacrotuberous ligament. It can also indicate a coexisting lumbar problem. The following guidelines are helpful in interpreting the results of the SLR test:

- Range of 0 to 30 degrees: hip pathologic condition or severely inflamed nerve root
- Range of 30 to 50 degrees: sciatic nerve involvement
- Range of 50 to 70 degrees: probable hamstring involvement
- Range of 70 to 90 degrees: SIJ is stressed

The patient is supine on the examining table. The clinician lifts one of the patient's knees slightly to dorsiflex the foot to neutral first, then he or she lets the knee extend and lifts the leg by supporting the heel while palpating the opposite ASIS. The leg is raised until the clinician can appreciate motion of the pelvis occurring under the fingertips of the palpating hand. This determines the hamstring length in the leg being raised. The other side is then similarly tested.

If the tester adds femoral adduction with internal rotation, then it will increase the stretch on the sciatic nerve and its roots.

Active Straight-Leg Raise Test

The patient lies supine and is asked to raise the affected leg about 8 inches or 20 degrees. The clinician checks for pain in the SIJ region and sees if weakness affects the patient's ability to lift the leg. If pain is felt, then the tester stabilizes the pelvis by compressing the ASIS medially or wraps a belt around the pelvis and repeats the test. The test is considered positive if no pain (or weakness) is felt with the pelvis compressed.[161] This test is helpful in diagnosing instability of the pelvic girdle and pregnancy-related posterior pelvic pain.[121,122] It is also used to assess the ability to transfer loads between the lumbosacral spine and the lower extremities.[43,136,162] If instability exists, then the clinician should not manipulate the joint unless it is locked.

Long Sit Test (Leg Length Test or Supine to Sit Test)

The long sit test indicates a pelvic rotation and helps determine the presence of either an anterior innominate or a posterior innominate by a change in the relative length of the legs during the test. The patient is instructed to lie supine with the knees bent. He or she is then asked to lift the hips to a bridge and return to the starting position. The examiner moves the knees into extension passively and evaluates the medial malleoli

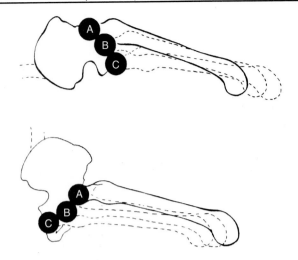

Figure 19-27 Mechanism of the long sitting test in posterior and anterior innominate dysfunctions. **A,** In the supine position, posterior rotation of the ilium on the sacrum appears to shorten the leg (*A*) and anterior rotation to lengthen it (*C*). **B,** In the sitting position, the reverse occurs: posterior rotation appears to lengthen the leg (*A*), and anterior rotation appears to shorten it (*C*). (From Saunders HD: Evaluation, treatment, and prevention of musculoskeletal disorders, ed 2, Minneapolis, 1985, H Duane Saunders.)

levels. The patient is next asked to perform a sit-up, keeping the legs straight. The clinician observes the change, if any, between the malleoli. The presence of a posterior innominate will make the leg in question (the side of the positive standing flexion test) appear to be getting longer from a position of relative shortness (short to long or equal to long). This phenomenon occurs because, in the posterior innominate, the posterior rotation of the innominate moves the acetabulum in a superior direction and carries the leg along with it. Thus the leg appears shortened. Just the opposite occurs in the anterior innominate. When the long sitting test is performed, the leg in question will appear to move from long to short or from equal to short. These mechanisms are shown in Figure 19-27. This test demonstrates poor reliability and questionable validity when used alone.[160]

Distraction Test (Ilium Dorsolateral Provocation Test in Neutral or Gapping Test)

Distraction and compression tests are used to ascertain the presence of joint irritability; hypermobility, instability, or locking; serious disease such as the active stage of an arthritis (ankylosing spondylitis, rheumatoid arthritis, Reiter's disease, gout); Paget's disease; or infection. The patient lies in supine with a pillow under the knees and the hands behind the low back to maintain physiologic lordosis (this positions the SIJs in neutral). The clinician may leave his or her arms parallel with the palms on the same ASISs or may cross them to opposite ASISs. The examiner may need to reposition the hands on the ASISs for patient comfort. The clinician then applies pressure down with the shoulders over the hands and the elbows

straight. The test should be held for 1 to 3 minutes (based on patient tolerance). If no symptoms are provoked, then the clinician should take up any slack and give a sudden, sharp spring to the ASISs. This action creates a nutation moment.[43,116] Pain in the upper inner gluteal quadrant as a result of either of these maneuvers is considered to be a positive sign, indicating SIJ pathologic condition. If the pain comes quickly, the tester should consider instability or ileitis; if the pain comes slowly, then the tester should consider hypomobility. This test is believed to have fair reliability and moderate specificity by itself.[160]

Compression Test (Ilium Ventromedial Provocation Test)

The patient is placed in side lying, with the painful side up and the pelvis vertical. The hips are flexed about 15 degrees, and the knees are in a comfortable position. The patient may need a small pillow or towel roll under the waist to keep the pelvis in neutral (especially for women). The clinician stands behind, with the patient close to the edge of the table. The clinician places flat or cupped palms (one of top of the other) over the ventrolateral aspect of the iliac crest. The patient's pelvis is rolled slightly forward, out of vertical, to get a better compression to both sides of the pelvis. Next, downward force is applied through the ilium and held for 30 seconds to 1 minute. The test is considered positive if the pressure reproduces the specific pain.

Pain can be felt in various areas because of the complex innervation of the sacroiliac capsuloligamentous structures. The pain can be anywhere from the paravertebral low-back area, the gluteal region, the groin, and/or lower abdomen. The pain can be anywhere from L3 to S2.[61] This test has fair reliability and specificity by itself and has been used to check for pelvis fracture.[160]

FABER (Patrick's) Test

The FABER test is useful in differentiating between hip and sacroiliac pain. The hip is flexed, abducted, and externally rotated, with the lateral malleolus resting on the opposite thigh above the knee (figure four position) in supine. The opposite ASIS is stabilized, and pressure is applied to the externally rotated leg through the knee. Pain located in the groin or anterior thigh is indicative of hip pathologic condition. Pain in the SIJ is indicative of sacroiliac involvement.

PIRIFORMIS TIGHTNESS OR PIRIFORMIS SYNDROME

Tightness of the piriformis muscle is easily checked by full flexion of the hip, adduction, and external rotation. Relative end feel and range of motion can be assessed. To check for pain from the piriformis contracting over the sciatic nerve, the patient is positioned as described previously and active, isometric hip internal rotation is assessed.[35,163]

Pubic Tubercles and Pubic Symphysis

The pubic tubercles are anterior, just lateral to the pubic symphysis. The pubic symphysis is part of the "pelvic ring" and can be influenced by the SIJs (or vice versa).

The pubic tubercles are assessed for their relative superoinferior and anteroposterior relationships. If unlevelness is detected, then the positive side is correlated to the side of the positive standing flexion and/or Gillet test. To avoid embarrassment and unnecessary probing in this region, it is recommended that the clinician slide the heel of his or her hand down the abdomen until contact is made with the pubic bone. It is also helpful to demonstrate the palpation to the patient on a model (or on the clinician), particularly for sensitive and/or modest patients.

The tubercles may then be easily located with the fingertips. In most men and some women—because of the strength of the abdominal muscles—it is sometimes helpful to ask the patient to flex the knees a little to relax these muscles. Palpation is further facilitated by asking the patient to inhale; on exhalation, the clinician slides his or her fingers over the top and presses down on the tubercles (see "Key Landmarks for Pelvic Girdle Evaluation").

Anterior Superior Iliac Spine

Positioning of the ASISs can be assessed for any change from the standing position. In assessing the superoinferior and mediolateral relationships, the clinician places his or her thumbs under the lip of the ASIS and looks from a position perpendicular to the midline. To determine the anteroposterior relationship of the ASISs, the clinician places the fingertips on the tips of the ASISs and looks along the plane of the abdomen. The umbilicus also becomes a reference point for the mediolateral positioning.

Prone Position

Ilium Cranial Provocation Test (Shear Test)

The patient is prone with a pillow under the pelvis to put the SIJ in the maximal loose-packed position. The arms should be kept at the patient's sides to keep the thoracolumbar fascia loose, and the toes should be off the end of the table. The tester should stand on the same side that is to be tested and stabilize the sacrum with the cranial hand, just medial to the PSIS. With the caudal palm, he or she should push craniolaterally on the ischial tuberosity and hold for 30 seconds, then apply overpressure if no pain is felt. This test is more provocative than the ilium caudal test. A positive test would reproduce posterior pain.[48]

Ilium Caudal Provocation Test (Shear Test)

The patient should be positioned as in the previous test, and the tester stabilizes the ILA with the caudal hand. The cranial hand is used to push the ilium caudally and medially, and the

tester holds the position for 30 seconds. If no pain is felt, overpressure is applied. A positive test would reproduce posterior pain.[48]

Sacral Thrust

The patient is prone, and the examiner palpates the second or third spinous process of the sacrum. The tester pushes down on S3 with the heel of the hand. The lumbar spine is less likely to hyperextend if the clinician pushes on the midpoint of the sacrum, which improves the specificity of the test. The tester applies a strong pressure downward (up to six times) to try to reproduce the patient's pain. Reproduction of pain would be a positive test.[157,160]

Prone Knee Flexion to 90 Degrees

The clinician stands at the foot of the examination table and holds the patient's feet in a symmetrical position, with the thumbs placed transversely across the soles of the feet just forward of the heel pad. Sighting through the plane of the heel with the eyes perpendicular to the malleoli, the clinician assesses the relative length of the legs in the prone position (the short side may not be the same as in the supine or standing position). If one leg appears shorter, then it may be the positive side. The knees are then simultaneously flexed to 90 degrees. Care must be taken to maintain the feet in the neutral position and to bring the feet up in the midline. Deviation to either side will cause a false impression. If the leg still appears short, then an anterior innominate should be considered a possibility. If the leg that seemed short now appears longer, then a posterior innominate should be suspected.

COMBINATION OF TESTS

Using a combination of at least three SIJ tests is the best approach for accurate diagnosis and successful intervention. The three combinations that have shown to provide the most accurate information are as follows[160]:

Combination		Indicator
1	Distraction test	2 of 4 positive
	Compression test	
	Thigh thrust	
	Patrick's test (Patrick's sign)	
	Gaenslen's test	
2	Distraction test	3 of 5 positive
	Compression test	
	Thigh thrust	
	Gaenslen's test	
	Sacral thrust	
3	Standing flexion	3 of 5 positive
	Sitting posterior	
	Superior iliac spine (PSIS) Palpation	
	Supine-to-sit test	
	Prone knee flexion test	

PROVOCATION TESTS

Pain provocation tests have better reproducibility and are more reliable than tests of mobility or configuration.[156,164] If the patient experiences immediate pain with these tests, then he or she could have instability or sacroiliitis. If the patient has a delayed response, then it is probably a mechanical dysfunction. Other afflictions that may result from SIJ instability include trochanteric bursitis and piriformis syndrome. It is important to hold the SIJ provocation tests for 1 to 3 minutes to initiate stepwise creep. In chronic sacroiliac pain, provocation should increase symptoms as a result of adaptive shortening of the soft tissues. If the patient has more pain with nutation, then counternutation should be used for treatment (and vice versa). Nutation is more commonly seen as provocative.[48]

Mobility tests are considered clinically relevant in combination with positive provocation tests.[165] It should be remembered that the painful side is not always the side with the pathologic condition.

When a negative lumbar examination and a combination of three or more positive provocation SIJ tests occur, in addition to no centralization or peripheralization, the patient is at least three to 20 times more likely to have positive diagnostic SIJ injections.[157]

The most reliable provocation tests include the following[48]:
- Ilium dorsolateral (distraction)
- Ilium ventromedial (compression)
- Thigh thrust (Oestgaard)
- Sacral thrust
- Modified Gaenslen's: nutation
- Modified Gaenslen's: counternutation

Extra tests for the SIJ include the following:
- Ilium cranial
- Ilium caudal

See each provocation test listed previously under "Sacroiliac Joint Examination."

PALPATION

Symmetry of the Sacrotuberous and Sacrospinous Ligaments

These ligaments must be palpated through the gluteal mass. The sacrotuberous ligament and the hamstrings attach to the ischial tuberosity. In addition, an ischial bursa is located here. With the patient prone, the clinician palpates the ischial tuberosities. He or she uses the thumbs to find the inferomedial part of the tuberosities and moves them up superolaterally to palpate the sacrotuberous ligaments. Then the fingertips are used to palpate transverse to the ligament. The clinician must assess changes in tension and springiness from one side to the other. If such changes are noted, then they may be because of positional changes of the ilium. If an anteriorly rotated innomi-

nate exists, then the ligament would feel firm; if posteriorly rotated, then it would feel taut. The sacrospinous ligament runs from the ischial spine to the lateral edge of the sacrum and coccyx, ventral to the sacrotuberous ligament. This ligament is usually not palpable.

Piriformis Tightness

The piriformis was tested in the supine position while on stretch. It is now tested prone while not on stretch by having the patient flex the knees to 90 degrees and internally rotate the hips by allowing the legs to move laterally.

PHYSICAL FINDINGS AND DIAGNOSIS OF PELVIC GIRDLE DYSFUNCTIONS

The following positive physical findings characterize the five most common pelvic girdle dysfunctions:
1. Posterior innominate
2. Anterior innominate
3. Superior pubis
4. Superior or inferior innominate shear (upslip, downslip)
5. Iliac outflare (innominate externally rotated)

Table 19-8 outlines the indications of each finding.

Posterior Innominate

A posterior innominate is a unilateral iliosacral dysfunction. It is by far the most common pelvic dysfunction.

Anterior Innominate

An anterior innominate is also a unilateral iliosacral dysfunction and is essentially the reverse of the posterior innominate.

Superior Pubis

Dysfunctions of the pubic symphysis are likely the most commonly overlooked lesions of the pelvis. These lesions are usually shear lesions, either in a superior or inferior direction. Anterior and posterior shears are rare and, if present, usually result from trauma. Both childbearing and trauma may cause the symphysis to become unstable. Such instability is very painful with any movement—especially in weight bearing—and local to the pubis. Such a lesion can be viewed objectively in unilateral weight-bearing radiographs.

Superior or Inferior Innominate Shear (Upslip, Downslip)

Usually considered uncommon, vertical shear lesions of an entire innominate have been shown to occur more frequently than was originally thought.

Table 19-8	Indications for Pelvic Girdle Examination Findings			
	Left Posterior Innominate	Right Anterior Innominate	Left Superior Pubis	Left Superior Shear
Iliac crests	High on the left	Low on the right	May be high on the left	High on the left
Posterior superior iliac spine (PSIS)	Low and posterior on the left	High and anterior on the right	Posterior in relation to the pelvic dorsal plane and anterior to the sacral base in the prone position	High on the left
Anterior superior iliac spine (ASIS)	High and anterior on the left	Low and posterior on the right	Superior on the left; may be slightly posterior	Positive on the left
Standing flexion test	Left PSIS moves first or farther superiorly	Right PSIS moves first and/or farther superiorly	Blocked side will move first; the side that is blocked (in this case the left, superior pubis) will indicate the type of pubic lesion (superior or inferior)	Positive on the left
Gillet test	Left PSIS moves inferiorly and laterally less than the right	Right PSIS moves less inferiorly and laterally compared with the left		Positive on the left, from short to long
Long sitting test	Left malleolus moves from short to long	Right medial malleolus moves from long to short	May be equal or shorter on the left before becoming longer	Positive on the left
Sitting flexion test	Negative (unless a sacral lesion coexists)	Usually negative (unless a sacral lesion coexists)	Probably negative	
Pubic symphysis	Negative (may be superior if also involved)	Usually normal	Left pubic tubercle will be superior and tender	High on the left
Hip	May lie in some external rotation	Right leg may lie in some internal rotation	Normal	Normal
Tensor fasciae latae (TFL)	Tight and/or tender on the right	May be tender on the left		
Piriformis				Normal
Other findings	Tense left sacrotuberous ligament, decreased lumbar lordosis, pain (usually well defined) in the sulcus and/or unilateral buttock pain	Possibly increased lumbar lordosis; possible complaint of cervical and/or lumbar symptoms	Almost all of these lesions occur simultaneously with the posterior innominate	High-left ischial tuberosity

Iliac Outflare (Innominate Externally Rotated)

Iliac outflare is essentially the opposite of an iliac inflare. The outflare occurs as part of a 3-D movement about an oblique axis with nutation because of the dorsal sacroiliac ligaments. With nutation the innominate moves posteriorly; with outflare the cranial innominate adducts and the caudal innominate abducts. Inflare occurs with counternutation, just the opposite movements of nutation: the innominate moves anteriorly; with inflare the cranial innominate abducts and the caudal innominate adducts. The outflare is a part of all SIJ motion that results from hip movement in a nonweight-bearing position.[53,166]

These pelvic dysfunctions are quite rare. Their combined occurrence may represent fewer than 5% to 10% of all pelvic dysfunctions. For the sake of completeness, however, their findings are included.

TREATMENT

Many of the tests for the SIJ have poor reliability when used in isolation. When two or three tests are all positive, the quality and outcomes are greatly improved. The success of treatment depends on the accuracy and quality of the examination combined with the patient history. Several different philosophies dictate the kind of treatment clinicians choose for SIJs. Regardless of which intervention the clinician selects, the principles behind it should be the same. A patient with a hypermobile or unstable joint should be educated on the diagnosis and treated with techniques and dynamic exercises that stabilize the joint (or balance the forces around it).[98] The patient may also require an sacroiliac belt to help stabilize the SIJs and/or symphysis pubis. The belt should be placed at

S3—below the lateral iliac crest and ASIS and above the greater trochanter.[167]

A hypomobile joint requires treatment techniques that include soft tissue mobilization to prepare the joint to be mobilized, manipulation, and exercises that help to restore mobility and normal alignment, as well as self-mobilization. Many factors may contribute to a hypomobile joint including shortened or hypertonic hip muscles, capsular limitation of the hip, rotated L5 and S1, leg length discrepancy, and/or weak sacrotuberous and sacrospinous ligaments. Restricted SIJ motion can be physiologic. For example, in men older than 50 years of age, a bony bridge can develop between the ilium and sacrum, which limits SIJ motion.[50]

Arthritis and sacroiliitis are two other categories to consider when deciding what treatment to use for the SIJ. Some disorders that can cause sacroiliitis are psoriatic arthritis, Crohn's disease, Reiter's disease, and ulcerating colitis.[50] Sacroiliitis may improve with a sacroiliac belt.

When deciding what exercises and techniques to use, the clinician must keep in mind patient tolerance, what stage of healing the patient is in, as well as the influences that the lumbar spine, hip, leg length, and sacroiliac ligaments have on the SIJ.

The age of the patient will affect the appearance of the SIJ and how smooth or rough the joint surfaces are. Hormones will also affect the stability of the joints (i.e., pregnancy and the hormone relaxin). The clinician should also consider whether or not trauma was involved.

The goals of treatment during the acute phase are as follows:
- Decrease inflammation, pain, and muscle spasm (may include modalities and isometrics).
- Increase tolerance to weight bearing as appropriate (may need to correct leg length discrepancy).
- Encourage healing of tissues with stabilization as needed.
- Increase pain-free range of motion in and around the SIJ.
- Restore soft tissue mobility around the pelvis and hip.
- Restore proper neuromuscular control.
- Start progressing to the functional stage with instruction in proper posture and body mechanics.

After pain and inflammation decrease, the strength, posture, and range of motion can be restored. It is helpful to start range-of-motion exercises (in the pain-free range) as soon as possible to encourage the joints to move more normally. Isometric exercises can be gradually progressed as strength and range of motion improve. Manual techniques—including soft tissue massage and/or modalities—help decrease pain. The patient should be educated on proper posture and body mechanics to decrease the nociceptive stresses to the area of injury. If the SIJ is locked, then a manipulation can be performed. It is recommended to start with the patient in a counternutated position, because the SIJ often gets locked in a nutated position. If pain occurs with this technique, then the clinician should revert to a nutated position. The patient should be educated to avoid positions that produce more counternutation and to substitute instead positions of nutation, so the collagenous structures can adapt to the nonpainful position after the manipulation.

The goals during the functional phase are as follows:

- Decrease or eliminate the patient's pain.
- Restore normal, pain-free range of motion.
- Integrate the entire body into the exercise program while actively stabilizing the pelvis.
- Normalize gait, if needed.
- Restore strength and neuromuscular control of the pelvis and lower extremities.

Many techniques are used to retrain the neuromuscular system (see chapter on neuromuscular control) including stabilization exercises, progressive resistive exercises, work hardening, Feldenkrais method, Tai Chi, Pilates, yoga, and several different physical training programs that emphasize balance and proprioceptive techniques.

Contraction of the TA also helps to stabilize the SIJs. The drawing-in maneuver activates the TA and the internal obliques.[74]

Table 19-9 reviews the different manual therapy techniques for treatment of the SIJ (discussed following).

Manipulation and Mobilization Techniques

Manipulation should be performed in counternutation first, because the SIJ is usually locked in nutation. If the first technique is not successful, then the clinician should manipulate the joint into nutation. To determine success, the clinician should repeat tests that were positive and/or reevaluate the patient's intensity of pain and symptoms.

Table 19-9	Manual Therapy Techniques for Treatment of Sacroiliac Joint
Manipulation/mobilization techniques	Counternutation mobilization/manipulation in prone
	Alternate counternutation mobilization/manipulation in side lying
	Nutation mobilization/manipulation in side lying
	Nutation mobilization/manipulation in supine
Self-mobilization of the sacroiliac joint (SIJ)	Nutation
	Counternutation
Muscle energy techniques (METs)	Superior or inferior pubic symphysis
	Superior pubic symphysis (right side) or superior pubic shear
	Inferior pubic symphysis (left side) or inferior pubic shear
	Superior iliac subluxation (upslip)
	Posterior rotation of the right innominate (or to restore anterior rotation)
	Anterior rotation of the right innominate (or to restore posterior rotation)
Management of SIJ instability Therapeutic exercise for the pelvis/SIJ	

To decrease the tendency of the symphysis pubis to dominate the motion, the involved side should be positioned first, then the opposite side should be positioned.[53] It is helpful to perform a transverse soft tissue mobilization (with hip internal rotation, passively) for approximately 5 minutes before manipulation to relax local muscles (including the piriformis).[48]

Counternutation Mobilization and Manipulation in Prone

Patient Position

The patient is in prone with one leg extended on the table and the other leg bearing weight through the floor. The table should be at the height necessary for the patient to have the weight-bearing foot on the floor. The patient's affected side is on the table, and the cranial end of the table is raised to put the patient in extension. The clinician should lift the head of the table until movement is felt at the sacrum (nutation), usually around 20 degrees. The bend in the table should be between T8 and the SIJ to allow movement and torsion in the lumbar spine while positioning the patient. The lumbar spine wants to give first, so it needs to be locked before performing SIJ techniques. To avoid movement at other joints in the lumbosacral region, the patient must be put in a position of trunk rotation and side bending toward the affected side. For example, if the right side is involved, then the patient is put in extension with right rotation and right side bending. When the patient is put into maximal rotation, the side bending occurs automatically because the inclined table puts the patient in extension. A pillow can be placed under the patient's shoulder and arm to stabilize this rotated position.

The uninvolved hip is positioned into flexion by moving the weight-bearing foot forward, so the ball of the patient's foot is on the ground. The therapist can keep the patient's foot in place by placing his or her forefoot under the patient's heel.

Therapist Position

The therapist stands on the uninvolved side next to the patient's thigh; it is helpful if the table can be at the level of the therapist's thigh (some may need to stand on a stool to perform the technique). The cranial hand is placed lateral to the involved PSIS and over the dorsal iliac crest. The caudal hand lifts the distal end of the anterolateral thigh of the involved side into hip extension and slight internal rotation with slight adduction.

When the sacrum starts to move forward with the ilium, the therapist moves the patient's uninvolved foot forward on the floor into full hip flexion, without losing the spinal extension.

Performance of Technique

With the ilium rotated forward (involved side), the therapist's cranial hand pushes the ilium ventrally while the caudal hand lifts the leg into more extension. Before the thrust, the patient takes a deep breath and exhales. The therapist starts to press down on the ilium gradually with exhalation until the end range of motion is reached; then quick but firm overpressure is applied.

Alternate Counternutation Mobilization and Manipulation in Side-Lying

Patient Position

The patient is in side lying with the involved side up, and his or her body is close to the edge of the table. It is important to lock the lumbar spine and to localize the manipulative movement to the involved SIJ. The lumbar spine is put into extension, combined with trunk rotation and side bending toward the involved side. This positioning will lock the lumbar facets and put the iliolumbar ligament on slack. To lock the lumbar spine, the patient is positioned in maximal trunk rotation; then the side bending is added by lifting the head of the table. The involved hip is moved into maximal extension, and the spinal extension is maintained as the uninvolved (bottom leg) is brought into flexion. (For example, if the left side is involved, then the patient is put into extension with left rotation and left side bending.)

Therapist Position

The table is at the level of the therapist's pelvis. The therapist stands in front of the patient's pelvis and holds the top leg in extension and abduction by resting the thigh on his or her caudal forearm. The therapist clasps his or her hands over the involved posterior iliac crest, while the cranial forearm rests on the top of the iliac crest. The heel of the caudal hand rests over the ischial tuberosity. The therapist puts the bottom leg around his or her iliac crest and trunk to stabilize it.

Performance of Technique

With the upper ilium rotated forward and the upper leg extended, the therapist moves the upper leg into more extension by using his or her upper arm along with rotating his or her trunk. Before the thrust maneuver, the patient is instructed to take a deep breath and exhale. The therapist starts to rotate the ilium forward and anterior gradually with exhalation until the end range of motion is reached; then a quick overpressure is applied. To get more movement with this technique, the therapist should flex the patient's lower hip by shifting his or her pelvis toward the patient's head.

Nutation Mobilization and Manipulation in Side-Lying

Patient Position

The patient is in side lying with the involved side up, with the patient's body close to the edge of the table. The table is at the level of the therapist's pelvis. The lumbar spine is put into flexion (nutation), then rotated in the opposite direction of the involved SIJ. The spine is side bent toward the involved side by raising the head of the table, to put the iliolumbar ligament on slack and to lock the lumbar spine. (For example, if the left SIJ is involved, the patient is put into right rotation and left side bend.) The lumbar spine lies on the inclined part of the table, and the pelvis is on the flat part of the table. The patient's top elbow is bent up by the head, and the bottom arm lies behind the back for stability.

Therapist Position

The therapist stands in front of the patient's pelvis and holds the top leg in hip and knee flexion. The therapist can hold this position by placing the patient's leg around his or her iliac crest and low back, so the thigh is fixed between his or her trunk and upper arm. The other way to position the patient's top leg is by holding it from underneath with the cranial forearm. The patient's hip should be allowed to go into external rotation to help with the technique. The clinician should not allow the top leg to adduct.

The cranial hand holds the ASIS, while the caudal hand holds the PSIS and PIIS and the forearm lies over the ischial tuberosity; thus both hands are holding the innominate. The therapist moves the ilium into maximal nutation with his or her hands and uses his or her trunk to move the patient's leg into more flexion. The patient's bottom leg can be fixed in extension with a belt or stabilized with the therapist's caudal knee. The pelvis must stay vertical, and the top ilium must not be pulled forward to maintain flexion in the lumbar spine.

Performance of Technique

The top ilium is manipulated and mobilized with a backward (dorsal) rotation, in relation to the sacrum, which is fixed by stabilizing the bottom leg in extension and locking the lumbar spine.

Nutation Mobilization and Manipulation in Supine

Patient Position

The patient lies supine with the uninvolved side close to the edge of the table. The table is at the level of the therapist's knees. The table is inclined, and the L5-S1 segment is positioned at the level of the hinge.

To localize the technique, a firm padding is placed under the sacrum, just medial to the PSIS of the involved side. The padding should support the lumbar spine as well.

Raise the head of the table to put the lumbar spine into a flexed position. Next, perform an axial rotation opposite to the involved side. (For example, if the left side is involved, the spine is rotated to the right). An automatic side bending opposite to the rotation occurs (because of the inclined table) and locks the lumbar spine. To maintain this position, the patient can grasp the edge of the table, or a pillow can be used for support.

First, the involved hip is brought into maximal flexion and slight external rotation. The other hip is extended (while maintaining lumbar flexion), by moving the uninvolved leg off the table with the foot on the floor.

Therapist Position

The therapist stands by the pelvis on the uninvolved side and grasps the involved ilium with both hands. The caudal hand is on the ischial tuberosity and the cranial hand is over the anterior ASIS and iliac crest. The patient's knee and shin on the involved side are supported against the therapist's chest/trunk.

Performance of Technique

The ilium is rotated backward (dorsal) by moving the cranial and caudal hands in opposite directions. (The cranial hand pushes the ASIS backward—toward the table—while the caudal hand pulls the ischial tuberosity away from the table). The therapist can reinforce the mobilization by bringing the hip into more flexion by moving his/her trunk cranial (relative to the patient).

SELF-MOBILIZATION OF THE SACROILIAC JOINT

Self mobilization of the SIJ would be indicated if patients experiences SIJ pain when they are at home or work or engaged in sports activities and a therapist is not available to perform the mobilization/manipulation technique. Self-mobilization can also be used as a part of a home exercise program to reinforce the technique the therapist performed in the clinic. Self-mobilization of the SIJ is done to encourage right SIJ nutation.

Nutation

Procedure for Patients That Prefer Lumbar Lordosis (Extension)—Posterior Rotation of the Right Innominate

1. The patient sits in a chair with a towel roll behind the lumbar spine, just above the ilia, to position the sacral base ventral.
2. The patient puts the right leg in a figure four position so that the right ankle is on top of the left knee. This moves the right ilium backward.
3. The patient then rotates the trunk to the left and hooks the left elbow behind the chair to hold in place. This moves the right sacrum more forward.
4. This technique can be done three times a day (holding 4 to 5 minutes) or when sore.

Procedure for Patients That Prefer Lumbar Flexion

1. The patient sits in the figure four position (as previously discussed) to move the right ilium backward.
2. The patient bends forward, pulling the base of the sacrum forward. Then he or she rotates the trunk to the left. This moves the right sacrum more forward. The patient then puts the right elbow on the right knee. The frequency and time would be the same as previously mentioned.

Counternutation

Anterior Rotation of the Right Innominate

1. The patient sits in a chair with the spine in extension, which moves the base of the sacrum backward.
2. The patient rotates the trunk to the right, which moves the right side of the sacrum further backward. The right elbow hooks behind the chair to maintain the rotated, extended position.
3. The right foot is placed just outside the right front chair leg, and the left leg is crossed over the right (left ankle over the right distal thigh). This position internally rotates the right leg and pulls the right ilium forward. This position can be held 4 to 5 minutes, three times a day or when sore.[48]

Some theorize that mobilization or manipulation of the uninvolved joint can decrease the stress to the involved, painful joint. Other interventions that have been used to treat the SIJ include manual therapy, soft tissue mobilization, therapeutic exercise, education, modalities, SIJ belts, and use of orthotic devices.

MUSCLE ENERGY TECHNIQUES

A muscle energy technique (MET) is any manipulative treatment procedure that uses a voluntary contraction of the patient's muscles against a distinctly controlled counterforce from a precise position and in a specific direction. MET is considered to be an active technique—as opposed to a passive technique in which the clinician does the work—and it requires direct positioning (where the motion restriction barrier is engaged but not stressed). MET may be used to lengthen shortened muscles, strengthen weakened muscles, reduce localized edema, and mobilize restricted joints. The focus of this section is on the use of MET in mobilization of joint restrictions.

Types of Muscle Contraction

MET may use different forms of muscle contraction for the purposes outlined previously. The contractions are usually isotonic and isometric but may also be isokinetic (Table 19-10).

For less stiff joints or subluxations, or when the mobilization and manipulation techniques are not helpful or appropri-

Table 19-10	Types of Muscle Contraction
Contraction Type	Description
Isotonic	The muscle exerts a constant tension as the proximal and distal attachments approximate (i.e., a shortening or concentric contraction). It may also occur when the proximal and distal attachments separate (i.e., a lengthening or eccentric contraction). An isotonic contraction can be thought of as muscle movement with a constant load; an example is raising and lowering a weight.
Isometric	The muscle is exerted against an unyielding resistance in which the proximal and distal attachments neither separate nor approximate (i.e., no joint motion is produced).
Isokinetic	The muscle is exerted against a resistance in which speed is the controlled variable. Specialized equipment is usually required to produce this type of exercise contraction, but it may be performed manually as well.

ate, METs may be used. The diagnoses that seem to have the most success with METs are pubic symphysis dysfunction and anterior or posterior innominate rotations.

Superior and Inferior Pubic Symphysis

Combined Treatment for Superior and Inferior Pubic Subluxations

This technique is a powerful mover of the pubic symphysis. It first uses the hip abductors to "gap" the joint and then the hip adductors to "reset" the joint in its normal position.

Patient Position

The patient is in supine, with the hips and knees flexed together and the feet resting so that the toes are near the end of the table.

Therapist Position

The therapist holds the patient's knees together while standing at the end of the table.

Performance of Technique

The therapist puts his or her hands on either side of the patient's knees and asks the patient to try and abduct (open or push apart) the knees against resistance by the therapist. The patient holds the maximal isometric contraction for about 5 to 10 seconds and then relaxes. Then the therapist abducts the patient's knees passively about 30 to 45 degrees (or asks the patient to allow the legs to fall apart). The previous step is then repeated by pushing the knees out (abducting) from this new position with maximal isometric contraction, holding 5 to 10 seconds. Immediately after the patient releases the contraction, the therapist rapidly adjusts his or her hands so that the forearm lies between the patient's knees (the therapist's hand and elbow make contact with the medial aspect of the patient's knees) and asks the patient to maximally adduct (close) the knees against resistance by the therapist. This position is held for 5 seconds, for two to three repetitions, and the patient is retested.

Many times, an audible *pop* is heard during this treatment. This sound may represent a separation of the pubic symphyses, allowing them to reset themselves. This technique can be used separately or in combination with the specific pubic subluxation techniques also described.

Home Program

This exercise can easily be performed at home by pushing the knees out against a belt, a towel, or the patient may use his or her own hands for resistance. The adduction component can be performed with a towel roll or the patient's fist, elbow, and/or hand between the knees for resistance.

Superior Pubic Symphysis (Right Side) or Superior Pubic Shear

Superior pubic shear is diagnosed by the following:
- Positive standing flexion test on one side
- Pubic tubercle superior on the same side as the positive standing flexion test
- Tense and/or tender inguinal ligament on the same side
- Muscular correction of this very common pelvic dysfunction uses combined forces of rectus femoris and hip adductor group

Patient Position

The patient is in supine near the right side of the table, while the right (involved) leg hangs off the right edge (ischial contact with the table).

Therapist Position

The therapist stands on the right (involved) side of the patient and holds his or her right leg with one hand, while stabilizing the left ASIS with the other hand. The therapist gradually lowers the right leg toward the floor, with slight abduction, until resistance is felt. The therapist can hold the patient's knee in place (in passive knee extension) between his or her legs.

Performance of Technique

The patient is asked to lift his or her knee up into the therapist's hand and in toward the table while the therapist resists. The isometric contraction is held for 5 to 10 seconds and then released. This is repeated three to five times, and then the patient is retested. If successful, then the patient will have decreased pain and improved position of the symphysis. Note: The forces generated are to be submaximal; 10 lb of resistance is likely sufficient to accomplish the task.

Inferior Pubic Symphysis (Left Side) or Inferior Pubic Shear

Inferior pubic shear is diagnosed by the following:
- Positive standing flexion test on one side
- Pubic tubercle inferior on the same side as the positive standing flexion test
- Possible tense and/or tender inguinal ligament on the same side
- Muscular correction of this pelvic dysfunction is similar to technique for the anterior innominate and uses action of gluteus maximus combined with direct pressure onto ischium from clinician (This allows the pubis to slide superiorly from the dysfunctional inferior position.)

Patient Position

The patient is in supine near the left (involved) side of the table.

Therapist Position

The therapist stands on the right (uninvolved) side of the patient and fully flexes the patient's left (involved) hip and knee. This knee can rest on the therapist's right shoulder or axilla. The therapist puts his or her closed, right fist under the patient's left ischial tuberosity and takes up all the slack.

Performance of Technique

The patient is asked to extend or straighten (submaximally) the left (involved) leg while the therapist resists isometrically. The contraction is held for 5 to 10 seconds and then released. This is repeated three to five times, and then the patient is retested.

Superior Iliac Subluxation (Upslip)

Superior iliac subluxation is diagnosed by the following:
- Superior iliac crest
- Superior ASIS on the same side
- Superior PSIS on the same side
- Superior pubic tubercle on the same side
- Superior ischial tuberosity on the same side

This technique is a direct action thrust technique but applies principles of closed-packed versus loose-packed joint mechanics to affect the mobilization.

Patient Position

The patient is prone.

Therapist Position

The therapist stands at the foot of the treatment table on the side of the lesion.

The therapist grasps the patient's distal lower leg above the ankle and raises the entire leg into approximately 30 degrees of hip and lumbar extension and 30 degrees of abduction. Then he or she internally rotates the leg. This approximates the closed-packed position of the hip as closely as possible.

Performance of Technique

The therapist instructs the patient to grasp the top table edge with his or her hands and proceeds to take up the slack by distracting the leg along its long axis until tightness is perceived along the kinetic chain. The therapist applies a quick caudal jerk on the leg. The patient is then retested, and treatment is repeated if necessary.

By using the closed-packed position of the hip, the effect of the distraction is applied to the innominate rather than the hip. Mobilization of the hip is performed supine in the loose-packed position.

Posterior Rotation of the Right Innominate (or to Restore Anterior Rotation)

- Pelvic examination (ASIS is high, PSIS is low)
- Positive standing flexion test
- Positive long sitting test: from short to long (on the side of the positive standing flexion test)
- Positive prone knee flexion test: from short to long
- Hip musculature is checked for symmetry
- Muscular correction of this positional fault involves muscles that can rotate innominate in anterior direction (In this case, the rectus femoris is the major mover.)

Patient Position

The patient is in supine, holding the left leg in hip flexion (until the opposite leg starts to come up), and the involved (right) leg is hanging free over the edge of the table. The hip is extended, and the knee is flexed. This technique may also be performed in prone or side lying.

Therapist Position

The therapist stands on the involved (right) side of the patient and may assist holding the flexed, uninvolved knee and hip. The therapist uses the other hand to extend the right hip by gently pushing down on the knee to take up the slack.

Performance of Technique

Once resistance is felt, the patient is asked to perform a submaximal isometric contraction into right hip flexion while the therapist resists. The patient is instructed to hold 5 to 10 seconds while breathing in a relaxed, smooth manner and then relax. The therapist then extends the leg into the new range of motion until resistance is felt again. He or she can assist the patient in pulling the flexed hip and knee up to the new barrier and to repeat the sequence.

Home Program

The patient lies in supine with the involved leg close to the edge of the table, and the uninvolved leg flexed up to the chest. The patient lowers the involved leg off the bed into hip extension with slight abduction until resistance is felt. The patient begins with an isometric contraction of hip adduction for 5 seconds. Slight hip flexion is then added for 5 seconds. After each contraction, the patient lowers the leg into more extension until the new resistance is felt. This exercise is repeated three to five times.

Anterior Rotation of the Right Innominate (or to Restore Posterior Rotation)

- Pelvic examination (ASIS is low, PSIS is high)
- Positive standing flexion test
- Positive long sitting test: from long to short (on the side of the positive standing flexion test)
- Positive prone knee flexion test: short to short
- Hip musculature id checked for symmetry
- Muscular correction of this positional fault uses muscles that can rotate the innominate in a posterior direction. In this case the major mover is the gluteus maximus.

Patient Position

The patient is supine near the end of the table with the uninvolved (left) leg hanging off the edge. A small towel roll may be placed under the lumbar spine if needed. This technique can also be performed in prone or side lying.

Therapist Position

The therapist stands on the right side. The therapist cups the right ischial tuberosity with his or her right hand and leans (with the shoulder/axilla) into the patient's right bent leg to flex the patient's hip toward his or her chest until resistance is felt. To encourage more posterior rotation of the innominate, the hip flexion is increased until movement is felt at the lumbosacral junction. The therapist palpates the lumbosacral junction and sacral sulcus with his or her left second and third fingers.

Performance of Technique

The therapist asks the patient to extend his or her right hip by pushing the knee into the therapist's shoulder/axilla. (Note: The hip does not actually move into extension; it remains in flexion.) The patient is asked to perform a submaximal isometric contraction while the therapist resists. The patient is instructed to hold the contraction for 5 to 10 seconds, with smooth breathing, and then relax. The therapist pushes the hip into more flexion to reach the new resistance and repeats the technique. This exercise is repeated three to five times, and the patient is retested with the long sitting or the standing flexion test.

Home Program

The patient lies prone with the involved leg flexed up to the chest and the uninvolved leg off the edge of the table, with the foot on the floor. The patient flexes the involved hip until he or she feels resistance, then gently performs an isometric contraction by extending the involved hip by pushing the leg into the table. This position is held for 5 seconds and then released. The patient pushes the hip into more flexion and rotates the innominate posteriorly to reach the new resistance; then the exercise is repeated three to five times.

This exercise can also be similarly performed in supine, with the patient holding the involved, flexed knee and hip close to the chest. The patient then pushes the bent leg out against the hands for the isometric contraction, while the uninvolved leg hangs off the edge of the bed or table.

This treatment may be prescribed for a patient to do as part of a home program two to three times per day for several days. This technique is a powerful rotator of the innominate and can be easily overdone unless specific guidelines are given.

Management of Sacroiliac Joint Instability

- The patient should avoid asymmetry of the hips and pelvis (e.g., jumping on one leg, taking long steps, running up and down stairs every other step).
- Asymmetry in postures should be maintained.
- Postures lasting longer than 30 minutes should be avoided.
- It should be remembered that internal and external oblique abdominal muscle activity is higher in standing than in sitting or supine positions. Decreased oblique abdominal muscle activity occurs when the legs are crossed (upper legs or figure four position), while sitting on a firm seat with use of back and arm rests. Leg crossing is physiologically valuable. It substitutes ligament support for abdominal muscle activity.[168]
- Initially, the patient should avoid sitting on the affected buttock (and sit on the unaffected buttock instead). When sitting in a symmetrical position, he or she should sit with the back straight and the hips abducted.
- Later the patient should sit with legs crossed. According to Snijders et al.,[168] decreased muscle activity and increased ligament tension occurs in this position. The involved leg should be crossed over to promote nutation; the uninvolved leg should be crossed over to promote counternutation.
- The patient should avoid standing on the affected leg if the problem is nutation but stand on that leg if counternutation is the problem.
- The patient should try to lie flat in supine, without putting the lumbar spine in hyperextension or the hips in hyperflexion.
- The patient should avoid maximal range of motion of the hips and lumbar spine.
- The sacroiliac belt should be worn with all exercises and activities initially. Depending on the severity of the injury, the belt may need to be worn 23 hours a day—except when bathing—especially if the patient has pain with turning in bed or changing positions.[48]

- The belt should be positioned just below the ASIS and above the greater trochanter.[169]
- Exercise recommendations include dynamic exercise. The patient should start first toward counternutation, then progress toward functional nutation.[80] In addition, he or she should gradually progress to walking while wearing the belt; 2 lb hand weights should be used with arm swing.[170]

Therapeutic Exercise for the Pelvis and Sacroiliac Joint

The general principles of exercise prescription are to lengthen any tight or shortened muscles, which may need to have the gamma bias reset with use of contract-relax techniques or MET, and to strengthen the weak muscles, starting with the local muscles to get the proper form and force closure, as well as improve motor control. The goal is for pelvic stabilization, correction of trunk and lower-extremity muscle imbalances, and normalization of gait. As the pain and inflammation are controlled, the exercises can be progressed to include more functional, activity-related, and sport-specific movements.

It is important to start the exercise program with training of proper motor control of the local and global muscles so that the underactive muscles can be activated. Therefore the movement must be performed with proper technique, and the therapist should educate the patient to increase his or her postural awareness.

The clinician should start by teaching the patient how to find neutral spinal alignment and to breathe from the diaphragm. The reader should refer to Diane Lee's book, *The Pelvic Girdle,* for a detailed description on how to instruct and progress the patient.

Once the patient finds a neutral spine, the therapist can teach him or her how to contract the pelvic floor muscles and TA-multifidus. Contracting the pelvic muscles and TA together is more effective in strengthening these muscles than contracting them in isolation.[79] A pressure biofeedback unit may be used to help isolate the TA in prone or supine. The TA exercise can be performed in side lying, as well as in four-point kneeling (whatever position is most relaxing for the patient). In prone, the cuff is placed under the abdomen and inflated to 70 mm Hg. When the patient is asked to slowly draw the navel up and in, away from the pubic bone, the pressure on the cuff should decrease up to 10 mm Hg. The patient should only use 10% to 15% effort, and should palpate the contraction with his or her fingers 2 cm or 1 inch inferior medial to the ASIS. The correct technique would feel like gentle tension under the fingers, not bulging out into the fingers (bulging indicates contraction of the internal obliques). The multifidus can also be palpated lateral to the spinous process and should feel like a swelling of the muscle. The patient should continue to breathe from the diaphragm, while keeping the global muscles relaxed. He or she should perform 10 repetitions, holding each for 10 seconds. Progression should include adding the global muscles with the local muscles with movement of the upper and lower extremities, as well as functional and rotational movements, while maintaining the pelvic floor, multifidus, and TA contractions.

SUMMARY

In summary, the best management of the pelvic-hip region requires performing a thorough examination with attention directed also toward the lumbar spine. The therapist must evaluate form (ligaments, joints, and bone) and force (muscle, tendon, and fascia) closure and motor control. He or she must be cognizant of how the subjective history and emotional state of the patient can affect all of these elements, as well as posture. The therapist uses manual therapy skills, exercise, and education—along with touch—to help the patient achieve mobile stability. The goal is to teach the patient a better way to move in daily life, without joint and muscle imbalance, so he or she can manage and decrease symptoms and return to desired activities.

Although this region is very complex, with determination, continued research, and experience, the clinician may develop an effective means to evaluate and treat this region.

Case Study

The following case is an example of a patient with lumbo-pelvic hip dysfunction. Variations of this scenario are common.

Subjective History

A 26-year-old woman presents for evaluation and treatment of left PSIS, buttock, and occasional posterior thigh pain (not further than the midthigh). She indicates that her problem began during her last trimester of pregnancy. This was her first pregnancy. Her pain continued after the birth. It is now 5 months later, and the pain persists. The pain is worse with standing and walking activities, and it is better with sitting. She also complains of pain with turning in bed. Other than this discomfort, which she describes as "dull and achy" with occasional "sharp twinges," her general health is excellent, with no significant history of disease or surgery. Her obstetrician-gynecologist said her pain was normal and it should go away. It is starting to interfere with her ADL and taking care of her child. She does not work outside the home and would like to get back to a workout routine to lose some of the "baby weight."

Objective Examination

Posture: Normal kyphosis-lordosis but with a tendency toward a forward head and protraction of the shoulder girdles.

Basic functional examination of the lumbar spine (only positive tests are listed):
- Lumbar flexion: minimal pain
- SIJ dorsal lateral test: moderate pain

SIJ provocation examination:
- Oestgaard (thigh thrust): moderate pain
- Sacral thrust: moderate pain
- ASLR test: positive on the left
- Palpation: tender over the LDSIL
- Neurologic examination: within normal limits (WNL)

Assessment

The patient was retested with the sacroiliac belt, and the SIJ tests were negative.

ASLR test was positive, but improved with the belt.

Treatment Plan

The patient was educated on the use of a sacroiliac belt and instructed to wear it at all times (for 3 months, possibly longer, depending on how long she breastfeeds), except when showering. She was instructed on a core-stabilization program, including the pelvic floor muscles.

Results

The patient's pain was almost completely relieved after her first treatment with the sacroiliac belt.

Discussion

The patient likely sustained an SIJ instability with pelvic ring involvement secondary to her pregnancy and delivery. A follow-up check 6 months after treatment revealed that she remained asymptomatic and was jogging 3 to 4 miles a day, 3 to 5 days per week. She continued to perform her stabilization exercises on a regular basis.

REFERENCES

1. Tschauner C: Die hufte, Stuttgart, 1997, Ferdinand Enke Verlag.
2. Agus H, Omeroglu H, Ucar H, et al: Evaluation of the risk factors of avascular necrosis of the femoral head in developmental dysplasia of the hip in infants younger than 18 months of age, J Pediatr Orthop 11:41-46, 2002.
3. Leonhart H, Tillman B, Tondury G, et al: Rauber/Kopsch Anatomie des Menschen, Lehrbuch und Atlas. Band III, Stuttgart, Germany, 1998, Georg Thieme.
4. Reichel H: Hip arthroses: prevention, diagnostics, and therapy, Stuttgart, 2000, Thieme Verlag.
5. Klaue K, Durnin CW, Ganz R: The acetabular rim syndrome: clinical presentation of dysplasia of the hip, J Bone Joint Surg 73B:423-429, 1991.

6. Kapandji IA: The physiology of the joints. II. The lower limb, ed 2, Edinburgh, 1970, Churchill Livingstone.

7. Tan V, Seides RM, Katz MA, et al: Contribution of acetabular labrum to articulating surface area and femoral head coverage in adult hip joints: an anatomic study in cadavera, Am J Orthop 30:809-812, 2001.

8. Shibutani N: Three-dimensional architecture of the acetabular labrum—a scanning electron microscopic study, J Jap Orthop Assoc 62:321-329, 1988.

9. Peterson F, Peterson W, Tillman B: Structure and vascularization of the acetabular labrum with regard to the pathogenesis and healing of labral lesions, Arch Orthop Trauma Surg 123(6):283-288, 2003.

10. Dihlmann W: Joint-vertebra connections: clinical radiology, including computer-tomographic diagnosis, differential diagnosis, ed 3, Stuttgart, 1987, Thieme Verlag.

11. Tonnis D, Heinecke A: Diminished femoral antetorsion syndrome: a cause of pain and osteoarthritis, J Pediatr Orthop 11:419-431, 1991.

12. Murphy SB, Ganz R, Muller ME: The prognosis in untreated dysplasia of the hip: a study of radiologic factors that predict the outcome, J Bone Joint Surg 77A:985-989, 1995.

13. Matthijs O, van Paridon-Edauw D, Winkel D: Manuele therapie van de perifere gewrichten. Deel 3: heup, knie, enkel en voet, kraakbeen, Houten, The Netherlands, 2004, Bohn Stafleu Van Lochem.

14. Cyriax J: Textbook of orthopaedic medicine, ed 7, vol 1, London, 1978, Bailliere-Tindall.

15. Simon SR, Alaranta H, An K-N, et al: Kinesiology. In Simon SR, editor: Orthopaedic basic science, Chicago, 1994, American Academy of Orthopaedic Surgeons.

16. Hewitt J, Glisson R, Guilak F, et al: The mechanical properties of the human hip capsule ligaments, J Arthroplasty 17:82-89, 2002.

17. Hewitt J, Guilak F, Glisson R, et al: Regional material properties of the human hip joint capsule ligaments, J Orthop Res 19:359-364, 2001.

18. Delee JC: Fractures and dislocations of the hip. In Rockwood CA, Green DP, Guchholz RW, et al, editors: Fractures in adults, vol 2, Baltimore, 1996, Lippincott-Raven.

19. Wettstein M, Garofolo R, Borens O, et al: Traumatic rupture of the ligamentum teres as a source of hip pain, Arthroscopy 20:385-391, 2004.

20. Grieve GP: Modern manual therapy of the vertebral column, Edinburgh, 1986, Churchill Livingstone.

21. Grieve GP: Common vertebral joint problems, Edinburgh, 1981, Churchill Livingstone.

22. Kagan A: Rotator cuff tears of the hip, Clin Orthop Relat Res 368:135-140, 1999.

23. International Academy of Orthopedic Medicine: US hip course notes, Denver, 2003.

24. Hall SJ: The biomechanics of the human lower extremity. In Basic giomechanics, New York, 1991, McGraw-Hill.

25. Kapandji A: The physiology of the joints, vol 2. The lower limb, ed 2, Edinburgh, 1991, Churchill Livingstone.

26. Harvey G, Bell S: Obturator neuropathy: An anatomic perspective, Clin Orthop 363:203-211, 1999.

27. More RC, Karras BT, Neiman R, et al: Hamstrings—an anterior cruciate ligament protagonist: an in vitro study, Am J Sports Med 21:231-237, 1993.

28. Anderson MA, Gieck JH, Perrin DH, et al: The relationship among isometric, isotonic, and isokinetic concentric and eccentric quadriceps and hamstrings force and three components of athletic performance, J Orthop Sports Phys Ther 14:114-120, 1991.

29. Vleeming A, Stoeckart R, Volkers ACW, et al: Relations between form and function in the sacroiliac joint. I. Clinical anatomic aspects, Spine 15:130-132, 1990.

30. Vleeming A, Volkers ACW, Snijders CJ, et al: Relations between form and function in the sacroiliac joint. II. Biomechanical aspects, Spine 15:133-136, 1990.

31. Hardy SL: Femoral nerve palsy associated with an associated posterior wall transverse acetabular fracture, J Orthop Trauma 11:40-42, 1997.

32. Warfel BS, Marini SG, Lachmann EA, et al: Delayed femoral nerve palsy following femoral vessel catheterization, Arch Phys Med Rehabil 74:1211-1215, 1993.

33. Papastefanou SL, Stevens K, Mulholland RC: Femoral nerve palsy: an unusual complication of anterior lumbar interbody fusion, Spine 19:2842-2844, 1994.

34. Synek VM: The piriformis syndrome: review and case presentation, Clin Exp Neurol 23:31-37, 1987.

35. Hughes S, Goldstein M, Hicks D, et al: Extrapelvic compression of the sciatic nerve, J Bone Joint Surg Br 74A:1553-1559, 1992.

36. McCrory P, Bell S: Nerve entrapment syndromes as a cause of pain in the hip, groin and buttock, Sports Med 27:261-272, 1999.

37. Filler AG, Haynes J, Jordan SE, et al: Sciatica of nondisc origin and piriformis syndrome: diagnosis by magnetic resonance neurography and interventional magnetic resonance imaging with outcome study of resulting treatment, J Neurosurg Spine 2(2):99-115, 2005.

38. Matthijis O, van Paridon D, Sizer P, et al: Diagnosis-specific orthopedic management of the hip, IAOM-US, OPTP 2007.

39. Puranan J, Orava S: The hamstring syndrome—a new gluteal sciatica, Ann Chir Gynaecol 80:212-214, 1991.

40. Orava S: Hamstring syndrome, Oper Tech Sports Med 5:143-149, 1997.

41. Bradshaw C, McCrory P, Bell S, et al: Obturator nerve entrapment: a cause of groin pain in athletes, Am J Sports Med 25:402-408, 1997.

42. Ivins GK: Meralgia paresthetica, the elusive diagnosis: clinical experience with 14 adult patients, Ann Surg 232:281-286, 2000.

43. Lee D: The pelvic girdle, New York, 2004, Churchill Livingstone.

44. Solonen KA: The sacroiliac joint in the light of anatomical roentgenological and clinical studies, Acta Orthop Scand (suppl) 27:1-127, 1957.

45. Vleeming A, Snijders CJ, Stoeckart R, et al: The role of the sacroiliac joints in coupling between spine, pelvis,

legs and arms. In Vleeming A, Mooney V, Dorman T, et al, editors: Movement, stability and low back pain, Edinburgh, 1997, Churchill Livingstone, p 53.

46. Snijders CJ, Vleeming A, Stoeckart R, et al: Biomechanics of the interface between spine and pelvis in different postures. In Vleeming A, Mooney V, Dorman T, et al, editors: Movement, stability and low back pain: the essential role of the pelvis, Edinburgh, 1997, Churchill Livingstone.

47. Smidt GL, Wei SH, McQuade K, et al: Sacroiliac motion for extreme hip positions: a fresh cadaver study, Spine 22(18):2073-2082, 1997.

48. International Academy of Orthopedic Medicine: US lumbar spine and sacroiliac joint course notes, Denver, 2003 and 2008.

49. Goode A, Hegedus EJ, Sizer P, et al: Three-dimensional movements of the sacroiliac joint: a systematic review of the literature and assessment of the clinical utility, J Man Manip Ther 16(1):25-38, 2008.

50. Winkel D: Diagnosis and treatment of the spine, Philadelphia, 1996, Aspen Publishers.

51. Kissling RO, Jacob HA: The mobility of the sacroiliac joint in healthy subjects, Bull Hops Jt Dis 54:158-164, 1996.

52. Sturesson B, Selvik G, Uden A: Movements of the sacroiliac joints. A roentgen stereophotogrammetric analysis, Spine 14:162-165, 1989.

53. Smidt GL, McQuade K, Wei S-H, et al: Sacroiliac kinematics for reciprocal straddle positions, Spine 20:1047-1054, 1995.

54. Vleeming A, Pool-Goudzwaard AL, Stoeckart R, et al: The posterior layer of the thoracolumbar fascia: its function in load transfer from spine to legs, Spine 20:753-758, 1995.

55. Williams PL: Gray's anatomy, ed 38, New York, 1995, Churchill Livingstone.

56. Salsibali N, Valorjerdy MR, Hogg DA: Variations in thickness of articular cartilage in the human sacroiliac joint, Clin Anat 8:388-390, 1995.

57. Bowen V, Cassidy JD: Macroscopic and microscopic anatomy of the sacroiliac joint from embryonic life until the eighth decade, Spine 6:620, 1981.

58. Dar G, Khamis S, Peleg S, et al: Sacroiliac joint fusion and the implications for manual therapy diagnosis and treatment, Man Ther 13(2):155-158, 2008.

59. Gerlach UJ, Lierse W: Functional construction of the sacroiliac ligamentous apparatus, Acta Anat (Basel) 144:97-102, 1992.

60. Vleeming A, van Wengerden JP, Dijkstra PF, et al: Mobility in the SI-joints in old people: a kinematic and radiologic study, Clin Biomech (Bristol, Avon) 7:170, 1992.

61. Jaovisidha S, Ryu KN, De Maeseneer M, et al: Ventral sacroiliac ligament: anatomic and pathologic considerations, Invest Radiol 31:532-541, 1996.

62. Schwarzer AC, Aprill CN, Bogduk N: The sacroiliac joint in chronic low back pain, Spine 20:31-37, 1995.

63. Vleeming A: The function of the long dorsal sacroiliac ligament: its implication for understanding low back pain, Spine 21:556, 1996.

64. Fortin JD, Pier J, Falco F: Sacroiliac joint injection: pain referral mapping and arthrographic findings. In Vleeming A, Mooney V, Dorman T, et al, editors: Movement, stability and low back pain, Edinburgh, 1997, Churchill Livingstone.

65. Fortin JD, Kissling RO, O'Connor BL, et al: Sacroiliac joint innervation and pain, Am J Orthop 28(12):687, 1999.

66. Willard FH: The muscular, ligamentous and neural structure of the low back and its relation to back pain. In Vleeming A, Mooney V, Dorman T, et al, editors: Movement, stability and low back pain, Edinburgh, 1997, Churchill Livingstone.

67. Vleeming A, Stoeckart R, Snijders CJ: The sacrotuberous ligament: a conceptual approach to its dynamic role in stabilizing the sacroiliac joint, Clin Biomech (Bristol, Avon) 4:201, 1989.

68. Vleeming A, van Wingerden JP, Snijders CJ, et al: Load application to the sacrotuberous ligament: influences on sacroiliac joint mechanics, Clin Biomech (Bristol, Avon) 4:204, 1989.

69. Pool-Goudzwaard AL, Kleinrensink GJ, Snijders CJ, et al: The sacroiliac part of the iliolumbar ligament, J Anat 457-463, 2001.

70. Bogduk NLT: Clinical anatomy of the lumbar spine and sacrum, ed 3, New York, 1997, Churchill Livingstone.

71. Dreyfuss P, Michaelsen M, Pauza K, et al: The value of medical history and physical examination in diagnosing sacroiliac joint pain, Spine 21:2594-2602, 1996.

72. Santaguida PL, McGill SM: The psoas major muscle: a three-dimensional geometric study, Clin Biomech (Bristol, Avon) 28:339-345, 1995.

73. Hodges PW, Richardson CA: Inefficient muscular stabilization of the lumbar spine associated with low back pain: a motor control evaluation of transverses abdominis, Spine 21(22):2640, 1996.

74. Richardson CA, Snijders CJ, Hides JA, et al: The relationship between the transversely oriented abdominal muscles, sacroiliac joint mechanics and low back pain, Spine 27(4):399, 2002.

75. Hodges PW, Richardson CA: Altered trunk muscle recruitment in people with low back pain with upper limb movement at different speeds, Arch Phys Med Rehabil 80(9):1005-1012, 1999.

76. Sapsford RR, Hodges PW, Richardson CA, et al: Co-activation of the abdominal and pelvic floor muscles during voluntary exercises, Neurourol Urodyn 20(1):31-42, 2001.

77. Richardson CA, Jull GA, Hodges PW, et al: Therapeutic exercise for spinal segmental stabilization in low back pain: scientific basis and clinical approach, Edinburgh, 1999, Churchill Livingstone.

78. Hodges PW, Kaigle Holm A, Holm S, et al: Intervertebral stiffness of the spine is increased by evoked contraction of the transverses abdominis and the diaphragm: in vivo porcine studies, Spine (submitted) 2003b.

79. Sapsford RR, Hodges PW, Richardson CA, et al: Co-activation of the abdominal and pelvic floor muscles during voluntary exercises, Neurourol Urodyn 20:31, 2001.

80. Sapsford RR, Hodges PW: Contraction of the pelvic floor muscles during abdominal maneuvers, Arch Phys Med Rehab 82:1081-1088, 2001.

81. Magee DJ: Orthopedic physical assessment, ed 5, St Louis, 2009, Saunders.

82. Maigne JY, Maigne R, Guerin-Surville H: Upper thoracic dorsal rami: anatomic study of their medial cutaneous branches, Surg Radiol Anat 13:109-112, 1991.

83. Moseley GL, Hodges PW, Gandevia SC: Deep and superficial fibers of the lumbar multifidus muscle are differentially active during voluntary arm movements, Spine 27(2):E29, 2002.

84. Shindo H: Anatomical study of the lumbar multifidus muscle and its innervation in human adults and fetuses, J Nippon Med School 62:439-446, 1995.

85. Van Wingerden JP, Vleeming A, Buyruk HM, et al: Muscular contribution to force closure: sacroiliac joint stabilization in vivo. In Proceedings from the 4th Interdisciplinary World Congress on Low Back and Pelvic Pain, Montreal, 2001, pp 153-159.

86. Cresswell A: Responses of intra-abdominal pressure and abdominal muscle activity during dynamic loading in man, Eur J Appl Physiol 66:315, 1993.

87. Hodges PW, Cresswell AG, Daggfeldt K, et al: In vivo measurement of the effect of intra-abdominal pressure on the human spine, J Biomech 34:347, 2001.

88. Hodges PW, Kaigle Holm A, et al: Intervertebral stiffness of the spine is increased by evoked contraction of transverses abdominis and the diaphragm: in vivo porcine studies. In International Society of the Study of the Lumbar Spine, (53)13-17, 2003.

89. Hodges PW, Gandevia SC, Richardson CA: Contractions of specific abdominal muscles in postural tasks are affected by respiratory maneuvers, J Appl Phyisol 83(3):753, 1997.

90. Waldron T, Rogers J: An epidemiologic study of sacroiliac fusion in some human skeletal remains, Am J Phys Anthropol 83(1):123-127, 1990.

91. Barakatt E, Smidt GL, Dawson JD, et al: Interinnominate motion and symmetry: comparison between gymnasts and nongymnasts, J Orthop Sports Phys Ther 23:309-319, 1996.

92. Zheng N, Watson LG, Yong-Hing K: Biomechanical modeling of the human sacroiliac joint, Med Biol Eng Comput 35:77-82, 1997.

93. Rydell N: Biomechanics of the hip joint, Clin Orthop 92:6-15, 1973.

94. Riezbos C, Lagerberg A: Over belasting, Versus, tijdschrift voor fysiotherapie 18(1):21-60, 2000.

95. Panjabi MM: The stabilizing system of the spine. II. Neutral zone and instability hypotheses, J Spinal Disord 5(4):390, 1992.

96. Snijders CJ, Vleeming A, Stoeckart R: Transfer of lumbosacral load to iliac bones and legs. II. Loading of the sacroiliac joints when lifting in a stooped posture, Clin Biomech (Bristol Avon) 8:295-301, 1993.

97. Snijders CJ, Vleeming A, Stoeckart R: Transfer of lumbosacral load to iliac bones and legs. I. Biomechanics of self-bracing of the sacroiliac joints and its significance for treatment and exercise, Clin Biomech (Bristol Avon) 8:285, 1993.

98. Franke BA: Formative dynamics: the pelvic girdle, J Man Manip Ther 11:12-40, 2003.

99. Shumway-Cook A, Wollacott MH: Motor control: theory and practical applications, ed 2, Philadelphia, 2001, Lippincott Williams & Wilkins.

100. Holstege G, Bandler R, Saper CB: The emotional motor system, Amsterdam, 1996, Elsevier.

101. Murphy M: The future of the body: explorations into the further evolution of human nature, New York, 1992, Tarcher Putnam.

102. Cailliett R: Low back pain syndrome, Philadelphia, 1988, FA Davis.

103. Tully EA, Prajakta B, Galea MP: Lumbofemoral rhythm during hip flexion in young adults and children, Spine 27(20):E432-E440, 2002.

104. Sturesson B, Uden A, Vleeming A: A radiosteriometric analysis of movements of the sacroiliac joints during the standing hip flexion test, Spine 25(3):364, 2000.

105. Hungerford BA: Patterns of intra-pelvic motion and muscle recruitment for pelvic instability, doctorial thesis, Sidney, Australia, 2002, University of Sydney.

106. Hungerford B, Gilleard W, Lee D: Alteration of sacroiliac joint motion patterns in subjects with pelvic motion asymmetry. In Proceedings from the 4th World Interdisciplinary Congress on Low Back And Pelvic Pain, Montreal, 2001.

107. Chamberlain WE: The symphysis pubis in the roentgen examination of the sacroiliac joint, AJR Am J Roentgenol 24:621, 1930.

108. Kristiansson P, Swardsudd K: Discriminatory power of tests applied in back pain during pregnancy, Spine 21:2337-2344, 1996.

109. Hagen R: Pelvic girdle relaxation from an orthopaedic point of view, Acta Orthop Scand 45:550, 1974.

110. Fortin JD, Apill CN, Ponthieux B, et al: Sacroiliac joint: pain referral maps upon applying a new injection/arthrography technique. II. Clinical evaluation, Spine 19:1475-1482, 1994.

111. LeBlanc KE: Sacroiliac sprain: an overlooked cause of back pain, Am Fam Physician 46:1459-1463, 1992.

112. Gracovetsky S, Farfan HF: The optimum spine, Spine 11:543, 1986.

113. Pearcy M, Tibrewal SB: Axial rotation and lateral bending in the normal lumbar spine measured by three-dimensional radiography, Spine 9:582, 1984.

114. Inman VT, Ralston HJ, Todd F: Human walking, Baltimore, 1981, Williams & Wilkins.

115. Gracovetsky S: Linking the spinal engine with the legs: a theory of human gait. In Vleeming A, Mooney V, Snijders CJ, et al, editors: Movement, stability and low back pain: the essential role of the pelvis, Edinburgh, 1997, Churchill Livingstone.

116. Levangie PK: The association between static pelvic asymmetry and low back pain, Spine 24:1234-1242, 1999.

117. Johnson AW, Weiss CB, Wheeler DL: Stress fractures of the femoral shaft in athletes—more common than expected, Am J Sports Med 22:248-256, 1994.

118. Melchione WE, Sullivan MS: Reliability of measurements obtained by the use of an instrument designed to indirectly measure ilio-tibial band length, J Orthop Sports Phys Ther 18:511-515, 1993.

119. Kendall FP, Kendall-McCreary E: Muscles, function and testing, ed 3, Baltimore, 1983, Williams & Wilkins.

120. Jull GA, Janda V: Muscle and motor control in low back pain. In Twomey LT, Taylor JR, editors: Physical therapy of the low back: clinics in physical therapy, New York, 1987, Churchill Livingstone.

121. Mens JM, Vleeming A, Snijders CJ, et al: Validity of the active straight leg raise test for measuring disease severity in patients with posterior pelvic pain after pregnancy, Spine 27:196-200, 2002.

122. Mens JM, Vleeming A, Snijders CJ, et al: The active straight-leg-raising test and mobility of the pelvic joints, Eur Spine J 8:468-473, 1999.

123. Norkin C, Levangie P: Joint structure and function: a comprehensive analysis, Philadelphia, 1992, FA Davis, pp 355-358.

124. Mont MA, Jones LC, Einhorn TA, et al: Osteonecrosis of the femoral head: potential treatment with growth and differentiation factors, Clin Orthop Rel Res 355S:S314-S335, 1998.

125. Martinez AG, Weinstein SL: Recurrent Legg-Calvé-Perthes disease, J Bone Joint Surg 73A:1081, 1991.

126. Wiig O, Svenningsen S, Terjesen T: Evaluation of the subchondral fracture in predicting the extent of femoral head necrosis in Perthes disease: a prospective study of 92 patients, J Pediatr Orthop B 13(5):293-298, 2004.

127. Yamamoto Y, Hamada Y, Ide T, et al: Arthroscopic surgery to treat intra-articular type snapping hip, Arthroscopy 21(9):1120-1125, 2005.

128. Yamamoto Y, Ide T, Hamada Y, et al: A case of intra-articular snapping hip caused by articular cartilage detachment from the deformed femoral head consequent to Perthes disease, Arthroscopy 20(6):650-653, 2004.

129. Guille JT, Lipton GE, Tsirikos AI, et al: Bilateral Legg-Calve-Perthes disease: presentation and outcome, J Pediatr Orthop 22(4):458-463, 2002.

130. Westhoff B, Petermann A, Hirsch MA, et al: Computerized gait analysis in Legg Calve Perthes disease—analysis of the frontal plane, Gait Posture 24(2):196-202, 2006.

131. Wenger DR, Ward WT, Herring JA: Current concepts review, Legg-Calvé-Perthes disease, J Bone Joint Surg 73A:778, 1991.

132. McCarthy JC, Noble PC, Schuck MR, et al: The role of labral lesions to development of early degenerative hip disease, Clin Orthop Relat Res 393:25-37, 2001.

133. Narvani AA, Tsiridis E, Tai C, et al: Acetabular labrum and its tears, Br J Sports Med 37:207-211, 2003.

134. Mason JB: Acetabular labral tears in the athlete, Clin Sports Med 20:779-790, 2001.

135. Fario LA, Glick JM, Sampson TG: Hip arthroscopy for acetabular labral tears, Arthroscopy 15:132-137, 1999.

136. Konrath GA, Hamel AJ, Olson SA, et al: The role of the acetabular labrum and the transverse acetabular ligament in load transmission in the hip, J Bone Joint Surg 80(12):1781-1788, 1998.

137. Leopold SS, Battista V, Oliverio JA: Safety and efficacy of intraarticular hip injection using anatomic landmarks, Clin Orthop Relat Res Oct 391:192-197, 2001.

138. Seldes RM, Tan V, Hunt J, et al: Anatomy, histologic features, and vascularity of the adult acetabular labrum, Clin Orthop Relat Res 382:232-240, 2001.

139. Hase T, Ueo T: Acetabular labral tear: arthroscopic diagnosis and treatment, Arthroscopy 15:138-141, 1999.

140. Leunig M, Werlen S, Ungersböck A, et al: Evaluation of the acetabulum labrum by MR Arthrography, J Bone Joint Surg 79B:230-234, 1997.

141. Fitzgerald RH: Acetabular labrum tears: diagnosis and treatment, Clin Orthop Relat Res 311:60-68, 1995.

142. Leunig M, Beck W, Woo A, et al: Acetabular rim degeneration: a constant finding in the aged hip, Clin Orthop Rel Res 413:201-207, 2003.

143. Pavlica P, Barozzi L, Salvarani C, et al: Magnetic resonance imaging in the diagnosis of PMR, Clin Exp Rheumatol 18(suppl 20):S38-S39, 2000.

144. Wank R, Miller TT, Shapiro JF: Sonographically guided injection of anesthetic for iliopsoas tendinopathy after total hip arthroplasty, J Clin Ultrasound 32(7):354-357, 2004.

145. Pelsser V, Cardinal E, Hobden R, et al: Extraarticular snapping hip: sonographic findings, Am J Roentgenol Radium Ther Nucl Med 176:67-73, 202-208, 2001.

146. Meyers WC, Foley DP, Garrett WE, et al: Management of severe lower abdominal or inguinal pain in high-performance athletes, Am J Sports Med 28:2-8, 2000.

147. Brennan D, O'Connell MJ, Ryan M, et al: Secondary cleft sign as a marker of injury in athletes with groin pain: MR image appearance and interpretation, Radiology 235:162-167, 2005.

148. Morelli V, Smith V: Groin injuries in athletes, Am Fam Physician 64:1405-1414, 2001.

149. Renstroem AF: Groin injuries: a true challenge in orthopaedic sports medicine, Sports Med Arthrosc 5:247-251, 1997.

150. Orchard JW, Cook JL, Halpin N: Stress-shielding as a cause of insertional tendinopathy: the operative tech-

nique of limited adductor tenotomy supports this theory, J Sci Med Sport 7(4):424-428, 2004.

151. Maitland GD: Vertebral manipulation, London, 1977, Butterworth Heinemann.

152. Elgafy H, Semaan HB, Ebraheim NA, et al: Computed tomography findings in patients with sacroiliac pain, Clin Orthop Relat Res 382:112-118, 2001.

153. Bellamy N, Newhook L, Rooney PJ, et al: Perception—a problem in the grading of sacroiliac joint radiographs, Scand J Rheumatol 13:113-120, 1984.

154. Bernard TN, Cassidy JD: The sacroiliac joint syndrome: pathophysiology, diagnosis and management. In Frymoyer JW, editor: The adult spine: principles and practice, New York, 1991, Raven Press Ltd, pp 2107-2130.

155. Buyruk HM, Snikders CJ, Vleeming A, et al: The measurements of sacroiliac joint stiffness with colour Doppler imaging: a study on healthy subjects, Eur J Radiol 21:117-121, 1995.

156. Maigne JY, Aivaliklik A, Pfefer F: Results of sacroiliac joint double block and value of sacroiliac pain provocation tests in 54 patients with low back pain, Spine 21:1889-1892, 1996.

157. Laslett M, Young SB, Aprill CN, et al: Diagnosing painful sacroiliac joints: a validity study of a McKenzie evaluation and sacroiliac provocation tests, Aus J Physiother 49:89-97, 2003.

158. Woerman AL, Binder-MacLeod S: Leg length discrepancy assessment: accuracy and precision in five clinical methods of evaluation, J Orthop Sports Phys Ther 5:230, 1984.

159. White KK, Williams SK, Mubarak SJ: Definition of two types of anterior superior iliac spine avulsion fractures, J Pediatr Orthop 22(5):578-582, 2002.

160. Cook C, Hegedus E: Orthopedic physical examination tests: an evidence-based approach, Upper Saddle River, NJ, 2008, Pearson Prentice Hall.

161. O'Sullivan PB, Beales DJ, Beetham JA, et al: Altered motor control strategies in subjects with sacroiliac joint pain during the active straight-leg-raise test, Spine 27:E1-E8, 2002.

162. Cowan SM, Schache AG, Brukner P, et al: Delayed onset of transversus abdominis in long standing groin pain, Med Sci Sports Exerc 36(12):2040-2045, 2004.

163. Broadhurst NA, Simmons DN, Bond MJ: Piriformis syndrome: correlation of muscle morphology with symptoms and signs, Arch Phys Med Rehabil 85(12): 2036-2039, 2004.

164. Laslett M, Williams W: The reliability of selected pain provocation tests for sacroiliac joint pathology, Spine 19(11):1243-1249, 1994.

165. Dreyfuss P, Dryer S, Griffing J, et al: Positive sacroiliac screening tests in asymptomatic adults, Spine 19(10):1138, 1994.

166. Lavignolle B, Vital JM, Senegas J, et al: An approach to the functional anatomy of the sacroiliac joints in vivo, Anat Clin 5(3):169-176, 1983.

167. Fortin JD: Sacroiliac joint dysfunction: a new perspective, J Back Musculoskeletal Rehabil 3:31-43, 1993.

168. Snijders CJ, Slagter AH, van Strik R, et al: Why leg crossing? The influence of common postures on abdominal muscle activity, Spine 20(18):1989-1993, 1995.

169. Damen L, Spoor CW, Snijders CJ, et al: Does a pelvic belt influence sacroiliac joint laxity? Clin Biomech (Bristol Avon) 17:495-498, 2002.

170. Monney V, Pozos R, Vleeming A, et al: Exercise treatment for sacroiliac pain, Orthopedics 24:29-32, 2001.

171. Fuss FK, Bacher A: New aspects of the morphology and function of the human hip joint ligaments, Am J Anat 192(1):1-13, 1991.

Surgical Treatment and Rehabilitation of the Hip Complex

Total hip arthroplasty (THA) has given many individuals suffering from end-stage joint disease and hip pain renewed life through dramatic functional improvements and pain relief. In fact, there has been a 46% increase in the number of total hip replacements from 1990 to 2002.[1] Some of this increase may be because of the aging baby boomer population, who are continuing to stay active. It is of utmost importance for a large number of the patients to maintain a good quality of life by continuing to participate in the recreational activities they enjoy. However, despite the increase in surgeries and the activity level of those having the surgeries, relatively little research exists regarding the specifics of returning to recreational activities and sports after a THA.

Traditionally, rehabilitation has focused on returning the patient to only the most basic functional goals such as walking, getting up from a chair or bed, and stair climbing. Unfortunately, for many patients this is not sufficient, and they express a desire to return to a higher level of activity and sports participation. In fact, patients often return to these activities regardless of whether they are in the proper physical condition to do so. Often they lack the informed guidance and conditioning necessary to help them achieve their higher goals. It may not be common practice yet for surgeons to suggest advanced physical therapy in the later stages post-THA; however, a number of physicians and health practitioners have remarked that a definite need exists for advanced rehabilitation at that time. Seyler et al.[1] published a review article that focused specifically on returning to sports after THA. In the article they stressed the importance of "extensive lower extremity rehabilitation before returning to high-activity sports after THA." Dubs et al.[2] elaborated on the importance of exercise to strengthen muscles, increase mobility, and improve neuromuscular coordination. He discussed the concept of a "muscle damping system," which serves to absorb the loads placed on the hip joint during higher-level activities such as sports. Brander and Stulberg went so far as to say that "current joint replacement rehabilitation protocols, which focus only on the achievement of basic functional goals, are inadequate."[3] Although some physicians tell patients that walking alone is adequate for strengthening, Sashika et al.[4] found that this was not the case. On examining THA patients 6 to 48 months after surgery, they found that the patients lacked sufficient strength

to achieve their functional goals. Likewise, Trudelle-Jackson et al.,[5] who examined patients receiving only the standard acute rehabilitation, found continued impairments at 4 to 12 months after THA. The patients in their study received physical therapy for up to 6 weeks during the initial stages of rehabilitation. The goal of this chapter is to present appropriate recommendations for the patient, physician, and physical therapist regarding postoperative THA rehabilitation.

More specifically, our objectives for this chapter are to address the following areas. The reader is given a clear overview of the different types of surgical approaches for THA, as well as a discussion of the pros and cons of each. The chapter looks at specific component features of the prosthesis and discusses what criteria are important for the surgeon to consider when making the appropriate choice for the patient. In addition, it takes a close look at the effect of these procedures on the musculoskeletal system of the patient and explains muscular deficits that exist postsurgery. A review of research is included on joint loading during various activities in an attempt to understand the rationale behind recommendations for when to return to higher-level activities, and current recommendations for THA precautions and for returning to higher-level activities such as sports are discussed. Finally, specific recommendations are made for rehabilitation after THA, with special emphasis on advanced training to help the patient return safely to higher-level activities and sports.

EXAMINATION OF LOADS PLACED ON HIP JOINT

Scientific Studies of Hip Biomechanics

Numerous scientific approaches have been developed to better understand the biomechanics of a prosthetic hip. One such approach is an in vitro study, literally translated as *in glass*. *In vitro* refers to a study that is done in an artificial environment such as a laboratory and may include the use of human cadavers, animal specimens, or synthetic material. *In vivo,* translated as *in living,* refers to a study that is performed using a living person (some in vivo studies are discussed in the following section). A third method of study involves using mathematic models to explain loads placed on a joint. Mathematic models are helpful in explaining general concepts and calculations but must be interpreted carefully because they do not always accurately reflect what actually occurs in a patient.

To understand the circumstances that can lead to failure of the hip prosthesis, it is necessary to examine the type of loads that are placed on the hip joint. These concepts will assist the health practitioner in understanding which activities are least damaging during the postoperative "healing" phase, as well as reveal why certain activities could lead to excessive wearing of the joint. Excessive wearing is important to understand and avoid, because it could ultimately decrease the normal lifespan of the prosthesis.

One of the first published in vivo experiments was reported by Rydell in 1966.[6] In an attempt to measure contact forces within the hip joint, he placed a specialized hip prosthesis containing strain gauges into a live patient. He then took measurements at 6 months postoperation and found that during gait, the contact forces on the prosthesis were 2.3 to 3.3 times the body weight. More recently, researchers have begun to perform in vivo experiments using prostheses containing telemeterized pressure-sensing transducers. Using these components, scientists have found that the contact forces during gait are actually even higher than those originally reported by Rydell.[6] Furthermore, during running, Rydell discovered increases in contact forces by 43%. He found that adding a cushioned heel insert decreases these forces and thus recommended a heel insert for his THA patients.[6] Lim et al.[7] also reported that there was a 10% decrease in contact forces during running with a soft heel. In contrast, during walking, the same level of load was placed on the joint regardless of the type of shoe or sole the patient was wearing. In fact, walking barefoot placed the least amount of stress on the joint. In addition, the authors also reported that softer floor material placed increased load on the hip compared with harder surfaces. They attributed this to the increase in antagonist activity necessary to stabilize the hip while walking on a softer, unstable surface. This may be especially relevant to the THA patient who wants to return to certain outdoor sports activities such as golf, in which walking on grass simulates such a softer surface. Incidentally, during the study when the patients stumbled without falling, the hip joint forces increased to up to 8.7 times the body weight.[7] In the rehabilitation section, the effect of THA surgery on postural stability is discussed and ways in which exercises can help to minimize such precarious losses of balance are described.

Some studies have focused on examining torsional forces rather than looking strictly at contact forces. The bone-implant interface stability is essential to the long-term survivability of the prosthesis. A torsional force is likely to be most destructive to this interface, especially during the early postoperative period. A study by Kotzar et al.[8] looked at peak torsional loads on the hip joint in early postoperative patients with activities of daily living (ADL). They found that greater torsional forces occurred with walking and single-leg stance than with stair climbing and rising from a chair. Despite the fact that the overall torsional force was less with stair-climbing and sit-to-

stand activities, the torque-to-contact pressure ratio was higher. In other words, there were decreased contact forces within the joint relative to torque on the joint; thus perhaps decreased stability during these activities. The less stable the joint is, the more inappropriate muscle activity is likely to be present to compensate. This may explain why it is more common for the patient to complain of increased pain with activities like stair climbing and rising from a chair.

Another area of focus has been to look at the level of activity in the muscles surrounding the joint with the assumptions that this would reflect the amount of load placed on the prosthesis. Because increased hip abductor activity is correlated to increased load in the hip joint, it may be that large hip abductor forces contribute to premature loosening of the prosthetic hip in the early postoperative stages when the bone-implant interface is still fragile. Thus it would be prudent to minimize abductor activity during this acute phase. Conversely, once the joint has healed, one would want to ensure that these same muscles are of sufficient strength. As one author wrote, "the main contributors to hip joint loading are the muscles of abduction, which may provide loads of up to three times the body weight during the stance phase of walking. As a result, any muscular weakness around the hip joint, especially the hip abductors, will change the hip joint forces and lead to instability."[9] In other words, the hip musculature affects loading of the joint approximating the femoral head with the acetabulum, and thus it determines the stability of the joint. Therefore weaker hip musculature decreases this joint approximation and results in a less stable joint.

A number of studies by Neuman[10] have looked at electromyography (EMG) of hip abductor activity during gait. The least amount of EMG hip abductor activity occurred with using a cane on the contralateral side to the prosthesis. In addition, carrying a load in both hands created less hip abductor activity than in just one hand. If it is necessary to carry an object using one hand, then it is preferable to carry the load on the side ipsilateral to the prosthesis to decrease the amount of load placed on the joint.

SURGICAL PROCEDURES

In general, the goals of total hip replacement include longevity, biocompatibility, restoration of normal anatomy, minimization of risk, and maximization of function. The surgeon must consider several factors that influence the postsurgical stability, function, and longevity of a THA. The most important decision includes the surgical approach and the bearing material used. Postoperative hip dislocation is one of the most feared complications of hip replacement surgery, with dislocation rates ranging from 0.4% to 11%.[11] Improved soft tissue management during surgery, coupled with improved materials and more anatomic femoral head sizes, have added to postoperative stability and decreases in dislocation rates.

An examination of the soft tissue structures that are violated during the surgical approach to THA can give us insight into the importance of adhering to precautions during the acute postoperative phase. In addition, understanding which soft tissues are involved dictates which muscle groups should be targeted in the advanced rehabilitative phase, especially in preparation for return to a sport. For example, golf requires a great deal of hip strength, specifically in the external rotators, gluteus medius, and maximus muscles. How these muscles are incised during surgery is discussed following. Care should be taken to protect injured tissue postoperatively to limit complications such as further muscle injury and hip dislocation.

The concept of internervous planes is important to muscle rehabilitation. A few distinct nerves innervate the muscles surrounding the hip joint. In general, if a muscle is incised, separated, or otherwise torn within its substance, then it runs the risk of becoming partially or wholly denervated, depending on the location of the injury with respect to the nerves' branches. Therefore when making surgical approaches, it is vital to know when it is appropriate to go through muscle bellies and when it is more prudent to avoid muscle injury. An internervous plane is a space created by dissection between two muscles that are innervated by different nerves, ensuring that neither is denervated, although still successfully dissecting more deeply.

Four common approaches to the hip are used for THA surgery. Each has its advantages and disadvantages, and it is important to appreciate the differences to understand postoperative limitations. The four approaches discussed include the (1) anterior, (2) anterolateral, (3) medial, and (4) posterior approaches. In addition to the classic descriptions, there exist variations on each of these approaches.

The anterior approach (or Smith-Peterson approach) is advocated for its sparing of the posterior hip soft tissues and superior stability with respect to posterior hip dislocations. However, this approach is technically demanding, requiring extensive detachment of tendinous insertions and muscle retraction, and it often requires specialized operating room equipment. The superficial incision is on the anterior aspect of the thigh, and the deep dissection continues through the deep fascia between the tensor fascia latae (superior gluteal nerve) laterally and sartorius and rectus femoris (both innervated by the femoral nerve) medially. The lateral femoral cutaneous nerve is at risk during this approach. Advantages include minimal neuromuscular disruption and posterior stability, but it can be difficult to adequately visualize the acetabulum without stripping a great deal of soft tissue.

A variation on the anterior approach, the anterolateral approach to the hip is the most commonly used approach in total hip replacement surgery. Popularized by Watson-Jones, this approach combines excellent exposure of the acetabulum with safe reaming of the femoral shaft. The skin incision is made lateral to that of the anterior approach, and the deep dissection exploits the intermuscular plane between the tensor fasciae latae (superior gluteal nerve) and the gluteus medius (superior gluteal nerve). This approach does not use a true internervous plane. However, because the superior gluteal nerve enters the tensor fascia latae very close to its origin at the iliac crest, it is not in danger as long as the plane between the gluteus medius and the tensor fascia latae is not developed to the origins of both muscles from the ilium. To fully present

the femur for reaming, part of the abductor mechanism must be detached to allow for maximum adduction. This may be accomplished by either cutting the bony attachment of the abductors and reflecting it or by sharply releasing part of the gluteus medius and all of the gluteus minimus. At the end of the procedure it is important to repair the abductor musculature. The femoral nerve is at risk during this approach, and the most common problem is compression neuropraxia.

The direct lateral or transgluteal approach prevents the need for trochanteric osteotomy (bony cut to release the abductors). The bulk of the gluteus medius muscle is left intact, allowing for early mobilization following THA surgery. This is particularly important because a complication of injury to the gluteus medius is abductor weakness postoperatively. This typically manifests as a limp, most notably an abductor lurch. A lack of wide exposure relative to the anterolateral approach makes this one technically difficult to use for revision arthroplasty. Again, no true internervous plane exists because this approach uses a muscle-splitting technique. The gluteus medius muscle is split along its line to the entry of the superior gluteal nerve, and the vastus lateralis is similarly split along its own line to the point of entry of the femoral nerve. As would be expected, both of these nerves are at risk during this operation. Both anterolateral and direct lateral approaches include incisions through the gluteus muscles and therefore may have a longer period of abductor weakness postoperatively.[11,3]

The final approach mentioned here is the posterior approach. Popularized by Moore, it is the most common and practical approach used to expose the hip. Importantly, the abductor mechanism is not violated in this approach, preventing the loss of abductor power in the postoperative period associated with the anterolateral approach.[11,3] Again, no true internervous plane exists, and the deep dissection is carried through the gluteus maximus along its fibers. The nerves innervating the gluteus maximus enter medial to the split; therefore surgical dissection does not result in significant denervation. Although the posterior approach spares the abductor mechanism, it is associated with a higher than average dislocation rate. A review of 13,203 patients undergoing THA demonstrated a combined dislocation rate of 1.27%, whereas the rate for those having a posterior approach was reported to be 3.23% (3.05% without a posterior repair and 2.03% with a posterior repair). When the posterior capsule, the piriformis, and short external rotator muscles are repaired, the rate of dislocation is reduced. In a study by Pellicci et al.,[12] the authors showed a 0.0% to 0.8% dislocation rate with the posterior approach coupled with repair of the capsule, piriformis, and the short external rotators. Ultrasonography studies have looked at the integrity of the repaired posterior soft tissues after THA and found that at 6 weeks and 12 weeks, 89% integrity of the external rotators and posterior capsule exists.[13] Instructions to the patients in this study were to weight bear as tolerated and to adhere to the THA precautions for 6 weeks. Repair of the posterior structures acts as a biologic scaffold for healing that may be important for long-term stability.[13]

Once the surgeon has decided on a surgical approach, he or she has a variety of options when it comes to THA implant materials and head sizes. Those patients wishing to return to playing golf and other sporting activities after a THA have several physical goals. To comfortably navigate a golf game and course, one must be able to walk pain free, have good range of motion (including the ability to squat and kneel), and have the freedom at the hip to rotate and transfer loads. Advances in reconstruction aside from the mastering of muscle-sparing surgical approaches include improved fixation, a variety of bearing materials, and more anatomic head sizes.

Dislocation has been a common complication of THA, which has led to a great deal of fear and perioperative limitations. The circumstances surrounding dislocation that may be the result of prosthetic impingement, bony impingement, or spontaneous dislocation are discussed in more detail later in the chapter. Prosthetic impingement has been addressed with the advent of larger, more anatomic head sizes. The harder, highly cross-linked polyethylene acetabular liners, as well as metal and ceramic liners, accommodate larger femoral heads. The larger the head is, the greater the range of motion is before the implant will impinge. Increasing the femoral head size from 22 mm to 40 mm increases the required displacement for dislocation by about 5 mm, with the acetabular component at 45 degrees of abduction (Figure 20-1).[14] Larger heads also allow for easier closed reductions if the hip dislocates. In addition to the increased range of motion to impingement, larger heads have been shown to offer an increased suction effect between the head and the cup, resulting in further stability and resistance to dislocation.

Osseous impingement may occur as the prosthetic neck affects the bony acetabulum. This is at particular risk if the acetabular component is in a more vertical position in the pelvis than is desirable. Although large heads offer increased stability and thus lower dislocation rates, they cannot compensate for a poorly positioned acetabular component.

The bearing materials currently in use today include conventional and highly cross-linked polyethylene acetabular components, a variety of metals, and ceramic material (Figure 20-2). Each material has distinct wear characteristics that affect longevity. Ceramic heads coupled with highly cross-linked polyethylene have improved wear characteristics, but the

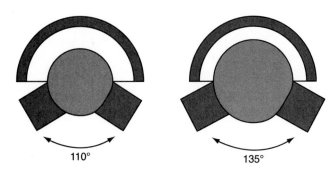

Figure 20-1 Effect of increasing the femoral head size on impingement. A larger head increases the impingement-free range of motion. (From Malik A, Maheshwari A, Dorr D: Impingement with total hip replacement, J Bone Joint Surg Am 89:1832-1842, 2007.)

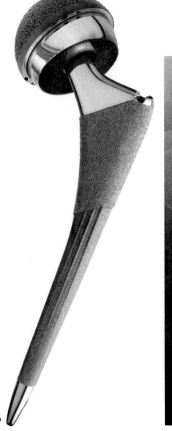

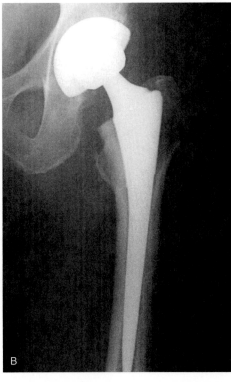

Figure 20-2 A, Metal head and cup with femoral stem attached (complete total hip arthroplasty [THA] prosthesis). **B,** Implanted THA with polyethylene liner on radiograph (ceramic on poly). (Courtesy Smith and Nephew, Memphis, Tenn.)

femoral head size is limited by the thickness of the polyethylene liner (Figure 20-3, *A*). Ceramic heads coupled with ceramic liners offer excellent wear properties, accommodate larger heads than highly cross-linked polyethylene liners, and have ideal wettability; however, they are limited by an increased fracture risk, ultimate size limitations, and an audible squeak with range of motion (Figure 20-3, *B*). Metal-on-metal bearings approximate anatomic head sizes and have excellent wear characteristics but also squeak and have a theoretical risk of metal ion release as a result of wear (Figure 20-3, *C*). Metal-on-metal implants have the additional benefit of resisting separation in vivo. In 20 subjects analyzed in vivo with video fluoroscopy evaluation of the femoral head, acetabular component separation during normal gait was shown to be 2 mm of average sliding during swing phase with metal-on-polyethylene components and 0 mm with metal-on-metal implants.[15]

Hip resurfacing arthroplasty is gaining popularity in those patients who are candidates for such a procedure. These patients include those who are relatively young, have good bone stock, and have limited femoral head and neck deformity. Hip resurfacing, although more technically demanding than total hip replacement surgery, is considered conservative treatment because it does not burn bridges with respect to future joint reconstruction, conserves bone stock, and offers a more anatomic option than total hip replacement. In addition, the larger heads used in resurfacing allow for increased stability and therefore fewer dislocations (Figure 20-4).

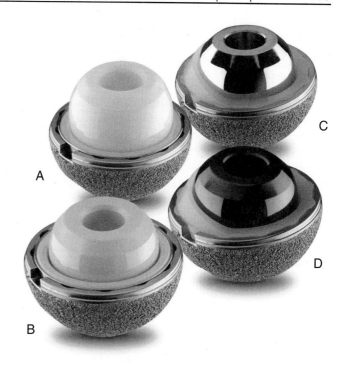

Figure 20-3 A, Ceramic head, ceramic liner, metal acetabular component. **B,** Ceramic head, ceramic liner, metal acetabular component. **C,** Metal head, polyethylene liner, metal acetabular component. **D,** Oxidized zirconium head, polyethylene liner, metal acetabular component. (Courtesy Smith and Nephew, Memphis, Tenn.)

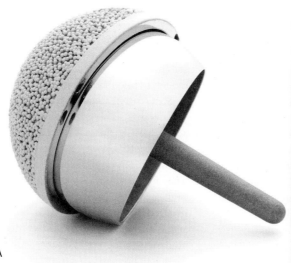

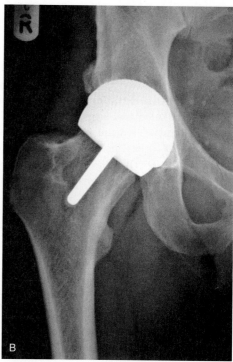

Figure 20-4 A, Hip resurfacing components, head in cup (metal on metal). **B,** Metal on metal hip resurfacing implanted (radiograph). (Courtesy Smith and Nephew, Memphis, Tenn.)

Postsurgery Precautions

Recommendations for the Protective Phase of Healing

During the early part of rehabilitation, it is important to protect the soft tissue structures to avoid overextension of the capsular and muscular structures and allow sufficient time for them to heal. For a straightforward THA (lateral approaches), the precautions are to avoid hip flexion beyond 90 degrees, internal rotation beyond neutral, and adduction beyond midline for 6 weeks.[3,13,16] For more complicated high-risk THA patients, the period may be extended to 3 months.[3] There may also be a recommendation for a hip abductor orthosis brace with range of motion stops, hip spica, or hip-knee-ankle orthosis in cases of recurrent or revision THA surgeries (usually worn around 6 weeks). In addition, some procedures such as trochanteric osteotomy have further restrictions of no resisted abduction or active isotonic hip abduction against gravity until the osteotomy has healed. In the case of an acetabular bone graft, the patient is usually restricted from weight bearing for the first few weeks.[3] The precautions for the anterior approach include no external rotation and extension to preserve the anterior structures during the healing period. Interestingly, Peak et al.[16] examined the effectiveness of additional restrictions (abduction pillow, no side lying, no driving or riding in car) on THA patients and found that patients with fewer restrictions (only no flexion >90 degrees, no adduction, and no internal or external rotation >45 degrees) returned to prior levels of function faster than the restricted group. Thus although certain precautions are necessary for healing, excessive restrictions may not be conducive to a quick, full return to function.

Early and Late Dislocations After Total Hip Arthroplasty

Meek et al.[17] describes dislocation as occurring mainly at two points: (1) immediately postoperatively during the healing phase or (2) much later. According to their study, after the first year, the incidence of dislocation increases with time. Berry[18] looked at the cumulative long-term risk of dislocation after a primary Charnley THA and came up with a formula to calculate the risk of dislocation. Figures given were a 1% risk at 1 month postoperatively, 1.9% risk at 1 year postoperatively, a 1% increase every 5 years, and a 7% increase at 25 years. The prevalence of redislocation after nonoperative management was 33%.

In the unlikely event of a dislocation, it is important for the therapist to recognize it and act quickly because of the time-sensitive nature of the injury. It is necessary for a closed reduction to be performed within the first few hours of the incident, or else it may be necessary to perform an open reduction because of soft tissue swelling and muscle shortening.[3] An acute dislocation will generally be associated with immediate pain, which is increased with weight bearing. The patient may also report hearing a *pop*. An anterior dislocation is usually found in external rotation, whereas a posterolateral dislocation will be in slight adduction and internal rotation.

It is quite evident that an isolated event of dislocation is quite traumatic. Moreover, repeated dislocations can lead to even greater complications. It appears that the rate of recurrent dislocations is most dependent on the following factors: late onset of dislocation (>3 months), soft tissue imbalances, a smaller femoral head size, and cup malposition in both anteversion and inclination.[19,20] Yuan and Shih[19] looked at 2728 THA (primary and revision) patients and found that the late dislocators in both groups had a higher rate of recurrent dislocations than the early dislocators. Von Knoch et al.[20] also found this to be true. Soft tissue imbalance, defined by Yuan as a leg length discrepancy or a Trendelenburg's gait, was another factor contributing to a higher rate of recurrent dislocation in patients.[19] Recurrent dislocations may lead to the need for a revision surgery, which has been shown to have a poorer prognosis for the individual than a primary THA. Revision THA surgeries have a higher mortality rate, a higher infection rate, a lower overall satisfaction for the patient, and a higher rate for more recurrent dislocations.[19]

Concerns About Surgical Revision and Aseptic Loosening With Activity

One of the greatest concerns of patients and surgeons postsurgery is the longevity and prognosis of the prosthesis. In 1999, Lim et al.[7] showed that total hip replacements had a 95% to 98% prospect of surviving 10 years. A number of factors affect wear and determine long-term outcomes of the surgery. Aseptic loosening of the prosthesis is one of the major causes of surgical failure. McGrory et al.[21] theorized that repeat load through the joint causes accelerated wearing of prosthetic parts, weakened bone because of an immune reaction to particulate debris from the prosthesis, and increased risk of fracture. They also stated that decreased sensory nerve input, proprioception, and pain cause decreased at-risk monitoring, leading to increased patient participation in potentially risky activities. However, the actual research on whether increased activity causes a higher rate of aseptic loosening is variable and contradictory.

Some studies have shown that a greater longevity of the prostheses is seen with less activity. Those patients who are less active have an increased amount of time before a revision is necessary. Kilgus et al.[22] performed a study comparing two types of hip procedures in a less active versus an active group. They found that revision rates because of aseptic loosening are higher in both active groups compared with the less active groups. The authors also found that in the conventional group, activity level and preoperative diagnosis are related to the amount of time before failure. Those who are less active and for whom osteoarthritis (OA) is the preoperative diagnosis have a decreased failure rate. However, those with OA in the high-activity group are at the greatest risk of revision because of their poor bone quality and poor potential for bone healing and remodeling. Similarly, a few other studies have shown a pattern of increased activity correlating to decreased prosthetic longevity. McGrory et al.[21] showed that for prostheses that lasted less

BOX 20-1	Activity After Total Hip Arthroplasty		
Recommended/Allowed	**Allowed With Experience**	**Not Recommended**	**No Conclusion**
Stationary bicycling	Low-impact aerobics	High-impact aerobics	Jazz dancing
Croquet	Road bicycling	Baseball/softball	Square dancing
Ballroom dancing	Bowling	Basketball	Fencing
Golf	Canoeing	Football	Ice skating
Horseshoes	Hiking	Gymnastics	Roller/inline skating
Shooting	Horseback riding	Handball	Rowing
Shuffleboard	Cross-country skiing	Hockey	Speed walking
Swimming		Jogging	Downhill skiing
Doubles tennis		Lacrosse	Stationary skiing
Walking		Racquetball	Weight lifting
		Squash	Weight machines
		Rock climbing	
		Soccer	
		Singles tennis	
		Volleyball	

From Healy, et al: Hip society survey, Am J Sport Med 29(3):382, 2001.

than 10 years, revision rate is twice as high in more active patients.

Likewise, a correlation also exists between the activity level and age of the patients. Older, more infirm patients and female patients tend to have a decreased revision rate compared with younger patients.[21-23] Perrin found those that developed loosening are younger than 55 years old and walk 50% more preoperatively. Chandler et al.[25] showed that in young patients (younger than 30 years old) nearly two thirds experience loosening, and Dorr et al.[25] showed an increased failure rate of 22% in young patients under 45 years old. This age difference in longevity of the prosthesis is surmised to be the result of the increased activity level of these younger patients.

However, a number of studies contradict the hypothesis that increased activity increases prosthetic wear. Dubs et al.[2] showed an increased revision rate in nonactive patients of 14.3% verses 1.6% in active patients. Another study by Widhalm et al.[26] demonstrates 18% component loosening in patients who participate in sports verses 57% in those who do not.[26] In addition, Ritter et al.[27] demonstrated a positive correlation between surgical outcomes and the amount of activity of the patient and attributed this improved outcome to the increased range of motion presurgery seen in those that were more active. The authors concluded that negative influences on hip replacement did not occur because of intelligent participation in activities such as walking, golfing, bowling, swimming, and biking during the 5.8-year follow-up study.

Although the literature is varied, it seems that younger and more active patients are at higher risk for earlier revision, but that intelligent participation in activities that do not place excess load on the hip joint may in fact be beneficial. In fact, the importance of exercise on joints and bone is also very clear in the literature to promote increased bone density. Some form of exercise is important both for the longevity of patients and their quality of living, as well as the success of any surgery they undergo. Healy et al.[23] published the results of a survey of physicians in the Hip Society about their recommendations for return to sports after THA (Box 20-1).

Muscular Deficits After Total Hip Arthroplasty Surgery

As mentioned earlier, the muscles that surround the hip joint serve a very important purpose in providing stability to the hip joint by approximating the femoral head to the acetabulum. The effect of muscular deficit around the hip after THA surgery is described as jeopardizing the implant fixation interface.[28] The more unstable the hip joint is, the more destructive it can be to the integrity and ultimately the lifespan of the prosthesis.

Studies have shown that an increase in hip strength occurs after THA likely because of the fact that the individual is more active as a result of having decreased pain. However, some debate exists as to how much and how quickly strength is gained. One of the elements that seems to have an influence on the degree to which the patient gains strength postoperatively is whether or not the patient undergoes a supervised progressive-strengthening program. Progressive strengthening and rehabilitation is discussed in more detail in the proceeding sections.

Several studies in which the patients did not attend physical therapy beyond the initial acute-care phase clearly show that these patients do not progress to their full potential. In one study, 56% of postsurgical hips with weakness at 3 months still had a positive Trendelenburg's gait after 12 months. A positive Trendelenburg's gait is generally indicative of hip abductor weakness but in some cases may indicate a loosening of the prosthesis.[28,29] There was no mention of patients receiving postoperative rehabilitation in this article.[29] Shih et al.[9] looked at strength of the hip flexors, extensors, and abductors 6 months and 12 months postoperatively. He found that although strength increased, the operated hip only achieved

80% to 90% of the strength of the nonoperated hip even after 1 year. Similarly, he found that symptoms only decreased to a significant level after 1 year. In addition, 1 year after surgery, the muscle torque of the operated hip still did not equal the muscle torque in the nonoperated hip in either group (men achieved 84% to 89% of healthy hip values, whereas women achieved 79% to 81%). In this study, patients received 1 week of physical therapy after which they were individually responsible for their own care and no longer under any particular guidance from a specialist. Force plates have also been used to measure lower-extremity weakness after THA surgery. In one such study by Long et al.,[28] they showed a difference between operated and nonoperated hips during gait, with the operated side showing a decreased force plate reading, indicating weakness on that side. Again no mention was made of the patients receiving any type of rehabilitation. In addition to evidence of continued hip weakness, Reardon et al.[30] found quadriceps muscle wasting that persisted after a THA. Patients were given predominantly nonweight-bearing exercises (hydrotherapy and exercise bike). The study found there to be significant atrophy and weakness of the quadriceps muscle on the operated side compared with the nonoperated side, which persisted 5 months postoperatively. They surmised that closed chain, weight-bearing exercise might have been more effective at strengthening than the nonweight-bearing exercises their subjects had performed.[30] Weight-bearing exercises are normally performed in an outpatient physical therapy session. Clearly, normal daily activity and exercises taught during inpatient therapy are not sufficient to achieve adequate strength gains.

Furthermore, studies that emphasize an advanced rehabilitation program show positive gains in strength, postural stability, and function. Bertocci et al.[21] shows equal strength in both legs 4 to 5 months postoperatively.[21] However, one difference between Bertocci et al.'s study and Shih et al.'s study[9] (mentioned previously) is that subjects had received acute and subacute rehabilitation followed by an average of 13 sessions of outpatient and home physical therapy, whereas the other studies had minimal physical therapy. This may explain why the nonoperated and operated sides had achieved equal strength at 4 to 5 months, whereas in the other two studies, the operated side remained weaker at 6 months. One point to note about Bertocci et al.'s study is that although the operated leg's strength achieved that of the nonoperated leg, a significant difference still existed between the strength of the THA and non-THA subjects. The THA subjects demonstrated significantly decreased toque, total work, and power in both legs compared with healthy age-matched subjects. The authors emphasize the need for continued rehabilitation even after 4 to 5 months to attain the patient's full potential.[31] More about the specifics of other studies that focus on advanced exercise is discussed in the rehabilitation section of this chapter.

Most of the studies that examine lower-extremity strength after THA look at the bigger muscle groups; however, in some of the surgical procedures, the deeper rotator muscles are also significantly damaged. We came across no research that examines the strength of the rotators after a THA. In Shih et al.'s study,[9] the authors explain that they did not test the hip internal rotator, hip external rotator, or adductor strength, because they consider them less important in the functional evaluation of the hip joint. However, these muscles play an important role in stabilizing the hip and pelvis in the majority of activities ranging from walking, turning, and stair climbing to popular sports such as golf and tennis. Numerous studies have found that the hip external rotators are of great importance to the function of the lower extremity.[32-34] Therefore we believe these locations should not be overlooked.

It is apparent from these studies that the strength of the hip muscles after THA is often not fully regained and that specific strengthening exercises are necessary for the full recovery of the patient.

Functional Deficits

In addition to strength and neuromuscular deficits, it is important to examine the degree to which functional deficits remain after a THA operation. Loizeau et al.[35] examined gait patterns of THA patients on average of 4 years postoperatively and found that their stride length and gait speed are decreased compared with the contralateral leg and with age-matched normals.[35] The THA patients are fairly active and participate in leisure activities such as fishing, golfing, and cross-country skiing, but no mention of any formal exercise training exists.

Sashika et al.[4] examinined THA patients 6 to 48 months postoperatively and found that they lack sufficient strength to achieve their functional goals. Although it is commonly thought that a progressive-ambulation program will bring about sufficient physiologic changes in strength, the author concludes from his results that walking alone is not adequate to strengthen the hip abductors and to prevent disability.

Another study by Trudelle-Jackson et al.[5] uses a twelve-item hip questionnaire to assess physical function in patients between 4 to 12 months postoperatively. They found continued impairments even after 1-year post-THA. They conclude that the traditional exercises that patients receive before they are discharged from rehabilitation are insufficient to achieve full function.

REHABILITATION

Rehabilitation after THA is extremely important to protect the joint and return the patient to their desired level of activity. Dubs et al.[2] described a two-part rehabilitation program, "the first 6 months postoperatively focusing mainly on mobility and strength" using "low-impact activities such as swimming, cycling, and rowing." After this stage, when the muscles are strong, the patient can return to higher-impact sports such as tennis, cross-country skiing, and hiking. In this section, a recommended postoperative exercise program is proposed, with guidelines concerning timing and specific exercises to properly return these patients to recreational activities. Similar to Dubs et al.'s recommendation, the first two phases focus on gaining strength and mobility during the first 6 months. Phase 3 focuses on increasing strength, neuromuscular control, and power to return the patients to their desired recreational activities.

Postoperative Physical Therapy

Specifics of this three-phase program can be found in Table 20-1.

Phase 1: Acute Inpatient

Directly after surgery, physical therapy plays a number of critical roles in both patient education and in gaining sufficient strength and mobility to effectively discharge the patient to his or her home. In fact, Freburger[36] found that increased use of physical therapy during acute-care hospitalization is associated with less than expected cost of care and greater chance of discharge to home. The reader should refer to Table 20-1 for the main goals of physical therapy during this phase.

As mentioned earlier, some differences exist in the type of precaution and length of time to adhere to the precautions based on the surgery type and the doctor's opinion. Youm et al.[37] received surveys from 363 members of American Academy of Hip and Knee Surgeons (AAHKS) listing the type and length of precaution, as well as when the surgeons would

Table 20-1	Goals of Physical Therapy and Exercise Prescription	

Phase	Goals	Exercise Prescription
1	Patient will demonstrate understanding of total hip precautions (refer to physician and type of surgery for specifics). Patient will be independent in home exercise program, with some understanding of proper progression. Patient will be independent in transfers and functional activities for safe discharge home. Patient will be able to safely ambulate appropriate distances (100 feet) and safely negotiate stairs based on the home situation.	Two times a day, 5 days a week Day 1-2: transfer training in the room Bedside exercises (10 repetitions every hour of each of the following exercises): 1. Quadriceps sets 2. Gluteal sets 3. Ankle pumps Day 2: discharge Gait training including steps Activities of daily living (ADL) training following hip precautions Exercises as follows, progressing as tolerated to 20 repetitions three times a day: 1. Same three previously mentioned 2. Active hip flexion (precautions maintained) and active abduction 3. Terminal knee extension 4. Isometric hip abduction (submaximally)
2	Patient will have minimal pain and edema. Patient will maintain hip precautions for 6-8 weeks (or as per physician) to allow for healing. Patient will regain lower-extremity range of motion and strength. Patient will demonstrate full weight bearing, with a normal and reciprocal gait pattern without an assistive device. Patient will be able to ascend and descend steps reciprocally. Patient will demonstrate fair balance and proprioception to decrease risk of falls.	Resistance and endurance muscular strength training: 60% to 80% of the maximum effort of the muscle Phase 1: 8-12 repetitions of weight that can be lifted eight times; last few reps should be difficult Phase 2: progress in repetitions/sets until 15 reps of three sets are reached Phase 3: after reaching 15 reps of three sets, drop back to 8-10 reps of 3 sets (add weight)

Exercises	Rationale
Exercise bike 15-30 minutes	Warm-up Increasing mobility and aerobic capacity
Prone hip internal/ external rotation (see Figure 20-5) A)	Hip rotation mobility, control, and strength
Standing hip flexion using pulley or band	Hip flexion strength is one of last muscle groups to return to full strength
Straight-leg raises 8 weeks postoperatively and once patient demonstrates 80% strength with previously mentioned exercise	As previously mentioned
Standing three-way hip with the pulley on operated leg until at least 8 weeks postoperatively, then with both legs (see Figure 20-5, B)	Stability during weight bearing, hip abduction, and extension strength
Prone hip extension with knee flexed (see Figure 20-5, C)	Hip extension mobility and strength
Hamstring curls	Hamstring strength

Continued

Table 20-1	Goals of Physical Therapy and Exercise Prescription—cont'd

Phase	Goals	Exercise Prescription	
		Knee extension	Quadriceps strength
		Leg press	Gross hip mobility and strength
		Calf raises	Calf strength for normalized gait
		Partial squat and lunge progressing deeper after 8 weeks	Gross hip mobility, strength, and neuromuscular control
		Step ups (4 inches progressing to 8 inches)	Gain reciprocal pattern on stairs
		Step downs (4 inches progressing to 8 inches)	Eccentric quadriceps strength with good hip control and biomechanical alignment
		Bridges (see Figure 20-5, *D*)	Hip and core strength and control
		Curl-up with one leg extended (see Figure 20-5, *E*)	Trunk stability
		Balance with narrow bilateral stance progressing to single-leg stance, with eyes closed (control level pelvis)	Beginning proprioception/balance
3	Patient will have full strength, endurance, and functional mobility.	Strength	
	Patient will be able to return to all desired and reasonable functional and recreational activities.	Squats/leg press	
		Hip external rotation (see Figure 20-6, *A*)	
		Hip extension	
	Patient will demonstrate good core and pelvic control during all functional and recreational activities.	Hip abduction (see Figure 20-6, *B*)	
		Knee extension	
		Standing pelvic drop (see Figure 20-6, *C*)	
	Patient will be able to demonstrate good, age-appropriate balance.	Week 1-3: three sets of 15 reps at 15 repetition maximum (RM)	
		Week 4-6: three sets of 10 reps at 10 RM	
	Patient has a good understanding of how to maintain and/or achieve the desired level of strength through a home exercise/gym routine.	Week 7-9: three sets of 8 reps at 8 RM	
		Core endurance training (see Figure 20-7, *A-C*)	
		(These exercises promote good trunk stability and control. Because of the stabilizing nature of these muscles, endurance is key.	
		Hold the exercises as long as possible with good form: three sets with rest in between. Then increase the time held each day to promote increased endurance.)	
		Balance and proprioception training (see Figure 20-7, *A-C*)	
		(Following are some options for exercises to promote coactivation of the lower-extremity muscles along with trunk stabilization. The unstable surfaces help train the mechanoreceptors to detect joint position and prepare the body to be active on unstable and variable surfaces. Perform each exercise for 1 minute or as long as good form is maintained. Increase the amount of time as the patient gets stronger.)	

allow return to certain activities. The five most common precautions or devices are a high toilet seat, restricted hip flexion during ADL, a reacher-grabber, an abduction pillow, and a high chair. The median length of use for all precautions and devices is 6 weeks, except for hip flexion, which is 8 weeks. Generally, if the patient has a cemented THA, then he or she is full weight–bearing 2 weeks earlier than an uncemented THA. However, one study found that no difference in function exists between immediate and late weight bearing using an uncemented THA prosthesis.[38]

Enloe et al.[39] used a panel of professionals to gain a consensus of the most common and beneficial exercise prescription for physical therapy for acute THA (this prescription is listed in Table 20-1). These authors found that many physical therapists avoid the straight-leg raise postoperatively, possibly because of the study by Rydell[6] using in vivo stain gauge measurements in which they found the straight-leg raise generates one to two times greater force than walking. Conversely, in an in vivo study by Krebs et al.,[40] the authors found that the straight-leg raise exercise has among the lowest peak hip pressures recorded (less than half of free-speed gait and only 10% more than the supine slide board abduction exercise). The authors question whether it is actually necessary to restrict straight-leg raise after THA. Additionally, they found that isometric hip abduction has the highest pressure recorded for all of the tested exercises. Thus one should cautiously decide when and if to add these exercises.

The authors of this chapter chose to include isometric abduction as per the consensus from Enloe et al.[39] but recommend performing it submaximally, as per the recommendations of Sashika et al.[4] Straight-leg raises are not be added until phase 2, along with gravity-resisted abduction, which also has higher pressures and is not recommended for acute postoperative patients with cementless hip prostheses.[41]

Phase 2: Outpatient Strength and Mobility Gaining

Not a great deal of literature discusses an appropriate THA program after the initial acute phases of rehabilitation. Brander and Stulberg propose some guidelines for physical therapy pre- and post-THA but qualify it by saying that, "there are no clear, prospective, randomized trials determining the most effective protocols."[3] They recommend rotational exercises and maximal hip internal and external rotation range of motion to successfully return to sports such as golf. In addition, the authors recommend that physical therapy that continues "well beyond the early (first 12-week) recovery period." They go on to say "postoperative rehabilitation protocols should be modified to include longer-term focus on strength and function. Patient-specific goals should be considered when prescribing exercise and other therapeutic interventions after hip arthroplasty." The importance of regaining hip strength, particularly in the gluteus medius, gluteus maximus, and the external rotators is evident after a THA. As the literature has shown, frequently these muscles are not strengthened to their preoperative capacity. Not only is it important for the nonathletic patient to regain full hip strength but also mandatory for the patient to strengthen the muscles around the joint before they return to sports to prevent component loosening during the higher level of activity. Specific patient goals during this phase are discussed in Table 20-1.

Trudelle-Jackson et al.[5] discuss the need for physical therapy at 4 or more months postoperatively to emphasize weight bearing and postural stability. They found that isometric and active range of motion (AROM) exercises are not enough to provide the proper strength for full functional return, which is dangerous because component loosening can occur at a higher rate if weakness exists in the lower extremity.[5] A correlation exists between the patient's own functional assessment and hip abduction and knee extension strength.[42] Similarly, Sashika et al.[4] found that THA patients show mild to moderate disability 6 to 48 months postoperatively. He found that walking alone does not strengthen the hips enough. Instead, patients need a formalized strengthening program to gain return of full function.

As for looking at which specific muscles do not return to full strength, Rossi et al.[43] found that presurgery hip extensor strength is decreased by 39% and hip flexor by 29%. After surgery, strength improves in hip extension by 50% and flexion by 27%. By 60 days after surgery, hip extension strength increases by 133% but is still only 61% of the uninvolved side. Likewise, hip flexor strength increases by 127% but is 71% of uninvolved side. Clearly, the largest strength gains happen initially, but strength is still not full by 60 days after surgery; therefore more therapy would be beneficial.

Patients with a diagnosis of OA who had therapy 8 weeks pre- and at least 12 weeks postoperatively show increased functional scores at 1 week presurgery, which continued postsurgically. The exercise protocol they used consisted of one to three sets of 10 isotonic exercises, plus hydrotherapy for 30 minutes.[44]

Bolgla and Uhl[41] performed EMG analyses of six different hip abduction strengthening exercises. They found that the least amount of hip abductor activity occurs with nonweight-bearing standing hip abduction and standing hip abduction with flexion. Weight-bearing exercises with contralateral hip abduction have the same amount of EMG activity as side-lying hip abduction. The most abductor activity is found with pelvic drop on contralateral side with weight bearing. Their recommendation is to begin with nonweight-bearing exercises before progressing to weight-bearing exercises or side-lying hip abduction. They only recommend the pelvic drop exercises for more advanced rehabilitation.

It is also reasonable to assume that proprioception is compromised postsurgery because of damages of the soft tissue and capsular structures that contain the mechanoreceptors. Some studies have shown that postural stability is decreased on the THA side compared with the nonoperated side. Thus it would seem to be important to focus on proprioception and neuromuscular and balance training in addition to strengthening.[42] Several studies have examined joint position sense after THA and have found there to be no significant differences between THA and non-THA subjects.[45-47] Joint position sense remains intact after THA. However, it seems that postural stability is affected. This supports the value of neuromuscular and balance training to maximize stability. This stability is particularly valuable while walking on an unstable surface, as is needed in the return to many recreational activities.

We took all of these considerations and used similar guidelines in the design of the strengthening exercise program in Table 20-1 (Figure 20-5).

Advanced Physical Therapy

Phase 3: Return to Full Function and Recreation

Once patients demonstrate the proper neuromuscular coordination and strength base, through the ability to perform high-repetition, low-weight exercises in phases 1 and 2, they are able to progress to a more aggressive strengthening program. This program emphasizes postural stability and control in weight-bearing exercises and targets specific muscle weakness for patients to achieve their functional and recreational goals. This program has three components: (1) strength, (2) endurance, and (3) postural stability and neuromuscular control.

Researchers have shown that the most successful way to gain strength and lean mass is through a periodized strength-training program for at least 8 weeks.[48] "Periodized strength training refers to varying the training program at regular time intervals in an attempt to bring about optimal gains in strength, power, motor performance, and/or muscle hypertrophy."[48] However, most of these studies were done on younger, male, trained athletes. The American College of Sports Medicine recommends against the high-weight, low-repetition exercises used in these studies for people over the age of 50 because of increased risk of orthopaedic injury.[49] Although the majority of THA patients are over 50 years old, the authors of this chapter recommend the use of periodized strength-training principle of manipulating training variables; however, low-to-moderate level of repetitions should be used.

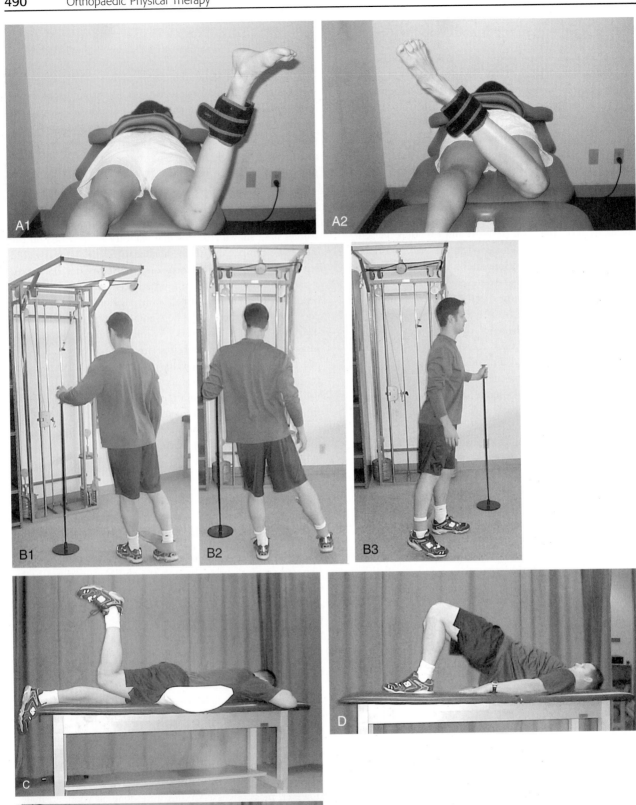

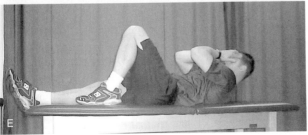

Figure 20-5 A, Prone hip internal and external rotation stretch. **B,** Standing three-way hip. **C,** Prone hip extension. **D,** Bridges. **E,** Curl-up with leg extended. (**B-E** from Donatelli R: Sports-specific rehabilitation, St Louis, 2007, Churchill Livingstone.)

An important area of discussion is the eccentric strength of trained muscles. Sashika et al.[4] showed significant strength gains in patients 6 to 48 months after THA using a 6-week training program emphasizing eccentric hip abductor control.[4] Eccentric strength is especially necessary because of the need for hip and pelvic control. Bechler et al.'s study[50] using EMG testing of the hip muscles during the golf swing emphasizes the importance of adequate strength in these muscles not only for producing power but also for controlling aberrant motion and stabilizing the hip for improved accuracy during the swing. Therefore to properly train these muscles, especially for the demands of golf and other recreational activities, eccentric and balance training are important components of the training program. To accomplish this training, the eccentric, lengthening, component of each strengthening exercise should be emphasized; it should take at least twice as long as the concentric, shortening component.

It is necessary to train the endurance and control of the hip muscles, as well as the core and trunk muscles, particularly for good postural control in all activities (particularly recreational activities).[51] Thompson[52] reported that golfers participating an 8-week core stabilization program showed significant improvement in maximum swing speed, as well as in general fitness. Many of the core training guidelines we use are those proposed by McGill et al.[53] for increasing activation of the key core muscles for lumbar stability, as well as postural stability exercises shown via an EMG study demonstrating the efficacy of the side bridge position for training both external oblique abdominal and gluteus medius muscles.[54] Although no studies have shown the amount of force this will place on the hip joint, we believe that the stresses will be similar to those of isometric hip abduction and weight-bearing hip exercises (appropriate at this time). However, is it important to monitor the position of the patient and provide appropriate modification and progression.

Finally, as mentioned previously, it is important to continue training postural stability and neuromuscular control. This aspect of the training is further progressed by performing many of the exercises on unsteady surfaces (e.g., bosu ball, foam pad, shuttle balance).

In the phase 3 section of Table 20-1, the training guidelines for a 9-week periodized strength-training program are provided. Examples of periodized strength-training exercises appear in Figure 20-6, followed by the endurance and core exercises in Figure 20-7. Figure 20-8 provides suggestions for advanced proprioception and balance training.

Maintaining Strength: Weight Lifting One Time per Week

The maintenance phase includes using similar exercises to those in phase 3, but patients only need to lift weights once a week. Patients should find a weight that they can lift eight times (the last few repetitions should be difficult). Patients should perform two sets of eight repetitions of each exercise once a week and continue with aerobic and recreational exercise as well.

Current Recommendations and Studies Concerning Golf and Tennis

Because returning to recreational activity is a large reason why many patients elect to have the surgery, it is not surprising that an increase is seen in overall activity level after total hip replacement.[55,56] However, a decrease is seen in the specific types of activities in which patients are involved, including golf.[55] This may be in part because of the uncertainty regarding recommendations concerning returning to these specific sports. Because of the variable conclusions of the general effects of activity on a total hip replacement, the authors of this chapter thought it would be important to look at specific studies directed toward the popular recreational sports of golf and tennis.

Mallon et al.[57,58] conducted notable studies concerning returning to golf after a total hip replacement. The authors distributed a hip survey to 47 surgeons, as well as to 187 amateur and six professional golfers. Of these golfers, two professionals and 20 amateurs had bilateral total hip replacements. The following interesting results were gathered from the surgeons: 95.7% of surgeons do not discourage playing golf after a THA, and only 21% feel it increases postsurgery complications. In addition, 68.3% would not discourage golf after hip revision, but 17.1% would. Many do not make specific recommendations concerning returning to golf, although 11.4% recommend changes in the stroke after a THA to a shorter and gentler swing. The average time before patients return to golf is 19.5 weeks, with a range of 12 to 52 weeks. The golfers report satisfaction with the results of the surgery, with improved performance and decreased pain. In general, their handicaps had increased by 1.1 strokes, but the drive length also increased by 3.3 yards. Eighty-seven percent reported no pain while playing and only a mild ache after playing.

Another good study of players returning to golf is a German study by Liem et al.[59] in which the authors studied golfers (mean age, 66.2 years) with bilateral THA.[59] Most returned to their preoperative golf level, playing about two to three times a week. Similar to Mallon et al.'s results,[57,58] the majority, 51.6%, returned to golf after about 3 months and 95.2% by 6 months, which most of them felt was the right amount of time. Even three patients who had revisions because of infection returned to golf about 4.5 months postrevision. However, interestingly, female subjects took longer to return to golf, about 4.5 months, verses male subjects, 3.5 months. One third of them thought they could have returned sooner but were following their doctors' advice. This may be an indication that doctors are more cautious with their female patients. When the golfers were asked about their pain level, 80.4% of patients reported being pain free; the others had pain during the swing (8.7%) or with walking (10.9%). In addition, 47.8% enjoyed golf more postsurgery, 50.0% enjoyed it the same, and 2.2% enjoyed it less. No difference was seen for outcomes based on the side of THA or whether it was bilateral verses unilateral. Liem et al.'s results[59] are different from Mallon et al's results[57,58] in one category, handicap score. These authors found that

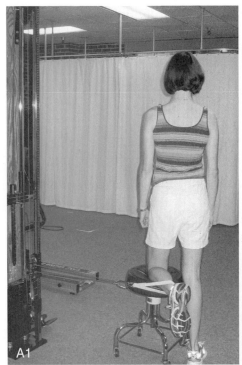

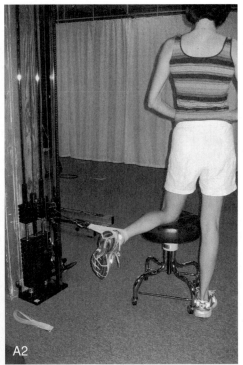

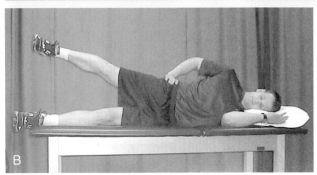

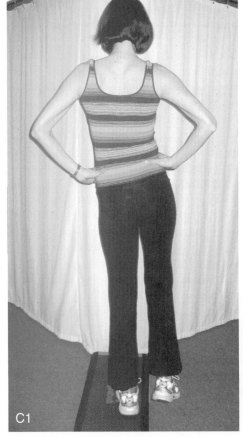

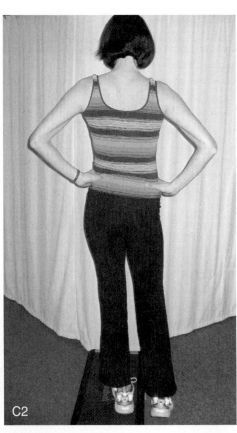

Figure 20-6 A, Resisted hip external rotation—two exercises. **B,** Hip abduction. **C,** Standing pelvic drop off of a step—eccentrically biased. (**A** and **B** from Donatelli R: Sports-specific rehabilitation, St Louis, 2007, Churchill Livingstone.)

golfers improved both their handicap (27.3 to 24.5), as well as their driving distance (169.8 to 176.6). This improvement was mainly seen in male subjects and did not reach a significant difference in female subjects. This difference was attributed to different medical systems. In Germany, all patients participate in physical therapy for 2 to 3 weeks in the hospital, which the authors felt led to their improvement in both handicap and driving distance. They found that the average rehabilitation was 19.2 days after release from hospital; those with no physical therapy were significantly less likely to increase their driving distance. The other difference between subjects in Germany and the United States that may have led to the various results is that, in Germany, golfers rarely use carts.

There have been a couple of recent, very good studies concerning returning to tennis after a THA. Seyler et al.[1] surveyed United States Tennis Association (USTA) members. They found that those who have had a THA return to compete between 1 and 12 months after surgery and feel like they have

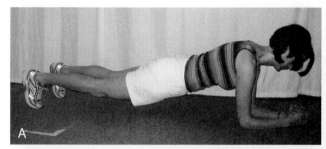

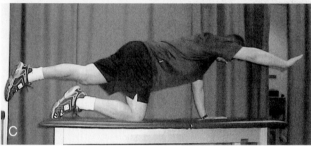

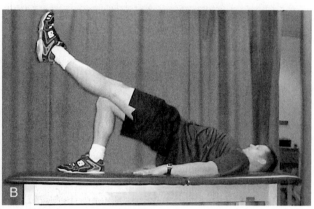

Figure 20-7 A, Side-bridge and plank. Begin on the knees, then progress to full leg extension. For advanced phases, rotate between the side-bridge and plank exercises, keeping the core and hips straight and in one line. **B,** Single-leg bridge. **C,** Quadruped with alternate arm and leg extension. (**A1** and **B** from Donatelli R: Sports-specific rehabilitation, St Louis, 2007, Churchill Livingstone.)

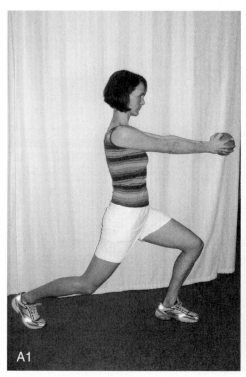

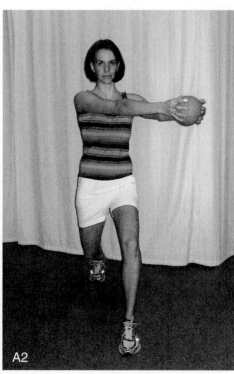

Figure 20-8 A, Trunk rotation with lunges.

Continued

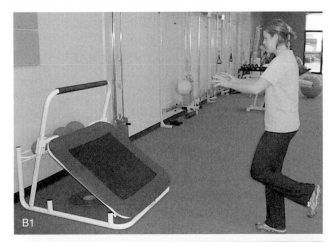

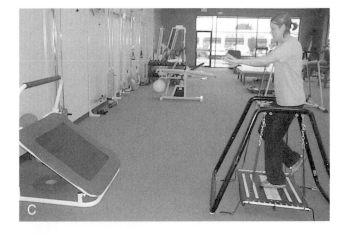

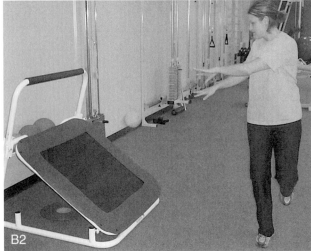

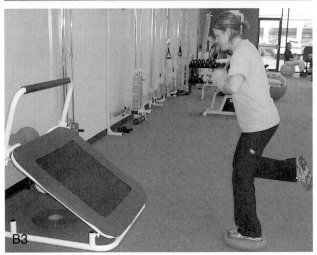

Figure 20-8, cont'd B, Single-leg balance medicine ball toss and variations. **C,** Single-leg balance on the shuttle balance with variations. (**B** and **C** from Donatelli R: Sports-specific rehabilitation, St Louis, 2007, Churchill Livingstone.)

near full return, which lasts for around 8 years after the surgery. Even though 1 year after THA 31% complain of stiffness during playing, they feel, overall, that many components of their game have improved. Mont et al.[60] sent a questionnaire to 50 men and eight women of the USTA after THA an average of 8 years postsurgery and found similar results: 100% of patients stated they had severe pain and stiffness before surgery, 31% 1 year after surgery, and 16% at the time of the survey (8 years later). In addition, a corresponding decrease was seen

in the use of nonsteroidal anti-inflammatory drugs (NSAIDs) of 90% to 26%. The authors found that only 14% of surgeons approve of this high-impact activity, 34% recommend only doubles tennis, and 52% are opposed to tennis altogether. When asked about their reasons for having the surgery, 21% of patients stated they had the operation specifically to return to playing tennis, 36% wanted to play and have decreased pain, and 43% wanted to play and have better motion. As those numbers show, returning to sports and activity is a large factor in patients making the decision to have the operation and should be considered during rehabilitation. Although the mobility of patients and their level of comfort are better after surgery, ball speed is significantly decreased and may be an indication of the need for further strengthening and rehabilitation.

The results of both the golf and tennis studies show that it is very reasonable to resume playing these activities after THA. Most patients showed increased satisfaction, improved pain levels, and even some positive changes in their game. However, individual differences exist, and possibly, as Liem et al.[59] suggested, some gender differences that may define the amount of

time it takes before it is safe to return to full participation in these sports. Yun summarizes it well: "Muscle mass, coordination, balance, and reflexes need to be developed before you play, and postoperative return may depend on preoperative proficiency."[61] It is important to work closely with medical professionals on the surgery and rehabilitation team who are able to assess when a patient is well healed and strong enough to begin returning to these sports, as well as to provide guidance as the patient progresses to full participation. Box 20-2 contains recommended suggestions for modifications one should consider when golfing.[58]

BOX 20-2 Specific Golf Recommendations

Many authors had specific recommendations based on their research, which we thought were valuable to include. As previously mentioned, Neumann[10] recommended that a load (e.g., golf bag) be carried on the ipsilateral side with a cane (or perhaps a golf club) on the contralateral side to decreased the stresses at the hip joint. In the case of someone at high risk of prosthesis loosening, he discouraged carrying a load altogether. Clifford[62] recommended that a golfer should practice chipping and putting first, before playing a full round of golf. Yun[61] recommended that patients returning to golf work with a professional and ride a cart for 6 months.

Mallon et al.'s recommendations[57,58] for golfers are as follows:
- Avoid playing golf in wet weather. Slipping and falling during a golf swing could be disastrous.
- The golfer may be able to play better without golf spikes. If the feet are not quite as stationary, then they can turn a bit during

the swing and take the stress off the knee and hip. The golfer must be cautious, however, that the chance of slipping and falling without spikes is slightly increased.
- Any golfer with a total joint replacement should learn to play more on the toes. Swinging flat-footed transfers torsional stress loads to the joint replacement. On the backswing, the left heel should be elevated. On the downswing, the right heel should come up off the ground.
- The golfer with a total hip arthroplasty (THA) should learn to play with a greater hip turn. The hip turn is primarily accomplished by the lower-back and trunk musculature. By rotating the trunk, muscles about the hip are stretched less, reducing the stresses at the hip. This must be accompanied by playing on the toes, or the stress of the trunk (hip) rotation will be transmitted to the hip or knee.

CASE STUDY

An 84-year-old male golfer was referred to physical therapy with a diagnosis of left abductor tendonitis. He had had THA revision surgery to his left hip 8 years ago after his initial THA had dislocated three times. Events that led to dislocation are as follows:
1. Bending forward to pick up a piece of paper from the ground near the end of the initial 6 to 7 weeks
2. Rising to get up from the toilet
3. Bending to put clothes onto clothing hook in his car

The patient reports wearing a brace for 3 months between each episode of dislocation. The revision was performed 11 months after the initial THA. The patient also had a right THA 10 years ago and a right total knee arthroplasty 3 years ago. Comorbidities included a history of heart disease and a heart attack, a pacemaker and stent placement, and a history of skin cancer.

The current symptoms had begun roughly 2 to 3 months prior and were most aggravated by activities such as sit to stand, initial ambulation on standing, ascending stairs, and walking distances longer than a block. The patient reported

that the pain level would increase to 8 out of 10 after walking 1 block and said he would try to ease the pain by bending forward. The patient pointed out that this still did not ease the pain completely. He took Tylenol to control his symptoms. The patient's goal was to return to golf without pain.

Recent radiographs show well-fixated acetabular and femoral components with no evidence of osteolysis, loosening, or infection.

Evaluation revealed a positive Trendelenburg's gait (left), with report of increased pain in the left hip when carrying a weight on the right side. Range of motion was roughly equal on both sides except for external rotation on the left, which was limited to 15 degrees versus 40 degrees on the right. Hip flexion was also slightly decreased on the left to 100 degrees versus 108 degrees on the right.

Strength measurements revealed significant weakness in the external rotators (3+/5 on the left, 4/ on the right), hip abduction was also weak (4− on the left, 4 on the right). Hip flexor, hip adductor, hip internal rotation, knee

Continued

CASE STUDY—cont'd

extension, and knee flexion strength were good. Hip extensor strength (tested later) was found to be weak (4−). Palpation revealed no tenderness at the lateral hip and greater trochanter area. However, there was increased hypertonicity in the gluteals and TFL muscles. Berg balance test: 54/56. Turning to look behind his back was the main difficulty in the test.

The patient was seen seven times during which he received strengthening exercises for his hip and trunk, range of motion exercises, gait-training exercises with emphasis on pelvic positioning, balance exercises, and manual treatment to address soft tissue and capsular restrictions. Therapeutic exercises included clamshells, hip hikes, standing hip abduction with Thera-Band along with side-lying hip abduction with weights, prone hip extensions, bridges, plank from knees, prone hip external and internal rotation with manual resistance and ankle weights, trunk rotations with pulleys in standing, hip rotations with pulleys, and balance exercises in single-leg stance.

During the course of treatment, the patient reported increased distances of ambulation before the onset of pain. He reported improved ease with climbing inclines and even reported that he was able to hit the golfball further than he had in 10 years (200 yards versus his usual 175 to 180 yards). His active range of motion for external rotation in the left hip increased to 30 degrees and his external rotation strength and abduction strength showed improvement. He was compliant with his home exercise program.

The patient was referred back to the physician after the seventh visit because of reports of exercise-induced angina. On follow-up, it turned out that patient had an occluded stent and had to undergo an angioplasty. Physical therapy was discontinued at that time for necessary recovery.

When he was contacted 1 month later, the patient said that he was recovering well from his surgery and that he planned to continue with his exercises independently. He was contacted 5 months later and said that he had undergone eye surgery and had discontinued golfing and exercising. Unfortunately, the authors were unable to accurately assess the long-term benefits of the exercise program because of the fact that patient had not been consistent with his exercise program. However, based on the benefits seen in the amount of time he was compliant, it appears that the selected exercises and activities were very beneficial both functionally and recreationally.

REFERENCES

1. Seyler TM, Mont MA, Ragland PS, et al: Sports activity after total hip and knee arthroplasty, Sports Med 36(7):571-583, 2006.
2. Dubs L, Gschwend N, Munzinger U: Sport after total hip arthroplasty, Arch Orthop Trauma Surg 101(3):161-169, 1983.
3. Brander V, Stulberg SD: Rehabilitation after hip- and knee-joint replacement: an experience- and evidence-based approach to care, Am J Phys Med Rehabil 85(suppl 11):S98-S118, 2006.
4. Sashika H, Yoshiko M, Watanabe Y: Home program of physical therapy: effect on disabilities of patients with total hip arthroplasty, Arch Phys Med Rehabil 77:273-277, 1996.
5. Trudelle-Jackson E, Emerson R, Smith S: Effects of a late-phase exercise program after a total hip arthroplasty, Arch Phys Med Rehabil 58:1056-1062, 2004.
6. Rydell NW: Forces acting on the femoral-head prosthesis: a study on strain gauge supplied prosthesis in living persons, Acta Orthop Scand 37(suppl 88):1-132, 1966.
7. Lim L, Carmichael SW, Cabanela ME: Biomechanics of total hip arthroplasty, Anat Rec B New Anat 257:110-116, 1999.
8. Kotzar GM, et al: Torsional loads in the early postoperative period following total hip replacement, J Orthop Res 13:945-955, 1995.
9. Shih CH, Du YK, Lin YH, et al: Muscular recovery around the hip joint after total hip arthroplasty, Clin Orthop Relat Res 302:115-120, 1994.
10. Neumann DA: An electromyographic study of the hip abductor muscles as subjects with a hip prosthesis walked with different methods of using a cane and carrying a load, Phys Ther 79(12):1163-1173, 1999.
11. Masonis JL, Bourne RB: Surgical approach, abductor function, and total hip arthroplasty dislocation, Clin Orthop Relat Res 406:46-53, 2002.
12. Pellicci PM, Bostrom M, Poss R: Posterior approach to total hip replacement using enhanced posterior soft tissue repair, Clin Orthop Relat Res 355:224-228, 1998.
13. Su EP, Mahoney CR, Adler RS, et al: Integrity of repaired posterior structures after THA, Clin Orthop Relat Res 447:43-47, 2006.
14. Crowninshield R, Maloney WJ, Wentz DH, et al: Biomechanics of large femoral heads: what they do and don't do, Clin Orthop Relat Res 429:102-107, 2004.
15. Komistek RD, Dennis DA, Ochoa JA, et al: In vivo comparison of hip separation after metal-on-metal or metal-on-polyethylene total hip arthroplasty, J Bone Joint Surg Am 84:1836-1841, 2002.
16. Peak EL, Parvizi J, Ciminiello M, et al: The role of patient restrictions in reducing the prevalence of early dislocation following total hip arthroplasty: a randomized, prospective study, J Bone Joint Surg 87-A(2):247-253, 2005.

17. Meek RM, Allan DB, McPhillips G, et al: Epidemiology of dislocation after total hip arthroplasty, Clin Orthop Relat Res 447:9-18, 2006.

18. Berry D: Effect of femoral head diameter and operative approach on risk of dislocation after primary total hip arthroplasty, J Bone Joint Surg Am 87:2456-2463, 2005.

19. Yuan LJ, Shih CH: Dislocation after total hip arthroplasty, Arch Orthop Trauma Surg 119:263-266, 1999.

20. von Knoch M, Berry DJ, Harmsen WS, et al: Late dislocation after total hip arthroplasty, J Bone Joint Surg 84-A(11):1949-1953, 2002.

21. McGrory BJ, Stuart MJ, Sim FH: Participation in sports after hip and knee arthroplasty, J Bone Joint Surg 70(4):342-348, 1995.

22. Kilgus DJ, Dorey FJ, Finerman GA, et al: Patient activity, sports participation, and impact loading on the durability of cemented total hip replacements, Clin Orthop Relat Res 269:25-31, 1991.

23. Healy WL, Iorio R, Lemos MJ: Athletic activity after joint replacement, Am J Sports Med 29(3):377-388, 2001.

24. Chandler HP, Reineck FT, Wixson RL, et al: Total hip replacement in patients younger than thirty years old: a five-year follow-up study, J Bone Joint Surg Am 63(9):1426-1434, 1981.

25. Dorr LD, Takei GK, Conaty JP: Total hip arthroplasties in patients less than forty-five years old, J Bone Joint Surg Am 65:474-479, 1983.

26. Widhalm R, Höfer G, Kruluger J, et al: Is there greater danger of sports injury or osteoporosis caused by inactivity in patients with hip prosthesis? Sequelae for long-term stability of prosthesis anchorage, Z Orthop Ihre Grenzgeb 128(2):139-143, 1990.

27. Ritter MA, Meding JB: Total hip arthroplasty: can the patient play sports again? Orthopedics 10(10):1447-1452, 1987.

28. Long WT, Dorr LD, Healy B, et al: Functional recovery of noncemented total hip arthroplasty, Clin Orthop Relat Res 288:73-77, 1992.

29. Baker AS, Bitounis VC: Abductor function after total hip replacement: an electromyographic and clinical review, J Bone Joint Surg 71(1):47-50, 1989.

30. Reardon K, Galea M, Dennett X, et al: Quadriceps muscle wasting persists 5 months after total hip arthroplasty for osteoarthritis of the hip: a pilot study, Intern Med J 31:7-14, 2001.

31. Bertocci GE, Munin MC, Frost KL, et al: Isokinetic performance after total hip replacement, Am J of Phys Med Rehabil 83:1-9, 2004.

32. Leetun DT, Ireland ML, Willson JD, et al: Core stability measures as risk factors for lower extremity injury in athletes, Med Sci Sports Exerc 36(6):926-934, 2004.

33. Zhang LQ, Nuber GW, Bowen MK, et al: Multiaxis muscle strength in ACL deficient and reconstructed knees: compensatory mechanism, Med Sci Sports Exerc 34(1):2-8, 2002.

34. Nadler SF, Malanga GA, DePrince M, et al: The relationship between lower extremity injury, low back pain, and

35. Loizeau J, Allard P, Duhaime M, et al: Bilateral gait patterns in subjects fitted with a total hip prosthesis, Arch Phys Med Rehabil 76:552-557, 1995.

36. Freburger J: An analysis of the relationship between the utilization of physical therapy services and outcomes of care for patients after total hip arthroplasty, Phys Ther 80(5):448-458, 2000.

37. Youm T, Maurer SG, Stuchin SA: Postoperative management after total hip and knee arthroplasty, J Arthroplasty 20(3):322-324, 2005.

38. Andersson L, Wesslau A, Bodén H, et al: Immediate or late weight bearing after uncemented total hip arthroplasty: a study of functional recovery, J Arthroplasty 16(8):1063-1065, 2001.

39. Enloe LJ, Shields RK, Smith K, et al: Total hip and knee replacement treatment programs: a report using consensus, J Orthop Sports Phys Ther 23(1):3-11, 1996.

40. Krebs DE, Elbaum L, Riley PO, et al: Exercise and gait effects on in vivo hip contact pressures, Phys Ther 71(4):301-309, 1991.

41. Bolgla LA, Uhl TL: Electromyographic analysis of hip rehabilitation exercises in a group of healthy subjects, J Orthop Sports Phys Ther 35(8):487-494, 2005.

42. Trudelle-Jackson E, Emerson R, Smith S: Outcomes of total hip arthroplasty: a study of patients one year post-surgery, J Orthop Sports Phys Ther 32(6):260-267, 2002.

43. Rossi MD, Brown LE, Whitehurst MA: Assessment of hip extensor and flexor strength two months after unilateral total hip arthroplasty, J Strength Cond Res 20(6):262-267, 2006.

44. Gilbey HJ, Ackland TR, Wang AW, et al: Exercise improves early functional recovery after total hip arthroplasty, Clin Orthop Relat Res 408:193-200, 2003.

45. Grigg P, Finerman GA, Riley LH: Joint position sense after total hip replacement, J Bone Joint Surg Am 55:1016-1025, 1973.

46. Karanjia PN, Ferguson JH: Passive joint position sense after total hip replacement surgery, Ann Neurol 13:654-657, 1983.

47. Stender BL, Drowatzky JN: Joint position sense in subjects with total hip replacements: the possible role of muscle afferents, Clin Kinesiol 48:10-24, 1994.

48. Fleck S: Periodized strength training: a critical review, J Strength Cond 13(1):82-89, 1999.

49. American College of Sports Medicine position stand: the recommended quantity and quality of exercise for developing and maintaining cardiorespiratory and muscular fitness, and flexibility in healthy adults, Med Sci Sports Exerc 30:975-991, 1998.

50. Bechler JR, Jobe FW, Pink M, et al: Electromyographic analysis of the hip and knee during the golf swing, Clin J Sport Med 5:162-166, 1995.

51. Watkins RG, Uppal GS, Perry J, et al: Dynamic electromyographic analysis of trunk musculature in professional golfers, Am J Sports Med 24(4):535-538, 1996.

hip muscle strength in male and female collegiate athletes, Clin J Sports Med 10(2):89-97, 2000.

52. Thompson C: Effect of core stabilization training on fitness, swing speed, and weight transfer in older male golfers, Med Sci Sports Exerc 36(suppl 5):2-4, 2004.

53. McGill SM, Childs A, Liebenson C: Endurance times for low back stabilization exercises: clinical targets for testing and training from a normal database, Arch Phys Med Rehab 80:941-944, 1999.

54. Ekstrom R, Donatelli R, Carp KC: Electromyographic analysis of core trunk, hip, and thigh muscles during commonly used rehabilitation exercises, Unpublished article.

55. Chatterji UF, Ashworth MJ, Lewis PL, et al: Effect of total hip arthroplasty on recreational and sporting activity, ANZ J Surgery 74(6):446-449, 2004.

56. Visuri T, Honkanen R: Total hip replacement: its influences on spontaneous recreation exercise habits, Arch Phys Med Rehabil 61(7):325-328, 1990.

57. Mallon WJ, Callaghan JJ: Total hip arthroplasty in active golfers, J Arthroplasty 7(suppl):339-346, 1992.

58. Mallon WJ, Liebelt RA, Mason JB: Total joint replacement and golf, Clin Sports Med 15(1):179-190, 1996.

59. Liem D, van Kabeck K, Poetzl W, et al: Golf after total hip arthroplasty: retrospective review of 46 patients, J Sports Rehabil 15:206-215, 2006.

60. Mont MA, LaPorte DM, Mullick T, et al: Tennis after total hip arthroplasty, Am J Sports Med 27(1):60-64, 1999.

61. Yun AG: Sports after total hip replacement, Clin Sports Med 25(2):359-364, 2006.

62. Clifford PE, Mallon WJ: Sports after total joint replacement, Clin Sports Med 24(1):175-186, 2005.

21

Robert M. Poole
and Turner A. Blackburn Jr.

Dysfunction, Evaluation, and Treatment of the Knee

ANATOMY OF THE KNEE

The foundation for understanding the knee joint is comprehension of its anatomy. Although individual variations may occur, the functional components of knee anatomy remain unchanged.

Structural Foundation

The knee joint lies between the femur and the tibia, two of the largest and strongest levers in the human body. It is exposed to severe angular and torsion stresses, especially in athletes. The knee is basically a ligament-controlled joint, reinforced by the quadriceps, hamstring, and gastrocnemius muscle groups. These structures provide the main stabilizing influences for the knee joint.[1-3]

The distal end of the femur has an expanded medial and lateral condyle. The proximal end of the tibia is flared to create a plateau with medial and lateral sections to accommodate the medial and lateral femoral condyles (Figure 21-1). The tibial spine divides these sections. Located in the medial and lateral sections are the menisci, which deepen the contour sections to ensure proper contact with the corresponding femoral condyle. The expanded femoral and tibial condyles are designed for weight bearing and to increase contact between the bones. The shape of the femoral condyles is also important in the movement of the tibia on the femur.

Besides the tibiofemoral joint, the patellofemoral joint, which consists of the patella and its articulating surface, is found on the femur. The patella, the largest sesamoid bone in the body, is embedded in the quadriceps tendon. Its location allows greater mechanical advantage for the extension of the knee. The patellar groove on the distal end of the femur covers the anterior surfaces of both condyles and takes the shape of an inverted U (Figure 21-2). The articular surface of the patella can be divided into a larger lateral part and a smaller medial part, which fit into the corresponding groove on the femur.[4]

Extensor Mechanism

The extensor mechanism of the knee consists of the quadriceps femoris muscle, which has four parts: (1) the rectus femoris, (2) the vastus intermedius, (3) the vastus lateralis, and (4) the vastus medialis. The vastus medialis muscle is further divided into the vastus medialis longus and the vastus medialis obliquus (Figure 21-3, *A*). These muscles come together to form a common tendon that continues from the quadriceps group to the tuberosity of the tibia and is called the *ligamentum patellae* or *patellar tendon*. The muscles use the patella to provide a greater mechanical advantage for the extension of the knee. The articularis genu muscle is also included in the extensor mechanism (Figure 21-3, *B*). This small muscle is attached to the suprapatellar bursa and synovial membrane of the knee and provides support for these structures during movements of the knee.

Other structures are included in the extensor mechanism. The patellar fat pad lies beneath the patellar tendon running from the inferior pole of the patella to the tibial tubercle. The patellofemoral and patellotibial ligaments, which are thickenings of the extensor retinaculum, also help to cover the anterior portion of the knee and stabilize the patella. A synovial membrane that is one of the most extensive and complex in the human body surrounds the entire knee joint.

Medial Compartment

The extensor retinaculum and the muscles of the thigh support the medial compartment of the knee. The pes anserinus group, composed of the sartorius, gracilis, and semitendinosus muscles (Figure 21-4), crosses the posteromedial aspect of the joint and attaches to the anteromedial part of the tibia at the level of the tibial tubercle. The adductor magnus muscle attaches to the medial femoral condyle at the adductor tubercle. The most important of these stabilizers is the semimembranosus muscle, which has five components; the principal component is attached to the tubercle on the posterior aspect of the medial tibial condyle. The semimembranosus is an important medial stabilizer of the knee; fibers from the other four slips of this muscle support the posterior capsule and posterior medial capsule and also attach to the medial meniscus to pull it posteriorly from the joint as the knee flexes (Figure 21-5).[5]

The *C*-shaped medial meniscus has an intimate attachment to the capsular ligament along its periphery. The capsular ligaments are divided into meniscofemoral and meniscotibial components.[6] The medial capsular ligaments can be further divided into anterior, middle, and posterior thirds (Figure 21-6). The posterior third is often referred to as the *posterior oblique ligament* and is important in controlling anteromedial rotatory instability.[7] Lying superficial to these ligaments is the tibial collateral ligament. It originates at the medial condyle of the femur, medially below the adductor tubercle, and it attaches distally to the medial condyle on the medial surface of the shaft of the tibia below the pes anserinus group.

The posterior cruciate ligament is also included in the medial compartment. It has often been referred to as the *key to the stability of the knee*.[8] It is attached to the posterior intercondylar area of the tibia and to the posterior extremity of the

lateral meniscus, passing upward, forward, and medially as a broad band to attach to the lateral surface of the medial condyle of the femur.

The ligament is composed of the main posterolateral band and a smaller anteromedial band. Tension within each band varies as the knee moves from flexion to extension (Figure 21-7).

Lateral Compartment

The structures of the lateral compartment of the knee are somewhat similar to those of the medial compartment. Muscular support for lateral structures is provided by the tensor

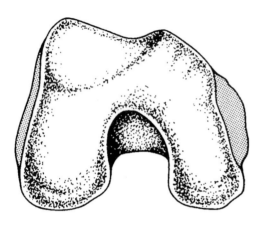

Figure 21-1 Distal end of femur with expanded medial and lateral condyles.

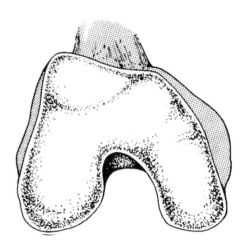

Figure 21-2 Distal end of femur showing patellar groove and anterior condylar surface.

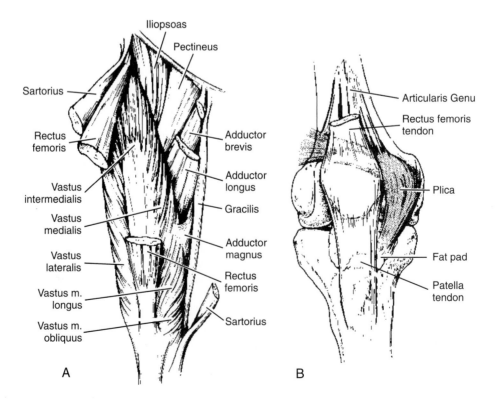

Figure 21-3 A, Muscles of the extensor mechanism. **B,** Patellar tendon (ligament) and articularis genu muscle.

fasciae latae, which can be separated into two functional components: (1) the iliopatellar band and (2) the iliotibial tract.[9] These structures attach anterolaterally to Gerdy's tubercle on the lateral aspect of the tibia (Figure 21-8). Also providing support for the lateral side are the two heads of the biceps femoris. The long head and the short head form a common tendon (lateral hamstring), which splits around the fibular collateral ligament and attaches to the head of the fibula.

The triangular and flat popliteus muscle forms the deep floor of the lower part of the popliteal fossa (Figure 21-9, A). The larger part of the fossa arises on the lateral condyle of the femur and helps support the fibrous lateral capsule adjacent to the lateral meniscus. The popliteus muscle inserts in the posteromedial edge of the tibia and serves to reinforce the posterior third of the lateral capsular ligament. The fibular collateral ligament appears on the lateral aspect of the knee as a large rounded cord, which is attached to the lateral epicondyle of the

femur and below to the head of the fibula; it has no attachment to the lateral meniscus (Figure 21-9, B).

The lateral capsular ligaments attach to the lateral meniscus in much the same way that the medial capsular ligaments attach to the medial meniscus. The lateral capsular ligaments can also be divided into meniscofemoral and meniscotibial sections. These can be further subdivided into anterior, medial, and posterior thirds. The middle third of the lateral capsular ligament provides support against anterior lateral rotatory instability. The posterolateral third of the lateral compartment is also supported by the arcuate ligament. The arcuate ligament consists of a Y-shaped system of capsular fibers, the stem of which is attached to the head of the fibula. The two branches of the upper portion extend medially to the posterior border of

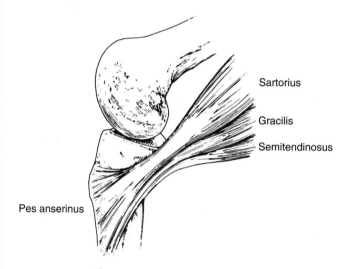

Figure 21-4 Muscles of the pes anserinus group, medial aspect of the knee.

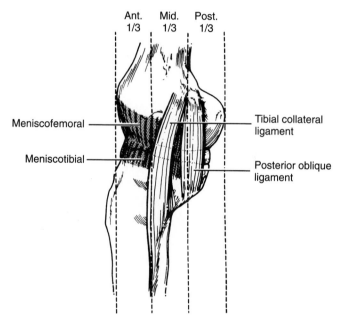

Figure 21-6 Divisions of the medial capsular ligaments.

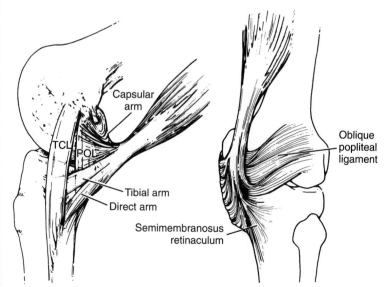

Figure 21-5 The five components of the semimembranosus muscle. *POL,* Posterior oblique ligament; *TCL,* tibial collateral ligament.

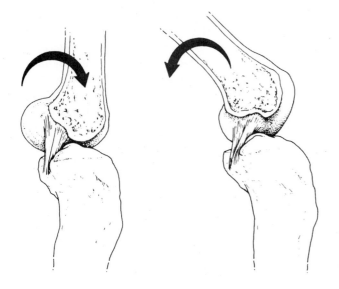

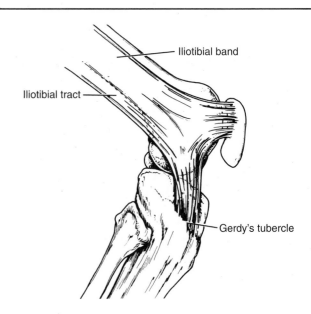

Figure 21-7 Attachment of the posterior cruciate ligament. The different bundles change in tension as the knee moves from extension to flexion.

Figure 21-8 Iliotibial band and iliotibial tract and their attachment to Gerdy's tubercle.

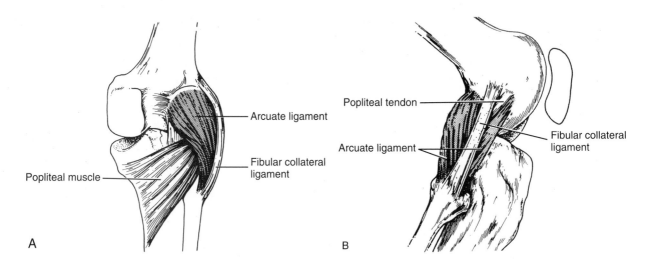

Figure 21-9 A, The popliteus muscle forms the deep floor of the popliteal fossa. **B,** The fibular collateral ligament and the arcuate ligament. Components of the arcuate complex.

the intercondylar area of the tibia and anteriorly to the lateral epicondyle of the femur (see Figure 21-9). Collectively, the posterior third of the lateral capsular ligament, the fibular collateral ligament, the arcuate ligament, and the aponeurosis of the popliteus muscle are known as the *arcuate complex.* The arcuate complex provides lateral support for the knee joint.

The anterior cruciate ligament (ACL) is also included in the lateral compartment. It consists of an anteromedial bundle, an intermediate bundle, and a posterolateral bundle. The anteromedial bundle originates on the posterior superior medial surface of the lateral femoral condyle and inserts on the medial aspect of the intercondylar eminence of the tibia. The posterolateral bundle lies more anterior and distal to the anteromedial bundle on the medial surface of the lateral femoral condyle and inserts laterally to the midline of the intercondylar eminence.

The intermediate bundle lies between these two bundles. Tension on these bundles is altered as the knee moves from flexion to extension (Figure 21-10).

EVALUATION OF THE ACUTELY INJURED KNEE

Evaluation of an acutely injured knee should be completed as soon as possible after injury.[8,10,11] A detailed history and description of the mechanism of injury are vital components of the initial evaluation. It is also very important to complete the evaluation before muscle spasm begins to determine accurately the extent of damage to the knee.

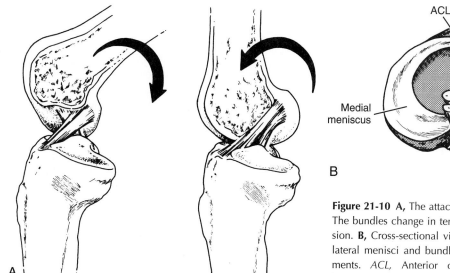

Figure 21-10 A, The attachments of the anterior cruciate ligament (ACL). The bundles change in tension as the knee moves from flexion to extension. **B,** Cross-sectional view of the knee joint showing the medial and lateral menisci and bundles of the anterior and posterior cruciate ligaments. *ACL,* Anterior cruciate ligaments; *PCL,* posterior cruciate ligament.

Table 21-1	Diagnostic Tests for Knee Instabilities	
Instability	**Tear**	**Test**
Straight medial	Medial compartment and posterior cruciate ligament	Abduction stress in full extension Posterior drawer
Straight lateral	Lateral compartment and posterior cruciate ligament	Adduction stress in full extension Posterior drawer
Straight posterior	Posterior cruciate ligament, posterior capsule	Posterior drawer
Straight anterior	Posterior cruciate ligament, ACL medial and lateral compartments	Anterior drawer and all straight instability tests
AMRI	Medial compartment, posterior oblique, MCL	Abduction stress at 30 degrees, anterior drawer with external rotation
ALRI	Middle-third lateral capsular ACL	Anterior drawer in neutral, Lachman's, jerk/pivot shift
PLRI	Arcuate complex	Adduction stress at 30 degrees, external rotation recurvatum, posterior lateral drawer
Combined ALRI/AMRI	Injury to anatomy of ALRI/AMRI	Tests for ALRI and AMRI
Combined AMRI/PLRI	Injury to anatomy of AMRI and PLRI	Tests for AMRI and PLRI
Combined ALRI/PLRI	Injury to anatomy of ALRI and PLRI	Tests for ALRI and PLRI
Combined ALRI/AMRI/PLRI	Injury to anatomy of ALRI/AMRI/PLRI	Tests for ALRI, AMRI, and PLRI

ACL, Anterior cruciate ligament; *ALRI,* anterolateral rotatory instability; *AMRI,* anteromedial rotatory instability; *MCL,* medial collateral ligament; *PLRI,* posterolateral rotatory instability.

Pain parameters—the existence of pain, the onset of pain, and whether the patient can walk without pain—are good indicators of the extent of injury. Another important indicator is the extent of fluid accumulation in the joint. Fluid accumulation within 2 hours of injury indicates the possibility of a hemarthrosis, which could result from an ACL tear, an osteochondral fracture, a peripheral meniscus tear, or an incomplete ligament sprain. Fluid accumulation that occurs 24 hours after injury is usually a synovial fluid buildup, which is indicative of meniscal tear, a tear of the capsular lining of the knee joint, or a subluxated patella. With a major tear of knee tissues, no fluid accumulation occurs; instead the fluid extravagates into the soft tissues. This is usually associated with extensive capsular tears or tears of the posterior cruciate ligament. Palpation of the knee for areas of tenderness or local edema may help to isolate the site of injury. It is always important to establish pulses and the status of sensation around the joint because surrounding neurovascular structures may be damaged in any knee injury.

Diagnostic Tests

Once the history and mechanism of injury have been determined, along with the neurovascular status, several special tests should be performed to complete the examination (Table 21-1). All tests should be performed on the normal knee first. This helps to establish a baseline of stability in a normal joint and helps to gain the patient's confidence and promote relaxation. The patient should be positioned comfortably supine on the examining table, head down on a pillow and hands relaxed.

Abduction Stress Test

The extremity is slightly abducted at the hip and extended so that the thigh is resting on the surface of the examination table. The knee should be flexed to 30 degrees over the side of the table, with one of the examiner's hands placed on the lateral aspect of the knee while the other hand grasps the foot. A gentle abduction stress is applied to the knee while the examiner's hand on the foot provides gentle external rotation. By repeating this test in a consistent manner, the examiner can gradually increase the stress up to the point of pain and maximum laxity without producing a muscle spasm. The injured and uninjured knees are compared. The abduction stress test is always performed with each knee in full extension and in 30 degrees of flexion (Figure 21-11).

A positive abduction stress test at full extension indicates injury to the posterior cruciate ligament and medial compartment; therefore a rotatory instability cannot be classified. A negative test at full extension but a positive test at 30 degrees of flexion indicates a tear of the ligaments of the medial compartment, and a diagnosis of anteromedial rotatory instability can be made.

Adduction Stress Test

By simply changing hands, moving the hand to the medial aspect of the knee, and applying an adduction force at both 30 degrees and full extension, the examiner can perform the adduction stress test. A positive adduction stress test at 30 degrees indicates posterolateral rotatory instability (Figure 21-12).

Anterior Drawer Test

In the anterior drawer test, the patient actively raising his or her head produces hamstring tightening, which can alter the results of the test. The lower extremity should be flexed at the hip to 45 degrees and the knee flexed to 80 or 90 degrees, with the foot flat on the table. The examiner sits on the table, positioning his or her buttocks on the dorsum of the foot to fix it firmly. The examiner's hands are placed about the upper part of the tibia, with the forefingers positioned to palpate the hamstrings to ensure that they are relaxed. The thumbs are positioned at the anterior joint line both medially and laterally. The examiner provides a gentle pull repeatedly in an anterior direction. This test should be performed first with the foot and leg externally rotated beyond the neutral position (Figure 21-13), then internally rotated as much as possible (Figure 21-14), and finally in the neutral position (Figure 21-15). Each lower extremity is tested, and results are compared.

A positive anterior drawer test with the foot in external rotation indicates anteromedial rotatory instability; with the foot in the neutral position, a positive test indicates anterolateral rotatory instability; and with the foot in internal rotation, it indicates a posterior cruciate tear.

Posterior Drawer Test

In the posterior drawer test, the hip is flexed to 45 degrees, the knee is flexed to 90 degrees, and the foot is placed flat on the table. Again, the examiner sits on the dorsum of the foot to fix it firmly. The hands are positioned so that the middle fingers can palpate the hamstrings; the thumbs are placed along the tibia at the joint line. The examiner pushes straight back gently. Movement of the tibia on the femur is noted with a positive posterior drawer test (Figure 21-16, *A*). A positive posterior drawer sign can often be misinterpreted as a positive anterior drawer sign. For additional clarification of the posterior instability test, a gravity test may be helpful. With the

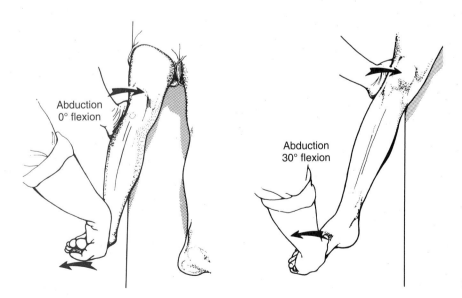

Abduction
0° flexion

Abduction
30° flexion

Figure 21-11 Abduction stress test.

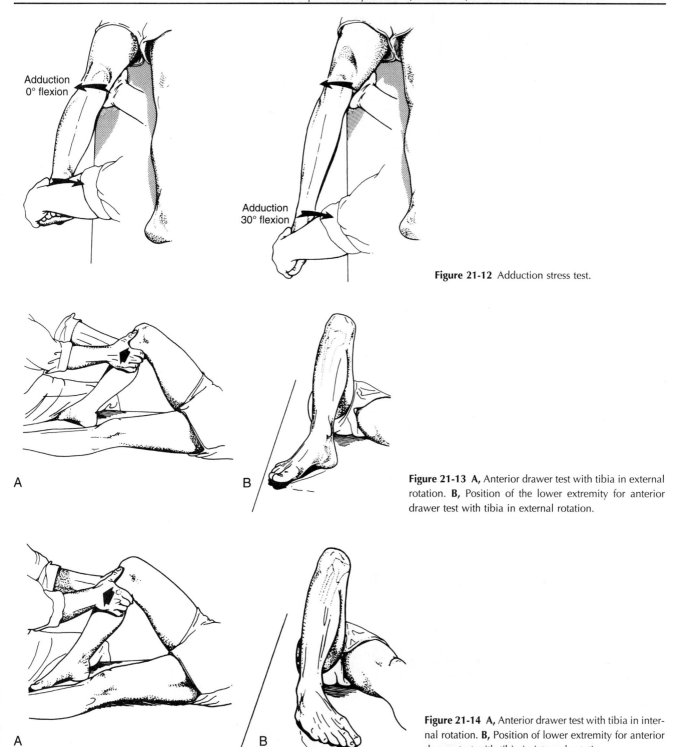

Adduction
0° flexion

Adduction
30° flexion

Figure 21-12 Adduction stress test.

A   B

Figure 21-13 A, Anterior drawer test with tibia in external rotation. **B,** Position of the lower extremity for anterior drawer test with tibia in external rotation.

A   B

Figure 21-14 A, Anterior drawer test with tibia in internal rotation. **B,** Position of lower extremity for anterior drawer test with tibia in internal rotation.

patient supine and the knees together and flexed to approximately 80 degrees and the feet planted together on the table, posterior displacement of the tibial tuberosity can be seen when viewed from the side (Figure 21-16, *B*).

Posterior Lateral Drawer Test

The patient is positioned as previously described (see Figure 21-16); the examiner will not see a posterior drawer but an

increased external rotation of the tibia as compared with the uninvolved side.

External Rotation Recurvatum Test

With the patient supine and legs extended and relaxed, the examiner lifts the leg off of the bed by grasping the great toe. The involved side will demonstrate the tibia rolling into exter-

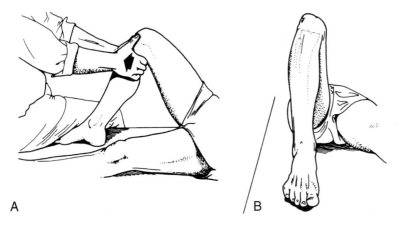

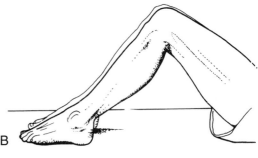

Figure 21-15 A, Anterior drawer test with tibia in neutral position. **B,** Position of lower extremity for anterior drawer test with tibia in neutral position.

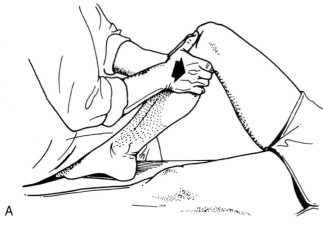

Figure 21-16 A, Posterior drawer test for posterolateral instability. **B,** Gravity test for posterolateral instability.

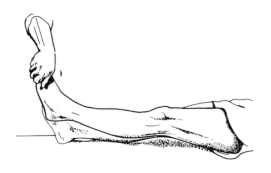

Figure 21-17 External rotation recurvatum test.

nal rotation as compared with the uninvolved side (Figure 21-17).

Jerk Test and Pivot Shift Test

The examiner supports the lower extremity and flexes the hip to about 45 degrees and the knee to 90 degrees, while at the same time internally rotating the tibia. If the right knee is being examined, then the foot should be in the examiner's right hand, internally rotating the tibia, while the left hand is placed over the proximal end of the tibia and fibula. The left hand is used to exert a valgus stress. The knee is gradually extended, maintaining the internal rotation and valgus stress. With a positive jerk test, a subluxation of the lateral femoral condyle

on the tibia occurs at about 20 degrees of flexion. With further extension, a spontaneous relocation occurs. This relocation is described in engineering terms as a *jerk,* a sudden change in the rate of acceleration between surfaces. In this case it is the change in the velocity of the tibia in relation to the femur (Figure 21-18). A positive jerk test indicates anterolateral rotatory instability. The pivot shift test is similar except that the knee is moved from extension to flexion. Great care should be taken to be gentle in this test because a dramatic shift can cause discomfort.

Anterior Drawer-in-Extension Test (Lachlan-Ritchey or Lachman's Test)

The anterior drawer-in-extension test is performed with the patient's knee in approximately 20 degrees of flexion.

The examiner uses one hand to stabilize the femur by grasping the distal thigh just proximal to the patella. With the other hand, the examiner grasps the tibia medially to the tibial tubercle. The tibia should be allowed to fall into external rotation as this test is performed. Firm pressure is applied to the posterior aspect of the tibia in an effort to produce anterior subluxation (Figure 21-19). The tibia and femur are moved anteriorly and posteriorly on one another. Increased translation and lack of ligament end feel are noted in the involved knee. This test is one of the most sensitive methods of diagnosing ACL injury.

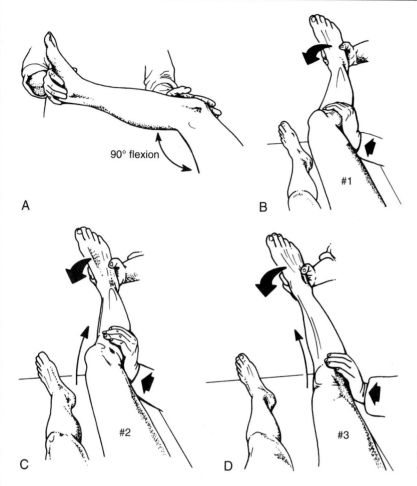

Figure 21-18 **A,** Starting position for performing the jerk test. **B** and **C,** Jerk test sequence. **D,** End position of jerk test.

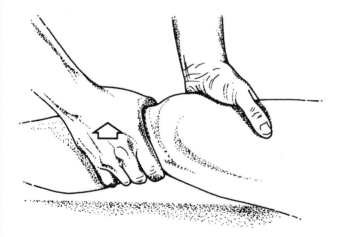

Figure 21-19 Anterior drawer in extension test.

CLASSIFICATION OF INSTABILITY

Given the clinical findings of the tests just described and using the system of classification of knee ligament instabilities of Hughston et al.,[8,12,13] knee ligament instabilities can be classified as either *straight* (nonrotatory) or *rotatory.* Rotatory instabilities may be further subclassified as *simple* or *combined.*

Straight Instability

Four types of instability involve no rotation of the tibia on the femur. These are called *straight instabilities* because if any rotation occurs, then it is not around the centrally located posterior cruciate ligament. They are as follows:

1. Medial instability—A tear in the medial compartment ligaments with an associated tear of the posterior cruciate ligament. It is demonstrated by a positive abduction stress test with the knee in full extension and a posterior drawer test.
2. Lateral instability—A tear in the lateral compartment ligaments and the posterior cruciate ligament. This is demonstrated by a positive adduction stress test with the knee in full extension and a posterior drawer test.
3. Posterior instability—A tear in the posterior cruciate ligament and laxity in both the posterior oblique ligament and the arcuate complex. This is demonstrated by a positive posterior drawer test in which both tibial condyles subluxate posteriorly by an equal amount with no rotation. If only the posterior cruciate ligament is torn, then a small posterior drawer translation will occur. This is called an *isolated posterior cruciate tear.*
4. Anterior instability—A torn ACL, torn medial and lateral capsular ligaments, and a torn posterior cruciate ligament. This is demonstrated by a positive anterior drawer sign in

which both tibial condyles subluxate anteriorly by an equal amount with no rotation.

Simple Rotatory Instability

Three types of simple rotatory instability exist. Each demonstrates a rotatory component of the tibia on the femur involving either the medial or the lateral tibial condyle. The rotation occurs around the centrally located posterior cruciate ligament.

1. Anteromedial rotatory instability—A tear of the medial compartment ligaments including the posterior oblique and/or the middle third of the medial capsular ligament, as well as the medial collateral ligament (MCL). The abduction stress test at 30 degrees of flexion is positive, as is the anterior drawer test with the tibia externally rotated.
2. Anterolateral rotatory instability—A tear of the middle third of the lateral capsular ligament and possibly the ACL. It is demonstrated by a positive jerk test and a positive anterior drawer test with the tibia in the neutral position. The Lachman's test is positive.
3. Posterolateral rotatory instability—A tear of the arcuate complex. The adduction stress test at 30 degrees of knee flexion, posterior lateral drawer test, and the external rotation recurvatum test are positive.

Combined Rotatory Instabilities

Four types of combined rotatory instability have been described.

1. Combined anterolateral and anteromedial rotatory instabilities—Tears of the MCL, and middle and posterior one third of the medial capsular ligaments and middle one third lateral capsular ligament and the ACL. The posterior cruciate ligament remains intact. The anterior drawer test with the tibia in the neutral and externally rotated positions, the abduction stress test at 30 degrees, the Lachman's test, and the jerk test are positive.
2. Combined anterolateral and posterolateral instability—A tear of the middle and posterior (arcuate ligament complex) one third of the lateral capsular ligaments and a tear of the ACL. The posterior cruciate ligament remains intact. The external rotation recurvatum test is positive, as is the adduction stress test at 30 degrees, the Lachman's test, the posterior lateral drawer test, the anterior drawer test with the tibia in neutral, and the jerk test.
3. Combined anteromedial and posterolateral instability—A tear of the MCL, the middle and posterior one third capsular ligaments and the posterior one third of the lateral capsular ligament (the arcuate complex). The anterior and posterior cruciate ligaments are intact. Positive tests include the external rotation recurvatum test, the posterior lateral drawer test, the abduction and adduction stress tests at 30 degrees, and the anterior drawer test with the tibia externally rotated.
4. Combined posterolateral, anterolateral, and anteromedial rotatory instability—Tears of the middle one third of the lateral capsular ligament, ACL, arcuate complex, medial

capsular ligaments, and MCL. The posterior cruciate ligament is intact. In a knee with these lesions, anterior drawer tests with the tibia in the neutral position and in external rotation are positive. A posterolateral drawer test is positive and causes the tibia to rotate externally and backward. The external rotation recurvatum test is positive. Adduction and abduction stress tests are positive with the knee at 30 degrees of flexion but negative with it at full extension. The jerk and Lachman's tests are also positive.

SURGICAL INTERVENTION FOR ROTATORY INSTABILITIES

Surgical treatment of rotatory instability should always be directed toward restoring the normal anatomy by correcting the pathologic anatomy. Far too many surgical procedures exist to attempt to review them in this work. Understanding surgical procedures and surgical philosophy provides a starting point for restoring normal function through an effective rehabilitation program in the knee-injured patient.[14]

Basic surgical philosophy mandates the repair of acutely torn structures.[15,16] Unfortunately, direct repair of the ACL is not successful. Acute repair of capsular ligaments may also be performed. In chronic situations, extraarticular reconstruction using capsular reefings, tendon transfers, and tenodesis, as well as anterior cruciate intraarticular grafts, is necessary. These materials may be composed of autografts (the body's own tissue [e.g., the patellar or semitendinosus tendon]), allografts (tissue from cadaver sources), or artificial materials.

Rehabilitation for Knees With Rotatory Instability

With the refinement of diagnostic skills and the addition of complex new surgical techniques, the rehabilitation of knee injuries has become more complex. Rehabilitation programs should always be based on sound biomechanical principles and directed toward restoring a functionally stable knee that will meet the demands of the patient's sport or activity. Proper strength, flexibility, endurance, proprioception, agility, skill, and speed should be combined in an exercise program to meet this goal.[17,18] Maintenance of strength in the uninjured leg and upper extremity should also be included in any rehabilitation program.[19]

Paulos et al.[20,21] state two principles of rehabilitation: First, the effects of immobility must be minimized; second, healing tissues must never be overloaded. Immobility of a joint can lead to contracture, histochemical changes, and a decrease in ligamentous strength. Joint contracture is manifested mechanically in the amount of torque required to move the knee joint. The torque may have to be increased 10 times over the force normally required to move the joint. The ligament-bone complex also reacts to immobility. Not only is the ligament itself weakened but also its bony attachment has been found to be weakened by as much as 40% after only 8 weeks of immobility. Noyes et al.[22] found that after 8 weeks of immobilization, the joint required reconditioning for at least 1 year before 90% of its strength returned. Histochemically, selective atrophy of type I fibers, which are slow-twitch or red muscle fibers, has been shown to decrease total muscle mass by as much as 30% to 47% with immobilization. Today, most surgical procedures for the knee allow for early motion.

The second principle concerns protecting the healing tissues from excessive overload. In the early phases of rehabilitation, healing tissues should be protected from abnormal joint displacement, such as twisting or falling on the knee. Subjecting the healing tissues to cyclic forces causes the second form of common mechanical failure. This causes a fatigue-like failure. Stretching the healing tissues past their elastic limit induces a third form of overload. Proper surgical technique is probably the most important means of preventing this type of ligamentous failure. However, high forces over an extended period of time can produce this type of failure; for example, when extending the knee rapidly from 30 degrees to full extension with high resistance, an anterior drawer effect creates a strain on the ACL and weakens the repair if sufficient healing has not occurred. For this reason, it is vitally important to consider the surgical procedure used along with the other variables when formulating the rehabilitation program.

In vivo strain gauge studies indicate that the stresses across the ACL in both open and closed chain are well below rupture stresses even with 10 lb of ankle weight on leg raises or rubber tube resisted squats.[26] So open and closed chain rehabilitation with light resistance is not a problem even early in the postoperative program. Protected weight bearing is also not a problem. Three studies[23-25] compared open and closed kinetic chain from 0 to 12 weeks, finding no difference in outcomes for either group. Cooper et al.[27] reported anatomy studies of young cadaver knees that the strength of the patella tendon is up to 100% the strength of the normal ACL. All that being said, rehabilitation for the postoperative ACL patient is straightforward and criteria or functional based.

The patient who has just undergone an intraarticular ACL reconstruction may be placed in a splint in full extension for several days until quadriceps control is obtained and then no brace is used. Electrical stimulation may aid the patient in gaining quadriceps control. Ambulation is weight bearing as tolerated with crutches. At postoperative day 1 flexion, range of motion is begun and passive extension is emphasized to gain full extension (for that patient) as soon as possible. Quadriceps sets, terminal knee extensions, straight-leg raises, hip flexion, hip abduction, hip extension, hip adduction and hamstring curls with light resistance (0 to 10 lb, five sets of 10 lifts over 10 to 12 weeks postoperatively) can be started as soon as possible. The therapist should not forget heel and toe lifts to keep the gastrocnemius and anterior tibialis strong. As noted earlier, the patient should be protected from overload of the healing structure. A slow progression is essential to produce a good end result with an intraarticular procedure. Therapeutic swimming may begin as soon as the stitches are removed. The patient may gradually increase weight bearing and wean off the crutches over a period of several weeks. Stationary bicycling may begin as soon as tolerated.

Once the patient has worked off his or her crutches (3 to 6 weeks), closed chain activities such as step-ups, minisquats, and rubber tubing squats can begin. Leg press activities can also be started. By 12 weeks status postoperative (SPO), the patient is working up to 10 lb on straight-leg raises, riding a bike for 30 minutes daily, walking 2 miles, and handling the closed chain activities well. Isokinetic testing may be performed now. Isokinetic workouts at low intensity may start as soon as the patella femoral joint has calmed down, as well as mild running and other closed chain activities. Once aggressive functional exercises are started, the patient may be placed in a functional brace.

The patient who has undergone an extraarticular reconstruction with iliotibial tract tenodesis may be in a cast for approximately 6 weeks. He or she is encouraged to do quadriceps setting and active-assisted straight-leg raises. Hamstring contraction and ankle pumps are begun as tolerated. Gait is nonweight bearing.

With extraarticular repairs, some patients are placed in a hinged immobilizer. Motion in the hinged immobilizer is limited to 40 to 70 degrees for the first 3 weeks. After 3 weeks, the flexion stop is eliminated, and the patient is allowed to gain as much flexion as possible. At 6 weeks, with the patient still nonweight bearing, active-assisted flexion range of motion exercises are begun in an attempt to reach full flexion. The patient is encouraged to continue to work on quadriceps setting with the addition of hamstring curls and hip flexion strengthening exercises. The patient will actively work toward full extension with terminal knee extension and straight-leg raise exercises in the period from 6 weeks to 12 weeks after surgery.

Twelve weeks after surgery, the patient gradually progresses from partial weight bearing to full weight bearing as tolerated. At full weight bearing, he or she is allowed to progress to advanced activities such as side step-ups and leg presses. The patient should use a toe-heel gait to encourage extension of the knee, but once full extension is reached, normal heel-toe gait is resumed. Bicycling and swimming may also start at this point. At 6 months postsurgery, the patient may begin agility and competitive preparation exercises. These are expected to help the patient progress back to his or her sport activities and should be designed to be the same types of activities the patient will use in his or her sport.

When prosthetic ligaments are used, the biomechanics and healing restraints that normally are a big factor in the postsurgical rehabilitation process are less important. The patient is again placed in a cast brace or a long leg brace, which is locked at 45 degrees for the first 3 days. The patient's gait is nonweight bearing. The patient is allowed to work on exercises out of the brace and work on active extension with straight-leg raises, terminal knee extensions, and flexion-to-extension exercises, as well as active-assisted flexion. Hamstring strengthening and hip strengthening begin during the first 3 weeks. After 1 week, the cast brace is reset to minus 15 degrees of extension, and partial weight bearing is allowed. At the end of 6 weeks, the brace is returned to full extension. At 12 weeks the patient is allowed to progress off the crutches but must continue to wear the cast brace until 4 months after surgery. No running is allowed until after muscle strength has returned to 80% of normal. Isokinetic testing is again helpful in making this assessment. Other functional guidelines for return to running would include the ability to do ride an exercise bike 30 minutes, walk two miles, and perform 50 8-inch side step-downs.

For the patient who will return to athletic endeavors, the advanced rehabilitation program should contain functional and specific exercises that will imitate the motions demanded of the patient by his or her sport. Bicycling is a good means of building endurance and aerobic capacities for the patient who will be returning to an active sport. Straight-leg raises should be continued until the patient can lift 10 lb; range of motion activities should continue until the range of motion in the operated leg is close to that of the normal extremity.

Once 10 lb can be lifted with a high number of repetitions, different weight machines can be used to supplement the high-repetition low-weight program. Hamstring curl and leg press machines are recommended for increasing the bulk of the leg. When an athlete can walk up and down stairs for 30 minutes, ride a bicycle for 1 hour, and has 80% of his or her quadriceps strength, as measured with isokinetic testing, and when proper healing has taken place, a running program can be initiated. When the patient can run 2 miles with no swelling, pain, or limp, he or she can begin to sprint. Once the athlete can sprint at nearly full speed, different cutting activities can be performed. These cutting activities promote agility and should be similar to the situations that the athlete would encounter in his or her sport.

Proprioception and balance are usually lost after major knee injury and/or surgery. Balancing activities such as standing on one foot with the eyes open and closed and standing on the toes with the eyes open and closed should be included in the advanced rehabilitation process.

One other factor is important in the advanced rehabilitation of the athlete. The athlete has to be psychologically ready to return to play. After any major knee injury and subsequent surgery, the rehabilitation process is never complete until the athlete is confident that he or she can again participate in his or her sport without being reinjured. A well-planned program of exercise with reasonably set goals will help the athlete return to the sport with the confidence needed to participate, without the lingering doubts caused by the previous injury.

The illustrations following the case studies (Figures 21-20 to 21-35) demonstrate the techniques discussed. As with any exercise program, a great deal depends on communication among the therapist, the surgeon, and the patient. Each must be aware of the biomechanical and healing restraints after an injury, and all must be willing to do their part to produce a good result after an injury.

CASE STUDIES

Case Study 1

The following case study illustrates rehabilitation after reconstruction of the ACL.

T.W. is a motorcycle policeman and an avid softball player who plays for several teams during the spring and summer seasons. During a late fall softball game, T.W. misjudged a fly ball, and as he was trying to change his direction of movement, he cut to the left and felt a pop, followed by a giving-way sensation in his left knee. It was quite uncomfortable, and he left the field limping. He applied ice to his knee, but it swelled immediately. Although he could still walk on it, he exhibited a severe limp.

He visited his orthopaedist the next day. With the examination and his history of cutting, the popping sound, the giving way, and the immediate swelling, it was obvious that he had torn his ACL. He was diagnosed with an anterior lateral rotatory instability. Given the options that he could follow for the care of his knee, T.W. elected to have surgical correction of his problem. It was clear that he wanted to maintain an active lifestyle and was going to continue playing amateur sports in the future.

Diagnostic classification: Musculoskeletal 4I: ACL Tear with Internal Derangement 717.8

T.W. was then started on a conservative program of quadriceps sets, terminal knee extensions, straight-leg raises, hamstring curls, and stationary biking as soon as he was comfortable. He was on crutches and partial weight bearing and elected not to use any type of immobilizer. He continued to use ice, compression, and elevation for his leg. In 1 week, his orthopaedist was able to complete a better examination because much of the swelling of the knee was gone. He was found to have a 2+ pivot shift, positive anterior drawer in extension, and 2+ anterior drawer at 90 degrees. The surgeon thought that the inflammatory process should calm down a bit before patella tendon graft surgery was performed. Six weeks after the injury, T.W. underwent patella tendon graft endoscopically performed ACL surgery. His menisci were found to be in good shape at the time of surgery.

A straight immobilizer was used postoperatively and a point was made to ensure that the immobilizer was in an extremely straight position. Ice and elevation were used initially. On postoperative day 1, the patient was up on crutches, in a chair, and working diligently on ankle pumps to decrease the chance of phlebitis. Quadriceps setting exercises were begun to decrease swelling and maintain quadriceps tone. On postoperative day 2, the patient ambulated with partial weigh bearing to the physical therapy department, where passive extension without immobilizer was begun with the heel propped up on pillows. Terminal knee

CASE STUDIES—cont'd

extensions with electrical stimulation, hamstring stretching, and active-assisted flexion were also performed.

T.W. lived locally and was discharged late on postoperative day 3, leaving the hospital with 0 degrees of extension, 10 degrees of active extension, and 90 degrees of active-assisted flexion. He continued to work hard on a home exercise program as instructed by the hospital's physical therapist.

At postoperative week 2, T.W. continued his passive extension stretching many times throughout the day. Aggressive knee flexion, terminal knee extension, straight-leg raises, hip abductors, hip flexors, and hamstring curls were performed, five sets of 10 twice a day to three times a day, working gradually up to 5 lb. Stationary bicycle exercise was started a couple of days later. Weight bearing was to tolerance, and the straight immobilizer was discarded at the 2-week mark because his quadriceps control was excellent.

At 1 month, crutches were discarded because T.W. had good control of his quadriceps. Range of motion was 0 to 130 degrees. There was very little swelling about the knee and no limp when walking. He continued with his earlier exercises but began gentle closed chain activities. These were performed using horizontal leg press machine, the Shuttle 2000, and rubber tubing minisquats. Step-ups were added at the 6-week mark, and by 8 weeks he began mini-trampoline running and slide board activities. Isokinetic activities at mild to moderate intensity were begun at a variety of speeds.

At the 3-month mark, T.W. had a 20% to 25% deficit in his quadriceps when the two legs were compared, as shown with isokinetic testing. He was allowed to begin 1-month progressive-running program, step-ups, and all activities in the weight room except heavy flexion to extension. He did work at heavier intensity in the 90 to 45 degrees range of motion . His patellofemoral joint was monitored closely. By the 4-month mark, he was performing these exercises quite aggressively. At 5 months, he began agility training, including figure-eight runs, hopping on one foot, and general plyometric jumping.

At 6 months, his isokinetic test showed equality between the two quadriceps. He was running, cutting with no problems, and was fitted with an ACL brace to allow for his softball activities.

One-year postoperatively, the patient was having no problems whatsoever. Range of motion was 0 to 140 degrees.

Case Study 2
The following case study illustrates rehabilitation after a surgical repair of a posterior lateral rotatory instability (PLRI).

S.K. is a 17-year-old defensive end on his high school football team. He is 6-feet 4-inches tall and weighs 265 lb.

During a first-round playoff game, S.K. sustained a non-contact posterior lateral injury to his knee. On the field he felt diffuse severe pain that did not allow full extension or flexion of the knee.

After being transported from the field, S.K. was thoroughly examined. There was little to no swelling, a positive external rotation recurvatum test, and adduction stress at 30 degrees. A compressive wrap was applied, and he was fitted with a hinged knee immobilizer locked at 45 degrees of flexion and allowed to ambulate without weight bearing with crutches.

S.K. was seen in the clinic by his orthopaedist the next morning. With his history and presentation, it was confirmed that S.K. has sustained a posterolateral injury that would require surgery to return him to function and sports. The following tests were positive during his physical examination: the reverse pivot shift test and the posterior drawer with external rotation test, as well as the external rotation recurvatum test. Magnetic resonance imaging (MRI) confirmed the results of the physical examination and also revealed no injury to the meniscus. S.K.'s surgery was scheduled within 1 week of the initial injury.

During surgery the following damaged tissues were repaired: biceps femoris long and short heads, deep and capsuloosseous layer of the iliotibial tract, arcuate ligament, head of the lateral gastrocnemius, and fibular collateral. Postoperatively, S.K. was placed in a hinged knee brace at 45 degrees, with a pelvic band attached to prevent external rotation. Because of his postoperative positioning, S.K. was started on ankle pumps to aid in the prevention of phlebitis, and he was educated on the importance of maintaining neutral rotation of the femur with no external rotation.

Diagnostic classification: Musculoskeletal 4I: Multiple Soft Tissue Tears 719.8

On postoperative day 1, the precautions of femoral rotation were reviewed. S.K. was instructed in quadriceps sets in the brace, with the brace locked at 45 degrees. He was instructed in and practiced proper transfer techniques and gait mechanics on all surfaces and stairs with crutches without weight bearing. These activities were performed twice a day to develop proper lower-extremity control.

On postoperative day 2, the dressing was changed to evaluate the wound. The wound consisted of a lateral "hockey stick" incision that was approximated with a sub-cutaneous stitch with surface closure using surgical staples. The wound was then redressed with 4 × 4 gauze dressing, secured with a white elastic wrap, and placed back in the brace. S.K. was then prepared for discharge from the hospital.

S.K. was scheduled for outpatient follow-up physical therapy during postoperative week 2. At this time, S.K. was instructed in the following exercises: active-assisted flexion, active extension over a bolster, quadriceps sets and leg raises

Continued

CASE STUDIES—cont'd

over a bolster, and pool activities to strengthen the hip. Extension was gained actively at a rate of 5 to 10 degrees per week, and the brace had to be adjusted accordingly. No hamstring stretches or passive extension were performed. Secondary to S.K.'s strong quadriceps, he was cautioned not to force extension and was reminded to gain extension of only 5 to 10 degrees per week to protect the repair.

The goals at this time were to gain range of motion and increase quadriceps strength for lower-extremity control. During postoperative weeks 5 to 9, S.K. finally began to see major improvement. He was progressed to ambulation with crutches, with weight bearing as tolerated. The aim of weight-bearing ambulation is to achieve full extension and lower-extremity control through functional exercise. Closed chain kinetic exercises such as hip shuttle, wall slides, and single-leg stance were introduced. Use of the stationary bike was also initiated, with close attention to seat height. If the seat is too high, then it can cause the patient to have an extension moment that is too forceful at the terminal end of the downstroke. Aquatic therapy was continued.

On postoperative weeks 10 to 15, S.K. progressed to ambulation with one crutch and quickly advanced to no crutches for ambulation, with weight bearing as tolerated. The previous exercise program continued, and more function-oriented exercises were added. The single-leg stance on firm and soft surfaces with perturbations for proprioceptive training was essential. Ankle strengthening with standing calf raises and posterior tibialis strengthening was added. Closed chain kinetic exercises were also advanced to include the minitrampoline, the stair climber, and elastic cord exercise backward and forward. Even though S.K. was advancing at the expected rate, constant counseling was provided to remind him of the final goals and of the need not to advance independently.

Postoperative months 5 to 7 began with careful assessment of strength, range of motion, and functional testing. The functional test used in this case was the triple-crossover hop test. S.K. was found to have full active range of motion (AROM), 5/5 strength with manual muscle testing (MMT), and absolutely no pain or swelling. Once functional criteria had been established, more intense weight room activities were performed and a walking-jogging-running program was added. When S.K.'s tolerance was established, functional and task (sport-specific and position-specific tasks [in this case, defensive-end specific]) training was also added.

On postoperative month 9, S.K. was prepared to return to full functional activities with the following presentation: 0/0/135 AROM, within 95% of that on the contralateral side on his isokinetic test, and less than $\frac{1}{4}$-inch quadriceps girth measurement difference when compared with the contralateral side. S.K. returned to two-a-day practice football camp that next summer without brace support and continued the season without limitations because of his injury.

Quadriceps Sets

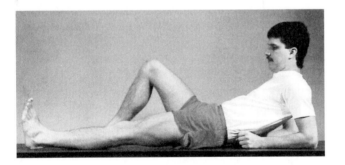

Figure 21-20 Quadriceps setting exercise. An isometric contraction of the quadriceps muscle. The leg should be straightened as much as possible, and the patella should track proximally. The patient should hold the contraction for at least five counts and perform the exercise about 50 times per hour.

Straight-Leg Raise

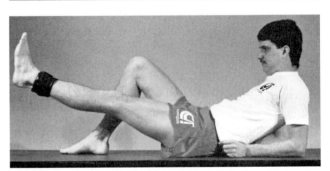

Figure 21-21 Straight-leg raise. The patient is positioned supine, with the opposite leg flexed to 90 degrees and the foot planted flat next to the involved knee. The quadriceps muscle is contracted and the leg lifted to approximately 45 degrees and no higher than the thigh of the opposite leg. The leg is held there for at least five counts and is then slowly lowered to the floor. The patient should relax for at lease two counts and repeat this exercise. Then sets of 10 lifts are completed, with a 1-minute rest between each set of 10. Straight-leg raises are performed three times a day. Once the patient can complete 10 sets of 10, three times a day, ankle weights are added for resistance. The patient should begin with a 1 lb weight and progress slowly to 5 lb, still maintaining 10 sets of 10 lifts. Weights are increased according to the patient's tolerance.

Terminal Knee Extension

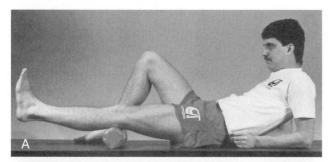
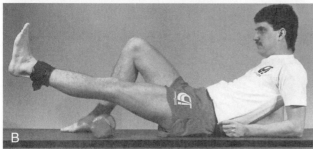

Figure 21-22 Terminal knee extension. **A,** A support is placed beneath the knee to be exercised. The quadriceps muscle is again contracted, and the heel is lifted from the floor in a short arc range of motion. Five sets of 10 of this exercise are completed three times a day. **B,** Resistance can be added as tolerated. The terminal knee extension can be incorporated with the straight-leg raise to assist in bringing the knee out to full extension.

Hamstring Stretching

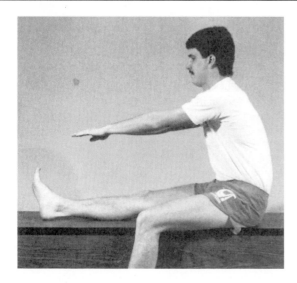

Figure 21-23 Hamstring stretching. The patient is in a sitting position, with one leg off the exercise table. The back is straight, and the leg to be stretched is straight. The patient reaches forward slowly and holds for a count of 10. At least 5 minutes of stretching is performed three times a day. The patient should be cautioned not to bounce when stretching.

Hamstring Curls

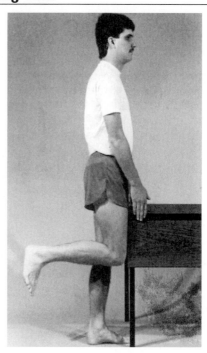

Figure 21-24 Hamstring curls. The patient stands with the thigh pressed against a wall or table to block hip flexion. The knee is flexed to its maximum position and held for a count of five. The foot is then lowered to the floor. Five sets of 10 of this exercise are performed three times a day. Resistance of 1 to 5 lb can be added progressively, according to the patient's tolerance.

Active Range of Motion for Flexion

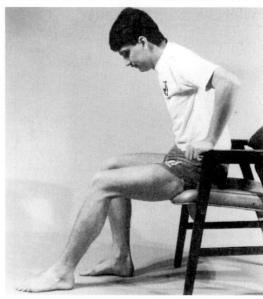

Figure 21-25 Active range of motion (AROM) for flexion. The patient is seated, with the feet flat on the floor. The injured leg is allowed to slide back actively along the floor, keeping the foot flat on the floor. The foot is planted, and the hips are allowed to slide forward over the affected leg, providing some extra stretch. This exercise may be repeated 30 times, three times a day. The stretch is held for at least a count of 10.

Hip Flexion Exercise

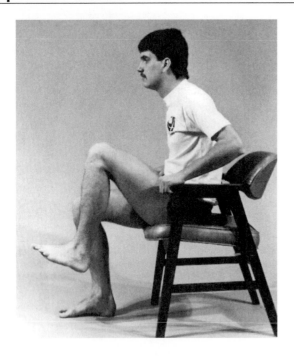

Figure 21-26 Hip flexion exercise. The patient is sitting, with the feet resting on the floor. The knee is lifted toward the chest at a 45-degree angle and held there for a count of five. The knee is lowered gently, and the foot is placed on the floor. Five sets of 10 repetitions of this exercise are performed three times a day, and resistance of 1 to 5 lb can be added at the knee as the patient tolerates it.

Flexion-to-Extension Exercise

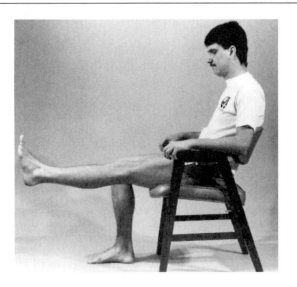

Figure 21-27 Flexion-to-extension exercise. In the starting position, the patient sits with the feet resting on the floor. The knee is then extended and held in as full extension as possible for a count of five and then gently lowered to the floor. This exercise can be repeated up to 10 sets of 10, three times a day. Resistance of 1 to 5 lb can be added as tolerated.

Hip Abduction Exercises

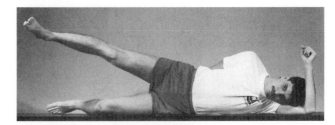

Figure 21-28 Hip abduction exercises. The patient is positioned side lying, with the unaffected knee flexed at 90 degrees and the hip flexed at 45 degrees. The affected leg is straight, and the body weight is shifted forward. The leg is lifted, held for a count of five, and gently lowered back to the starting position. Resistance of 1 to 5 lb can be added at the ankle. This exercise should be performed in five sets of 10, three times a day.

Adductor Stretching

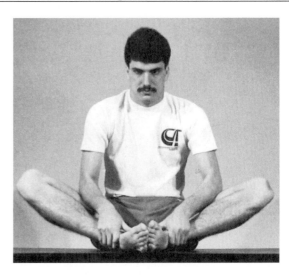

Figure 21-29 Adductor stretching. The patient should sit with the soles of the feet together and slide them back toward the buttocks as far as possible. With the elbows positioned on the leg, the patient pushes down toward the floor and holds for a count of 10. This should be repeated for approximately 5 minutes, three times a day.

Heel Cord Stretching

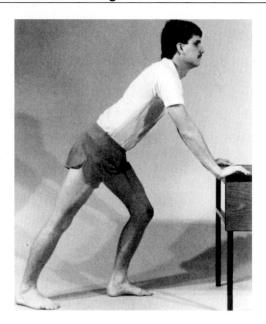

Figure 21-30 Heel cord stretching. The patient stands with the toes slightly pointed in and the heels on the floor. The knees are kept straight. The patient leans forward, stretching the muscles. The stretch should be held for a count of 10 and repeated for 5 minutes, three times a day. The soleus muscle can also be stretched in this position.

Adductor Leg Raise

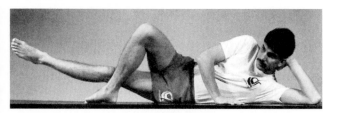

Figure 21-31 Adduction leg raise. The patient is again side lying, with the affected leg against the table. The leg is lifted into adduction and held for a count of five. This exercise can be repeated in five sets of 10 and resistance of 1 to 5 lb added as tolerated.

Quadriceps Femoris Stretching

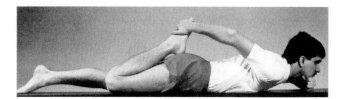

Figure 21-32 Quadriceps femoris stretching. The patient is positioned prone, and the heel is pulled toward the buttocks. The position is held for a count of 10 and then released. The patient should stretch for 5 minutes, three times a day.

Hip Flexor Stretching

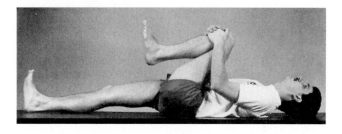

Figure 21-33 Hip flexor stretching. With the patient lying supine, one knee is pulled toward the chest while the opposite leg is held as straight as possible. The patient should hold this stretch for a count of 10 and then release; 5 minutes, three times a day is preferred.

Side Step-Up

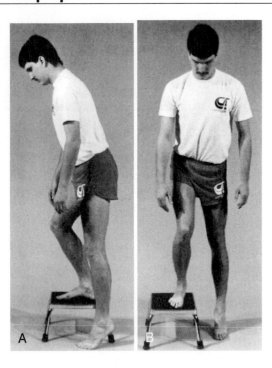

Figure 21-34 Side step-up. The patient should stand sideways, with the involved foot flat on a step. The body weight is lifted with the involved leg. The patient is allowed to push off with the uninvolved foot. Once the patient is able to complete this exercise 100 times once a day, the patient is progressed from a 4-inch step to a 7-inch step.

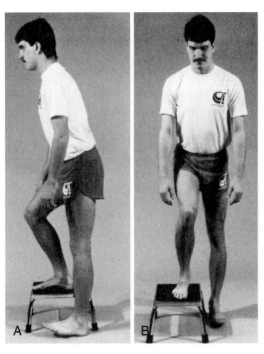

Figure 21-35 Side step-up. The progression of the side step-up exercise shows the patient again standing, with the involved leg on the step. However, in this exercise the patient is now allowed to push off the uninvolved foot. The patient must push off with the uninvolved heel touching the floor only. Again, 100 of these exercises, or 10 sets of 10, should be performed once a day.

ACKNOWLEDGMENTS

The authors thank Mark Baker, PT (Hughston Sports Medicine Hospital, Columbus, GA), and Sammy Bonfim, SPT (North Georgia College and State University), for their assistance in revising this chapter.

REFERENCES

1. Blackburn T, Craig E: Knee anatomy: a brief review, Phys Ther 60:1556, 1980.
2. Harty M, Joyce J: Surgical anatomy and exposure of the knee joint. In AAOS instructional course lectures, vol 20, St Louis, 1971, Mosby.
3. Kaplan E: Some aspects of functional anatomy of the human knee joint, Clin Orthop 23:18, 1962.
4. Williams P, Warwick R, editors: Gray's anatomy, ed 36, Edinburgh, 1980, Churchill Livingstone.
5. Brantigan O, Voshell A: The mechanics of the ligaments and menisci of the knee joint, J Bone Joint Surg 23:1, 1941.
6. Heller L, Langman J: The meniscofemoral ligaments of the human knee, J Bone Joint Surg 46:2, 1964.
7. Hughston J, Eilers A: The role of the posterior oblique ligament in repairs of acute medial collateral ligament tears of the knee, J Bone Joint Surg 55:5, 1973.
8. Hughston J, Andrews J, Cross M, et al: Classification of knee ligament instabilities. I. The medial compartment and cruciate ligaments, J Bone Joint Surg 58:2, 1976.
9. Terry G, Hughston J, Norwood L: The anatomy of the iliopatellar band and iliotibial tract, Am J Sports Med 14:1, 1986.
10. Bonnarens F, Drez D: Clinical examination of the knee for anterior cruciate ligament laxity. In Jackson D, Drez D, editors: The anterior cruciate deficient knee, St Louis, 1987, Mosby.
11. Hughston J: Acute knee injuries in athletes, Clin Orthop 23:114, 1962.
12. Hughston J, Norwood L: The posterolateral drawer test and external rotational recurvation test for posterolateral rotatory instability of the knee, Clin Orthop 147:82, 1980.
13. Hughston J, Andrews J, Cross M, et al: Classifications of knee ligament instabilities. II. The lateral compartment, J Bone Joint Surg 58:173, 1976.
14. Hughston J: Knee surgery: A philosophy, Phys Ther 60:63, 1980.
15. Hughston J, Barrett G: Acute anteromedial rotatory instability: long term results for surgical repair, J Bone Joint Surg 65:2, 1983.
16. Hughston J, Bowden J, Andrews J, et al: Acute tears of the posterior cruciate ligament: Results of operative treatment, J Bone Joint Surg 62:438, 1980.
17. Blackburn T: Rehabilitation of anterior cruciate ligament injuries, Orthop Clin North Am 16:241, 1985.
18. Montgomery J, Steadman J: Rehabilitation of the injured knee, Clin Sports Med 4:333, 1985.

19. Malone T, Blackburn T, Wallace L: Knee rehabilitation, Phys Ther 66:54, 1980.

20. Paulos L, Noyes F, Grood E, et al: Knee rehabilitation after anterior cruciate ligament reconstruction and repair, Am J Sports Med 9:140, 1981.

21. Paulos L, Payne F, Rosenburg T: Rehabilitation after anterior cruciate ligament surgery. In Jackson D, Drez D, editors: The anterior cruciate deficient knee, St Louis, 1987, Mosby.

22. Noyes F, Torvik P, Hyde W, et al: Biomechanics of ligament failure. II. An analysis of immobilization, exercise, and reconditioning effects in primates, J Bone Joint Surg 56:1406, 1974.

23. Mikkelsen C, Werner S, Eriksson E: Closed kinetic chain alone compared to combined open and closed kinetic chain exercises for quadriceps strengthening after anterior cruciate ligament reconstruction with respect to return to sports: a prospective, matched, follow-up study, Knee Surg Sports Traumatol Arthrosc 8(6):337-342, 2000.

24. Morrissey MC, Hudson ZL, Dreschler WI, et al: Effects of open versus closed kinetic chain training on knee laxity in the early period after anterior cruciate ligament reconstruction, SSTA, Knee Surg Sports Traumatol Arthrosc, 8(6):343-348, 2000.

25. Fleming BC, Oksendahl H, Beynnon B: Open- or closed-kinetic-chain exercises after anterior cruciate ligament reconstruction? Exerc Sport Sci Rev 33(3):134-140, 2005.

26. Beynnon BD, Johnson RJ, Fleming BC, et al: The strain behavior of the anterior cruciate ligament during squatting and active flexion extension: a comparison of an open and a closed kinetic chain exercise, Am J Sports Med 25:823-829, 1997.

27. Cooper DE, Deng XH, Burstein AL, Warren RF: The strength of the central third patellar tendon graft: a biomechanical study, Am J Sports Med 21(6):818-824, 1993.

28. Reed A, Birmingham TB, Stratford PW, et al: Hope testing provides a reliable and valid outcome measure during rehabilitation after anterior cruciate ligament reconstruction, Phys Ther 87(3):337-341, 2007.

SUGGESTED READINGS

Albert M: Eccentric muscle training in sports and orthopaedics, New York, 1991, Churchill Livingstone.

Baker CI, editor: The Hughston Clinic sports medicine book, Baltimore, 1995, Lippincott Williams & Wilkins.

Hughston J: Knee ligaments: injury and repair, St Louis, 1993, Mosby.

Jackson DW, editor: The anterior cruciate deficient knee, St Louis, 1990, Mosby.

Jackson DW: The anterior ligament: current and future concepts, New York, 1993, Raven Press.

Kennedy JC: The injured adolescent knee, Baltimore, 1979, Lippincott Williams & Wilkins.

Scott WN: Ligaments and extensor mechanism of the knee: diagnosis and treatment, St Louis, 1991, Mosby.

22

William Jay Bryan,
Matt Holland,
and Scott Moorhead

Surgery of the Knee and Rehabilitation Principles

The spectrum of differential diagnoses of the knee is significantly broad and demands, of surgeon and therapist alike, an intimate understanding of the anatomy, surgical techniques, and rehabilitation recommendations. This edition emphasizes the need for solid rapport between physician and therapist, as well as profound and consistent consultation of the literature, with an eye toward more recent developments in surgical technique and treatment approaches. We have chosen to present topics according to three broad injury-related areas: (1) sports medicine, (2) traumatic injuries, and (3) degenerative conditions.

A proper course of treatment begins with the physician and hinges on his or her ability to properly evaluate and direct subsequent options. Appropriate mediation of the transition from operative and nonoperative treatment to rehabilitation can ensure optimal care of the patient and ranges from prescribing appropriate analgesia to effectively communicating to the therapist key elements of the surgery, such as the quality of the tissues involved, the techniques used, and the relative success of the procedure. As the therapist assumes increasing prominence in the patient's care and frequently becomes the primary professional touchstone for the patient during recovery, mutual confidence between physician and therapist is critical.

Arguably, the success of professional rehabilitation hinges on the physical therapist's ability to keep the patient engaged and compliant (which can be a rather arduous task). A potent algorithm incorporates a command of current concepts, as well as access to the various weapons in the prepared therapist's arsenal. In recent years a significant increase has occurred in rehabilitative research, especially within the sports medicine realm, which is increasingly leading to evidence-based rehabilitation to promote successful outcomes. Therapists have at their disposal a variety of tools, such as manual muscle testing (MMT), isokinetic exercise and testing, and endurance testing, in addition to a bevy of modalities (e.g., heat and cold, electrical stimulation, cold laser, ultrasound, cooled compression devices, perturbation boards, acupuncture, braces, and of course, proper exercise prescription). Table 22-1 describes

some of the more common therapeutic modalities physical therapists use in the treatment of knee injuries.

ANTERIOR KNEE PAIN

Patellofemoral pain syndrome has become the most common knee condition treated by orthopaedic knee surgeons and sports medicine physical therapists alike. The term *patellofemoral pain syndrome* is indeed vague, and the pain generators may be either strain of the tissue surrounding the patella, acute contusions of patellar and trochlear articular cartilage, or varying degrees of patellar and trochlear articular cartilage breakdown. It is estimated that anterior knee pain will beset anywhere from 7% to 9% of the general population.[1] Because anterior knee pain may be attributable to a multitude of causes (Box 22-1),[1] a proper course of treatment requires understanding all the possibilities. Some of the most common causes are outlined in the following paragraphs.

When faced with constant, nonactivity-related anterior knee pain, the surgeon must consider sympathetic mediated pain, postoperative neuromas, referred radicular pain, and symptom magnification for secondary gain.[1] Sharp, intermittent pain is believed to be the result of loose bodies or unstable articular cartilage pathologic condition. Activity-related pain, on the other hand, could be the result of any number of phenomena: soft tissue overload with patellar malalignment, patellar tendonitis, quadriceps tendonitis, pathologic plica syndrome, fat pad syndrome, iliotibial band syndrome, or early lateral patellar compression syndrome. Posttraumatic chondromalacia patellae or arthrosis may cause articular tissue overload, or it may be the result of degenerative arthrosis from chronic malalignment.

Inflammatory arthritis is also responsible for activity-related pain, as are systemic diseases, which produce weakness, general deconditioning, and increased loads within the knee joint. Thus the therapist should be attuned to a multitude of conditions and approach each rehabilitation patient with a fresh view—irrespective of the referring physician's diagnosis.

Table 22-1   Common Modalities Used in Knee Injury Rehabilitation

Modality	Inflammation	Tendonitis	Bursitis	Pain Control	Muscle Reeducation	Scar Tissue	Joint Restriction
Iontophoresis	X	X	X				
Transcutaneous electrical nerve stimulation (TENS)				X			
Inferential electrical stimulation	X	X	X	X			
Neuromuscular electrical stimulation					X		
Biofeedback					X		
Ultrasound	X	X	X	X		X	
Manual therapy				X		X	X
Cold laser	X	X	X	X		X	

Box 22-1   All Knee Pain is Not a Knee Injury!

In adolescent athletes, hip pathologic condition, such slip capital femoral epiphyses, may present as anterior or deep knee pain. This fact underscores the importance of carrying out a basic hip examination when examining any adolescent athlete with knee pain.

Young athletes who report their kneecaps "slipping," as well as anterior knee pain and a tense effusion from hemarthrosis, may have sustained either a distal femoral metaphyseal Salter fracture or an anterior cruciate ligament (ACL) tear.

CLASSIFYING PATELLOFEMORAL PAIN

Physicians tend to sort patellofemoral problems into two general categories: (1) those accompanying patellar tilt and subluxation versus (2) those involving stable patellae. This is more than an academic division, for it often dictates bracing and surgical approach. Patients—male and female subjects with a generalized ligamentous laxity—often have unstable patellae, which variably tilt and subluxate. When ligamentous laxity syndrome is combined with the natural increased knee valgus in female subjects, the potential for anterior knee pain secondary to patellar instability (leading to a proclivity for patellar dislocation) increases significantly. Physicians include information from knee radiographs—particularly patellar sunrise and merchant views—and the powerful cartilage-imaging information from magnetic resonance imaging (MRI) scans to direct physical therapy care.

Unstable Patellae: Research

Studies have demonstrated that patients with patellar tilt and subluxation must be evaluated for entities such as increased Q angle, whereupon extreme cases may only do well with consideration of proximal and distal realignment procedures or with medial augmentation. Patients with normal Q angles and symptomatic patellar tilt and subluxation—either because of ligamentous laxity syndrome or history of recurrent patellar subluxation and dislocation—are considered candidates for medial patellofemoral ligament (MPFL) reconstruction. When either MRI or arthroscopic examination reveals significant patellofemoral chondromalacia, a series of joint fluid therapy injections may precede physical therapy. In younger patients with defined patellar or trochlear cartilage defects, trials have

been undertaken with autologous cartilage inserts. These types of procedures have been compared against both microfracture and osteochondral autograft transfer (OATS) procedures, with no general agreement as to the superior surgical approach.

Ligamentous Laxity

Patients with defined patellar tilt and subluxation must be examined for generalized ligamentous laxity. In such cases, stretching plays a minor role in rehabilitation. If the patella demonstrates increased lateral mobility with the ability to recenter the patella, then McConnell taping may be considered. As we mentioned, a variety of patella-stabilizing braces have evolved and may be used in substitution of McConnell taping. The role of these modalities is to mediate patellofemoral pain while allowing the patient to participate in exercises to improve quadriceps and vastus medialis oblique (VMO) strength.[2] Patients with rigid patellar tilt and subluxation more than likely have an increased Q angle; although rehabilitation may decrease their discomfort, lofty athletic goals may be difficult unless surgical realignment procedures are considered where conservative treatment fails. Patients who undergo proximal and distal realignment procedures will present rehab challenges as initial strengthening activities are limited because of pain.

Bracing

A wide variety of patellofemoral braces exist when dealing with those patients who demonstrate (either clinically or on MRI scan) patellar tilt and subluxation. The theory of these braces is to decrease pain by retracking patellar alignment. Powers et al.[3] evaluated a simple elastic sleeve during which time MRI

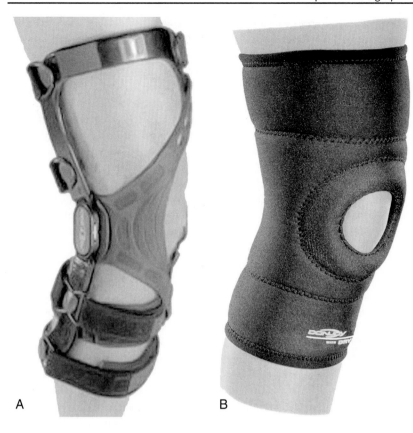

A   B

Figure 22-1 Examples of patella-stabilizing braces manufactured by DonJoy.

scans were taken with and without a patellofemoral joint brace. They concluded that there were no significant differences in medial-lateral patellar displacement or in patellar tilt between the braced and nonbraced conditions at all knee flexion angles.[3] Of course, since the 1999 study, more sophisticated patella femoral braces have appeared (Figure 22-1).

In 2004, Powers et al.[4] conducted a new study of dynamic patella femoral braces. MRI scan showed that these braces would increase total patellofemoral joint contact area between 21% to 24% when compared with the no brace condition. The conclusions were that large changes in pain in the contact area occur without sizable changes in patellar alignment, but the braces were indeed effective because patients enjoyed 44% to 50% reduction in knee symptoms while in the braces.[4] The use of taping or bracing in patients during exercise may promote a decrease in quadriceps inhibition because of pain; it also allows the patient to better perform exercises during physical therapy treatments or home exercises.

CORE STRENGTHENING TO IMPROVE KNEE OUTCOMES IN PATIENTS WITH STABLE PATELLAE

Many patients come to the physical therapist without the defined evidence of patellar tilt and subluxation or physical disruption of articular cartilage. In cases in which no anatomic abnormalities have been identified, the physical therapist must always start with core strengthening. Several studies have demonstrated that a weak gluteus medius muscle will promote

functional valgus knee collapse and secondary anterior knee pain. To effectively treat patellofemoral pain, the therapist must thoroughly evaluate the entire kinetic chain, including the foot and ankle, for excessive pronation, as well as hip abduction and external rotation strength. Initial patellofemoral pain syndrome regimens must strive to increase neuromuscular function, while decreasing stresses on both the soft tissues about the patella and the patellar trochlear cartilage. This generally means short arc quadriceps work, which may then evolve to more aggressive range of motion and closed chain exercises as symptoms decrease. Functional and plyometric exercises should begin only after all basic programs are well tolerated, and as quadriceps, hip, and core strength allow the patient to control functional knee valgus.

Finally, every effort should be made to maintain leg strength throughout all phases of rehabilitation. Patients with defined chondromalacia patella must be confined to short arc quadriceps work for several weeks to months based on physician recommendations; generally a series of joint fluid therapy injections is also in order. By and large, patient comfort is the guide to increasing activity level, although more often, physicians will also obtain follow-up MRI scans to measure articular cartilage healing.

Surgically Retracking the Patella by Medial Patellofemoral Ligament Reconstruction

Historically, surgeons seeking to improve patellar tracking have experimented with a number of procedures. Until recently, a simple arthroscopic lateral release was popular, but minimal gains from such procedures have dampened surgeon enthusiasm. The failure of isolated arthroscopic lateral retinacular releases to garner improvements under conditions beyond the activities of daily living (ADL) has given rise to new interest in retracking the patella by reconstructing the sometimes-compromised MPFL. In cases of single or repetitive patellar dislocation, the MPFL is often deficient and clearly deserves reconstruction. When dealing with tilt and subluxation, lateral release frequently accompanies MPFL reconstruction. Patellofemoral arthrosis—not easily treated, even with patellofemoral prosthetic replacement—also can be significantly improved with a lateral retinacular release and MPFL reconstruction. Table 22-2 summarizes the rehabilitation program for patients with MPFL reconstructions.

Patellar Tendinopathy (Jumper's Knee)

Patellar tendonitis (jumper's knee) is a chronic and often disabling condition for young and old athletes. Repetitive strain creates recurring microtears, which heal with less than ideal collagen and scar tissue. Plyometric exercises are to be avoided, whereas short arc quadriceps work should be the initial rehabilitation effort. Jumper's knee has significant prevalence in sports characterized by high demands on leg extensor speed and power, such as basketball, soccer, volleyball, and track and field events, where as many as 50% of participants are affected. Studies have shown that eccentric quadriceps strengthening can be beneficial and well tolerated. Research has centered on the use of nitrous oxide–producing nitrates, which seem to reduce the chronic inflammatory response seen in patellar tendonitis. Recalcitrant cases may come to surgery, in which open resection of inflamed granulomatous tissue has given rise to arthroscopic approaches where offending tissue and distal patellar bone is resected.

The pathogenesis of acute and chronic patellar tendon pain is under active investigation. It seems to be best described as a combination of tendon degeneration with overlying inflammation. Active rest from activity will always remain the center point for treating patellar tendinopathy, whereas the use of modalities are meant to facilitate tissue healing and recovery and allow patients to participate more in a rehabilitative program, as opposed to speeding a "return to play."

In a landmark 1986 study, Stanish et al.[5] showed that eccentric training was a vital part of their patellar tendinopathy treatment program. Eccentric drop squats were key; when training became pain free, the load was increased by adding weight and increasing the speed of the eccentric phase. Alfredson et al.[6] published their paper on Achilles tendinopathy and differed from the Kerwin and Stanish approach by progressing treatment in adding load (but not speed). Patients were instructed to exercise despite pain during the eccentric motion.

Visnes and Bahr[7] also published an excellent review on the use of eccentric training to treat patellar tendinopathy. These Norwegian authors concluded that although most studies included eccentric training for a positive patellar tendinopathy treatment effect, it remained to prove which type of eccentric protocol was responsible for the observed effects. All successful programs reviewed included a decline board (Figure 22-2) and allowed for some level of discomfort. Removing athletes from sports activities during treatment was common to all programs.

Crossley et al.[8] has recently reviewed the clinical features of patellar tendinopathy and their implications for rehabilitation, showing that the pathogenesis of patellar tendinopathy develops from the interplay of both extrinsic and intrinsic factors. The extrinsic factor, simply put, is mechanical overload, and it can be directly controlled during rehabilitation. It must be noted, however, that the presence of patellar tendinopathy is not consistent across individuals exposed to equivalent loading levels, suggesting that intrinsic factors also contribute. This exhaustive study of patients with patellar tendonitis showed that the therapist would do well to increase thigh flexibility, because decreased thigh flexibility correlated with increased incidence of patellar tendonitis.[8] Leg length discrepancy was also factorial, whereupon an appropriate heel and sole lift should be instituted. Neither arch height nor ankle dorsiflexion parameters have any significance. The negative correlative

Table 22-2	Rehabilitation Guidelines for MPFL Reconstruction	
Timeline	**Guidelines**	
Considerations	Limit flexion to less than 90 degrees during first 4 weeks, then gradually increase	
	Maintain patellar mobility throughout program	
	Continue to build quadriceps strength, especially vastus medialis oblique (VMO)	
Phase 1: Weeks 1 to 2	Quadriceps sets	
	Straight-leg raises	
	Patella glides	
	Weight bear as tolerated, limit flexion to 0 to 70 degrees	
	Hip abduction and adduction	
	Begin working on gastrocnemius strengthening	
Phase 2: Weeks 3 to 4	Closed chain work from 0 to 60 degrees	
	Step-ups	
	Iliotibial band stretching	
	Begin hip abduction at week 4 (i.e., Thera-Band sidestepping)	
	Begin proprioceptive training with balance board at week 4	
Phase 3: Weeks 5 to 6	Closed chain work from 0 to 90 degrees	
	General strength program	
	Hamstring exercises	
	Multihip exercises	
	Heel raises	
	Lunges	
	Squats, lunges, and leg presses from 0 to 90 degrees	
	Patient may be able to begin riding exercise bike but must have at least 110-degrees flexion	
Phase 4: Week 12	Begin jogging	
Phase 5: Week 16	Begin jumping and other plyometric exercises	

MPFL, Medial patellofemoral ligament.

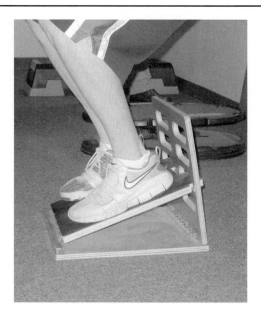

Figure 22-2 A decline board.

results should prove instructive, because wasting time on foot orthotic devices or ankle-stretching exercises appear to be of no avail in this patient population.[8]

PATELLAR TENDON RUPTURE

Patellar tendon rupture is a disabling injury that is most commonly seen in patients under 40 years old who participate in athletic activities demanding violent quadriceps muscle contraction in a flexed knee position. The prognosis after a patellar tendon rupture depends in large part on the interval between the injury and repair. Surgery soon after injury is recommended for optimal results. Most surgeons will reapproximate the ruptured tendon ends, carefully repair any associated medial and lateral retinacular tears, and most importantly, place a reinforcing cerclage suture, which may be either metal wire or high-tech suture, such as FiberWire. Postsurgical care involves the use of a hinged variable locked brace, progressive weight bearing, and immediate attention to controlled quadriceps strengthening. The tensile strength of the repair progresses in a linear fashion, such that between 8 to 12 weeks, both the intensity and the frequency of extensor-strengthening activities may be progressively expanded.

 Patellar Tendon Rupture Case Study

History

The patient is a 30-year-old man who was playing basketball on Feb 22, 2007. During initial push-off for an explosive jump, the patient heard and felt a loud pop, followed by the left knee giving way; the patient fell to the floor. The patella was observed to be sitting in the distal portion of the thigh, about 4 inches above its normal resting position.

Prior Medical History

The patient had a history of bilateral Osgood-Schlatter disease in his teenage years and a prior patellar tendon rupture and repair on the right knee in March of 2004.

Surgery

The patient underwent surgical repair for a complete patellar tendon rupture on February 27, 2007, with repair using four limbs of FiberWire sutures, as well as repair of the lateral retinaculum (Figure 22-3).

Diagnostic classification: Impaired Joint Mobility, Motor Function, Muscle Performance, and Range of Motion Associated with Bony or Soft Tissue Surgery, (4I)

Rehabilitation Considerations for Patellar Tendon Repair

- Week 0 to 2: Nonweight bearing with postoperative brace locked at 0 degrees. Full extension and no exercise to be done.

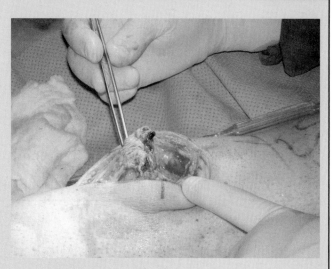

Figure 22-3 Exposure of the lateral retinaculum.

- Week 2: Touchdown weight bearing. Brace locked at 0 degrees. Begin heel slides to 30 degrees of flexion and initiate quadriceps sets and straight-leg raises in four planes with brace on
- Week 3: 25% Weight bearing allowed with brace opened to 30 degrees. Flexion. Heel slides to 60 degrees. Continue with quadriceps sets and straight-leg raises.

Continued

Patellar Tendon Rupture Case Study—cont'd

- Week 4: 50% Weight-bearing brace open to 60 degrees, and range of motion allowed to 90 degrees of flexion. Add patellar mobs and scar massage, especially in this case, with lateral retinacular repair. Begin multihip weight machine for hip strengthening.
- Week 5: 50% Weight-bearing brace open to 90 degrees and range of motion progression to 120 degrees of flexion. Begin light closed chain leg press within weight-bearing restrictions and wall slides for further range of motion gains.
- Week 6: 75% Weight-bearing brace open to 120 degrees. Work toward full range of motion of flexion, and continue with leg extension strengthening exercises.
- Week 7: Full weight bearing, brace unlocked, and continue with strength work. Begin step-ups forward and lateral. Gait training, and begin work on neuromuscular and proprioceptive exercises (Figure 22-4).

- Week 8: Discharge crutches. Begin hamstring strengthening and continued quadriceps strengthening.
- Weeks 8 to 12: Progression of leg extension strength and balance work to promote return to higher-level activity.
- Week 12 to 16: Begin light running when normal strength of the extensor mechanism and leg extension has returned to normal.
- Week 20: May begin jump program including Sportsmetrics.
- 6 to 9 months after surgery: Return to sports.

The patient had no complications during rehabilitation and performed exercises 5 days a week initially; as strength program progressed, the patient continued with three times per week. The patient did not return to basketball (because of having bilateral patellar tendon ruptures playing basketball), but in October of 2007 he returned to playing recreational soccer 8 months after surgery.

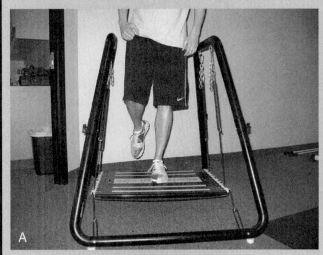
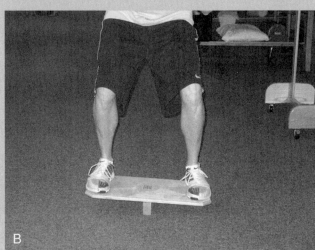

Figure 22-4 The patient conducting proprioceptive exercises 7 weeks after surgery.

ANTERIOR CRUCIATE LIGAMENT INJURIES

Rehabilitation after anterior cruciate ligament (ACL) reconstruction has significantly evolved over the last 30 years. Numerous studies show that rehabilitation protocols of the past 20+ years, which promoted immobilization for 6 weeks or longer (although inflammation diminished and the graft healed), have proven to be detrimental to the ACL-reconstructed patient's success. Numerous animal model studies have demonstrated adverse effects of immobilization, including subsequent problems with articular cartilage, ligaments, capsular structures, musculature, and osteopenic changes of the surrounding bony structures.[9-12]

With the advancement of surgical techniques, graft fixation, and graft choices, as well as a better understanding of the biology and biomechanics of the knee, clinicians can promote early stress and earlier range of motion, in addition to weight bearing on the reconstructed knee, with the goal of returning the patient back to complete level of function in as short a time as possible. Tellingly, debate still arises as to whether ACL reconstruction needs to be performed in every patient with an ACL tear. Agberg et al.[13] recently provided data with a 15-year follow-up in patients with a unilateral nonreconstructed ACL injury treated with rehabilitation and activity modification. Patients were followed at 1, 3, and 15 years after injury. Of the initial 100 consecutive patients who were observed at the

15-year follow-up, 67 (or 71%) continued with the unilateral nonreconstructed ACL injury, whereas 22 (or 23%) had undergone ACL reconstruction. The remaining 11 subjects did not attend the assessment of neurovascular function at the 15-year follow-up. Their results show that a majority (69% to 85%) of the patients at the 15-year follow-up had good functional performance and knee muscle strength. However, all these injuries were of nonprofessional, recreational, or competitive activity level patients, and they were advised to modify activity level, especially by avoiding contact sports. These patients also had no significant meniscal injuries at the time of evaluation. Thus patients who are younger, more competitive, playing on a professional level, or who are unwilling to modify their activities would likely fare differently from this cohort.

With recent advances in ACL reconstruction surgical techniques, from open to arthroscopic to "all inside" one incision techniques, comes significant progress in graft fixation, and many options are available to today's orthopaedic surgeons. Additionally, the types of graft available are numerous, with the pendulum swinging from a several autograft choices to increasing patient and physician preference for allograft (cadaver) tissue. Autograft choices include the gold standard bone-patellar tendon-bone graft, as well as quadriceps and hamstring tendon autografts. Allograft choices include posterior and anterior tibialis tendons, bone-patellar tendon-bone, and Achilles tendon.

The advantages of allograft tissue can be significant. Among others, they include decreased morbidity from harvest site, preservation of extensor and flexor mechanisms, decreased operative time, generally large availability of graft sources, and improved cosmetic appearance. However, potential disadvantages or concerns do arise with the risk of infection (although extremely low, some showing rates of perhaps 1 in 1.5 million), remodeling of the graft, higher costs of the graft, alteration of graft structural properties because of sterilization and storage procedures, and slow and possibly incomplete incorporation of the graft. These concerns continue to inspire debate among surgeons regarding graft superiority.

The literature shows support on both sides. Shino et al.[14] showed that allograft tissue corrected anterior laxity better than autograft tissue in knees undergoing ACL reconstruction. Conversely, Victor et al.[15] conducted an evaluation of a series of allografts compared with autografts, finding that anterior laxity was increased in the allograft group. Significant data show slower incorporation of soft tissue grafts versus bony grafts, but whether this should change postoperative rehabilitation or limitations is in controversy (Table 22-3).

To illustrate, Friedman et al.[16] performed a metaanalysis of 21 studies and reported a significantly lower rate of failures in patellar tendon autograft versus hamstring tendon autograft. This team used a KT-1000 arthrometer and pivot shift testing to measure laxity between the two groups. A higher proportion (79%) of the patellar tendon group had a side-to-side difference of less than 3 mm, compared with the hamstring group (74%). The patellar group also demonstrated a higher incidence of anterior knee pain (17.4% compared with 11.5% in the hamstring group).

Table 22-3	Biomechanical Properties of Selected ACL Graft Tissues		
Tissue	Ultimate tensile load (N)	Stiffness (N/mm)	Cross-Sectional Area (mm²)
Intact ACL	2160	242	44
Bone-patellar tendon-bone (10 mm)	2977	620	35
Quadruple hamstring	4090	776	53
Quadriceps tendon (10 mm)	2352	463	62

ACL, Anterior cruciate ligament.
From West RV, Harner C: Graft selection in anterior cruciate ligament reconstruction, Am Acad Orthop Surg 13(3):197-207, 2005.

Double Bundle

Double-bundle ACL reconstruction has also generated interest. This has been ongoing in European countries for some time and continues to gain favor with physicians in the United States. Obvious anatomic correlation exists, because the natural presentation of the two-bundled ACL consists of anteromedial and posterolateral strands. Traditional ACL reconstruction is used to mainly reproduce the anteromedial bundle, which does provide excellent stability with anterior-posterior translation; however, there continues to be some rotational factor that is more adequately controlled by the posterolateral bundle. Importantly, numerous studies have shown a continued rotatory deficiency with traditional single-bundle ACL reconstruction, particularly if graft placement is not in anatomic position.[17-20] Accordingly, long-term follow-up of those patients invested with the double-bundle technique remains an important future step in the orthopaedics field.

As it now stands, rehabilitation after double-bundle ACL reconstruction is similar to single-bundle ACL, with the overall goal to restore more normal kinematics in regards to anterior-posterior translation while controlling rotatory motion.

Return to Sports

Return to sports is always at the forefront of athletes' minds after ACL reconstruction. Certainly differences exist with respect to the patient's injury, concomitant injuries, reconstruction techniques, graft choices and fixation devices, as well as surgeon experience and skill. These considerations, again, must be reviewed thoroughly by the surgeon and therapist. As each situation may be unique, however, certain guidelines have been developed. Noyes et al.[21] developed a battery of functional tests, consisting of a single-leg hop for distance, a triple hop for distance, a crossover hop for distance, and a 6 m timed hop. Subsequent independent testing showed good reliability and reproducibility for this combination of tests. Other important clinical criteria are listed in Table 22-4.

Table 22-4	Criteria for Return to Sports

Test	Range
Full range of motion	
KT1000 side-to-side difference	<3 mm
Quadriceps strength	85% or greater compared with contralateral side
Hamstring strength	100% of contralateral side
Hamstring-to-quadriceps strength ratio	70% or greater
Functional testing	85% or greater compared with contralateral side

From DeLee JC, Drez D: Delee and Drez's orthopaedic sports medicine: principles and practice, ed 2, Philadelphia, 2003, Saunders.

Table 22-5	Factors That Can Cause Limitation of Knee Motion After ACL Reconstruction

Surgical	Inappropriate graft placement/tensioning
	Acute surgery on a swollen knee
	Concomitant medical collateral ligament repair
Medical	Arthrofibrosis, intrapatellar contracture syndrome, and patella infera
	Cyclops syndrome
	Reflex sympathetic dystrophy
Rehabilitative	Poorly supervised or poorly designed rehabilitation program, prolonged immobilization

From Shelbourne KD, Patel DV: Treatment of limited motion after anterior cruciate ligament reconstruction, Knee Surg Sports Traumatol Arthrosc 7(2):85-92, 1999.
ACL, Anterior cruciate ligament.

Pain and Swelling

Pain and swelling are common after most surgical interventions, especially with the invasiveness of ACL reconstructions, which can be variable per patient, technique, and graft used. However, certain modalities are common in controlling these postoperatively, including cryotherapy, compressive wraps, elevation, and antiinflammatory agent (as well as narcotic agent) use in the immediate postoperative period. Use of cryotherapy has been shown to decrease some subjective pain scores, reducing the need for analgesia.[22] The addition of immediate motion has also improved postoperative rehabilitation. In contrast to early years of rehabilitation, in which the knee was immobilized or even placed in a cylinder cast for 5 to 6 weeks, there appears to be a more reasonable consensus now that early motion is more conducive to graft healing and more rapid return to function. Although the surgeon should obtain full motion before leaving the operating suite, postoperatively it is up to the rehabilitation team (which includes the patient) to institute and commence motion-restoring measures. Occasionally, these can be augmented with the use of a continuous passive motion (CPM) machine; however, in light of advances in arthroscopic reconstruction techniques and accelerated rehabilitation, CPM machines have fallen out of favor somewhat in the standard primary ACL reconstruction protocol. It is worth mentioning that fears of causing increased laxity in the graft or decreased incorporation of the graft by encouraging early motion have been allayed by numerous studies that do not support this theory. The benefits of increasing early range of motion significantly outweigh these fears and lead to reductions in pain, lessen adverse changes in articular cartilage, and help to prevent scarring and capsular contractures (Table 22-5).

Immediate versus Delayed Weight Bearing

Historically, concerns about graft fixation and development of graft laxity led physicians to keep patients from early weight bearing after ACL reconstruction. Advantages of early weight bearing have been shown to improve cartilage nutrition and decrease disuse osteopenia. In randomized, controlled trials by

Tyler et al.,[23] comparisons were made between rehabilitation with nonweight bearing for 2 weeks versus immediate weight bearing. They found no evidence of increased range of motion of the knee, VMO function, or anterior-posterior knee laxity. However, those patients treated with immediate weight bearing showed significant decrease in anterior knee pain, from 35% in the nonweight-bearing patients down to 8% in immediate weight-bearing patients. Thus with no evidence of detrimental effects on the ACL reconstruction or graft and the indication of decreased anterior knee pain, full immediate weight bearing has been safely recommended. In 2005, Beynnon et al.[24] published level-one evidence findings on patients randomized to one of two postoperative ACL rehabilitation programs: one "accelerated" and the other "nonaccelerated." The two programs consisted of identical goals, restrictions, exercises, and activities but initiated these benchmarks at different times during the follow-up. The accelerated group performed tasks anywhere from 1 to 6 weeks before the nonaccelerated group. The study revealed no significant difference at 2 years in the increase of anterior knee laxity relative to baseline values obtained immediately after surgery between the two groups. In fact, the accelerated group experienced less anterior laxity at 2 years than the nonaccelerated cohort. Moreover, the groups were similar in terms of clinical assessment, patient satisfaction, activity level, and function (Table 22-6).

Open versus Closed Chain Exercises

Debate ensues in regards to open versus closed chain exercises after ACL construction. Some argue that closed kinetic chain exercises can provide more compression forces across the knee while activating the hamstring muscle group. These two factors could possibly decrease anterior shear forces in the knee that might otherwise be taken up by the reconstructed ACL. In a prospective, randomized controlled trial by Bynum et al.,[25] patients were randomly selected into either open or closed kinetic chain rehabilitation programs with follow-up measurements at 1 year after surgery. The subjects in the closed kinetic

Table 22-6 Accelerated and Nonaccelerated Rehabilitation Protocols

	Accelerated Protocols	Nonaccelerated Protocols
Rehabilitation Goals		
Range of Motion		
0 to 70 degrees	Week 1	Week 2 to 3
0 to 90 degrees	Week 2	Week 4
0 to 120 degrees	Week 3	Week 6
Full range of motion	Week 4	Week 8
Weight bearing		
Toe touch	Week 1	Week 1
Partial (with toe touch only using crutches)		Week 2 to 3
Full, no crutches	Week 2	Week 4
Restrictions		
Brace		
Locked at 0 degrees		Week 1
0 to 70 degrees	Week 1	Week 2 to 3
0 to 90 degrees	Week 2	Week 4
Wean from brace	Week 2 to 6	Week 4 to 6
Crutch use	Week 1 to 3	Week 1 to 4
Sports	Possible 24 weeks	Possible 32 weeks
Protocol exercises		
Open Kinetic Chain		
Quadriceps sets 0 degrees	Week 1 to 4	Week 1 to 7
Cocontraction Quadriceps/Hamstrings		
At 0 degrees	Week 1	Week 1
At 30 degrees	Week 2 to 4	Week 2 to 4
Patella mobilization	Week 2 to 7	Week 2 to 7
Partial leg extension, 45 to 70 degrees	N/A*	Week 2 to 3
Partial leg extension, 45 to 90 degrees	Week 2 to 4	Week 4 to 11
Full knee extension, 0 to 90 degrees	Week 6 to end	Week 12 to end
Short arc quadriceps, 0 to 30 degrees	Week 5 to end	Week 12 to end
Straight-Leg Raise	Week 2 to end	Week 12 to end
Isotonic Hip Exercise		
Flexion	Week 2 to end	Week 4 to end
Extension	Week 2 to end	Week 2 to end
Abduction	Week 2 to end	Week 2 to end
Adduction	Week 2 to end	Week 2 to end
Closed kinetic chain		
Partial squats, 45 to 90 degrees with body weight	Week 6 to 8	Week 8 to 11
Squats 0 to 90 degrees with weight	Week 8	Week 12
Wall slides to 70 degrees	Week 6 to end	Week 8 to end
Sport cord forward/backward single line	Week 5	Week 8
Sport cord lunges	Week 12	Week 12
Sport cord step-ups	Week 6	Week 12
Step-ups	Week 6	Week 12
Toe raises	Week 5	Week 5
Functional Activities		
Stationary Bike		
No resistance, 120 rpm	Week 3	Week 3
Low resistance, 90 rpm	Week 5	Week 5
Moderate resistance, 60 to 90 rpm	Week 8	Week 8
Upper-extremity weight program	Week 3	Week 3
Swimming, upper extremity only	N/A	Week 3

Continued

Table 22-6   Accelerated and Nonaccelerated Rehabilitation Protocols—cont'd

	Accelerated Protocols	Nonaccelerated Protocols
Swimming with flutter kick	Week 2	Week 4
Stair-climbing machine	Week 5	Week 8
Cross-country skiing machine	Week 8	Week 8
Bike outdoors	Week 8	Week 12
Jog on flat surface	Week 8	Week 12
Sport-Specific		
Drills		
Lateral shuffles and backward run	Week 12	Week 12
Figure-eight runs	Week 16	Week 24
Jumping rope	Week 12	Week 12
Plyometric exercises	Week 16	Week 24

From Beynnon BD, Uh BS, Johnson RJ, et al: Rehabilitation after anterior cruciate ligament reconstruction: a prospective, randomized double-blind comparison of programs administered over 2 different time intervals, Am J Sports Med 33(3):347-359, 2005.
*N/A, Not applicable; *rpm*, revolution per minute.

chain group had KT-1000 measurements that were closer to normal, in addition to less anterior knee pain, earlier return to normal activities, and greater satisfaction compared with the open chain group. Closed chain kinetic exercise appears to be more in favor, because multiple authors have found open kinetic chain exercises to have more anterior tibial translation compared with closed kinetic chain exercises (in side-to-side comparisons). This is generally more evident in the lower degrees of flexion from 0 to 60 degrees.[26,27]

Patellofemoral joint problems are important to consider when comparing open and closed kinetic chain exercises. Closed chain exercises place lower stress on the patellofemoral joint at lower flexion angles, whereas open chain quadriceps exercises place a higher stress on the patellofemoral joint at lower flexion angles. Thus open chain quadriceps exercises should be avoided or reduced with patellofemoral symptoms, particularly if a patient is already experiencing these, which can interfere with progression of therapy. Recently, Gerber et al.[28] implemented eccentric resistance training to induce considerable gains in muscle size and strength to allow further benefit of postoperative rehabilitation. In their study, 40 patients were divided into two groups of 20 each. Both groups completed 2 to 3 weeks of phase-one exercises focused on controlling pain and effusion, regaining range of motion, and obtaining basic quadriceps function. Beginning 3 weeks after surgery, one group began an eccentric exercise program for 12 weeks, consisting of progressing negative work using one of two recumbent eccentric ergometers. They evaluated changes in muscle structure with MRI of the involved and uninvolved thighs, both before and after training. The volume in peak cross-sectional areas of the quadriceps, hamstrings, and gracilis in proportion to the gluteus maximus were calculated from these images. These volumes increased significantly with both the eccentric and the standard rehabilitation programs; however, the increases in quadriceps volume and peak cross-sectional area were significantly greater, by more than two thirds, in the eccentric group. The conclusion was that progressive, eccentric resistance exercise can induce changes in the

structure of the quadriceps and gluteus maximus by more than twofold, or it can greatly exceed (by more than twofold) those changes after an institutional standard rehabilitation program. Arguably, this may be ideal for mitigating the persistent muscle impairments commonly observed after ACL reconstruction.

Bracing

The rationale for using postoperative bracing in ACL reconstruction continues to be somewhat controversial. Two main types of bracing are available: (1) the rehabilitation brace and (2) the functional brace. The immediate postoperative period uses a rehabilitation brace, which is thought to protect the ACL reconstruction and/or donor site while range of motion, weight bearing, and muscle activity are initiated. Once the patient has regained full motion, is able to bear weight without difficulty, and has regained some muscle control, the rehabilitation brace is generally discontinued. Functional bracing is generally used further along into rehabilitation or to facilitate a return to sports. Although no adequate long-term studies have shown the benefits of bracing, a recent study of orthopaedic surgeons in 2003 showed that in a survey of the American Orthopaedic Society of Sports Medicine, 87% of respondents always or sometimes continued to brace the ACL reconstructed knee.[29] Wright et al.[30] conducted a systematic review of level-one evidence of 12 randomized controlled trials to determine if appropriate evidence existed to support bracing. In their review, they discussed each of the randomized controlled trials, and they found that the evidence does not demonstrate improved range of motion, decreased pain, improved graft stability, or decreased incidence of reinjury among the braced cohort compared with the nonbraced control groups. Thus they concluded use of these functional braces is not supported by currently available evidence. However, Fleming et al.[31] evaluated a particular brace (Legend, DJ Ortho) and showed a significant reduction in strain values compared with the nonbraced group for anterior shear load up to 130 N in nonweight-bearing and weight-bearing conditions. They also evaluated internal tibial torque up to 9 N/mm strained in a braced knee; this was significantly less than the nonbraced knee when the knee was nonweight bearing only. However, the brace did not reduce strain values when the knee was subjected to external torques or varus and valgus moments in the weight-bearing and nonweight-bearing knees. This study concludes that a brace can provide some protection to the ACL-ACL graft under those specific loading conditions. (Although the directions of loading used are known to injure the ACL, the loads that were tested were well below those that cause injury or that the athlete might experience during sport.) In any case, care must be taken to differentiate this population from others, because those with concomitant ligamentous or meniscal repair may require a different course of care.

The question of whether patients engaged in high-demand activities deserve prophylactic or protective bracing continues to stoke debate. Sterett et al.[32] specifically addressed injuries in skiers with ACL reconstruction. In an evaluation of 257 skier employees with ACL reconstruction that wore braces compared with 563 skier employees with ACL reconstruction that did not, they found that nonbraced skiers were 2.74 times more likely to suffer subsequent injury than were braced skiers.[32] Because of the increased risk of reinjury in nonbraced skiers, the authors recommend functional bracing for skiers with ACL reconstruction. It is reasonable to question whether one could extrapolate the results of this study to apply to other patients engaged in aggressive, high-demand activity. Regardless, communication between the physical therapist and the orthopaedic surgeon remains paramount to determine the length of time that the brace is needed, goals that need to be obtained before advancing or graduating out of the brace, and the individual preferences of the orthopaedic surgeon involved. Most importantly, expectations for what the brace will allow the patient to do and not do must be clear from the beginning. Many patients view bracing as an infallible panacea for injury and reinjury, and this is clearly not the case.

Gender issues continue to play a role in ACL injuries. Female subjects experience ACL tears more frequently than male subjects, with an incidence rate between 2.4 and 9.7 times greater than that of male athletes competing in similar activities. Potential reasons for the greater frequency of ACL tears in women include a smaller intercondylar notch, generalized joint laxity, higher body mass index (BMI), hormonal fluctuations, and altered neuromuscular firing patterns. Female subjects, both adult and children, also have higher knee valgus angles and moments during the variety of cutting, landing, and squatting tasks.[33-35] Other findings show female subjects demonstrate decreased hip flexion, as well as knee flexion stiffness during cutting tasks. In addition, evidence indicates that hip adduction angles during a variety of activities are greater in female subjects and are positively related to knee valgus angles.[36-38] Some of these factors can be found in Table 22-7. Increasing evidence suggests that core and trunk strengthening will significantly help with female ACL rehabilitation in all patients. Further specific training programs have been thoroughly evaluated and scientifically proven to decrease serious

Table 22-7	Factors to Consider in ACL Rehabilitation of the Female Athlete	
Factor	**Rehabilitation**
Female subjects exhibit wider pelvis and increased genu valgum	Dynamic control of valgus moment at knee joint
Female athletes recruit quadriceps muscle to stabilize knee	Retrain neuromuscular pattern for female athlete to use hamstrings
Female subjects generate muscular force more slowly than male subjects	Train for fast speeds and reaction timing
Jumping athletes lose hip control on landing	Train hip and trunk control
Less-developed thigh musculature	Train hip musculature to assist in stabilization
Genu recurvatum and increased knee laxity	Train athlete to control knee extension (stability position)
Exhibit less-effective dynamic stabilization	Enhance neuromuscular control and protective pattern reflexes
Poorer muscular endurance rates	Train female athlete to enhance muscular endurance

From Wilk KE, Arrigo C, Andrews Jr, et al: Rehabilitation after anterior cruciate ligament reconstruction in the female athlete, J Athl Train 34:177-193, 1999.
ACL, Anterior cruciate ligament.

knee ligament injury in the female athlete (Table 22-8). In particular, Sportsmetrics developed by Cincinnati Sports Medicine, is a plyometric-type training program designed to teach the athlete to preposition the entire body safely when accelerating (jumping) or decelerating (landing). The program uses a series of jumping and complex multidirectional motions. These help provide neuromuscular retraining and reeducation. Therefore at the completion of the program, acceleration, deceleration, and multidirectional movements are safely programmed into the body to establish a foundation of strength, coordination, and overall physical conditioning to help prevent injury.

Neuromuscular electrical stimulation and volitional muscle contractions also have been thoroughly evaluated. Consensus now shows that patients who undergo neuromuscular electrical stimulation and biofeedback combined with volitional exercises achieve more normal gait parameters and better restoration of extensor strength compared with rehabilitation with volitional exercises alone. Schneider-Mackler et al.[39] showed this in a randomized controlled trial of rehabilitation after ACL reconstruction using electrical stimulation and volitional exercises in combination therapy versus volitional exercises alone. They found that patients who underwent the combined therapy had more normal gait parameters and stronger quadriceps muscles compared with patients who underwent volitional exercises alone.

Studies have also indicated that balance, coordination, and perturbation training is vital in the rehabilitation of ACL injuries. Floyd et al.[40] demonstrated that stability and balance

Table 22-8   ACL Rehabilitation in Women: Eight Special Considerations and Specific Exercise Drills

Considerations	Exercise Drills
Hip musculature to stabilize knee	Lateral step-overs (regular, fast, very slow)
	Step-overs with ball catches
	Step-overs with rotation
	Lateral step-ups on foam
	Dip walk
	Squats (foam) (Balance Master)
	Front diagonal lunges onto foam
Retrain neuromuscular pattern hamstring control	Lateral lunges straight
	Lateral lunges
	Lateral lunges with rotation
	Lateral lunges onto foam
	Lateral lunges with ball catches
	Squats unstable pattern
	Lateral lunges jumping
	Lateral unstable pattern
	Coactivation balance through biofeedback
	Slide board
	Fitter (Fitter International, Calgary, Alberta, Canada)
Control valgus movement	Front step-downs
	Lateral step-ups with Thera-Band (The Hygienic Corporation, Akron, OH)
	Tilt board balance throws
Control hyperextension	Plyometric leg press
	Plyometric leg press with four corners
	Plyometric jumps
	• One box
	• Two boxes
	• Four boxes
	Three boxes rotation
	Four boxes with catches
	Bounding drills
	Forward and backward step-over drills
High-speed training, especially hamstrings	Isokinetic exercises
	Backward lunging
	Shuttle
	Lateral lunges (fast jumps)
	Resistance tubing for hamstring
	Backward running
Neuromuscular reaction	Squats on tilt board
	Balance beam with cords
	Dip walk with cords
	Balance throws
	Balance throws perturbations
	Lateral lunges with perturbations onto tilt board
Less-developed thigh musculature	Knee extensor and flexor-strengthening exercises
	Squats
	Leg press
	Wall squats
	Bicycling
Poorer musculature endurance	Stair climbing
	Bicycling
	Weight training (low weights, high repetitions)
	Cardiovascular training
	Balance drills for longer durations

From Wilk KE, Arrigo C, Andrews Jr, et al: Rehabilitation after anterior cruciate ligament reconstruction in the female athlete, J Athl Train 34:177-193, 1999.
ACL, Anterior cruciate ligament.

training stimulated ligament and capsular proprioceptors, reinforcing cocontraction of muscles, leading to improvement in joint stability. This has also shown to be beneficial in patients who have had nonoperative treatment of ACL injuries. Chmielewski et al.[41] demonstrated that subjects with nonoperative ACL injuries are five times more likely to successfully return to high-level physical activities if they receive perturbation training than if they received standard strengthening and conditioning alone. Based on this information, a thorough program of rehabilitation after ACL reconstruction includes the standard exercises of increasing motion and strengthening, as well as perturbation exercises that stimulate the knee joint, ligament, and capsular mechanical receptors, as well as plyometric exercises to improve voluntary inactivation times and strength (Table 22-9).

Complications

Complications have significantly decreased in recent years with improved surgical techniques, graft choices, and graft fixation; however, they still must be thoroughly evaluated quickly and brought to the surgeon's attention as soon as concern arises. Loss of motion is often cited as the most common complication after ACL reconstruction. Once the physician or therapist rec-

Table 22-9	**Postoperative ACL Rehabilitation Program to Achieve Full Range of Motion**

Time After Surgery	Prescribed Program
Day of surgery	Continuous passive motion (CPM) machine for elevation and gentle motion
	Cryocuff for compression and cold therapy
	Full passive extension exercises for 10 minutes every waking hour
	Static flexion to at least 90 degrees in the CPM machine three times a day
	Active quadriceps contractions; actively lift leg out of the CPM machine
Day after surgery	Same exercises as day of surgery
	Discharged to home if goals are met: full hyperextension equal to normal knee, flexion to at least 90 degrees, good quadriceps leg control, minimal swelling
First week after surgery	Continue with prescribed exercises
	Limit activities to eating and bathroom privileges
Second week after surgery	Additional exercises added to program: prong hangs, wall slides
	Extension board used if needed
	Full weight-bearing with normal gait
2 to 5 weeks after surgery	Additional exercises added to program: heel slides, stationary bicycle, Stairmaster

From Shelbourne KD, Patel DV: Treatment of limited motion after anterior cruciate ligament reconstruction, Knee Surg Sports Traumatol Arthrosc 7(2):85-92, 1999.
ACL, Anterior cruciate ligament.

ognizes that a problem with motion exists, aggressive countermeasures should be implemented to try and prevent a fixed motion loss. Prone hangs, extension boards, and manual pressure can be used to help with extension lags. Wall slides, leg slides, and manual pressure can help improve flexion deficits. If the loss of motion progresses to a fixed state, then surgical intervention is often required. Once this has been completed, aggressive rehabilitation afterwards to maintain the motion can be instituted after the acute inflammatory phase has resolved. Another cited problem after ACL reconstruction involves anterior knee pain, the patellofemoral joint being the most common source. The literature remains somewhat equivocal in providing good evidence that graft selection plays a significant role; however, in a multistudy analysis, there was shown to be a higher incidence of anterior knee pain with the patellar tendon group at 17% versus the hamstring group at 12%. Sachs et al.[42] showed a correlation between development of patellofemoral symptoms and the presence of flexion contracture and quadriceps weakness, thus leading to early initiation of rehabilitation and range of motion and patellar mobilization techniques. In patients who begin to demonstrate patellofemoral symptoms or anterior knee pain, the rehabilitation program should be modified to eliminate exercises that might cause further aggravation. Additional, although rare, complications after an ACL reconstruction, particularly after central-third patellar tendon autografts, include extensor mechanism problems, patellar fractures, patellar tendon rupture, and even quadriceps rupture. Although these are extremely rare, they do require immediate attention and should be thoroughly evaluated. Infection is another potential but fortunately a rare complication, affecting less than 0.2% of patients after ACL reconstruction (Box 22-2).[43]

TRAUMA (EXCLUDING EXTENSOR MECHANISM ISSUES)

Knee rehabilitation after an intraarticular fracture of the knee has many variables. In general, the principle of early motion still prevails.[44,45] The major modification concerns the weight-bearing status. The main goal in fixation of these types of fractures is anatomic alignment of the articular surface. This can be accomplished through a variety of surgical interventions, ranging from minimally invasive techniques to large open procedures. External fixators, contoured plates, and cannulated screws are some of the choices available. Fracture stability is dependent on fracture pattern, fixation techniques, patient bone quality, and comorbid conditions. Initially there will be a period of limited weight bearing (nonweight bearing or touch toe). This usually will progress to full weight bearing over 8 to 12 weeks. However, this is surgeon dependent, with the previously mentioned factors playing a role on the individual patient's fracture healing. In addition, attention must be given to the foot and ankle to help prevent an equinus contracture during the limited weight-bearing period. Early range of motion will generally be started within the first postoperative week; CPM machines can be used to help facilitate

Magnetic resonance imaging (MRI) scans done after knee injuries have brought attention to so-called bone bruises. The MRI scan will show an area of increased bony water uptake beneath the injured chondral surface. The concern is that the level of impact creating bony bruises has concurrently injured the overlying cartilage. A landmark study demonstrated that the inflammation occurring after chondral injury and bone bruises was in itself deleterious to the injured tissues. Most orthopedic knee surgeons feel that the recognition of a bone bruise implies a significant articular injury, and that for proper chondral protection, the athlete should be guarded against weight bearing, allowing articular cartilage to heal. The quandary is the time articular cartilage deserves for healing. It is reasonable that for 6 to 8 weeks after recognition of a bone bruise, the athlete is either kept on crutches or kept to slow

walking without increasing joint loads. However, follow-up MRI scans are becoming more popular to assess bone bruises, and recommendations for more accurate guarded weight bearing will appear in the literature within the next 5 years.

The previously mentioned study's focus on accompanying inflammation also raises questions as to whether oral antiinflammatory medicines or intraarticular cortisone injections might have a beneficial effect on healing cartilage, although these agents are also known to slow tissue healing. A great deal of research is needed to help clinicians advance articular cartilage healing. Recent studies in Asia have shown that hyaluronate (joint fluid therapy injections) may also prove chondroprotective. These injections will be given soon after injury recognition.

Box 22-3   Regaining Knee Motion

In patients that have difficulty regaining knee extension, the clinician should consider prone stretching, manual overpressure, extension boards, applying heating pads to the hamstrings and posterior thigh structures, and bicycling with a high seat. With patients who have difficulty achieving knee flexion, one should consider controlled squats, manual overpressure, bicycling with a low seat, applying heating pads to quadriceps, and using devices such as a Flexionator (ERMI, Inc., Atlanta, Ga) (Figure 22-5).

motion (Box 22-3). At no time, however, is motion performed at the expense of loss of fracture reduction.

Subsequently, mobilization in a hinged brace is often preferred.[3] Function should progress throughout the healing stage, with the goal of full functional range of motion. Patella mobilization techniques are instituted as well. Passive, active, and active-assisted quadriceps and hamstring exercises can also begin at this time. Return to full activity is in the 3- to 6-month range, depending on fracture healing and return of motion and strength (Box 22-4).

Rehabilitation After Articular Cartilage Repair Procedures

Reinhold et al.[46] have published an excellent review of current concepts in the rehabilitation after articular cartilage repair procedures in the knee. They emphasize the physical therapist must create an environment that facilitates the healing process while avoiding potentially harmful forces to the repair site. The two canons of rehabilitation of articular cartilage procedures are weight-bearing restrictions and prescribed range of motion limitation. Individual approach is of course necessary, given the variety of articular cartilage procedures that are often done in combination with other surgical repairs. A gradual progression in weight bearing and range of motion will not only protect the healing cartilage but also has been shown to stimu-

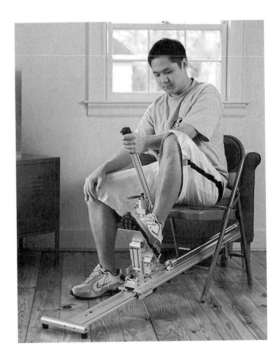

Figure 22-5 Devices such as the Flexionator can enable patients to restore range of motion. (Courtesy ERMI, Inc., Atlanta, Ga.)

late matrix production and improve mechanical properties. CPM machines and adherence to bicycling programs will achieve prescribed range of motion while preventing arthrofibrosis. Controlled weight-bearing activities are facilitated by use of assistive devices, pool therapy, and force platforms, which provide patients with weight-bearing biofeedback. Physical therapy monitoring of articular cartilage repair patients is one of the most demanding types of knee rehabilitation. Gradually increasing the amount of stress applied to the injured knee must be constantly reevaluated. Patients who develop inordinate pain or effusion during rehabilitation provide a surefire sign that the tissues are being overloaded, and it is wise to avoid the painful swollen knee.

Box 22-4   Red Flags in Knee Rehabilitation

Sympathetic Mediated Pain

Untoward pain with joint stiffness and red and/or shiny skin should give concern for impending reflex sympathetic dystrophy. Early intervention by pain control physicians should be invoked. Treatment involves not only increasing pain medications but also a slow, cautious approach to physical therapy during the initial phases. In addition, it is often accompanied by assessment of the patient's mental health and any effect that chronic disabling pain may have. Recent approaches have featured the use of neurotrophic medications and psychiatric and psychologic counseling.

Infection

Most knee injuries will create erythema and warmth. Postsurgical patients are no different. Most postsurgical infections may not become apparent immediately after surgery. Instead they are noted in the weeks after surgery as the effects of preventative antibiotic agents given at surgery wane and bacteria gain a foothold into injured or surgically operated tissues. A sudden report of increased pain, along with decreased joint motion, should raise therapy concern. Not all patients demonstrate fever, but the warmth of infected tissues is often dramatic. Immediate medical attention is in order, and oral antibiotic agents may unwittingly mask a serious, deep infection, whereupon medical attention is required as soon as possible to obtain relevant aspirated cultures. Patients with deep infection will require surgical attention and, perhaps, prolonged intravenous antibiotic agents. The situation becomes complicated when patients are placed on suppressive oral antibiotic agents, which are not curative but rather suppress and mask an insidious process that could result in permanent joint destruction.

According to Reinhold et al.,[46] cartilage repair rehabilitation is based on four biologic phases. During phase 1—the proliferation phase—cartilage healing requires absolute protection against any excessive load during the first 4 to 6 weeks. The role of the physical therapist is to maintain prescribed range of motion and muscle strength. During phase 2—the transition phase—which usually consists of weeks 4 to 12 after surgery, the repaired tissue is gaining strength, which allows for progression of rehabilitation exercises. During this time, muscle strengthening and endurance are featured, although weight-bearing status may still be restricted. In phase 3—the remodeling phase—the activities that take place from 3 to 6 months postoperatively allow for more functional training while curtailing vigorous activity in light of pain or effusion. Low- to moderate-impact activities will be allowed, but running, jumping, or twisting must remain prohibited during the cartilage healing and remodeling phase. In the final and fourth phase—the maturation phase—rehabilitation continues from 4 to 18 months after surgery. It is assumed that any cartilage healing has occurred and that the patient may return to impact-loading activities.[46]

Many authors have demonstrated that a return to competitive athletics can occur for microfracture, OATS, and ACI procedures. Chondral débridement and microfracture procedures should allow for return to sport in 4 to 6 months after surgery, whereupon cartilage transfer procedures, such as ACI or OATS, demand a minimum of 10 to 18 months before sports activity loads are permitted. Although it would be ideal to know the exact extent of articular cartilage healing, clinicians' understanding is hampered by the fact that MRI is incapable of making such a fine distinction, and surgically reexamining the tissues (so-called second-look surgery) is unethical. Much knowledge has been gained about anticipated healing when athletes have sustained a subsequent injury and arthroscopy has documented the extent of articular cartilage healing, allowing orthopaedic surgeons to make broad recommendations for cartilage repair rehabilitation procedures.

Acupuncture

Acupuncture remains a controversial adjunct in treating injured or arthritic knees. Manheimer et al.[47] treated patients with osteoarthritis over 26 weeks, comparing a true acupuncture group with a sham group. Acupuncture seemed to provide improvement in function and pain relief when compared with credible sham acupuncture. The mechanism of action proves elusive. Optimal effects took a minimum of 8 weeks for functional improvement and 14 weeks for maximal pain reduction. From a physiologic perspective, this delayed response is not consistent with the most commonly proposed mechanisms of acupuncture (gate control or neuropeptide release). This study was additionally flawed because patients were not controlled in pursuing any other physical therapy or using nonsteroidal anti-inflammatory drugs (NSAIDs) or Cox-2 inhibitors.[47]

CONCLUSION

This chapter outlines many of the more common knee conditions treated by the orthopaedic physical therapist. The physical therapist must have a thorough understanding of the pathologic condition and a solid understanding of the current literature and research regarding these injuries to effectively treat the knee patient in an evidence-based manner and to promote optimal outcomes.

REFERENCES

1. Post WR: Anterior knee pain: diagnosis and treatment, J Am Acad Orthop Surg 13:534-543, 2005.
2. Powers CM, et al: Effect of bracing on patellar kinematics in patients with patellofemoral joint pain, Med Sci Sports Exerc 31(12):1714-1720, 1999.
3. Powers CM, Ward SR, Chan LD, et al: The effect of bracing on patella alignment and patellofemoral joint contact area, Med Sci Sports Exerc 36(7):1226-1232, 2004.

4. Whittingham M, Palmer S, Macmillan F: Effects of taping on pain and function in patellofemoral pain syndrome: a randomized controlled trial, J Orthop Sports Phys Ther 4(9):504-510, 2004.

5. Stanish WD, Rubinovich RM, Curwin S: Eccentric exercise in chronic tendonitis, Clin Orthop Relat Res 208:65-68, 1986.

6. Alfredson H, Cook J: A treatment algorithm for managing Achilles tendinopathy: new treatment options, Br J Sports Med 41(4):211-216, 2007.

7. Visnes H, Bahr R: The evolution of eccentric training as treatment for patellar tendinopathy (jumper's knee): a critical review of exercise programmes, Br J Sports Med 41(4):217-223, 2007.

8. Crossley KM, Thancanamootoo K, Metcalf BR, et al: Clinical features of patellar tendinopathy and their implications for rehabilitation, J Orthop Res 25(9):1164-1175, 2007.

9. Akeson WH, Amiel D, Woo SL: Immobility effects on synovial joints the pathomechanics of joint contracture, Biorheology 17:95-110, 1980.

10. Haggmark T, Eriksson E: Cylinder or mobile cast brace after knee ligament surgery: a clinical analysis and morphologic and enzymatic studies of changes in the quadriceps muscle, Am J Sports Med 7:48-56, 1979.

11. Jozsa L et al: Quantitative alterations in intramuscular connective tissue following immobilization: an experimental study in rat calf muscle, Exp Mol Pathol 49:67-78, 1988.

12. Noyes FR: Functional properties of knee ligaments and alterations induced by immobilization: a correlative biomechanical and histological study in primates, Clin Orthop Rel Res 123:210-241, 1977.

13. Agberg E, et al: 15-year follow-up of neuromuscular function in patients with unilateral non-reconstructed anterior cruciate ligament injury initially treated with rehabilitation and activity modification: a longitudinal prospective study, Am J Sports Med 35:2109-2117, 2007.

14. Shino K, et al: Quantitative evaluation after arthroscopic anterior cruciate ligament reconstruction: allograft versus autograft, Am J Sports Med 21:609-616, 1993.

15. Victor J, et al: Graft selection in anterior cruciate ligament reconstruction—prospective analysis of patellar tendon autografts compared with allografts, Int Orthop 21:93-97, 1997.

16. Friedman, et al: Arthroscopic anterior cruciate ligament reconstruction: a meta-analysis, Am J Sports Med 31:2-11, 2003.

17. Yogi, et al: Biomechanical analysis of an anatomic anterior cruciate ligament reconstruction, Am J Sports Med 30:660-666, 2002.

18. Tasman, et al: Abnormal rotational knee motion during running after anterior cruciate ligament reconstruction, Am J Sports Med 32: 975-983, 2004.

19. Deleted in pages.

20. Yagi, et al: Double-bundle ACL reconstruction can improve rotational stability, Clin Orthop Relat Res 454:100-107, 2007.

21. Noyes FR, Barber SD, Mangine RE: Abnormal lower limb symmetry determined by function hop tests after anterior cruciate ligament rupture, Am J Sports Med 19:513-518, 1991.

22. Ohkoshi Y, et al: The effect of cryotherapy on intra-articular temperature and postoperative care after anterior cruciate ligament reconstruction, Am J Sports Med 27: 357-362, 1999.

23. Tyler TF, et al: The effect of immediate weight bearing after anterior cruciate ligament reconstruction, Clin Orthop Relat Res 357:141-148, 1998.

24. Beynnon B, et al: Rehabilitation after anterior cruciate ligament reconstruction: a prospective, randomized, double-blind comparison of programs administered over 2 different time intervals, Am J Sports Med 33(3):347-359, 2005.

25. Bynum EB, Barrack RL, Alexander AH: Open versus closed chain kinetic exercises after anterior cruciate ligament reconstruction: a prospective randomized study, Am J Sports Med 23:401-406, 1995.

26. Jenkins WL: A measurement of anterior tibial displacement in the closed and open kinetic chain, J Orthop Sports Phys Ther 25:49-56, 1997.

27. Yack HJ, Collins CE, Whieldon TJ: Comparison of closed and open kinetic chain exercise in the anterior cruciate ligament-deficient knee, Am J Sports Med 21:49-54, 1993.

28. Gerber JP, et al: Effects of early progressive eccentric exercise on muscle structure after anterior cruciate ligament reconstruction, J Bone Joint Surg Am 89(3):559-570, 2007.

29. Decoster LC, Vailis JC: Functional anterior cruciate ligament bracing: a survey of current brace prescription patterns, Orthopedics 26(7):701-706, 2003.

30. Wright RW, Fetzer GB: Bracing after ACL reconstruction: a systematic review, Clin Orthop Relat Res 455:162-168, 2007.

31. Fleming BC, et al: The influence of functional knee bracing on the anterior cruciate ligament strain biomechanics in weight bearing and non-weight bearing knees, Am J Sports Med 28:815-824, 2000.

32. Sterett WI, et al: Effect of functional bracing on knee injury in skiers with anterior cruciate ligament reconstruction: a prospective cohort study (case studies), Am J Sports Med 34:1581-1585, 2006.

33. Malinzak RA, et al: A comparison of knee joint motion patterns between men and women in selected athletic tasks, Clin Biomech (Bristol, Avon) 16(5):438-445, 2001.

34. McKean KA: ACL Injuries—the gender bias, J Orthop Sports Phys Ther 33:A1-30, 2003 (abstract).

35. Sigward S: The influence of experience on knee mechanics during side-step cutting in females, Clin Biomech (Bristol, Avon) 21:740-747, 2006.

36. Ferber R, Davis IM, Williams DS 3rd: Gender differences in lower extremity mechanics during running, Clin Biomech (Bristol, Avon) 18(4):350-357, 2003.

37. Ford KR, Myer GD, Toms HE, et al: Gender differences in the kinematics of unanticipated cutting in young athletes, Med Sci Sports Exerc 37:124-129, 2005.

38. Pollard CD, Heiderscheit BC, van Emmerik RE, et al: Gender differences in lower extremity coupling variability during an unanticipated cutting maneuver, J Appl Biomech 21(2):143-152, 2005.

39. Schneider-Mackler L, Ladin Z, Schepsis A, Young J: Electrical stimulation of the thigh muscles after reconstruction of the anterior cruciate ligament: effects of electrically elicited contraction of the quadriceps femoris and hamstring muscles on gait and on strength of the thigh muscles, J Bone Joint Surg Am 73(7):1025-1036, 1991.

40. Floyd D: Rationale for training programs to reduce anterior cruciate ligament injuries in Australian football, J Orthop Sports Phys Ther 31(11):645-654, 2001.

41. Chmielewski TL, et al: Perturbation training improves knee kinematics and reduces muscle co-contraction after complete unilateral anterior cruciate ligament rupture, Phys Ther 85:740-754, 2005.

42. Sachs RA, et al: Patellofemoral problems after anterior cruciate ligament reconstruction, Am J Sports Med 17:760-765, 1989.

43. Matava M, et al: Septic arthritis of the knee following anterior cruciate ligament reconstruction: results of a survey of sports medicine fellowship directors, Arthroscopy 14:717-725, 1998.

44. Koval KJ, Helfet DL: Tibial plateau fractures: evaluation and treatment, J Am Acad Orthop Surg 3:86-94, 1995.

45. Berkson EM, Virkus WW: High-energy tibial plateau fractures, J Am Acad Orthop Surg 14:20-31, 2006.

46. Reinhold et al: Current concepts in the rehabilitation following articular cartilage repair procedures in the knee, J Orthop Sports Phys Ther 36:774-794, 2006.

47. Manheimer E, et al: Acupuncture for knee osteoarthritis—a randomized trial using a novel sham, Acupunct Med 24(suppl):S7-S14, 2006.

23

Allen Carpenter
and Robert A. Donatelli

Dysfunction, Evaluation, and Treatment of the Foot and Ankle

This chapter briefly reviews the anatomy and normal and abnormal biomechanics of the foot and ankle. Various foot and ankle pathologic conditions are also discussed with respect to pathomechanics, evaluation, and treatment. The pathologic conditions include entrapment syndromes, traumatic injuries to the foot and ankle, and foot deformities. The biomechanical evaluation of the foot and ankle is also described.

NORMAL BIOMECHANICS

Anatomy

Some 30 bones comprise the skeletal structure of the foot and ankle.[1-5] This osseous structure can be broken down into a forefoot, a midfoot, and a rearfoot section. In the rearfoot, the osseous structures of clinical importance are the distal ends of the fibula and tibia, the talus, and the calcaneus. These four bones interact to serve as supportive structures and pulley systems for the various tendons that pass over the bones.[6] The tibia, fibula, and talus together form a hinge joint: the talocrural joint. Two types of motion occur at this joint: (1) osteokinematic and (2) arthrokinematic.[2-7] Osteokinematic movement is the overall movement of two bones without reference to the motion occurring between the joint surfaces (i.e., flexion and extension). Arthrokinematic movement is the motion actually occurring between the two joint surfaces (i.e., roll and spin).[5]

Plantar flexion and dorsiflexion are the osteokinematic motions occurring at the talocrural joint. Osteokinematic movement at the talocrural joint is governed and restricted primarily by the bony configuration of the joint surfaces. The primary arthrokinematic joint motions of the talocrural joint are roll and slide. Several ligaments help restrict the arthrokinematic movements found at the talocrural joint. These are the anterior tibiofibular, the anterior and posterior talofibular, the deltoid, and the calcaneofibular ligaments.[2-7]

A second joint found in the rearfoot, the subtalar joint, is composed of the calcaneus inferiorly and the talus superiorly.[2-8] Because the axis of the subtalar joint is triplanar (movement occurs in all three body planes simultaneously), a complex series of supination and pronation motions occurs there.[6] In the open kinetic chain, supination is defined as inversion, plantar flexion, and adduction of the calcaneus on the talus; whereas pronation is defined as eversion, dorsiflexion, and abduction of the calcaneus on the talus.[4-8] These joint motions are governed by ligamentous tension and bony restraint mechanisms. The deltoid, anterior and posterior talofibular, and calcaneofibular ligaments prevent excessive motion from occurring at the subtalar joint.[3-5,7,9]

The rearfoot is separated from the forefoot by the midfoot, which is made up of the navicular and cuboid bones. The midtarsal joint is the major articulation of the midfoot, and it is composed of the approximation of the navicular and cuboid to the talus and calcaneus, respectively.[1-5] As in the subtalar joint, the triplanar motions of supination and pronation occur at the midtarsal joint. These triplanar motions at the midtarsal joint occur about two joint axes: (1) longitudinal and (2) oblique. The longitudinal axis extends lengthwise through the foot and slopes upward and medially.[10] The motions of eversion during pronation and inversion during supination in an open kinetic chain occur about the longitudinal axis. Clinically, inversion and eversion about the midtarsal joint can be observed in the normal rise and drop of the medial arch of the foot in the weight-bearing position.[10] The oblique axis of the midtarsal joint is described by several authors as being inclined 52 degrees above the horizontal and 57 degrees from the frontal plane.[10] About the oblique midtarsal joint axis, the open kinetic chain motions of plantar flexion and adduction occur during supination, whereas dorsiflexion and abduction occur during pronation.[6,7,11] Ligamentous structures restraining the motions of supination and pronation are the bifurcate, spring (calcaneonavicular), short and long plantar ligaments, and the plantar aponeurosis.[3-6]

The osseous structures of the forefoot are the three cuneiforms, the five metatarsals, the two plantar sesamoids of the first metatarsal, as well as the 14 phalanges. These bones form several joints, of which only the metatarsophalangeal (MTP) and interphalangeal (IP) joints will be briefly discussed because it is the normal mobility of these joints that enables normal movement and stability of the forefoot. The metatarsal heads tolerate the vertical forces of weight bearing while the toes stabilize the forefoot dynamically. The MTP joint is an ellipsoidal joint that allows the osteokinematic motions of abduction, adduction, flexion, and extension to occur. The IP joints are pure hinge joints that allow the osteokinematic motions of flexion and extension to occur. Both joints have proper joint capsules with accompanying supportive ligamentous structures.[1-5,7]

The foot has several muscles of clinical importance. The role many of these muscles play in the production of pathologic condition in the foot is covered in the discussion of foot pathologic conditions. Some of these muscles are the gastrocsoleustendoachilles complex, the peroneus brevis and longus, and the tibialis posterior and anterior.[2-5] These muscles are crucial in the rehabilitation of the foot and ankle.

Important neurovascular structures passing through and terminating in the foot are the posterior (which divides into the medial and lateral plantar nerves) and anterior tibial nerves, the musculocutaneous nerve, the sural nerve, the dorsalis pedis artery, and the posterior tibial artery (which divides into the medial and lateral plantar arteries).[2-5] The effect these structures have on foot pathologic condition is further discussed in the section on entrapments.

Nonweight-Bearing Motion

During nonweight-bearing lower-extremity motion at the subtalar joint, movement occurs about a fixed talus during pronation and supination, respectively.[5,12-18] The calcaneus will evert, dorsiflex, and abduct and invert, plantar flex, and adduct about the talus during pronation and supination, respectively.[6,12,14-18] The lack of talar motion in the nonweight-bearing lower extremity is due to the absence of direct muscular attachments to the talus.[4,6,16]

During nonweight-bearing pronation, lower-extremity motion at the midtarsal joint consists of eversion about the longitudinal axis and abduction and dorsiflexion about the oblique axis. During supination, inversion occurs about the longitudinal axis and adduction and plantar flexion occur about the oblique axis.* The extent of permissible movement at the midtarsal joint depends on the position of the subtalar joint. The position of the subtalar joint dictates the amount of available motion of the joints at the midfoot and forefoot. Supination of the subtalar joint causes a decrease in the available motion of the midtarsal joint; pronation at the subtalar joint causes an increase of available motion.[6,12,13,19-21]

MTP joint motion in the nonweight-bearing lower extremity can affect the amount of joint motion seen in the forefoot and rearfoot joints. MTP joint extension will cause the forefoot and rearfoot joints to be placed in a closed-packed position. Therefore a cinching up of the joints of the foot occurs. This cinching up is described as the *windlass effect*.[4,17,22-24] It is produced by the increased tension of the plantar fascia between the bases of the MTP joints and the calcaneus.[4,22] A minimum

of 60 degrees of MTP extension is needed for normal MTP function during gait.[4,6,17,25]

Weight-Bearing Motion

Some differences exist between weight-bearing and nonweight-bearing motion in the foot and ankle. These differences are a result of the gravitational and ground reaction forces imparted to the foot and ankle during weight bearing.[6,17,18,24]

One such difference between the weight-bearing conditions is in the motion occurring at the subtalar joint. During supination in the weight-bearing condition, the calcaneus inverts while the talus dorsiflexes and abducts.[6,14,15,18,24] During pronation the calcaneus everts while the talus plantar flexes and adducts.[6,14,15,18,24] The chief difference between the two weight-bearing conditions is the presence of talar motion in the weight-bearing condition and its absence in the nonweight-bearing condition.

During the gait cycle, the previously cited events of lower-extremity weight-bearing motion can be observed. At heel-strike, the subtalar joint is in a neutral to slightly supinated position, creating stability for weight acceptance while the talocrural joint is in dorsiflexion. As the talocrural joint begins to plantar flex from initial contact to weight acceptance, the subtalar joint begins pronating. Both of these motions occur as a result of the body weight and ground reaction forces during weight acceptance and allow for shock absorption. Eccentric action of the invertors and dorsiflexors of the talocrural and subtalar joints controls this pronation motion. When the gait cycle progresses from weight acceptance to midstance, the subtalar joint is fully pronated and the talocrural joint is progressing into closed kinetic chain dorsiflexion.[4,6,8,18,24]

As the gait cycle continues from midstance to propulsion, the subtalar joint begins to resupinate at the end of midstance, reaching maximum supination at toe-off. Again, this supination of the subtalar joint creates increased stability of the midfoot and forefoot for propulsion. Resupination activity at the subtalar joint results from concentric muscle activity of the plantar flexors and invertors of the subtalar joint and external rotation of the lower limb. The talocrural joint goes through a cycle of dorsiflexion-plantar flexion-dorsiflexion from midstance through the swing phase of gait. From midstance to toe-off, the talocrural joint is in closed kinetic chain dorsiflexion because of the tibia advancing over the talus. Talocrural plantar flexion then occurs as propulsion takes place. Lastly, the ankle joint must dorsiflex the foot again to clear the foot from the ground during the swing phase. This plantar flexion-dorsiflexion activity of the talocrural joint is due to the eccentric and concentric activity of the plantar flexors.[4,6,8,18,24]

Midtarsal joint motion, as in the nonweight-bearing condition, is dependent on the position of the subtalar joint. Supination at the subtalar joint decreases the amount of available motion at the midtarsal joint. Therefore the midtarsal joint locks with subtalar joint supination, creating stability in the rearfoot for initial contact and weight acceptance. As the gait cycle progresses to midstance and the midfoot and forefoot come into contact with the ground, pronation of the subtalar

---

*References 6, 7, 11, 12, 15, and 19.

joint unlocks the midtarsal joint, causing the foot to become an unstable "loose bag of bones," allowing it to adapt to the ground surface below.[4,6,8,13,18-21] This pronation motion of the midtarsal joint consists of eversion along the longitudinal axis and dorsiflexion and abduction along the oblique axis. Supination of the midtarsal joint is again seen from just after midstance to propulsion and toe-off in the gait cycle. During midtarsal supination, inversion about the longitudinal axis and plantar flexion and adduction along the oblique axis are demonstrated.[4,6,8,18,24]

Eccentric muscle action of the invertors of the foot control midtarsal joint pronation as it occurs. Concentric muscle activity of the invertors of the foot and ankle cause the supination motions observed at initial contact and toe-off.[4,6] As previously stated, the extent of supination and pronation movements also depends on the subtalar joint position.

Both supination and pronation are necessary for normal function of the lower extremity. As described previously, concurrent pronation of the midtarsal and subtalar joints allows the foot to adapt to uneven surfaces and to dissipate and transmit ground reaction forces.[4,6,17,18,24] Supination transforms the foot and ankle into a rigid lever to transfer the vertical forces of propulsion to the ground from the lower extremity, thus reducing the shear forces transmitted directly to the forefoot during propulsion.[4,6,17,18,24] A rigid foot during propulsion enables the muscle pulleys of the posterior tibialis and peroneus longus to be established, thus increasing the efficiency of global muscle function. Supination and pronation of the subtalar joint also serve to convert the transverse plane rotations of the trunk and lower extremity into sagittal plane rotations.[8,17] During normal gait activity, the trunk and lower limb rotate internally at initial contact and externally at heel-off. The subtalar joint, in response to these transverse plane rotations, pronates during internal rotation of the tibia and supinates during tibial external rotation, thus acting as a torque converter for the lower extremity.[6,17]

The chief activity at the MTP joints during weight-bearing activity is the dorsiflexion-plantar flexion motion of the toes. As heel-off occurs, the toes passively dorsiflex, which tightens the plantar aponeurosis and cinches up the tarsal and metatarsal bones. This cinching up of the plantar aponeurosis assists in the transduction of the foot into a rigid lever for propulsive activities, creating the windlass effect described earlier. Plantar flexion of the phalanges, mainly the hallux, during toe-off acts as the chief propeller of the lower extremity.[4,6,22,24] The toes then actively plantarflex as toe-off occurs. Several sources in the literature provide in-depth discussions of the normal mechanics of the foot.[6,16,17,24]

ABNORMAL BIOMECHANICS

Abnormal biomechanics are discussed in reference to the weight-bearing condition. The adverse effects of abnormal biomechanics are usually seen during the stance phase of gait. In the foot and ankle, these adverse effects are usually the result of either excessive pronation or excessive supination.[6]

Excessive Pronation

Excessive pronation is defined as pronation that either occurs for too long a time or is excessive.[6] This excessive pronation takes place at the subtalar joint. When pronation occurs for too long a time, the subtalar joint remains pronated after the weight acceptance phase of gait. If the subtalar joint exhibits more than 30 degrees of calcaneal eversion from weight acceptance to the midstance phase of gait, then too much pronation is present.[6]

Excessive pronation can be attributed to congenital, neuromuscular, and/or acquired factors. Only the acquired factors are discussed in this chapter. For further information on neuromuscular or congenital factors, see Jahss' textbook on disorders of the foot.[26]

Acquired factors causing excessive pronation can be divided into extrinsic and intrinsic causes. Extrinsic causes are those because of events occurring outside of the foot and ankle region, in the lower leg or knee.[6] Examples of extrinsic causes are gastrocsoleus tightness, rotational deformities of the lower extremity (e.g., femoral anteversion and tibial varum), and leg length discrepancies.

Intrinsic causes of excessive pronation are those that occur within the foot and ankle region.[6] Most intrinsic causes are usually fixed deformities of the subtalar and midtarsal joints.[6] Examples of intrinsic causes of acquired flatfoot include trauma, ligament laxity, bony abnormalities of the subtalar joint, forefoot varus, forefoot supinatus, rearfoot varus, and ankle joint equinus.[27]

Both intrinsic and extrinsic causes can produce excessive compensatory subtalar joint pronation. The response to the extrinsic or intrinsic cause of excessive pronation varies from person to person, depending on the number of intrinsic and extrinsic factors present and the mobility of the subtalar, midtarsal, and other foot joints.

An alteration in the normal mechanics of the lower extremity occurs with excessive pronation at the subtalar joint. When the subtalar joint compensates for a deformity by pronation, it occurs in addition to the normal amount of pronation necessary for gait.[27] It has been reported that pronation is most destructive to the foot when it occurs during the push-off phase of gait.[6] Pronation during the push-off portion of gait causes the foot to be unstable at a time when the foot needs to be a rigid lever.[4,6,15,19,24] If unstable, then the foot will be unable to transmit the forces encountered during push-off.[4,6,24] This inability to transmit forces may lead to tissue breakdown within the foot (e.g., Morton's neuroma).[6] An added effect of an excessively long pronatory phase is disruption of the normal transverse rotatory cycle of the lower extremity, possibly leading to pathologic condition at the knee and hip.[4,6,20,24]

Excessive Supination

Abnormal supination is the inability of the foot to pronate effectively throughout the stance phase of gait.[27] It is commonly known as the *pes cavus* or *high-arched foot*. Excessive supination is much the same as excessive pronation; supination can occur for too long a time period or can be excessive.[6] As in excessive pronation, a myriad of causes ranging from congenital to acquired deformities may result in excessive supination.

An excessively supinated foot prevents the foot and ankle from absorbing shock by altering the normal transverse rotational events of the lower extremity.[4,6,20,24] The foot and ankle therefore transmit this stress up the lower extremity to the knee, hip, or back, possibly causing a pathologic condition.[6,13,14] In addition, the foot remains rigid at a time when it needs to become mobile and adaptable (i.e., from heel-strike to weight acceptance). Therefore the foot is unable to adapt to uneven terrain, and the result is a loss of equilibrium (a possible perpetuating factor in repeated ankle sprains in the athlete).[6] Unlike excessive pronation, the excessive supinator does not usually demonstrate a breakdown of tissue in a progressive nature, which leads to a hypermobile foot. Rather, it is an inflexible foot that causes tissue inflammation and possible joint destruction.[27]

DYSFUNCTIONS AND PATHOLOGIC CONDITIONS

Entrapments

Tarsal Tunnel Syndrome

Tarsal tunnel syndrome is an entrapment of the posterior tibial nerve and artery as they pass through a fibrous osseous tunnel located posteromedial to the medial malleolus.[28-33] The roof of the tunnel is composed of the flexor retinaculum (the laciniate ligament), and the floor is composed of the underlying bony structures. A decrease in the diameter of the tunnel may cause compression of the posterior tibial nerve and artery, resulting in symptoms including, but not limited to, burning pain and numbness in the medial foot and ankle.[30,31,33] The decrease in diameter may be caused by an external or internal pathologic condition.

The most commonly reported causes of tarsal tunnel syndrome are posttraumatic fibrosis (secondary to sprains or fractures); space-occupying lesions such as bony exostoses, tendon sheath ganglions, tenosynovitis, or nerve tumors; and structural abnormalities of the foot such as excessive pronation.[33] Excessive pronation of the subtalar joint is an external pathologic condition that tends to compress the tunnel. The laciniate ligament is stretched during excessive pronation, thereby decreasing the diameter of the tunnel.[29-31] Tendinitis of the posterior tibial, the flexor digitorum longus, and/or the flexor hallucis longus tendon is an example of an internal pathologic condition causing a decrease in the diameter of the tarsal tunnel.[28,30,31] Misalignment of the bony structures of the talocrural joint secondary to trauma and fracture can be considered a combination of internal and external pathologic conditions causing a diminished tarsal tunnel diameter. All of these pathologic conditions may compromise the tunnel either by occupying or by decreasing its space.[28,31]

Another reported cause of tarsal tunnel symptoms is entrapment of the posterior tibial nerve by the abductor hallucis muscle as the nerve enters the plantar aspect of the foot. A tethering of the nerve by the abductor hallucis tendon causes the entrapment and the underlying bone as the nerve enters the foot.[32,34] This tethering stretches the posterior tibial nerve during gait activities.

Neuromas

Neuromas are fibrotic proliferations of the tissue surrounding the neurovascular bundles located between the metatarsals. Abnormal shearing forces between the metatarsal heads and the underlying tissues usually cause the fibrotic proliferation. An ischemic response of the neurovascular bundles is the end result of the tissue proliferation, ultimately leading to the symptoms felt by the patient.[6,28,32]

The pathomechanics involved in the formation of a neuroma are usually the result of abnormal pronation during the propulsive phase of gait.[6] Normally the neurovascular bundles lie plantar to and between the metatarsals. During abnormal pronation, the metatarsal heads of the first, second, and third metatarsals move in a lateroplantar direction while the fifth metatarsal head moves in a dorsomedial direction.[6,35] At the same time, ground reaction forces and the patient's shoe fix the soft tissues on the plantar surface of the foot. The metatarsal head motion establishes a shear and a compressive force. The compressive force is due to the metatarsal heads lying over the neurovascular bundles.[6] The result of these compressive and shear forces is fibrotic proliferation of the surrounding tissue in an effort to protect the neurovascular bundles.[6,8,32]

Trauma

Fractures

Talocrural fractures are the result of four basic types of abnormal force: (1) compression, (2) inversion, (3) eversion, and (4) torsion.[33-35] Inversion or eversion fractures are usually accompanied by a torsional component.[36-38] An inversion or eversion fracture, with or without a torsional component, results in damage to the soft tissues and osseous structures about the talocrural and subtalar joints.[29,36-38] Depending on the severity of the injury and on whether the forefoot is in supination or pronation, a fracture of the medial and/or the lateral malleolus can be seen.[37-39] A possible concomitant injury is an osteochondral fracture of the talar dome.[36-38] Disruption of the inferior tibiofibular syndesmosis may also be a consequence of an inversion or eversion fracture.[36-38]

Compression fractures of the talocrural joint are usually the result of a jumping incident.[29,36,39] In this type of fracture, direct damage occurs to the talus as a result of the applied force. A secondary event may be disruption of the inferior tibiofibular syndesmosis as in an inversion or eversion injury.[36,39]

Metatarsal fractures generally involve either the first or the fifth metatarsal and can be a result of either trauma or excessive stress.[40] The mechanism of injury in a traumatic fracture of the first metatarsal usually involves an abduction and hyperflexion or hyperextension force.[29,36] In a traumatic fracture of the fifth metatarsal, the mechanism of injury usually involves inversion of the foot. The peroneus brevis contracts forcefully to prevent the excessive inversion, thus avulsing the styloid process of the fifth metatarsal.[29,36]

Stress fractures are usually the result of hyperpronation of the midtarsal and subtalar joints.[6,29,41] The hyperpronation prevents the foot from locking because of the lack of subtalar joint supination. Instead of being transmitted up the kinetic chain, the forces of propulsion are dissipated within the foot, which is incapable of handling the extra stress of the propulsive forces.[6,41] However, stress fractures can also be a result of a lack of pronation in the subtalar joint (the supinated foot). If the subtalar joint is unable to pronate, then proper shock absorption of the forces of compression does not take place, which places excess stress on the osseous structures.[6]

Sprains

The mechanism of a talocrural sprain is either lateral or medial, with or without a torsional force component. In a lateral injury, the mechanism involves an inversion force. The injury may involve ligamentous damage occurring in the following order: the anterior talofibular, calcaneofibular, posterior talofibular, and posterior tibiofibular ligaments. As more ligaments become involved, the severity of the injury increases.[28,29,31]

Medial mechanisms of injury are the result of eversion forces. The deltoid and tibiofibular ligaments are usually torn in this type of injury.[28,29,42] An associated fracture of the fibula is the usual complication of an eversion injury.[28,29,36,39,42] Medial injuries are rare compared with lateral injuries.

MTP sprains normally involve a hyperflexion injury to the joint. Capsular tearing, articular cartilage damage, and possible fracturing of the tibial sesamoid are seen in MTP joint sprains.[28,29] This type of injury is thought to be a cause in hallux limitus deformities.[6]

Tibiofibular sprains are frequently a secondary involvement of talocrural injuries or a result of a compression injury.[28] Fracture of the dome of the talus or of the distal end of the fibula is a possible complication.[28,39] The mechanism of injury often involves a rotational or compressive force with a concomitant dorsiflexion force.[28,29,39]

Pathomechanics

Hallux Abductovalgus

By definition, hallux abductovalgus is adduction of the first metatarsal with a valgus deformity of the proximal and distal phalanges of the hallux.[6,43] Hallux abductovalgus may be a result of hypermobility of the first metatarsal in a forefoot adductus, rheumatoid inflammatory disease, neuromuscular disease, or a result of postsurgical malfunction.[6,44,45] In all of these conditions, a subluxation of the first MTP joint occurs initially, followed by dislocation.[6,44,45]

Classically, four stages occur in the progression of this hallux deformity. The predisposing factor is a hypermobility of the first metatarsal.[6,44,45] This hypermobility allows the hallux to abduct and the first metatarsal to adduct and invert on the tarsus and the hallux. Abnormal pronation is usually the cause of the hypermobility of the first metatarsal.[6,43-45] Any structural or neuromuscular problem causing abnormal pronation or a laterally directed muscular force may lead to a hallux abductovalgus deformity.[6,44,45]

In stage one a lateral subluxation of the base of the proximal phalanx is seen on the roentgenogram. Abduction of the hallux, with indentation of the soft tissues laterally, is seen once stage two is reached. Metatarsus adductus primus, an increase of the adduction angle between the first and second metatarsals, is the hallmark of stage three of the deformity. A subluxation or dislocation of the first MTP joint characterizes stage four, with the hallux riding over or under the second toe.[6] Once stage four is reached, secondary complications can include the development of a hammertoe deformity of the second toe, all the lesser toes may be dictated into valgus, and/or the entire forefoot can fail, allowing excessive loads to be transferred onto the lesser metatarsal heads.[46] If forefoot failure occurs, then transverse metatarsalgia is likely with concurrent increased risk of stress fractures.[46]

Hallux Rigidus and Hallux Limitus

Hallux rigidus is a hypomobility of the first MTP joint. Hallux limitus is an ankylosing of the first MTP joint. A rigidus deformity may be a precursor to a limitus deformity.[6,29,43]

Several causes of hallux limitus deformity exist. Hypermobility of the first ray associated with abnormal pronation and calcaneal eversion, immobilization of the first MTP joint, degenerative joint disease of the first MTP joint, trauma causing an inflammatory response of the joint, metatarsus primus elevatus, and an excessively long first metatarsal may all be precursors.[6,28,29] All of these precursors cause immobilization of the first MTP joint. As a result of this immobilization of a synovial joint, a limitus deformity occurs.[47-50]

The pathomechanics of a hallux limitus deformity are due to two problems: (1) an inability of the first metatarsal to plantar flex or (2) an inability of the first MTP joint to dorsiflex. Abnormal pronation of the subtalar joint prevents the first metatarsal from plantar flexing because of the effect of ground reaction forces on the metatarsal. Ground reaction forces dorsiflex the first metatarsal during abnormal pronation. An excessively long first metatarsal can also prevent the metatarsal from plantar flexing. Any trauma or inflammatory disease that causes bony deformation of the first MTP joint can prevent normal MTP joint motion. If this type of immobilization continues untreated, then the end result will be a rigidus (or ankylosed) deformity of the first MTP joint.[6,28,51]

Tailor's Bunion

Tailor's bunion is the mirror image of an abductovalgus deformity of the first ray occurring at the fifth MTP joint.[6] Adduction of the fifth toe and abduction of the fifth metatarsal are seen in this deformity.[6,34] The cause of a tailor's bunion can be broadly grouped as either structural or biomechanical.[52] Structural causes can include pressure over the lateral aspect of the fifth metatarsal head from tight shoes, static foot posturing (as in Tailor's), or a prominent lateral condyle.[52] Four biomechanical causes of Tailor's bunion are (1) abnormal pronation, (2) uncompensated forefoot varus, (3) congenital dorsiflexed fifth metatarsal, and (4) congenitally plantar flexed fifth metatarsal.[52]

Abnormal pronation is reported to be a factor in the cause of Tailor's bunion.[6,52] For abnormal pronation to cause a Tailor's bunion, one of the other causative factors noted previously must also be present.[6] Abnormal pronation causes hypermobility of the fifth metatarsal. This hypermobility produces internal shearing between the metatarsal and the overlying soft tissue. As the deformity progresses, the events described in the hallux abductovalgus deformity occur.[6]

Uncompensated forefoot varus, exceeding the range of motion of pronation of the subtalar joint, causes the fifth metatarsal to bear excessive weight. This excessive weight-bearing forces the fifth metatarsal to dorsiflex and evert. The dorsiflexion and eversion cause the fifth metatarsal to abduct and the proximal phalanx of the fifth toe to adduct, resulting in a Tailor's bunion.[6]

Congenital plantar flexion of the fifth metatarsal prevents the fifth metatarsal from dorsiflexing beyond the transverse plane of the other metatarsal heads. This plantar flexed attitude and abnormally pronating foot cause the fifth metatarsal to become unstable. Ground reaction forces force the fifth metatarsal to evert, abduct, and dorsiflex. Eventually the fifth metatarsal subluxates and is no longer functional.[6]

The last cause of a Tailor's bunion is a congenitally dorsiflexed fifth metatarsal. The only visual abnormality present is a dorsally located bunion. The dorsal attitude of the fifth toe causes abnormal shearing between the bone and the overlying dorsal soft tissues. This abnormal shearing is due to the firm fixation of the soft tissues by the shoe.[6]

Hammer Toes

In a hammer toe deformity, the MTP and distal interphalangeal (DIP) joints are in extension while the proximal interphalangeal joint (PIP) is in flexion.[6,31,52,53] Hammer toe can be classified into two categories: (1) flexible (dynamic) and (2) fixed (static). The determinant between the two classifications is dependent on whether available motion exists at the PIP joint.[26] Plantar flexed metatarsals, loss of lumbrical function, imbalance of interossei function, paralysis of the extensors of the toes, shortness of a metatarsal, forefoot valgus, hallux abductovalgus, trauma to the MTP joint causing instability, and subluxation of the fifth toe into pronation are all possible causes of a hammer toe deformity.[6,31] The common denominator among all of these pathologic conditions is the production of a force imbalance across the MTP joint. This force imbalance may lead to a joint instability of the MTP or an imbalance of the muscles crossing the MTP joint.[4,6,31]

Claw Toes

A claw toe deformity occurs when the MTP joint is in extension and the DIP and PIP joints are in flexion.[6,32,53-55] The possible causes are forefoot adductus, congenitally plantar flexed first metatarsal, arthritis, spasm of the long and short toe flexors, weak gastrocnemius, forefoot supinatus, and pes cavus.[6,32]

Forefoot adductus, congenitally plantar flexed first ray, forefoot supinatus, and pes cavus all have the same pathomechanical effect on the toes.[6] The adduction angle of the metatarsals and the abduction angle of the phalanges increase. Instability of the MTP joints occurs as a result of this malalignment. The function of the lumbricals and flexors of the toes is altered as a result of the combined effect of instability and poor joint position. The alteration of these muscle groups instigates extension of the MTP and flexion of the DIP and PIP joints of all the digits of the foot.[6]

Arthritis of the MTPs leads to an overstretching of the restraining mechanisms of the extensor tendons of the toes, much the same as in arthritic conditions of the hand. This overstretching allows the tendons to drift laterally and alter their line of pull. Again, the alteration of the line of pull causes the toes to be abducted, and the claw toe deformity ensues.[6,32]

During heel-off and toe-off, the activity of the long toe flexors increases to compensate for a weak gastrocnemius. The increased toe flexor activity overpowers the extensors of the toes, resulting in a claw toe deformity. Spasm of the long and short toe flexors can cause a claw toe deformity in a similar fashion.[6]

Mallet Toes

Mallet toe refers to a flexion deformity of the DIP of one or more of the lesser toes.[56] The flexed attitude may be fixed or malleable. The cause of mallet toe deformity is uncertain.[56-58] Some authors speculate that the condition is congenital or the result of wearing shoes that are not long enough.[6,32,56] Other proposed causes include traumatic, idiopathic, and neuromuscular disorders, increased length of the lesser toe involved, and use of high-heeled shoes with a narrow toe box.[56-58]

Plantar Fasciitis

Plantar fasciitis involves an overstretching of the plantar fascia causing an inflammatory reaction, usually near the fascia's calcaneal attachment. The cause is multifactorial, with mechanical overload generally believed to be fundamental in the development of the condition.[59] Excessive pronation has been found to be an important mechanical cause of the structural strain, which results in plantar fasciitis.[60] However, work-related, weight-bearing, training errors in athletes and biomechanical abnormalities including, but not limited to, a tight Achilles tendon and reduced talocrural dorsiflexion are common predisposing factors.[61,62] Without regard to the mechanical reason for decreased dorsiflexion (bony abnormality or tight Achilles tendon) at the talocrural joint, the result is compensatory excessive pronation. During gait, the plantar fascia is overstretched, with excessive pronation and extension of the MTP joint occurring simultaneously. Therefore any individual who abnormally pronates during the push-off phase of gait is at risk of developing plantar fasciitis. The presence of a pes cavus foot also predisposes the individual to this condition, because in pes cavus the plantar fascia is already tight even when the foot is at rest.[53,64-66] These factors result in repetitive microtrauma and microtears, which impede the normal healing processes and result in the inflammatory reaction.[59]

GENERAL EVALUATION

Musculoskeletal Evaluation

A foot and ankle evaluation begins with a visual inspection of the lower extremity as a whole. Any muscular imbalances affecting structural alignment and possibly altering normal mechanics are noted. The examiner then focuses on the foot and ankle. Areas of redness, ecchymosis, effusion, edema, bony angulation, and callus formation are noted.[9,53,54] The visual inspection is followed by a palpatory examination. Any areas of tenderness and increased tissue tension are discerned.[9,53,54]

Next a range-of-motion evaluation noting the amount of dorsiflexion and plantar flexion of the talocrural and MTP joints is performed.[9,53,54,67] For normal function of the lower extremity, at least 10 degrees of dorsiflexion and 30 degrees of plantar flexion of the talocrural joint should be seen.[6,9,68] In addition, at least 60 degrees of dorsiflexion should be present for normal function of the first MTP joint.[17,25,69]

A gross manual muscle test (MMT) of the musculature about the ankle is performed next.[9,53,54] Consideration should be given to evaluating the strength of the ipsilateral hip and knee musculature as well, given their contribution to lower kinetic chain mechanics. For a more quantitative test of ankle muscle strength, an isokinetic evaluation can be performed. The examiner should expect to see normal absolute peak torque values at 30 degrees/second and at 120 degrees/second for all muscle groups tested. Peak torque values for ankle evertors and invertors should be around 21 feet/lb for men and 15 feet/lb OK MJW for women at 30 degrees/second. At 120 degrees/second, the torque values should be around 15 feet/lb for men and 10 feet/lb for women.[70,71]

A general overview of the neurovascular structure ends the general screening evaluation. Areas of decreased sensation and areas of hyperesthesia are noted. A general circulatory examination is performed to establish circulatory integrity of the arterial supply to the foot and ankle. The dorsalis pedis and posterior tibial pulses are established.[9,53,54]

Specific Evaluative Procedures

Tarsal tunnel entrapment may be discerned by two specific manual tests: (1) hyperpronation and (2) Tinel's sign.[29,31,53] Hyperpronation of the subtalar joint decreases the diameter of

the tarsal tunnel. During the hyperpronation test, the subtalar joint is maintained in excessive pronation for 30 to 60 seconds.[31] A positive test results in the reproduction of the patient's symptoms on a consistent basis. In Tinel's sign the examiner taps the posterior tibial nerve proximal to its entrance to the tarsal tunnel. A positive test again results in the reproduction of the patient's symptoms.

Along with these two manual tests, MMT and sensory testing are performed to determine the extent of nerve trunk compression. Weakness, as determined by a MMT, of the muscles innervated by the medial and lateral plantar nerves may be indicative of a peripheral nerve entrapment at the tarsal tunnel.[29,31] Sensory tests are performed to determine the presence and extent of areas of hypoesthesia. These areas should correspond to the particular areas of innervation of the involved nerves.[28,29,31]

Electromyography (EMG) studies can also be performed to further document the presence of tarsal tunnel entrapment. Latencies greater than 6.2 and 7.0 seconds to the abductor hallucis and the abductor digiti quinti, respectively, are indicative of entrapment of the posterior tibial nerve at the tarsal tunnel.[28]

The history obtained by the clinician will usually elicit complaints of burning, tingling, or pain in the medial arch or the plantar aspect of foot. These symptoms usually are aggravated by increased activity. The patient may complain of nocturnal pain with proximal or distal radiation of symptoms.[28,29,31]

During the general evaluation, the clinician may notice a valgus attitude of the calcaneus during static standing. This position of the calcaneus may be a predisposing, perpetuating, or precipitating factor in tarsal tunnel entrapment. One other evaluative procedure, a biomechanical foot evaluation, is also performed. In this evaluation other predisposing, perpetuating, or precipitating factors of tarsal tunnel may be discovered (e.g., excessive subtalar joint motion).[6,28,29,31] This portion of the evaluation is discussed in detail later in this chapter.

Patients with neuroma typically present a history of acute episodes of radiating pains and/or paresthesias into the toes. The onset of the pain is sudden and cramplike. Initially, the symptoms occur only when the patient is wearing shoes that compress the toes; with time the pain may become intractable. The patient reports that the symptoms are or were alleviated by the removal of shoes and massaging of the toes.[6,28-32] Clinical signs can include tenderness within the affected interdigital space, pain on metatarsal head approximation, and/or Mulder's click (felt by the examiner as the heads of the metatarsals are compressed and the plantar tissues are pushed dorsally into the space).[72,73]

Fractures and sprains of the talocrural joint are evaluated in much the same manner. The major difference is that the clinician must wait until a fracture has healed sufficiently before proceeding with any evaluative tests, whereas in a patient who has sustained a sprain, the clinician may apply the evaluative tests immediately. The evaluation generally consists of obtaining a history, performing range-of-motion measurements, strength testing, noting the presence of edema or effusion, and noting the presence of any residual deformity in the foot and ankle.[29,36,39]

Range-of-motion testing first assesses the osteokinematic motion of the involved joint. The joint itself, as well as the joints proximal and distal to it, are assessed. For example, in a talocrural fracture, the range of motion of the MTP joints, the hip and knee, as well as of the ankle is evaluated. Once the osteokinematic movements of any joints have been assessed, the arthrokinematic movements of any restricted joints are evaluated.[29,36,39,74,75] Additionally, intermetatarsal joint play motion should be assessed to determine any lack of mobility secondary to immobilization.

Strength is evaluated using MMT techniques and/or isokinetic procedures. As in the range-of-motion testing, the joints proximal to, distal to, and at the site of injury are all tested.[29] If isokinetic tests are performed, then the involved joint is tested at both slow and fast speeds.[71]

Circumferential measurements of the foot and ankle are taken to document the presence of effusion or edema. The flexibility of the heel cord is assessed to rule out Achilles tightness.

A biomechanical foot evaluation will also be beneficial in assessing the effect of any foot deformities may have on the patient's lower extremity.[29,36,39]

Two added components are found in the evaluation of talocrural and tibiofibular sprains: (1) ligamentous laxity and (2) talar mobility tests. Three ligamentous laxity tests are used to evaluate the integrity of the talocrural ligaments. The first is the anterior and posterior drawer test (Figure 23-1) to determine the integrity of the anterior and posterior talofibular ligaments.[9,29] The others are the inversion and eversion stress tests (Figure 23-2). These tests evaluate the integrity of the calcaneofibular and deltoid ligaments.[9,29] Talar mobility tests consist of medial and lateral stress tests (Figure 23-3). These tests evaluate the integrity of the inferior talofibular syndesmosis. Palpation may also be helpful in isolating the ligamentous tissues at fault.[9,29]

In pathomechanical conditions, the major portion of the assessment consists of a biomechanical foot and ankle evaluation and a proper medical workup. The medical workup is necessary to rule out systemic or neurologic causes for the

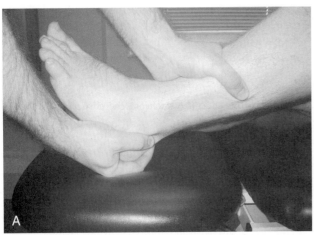
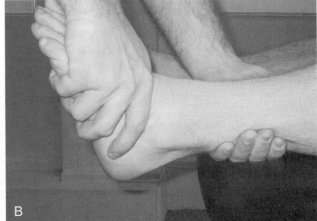

Figure 23-1 A, Anterior drawer test. **B,** Posterior drawer test.

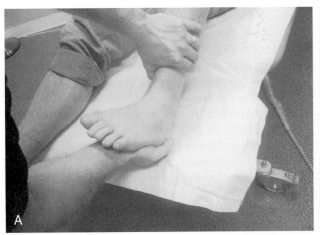
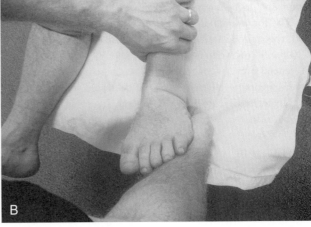

Figure 23-2 A, Inversion stress test. **B,** Eversion stress test.

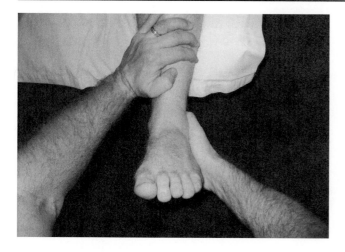

Figure 23-3 Medial talocrural stress test.

presenting deformity.[6] Obtaining a good history from the patient may be helpful initially and later on when assessing the effects of any treatments.

One pathomechanical entity requiring a slightly different evaluative procedure is plantar fasciitis. Along with a history, medical workup, and biomechanical evaluation, the clinician needs to perform a specific palpatory evaluation of the plantar fascia and calcaneal area. In the history, the patient will complain of pain and tenderness localized to the plantar aspect of the foot. The pain may radiate forward along the plantar aspect of the foot. Usually the pain is noted on standing after waking in the morning or after a period of sustained nonweight bearing, and it worsens as the client increases the distance he or she walks or runs.

On visual inspection of a patient with plantar fasciitis, the clinician may note the presence of a cavus foot. Edema of the medial plantar aspect of the heel may also be seen on visual inspection. Palpation may reveal point tenderness localized to the medial aspect of the calcaneus.[29,63-65] Passive toe extension may also reproduce the patient's pain.[53]

The chief physical therapy evaluative procedures for all of these conditions are a biomechanical gait analysis and a general lower kinetic chain evaluation including the ankle-foot, knee, and hip range-of-motion and strength testing to determine any perpetuating, predisposing, or precipitating factors to the development of these conditions. For a more detailed description of proximal joint contributions to lower-extremity dysfunctions, the reader should refer to the chapter on *Evaluation and Training of the Core* (Chapter 15).

Biomechanical Evaluation

The biomechanical assessment of the foot involves several steps. The evaluation begins with the visual inspection of the patient in a static standing posture, followed by static supine-lying, static prone-lying, static standing, and dynamic gait analyses.

Visual Inspection

The biomechanical evaluation begins with a visual inspection of the lower extremities while the patient is standing with the feet shoulder-width apart. The clinician needs to have visual access to the patient's entire lower quarter. The examiner observes for postural deviations or for signs of lower-extremity deviations.[76] Transverse plane rotations or torsions from the hip, femurs, knees, or tibias can be viewed from the front or from behind. Frontal plane deviations of varus or valgus of the tibias are viewed from behind; the examiner can view sagittal plane deviations from hip flexor or extensor tightness (or genu recurvatum) laterally.[76]

Static Supine-Lying Evaluation

During the supine-lying portion of the evaluation, the first step is to observe the foot for the presence of any callosities or deformities. Midfoot mobility is tested by a supination and pronation twist. The calcaneus is stabilized with one hand while a supination and pronation force to the forefoot is applied with the other (Figure 23-4). Next the range of motion of the first MTP joint is noted (Figure 23-5). The amount of intermetatarsal mobility is evaluated by applying inferior and superior forces and assessing the degree of resistance that is met by the clinician's hands. Finally, the angle of pull of the quadriceps muscle (Q angle) can further be measured. This angle is measured by placing the axis of a goniometer over the center of the patella, with the stationary arm aimed at the anterior superior iliac spine of the pelvis and the mobile arm in line with the tubercle of the tibia. The previous measurements are compared with those of the other limb for any dissimilarities.[6,29,53,75,77] Measurement results should be compared with the uninvolved lower extremity.

Static Prone-Lying Evaluation

The patient is positioned in a prone-lying attitude, with both lower extremities over the edge of a supporting surface so that the malleoli of the ankles are even with the edge of the surface. Visual inspection of the lower extremity consists of noting the presence of callosities and bony deformities of the foot and ankle.[6,29,53] Next the range of motion of talocrural dorsiflexion and plantar flexion is evaluated with the knee in extension (Figure 23-6).

One of the client's lower extremities is placed in slight knee flexion and abduction, with flexion and external rotation of the hip (Figure 23-7). This posture ensures that the opposite extremity is in a plane parallel with the ground and the supporting surface, keeping the foot at a right angle to the floor. Longitudinal bisection lines are now drawn with a fine-tip marker along the posterior aspect of the lower third of the calf and heel of the lower extremity.[77,78] It is extremely important to draw these bisection lines accurately. The clinician should make every effort to choose the same anatomic landmarks consistently to ensure the reliability of present and future measurements. If the clinician ensures the consistency of the location

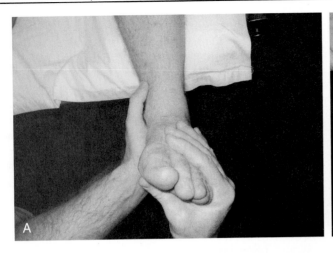

Figure 23-4 **A,** Midfoot supination twist. **B,** Midfoot pronation twist.

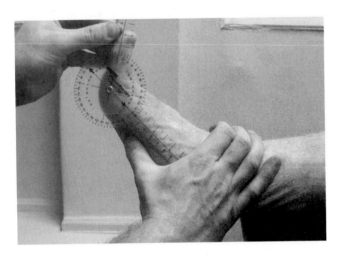

Figure 23-5 Goniometric measurement of metatarsophalangeal (MTP) joint flexion.

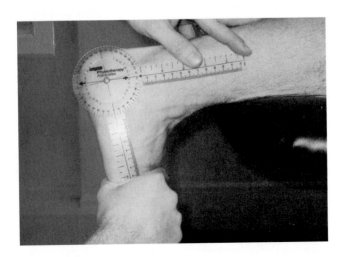

Figure 23-6 Goniometric measurement of talocrural joint dorsiflexion.

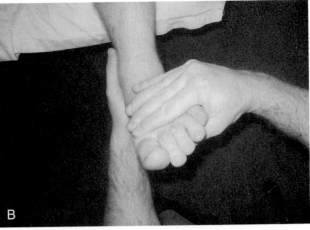

Figure 23-7 Prone-lying measurement position.

and use of the appropriate anatomic landmarks, then this procedure is reliable.[78]

Using the bisection lines, the clinician then measures the amount of subtalar joint range of motion. The clinician grasps the heel and the calf as indicated in Figure 23-8. The heel is moved in one direction (into inversion or eversion) until maximal resistance is felt, and the angular displacement of the heel is recorded. The same method is repeated in the opposite direction.[77,78] The eversion and inversion angles are summed to give the total subtalar joint range of motion.

The subtalar joint should pronate and supinate only a few degrees from the neutral position during normal gait. The most common method of finding the neutral position of the subtalar joint is by palpation, which is highly variable.[79-81] The anterior

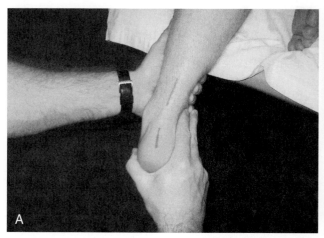
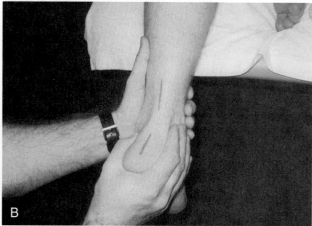

Figure 23-8 A, Calcaneal inversion. **B,** Subtalar inversion.

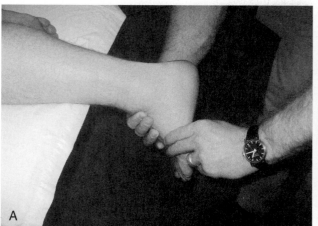
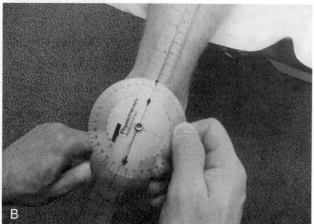

Figure 23-9 A, Paplation for subtalar joint neutral. **B,** Measurement of subtalar joint neutral.

aspect of the head of the talus is palpated with the thumb and middle finger of the medial hand (Figure 23-9, *A*). The examiner's lateral hand grasps the foot at the base of the fourth and fifth metatarsals and applies a downward distracting force to remove any resting ankle dorsiflexion. The foot is then passively inverted and everted as talar protrusion (laterally with inversion and medially with eversion) is palpated. The neutral position is the point at which talar protrusion is felt equally on both sides. Using the bisection lines, the neutral position is measured with a goniometer and documented in degrees of varus or valgus (Figure 23-9, *B*).[76] From the subtalar neutral position, a minimum of 4 degrees of eversion and 8 degrees of inversion of the calcaneus in the frontal plane (or total subtalar joint motion) are needed for normal function of the foot.[23,77,78]

Once the subtalar joint is in the neutral position, the frontal plane forefoot to rearfoot posture is determined by aligning one of the arms of a goniometer along the plane of the metatarsal heads and the other arm perpendicular to the bisection line of the heel (Figure 23-10).[77,78] The most prevalent forefoot to

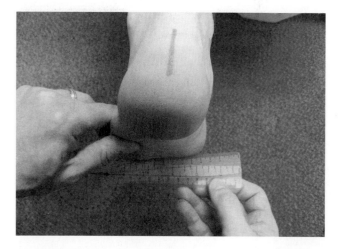

Figure 23-10 Measurement of forefoot to rearfoot posture.

rearfoot attitude in an asymptomatic population has been reported to be a varus attitude. The least common attitude is the neutral condition. A normal forefoot varus attitude, as measured by a goniometer, is 7.8 degrees, and a normal valgus attitude is 4.7 degrees.[78]

The possible influence of the gastrocsoleus complex on the subtalar joint can also be determined in the prone-lying position. Dorsiflexion at the talocrural joint with the knee in extension is compared with dorsiflexion with the knee in flexion. A dramatic increase in the range of motion of the talocrural joint, with the knee in flexion compared with extension, is an indication that the gastrocsoleus complex may be affecting subtalar joint mechanics.[6]

Static Standing Evaluation

The amount of tibial and calcaneal valgus or varus is measured with the patient in the static standing position and the feet shoulder-width apart, with equal weight on each leg. The clinician uses a goniometer to measure the angle of the calcaneal varus or valgus. The arms of the goniometer are aligned with the longitudinal bisection line of the calcaneus and parallel to the ground to measure the amount of calcaneal varus or valgus. To measure the amount of tibial varus or valgus, the arms of the goniometer are aligned with the longitudinal bisection line on the posterior aspect of the tibia and parallel to the ground (Figure 23-11).[6,29,53,77,82]

Gait Analysis

All of the previous information is correlated with a dynamic gait analysis. The patient is instructed to ambulate on a treadmill or the floor, with or without shoes. The speed of the gait should be slow at first and progressively increased to a normal pace. The markings on the heel allow the clinician to observe the patient for variances from the normal sequence of gait. The reader will recall that from heel-strike to foot-flat the subtalar joint pronates (the calcaneus everts). From midstance to heel-off, the subtalar joint resupinates (the calcaneus inverts). Close

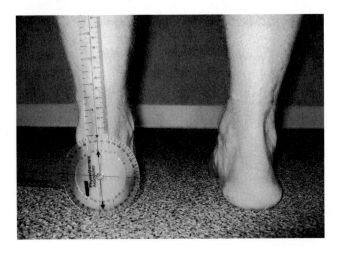

Figure 23-11 Measurement of tibial varum.

attention to the knee and hip joints should also be observed. Excessive genu varum or valgum or excessive hip internal or external rotation, as well as any limited motion, should be noted. This should correlate with the evaluated objective findings of these joints. The relationship of the lower extremity to the body should also be noted. The pelvis transfers energy between the lower and upper extremities. Therefore it should not move but ±5 degrees (anteroposterior and lateral tilt, rotation) throughout the gait cycle to assist in energy conservation.

SUMMARY OF EVALUATIVE PROCEDURES

The presence of a particular pathologic condition is not based solely on the findings from any one of the previous evaluative procedures. Instead the findings from all of the procedures should be correlated. Combining the results of the biomechanical and musculoskeletal examination of the entire lower kinetic chain with a detailed gait assessment provides the clinician with a comprehensive outlook of the possibilities of dysfunction. With these compounded results, a decision on the particular type of or approach to treatment should then be made. For instance, the presence of a forefoot deformity (e.g., forefoot valgus or varus) by itself is not indicative of a pathologic condition. The subtalar joint may be capable of compensating for this deformity. When the forefoot deformity is present along with some other factor (e.g., tight gastrocsoleus complex), the subtalar joint may be unable to compensate for the deformity. At this time, the decision to treat the forefoot deformity by the use of biomechanical orthotic devices is made.[69,78,83]

Treatment

Entrapments

Treatment for tarsal tunnel entrapment should address the predisposing and perpetuating causes of the entrapment. Permanent biomechanical orthotic devices to control the perpetuating and predisposing factors of excessive pronation are an effective method of treatment. In addition, lower-extremity muscle strengthening to correct the observed faulty mechanical components is of further use. In cases in which the tarsal tunnel symptoms are the result of internal causes (e.g., tendonitis of the posterior tibialis tendon), the physician may prescribe antiinflammatory medicine. The physician may opt to inject the area with medication or prescribe the use of iontophoresis and/ or phonophoresis with an antiinflammatory cream (such as 1% hydrocortisone cream).[84,85]

Conservative treatment of patients with neuromas of the foot consists of proper shoe wear. The patient is advised to wear wider shoes. Accommodative orthotic agents may be prescribed to relieve metatarsal head pressure on the neuroma and to correct the precipitating factor of abnormal pronation. Nonconservative treatment consists of surgical removal of the neuroma. For optimal results, nonconservative measures should be combined with treatments addressing the precipitating or perpetuating factors.[6,28,29,32] The use of orthotic agents, gastroc-soleus stretching to reverse possible overpronation because of a tight Achilles tendon, and/or lower-extremity strengthening in attempts to change other possible abnormal lower kinetic chain mechanics may all be warranted based on the findings of examination.

Trauma

Treatment of traumatic injuries consists of three phases: (1) acute, (2) subacute, and (3) postacute rehabilitation.

The acute phase of treatment follows the basic principles of protection from further injury: rest, ice, compression, and elevation of the injured site.[29,71,86] For the most part, the acute phase of treatment is a passive stage for the patient. This phase of treatment begins immediately after injury. Its duration is roughly the same for both fractures and sprains of the foot and ankle: 24 to 48 hours. Control and reduction of the inflammatory process are of the utmost importance during the acute stage. The maintenance of strength and range of motion of the proximal and distal joints to the site of the injury can further be a focus of the acute stage.

The subacute phase of treatment is slightly different for fractures and sprains of the foot and ankle. With fractures, the stability of the fracture site is of paramount importance. Control and reduction of edema and effusion, prevention of muscle atrophy, and maintenance of cardiovascular fitness are key goals for the rehabilitation program during this phase of treatment of foot and ankle fractures. Elevation of the involved extremity, isometric exercises of the immobilized muscles, and the use of upper-extremity ergometers are all recommended. Strengthening of the available adjacent joints remains important.[29,71,87]

Treatment of sprains differs from that of fractures in that mobility is encouraged during the subacute phase of the rehabilitation program.[29,71] With fractures, the patient is encouraged to begin sagittal plane exercises and movement. The exercises promote increased circulation and prevent excessive joint stiffness. Compressive supports (i.e., air splints) can be used to provide stability and prevent an increase in edema when the involved lower extremity is in a dependent position. Partial weight bearing using axillary crutches is also encouraged and progressed according to tolerance. Isometric exercises with the ankle muscles will be of benefit to reduce atrophy and assist with edema reduction. As in the subacute phase of traumatic fractures, the control of effusion and edema, maintenance of cardiovascular fitness, and lower-extremity strengthening of the adjacent joints are emphasized during the subacute phase of sprains.[29,71,86]

The postacute phase of traumatic injuries to the foot and ankle emphasizes the improvement of mobility and strength of the involved joints and muscles. Once again, the treatment of fractures and the treatment of sprains parallel each other. The only difference between the two types of injury is in the areas of emphasis in the initial period of treatment. The initial emphasis with fractures is on the improvement of range of motion, both osteokinematic and arthrokinematic, of the

involved joint, whereas the initial emphasis with sprains during the postacute phase is on improving the strength of the surrounding musculature and the proprioceptive ability of the injured joint. The strength of the invertors, evertors, dorsiflexors, and plantar flexors of the ankle is increased by the use of resistive exercises progressed according to tolerance and performance. The progression of balance and proprioceptive exercises should be incorporated from single-leg stance on various surfaces (floor, on foam), with eyes open and eyes closed to challenge the three components of balance. As previously mentioned, other involved muscle groups of the lower kinetic chain (knee and hip musculature) may also need further strengthening. The final rehabilitation stage of both types of injury is a progression to functional activities. For the athlete, the final stage is a progression to sport-specific skill and agility exercises (e.g., figure-eight exercises, lateral slides).[29,71,88-90]

Specific treatments of talocrural fractures include mobilization of the talocrural, inferior tibiofibular, midtarsal intermetatarsal, and MTP joints. Initially, the arthrokinematic motions of roll and glide are restored through various mobilization techniques.[29,71,91] Two mobilization techniques used in treating the talocrural joint are (1) posterior glide of the tibia and fibula on the talus and (2) long axis distraction of the talocrural joint[74,75,91] (see Chapter 26). The glide technique is used to assist in restoring the osteokinematic motion of dorsiflexion and plantar flexion. A general capsular stretch is provided by the distractive technique. Osteokinematic motions are also performed along with the arthrokinematic motions. Usually the osteokinematic motions can be performed while the patient is in a whirlpool or after application of moist heat. The warmth can assist pain control and promote tissue plasticity. Heel cord stretching is also emphasized during treatment.[29,71,91]

Along with the improvement of movement and strength, the joint proprioceptors must also be retrained. This retraining consists of tilt board and progression of unilateral weight-bearing and balance exercises on varying surfaces (on floor, on foam) with the eyes open and shut (with and without the visual component of balance).[88-90] Finally, in some cases, the prescription of a biomechanical orthotic device may be of assistance in controlling any abnormal pronatory or supinatory forces that may be present. The use of orthotic devices may be of most use in those patients who have experienced a stress fracture of the metatarsals.

Specific treatment of MTP sprains consists of icing to reduce the inflammatory process, protective wrapping, and a non-weight-bearing gait initially. Exercises that do not increase discomfort in conjunction with a graduated return to a pain-free activity program will follow. Mobilization of the MTP joint is performed when stiffness indicates this procedure to be of value.

Pathomechanical Conditions

As with entrapments, the treatments of pathomechanical conditions address the predisposing and perpetuating factors. These two factors are usually handled by the use of strengthening exercises to control abnormal transverse and frontal plane motions in the lower extremities, as well as biomechanical orthotic devices that assist in controlling the abnormal pronation or supination occurring at the subtalar joint. The orthotic devices will also support varus or valgus deformities of the forefoot if present.[6]

Other forms of treatment that accommodate or attempt to control the predisposing or perpetuating factors are heel lifts and accommodative shoes. For instance, decreasing the height of heels has been recommended for individuals who abnormally pronate because of intrinsic factors. Increasing the heel height has been recommended for individuals who abnormally pronate to compensate for extrinsic muscle problems (e.g., gastrocnemius tightness). Both of these heel height corrections have been recommended in the treatment of hallux abductovalgus conditions.[6,45,64]

Some pathomechanical conditions may require other forms of treatment in addition to the use of lower-extremity strengthening and flexibility and biomechanical orthotic devices. Mobilization of any joints exhibiting limitation of movement, thereby causing abnormal pronation or supination, may be needed. Such techniques may be useful in the treatment of a plantar flexed fifth metatarsal in a Tailor's bunion, a limitus deformity of the first MTP joint, and a mallet toe deformity. In conjunction with the mobilization techniques, the use of appropriate heating modalities has been shown to be effective in the treatment of joint hypomobility.[6,64]

Adjunctive treatments for inflammatory conditions of the foot and ankle include the use of cryotherapy to control any edema present. Iontophoresis or phonophoresis with 10% hydrocortisone cream can also be used to control the inflammatory reaction that is present with plantar fasciitis and to alleviate the presenting symptoms.[29,84]

Surgical correction of any deformities that are present is a promising alternative.[6,28] Surgery may also be the most effective treatment in cases in which the predisposing factor is an excessively long metatarsal or elevatus condition.[6,47] Tenotomies of the flexor tendon with relocation of the tendon onto the dorsal surface of the foot are alternative forms of treatment in such conditions as mallet toes.[6] Strengthening exercises of the uninvolved joints of the affected lower extremity will also be of benefit for patients requiring surgery to prevent disuse atrophy from occurring during the recuperative period.

 CASE STUDIES

Case Study 26-1

M.M. is a 35-year-old competitive runner (masters level) with a diagnosis of plantar fasciitis of the left foot. His pain began 4 weeks earlier after a training run. The pain was centered over the medial plantar aspect of his left heel, radiating distally to the first and second metatarsal heads and proximally to the insertion of the tendoachilles. Initially, the pain was localized to the plantar aspect of the foot. The heel pain was worse in the morning, improved by midday, and worsened by the evening. When M.M. trained, he was able to run approximately 6 minutes before he noticed an increase in the heel pain. He was able to continue to run for another 6 minutes before he had to stop. The pain remained elevated for approximately 30 minutes after he stopped running.

The past medical history was insignificant. Radiographs taken 2 weeks earlier were negative. M.M. stated that he was currently taking a prescription antiinflammatory drug. His orthopaedist had injected a prednisone-lidocaine mixture into the plantar aspect of the left heel approximately 2 weeks earlier. The patient also stated that he was continuing to run but only for 2 miles. In the previous 2 weeks, his symptoms remained unchanged.

Visual inspection was unremarkable, except for a slight tibial varus bilaterally (calcanei are in neutral position). Palpation of the left heel revealed an area of marked tenderness located over the insertion of the plantar aponeurosis. Extension of the MTPs, with concomitant deep pressure applied over the insertion of the plantar aponeurosis, increased M.M.'s symptoms. A slight decrease in the inter-metatarsal motion was noted during accessory joint testing of the left foot and ankle. Passive joint testing was within normal limits, except for a decrease in dorsiflexion of the left ankle with the knee extended. The left ankle dorsiflexed to 0 degrees and 20 degrees with the knee extended and flexed, respectively. Isometric break testing of the lower extremities was within normal limits (WNL).

The static biomechanical evaluation was significant for a decrease in left subtalar joint motion, bilateral forefoot varus, and bilateral tibial varum (Figure 23-12). The dynamic biomechanical evaluation was significant for abnormal pronation of the left foot (foot pronated from midstance to toe-off). The extent of pronation (in terms of quantity, not duration) increased with the speed of gait.

Given the patient's area and behavior of pain, he appeared to be experiencing an acute inflammatory condition of a mechanical nature. The source of M.M.'s problem was not single but multiple, involving several structural and functional deficiencies that were acting conjointly to decrease his ability to adapt to the different stresses his left foot and ankle were undergoing during running. The functional factors were the limited intermetatarsal joint play, gastrocnemius tightness (limited talocrural joint dorsiflexion), and limited subtalar joint motion. The structural factors were the forefoot varus and tibial varus.

The interrelationship between the structural and functional deficiencies can best be highlighted by a hypothesized effect of tibial varus on subtalar joint mechanics of the left foot. To have the foot in contact with the ground during the foot-flat, midstance, and heel-off phases of gait, the

CASE STUDIES—cont'd

subtalar joint must pronate to compensate for the degree of forefoot and tibial varus present. Unfortunately, no subtalar range of motion occurred, which prevented the subtalar joint from compensating for the combined amount of forefoot varus and tibial varus. This lack of compensation was compounded by the inability of the metatarsals to compensate for the forefoot varus by plantar flexing secondary to limited intermetatarsal motion. This lack of compensation on the part of the forefoot and rearfoot may place increased stress on the medial plantar structures (i.e., plantar aponeurosis), possibly causing damage to the tissues located there.[6]

Because M.M.'s problem was multifaceted, the treatment plan that was initiated attempted to address several of the functional and structural deficiencies noted. A home exercise program was implemented, with the goal of decreasing the abnormal stress imparted to the foot, controlling any inflammatory reaction occurring in the foot, and improving the flexibility of the posterior lower-leg musculature. The patient was instructed to discontinue running for 2 weeks, substituting a walking and cycling program, to apply ice packs to the left heel at night and after workouts, and to perform posterior lower-leg stretches (Figure 23-13). The

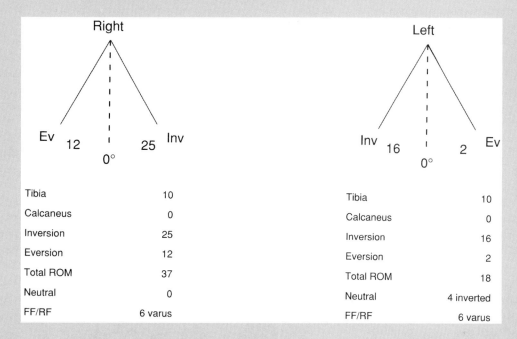

Right		Left	
Ev 12	25 Inv	Inv 16	2 Ev
0°		0°	
Tibia	10	Tibia	10
Calcaneus	0	Calcaneus	0
Inversion	25	Inversion	16
Eversion	12	Eversion	2
Total ROM	37	Total ROM	18
Neutral	0	Neutral	4 inverted
FF/RF	6 varus	FF/RF	6 varus

Figure 23-12 Static biomechanical evaluation form. *Ev,* Eversion; *FF,* forefoot; *Inv,* inversion; *RF,* rearfoot; *ROM,* range of motion.

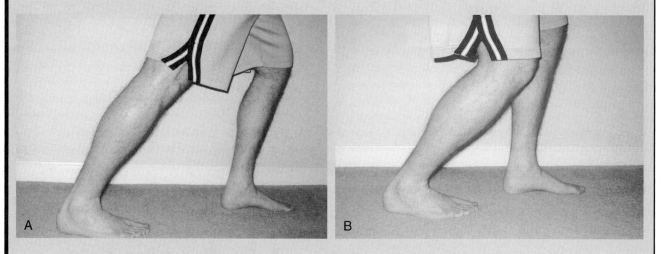

Figure 23-13 A, Gastrocnemius stretch. **B,** Soleus stretch.

Continued

CASE STUDIES—cont'd

walking and cycling program consisted of 30-minute pain-free workouts. If M.M. experienced any pain in his left foot, then he was to stop the activity and apply ice to the left foot. Return to this low-level activity could begin if by the next workout no further increase in M.M.'s symptoms occurred.

An office-based treatment program was also implemented to help reduce the inflammatory reaction in the left heel with modalities, improve the mobility of the forefoot area with joint mobilizations, and reduce the abnormal biomechanical stresses in the left foot with lower-extremity stretching and strengthening to correct abnormal mechanics. The patient was seen three times per week for the first 2 weeks. In addition to manual treatment and therapeutic exercise, the patient received 10-minute treatments of phonophoresis at 1.5 W/cm^2, using 10% hydrocortisone cream to the medial plantar surface of the left heel. The phonophoresis treatments were immediately followed by ice massage over the same area to which the phonophoresis was applied. At the initial office visit, a pair of temporary biomechanical orthotic devices was constructed using a 6-degree medial forefoot post and a 3-degree rearfoot post in an attempt to control the abnormal pronation. The patient was instructed to wear the orthotic devices for 1-hour periods, alternating with 1-hour rest periods on the day he received the orthotic devices. He was to double the period of wearing his orthotic device while keeping the rest period constant until he was able to wear the orthotic devices for an 8-hour period, after which he no longer needed a rest period. If at any time during this phase of treatment M.M. experienced any increase in his symptoms secondary to wearing an orthotic device, then he was to discontinue their use, ice the left foot, and inform the therapist.

After 2 weeks the patient reported a significant reduction in symptoms. A return to a running program was now instituted. M.M. was instructed to start running approximately one fourth of a mile during his first training session and walk one fourth of a mile. He was to increase the distance by doubling his previous workout as long as he was pain free for two consecutive workouts. Once he was able to run for 1 mile pain free, he could continue to increase the distance of the run by half-mile increments while decreasing the walking by half-mile increments until he achieved his desired training level. Permanent semirigid orthotic devices were constructed with a medial 6-degree forefoot post bilaterally and a 3-degree medial rearfoot post with 2 degrees of motion. The rearfoot post incorporated 2 degrees of motion to help compensate for the decreased subtalar joint motion and tibial varus. At the 6-month follow-up examination, M.M. stated that he was pain free.

Case Study 26-2

M.L. is a 35-year-old female patient who has primary complaints of pain posterior and superior to the medial malleolus bilaterally. The symptoms on the right are more severe than those on the left side. She is a recreational runner, who runs 5 miles four times per week. Recently, she has started experiencing pain during her runs. Initially, her symptoms commenced after running for 2 miles. Currently, they begin after running for 1 mile. The pain persists for 2 hours after she finishes running. Additionally, M.L. has begun experiencing pain when ascending and descending stairs, as well as if she is on her feet for more than half an hour. Her past medical history is significant for a minor ankle sprain that she suffered approximately 1 year ago. She did not receive any medical treatment, and the sprain healed satisfactorily within a reasonable amount of time.

Visual inspection of M.L. was unremarkable. The patient reported tenderness to palpation along the posterior tibialis just superior to the medial malleolus. All resisted ankle movements were 5/5 in strength. Repeated resisted ankle inversion reproduced her symptoms. Goniometric assessment of the talocrural joint range of motion was unremarkable except for ankle dorsiflexion, which was limited bilaterally. M.L. exhibited 5 degrees and 7 degrees of dorsiflexion passively in the left and right talocrural joints, respectively. Passive ankle movements in all planes did not reproduce M.L.'s symptoms.

A static and dynamic biomechanical foot and ankle assessment was performed. M.L. was positioned prone lying, and the subtalar joint neutral position was determined. The neutral position of the subtalar joint was 10 degrees inverted for the right and 12 degrees inverted for the left lower extremity, respectively. With the rearfoot in this posture, a forefoot varus of 10 degrees was noted bilaterally. When M.L. was examined in weight bearing, the orientation of the calcaneus with respect to the floor was determined in two standing postures. With M.L. standing in an erect posture and the subtalar joints in a neutral position, a calcaneal position of 0 degrees with respect to the floor was determined bilaterally. M.L. was now instructed to stand in a relaxed upright posture, and a calcaneal varum attitude of 7 degrees on the left and 4 degrees on the right was measured. M.L.'s tibial varum was also measured with the subtalar joint in its neutral position while in double- and single-limb stance. Measurement of this angle during single-limb stance is especially important for runners because of the increased time in unilateral weight bearing during running gait. Tibia varum with the subtalar joint in its neutral position when in double-leg stance was 0 degrees bilaterally. In single-leg stance, M.L. had 8 degrees and 6 degrees of tibial varum on the left and right lower extremities, respectively.

A visual inspection of M.L.'s lower-extremity biomechanics while walking and running was also conducted. During the initial contact to loading response phases of walking and running gaits, M.L. demonstrated excessive pronation of the subtalar joint bilaterally. The excessive

CASE STUDIES—cont'd

pronation appeared to be off a greater amount during running.

Given the location of the patient's symptoms—provocation of pain with resisted inversion and palpation along the posterior tibialis—M.L. appeared to be experiencing tendinitis of the posterior tibialis. The excessive pronation seen during M.L.'s walking and running gaits is an attempt by the lower extremity to compensate for the loss of ankle motion and skeletal malalignment noted during the physical evaluation. The excessive pronation has placed abnormal stress on the posterior tibialis, creating the tendinitis. The control of pain and of the existing inflammatory process was the primary goal of M.L.'s initial treatment program. During the first week of formal treatment, modalities and manual techniques were used to facilitate healing of M.L.'s tendon. Ice massage and deep friction massage were applied to the tendon during the first week of treatment.[92,93] After the massage, phonophoresis was administered at 3.0 MHz, 20% duty cycle, 0.75 W/cm^2 for 5 to 10 minutes to the tendon.[94] The physician was contacted to prescribe an anti-inflammatory medication to assist in the control of the inflammatory process. Additionally, M.L. was instructed to self-administer ice massages whenever her symptoms increased.

To address the loss of dorsiflexion noted during the passive range-of-motion examination, a mobilization program to the posterior talocrural joint capsule was instituted during the first week of treatment. In addition to the mobilization program, a home exercise program consisting of passive talocrural joint dorsiflexion stretches while in a nonweight-bearing posture were instituted. (Note: The therapist must take the time to educate the patient about the correct form in which this stretch should be performed to ensure the avoidance of pronation of the subtalar joint during the stretch.)

Excessive stresses must not be placed on the tendon. Therefore the patient was advised to discontinue running for at least 3 weeks. Alternate forms of cardiovascular training were suggested to M.L., including bicycling, swimming, or running in a gravity-reduced environment (e.g., in a pool using a flotation vest).

During the second and third weeks of treatment, once M.L. reported less pain with walking activities, weight-bearing heel cord stretching was initiated. Excessive pronation is prevented during this stretch by placing a wedge under the medial aspect of the foot. Lower-extremity strengthening exercises were initiated for control of movement of the kinetic chain. Ankle strengthening was emphasized in all movement directions except for ankle inversion. Concentric and eccentric ankle inversion exercises were added to the program once M.L. demonstrated that she could invert her foot without provoking her symptoms. Eccentric exercises during this phase of rehabilitation were emphasized, because they have been shown to prevent the recurrence of tendinitis.[95,96]

By the third week of treatment, when M.L. was able to perform resistive exercises without provoking symptoms, a home exercise program was implemented that incorporated more functional demands of the lower extremity. The program included directions to discontinue these exercises if they provoked any of her symptoms. The home exercises consisted of light hopping on a compliant surface, as well as single-leg balance activities on varying surfaces (with eyes open and with eyes closed) to prepare the patient for increased weight-bearing demands. If M.L. remained asymptomatic during these activities, then a fast-walking program with progression to running would be initiated.

The other aspect of this patient's management was the prescription of a biomechanical orthotic device.[79,97,98] A semirigid orthotic device with a 4-degree medial rearfoot post and a 5-degree medial forefoot post was fabricated. The instructions for use and wear of the orthotic device were the same as in the previous case. The initial examination revealed that M.L. had excessive forefoot and calcaneal varus and diminished talocrural joint dorsiflexion. This combination of skeletal alignment and soft tissue tightness contributed to the compensatory excessive pronation that was present. Therefore an orthotic device was given to the patient to decrease the abnormal stresses that were being sustained by the posterior tibialis tendon. At the 4-month follow-up examination, M.L. continued to be pain free and returned to her previous level of recreational running.

SUMMARY

This chapter provides a review of the anatomy and biomechanics of the foot and ankle, both abnormal and normal. Different pathologic entities, with their pathophysiologic conditions, evaluations, and treatments are described. A common bond between all the entities is in the areas of treatment and evaluation. When treating these conditions, the clinician must be aware of adjacent areas that may require treatment. These adjacent areas are discovered through a comprehensive evaluation of the lower kinetic chain.

Much research, both demographic and cause and effect, needs to be performed in the area of the foot and ankle. Future research should address the effectiveness of different treatments of the pathologic entities. An attempt should also be made to establish normative data regarding the different lower-extremity relationships and strength values. The foundation for a sound treatment program is sound research.

REFERENCES

1. Bojsen-Moller F: Anatomy of the forefoot, normal and pathological, Clin Orthop Relat Res 142:10, 1979.

2. Jaffe WL, Laitman JT: The evolution and anatomy of the human foot. In Jahss M, editor: Disorders of the foot, vol 1, Philadelphia, 1982, WB Saunders, p 1.

3. Moore KL: The lower limb. In Clinically oriented anatomy, Baltimore, 1980, Williams & Wilkins, p 491.

4. Sarafian SK: Anatomy of the foot and ankle: descriptive topographic functional, Philadelphia, 1983, JB Lippincott.

5. Warwick R, Williams PL: Gray's anatomy, Philadelphia, 1973, WB Saunders.

6. Root ML, Orien WP, Weed JH: Normal and abnormal function of the foot: clinical biomechanics, vol 2, Los Angeles, 1977, Clinical Biomechanics Corp.

7. Steindler A: The mechanics of the foot and ankle. In Kinesiology of the human body under normal and pathological conditions, Springfield, Ill, 1973, Charles C Thomas, p 373.

8. Perry J: Anatomy and biomechanics of the hindfoot, Clin Orthop Relat Res 177:9, 1983.

9. Fetto JF: Anatomy and examination of the foot and ankle. In Nicholas JA, Hershman EB, editors: The lower extremity and spine in sports medicine, vol 1, St Louis, 1986, Mosby, p 371.

10. Donatelli R: Normal anatomy and biomechanics. In Donatelli RA, editor: The biomechanics of the foot and ankle, 2 ed, Philadelphia, 1996, FA Davis Company, pp 20-21.

11. Elftman H: The transverse tarsal joint and its control, Clin Orthop Relat Res 16:41, 1960.

12. Manter JT: Movements of the subtalar and transverse tarsal joints, Anat Rec 80:397, 1941.

13. Phillips RD, Phillips RL: Quantitative analysis of the locking position of the midtarsal joint, J Am Podiatry Assoc 73:518, 1983.

14. Subotnick SI: Biomechanics of the subtalar and midtarsal joints, J Am Podiatry Assoc 65:756, 1975.

15. Green DR, Whitney AK, Walters P: Subtalar joint motion: a simplified view, J Am Podiatry Assoc 69:83, 1979.

16. Digiovani JE, Smith SD: Normal biomechanics of the adult rearfoot: a radiographic analysis, J Am Podiatry Assoc 66:812, 1976.

17. Donatelli R: Normal biomechanics of the foot and ankle, J Orthop Sports Phys Ther 7:91, 1985.

18. McPoil TG, Knecht HG: Biomechanics of the foot in walking: a functional approach, J Orthop Sports Phys Ther 7:69, 1985.

19. Hicks JH: The mechanics of the foot I: the joints, J Anat 87:345, 1953.

20. Morris JM: Biomechanics of the foot and ankle, Clin Orthop Relat Res 122:10, 1977.

21. Inman VT: UC-BL dual axis ankle control system and UC-BL shoe insert: biomechanical considerations, Bull Prosthet Res 10-11:130, 1969.

22. Hicks JH: The mechanics of the foot II: the plantar aponeurosis and the arch, J Anat 88:25, 1954.

23. Wright DG, Desai SM, Henderson WH: Action of the subtalar ankle joint complex during the stance phase of walking, J Bone Joint Surg 48(A):361, 1964.

24. Mann RA: Biomechanics of the foot and ankle. In Mann RA, editor: Surgery of the foot, ed 5, St Louis, 1986, Mosby, p 1.

25. Bojsen-Moller F, Lamoreux L: Significance of free dorsiflexion of the toes in walking, Acta Orthop Scand 50:471, 1979.

26. Jahss M, editor: Disorders of the foot, vol 1 and 2, Philadelphia, 1982, WB Saunders.

27. Donatelli R: Abnormal biomechanics. In Donatelli RA, editor: The biomechanics of the foot and ankle, ed 2, Philadelphia, 1996, FA Davis Company, pp 44-52, 60.

28. Singer KM, Jones DC: Soft tissue conditions of the ankle and foot. In Nicholas JA, Hershman EB, editors: The lower extremity and spine in sports medicine, vol 1, Philadelphia, 1986, Mosby, p 498.

29. Roy S, Irwin R: Sports medicine: prevention, evaluation, management, and rehabilitation, Englewood Cliffs, NJ, 1983, Prentice-Hall.

30. Koppell HP, Thompson WAL: Peripheral entrapment neuropathies, ed 2, Malabar, FL, 1976, Robert E Krieger.

31. Kushner S, Reid DC: Medial tarsal tunnel syndrome: a review, J Orthop Sports Phys Ther 6:39, 1984.

32. Viladot A: The metatarsals. In Jahss M, editor: Disorders of the foot, vol 1, Philadelphia, 1982, WB Saunders, p 659.

33. Stull P, Hunter R: Posterior tibial nerve entrapment at the ankle, Oper Tech Sports Med 4(1):54-60, 1996.

34. Hendrix CL, Jolly G, Garbalosa JC, et al: Entrapment neuropathy: the etiology of intractable chronic heel pain syndrome, J Foot Ankle Surg 37(4):273, 1998.

35. Oldenbrook LL, Smith CE: Metatarsal head motion secondary to rearfoot pronation and supination: an anatomical investigation, J Am Podiatry Assoc 69:24, 1979.

36. Glick J, Sampson TG: Ankle and foot fractures in athletics. In Nicholas JA, Hershman EB, editors: The lower extremity and spine in sports medicine, vol 1, Philadelphia, 1986, Mosby, p. 526.

37. Segal D, Yablon IG: Bimalleolar fractures. In Yablon IG, Segal D, Leach RE, editors: Ankle injuries, New York, 1983, Churchill Livingstone, p 31.

38. Lauge-Hansen N: Fractures of the ankle. II. Combined exploration-surgical and exploration-roentgenographic investigation, Arch Surg 60:957, 1950.

39. Turco VJ, Spinella AJ: Occult trauma and unusual injuries in the foot and ankle. In Nicholas JA, Hershman EB, editors: The lower extremity and spine in sports medicine, vol 1, Philadelphia, 1986, Mosby, p 541.

40. O'Donoghue DH, editor: Injuries of the foot. In Treatment of injuries to athletes, ed 3, Philadelphia, 1976, WB Saunders, p 747.

41. Hughes LY: Biomechanical analysis of the foot and ankle for predisposition to developing stress fractures, J Orthop Sports Phys Ther 7:96, 1985.

42. Leach RE, Schepsis A: Ligamentous injuries. In Yablon IG, Segal D, Leach RE, editors: Ankle injuries, New York, 1983, Churchill Livingstone, p 193.

43. Mann RA, Coughlin MJ: Hallux valgus and complications of hallux valgus. In Mann RA, editor: Surgery of the foot, ed 5, St Louis, 1986, Mosby, p 65.

44. Greensburg GS: Relationship of hallux abductus angle and first metatarsal angle to severity of pronation, J Am Podiatry Assoc 69:29, 1979.

45. Subotnick SI: Equinus deformity as it affects the forefoot, J Am Podiatry Assoc 61:423, 1971.

46. Thomas S, Barrington R: Hallux valgus, Curr Orthop 17:4, 2003.

47. Akeson WH, Amiel D, Woo S: Immobility effects of synovial joints: the pathomechanics of joint contracture, Biorheology 17:95, 1980.

48. Enneking W, Horowitz M: The intraarticular effects of immobilization on the human knee, J Bone Joint Surg 54(A):973, 1972.

49. Woo S, Matthews JV, Akeson WH, et al: Connective tissue response to immobility: correlative study of biomechanical and biochemical measurements of normal and immobilized rabbit knees, Arthritis Rheum 18:257, 1975.

50. Donatelli R, Owens-Burkart H: Effects of immobilization on the extensibility of periarticular connective tissue, J Orthop Sports Phys Ther 3:67, 1981.

51. Kelikan H: The hallux. In Mann RA, editor: Surgery of the foot, ed 5, St Louis, 1986, Mosby, p 539.

52. Ajis A, Koti M, et al: Tailor's bunion: a review, J Foot Ankle Surg 44:3, 2005.

53. Hoppenfeld S: Physical examination of the foot and ankle. In Hoppenfeld S, editor: Physical examination of the spine and extremities, New York, 1976, Appleton-Century-Crofts, p 197.

54. Mann RA: Principles of examination of the foot and ankle. In Mann RA, editor: Surgery of the foot, ed 5, St Louis, 1986, Mosby, p 31.

55. Spiegl P, Seale K: Surgical intervention. In Donatelli RA, editor: The biomechanics of the foot and ankle, ed 3, Philadelphia, 1996, FA Davis Company, p 367.

56. Raja S, Barrie J, Henderson AA: Distal phalangectomy for mallet toe, J Foot Ankle Surg 9:4, 2003.

57. Coughlin M: Operative repair of a mallet toe deformity, Foot Ankle 16:3, 1995.

58. Coughlin M: Lesser toe deformities. In Operative orthopaedics, ed 8, Philadelphia, 1992, JB Lippincott, pp 221-222.

59. Puttaswamaiah R, Chandran P: Degenerative plantar fasciitis: a review of current concepts, The Foot 17(1):3-9, 2007.

60. Kwong P, Kay D, et al: Plantar fasciitis: mechanics and pathomechanics of treatment, Clin Sports Med 7:1, 1988.

61. Gill L: Plantar fasciitis: diagnosis and conservative management, J Am Acad Orthop Surg 5:2, 1997.

62. Riddle D, Pulisic M, et al: Risk factors for plantar fasciitis: a matched case-control study, J Bone Joint Surg 85:A5, 2003.

63. Marshall RN: Foot mechanics and joggers' injuries, N Z Med J 88:288, 1978.

64. Aronson NG, Winston L, Cohen RI, et al: Some aspects of problems in runners: treatment and prevention, J Am Podiatry Assoc 67:595, 1977.

65. Leach RE, DiIorio E, Harney RA: Pathologic hindfoot conditions in the athlete, Clin Orthop Relat Res 177:116, 1983.

66. Turek SL: The foot and ankle. In Orthopaedics: principles and their applications, ed 4, vol 2, Philadelphia, 1984, JB Lippincott, p 1407.

67. Stolov WC, Cole TM, Tobis JS: Evaluation of the patient: goniometry; muscle testing. In Krusen FH, Kottke FJ, Ellwood PM, editors: Physical medicine and rehabilitation, Philadelphia, 1971, WB Saunders, p 17.

68. Adelaar RS: The practical biomechanics of running, Am J Sports Med 14:497, 1986.

69. Boissonnault W, Donatelli R: The influence of hallux extension on the foot during ambulation, J Orthop Sports Phys Ther 5:240, 1984.

70. Wong DLK, Glasheen-Wray M, Andrew LF: Isokinetic evaluation of the ankle invertors and evertors, J Orthop Sports Phys Ther 5:246, 1984.

71. Davies GJ: Subtalar joint, ankle joint, and shin pain testing and rehabilitation. In Davies GJ, editor: A compendium of isokinetics in clinical usage and clinical notes, LaCrosse, Wis, 1984, S&S Publishers, p 123.

72. Cloke D, Greiss M: The digital nerve stretch test: a sensitive indicator in Morton's neuroma and neuritis, J Foot Ankle Surg 12:4, 2006.

73. Mulder J: The causative mechanism in Morton's metatarsalgia, J Bone Joint Surg 33B:94-95, 1951.

74. Maitland GD: Peripheral manipulation, ed 2, Boston, 1977, Butterworths.

75. Mennell JM: Joint pain: diagnosis and treatment using manipulative techniques, Boston, 1964, Little, Brown.

76. Wooden M: Biomechanical evaluation for functional orthotics. In Donatelli RA, editor: The biomechanics of the foot and ankle, ed 2, Philadelphia, 1996, FA Davis Company, p 169.

77. Root ML, Orien WP, Weed JH: Biomechanical examination of the foot, vol 1, Los Angeles, 1971, Clinical Biomechanics Corp.

78. Garbalosa JC, McClure M, Catlin PA, et al: Normal angular relationship of the forefoot to the rearfoot in the frontal plane, J Orthop Sports Phys Ther 20(4):200, 1994.

79. Johanson MA, Donatelli R, Wooden M, et al: Effects of three different posting methods on controlling abnormal subtalar pronation, Phys Ther 74(2):149, 1994.

80. Elvaru R, Rothstein J, et al: Goniometric reliability in a clinical setting: subtalar and ankle joint measurements, Phys Ther 68:672, 1988.

81. Wooden M, Catlin P, et al: An examination of subtalar joint motion during the stance phase of gait, Poster presentation, New Orleans, 1994, APTA.

82. Murphy P: Orthoses: not the sole solution for running ailments, Phys Sportsmed 14:164, 1986.

83. Harris PR: Iontophorsesis: clinical research in musculoskeletal inflammatory conditions, J Orthop Sports Phys Ther 4:109, 1982.

84. Boone DC: Applications of iontophoresis. In Wolf S, editor: Clinics in physical therapy: electrotherapy, New York, 1986, Churchill Livingstone, p 99.

85. Sims D: Effects of positioning on ankle edema, J Orthop Sports Phys Ther 8:30, 1986.

86. Nicholas JA, Hershman EB, editors: The lower extremity and spine in sports medicine, vol 1 and 2, Philadelphia, 1986, Mosby.

87. DeCarlo MS, Talbot RW: Evaluation of ankle joint proprioception following injection of the anterior talofibular ligament, J Orthop Sports Phys Ther 8:70, 1986.

88. Rebman LW: Ankle injuries: clinical observations, J Orthop Sports Phys Ther 8:153, 1986.

89. Smith RW, Reischl SF: Treatment of ankle sprains in young athletes, Am J Sports Med 14:465, 1986.

90. Kessler RM, Herding D: The ankle and hindfoot. In Kessler RM, Herding D, editors: Management of common musculoskeletal disorders: physical therapy principles and methods, Philadelphia, 1983, Harper & Row, p 448.

91. Cummings GS: Orthopedic series, vol 1, Atlanta, 1992, Stokesville Publishing Co.

92. Davidson CJ, Ganion LR, Gehlsen GM, et al: Rat tendon morphologic and functional changes resulting from soft tissue mobilization, Med Sci Sports Exerc 29(3):313, 1997.

93. Cyriax J, Coldham M: Textbook of orthopaedic medicine, London, 1984, Bailliere Tindall.

94. Cameron MH: Physical agents in rehabilitation. From research to practice, Philadelphia, 1999, WB Saunders.

95. Alfredson H, Picteila T, Jonsson P, et al: Heavy-load eccentric calf muscle training for treatment of chronic Achilles tendinosis, Am J Sports Med 26(3):360, 1998.

96. Fyfe L, Stanish WD: The use of eccentric training and stretching in the treatment and prevention of tendon injuries, Clin Sports Med 11(3):601, 1992.

97. McPoil TG, Hunt GC: Evaluation and management of foot and ankle disorders: present problems and future directions, J Orthop Sports Phys Ther 21(6):381, 1995.

98. Gross MT: Lower quarter screening for skeletal malalignment-suggestions for orthotics and shoewear, J Orthop Sports Phys Ther 21(6): 389, 1995.

Overview of Foot Orthotics and Prescription

Our objectives when writing this chapter were to update old information and to present and review new information. To that end, we have updated concepts regarding the use of foot orthotics for treating a variety of injuries and pathologies. New information that will be reviewed includes concepts in foot and ankle evaluation that will assist the clinician with the fabrication of foot orthotics, and a review of new theories on soft tissue stress and how to assess instability of the mid-foot and forefoot. As a review of basic concepts, the chapter will review the mechanical principles for evaluation of the foot and ankle, and also the influence of foot orthotics on muscle activity throughout the lower extremity and lumbar spine.

WHAT IS THE PROBLEM?

Musculoskeletal and other disorders of human function related to dysfunction of the lower extremity are frequent, distressing, and debilitating. Increasing numbers of people are suffering from nontraumatic disorders of the musculoskeletal system that are not readily diagnosed or effectively treated by conventionally trained health professionals. The diagnostic methods (i.e., physical examination, laboratory tests, imaging techniques) used to identify structural disease or deformities are largely useless in defining these disorders. Therapies such as rest, medication, and surgery are relatively ineffective or provide only temporary relief of symptoms. These problems tend to be chronic and recurrent; frequently they result in degeneration or deformity in isolated joints or other tissues. The lack of understanding of the pathophysiologic condition of these common disorders causes them to be labeled simply as products of "overuse" or "syndromes" in an attempt to hide the inability of current medical paradigms to comprehend them.

WHY DO PEOPLE HAVE THESE PROBLEMS?

The structural and traumatic medical paradigm does not enable the understanding of these problems because they are due to normal anatomy that is functioning abnormally. The source of these problems lies outside of the body, not within it.

These disorders are related to the environment in which humans function. Our anatomic structures evolved over millennia to function efficiently in a primitive natural world. The 300 homeobox genes that determine the segmental structure of the human body are unchanged since the time of *Homo erectus*, 1.8 million years ago. Our current species, *Homo sapiens*, has successfully inhabited the earth for 195,000 years. For most of our evolutionary history, humans have existed in nature as nomadic hunter-gatherers for whom the integrity and efficiency of the musculoskeletal system was essential to survival. The development of agriculture and the domestication of animals began about 10,000 years ago, but people still walked, ran, and moved about on natural walking surfaces. The invention of machines and the beginning of the industrial revolution about 200 years ago led to urbanization and a radical change in the environment under the human foot. The irregular, variable textures and inclinations of natural walking surfaces began to be replaced by flat, level, paved ones. It is no coincidence that people began to complain about aching feet around the time that they began to wear modern types of shoes. Now, in the information age, we live and work in an environment that is different from that which we genetically evolved to inhabit. What consequences will this have?

Natural surfaces accept the shape of the human foot and allow the body to align itself and function in a stress-free way. These surfaces also stimulate the neuroreceptors in the soles of the feet with total contact and a wide variety of inputs.

Modern walking surfaces force the foot into an adaptive posture, called *excessive pronation of the subtalar joint* (STJ), which induces malalignment in the entire musculoskeletal system. They also produce excessive loading on small areas of the foot and inadequate stimulation and variety of sensory inputs (perturbations) when compared with natural surfaces.

Humans are victims of genetic success. We have altered our environment to induce injurious loading and adaptive stresses that cannot be indefinitely attenuated or compensated for.

Mechanical Effects

- The STJ pronates to the end of its range of motion. The leg internally rotates. The knee is malaligned and the patella

*Portions of this chapter courtesy Foot Science International, Christchurch, New Zealand.

maltracks. The hip anteverts. The pelvis anteverts and tilts. The spine and higher structures are all malaligned.

- The sole of the foot shows signs of overloading in specific locations (e.g., corns, calluses, hallux valgus).
- Malalignment induces stressful forces in tissues, stimulating the release of chemical pain mediators.
- Muscles and their associated attachments are overloaded by attempting to compensate for these mechanical alignments; eventually they malfunction.
- Oblique force vectors acting on joints lead to ligamentous stress, degeneration, susceptibility to failure, and eventual osteoarthritis.
- Gait is dysfunctional, and its sequence and determinants (as described by Inman[1]) become inefficient, further overloading all lower-extremity structures from T5 to the sole of the foot. Mobility and independence are impaired.
- The total posture of the body (which has adverse effects on internal organs and the musculoskeletal system) is liable to be abnormal.

Neuromotor Effects

- Unnatural stimulation of the foot and malalignment in the body results in inappropriate stimulation of mechanoreceptors with disordered proprioception, balance, and stability.
- Muscle imbalances (abnormal weakness or tightness) develops because of incorrect posture and dysfunctional myotatic reflexes related to compensating for malaligned forces in the body. Studies increasingly show the potential for foot orthotic devices to change the electromyographic (EMG) activity of muscles, even those in the hip and back.
- Dysfunctional motor patterns evolve in response to the abnormal neural input from mechanoreceptors in the foot and other structures. These patterns are attempting to compensate for the abnormal environment but do so at the expense of efficient locomotion.
- Muscles are overloaded and fatigue from attempting to attenuate abnormal impact vibrations.

Cardiovascular Effects

- Inadequate compression of the venous plexus fails to activate the venous foot pump and initiate the flow of blood to the heart during midstance.
- Failure of the venous foot pump impairs the efficiency of the contraction of the leg muscles during propulsion to return blood up the leg.
- The venous plexus is not effectively emptied, resulting in increased resistance to the inflow of arterial blood in the capillaries.
- Venous congestion and poor arterial blood flow are seen in the foot, leading to swelling, edema, reduced tissue oxygenation, degeneration, and ulceration. This is especially relevant to diabetes.
- Reduced cardiac return causes reduced stroke volume and cardiac inefficiency.

- A chain of adverse events begins. Lower-extremity dysfunction leads to musculoskeletal discomfort (aches and pains that are often ignored), which results in reduced physical activity, decreasing physical resilience. Later various disabilities, degeneration, disease, and changing postures develop.

NEW CONCEPTS REGARDING USE OF ORTHOTIC DEVICES

Foot orthotic devices have been successful in treating a variety of injuries and pathologic conditions. Research has shown orthotic devices help prevent back and lower-leg musculoskeletal problems,[2] patellofemoral pain,[3] ankle instability,[4] and various other lower-extremity injuries.[5-10]

Why and how the orthotic devices are effective continues to be researched to assist with the prescription of the devices. The Root method has been widely accepted and effective in orthotic fabrication. However, recent research has found some problems with Root's theory of the location of the subtalar joint axis (STJA). (In addition to the STJA, the midtarsal joint and forefoot are discussed.) In addition, research is proposing foot orthotic devices may alter motor control, affect shock absorbency, enhance sensory input, and affect tibial rotation. These new concepts (reviewed in this chapter), give other considerations to apply when evaluating and designing orthotic devices.

Subtalar Joint Axis Location

Manter,[11] Hicks,[12] and Root et al.[13] proposed that the STJA is a solitary axis that passes through the talocalcaneal joint in an oblique direction (posterior-lateral-plantar to anterior-medial-dorsal). Current research by Van Langelaan,[14] Benink,[15] and Lundberg and Svensson[16] has found (using more accurate methods of roentgen stereophotogrammetry) a number of discrete axes of rotation. Each spatial location of the STJA is dependent of the rotational position of the STJA. Based on the recent finding, Kirby hypothesized that "feet that function the most normally also would have a normal STJA spatial location."[17] Based on 16 years of work on over 2000 feet, Kirby devised an STJA palpation method to determine the STJA location. To locate the axis, palpation starts at the heel, with the thumb pushing the foot and marking the heel if no rotation occurs. The other hand and thumb is palpating the fifth metatarsal head to sense if any rotation occurs. After making the first mark on heel, the thumb is moved up and the points of no rotation are marked at 1 to 2 cm intervals. The line of no rotation is the plantar representation of the STJA (Figure 24-1).

Kirby[17] has consistently found a "normally" located STJA passes through the posterior-lateral heel posteriorly and through the first intermetatarsal space area of the plantar forefoot anteriorly (Figure 24-2, A). If the axis is palpated more medially, then pronation is noted in stance and the subject resists supination when needed in gait. If the axis is lateral

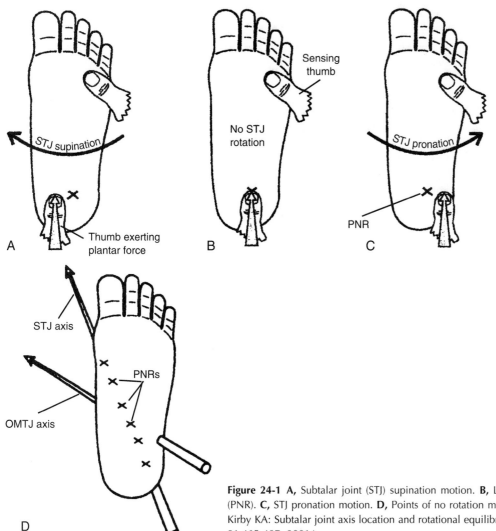

Figure 24-1 **A,** Subtalar joint (STJ) supination motion. **B,** Location of the point of no rotation (PNR). **C,** STJ pronation motion. **D,** Points of no rotation marked at 1- to 2-cm intervals. (From Kirby KA: Subtalar joint axis location and rotational equilibrium theory of foot function, JAPMA 91:465-487, 2001.)

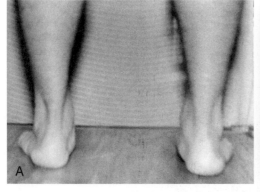 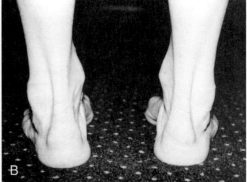

Figure 24-2 **A,** Compensated forefoot varus. **B,** Rigid forefoot valgus.

located with palpation, then supination is noted and pronation is resisted in gait. Payne et al.,[18] agrees with Kirby's STJA palpation method. Clinically, the posterior view of the weight-bearing foot with the medially deviated STJA displays excessive medial convexity in the medial midfoot just inferior to the medial malleolus. When viewing a foot posteriorly with a lateral deviation of the STJA, abnormal medial concavity is noted in the medial foot just inferior to the medial malleolus (Figure 24-2, *B*).

Midtarsal Joint and Forefoot

Other current studies propose the midtarsal joint may not be accurate in determining the motion of the forefoot on the rearfoot during weight bearing.[14-16,19] Payne[20] also agrees the two-axis model of the midtarsal joint needs to be improved. Kirby[17] looked at the transverse structure of the foot to determine the relationship of the forefoot to the rearfoot. A normal forefoot adductus is 8 to 10 degrees.[21] If the forefoot adductus is 20 degrees, then an increase in the STJ supination moment occurs in weight bearing. If the forefoot adductus is 0 degrees (forefoot rectus), then increased STJ pronation moment occurs during weight bearing.

The biomechanical or podiatric model of lower-limb function has been particularly useful in the prescription of devices that reliably relieve symptoms in a large number of lower-limb "overuse" conditions.[22] This has supported the belief that foot orthotic devices restrict and alter motion; however, more recent scientific publications indicate that this is not the case. Several authors have now provided evidence that orthotic devices do not significantly change the kinematics of the STJ, and studies using intracortical bone markers[23,24] have shown that orthotic devices produce an insignificant effect (0 to 1 degree) on calcaneal eversion.

Stacoff et al.[24] has concluded that successful treatment outcomes can be achieved with flexible, semirigid or rigid orthotic devices; however, the exact mechanism by which they work is unclear. Stacoff et al.[24] and Nigg[25] have proposed that the effect of orthotic devices is mediated by neuromotor processes rather than mechanical effects and may vary greatly from one person to another.

Some evidence[3] indicates that orthotic devices do affect tibial rotation, but this is not necessarily coupled to a corresponding change in talocalcaneal motion as was once thought. Many authors now believe that the effects of orthotic devices are much more variable and complicated than Root theorized in the 1960s and 1970s. Stacoff et al.[24] used intracortical pins inserted into the posterolateral aspect of the calcaneus and the anterolateral aspect of the tibial condyle.[24] They found decreased tibial internal rotation with the orthotic group compared with a control group. Numerous studies reported success with a variety of foot orthotic devices for patellofemoral pain.[3]

Nevertheless it is still quite likely that orthotic devices do alter foot and leg function, whatever the mechanism. The tissue stress theory provides a good explanation of how symptoms are relieved.[26] Forces that acutely or repeatedly deform human tissues to the limit of their elastic capability (in relation to the load deformation curve of a particular tissue structure) will produce pain with or without significant structural pathologic condition. The alteration of function produced by an orthotic device, even if it is very small, can alter the direction or magnitude of the force acting on the affected tissue and this reduction of loading or "tissue stress" results in the resolution of pain. Local therapies and rehabilitation also increase the resilience of tissues to accept loading without overloading.

Another interesting relationship between orthotic devices and force is that certain orthotic modifications such as a lateral forefoot post have been shown to reduce the force required to supinate the foot[17,27] or to dorsiflex the great toe to activate the windlass mechanism.[28] Reviews of the literature about foot orthotic devices indicates that "studies of the effects of orthoses are generally of poor quality" and "no trials have investigated long-term effectiveness."[8] In their study of the effects of foot orthotic devices in the treatment of plantar fasciitis, Landorf et al.[8] concluded that they produced small short-term improvements in function and reduction in pain but did not have beneficial long-term effects in comparison to a sham device. The authors also concluded that there was no difference in effectiveness between expensive custom devices and less costly prefabricated devices (Formthotics) custom fitted by heat molding.

PRESCRIBING FOOT ORTHOTIC DEVICES

Before 1990 most of the podiatric literature was descriptive, theoretical, or anecdotal. It generally accepted the biomechanical model as an explanation of observed patient outcomes. There were few attempts at high-quality RCT studies. Research[3,23-25] has now shown that results using surface markers (on the leg, heel, or shoe) grossly overestimate the potential of orthotic devices to change the kinematics of gait. Other theories explaining the effects of orthotic devices by way of neuromotor mechanisms have been proposed.[3,17,25,26,28] Some people now believe that orthotic devices exert their effects by altering the stimulation of mechanoreceptors in the foot and leg, with a consequent change in muscle activity, and orthotic devices have been shown to be able to improve proprioception and balance. Others contend that the devices apply a force to the sole of the foot in such a way that the muscles can more easily supinate the foot with less strain developing in the soft tissues.[17,27] It has even been suggested that pain relief and improvement of function may be quite independent of each other, with pain being relieved even if function is not improved.

Motor Control

Current research is finding foot orthotic devices may alter muscle activity from the back musculature to the foot. Murley and Bird[29] found increased peroneus longus EMG amplitude with rigid custom-made orthotic devices compared with footwear alone. This may improve lateral ankle stability. For example, Santilli et al.[30] found a significant decrease in peroneus longus activity with athletes with unilateral chronic ankle instability. Nawoczenski and Ludewig,[31] using semirigid foot orthotic devices, reported decreased biceps femoris activity and increased anterior tibialis activity with running. With use of a rigid custom device in running, Mundermann et al.[32] found increased EMG activity of the anterior tibialis, peroneus longus, and biceps femoris. Kudig et al.[33] found increased EMG activity of the posterior tibialis with use of a semirigid orthotic. Bird et al.[34] found the erector spinae had an earlier onset, and the gluteus medius had a later onset, during the gait cycle when bilateral heel lifts and bilateral lateral forefoot wedging occurred.

Nurse et al.[35] and Romkes et al.[36] found decreased anterior tibialis activity with the use of foot orthotic devices with walking. Nurse et al. also found decreased soleus EMG activity.

The authors believe this may mean greater fatigue resistance of the muscles because of the reduced work of the rearfoot inverters. Others also found that foot orthotic devices may decrease muscle fatigue and improve postural stability.[32,37-39]

Shock Absorption

Soft tissue will vibrate in response to impact force when the foot contacts the ground. Continued exposure to vibrations has been shown to be detrimental to soft tissues.[40-43] Nigg's review[25] of the literature suggests the concept of aligning the skeleton with shoe inserts should be reconsidered. He proposes that muscle tuning occurs with input signals from impact forces into the human body. This tuning occurs shortly before the next ground contact and minimizes soft tissue vibrations during impact loading. This is important because the impact forces affect fatigue, comfort, work, and performance during physical activity.[25] Thus shoe inserts (i.e., orthotic devices) may affect general muscle activity versus aligning the skeleton. The foot orthotic devices may dampen the soft tissue vibration in the lower extremity, indicated by the EMG change.[32]

Sensory Afferent Input

Studies suggest various foot orthotic devices may change the rate of discharge from mechanoreceptors of the firing pattern of sensory afferents.[32,35] Hertel et al. proposes that plantar afferent patterns may be altered by the use of foot orthotic devices that would influence muscle activity during functional tasks.[63] In a review of current research for chronic ankle instability, it was noted that loss of balance or postural control occurred in athletes with chronic ankle instability.[25] Multiple studies demonstrated that orthotic devices improved balance and postural control with ankle injuries or muscle fatigue. Research indicates that this may be because foot devices improve tactile sensation or position of the STJ.[4]

Various pressure-mapping systems have been promoted for gathering static and dynamic data from which superior foot orthotic devices can be made; however, recent research[44] has shown that plantar pressure contact area measurement can estimate only 27% of the height of the medical longitudinal arch.

The prevalence of forefoot varus "deformity" and the use of medial wedges under the great toe are being looked at more critically because of the findings[28] that forefoot varus wedges increase the force required to dorsiflex the great toe and consequently increase the loading on and strain within the plantar fascia. Payne[28] and others are now recommending posting on the lateral side of the forefoot. The use of moderate wedges of 6 degrees or less under the medial heel (rearfoot varus post) is favored, and both Kirby[17] and Payne[28] have shown it to reduce the force required to supinate the foot.

Given the likelihood that even simple orthotic devices are quite likely to reduce the loading on painful tissues, as well as the lack of validation for the functional effects of these devices, it seems best to use the basic concepts of a shell and posts. One method of doing this is through a system of prefabricated devices, such as the Formthotics mentioned following, which can be custom molded to the shape of the undersurface of the foot in a balanced "neutral" position and easily adjusted with wedges.

ASSESSMENT FOR ORTHOTIC DEVICES

Leg-Length Assessment

A thorough history is essential with orthotic prescription. Once a history is completed, a lower-extremity evaluation should be completed that covers sacroiliac assessment and leg-length issues ("functional versus structural"). Sahrmann[45] assesses leg length by palpation of the iliac crests with feet together and apart (Figure 24-3). She found that with the feet together, the side with the elevated iliac crest is in adduction and the other hip is in abduction. With feet apart, the iliac crests are even because the abductors are not stretched. The difference between the iliac crests' height should be at least one-half inch to be clinically significant. Individuals with true

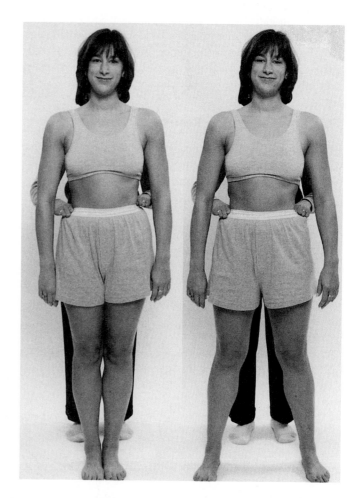

Figure 24-3 Apparent leg length discrepancy (iliac crest asymmetry). The left iliac crest is higher than the right iliac crest when the feet are together. Thus the right hip abductors are stiffer than the left hip abductors. Abduction of the hips levels the iliac crests because the abductors are not stretched. (From Sahrmann S: Diagnosis and treatment of movement impairment syndromes, St Louis, 2002, Mosby.)

structural differences report a history of congenital deformity or trauma resulting in bone loss.[45] In addition, any muscle imbalances and joint-soft tissue restrictions of the pelvic lower extremity should be addressed.

Subtalar Joint Motion

STJ motion is measured by the angle between the posterior longitudinal bisection of the lower one third of the leg and the bisection of the posterior calcaneus. The clinician should manually invert the calcaneus to measure inversion with a goniometer (Figure 24-4, *A*), and evert the foot for eversion (Figure 24-4, *B*). Twenty degrees of inversion to 10 degrees of eversion are within normal limits.[46]

Resting Calcaneal Stance

In a relaxed stance, the calcaneal resting position is measured by the angle of bisection of the lower one third of the leg to the longitudinal bisection line along the calcaneus. Calcaneal eversion greater than 6 degrees is related to excessive pronation.[47-50] In addition, as previously mentioned, Kirby[17] reported that with excessive pronation in relaxed stance, a medial bulge can be observed from the posterior view (see Figure 24-2 *A*). The medial bulge resembles an excessive medial convexity directly under the medial malleolus.

Manual Supination Resistance Test

Having the clinician place two fingers under the talonavicular joint or medial aspect of the plantar navicular bone completes the supination resistance test. Force is applied in an upward direction and is rated from 0 to 5, with 0 being very low resistance to supinate the foot and 5 very high resistance or nearly impossible to supinate the foot. It is assumed the greater the force needed to supinate the foot, the greater the force needed from the foot orthotic devices. Noakes and Payne[51] found the resistance test to be a reliable and clinically useful tool.

Jack's Test

The clinician manually dorsiflexes the hallux and grades the force from 1 to 5, with 1 being minimal resistance needed and 5 being excessive resistance to dorsiflexion. Regarding the windlass mechanism, as the hallux dorsiflexes it pulls on the plantar aponeurosis that can raise the arch and supinate the foot. This is one way the foot counters excessive pronation. Orthotic devices have been found to reduce the force needed to establish the windlass mechanism and decrease stress to the plantar fascia.[52] Murley and Bird[29] found that rigid foot orthotic devices may assist the windlass mechanism.

Balance Test

A modified Balance Error Scoring System (BESS) assessing single-leg stance only can be used. The clinician observes single-leg stance for 20 seconds, with the patient's eyes closed, hands on hips, and the contralateral leg flexed approximately 90 degrees. Healthy athletes should be tested for 30 seconds.[53] A balance error occurs if (1) the eyes open; (2) the hands come off the hips; (3) touchdown of the nonstance foot occurs; (4) step, hop, or other movement of the stance foot takes place;

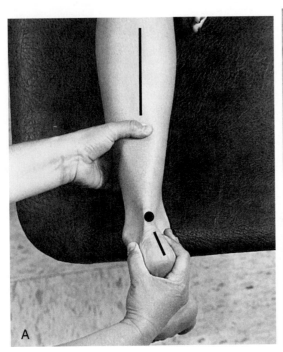
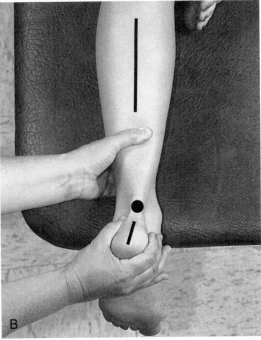

Figure 24-4 A, Forefoot varus. **B,** Forefoot valgus. (From Reese NB: Joint range of motion and muscle length testing, St Louis, 2003, Saunders.)

(5) the hips move into 30 degrees or more of abduction or flexion; (6) the forefoot or heel is lifted; or (7) the patient remains out of test position for more than 5 seconds.[54] The score is calculated by 1 point for each error. Orthotic devices should improve the stability and decrease the error rate. Foot orthotic devices have been shown to affect position and motion.[55] Research has reported high intertester reliability and fair to good validity for the BESS.[54]

Forefoot Stability Test

Another modification of the BESS helps to determine how forefoot proprioceptors function. In this case the clinician observes the patient's ability to rise on the toes in single-leg stance. If the patient has difficulty maintaining inversion, then poor efficiency with propulsion may exist. Foot orthotic devices should improve the stability and prevent inversion instability. Hicks[12] described nonweight-bearing assessment of passive mobility of the forefoot as a supination and pronation twist. Bordelon[56] describes 25 degrees of a supination and pronation twist to be normal mobility.

The authors of this chapter have observed significant asymmetries of forefoot supination and pronation twist. For the purposes of this chapter, instability of the forefoot is described as an excessive supination twist resulting from soft tissue stress and breakdown within the midtarsal joint and supporting ligaments to the medial arch. The supporting ligaments to the medial arch include the short and long plantar ligaments, the spring ligament, and the tendon of the posterior tibialis as it splits into several ligament-like structures after passing under the navicular. Often patients demonstrate excessive supination of the forefoot with passive pronation. Forefoot and midfoot stability may be assessed manually by holding the calcaneus with one hand and the distal region of the second through fifth metatarsals with the other hand (Figure 24-5). While inverting and holding the calcaneus, the clinician moves the forefoot through supination twist and then everts the forefoot into a pronation twist.

The supination and pronation movements of the forefoot are repeated, with the calcaneus held in neutral, and the clinician compares the amount of motion in both positions. If excessive movement is noted, then laxity exists along the midfoot. Laxity or hypermobility of the midfoot joint can be a factor in excessive pronation, causing poor stability with the push-off phase of gait during propulsion.[57]

SUBTALAR JOINT NEUTRAL

The subtalar joint neutral (STJN) position is still the standard used with neutral casting. To assess STJN, in prone position, the foot is positioned perpendicular to the ground. STJ motion is measured by the angle between the posterior longitudinal bisection of the lower one third of the leg and the bisection of the posterior calcaneus. The clinician palpates the medial aspect of the talus with the thumb and the lateral aspect of the talus with the index finger. While holding the fourth and fifth metatarsals, the clinician supinates and pronates the foot manually with the other hand. STJN is the position in which the talus is felt equally on the medial and lateral sides (Figure 24-6). Using a mathematic method to determine STJN, one study found that the mean neutral rearfoot position was approximately 2.5 degrees of inversion in 240 asymptomatic feet.[58]

Forefoot Position in Subtalar Joint Neutral

Once STJN is determined, the forefoot relationship is assessed. With the rearfoot maintained in STJN, the forefoot position is determined by aligning one arm of the goniometer along the plane of the metatarsal heads and aligning the other arm perpendicular to the calcaneal bisection line, as previously described. The goniometer axis is held laterally for a forefoot varus measurement, and the axis is placed medially if a forefoot valgus is present (see Figure 24-4). Zero to 2 degrees of forefoot varus is within normal limits.[59] Garbalosa et al.[58] found that

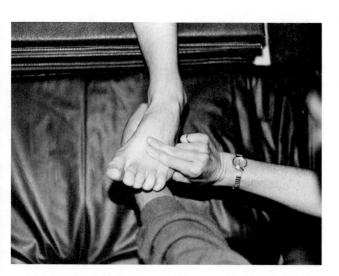

Figure 24-5 Midtarsal joint mobility.

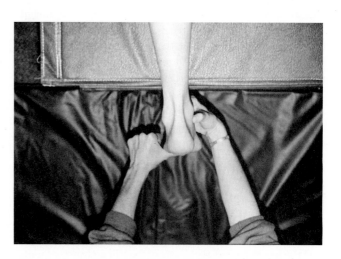

Figure 24-6 Subtalar joint neutral (STJN).

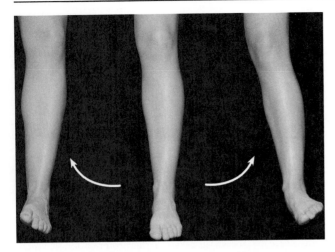

Figure 24-7 Assessment of biomechanics and joint function. (Courtesy Foot Science International, Christchurch, New Zealand.)

the average forefoot varus angle was 7.82 degrees in 86% of 240 asymptomatic feet studied.

REVIEW OF NEW FUNCTIONAL ASSESSMENT

Functional Assessment: Six Tests

Test One: Subtalar Motion Test

Manual therapy techniques are used to assess joint motion and mobilize any restrictions. Range of motion, quality of motion, end feel, and restriction of motion are examined, and restrictions are mobilized. The range of pronation and supination and the neutral subtalar position are identified. Deviations from the mechanically ideal alignment are noted. The foot is examined in stance to determine the difference between its relaxed posture and the neutral calcaneal stance alignment (Figure 24-7).

Test Two: Alignment Test

Biomechanical principles are used to assess skeletal alignment. The patient is examined in stance, from both the front and the back, and malalignments from the theoretically ideal are noted. The examination is from head to toe. Numerous reasons exist for asymmetry or malalignment of musculoskeletal structures. They are frequently related to dysfunction of the foot and leg. However, apparent mechanical "deformity" in the foot may be a compensation for joint and/or soft tissue restrictions in structures of the spine, pelvis, hips, or knees. The assessment is done in resting and neutral calcaneal stance (Figure 24-8).

Test Three: Supination Resistance Test

The examiner manually supinates the foot and grades the force required from 1 to 5 (Figure 24-9). The force required to supinate the foot is related to the axis of the STJ and varies significantly from person to person. The gait muscles in the foot and

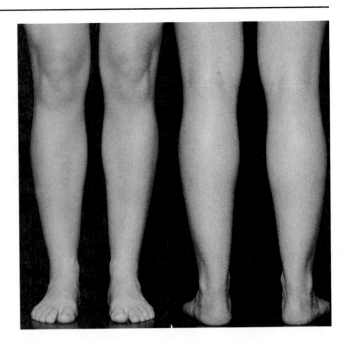

Figure 24-8 Assessment of closed kinetic chain mechanics. (Courtesy Foot Science International, Christchurch, New Zealand.)

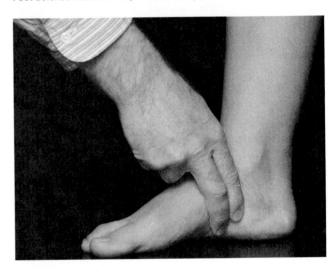

Figure 24-9 Assessment of the STJ axis. (Courtesy Foot Science International, Christchurch, New Zealand.)

leg generate this force. The higher the supination resistance is, the greater is the loading on these muscles and associated structures (and the more likely it is that overuse symptoms will occur). Orthotic devices that reduce supination resistance decrease this loading and therefore can relieve or prevent symptoms.

Test Four: Jack's Test

This clinical test assesses the tension in the plantar fascia associated with heel lift and propulsion. The way in which the terminal slips of the plantar fascia wind around the metatarsal heads has been called the *windlass mechanism*.[60] The STJ must supinate for the toes to dorsiflex. People vary greatly in the force required to dorsiflex the great toe to activate the windlass

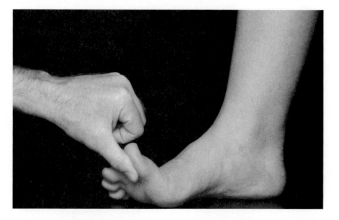

Figure 24-10 Assessment of the windlass mechanism. (Courtesy Foot Science International, Christchurch, New Zealand.)

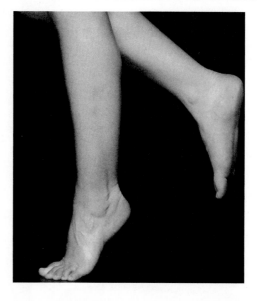

Figure 24-12 Assessment of propulsion. (Courtesy Foot Science International, Christchurch, New Zealand.)

Test Six: Forefoot Stability Test

Efficient propulsion requires a stable base. The patient is instructed to stand on one foot and then rise up onto the toes. The examiner observes the ease of rising onto the toes, the stability, and the tendency to inversion instability (Figure 24-12). The orthotic devices should improve stability and prevent inversion instability.

TYPES OF FOOT ORTHOTIC DEVICES

Many different materials and methods have been used to make orthotic devices; most of these have been shown to be effective. Orthotic devices can be full length, three-quarter length, or even very slim fitting, depending on the interior volume of the shoes in which they are intended to be worn. In addition, different types of devices exist for different types of footwear and activities. Two main classifications exist: (1) total-contact devices and (2) balanced-contact devices. Both types have been shown to be equally effective in relieving symptoms and improving function.[38]

Total-Contact Foot Orthotic Devices

Total-contact foot orthotic devices are made from a flexible, resilient material that is heated and molded to the shape of the undersurface of the foot. This molding can be done either directly onto the foot or on a plaster cast of the foot taken in the neutral subtalar position. The neutral casting method consists of applying plaster to the foot while maintaining a STJN position. The technique reviewed involves casting the foot in STJN while the patient is lying prone (Figure 24-13). This method produces a neutral foot impression, which is sent to a laboratory for orthotic fabrication. On completion and drying, the patient's name should be labeled on the cast. The molded

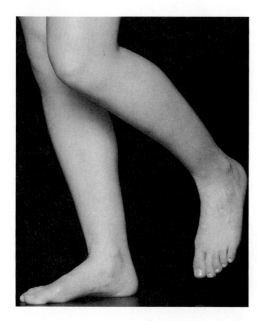

Figure 24-11 Assessment of proprioception and postural stability. (Courtesy Foot Science International, Christchurch, New Zealand.)

mechanism. The examiner manually dorsiflexes the great toe until the foot supinates and grades the force required from 1 to 5 (Figure 24-10). Orthotic devices that decrease this force reduce strain in the plantar fascia and improve the efficiency of gait.

Test Five: Balance Test

The patient stands on one leg, establishes balance, and then closes the eyes. The arch rises, and the foot seeks a functional neutral position. It then oscillates about this position. Balance is eventually lost, either medially or laterally. The examiner observes the stability of balance, the duration of balance, the functional neutral position, and the loss of balance (medial or lateral) (Figure 24-11). The orthotic devices should improve the stability and duration of balance but should not induce lateral instability.

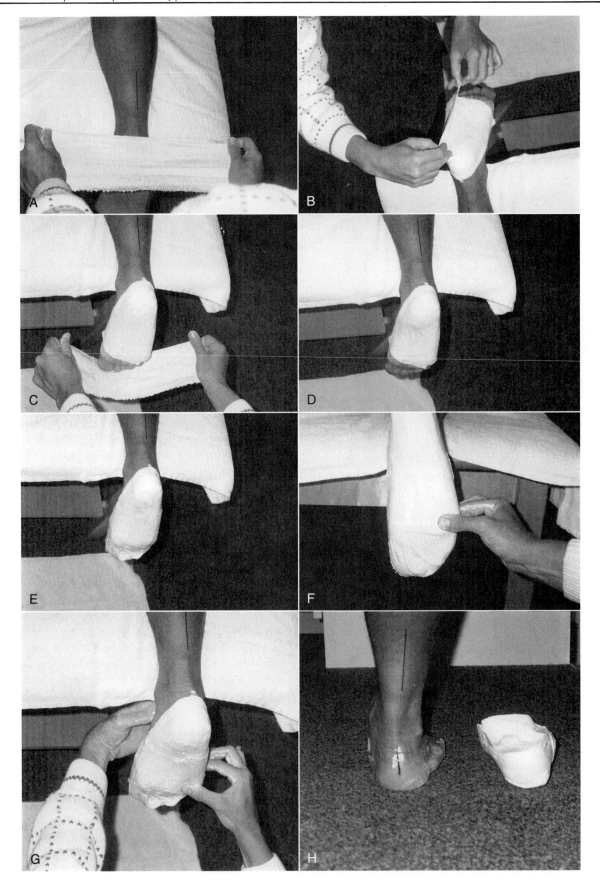

Figure 24-13 The patient lies prone, with the foot off the edge of the treatment table. Use two strips of quick-drying plaster doubled in length. Dip the plaster in water and ring out most of the liquid. **A,** Lay the first strip of wet plaster down from the heel downward, creating a one fourth–inch edge superiorly. **B,** Fold over the plaster and smooth it down to the arch of the foot. **C,** Lay the second strip of wet plaster from the toes upward, creating a one quarter–inch edge superiorly. Fold over the plaster and smooth it down to the arch of the foot, covering the toes. **D,** Smooth out the entire arch of the foot, releasing any air bubbles and ensuring total foot contact with the plaster **(E)**. **F,** Align the foot in subtalar joint neutral (STJN) and hold it in this position until the plaster is dry and hard. **G,** Gently break the seal around the edges by pulling the skin away from the plaster. **H,** Pop the seal off an outward direction and then pull downward to remove the cast from the foot. The cast should resemble the deformity.

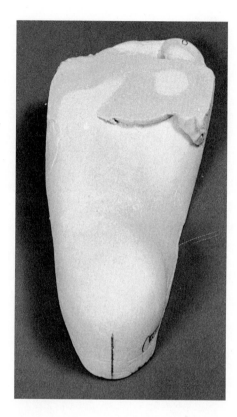

Figure 24-14 The modification process of forefront position on a positive cast. (From Lusardi MM: Orthotics and prosthetics in rehabilitation, ed 2, St Louis, 2007, WB Saunders.)

footprint then has to be shaped by grinding to a form that can be fitted comfortably into the shoe. The flexibility and resilience of these devices allows them to accommodate STJ pronation and supination during the three periods of the stance phase of gait (i.e., contact, midstance, and propulsion).

Balanced-Foot Orthotic Devices

Balanced-foot orthotic devices are made of harder thermoplastic materials and are generally favored by podiatrists. A negative cast of the neutral foot is taken and sent to a lab, where it is filled with plaster to make a positive model of the patient's foot (see Figure 24-12). Other changes related to the prescription are sent to the lab with the negative cast, and the positive cast is then modified with some infilling of the arch (Figure 24-14). A hard plastic material is heated to a high temperature and molded to the plaster replica of the foot to form the shell

and posts, either incorporated into the cast or added to the undersurface of the shell. The arch area of the cast is infilled to allow the STJ to move during gait. The theory behind balanced-foot orthotic devices is that the posts control undesirable motion of the STJ and total contact under the arch is not necessary.

Computer-Milled Orthotic Devices

The production of these orthotic devices involves the use scanners to collect data about the foot and digitize it to program a computer-controlled milling machine. The machine then mills blocks of foam or other material to match the contours of the undersurface of the foot or to form a positive cast on which material may be molded to form an orthotic shell. This provides a way of making a balanced orthotic by substituting sophisticated technology for messy plaster or foam-filled boxes for taking a cast of the foot. Some of these systems (e.g., Pedalign technology) use an optical scanner instead of pressure sensors to produce very comfortable and effective devices.

Formthotics

The Formthotics orthotic devices, developed by Dr. Charlie Baycroft, were designed to combine the benefits of total-contact and balanced-foot orthotic devices and also to enable the devices to be custom fitted and modified in the clinic to both the patient's feet and the shoes in which they are to be worn. A special type of foam is heated and molded to a new shape in the shoes, and it reacts to the patient's own body weight in a neutral stance position. This material is milled to a unique form to avoid the necessity of taking a mold in a sheet of material and then having to grind the footprint to fit the shoe. These devices are called *Formthotics* because they were "orthotics that can be formed to the correct shape of the foot and shoe in stance and in the therapist's office"[61] without the need for casts grinders or other expensive manufacturing facilities. Wedges, met domes, and arch pads are also provided to enable the Formthotics to be conveniently and easily adjusted as required.

The advantages of Formthotics is that they are light, quick, and inexpensive to make; dispensed to the patient on the same day; and easily modified by remolding and/or posting. Their fitting and adjustment is done under the control of the therapist that is treating the patient, rather than in a lab by technicians who have not seen the patient. A brief explanation of the manufacturing process follows.

Stage	Description
Fabrication and posting	A flexible shell is custom formed to the shape of the sole of the neutral foot using heat. The effect of so forming the device is to create a total-contact foot orthosis that distributes weight bearing over the entire sole of the foot and properly stimulates neuroreceptors (Figure 24-15, A).
The break-in period	The effect of a therapy is related to the patient's adaptation to it. Dynamic foot pressure will slightly deform thermoplastic foam orthotic devices to adapt to the patient's dynamics. This break-in period should not be omitted. The patient should use the devices for about 1 week before adjustments are made. Usually a significant improvement in pain and function occur during this period.
	The rearfoot or forefoot is adjusted by functional posting. Wedges are used as a means of applying force. The depth of insertion and angle of the wedge determine how much force is applied, but the patient should verify the improvement of function. A rearfoot varus (medial) wedge will usually improve balance and reduce supination resistance (Figure 24-15, B). A forefoot valgus (lateral) wedge most often decreases the force required to dorsiflex the great toe (Figure 24-15, C). The finished orthotic devices can be seen in Figure 24-15, D.
In-shoe testing	The six tests should be performed with the devices in the shoes. Changing shoes can also alter the functional effect of the devices.
Ongoing adjustment	The patient's adaptation and functional response to the devices varies over time. The devices should be checked and modified periodically, especially if symptoms recur or new ones develop.

PREFABRICATED FOOT ORTHOTIC DEVICES

Prefabricated foot orthotic devices are now becoming quite common. These are generally made from compression-formed ethylene vinyl acetate (EVA), molded under relatively high pressures and temperatures (about 140° C) or by injection molding. They are essentially like the innersoles supplied in shoes but more sturdy and with a higher arch profile. Some of these devices also incorporate various amounts of rearfoot or forefoot wedging in the design. They are meant to provide a generic shell reasonably approximating the average neutral foot and can be adjusted with wedges (Figure 24-16). These inexpensive and simple devices can be very effective in reducing symptoms.

Insoles

Simple insoles can be modified by the addition of arch cookies and wedges to make reasonably effective devices (Figure 24-17). Insoles are not formed to a custom shell and tend not to last as long as custom orthotic devices, but they can be successfully used in some patients with minor complaints.

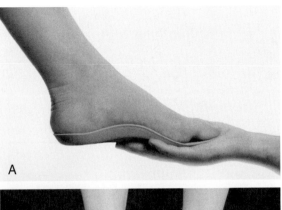

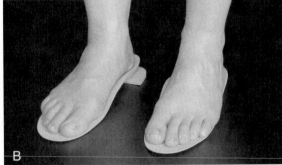

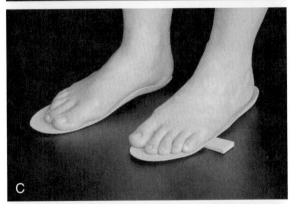

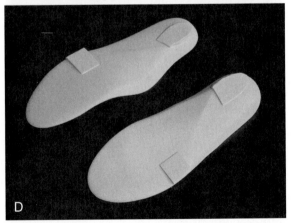

Figure 24-15 **A,** Molding a heated form to the shape of the individual foot. **B,** Fitting a rearfoot varus wedge. **C,** Fitting a forefoot valgus post. **D,** The finished orthotic devices. (Courtesy Foot Science International, Christchurch, New Zealand.)

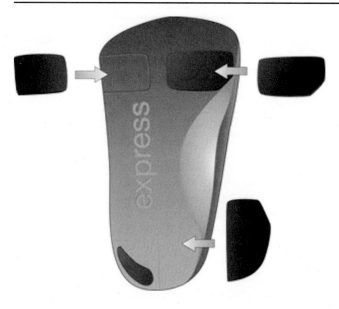

Figure 24-16 Express orthotic devices are an example of prefabricated devices that have been designed to facilitate reductions in supination resistance and activation of the windlass mechanism. They are provided in a kit form, with the devices and convenient wedges for adjusting them. (Courtesy Foot Science International, Christchurch, New Zealand.)

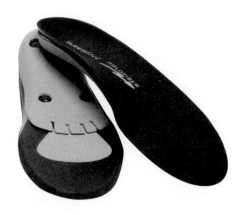

Figure 24-17 Prefabricated insoles. (Courtesy Superfeet, Ferndale, Wash.)

Corrective Additions

Posts

A post is material added to an orthotic shell or the prefabricated orthotic device. The shell can be fabricated from a patient's foot in STJN. The shell can be made at the office or sent to a custom orthotic laboratory after a negative-impression cast is made at the office. The amount and type of correction provided, as well as the type of device and the laboratories used, vary greatly among clinicians. An extrinsic post

is a correction applied to the outside of the orthotic shell. By contrast, an intrinsic post is applied within the orthotic shell. Some clinicians and laboratories prefer to use intrinsic posting as a correction to the forefoot and extrinsic posting for the rearfoot. The authors of this chapter believe that extrinsic posting may provide greater control of compensatory pronation. This may add bulk to the orthotic device, which may limit the types of footwear. The intrinsic post is useful with tight footwear, such as a woman's dress shoe, but it provides less control of compensatory pronation. Both types of posting are used to decrease compensatory motion and improve afferent input.

Rearfoot Extrinsic Post

A rearfoot extrinsic post consists of material applied along the calcaneal region of an orthotic shell. If the post is for a rearfoot varus deformity, the material is higher medial and tapers down laterally. The rearfoot varus post brings the ground closer to the medial calcaneal surface, decreasing excessive pronation during early midstance. This improves lower-extremity stability and muscle efficiency during midstance.

Forefoot Extrinsic Post

A forefoot post is material applied proximal to the metatarsal head region of an orthotic shell. A forefoot varus deformity post has more material medially and then tapers laterally to reduce excessive pronation during forefoot loading. This increases stability for effective propulsion. If both a rearfoot and a forefoot varus deformity are present, a medial rearfoot and forefoot post is applied.

Forefoot Valgus Post

A forefoot valgus post is material built up along the lateral orthotic shell, tapering medially to reduce excessive supination. This brings the ground up to the lateral component of the foot, preventing compensatory pronation and/or supination.

First-Ray Cutout

This relief cutout allows a plantar-flexed first ray to decompress the first metatarsal joint. With a rigid plantar flexed first ray, the first metatarsal hits the ground immediately after heel-strike, followed by supination to bring the lateral aspect of the foot to the floor.[62] This compensatory supination can be avoided by assisting the first ray to be more mobile. Another method used to relieve the plantar-flexed first ray consists of a metatarsal bar or pad placed proximal to the metatarsal heads. This is used to distribute the forces more evenly across the metatarsals, thus relieving metatarsalgia.

CASE STUDY: KNEE PAIN

Mr. J.C, an enthusiastic runner, arrived at the clinic late one Friday afternoon asking if someone might have a look at his sore knee.

The history was of generalized aching around the front of the left knee that was worse in the morning, when running, or standing up after sitting. J.C. was an avid runner who trained 60 to 80 miles per week and completed three or four marathons each year. His training had been reduced to around 20 miles per week over the past 8 weeks because his knee became sore. He had not been running for the past 5 days.

The past history was not remarkable. Mr. J.C. said he was always in good health and had only suffered from occasional aches and pains related to his sport. He said that he had tried changing his shoes a couple of times and had been treated for 3 weeks by a physiotherapist with ice, ultrasound, exercise, and some tape on his knee. He said the physiotherapist had advised that he stop running until the knee felt better, but he had ignored this advice.

Examination revealed slight tenderness along the medial border of the left patella and some retropatellar crepitus.

Six-Test Assessment of Lower-Extremity Function

Test One: Subtalar Motion Test

After passive assessment of STJ mobility by inversion and eversion range of motion testing, as well as testing of the midtarsal joint mobility by passive movement of the talonavicular and calcaneal cuboid, a restriction of the talonavicular joint of the left foot was found and mobilized.

Passive testing of rearfoot eversion was noted to be approximately 5 degrees on the right and 9 degrees on the left. After mobilization of the talonavicular joint, the forefoot was in a neutral position.

Test Two: Alignment Test

Slight asymmetry with the left iliac crest and shoulder slightly lower than the right in relaxed stance became symmetrical in subtalar neutral stance.

Test Three: Supination Resistance Test

Left-leg supination resistance was 4, and right-leg supination resistance was 3, indicating that the muscles of the left leg had to overcome more resistance to supinate the foot for efficient gait. During walking, prolonged pronation of both feet occurred during the stance phase. Resupination of the left STJ occurred at toe-off, which was substantially delayed. This test was positive for an overpronator.

Test Four: Jack's Test

Jack's test assesses the force required to activate the windlass mechanism. The arch must rise to shorten the distance between the origin and insertion of the plantar fascia. Excessive resistance to dorsiflexion of the toes impedes the forward progression of gait and impairs the efficiency of walking and running. Resupination of the STJ and dorsiflexion of the toes are interrelated. In this case the resistance to Jack's test was increased in the left foot. Once again indicating an overpronator.

Test Five: Balance Test

The single leg stance with the eyes open is a quick balance test. The patient should be able to stand on one leg, with hands on hips for 20 seconds, without any movements that might compensate for loss of balance. This patient's balance was better on the right leg than the left.

Test Six: Forefoot Stability Test

A quick test for forefoot stability is a single-leg stance up on the forefoot. Once again the patient should be able to stand up on the forefoot for 20 seconds. In this patient, forefoot stability was normal on both sides.

A provisional diagnosis of patellofemoral syndrome was made. Mr. J.C. was fitted with a pair of firm-density Formthotics by heating them in the shoes and custom forming them to the feet (with the patient standing in a neutral position with the center of the patella in line with the second toe). He was advised to try some short runs over the weekend and to return for a full examination and further treatment the next week.

Mr. J.C returned to the clinic 5 years later. When asked why he had not come back as requested, he replied that there was no need because the pain had completely resolved over the first weekend of wearing the Formthotics and had not recurred. He said that the orthotic devices were now severely worn out and he would like some new ones. He said that he had been training and competing without problems and had also improved his running times. He had worn the Formthotics at all times, changing them from one pair of shoes to another. "However," he said, "they are falling to pieces now, and I have to use tape to hold them together. I've tried running without them, but after a week or two my knee gets sore, so I put them back in the shoes and the pain goes away."

Comment: Patellofemoral pain is a common problem that responds well to treatment with foot orthotic devices. Simple flexible devices reduce stress in the affected area and can improve lower-extremity function without altering kinematics. Treating this condition without foot orthotic devices (e.g., exercises, taping) can be a slow and frustrating process for the therapist and the patient. If inadequately treated, this condition can resolve over time but may also go on to cause chondromalacia patella, degeneration, and softening of the retropatellar cartilage.

In this case the examination suggested that the orthotic devices should have been modified by the addition of wedges to make them more theoretically correct. A wedge or post applied under the heel on the medial side (rearfoot varus post) could have been used bilaterally to reduce the rearfoot eversion, reducing the supination resistance and also improving the balance.

CASE STUDY: KNEE PAIN–cont'd

However, more recent literature about foot orthotic devices supports the opinion that total contact devices (of soft but resilient materials custom formed to the precise shape of the patient's foot in a neutral posture) are as effective as balanced-foot orthotic devices, prescribed with wedges that are assumed to control motion of parts of the foot. In addition, excellent evidence indicates that custom thermoformed Formthotics are as effective as a hard plastic prescribed devices with posts that are made in a lab.[8]

Whatever orthotic theories might suggest, the reality in this case was that the patient had a rapid and extremely satisfactory outcome without further modifications of the orthotic devices; therefore no further adjustments were considered necessary.

SUMMARY

Research has proven that patients with numerous pathologic conditions are generally very satisfied with their orthotic devices. Studies have shown that foot orthotic devices affect the amount and rate of pronation. New research proposes that the benefits of orthotic devices are not necessarily the result of significant foot and ankle skeletal positional modifications; instead, they are the result of alterations in motor control through soft tissue vibration and changes in afferent input. These devices can affect fatigue, comfort, work, and performance with activities. The current evidence-based research should help the health care provider complete an efficient evaluation and produce cost-effective and beneficial orthotic devices.

REFERENCES

1. Inman V, Ralston H, Todd F: Human walking, Baltimore, 1981, Williams & Wilkins.
2. Larsen K, Weidich F, Leboeuf-Yde C: Can custom made biomechanical shoe orthoses prevent problems in the back and lower extremities? A randomized, controlled intervention trial of 146 military conscripts, J Manipulative Physiol Ther 25:326, 2002.
3. Bartold SJ: The role of orthoses in the treatment of patellofemoral pain in runners, J Sci Med Sport 2(1):1-10, 2001.
4. Richie DH Jr: Effects of foot orthoses on patients with chronic ankle instability, JAPMA 97:19-30, 2007.
5. Wallace RG, Traynor IE, Kernohan WG, et al: Combined conservative and orthotic management of acute ruptures of the Achilles tendon, J Bone Joint Surg Am 86-A:1198-1202, 2004.
6. Gross ML, Napoli RC: Treatment of lower extremity injuries with orthotic shoe inserts an overview, Sports Med 15:66-70, 1993.
7. Saxena A, Haddad J: The effect of foot orthoses on patellofemoral pain syndrome, JAPMA 93:264-271, 2003.
8. Landorf KB, Keenan A, Herbert MD: Effectiveness of foot orthoses to treat plantar fasciitis: a randomized trial, Arch Intern Med 166:1305-1310, 2006.
9. Alvarez RG, Marini A, Schmitt C, et al: Stage I and II posterior tibial tendon dysfunction treated by a structured non-operative management protocol: an orthosis and exercise program, Foot Ankle 27:2-8, 2006.
10. Rome K, Handoll HG, Ashford R: Interventions for preventing and treating stress fractures of bone of the lower limbs in young adults, Cochrane Database Syst Rev 2, 2005.
11. Manter JT: Movements of the subtalar and transverse tarsal joints, Anat Rec 80:397, 1941.
12. Hicks JH: The mechanics of the foot: the joints, J Anat 87:345,1953.
13. Root ML, Weed JH, Sgarlato TE, et al: Axis of motion of the subtalar joint, JAPMA 56:149, 1966.
14. Van Langelaan EJ: A kinematical analysis of the tarsal joints: an x-ray photogrammetric study, Acta Orthop Scand 54(suppl):204, 1983.
15. Benink RJ: The constraint mechanism of the human tarsus, Acta Orthop Scand 56(suppl):215, 1985.
16. Lundberg A, Svensson OK: The axes of rotation of the talocalcaneal and talonavicular joints, Foot 3:65, 1993.
17. Kirby KA: Subtalar joint axis location and rotational equilibrium theory of foot function, JAPMA 91:465-487, 2001.
18. Payne C, Noakes H, Oates M, et al: Resistance of the foot to supination, Victoria, Australia, 2002, Department of Podiatry School of Human Bioscience, La Trobe University.
19. Huson A: Functional anatomy of the foot. In Jahss MH, editor: Disorders of the foot and ankle, Philadelphia, 1991, WB Saunders, p 409.
20. Payne CB: The role of theory in understanding the midtarsal joint (commentary), JAPMA 90:377, 2000.
21. Weissman SD: Radiology of the foot, Baltimore, 1983, Williams & Wilkins, p 55.
22. Deleted in pages.
23. Deleted in pages.
24. Stacoff A, Reinschmidt C, Nigg BM, et al: Effects of foot orthoses on skeletal motion during running, Clin Biomech 15:54-64, 2000.
25. Nigg BM: The role of impact forces and foot pronation: a new paradigm, Clin J Sport Med 11:2-9, 2001.
26. McPoil TG, Hunt MA: Evolution and management of foot and ankle disorders: present problems and future directions, J Orthop Sports Phys Ther 21(6):381-388, 1995.
27. Payne C, Noakes H: The reliability of the manual supination resistance test, J Am Podiatr Med Assoc 93(3):185-189, 2003.

28. Payne C: Foot orthoses reduce the force needed to establish the windlass mechanism but do not change calcaneal angle, J Am Podiatr Med Assoc 93(3):187-188, 2003.

29. Murley GS, Bird AR: The effect of three levels of foot orthotic wedging on the surface electromyographic activity of selected lower limb muscles during gait, Clin Biomech 21:1074-1080, 2006.

30. Santilli V, et al: Peroneus longus muscle activation pattern during gait cycle in athletes affected by functional ankle instability, Am J Sports Med 33:1183-1187, 2005.

31. Nawoczenski DA, Ludewig PM: Electromyographic effects of foot orthotics on selected lower extremity muscles during running, Arch Phys Med Rehab 80:540-544, 1999.

32. Mundermann A, Wakeling JM, Nigg BM, et al: Foot orthoses affect frequency components of muscle activity in the lower extremity, Gait Posture 23:295-302, 2006.

33. Kulig K, Burnfield JM, Reischl S, et al: Effect of foot orthoses on tibialis posterior activation in persons with pes planus, Med Sci Sports Exerc 37:24-29, 2005.

34. Bird AR, Bendrups AP, Payne CB: The effect of foot wedging on electromyographic activity in the erector spinae and gluteus medius muscles during walking, Gait Posture 18:81-91, 2003.

35. Nurse MA, Hulliger M, Wakeling JM, et al: Changing the texture of footwear can alter gait patterns, J Electromyogr Kinesiol 15:496-506, 2005.

36. Romkes J, Rudmann C, Brunner R: Changes in gait and EMG when walking with the Masai barefoot technology, Clin Biomech 21:75-81, 2006.

37. Tomaro J, Burdett RG: The effects of foot orthotics on the EMG activity of selected leg muscles during gait, J Orthop Sports Phys Ther 21:317-327, 1993.

38. Vanicek N, Kingman J, Hencken C: The effect of foot orthotics on myoelectric fatigue in the vastus lateralis during a simulated skier's squat, J Electromyogr Kinesiol 14:693-698, 2004.

39. Ochsendorf DT, Mattacola CG, Arnold BL: Effect of orthotics on postural sway after fatigue of the plantar flexors and dorsiflexors, J Athl Train 35:26-30, 2000.

40. Wakeling JM, Nigg BM: Modification of soft tissue vibrations in the leg by muscular activity, J Appl Physiol 90:412-420, 2001.

41. Wakeling JM, Liphardt AM, Nigg BM: Muscle activity reduces sort tissue resonance at heel strike during walking, J Biomech 36:1761-1769, 2003.

42. Yoshitake Y, Shinohara M, Kouzaki M, et al: Fluctuations in plantar flexion force are reduced after prolonged tendon vibration, J Appl Physiol 97:2090-2097, 2004.

43. Bongiovanni LG, Hagbarth KE, Stjernberg L: Prolonged muscle vibration reducing motor output in maximal voluntary contractions in man, J Physiol 423:15-26, 1990.

44. McPoil TG, Cornwall MW: Use of plantar contact area to predict longitudinal arch height during walking, J Am Podiatr Med Assoc 96(6):489-498, 2006.

45. Sahrmann SA: Diagnosis and treatment of movement impairment syndromes, St Louis, 2002, Mosby.

46. Donatelli R: The biomechanics of the foot and ankle, Philadelphia, 1990, FA Davis.

47. Donatelli R, et al: Relationship between static and dynamic foot positions in professional baseball players, J Orthop Sports Phys Ther 29:316-330, 1999.

48. Eng JJ, Pierrynowski MR: The effect of soft foot orthotics on three dimensional lower limb kinematics during walking and running, Phys Ther 74:836-843,1994.

49. Eng JJ, Pierrynowski MR: Evaluation of soft foot orthotics in the treatment of patellofemoral pain syndrome, Phys Ther 73:62-69, 1993.

50. Johanson MA, et al: Effects of three different posting methods on controlling abnormal subtalar pronation, Phys Ther 74:149-158, 1994.

51. Noakes H, Payne C: The reliability of the manual supination resistance test, JAPMA 93:185-189, 2003.

52. Bolgla LA, Malone TR: Plantar fasciitis and the windlass mechanism: biomechanical link to clinical practice, J Athl Train 39:77-82, 2004.

53. Ekdahl C, Jarnlo GB, Anderson SI: Standing balance in healthy subjects, Scand J Rehab Med 21(4):187-195, 1989.

54. Bressel E, et al: Comparison of static and dynamic balance in female collegiate soccer, basketball, and gymnastics athletes, J Athl Train 42:42-46, 2007.

55. Landorf KB, Keenan A: Efficacy of foot orthoses: what does the literature tell us? AJPM 32:105-113, 1998.

56. Bordelon L: Clinical assessment of the foot. In Donatelli RA, editor: The biomechanics of the foot and ankle, ed 2, Philadelphia, 1996, FA Davis.

57. Donatelli R: Abnormal biomechanics of the foot and ankle, J Orthop Sports Phys Ther 9(1):11-16, 1987.

58. Garbalosa JC, McClure MH, Catlain PA et al: The frontal plane relationship of the forefoot to the rearfoot in an asymptomatic population, J Orthop Sports Phys Ther 20(4):200-206, 1994.

59. Riegger-Krugh C, Keysor JJ: Skeletal malalignments of the lower quarter: correlated and compensatory motions and postures, J Orthop Sports Phys Ther 23(2):106-170, 1996.

60. Hicks JH: Mechanics of the foot. II. The plantar aponeurosis, J Anat 88:25, 1954.

61. Charlie Baycroft. Foot Science International Ltd.

62. Inman UT: The joints of the ankle, Baltimore, 1976, Williams & Wilkins.

63. Hertel J, Sloss BR, Earl JE: Effect of foot orthotics on quadriceps and gluteus medius electromyographic activity during selected exercises, Ach Phys Med Rehab 86:26-30, 2005.

25

Kenneth H. Akizuki,
Lawrence M. Oloff,
and Lisa M. Giannone

New Advances in Foot and Ankle Surgery and Rehabilitation

The following chapter describes some of the more common surgical procedures of the foot and ankle. The subject matter is presented as a collaborative effort between the surgeon and the physical therapist. It is important that the therapist understands the nuances of the surgical procedure and that the surgeon understands the physical therapy needs brought on by their procedure. This professional partnership ultimately results in the very best care to the patient.

ACHILLES TENDON SURGERY

Achilles tendon injuries can be divided into acute and chronic. Ruptures of the Achilles tendon constitute the majority of those acute injuries that require surgical intervention. Surgery is generally recommended for the vast majority of Achilles tendon tears because of the potential for a better functional outcome and lowered risk of rerupture.[1] Ruptures typically occur in the midsection of the tendon (in the area sometimes referred to as the *hypovascular section of the tendon*) because of the diminished blood supply to this region. This diminished blood supply is thought to play a key role in the prevalence of ruptures in this area of the tendon. It also makes repair somewhat problematic because of the degenerative nature of this tissue. Sometimes tissue is imported to supplement the repair.[2]

The technical aspects of an Achilles tendon rupture repair are fairly straightforward. The tendon ends are brought into approximation after devitalized torn tendon ends are débrided. Usually some form of modified Kessler suture is used to lessen ischemia to the tendon repair site and to provide security to the repair.[3] Some surgeons favor a percutaneous repair to be less invasive, which can potentially speed up the recovery process.[4] The negative aspect of percutaneous repair includes the higher potential for sural nerve entrapment because of the blind nature of the procedure. In addition, the surgeon loses the ability to débride devitalized tendon tissue with percutaneous repairs. The last consideration is that estimating appropriate physiologic tension is simpler with open repairs.

The surgeon's confidence of the repair, the status of the tissues that are repaired, and the overall physiologic status of the patient are but a few of the factors that are taken into consideration in determining rehabilitation protocols after Achilles tendon repair. A basic understanding of tendon healing helps in deciding therapy protocols.[5] Right after the repair, tensile strength is good. Around 12 days after the repair, the tendon exhibits a weaker physical state, sometimes referred to as *tendomalacia*. This transient period of weakness can be potentially concerning.

Chronic Achilles tendon surgery can be more problematic. With chronic Achilles tendon pathologic condition, some form of tendon degeneration or tendinopathy typically occurs (Figure 25-1). The tendon goes through sequential degeneration, which weakens the tendon and eventually leads to rupture. Surgery is contemplated before rupture, particularly if symptoms are painful and functionally limiting. The surgery involves two approaches. The first approach is to débride the tendon (a newer approach is to not only débride the tendon but also to inject growth factors to enhance repair at the site).[6] The second approach is to import tissues because of the unhealthy nature of the involved tissues. The flexor hallucis longus tendon is the usual tissue imported.[7] In either of the two surgical approaches, one must consider the questionable integrity of these tissues in the rehabilitation process.

ACHILLES TENDON REHABILITATION

In the rehabilitation of Achilles tendon surgery, one needs to know the mechanism of the injury and whether a component of chronic preoperative tendonosis exists. This information will nuance the rehabilitation strategy and guide the pace and volume decisions in reloading the limb.

Although the patient will be protected with immobilization and nonweight bearing for some weeks after surgery per the surgeon's protocol, early rehabilitation efforts will be oriented at preventing stiffness in the forefoot and midfoot, as well as gentle subtalar mobilization. In addition, activation (as appropriate) of all leg muscle groups in neutral ankle positions can be done.

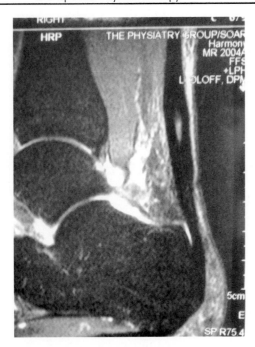

Figure 25-1 The sagittal short T_1 inversion recovery (STIR) sequence shows an area of high signal in the midsection of the tendon, indicating early degeneration.

Once early-phase motion is allowed, rehabilitation is targeted at gaining neuromuscular control of the muscles about the ankle in nonweight-bearing positions. Manual resistive exercise can move from isometric to work through gentle ranges as tolerated. Care should be taken with all range and muscle work not to overstretch the repair because an abnormal length tension relationship will compromise the patient's ability to regain normal plantarflexion strength.[8] This level of therapeutic and manual exercise continues through approximately 6 to 8 weeks postoperative, at which time weight-bearing restrictions are being reduced.

Once axial loading is allowed, closed kinetic chain exercise can be introduced at subbody weight load levels. All neuromuscular reeducation and subsequent strengthening of the calf complex should be performed from ranges of 0 degrees of dorsiflexion into ranges of plantarflexion, thereby avoiding loading the tendon in a stretched position (beyond neutral dorsiflexion) because these muscle loads produce higher levels of stress to the repaired tendon.[9] This phase of protected, nonweight-bearing strengthening is often prolonged to ensure that patients gain complete neuromuscular control and full recruitment of the gastrocnemius-soleus complex and the secondary medial and lateral compartment plantar flexors before progressing to full weight–bearing exercise.

Manual techniques and low-volume partial weight-bearing loads are the primary means of developing this level of muscle function and, in general, avoiding overload to the gastrocnemius-soleus complex before development of significant tendon healing and strength. Because complete development of tendon tensile strength occurs during approximately 1 year, the patient should expect recovery of full strength and functional load tolerance to parallel this time line.

Throughout all weight-bearing phases of rehabilitation, be sure to analyze the mechanics of the foot and ankle in standing. Assess the patient's ability to control pronation-supination motions so that a lack of control and coordination can be addressed in the rehabilitation process. Pronation and supination motions can create abnormal loads into the Achilles during function.[10] Thus the medial and lateral muscle groups must be trained in non-, partial, and full weight bearing to gain stability with activities of daily living (ADL) and sport-specific function.

Offer the patient creative ways to cross-train with increasing cardiovascular and strength volumes but, from a strength development perspective, in positions and with loads that are less than full body weight. Beware of traditional exercise equipment that may overload the healing tendon. Being creative and knowing the status of the tendon's healing maturity, as well as the status of the patient's muscular function, can help one design a program using common equipment in nontraditional ways that gradually and safely brings normal strength and function without overstretching or inflammatory setbacks.

If the patient has adequate strength, coordination, and can decelerate well at heel strike, impact and lateral training can sometimes be introduced and progressed as early as 4 months postoperative. Often, however, even in a normal course of Achilles rehabilitation, these loads are not tolerated well until after 6 months postoperative. Therapy should proceed with an awareness of these timelines and expect a somewhat slow but steady return of full muscular recruitment, control, and functional strength.

PERONEAL TENDON SURGERY

Peroneal tendon injuries are relatively common.[11] The peroneal tendon conditions that may require surgery take many forms. These include tendon tear, stenosing tenosynovitis, and subluxating tendons.

Peroneal tendon tears can occur with or without subluxation. These tears most commonly involve the peroneus brevis tendon. They are thought to be the consequence of sprains or attritional wear because of luxation tendencies. In either case the peroneus brevis tendon tears because of its closer proximity to the lateral malleolus, one of the pulley mechanisms for this tendon muscle complex. Sobel et al.[12] has described a classification system for these tendon tears, essentially dividing them into *partial* and *full-thickness tears*. These tears are typically longitudinal in orientation (Figure 25-2). When symptomatic, these tears are repaired, tubularizing if necessary. As with all tendon repairs, the tendon is protected for ample time in order not to jeopardize the repair site. Chronic subluxation of the peroneal tendons can contribute to abnormal tendon wear and tear. It can also produce symptoms such as pain and/or instability. Repair of these tendons has multiple procedural approaches, including tightening of the peroneal retinaculum, deepening of the retrolateral malleolar groove, and fibular osteotomy.[13] Physical therapy gets even more complex in these scenarios

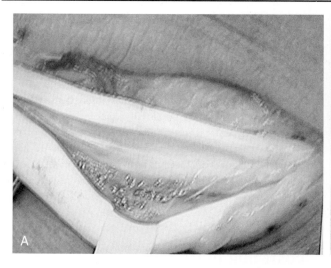
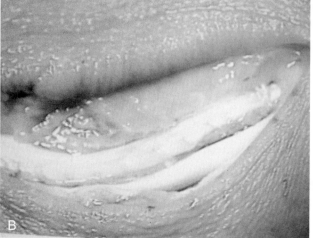

Figure 25-2 A, Longitudinal tear of the peroneus brevis tendon. **B,** The peroneal tendon tear has been repaired by tubularizing it.

because care must be taken not to jeopardize the reconstructed or tightened pulley system.

Stenosing tenosynovitis is somewhat less complex. In this condition, motion of the tendon within the tendon sheath is prohibited by adhesions that formed from long-term abnormal mechanics or injury.[14] The sheath is opened, and all adhesions are identified and released. If a low-lying muscle belly is present, then this is sometimes débrided proximal to the tunnel. Motion is encouraged early postoperatively to limit the possibility of recurrence.

PERONEAL TENDON REHABILITATION

With peroneal tendon rehabilitation, be precise about the exact surgical procedure performed. Identify whether the tendon sheath was released as in stenosing tenosynovitis or whether there was repair of a chronic or acute tendon tear. Know all alteration in bony anatomy that can occur as part of the procedure or repair of a retinaculum or tendon, because these factors will control the pace and reloading of the limb. In addition, identify the probable mechanism of injury and provocative activities that existed preoperatively. In this way, rehabilitation can be planned and designed to address those mechanical issues and muscular deficiencies that may have created the dysfunction and predisposed the patient to the injury. Motions that created stress and irritation preoperatively should be "trained for" in the rehabilitation process to restore full postoperative and lasting function.

Stenosing tendons that have had adhesions released will be moved early and through full ranges postoperatively. Restrengthening and reloading can occur methodically by developing neuromuscular control of the peroneal muscles, along with the gastrocnemius-soleus complex in both open and nonfull weight–bearing closed kinetic chain positions. Chronic instability and weakness of the lateral ankle and/or excessive use of the peroneal muscles as plantar flexors can lead to wear and stress to the peroneals.[15] Rehabilitation should address these tendencies in motion by identifying potentially stressful mechanics and training the appropriate muscles with both open and closed kinetic chain exercise to work as active stabilizers and/or movers of the joint.

In the case of tendon repair or stabilization, early rehabilitation will be much more guarded, allowing bony, tendon, and/or retinacular tissues to heal. Early rehabilitation will involve gentle dorsiflexion and plantarflexion range of motion. Care should be taken to avoid extremes of inversion and eversion motion. These motions, especially when combined with plantarflexion or dorsiflexion, can create stress across the pulley system of the peroneal muscles because they pass posterior to the lateral malleolus. Perform all therapeutic exercise with the ankle in neutral as it relates to the frontal and axial planes of motion. This precaution will allow isometric exercise to the invertors group with the ankle held at neutral and gentle work through the ranges of dorsiflexion and plantarflexion. Exercise for the peroneal muscles directly (when appropriate, several weeks postoperatively) should first be done isometrically, then from positions of mild inversion to positions of neutral motion at the ankle and subtalar joints. Only in the later stages of rehabilitation, once the tendon repair or bony stabilization is well healed, will the peroneal group be worked through a full range of concentric and eccentric motion. Be sure that the gastrocnemius-soleus complex is adequately strong so that the peroneal muscles are not required to overwork as plantar flexors when returning to full function.

Once neuromuscular control and strength is restored through the foot and ankle in open and nonfull weight–bearing positions, rehabilitation work can proceed into full weight bearing. Cue and train the patient to move with normal mechanics at the foot and ankle with all closed kinetic chain therapeutic exercise, ADL, and function. This can be accomplished by having the patient weight shift through the foot, either medially or laterally, to reduce eversion or inversion moments that may create stress to the newly repaired or stabilized tendon. In this way, rehabilitation has the best chance to correct mechanics in the foot and ankle motion that can predispose the tendon to postoperative wear and tear.

POSTERIOR TIBIAL TENDON SURGERY

Surgery of the posterior tibial tendon is indicated for three conditions: (1) stenosing tenosynovitis, (2) accessory navicular problems, and (3) tendinopathy. Each of these conditions is distinctly unique from both a surgical and a physical therapy perspective.

The least complex is stenosing tenosynovitis. As with the peroneal tendon described previously, the condition can originate either from trauma or abnormal mechanics. Distinguishing this condition from tendinopathy is critical in the decision process of surgery. Magnetic resonance imaging (MRI) is useful in determining the presence and extent of tendon degeneration or so-called tendinopathy or tendinosis.[16,17] The presence of tendinopathy may warrant tendon reconstruction. Adhesions within the sheath are not typically appreciated on MRI. To appreciate adhesions, ultrasound may indicate limited tendon movement. Alternatively, tenography is used.[14] Tenography uses an intrasheath injection of lidocaine, contrast dye, and a steroid agent. Diminished flow of contrast dye enables the detection of tendon-to-sheath adhesions. This study is performed in real time using fluoroscopy. On rare occasions, the study may prove therapeutic by virtue of the adhesiolysis effect of the injection itself. The surgical approach, once confirmed, involves opening the tendon sheath and release of adhesions. The amount of immobilization postoperatively is dictated by the extent that the laciniate ligament is released. If it is released completely to gain access to the tendon, then 3 weeks of crutch-assisted nonweight-bearing status is used. Continuous passive motion (CPM) machines may be used during that phase to help lessen the recurrence of the adhesions released at the time of surgery.

The presence of tendinopathy adds significant complexity to the surgery and the therapy. Tendinosis seems to be prevalent in the area behind and below the medial malleolus because of an anatomically consistent hypovascular zone.[18] This zone, coupled with a pronounced pronated foot type, is a formula for tendinosis and tear. When detected in earlier phases, reconstruction is accomplished using the flexor digitorum longus to augment the degenerated posterior tibial tendon.[19] Some form of foot realigning procedure, such as calcaneal osteotomy, may be used to lessen pronatory influence on the repaired tendon in the future. Longer-standing cases of tendon degeneration may be more complex because of eventual arthrosis that develops in the hindfoot joints from long-standing severe pronation. In such cases reconstruction uses arthrodesis of one or more hindfoot joints.

The last form of posterior tibial tendon surgery in this discussion involves cases using an accessory navicular bone, sometimes referred to as an *os tibiale externum*. This accessory bone is not uncommon. It can cause symptoms as the result of prominence. It can also become symptomatic after injuries,

typically eversion mechanism of injuries.[20] Patients in this later category can develop a painful diastasis. High signal at the junction of the accessory bone and the navicular on MRI can help support the diagnosis.[21] In recalcitrant cases of either mechanism, removal of the accessory bone is considered.[22] In such cases the surgeon will sometimes insert some form of anchor to supplement the potentially weakened tendon insertion or consider relocating the tendon insertion more plantar to the navicular bone. This portion of the procedure has a profound influence of the physical therapy protocols that follow. In such cases the surgical sire must be respected and protected postoperatively as the surgeon would for any tendon transfer.

POSTERIOR TIBIAL TENDON REHABILITATION

With the rehabilitation of posterior tibialis tendon surgery, therapy should immediately appreciate that preoperative anatomy and mechanics have a major role in injury.[23] Because most posterior tibialis stress and injury is caused by excessive pronation force through the medial foot, ankle, and arch, either chronically or acutely, rehabilitation efforts will focus on creating a medially "stabilized" foot and ankle.[24] By creating a dynamic arch with active muscle tension throughout the rehabilitation process, therapy has its best chances of creating a mechanically sound and functionally prepared foot and ankle.

Therapy must respect the surgical process, identifying degree of bony repair and/or tendon repair or transfer. These procedures require longer immobilization and protection to allow bone and tendon healing. Early rehabilitation targets gentle dorsiflexion, plantarflexion, and inversion range of motion, as well as the strict avoidance of any eversion ranging (because this places significant stress on healing bone or repaired and/or transferred tendon, disrupting or compromising the repair).

As healing progresses and the patient is able to load muscle tissue, neuromuscular reeducation is focused at the muscles of the medial foot, arch, and ankle. Manual techniques should be used to recruit and retrain not only posterior tibialis but also flexor hallucis longus, flexor digitorum longus, and the intrinsic muscles of the arch. When trained, these muscles combine to help stabilize the medial foot and create a "dynamic arch." This muscle training allows the patient to actively control and reduce pronation forces that were stressful preoperatively and need to be corrected to maximize postoperative success.

This same focus on recruiting and ensuring muscle activity of the medial foot and ankle groups is applied from early manual resistive phases of open-chain training, through non- and full weight–bearing closed kinetic chain training. The patient should be cued to use and maintain a dynamic arch with all functional ADL and sport-specific therapeutic exercises. The therapist can do this by instructing the patient to shift weight toward the lateral aspect of the foot, cupping the arch, with closed kinetic chain exercise and activity.

By exercising and training the patient to use the medial muscle groups, therapy offers the best opportunity for successful return to function because preoperative muscle deficiencies and mechanical tendencies for hyperpronation are thusly addressed.

The use of a medially supportive orthotic device and shoe wear that prevents pronation can be helpful throughout the rehabilitation process. These passive restraints provide relative rest to the tendon and medial foot during weight bearing and help support rehabilitation efforts that address the dynamic aspects of stabilizing the medial foot.[25] Patients, when returning to sport, should be counseled on shoe wear that provides support and control of pronation. Orthotic agents will supplement but should not replace efforts to use muscle activity as medial foot and ankle stabilization.

FASCIA SURGERY

Surgery for plantar fasciitis is less commonly used than in previous years. It is generally accepted that the vast majority of plantar fasciitis patients will respond to conservative care measures if all parties can be patient to undergo what can sometimes be a protracted recovery time for this condition. In those cases requiring surgery, partial plantar fascia release is most commonly used.[26] The procedure has evolved from a total to partial release to mitigate the chances of overlengthening that can lead to lateral column stress and further surgery. Flattening of the arch has also been observed in cases of fascia release.[27] Another benefit of relatively recent advances in this procedure is that it can be effectively carried out by endoscopic means, thereby lessening the convalescence (Figure 25-3). Whether the procedure is done endoscopically or by open approach, therapy precautions need to be undertaken to avoid stretching out what portions of the fascia remains. Undo stress to the calcaneocuboid joint in such cases may necessitate arthrodesis of this joint to resolve such complaints.

PLANTAR FASCIA REHABILITATION

When considering plantar fascia injury and surgery from a mechanical point of view, when rehabilitating, one should assume that there was an element of acute or chronic pronation that predisposed the injury. Explore preoperative movement habits and activities to identify mechanical tendencies into the ranges of pronation that may have existed. Postoperatively, the medial foot and arch become additionally vulnerable to losing normal support and medial "posting" based on the injury and release.[28] Be sure to not overstretch the released area in the first several weeks because this can contribute to further collapse medially as weight bearing proceeds through the limb. Additionally, an ineffective arch can lead to lateral column compression, overload to the lateral foot, and subsequent dysfunction.[29] Rehabilitation efforts throughout should be focused at creating dynamic support to the medial foot, arch, and ankle to prevent this potential complication.

Developing the musculature of the medial foot, ankle, and arch requires that the posterior tibialis, flexor hallucis longus, flexor digitorum longus, and the intrinsic muscles of the foot are all activated. This training is done open chained and manually in the early phases of rehabilitation. It can then be advanced to closed kinetic chain exercise. The therapist can be creative in designing partial and full weight–bearing exercise that recruits those muscles of the medial foot, ankle, and arch. Cueing to shift weight to the lateral weight-bearing side of the foot, actively and consciously, during exercise in which the foot is in contact with a platform, surface, or floor, can help recruit the musculature of the medial side and develop this dynamic arch. Muscle reeducation and recruitment starts from the floor up and affects the entire kinetic chain. This effort to maintain focus on the development of medial foot, ankle, and arch control should be maintained through the entire rehabilitation process and is combined with the more obvious elements of restoring full range, flexibility, and mobility of the foot, ankle, and subtalar joints.

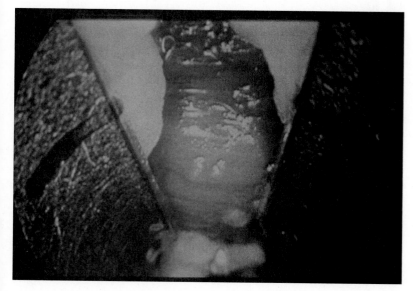

Figure 25-3 This fascia release is being performed endoscopically. Once released, the underlying muscle belly is visualized.

In this way rehabilitation efforts are focused on treating the mechanics of injury and/or overuse patterns and have the greatest chances of restoring pain-free and lasting function. As with other medial foot and arch dysfunction, the use of a basic medially supportive orthotic device can be helpful in the return to full weight–bearing activity and function. This passive restraint should be used only as a compliment to excellent neuromuscular control, strength, and endurance of the medially stabilizing musculature of the lower limb.

ARTHROSCOPY OF THE ANKLE AND SUBTALAR JOINT

The range of potential interventions possible by small joint arthroscopic techniques has evolved during the past 15 years.[30] Common techniques for the ankle joint include synovectomies, débridement, removal of loose bodies, reduction of impinging exostoses, revision and microfracture of osteochondral defects, and thermal stabilization techniques. Aftercare is critical to the success of the procedure and differs with each of the described approaches.

Certain general considerations apply to all ankle arthroscopy techniques. Typically two anterior portals are used, one medial the other lateral. Care is taken in portal placement to avoid injury to the overlying nerves.[31] Care is likewise taken in the manipulation of these portals postoperatively to avoid irritation. The development of neuritis by the surgeon or therapist can hinder therapeutic approaches and prolong recovery time. Weight-bearing status can differ significantly with each type of arthroscopic intervention. Removing loose bodies alone usually has the quickest return to weight-bearing status, whereas microfracture the slowest (Figure 25-4). In the case of microfracture, drilling or use of awls creates limited defects the subchondral bone to promote a fibrocartilage formation (Figure 25-5).[32] What is initially created is, in essence, a scab on the surface of the bone that converts to its target tissue over time. The initial scab is friable and not sturdy to mechanical irritation. It is generally recommended that 6 weeks of nonweight bearing be observed in such patients. Special considerations also exist with thermal stabilization techniques.[33] Radio frequency surgical wands, holmium lasers, and other heat instrumentation can be used to take advantage of the structure of collagen, which causes it to shrink when subjected to certain temperatures. Weight bearing is again limited and protected for the first 6 weeks, and side-to-side stressful motion is to be avoided for 3 months after the procedure.

Subtalar joint arthroscopy is not as universally used because of the anatomic constraints imposed by this joint. The procedure approaches are limited to the larger and more easily accessible posterior facet of the subtalar complex. The most common application of this procedure is in cases of impingement com-

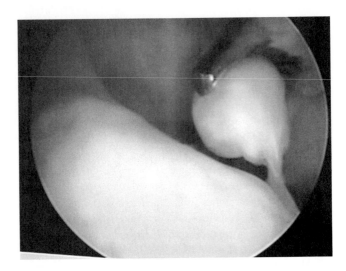

Figure 25-4 The loose body will be removed arthroscopically. Function is returned quickly.

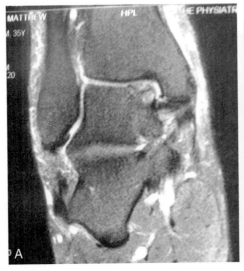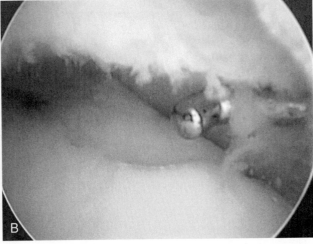

Figure 25-5 A, Magnetic resonance imaging (MRI) scan of a medial talar dome osteochondral lesion. **B,** Defect is visualized arthroscopically and will be treated with débridement and microfracture. No weight bearing is allowed for 6 weeks.

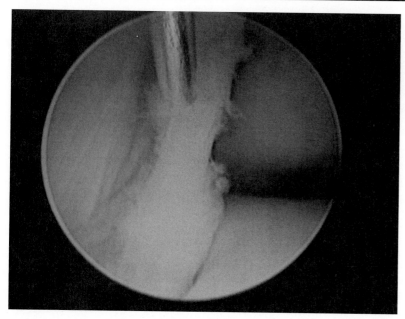

Figure 25-6 This is an arthroscopy of the subtalar joint. Partial tear of the interosseous ligament should be noted.

plaints after ankle sprain, more commonly referred to as *sinus tarsi syndrome.*[34] Two lateral portals are used, which allow access to the anterior and lateral margin of the posterior facet. A third posterior lateral portal can allow visualization of the posterior aspect of the joint. Typically, these posttraumatic conditions manifest as overproduction of fibrosynovial tissues at the margins of the joint. In sinus tarsi syndrome, most of this abnormal tissue is seen at the anterior margin of the posterior facet of the subtalar joint. This tissue is readily approached and evacuated by arthroscopic means. Tears of the interosseous ligament have been described.[35] These tears are usually incomplete, and repair is not necessitated (Figure 25-6). Although the intervention is relatively low-key, nonweight-bearing status is advised for 3 weeks. To prevent recurrent scar tissues, a CPM machine is helpful until the patient initiates conventional physical therapy.

REHABILITATION OF ANKLE ARTHROSCOPIC PROCEDURES

Ankle arthroscopy allows a rapid onset and progression of rehabilitation with the procedures that remove scar, fibrous tissue, or loose bodies. Because its purpose is to remove binding or irritating tissue, the ankle, subtalar, and foot joints are moved soon after surgery. Once the surgeon allows motion and the portals are adequately healed, continuous and frequent motion in as full a range as tolerated, with minimal amounts of immobilization, helps to prevent the reformation of scar and fibrous tissue growth that may again restrict motion and cause pain.

Arthroscopic techniques performed to repair cartilage defects or stabilize the ankle by shrinking collagen tissues require a more mechanically nuanced approach in rehabilitation. Weight-bearing loads will be strictly avoided for 6 to 8 weeks. In the case of cartilage repair in which subchondral bone

has been intentionally disturbed to create fibrocartilage scar, early continuous range of motion allows the most "organized" remodeling of the fibrocartilage scar, whereas compressive forces may disrupt that same healing.[36] Similarly, the collagen tissues shortened under the influence of heat need adequate time to "set" at their new length and should not be exposed to range or loading techniques for a similar amount of time. Muscle activation techniques, done manually and with the surrounding muscles held isometrically, can help reduce the degree of inhibition that can develop in the postoperative immobilization and protection phase.

Once loading is allowed, the rehabilitation specialist should be acutely aware of precise areas of the joint surface that have been repaired. In this way, partial and full weight–bearing training can be designed to control joint compressive forces through that area of the joint surface. Consider the patients weight-bearing mechanics, their preoperative provocative activities or exercises, along with precise knowledge about the area of the joint surface manipulated to position the foot, ankle, and limb when doing closed kinetic chain exercise. Correcting tendencies to pronate or supinate "into" the lesion will help relocate and reduce the joint reaction forces away from the surgical site. In addition, the clinician should be aware of motion in the sagittal plane that may increase or decrease compressive loading through the surgical site and select exercise positions accordingly to work the limb without simultaneously overloading the lesion. In this way the patient is neuromuscularly trained, from the foot up through the entire kinetic chain, to use muscle function that supports favorable limb alignment.

Similarly, with thermal stabilization procedures, the patient should be cued to maintain a foot and ankle position that holds the lateral, repaired collagen tissues in a neutral to shortened range for all closed kinetic chain activities. Range-of-motion activities to encourage normal flexibility are not avoided in total; however, they are reserved for the later phases of reha-

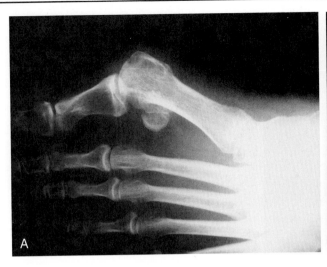

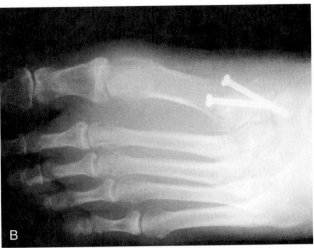

Figure 25-7 A, Lapidus procedures work well for patients with high intermetatarsal angles. **B,** In this same patient, a Lapidus procedure was performed. A Lapidus procedure involves arthrodesis of the first metatarsal-cuneiform joint. Immobilization is important with this form of hallux valgus correction.

bilitation and are measured—creating adequate but not excessive mobility of the tissues repaired.

With both of the more complicated arthroscopic procedures, functional, impact, and lateral loads are not added until approximately 4 months after surgery. All mechanical nuance applied in the early and midphases that focused on neuromuscular control, muscular strength, and muscular endurance continue to be applied through the progression into full function. The muscles of the lower leg, foot, and ankle must be well trained as "shock absorbers" and highly effective at decelerating load through the joint to appreciate a lasting functional result.

HALLUX VALGUS SURGERY

Numerous procedures address the different components that constitute hallux valgus deformity. The trend has been to concentrate the correction on some form of distal metatarsal osteotomy, proximal metatarsal osteotomy, and/or first metatarsal-cuneiform arthrodesis to restore alignment to these deformities.[37] The determination as to which procedure is most appropriate is arrived at by a combination of factors including radiographic angles, flexibility of the deformity, nature and stability of the foot type, and procedural preference of the operating surgeon.

The type of procedure materially affects the nature of the recovery time and follow-up care used. The postoperative restrictions are most severe for arthrodesis procedures of the first metatarsal-cuneiform joint, referred to as the *Lapidus procedure* (Figure 25-7). This procedure has enjoyed increasing popularity in recent years because of its stability over time, but the convalescence is extreme.[38] Eight to 12 weeks of cast immobilization is used. Half of that time is spent in a nonweight-bearing cast. Accelerated programs will potentially carry a higher risk for nonunion of the arthrodesis site that not only prolongs recovery but also can potentially necessitate revision

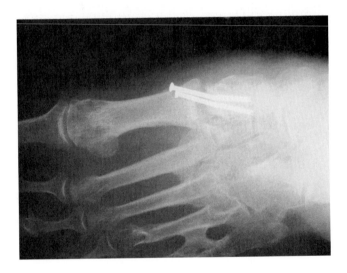

Figure 25-8 Early mobilization or premature aggressive therapy and breakdown of a Lapidus arthrodesis site.

surgery (Figure 25-8). Because of the long convalescence protocols to regain functional use of the extremity, encouraging range of motion of the first metatarsophalangeal (MTP) joint is beneficial.

Base wedge osteotomies have similar indications and postoperative management issues as a Lapidus procedure.[38] They are most commonly used for the more severe hallux valgus deformity in which a marked divergence of the first and second metatarsals occurs. The angle between the first and second metatarsals is sometimes referred to as the *intermetatarsal angle*. Six to 8 weeks of protected weight-bearing status by cast and/or cast boot is used.

The most common bunion operations performed are distal osteotomy procedures.[39] The most common of these are sometimes referred to as a *chevron* or *Austin type of bunionectomy* (Figure 25-9). This procedure involves not only reduction of

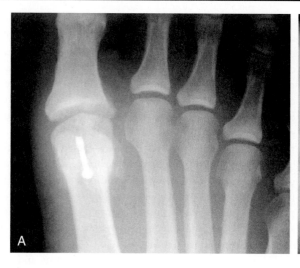
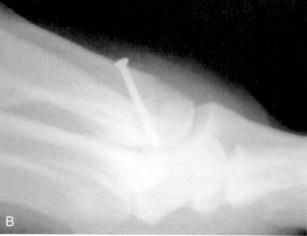

Figure 25-9 With an Austin or chevron type of bunionectomy, the osteotomy is made distally. The osteotomy is stable for weight bearing. Rigid fixation further enhances the stability of the procedure.

the enlarged medial first metatarsal head but also includes making a V-shaped cut in the distal metaphysis of the first metatarsal. The first metatarsal is then transposed an appropriate number of millimeters to reduce the deformity and the divergence of the first and second metatarsal. Fixation is usually used, making the osteotomy stable for weight bearing and early motion exercises. A stiff-soled postoperative shoe is used for 4 to 6 weeks, then one transitions to reasonable shoe gear thereafter.

With all the bunion procedures described, ancillary portions of the procedure are additional considerations for how aggressive the care can be postoperatively. For example, various medial capsular tightening procedures are used, so one needs to be cautious to keep the toe in a centralized position when any range-of-motion exercises are initiated postoperatively. Excessive abduction stress on the first MTP joint can lead to recurrence of deformity. The type of fixation used can influence postoperative care. Kirschner wire (also known as *K wire*) fixation is not as stable as screw fixation. Loosening of hardware and destabilization can result from premature excessive activity on an osteotomy or fusion site that has lesser forms of fixation. In addition, many long-standing hallux valgus deformities have varying degrees of arthrosis. Degenerative joints may not tolerate the same degree of rehabilitation protocol measures postoperatively (Figure 25-10).

HALLUX VALGUS REHABILITATION

Anatomically and mechanically, hallux valgus is the result of stress to the foot in ranges of plantarflexion, hyperpronation, and hyperabduction.[40] All procedures that correct this deformity involve bony manipulation and repair and may also involve ligamentous repair. Depending on the procedure, early weight bearing will be allowed or protected and rehabilitation will proceed accordingly. Early range efforts will target gentle flexion and extension at the first MTP joint and dorsiflexion

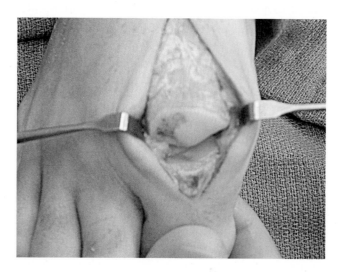

Figure 25-10 Many long-standing bunion deformities have wear of the articular cartilage. Sometimes microfracture type of procedures are performed at the same time. This would limit the type of therapy that is used postoperatively.

and plantarflexion at the ankle joint. Some element of inversion range of motion can be performed. Ranges that stress the medial aspect of the great toe and/or arch should be strictly avoided throughout the rehabilitation process. Do not range or load the foot, particularly the midfoot and forefoot, into any degree of eversion and/or abduction.

As with the rehabilitation of the plantar fascia and posterior tibialis injury and surgery, significant focus is placed on establishing a medially stabilized foot and arch dynamically. Use manual techniques to recruit all medial foot, ankle, and arch stabilizers—posterior tibialis, flexor digitorum longus, flexor hallucis longus, and intrinsic muscles of the foot. Because the vulnerable joint is distal in the kinetic chain, care should be taken not to create large levers across the MTP joint or the first metatarsal when working those muscle groups. Patients should be worked from a neutral position at the foot and ankle into inverted, adducted, and supinated ranges.

When proceeding to partial and full weight–bearing therapeutic exercise, be sure to set the patient up in foot and ankle positions that hold against hyperpronation, abduction, and eversion. This cueing allows the patient to recruit and use the muscles of the medial foot, arch, and ankle to stabilize stressful pronation forces while working in weight bearing. This training helps reduce stress to the repaired and/or reconstructed metatarsal or MTP joint, thus addressing predisposing stressful mechanics and muscle deficiencies.

Orthotic support for the arch may be helpful to passively support the foot while dynamic support is being developed. Assist the patient in selecting shoe wear that can do the same and may also reduce flexion moments across the first MTP joint.

Be sure to restore as much flexion and extension range at the MTP joint (and through the midfoot) as possible, because elements of degenerative joint disease may also exist at the joint. This flexibility and range can decompress joint reaction forces with movement required for pain-free ambulation and other functional activity.

ANKLE STABILIZATION SURGERY

Surgical stabilization of the ankle is considered in the active individual who has chronic instability of the ankle (as a result of one or more previous injuries) that created attenuation or insufficiency of the lateral ligaments. Although ankle bracing and strengthening of the ankle-supporting musculature can provide adequate functionality in many patients with chronic instability, such measures fall short in many more active patients. A case can be made for more aggressive approaches in such patients because chronic instability and repetitive injuries do create theoretical concerns of developing premature arthritis.[41]

Dozens of procedural approaches exist for the chronic unstable ankle patient. The best way to approach the procedural types is by dividing them into categories: tenodesis, delayed primary repair, ligament reconstruction, and thermal stabilization. The tenodesis operations generally use a portion of the peroneal tendons, which is rerouted into the fibular (thereby providing a restraint to inversion of the ankle). Most of these procedures do not selectively restrict motion of the ankle joint alone, but also restrict motion of the subtalar joint.[42] These methods have the longest track record and are generally successful. One theoretical shortcoming is that they also block subtalar joint motion. In those patients exhibiting subtalar instability, this may prove beneficial. In most, this additional limitation of motion on a neighboring joint is superfluous. The delayed primary repair, sometimes referred to as the *Brostrom procedure*, plicates the lateral collateral ligaments that have been attenuated or stretched out from prior trauma. It is more selective than the tenodesing operation in terms of its restriction of motion.[43] A shortcoming is that it is dependent on the quality of the tissues that are tightened. Ligament reconstruction gen-

erally imports other tissues, such as allograft, and replicates the course of the previously damaged lateral ligaments. Again it is more selective in limiting motion of the ankle alone. Healing can be longer, depending on the nature of the tissues that are imported. The thermal stabilization procedure is the newest of the procedures. First done on shoulders, thermal stabilizations offer an arthroscopic alternative to the stabilization group of procedures. It has been demonstrated that heat, applied by a radio frequency probe or laser, can cause the collagen to shrink because of its helical configuration. Arthroscopic procedures are preferred because of the lower morbidity and shorter healing times generally associated with these procedures when compared with their open-technique counterparts. However, these arthroscopic alternatives are relatively new, and the long-term outcomes still require scrutiny.

The majority of the lateral ligament tightening and reconstructive techniques require fairly long convalescences and cast immobilization postprocedure. Obvious concerns exist regarding causing premature or excessive inversion motion postoperatively in these patients because it may compromise the operative results. As a result, therapy is often initiated at the end of the postoperative repair process versus at the beginning.

ANKLE STABILIZATION REHABILITATION

As with the other rehabilitation procedures discussed in this chapter, preoperative mechanics and muscle deficiencies in the ability to add support and stabilize the ankle joint have a major influence on the postoperative rehabilitation programs for ankle stabilization procedures. After identifying the precise procedures chosen by the surgeon for repair and appropriately protecting the joint in terms of range and joint loading according to those tissues manipulated, therapy will address preoperative mechanical and muscular deficiencies.

Most ankle stabilization procedures will require approximately 6 to 8 weeks of protection, whether tendon was relocated or ligament was repaired and reinforced.[44] This allows adequate time for tissue healing to occur. Any therapeutic procedures allowed during that period would strictly avoid all ranging into inversion and would primarily target generating muscular recruitment in the dorsiflexor, plantar flexor, and invertor groups isometrically. Tension of the evertor (peroneal) muscle groups should be avoided, especially with procedures in which peroneal tendon was used as the stabilizer.

Once allowed, neuromuscular recruitment techniques should address all planes of the ankle, but especially address the retraining of the lateral ankle musculature. This work would proceed through ranges of neutral ankle motion into ranges of eversion. Eccentric or loaded motion into ranges of inversion should be reserved for the later phases of rehabilitation.

As with arthroscopic stabilization procedures, the patient should be cued and positioned with all non- and full weight–bearing closed kinetic chain exercise to hold the ankle in a position that avoids inversion and/or supination moments. The patient is thusly trained to actively recruit peroneal muscle concurrent with all pressing, calf-raising, and squatting movements, as well as other functional exercises. This type of cueing and training not only addresses muscle deficiencies preoperatively that will help support the procedure performed but also has elements of proprioceptive training that become important in the total rehabilitation of the ankle and limb.

Impact and lateral motion should not be introduced in the rehabilitation process until approximately 4 months postoperative. The patient should demonstrate adequate muscle function and range before proceeding to these final phases of functional rehabilitation. Early return to activity may be supported with some type of external restraint in the form of ankle bracing or a laterally elevated shoe wedge as additional protection to inversion/supination loads.

REFERENCES

1. Khan RJK, Fick D, Keogh A, et al: Treatment of acute Achilles tendon ruptures: a meta-analysis of randomized, controlled trials, J Bone Joint Surg 87(10):2202-2210, 2005.

2. Barber FA, Herbert MA, Coons DA: Tendon augmentation grafts: biomechanical failure loads and failure patterns, Arthroscopy 22(5):534-538, 2006.

3. Gebauer M, Beil FT, Beckmann J, et al: Mechanical evaluation of different techniques for Achilles tendon repair, Arch Orthop Trauma Surg 127(9):795-799, 2007.

4. Bradley JP, Tibone JE: Percutaneous and open surgical repairs of Achilles tendon ruptures: a comparative study, Am J Sports Med 18(2):188-195, 1990.

5. Aoki M, Ogiwara N, Ohta T, et al: Early active motion and weight bearing after cross-stitch Achilles tendon repair, Am J Sports Med 26(6):794-800, 1998.

6. Maestro Fernández A, Martínez Renobales J, Sánchez Zapirain I, et al: Open surgery with plasma rich in growth factors (PRGF) in acute ruptures of the Achilles tendon, Patologia del Aparato Locomotor 5(suppl 1):79-82, 2007.

7. Wapner KL, Pavlock GS, Hecht PJ, et al: Repair of chronic Achilles tendon rupture with flexor hallucis longus tendon transfer, Foot Ankle 14(8):443-449, 1993.

8. Mullaney M, McHugh MP, Tyler TF, et al: Weakness in end-range plantar flexion after Achilles tendon repair, Am J Sports Med 34(7):1120-1125, 2006.

9. Akizuki KH, Gartman, EJ, Nisonson B, et al: The relative stress on the Achilles tendon during ambulation in an ankle immobilizer: implications for rehabilitation after Achilles tendon repair, Br J Sports Med 35:329-334, 2001.

10. Bruggemann GP, Potthast W, Segesser B, et al: Achilles tendon strain distribution is related to foot and shank kinematics and muscle forces, J Biomech 40(suppl 2):S139, 2007.

11. Dombek MF, Lamm BM, Saltrick K, et al: Peroneal tendon tears: a retrospective review, J Foot Ankle Surg 42(5):250-258, 2003.

12. Sobel M, Geppert MJ, Olson EJ, et al: The dynamics of peroneus brevis tendon splits: a proposed mechanism,

13. Ogawa BK, Thordarson DB: Current concepts review: peroneal tendon subluxation and dislocation, Foot Ankle 28(9):1034-1040, 2007.

14. Gilula LA, Oloff L, Caputi R: Ankle tenography: a key to unexplained symptomatology. II. Diagnosis of chronic tendon disabilities, Radiology 151(3):581-587, 1984.

15. Sobel M, Geppert MJ, Warren RF: Chronic ankle instability as a cause of peroneal tendon injury, Clin Orthop Relat Res (296):187-191, 1993.

16. Nallamshetty L, Nazarian LN, Schweitzer ME, et al: Evaluation of posterior tibial pathology: comparison of sonography and MR imaging, Skeletal Radiol 34(7):375-380, 2005.

17. Wainwright AM, Kelly AJ, Glew D, et al: Classification and management of tibialis posterior tendon injuries according to magnetic resonance imaging findings, Foot Ankle 6(2):66-70, 1996.

18. Frey C, Shereff M, Greenidge N: Vascularity of the posterior tibial tendon, J Bone Joint Surg Am 72(6):884-888, 1990.

19. Feldman NJ, Oloff LM, Schulhofer SD: In situ tibialis posterior to flexor digitorum longus tendon transfer for tibialis posterior tendon dysfunction: a simplified surgical approach with outcome of 11 patients, J Foot Ankle Surg 40(1):2-7, 2001.

20. Ugolini PA, Raikin SM: The accessory navicular, Foot Ankle Clin 9(1):165-180, 2004.

21. Yun SC, Kyung TL, Heung SK, et al: MR imaging findings of painful type II accessory navicular bone: correlation with surgical and pathologic studies, Korean J Radiol 5(4):274-279, 2004.

22. Kopp FJ, Marcus RE: Clinical outcome of surgical treatment of the symptomatic accessory navicular, Foot Ankle Int 25(1):27-30, 2004.

23. Cheun JT, An KN, Zhang M: Consequences of partial and total plantar fascia release: a finite element study, Foot Ankle Int 27(2):125-132, 2006.

24. Brugh AM, Fallat LM, Savoy-Moore RT: Lateral column symptomatology following plantar fascial release: a prospective study, J Foot Ankle Surg 41(6):365-371, 2002.

25. Imhauser CW, Siegler S, Abidi NA, et al: The effect of posterior tibialis tendon dysfunction on the plantar pressure characteristics and the kinematics of the arch and forefoot, Clin Biomech 19:161-169, 2004.

26. Barrett SL, Day SV, Pignetti TT, et al: Endoscopic plantar fasciotomy: a multi-surgeon prospective analysis of 652 cases, J Foot Ankle Surg 34(4):400-406, 1995.

27. Cheung JT, An K, Zhang M, et al: Consequences of partial and total plantar fascia release: a finite element study, Foot Ankle Int 27(2):125-132, 2006.

28. Hinterman B: Tibialis posterior dysfunction: a review of the problem and personal experience, Foot Ankle Surg 3(3):61-70, 1997.

29. Dixon SJ, McNally K: Influence of orthotic devices prescribed using pressure data on lower extremity kinematics

and pressures beneath the shoe during running, Clin Biomech, 23(5):593-600, 2008.

30. Lui TH: Arthroscopy and endoscopy of the foot and ankle: indications for new techniques, Arthroscopy 23(8):889-902, 2007.

31. Ferkel RD, Heath DD, Guhl JF: Neurological complications of ankle arthroscopy, Arthroscopy 12(2):200-208, 1996.

32. Chuckpaiwong B, Berkson EM, Theodore GH: Microfracture for osteochondral lesions of the ankle: outcome analysis and outcome predictors of 105 cases, Arthroscopy 24(1):106-112, 2008.

33. Oloff LM, Bocko AP, Fanton G: Arthroscopic monopolar radio frequency thermal stabilization for chronic lateral ankle instability: a preliminary report on 10 cases, J Foot Ankle Surg 39(3):144-153, 2000.

34. Oloff LM, Schulhofer SD, Bocko AP: Subtalar joint arthroscopy for sinus tarsi syndrome: a review of 29 cases, J Foot Ankle Surg 40(3):152-157, 2001.

35. Frey C, Roberts NE: Sinus tarsi dysfunction: what is it and how is it treated? Sports Med Arthrosc 8(4):336-342, 2000.

36. Rush J: The pathology of bunions, Curr Orthop 12(4):258-261, 1998.

37. Easley ME, Trnka H: Current concepts review: hallux valgus. II. Operative treatment, Foot Ankle Int 28(6):748-758, 2007.

38. Haas Z, Hamilton G, Sundstrom D, et al: Maintenance of correction of first metatarsal closing base wedge osteotomies versus modified Lapidus arthrodesis for moderate to severe hallux valgus deformity, J Foot Ankle Surg 46(5):358-365, 2007.

39. Pinney S, Song K, Chou L: Surgical treatment of mild hallux valgus deformity: the state of practice among academic foot and ankle surgeons, Foot Ankle Int 27(11):970-973, 2006.

40. Salter RB, Simmonds DF, Malcolm BW, et al: The biological effect of continuous passive motion on the healing of full-thickness defects in articular cartilage: an experimental investigation in the rabbit, J Bone Joint Surg 62(8):1232-1251, 1980.

41. Saltrick KR: Lateral ankle stabilization, modified Lee and Chrisman-Snook, Clin Podiatr Med Surg 8(3):579-600, 1991.

42. Catanzariti AR, Mendicino RW: Tenodesis for chronic lateral ankle instability, Clin Podiatr Med Surg 18(3):429-442, 2001.

43. DiGiovanni CW, Brodsky A: Current concepts: lateral ankle instability, Foot Ankle Int 27(10):854-866, 2006.

44. Hyer CF, VanCourt R: Arthroscopic repair of lateral ankle instability by using the thermal-assisted capsular shift procedure: a review of 4 cases, J Foot Ankle Surg 43(2):104-109, 2004.

Mobilization of the Lower Extremity

The lower-extremity mobilization techniques described in this chapter are by no means all that exist. Rather, these are the techniques that the authors have found to be safe, easy to apply, and effective.

The reader is referred to Chapter 14 for a discussion of the definitions, indications, and contraindications of mobilization. In addition, Chapters 20 through 25 contain descriptions of anatomy, mechanics, pathologic condition, and evaluation of the lower-limb joints.

TECHNIQUES

For each technique illustrated, patient position, the therapist's hand contacts, and the direction of movement are described. Table 26-1 lists each technique along with the physiologic movement it theoretically enhances.

Hip

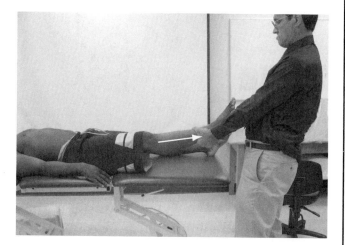

Figure 26-1 Long axis distraction. Patient position: Supine, leg extended. Contacts: Grasp the leg with both hands around the malleoli, elbows flexed; the leg is held in slight flexion and abduction. Direction of movement: The therapist leans backward and pulls along the long axis of the leg.

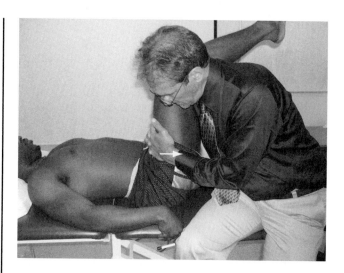

Figure 26-2 Distraction in flexion. Patient position: Supine, hip and knee flexed to 90 degrees. Contacts: The back of the knee rests on the therapist's shoulder; hands grasp the anterior aspect of the proximal thigh with fingers interlocked. Direction of movement: The femoral head is pulled inferiorly.

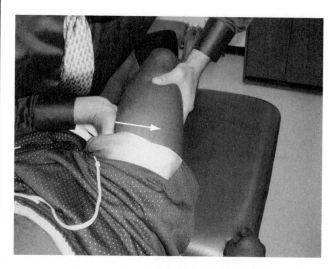

Figure 26-3 Lateral distraction. Patient position: Supine, leg extended. Contacts: One hand stabilizes the lateral aspect of the femur above the knee; the other hand contacts the first web space against the medial aspect of the proximal femur. Direction of movement: The femoral head is distracted laterally.

Table 26-1 Summary of Lower-Extremity Techniques

Joint	Mobilization Technique	Movement Promoted	Figure Number
Hip	Long-axis distraction	General	Figure 26-1
	Distraction in flexion	Flexion	Figure 26-2
	Lateral distraction	General	Figure 26-3
	Lateral distraction in flexion	Flexion	Figure 26-4
	Posterior capsule stretch	Flexion	Figure 26-5
	Anterior capsule stretch	Extension	Figure 26-6
	Medial capsule stretch	Abduction	Figure 26-7
Patellofemoral	Superior glide	Extension	Figure 26-8, *A*
	Interior glide	Flexion	Figure 26-8, *B*
	Lateromedial glide	General	Figure 26-9
Tibiofemoral	Anterior glide	Extension	Figure 26-10, Figure 26-11, Figure 26-14
	Posterior glide	Flexion	Figure 26-12, Figure 26-13, Figure 26-14
	Medial rotation	Medial rotation, flexion	Figure 26-15, *A* and *C*
	Lateral rotation	Lateral rotation, extension	Figure 26-15, *A* and *B*
	Distraction in flexion (prone)	General	Figure 26-17
	Distraction in flexion (sitting)	Flexion	Figure 26-16
	Distraction	Side lying	Figure 26-18
	Anteroposterior glides	General	Figure 26-19, *A* and *B*
Inferior tibiofibular	Tib-fib glide	Fibular movement, ankle plantar flexion and dorsiflexion	Figure 26-20, *A* and *B*
Ankle mortise	Distraction	General	Figure 26-21, Figure 26-22
		Anterior Glide *Posterior Glide*	**Plantar Flexion** *Dorsiflexion*
Subtalar	Distraction	General	Figure 26-28, Figure 26-29
	Distraction with calcaneal rocking	Inversion, eversion	Figure 26-30
Midtarsal	Talonavicular glide	Pronation, supination	Figure 26-31
	Calcaneocuboid glide	Pronation, supination	Figure 26-32, Figure 26-33
Intermetatarsal (anterior arch)	Glides	General	Figure 26-34
Metatarsophalangeal	Distraction	General	Figure 26-35
	Dorsal glide	Dorsiflexion	Figure 26-36
Plantar glide	Plantar flexion		Figure 26-36
	Mediolateral glide and tilt	General	Figure 26-37

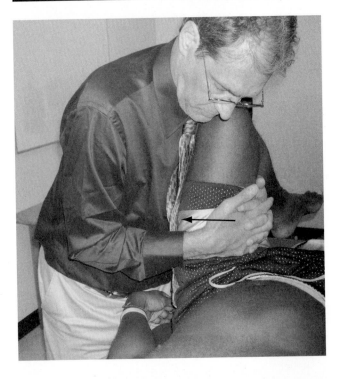

Figure 26-4 Lateral distraction in flexion. Patient position: Supine, hip and knee flexed to 90 degrees. Contacts: The back of the knee rests on the therapist's shoulder; hands grasp the medial aspect of the proximal thigh with fingers interlocked. Direction of movement: The femoral head is distracted laterally.

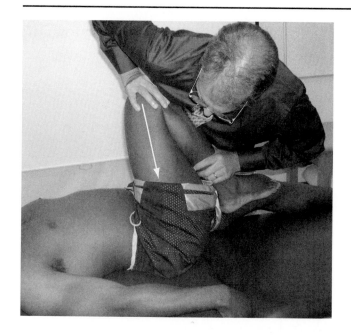

Figure 26-5 Posterior capsule stretch. Patient position: Supine, hip flexed to at least 100 degrees. Contacts: The medial aspect of the knee rests against the therapist's chest; hands grasp the distal femur and over the patella. Direction of movement: Push downward along the long axis of the femur posteriorly, inferiorly, and slightly laterally.

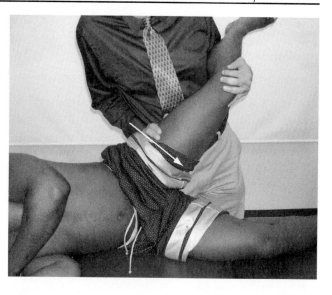

Figure 26-7 Medial capsule stretch. Patient position: Side lying, hip at end-range abduction. Contacts: One hand cradles the medial aspect of the knee to stabilize; the heel of the other hand contacts the lateral aspect of the hip at the greater trochanter. Direction of movement: Push the femoral head inferiorly.

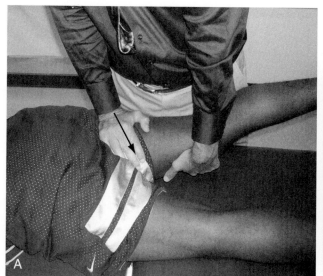
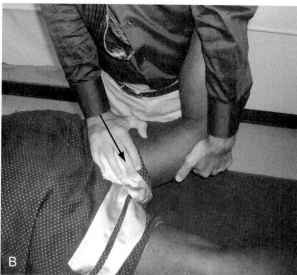

Figure 26-6 Anterior capsule stretch. Patient position: Prone, leg extended, small towel roll under the anterior superior iliac spine. Direction of movement: **A,** Simultaneously lift the knee while pushing the femoral head anteriorly; **B,** with the knee flexed, the same maneuver also stretches the rectus femoris.

Knee

Patellofemoral Joint

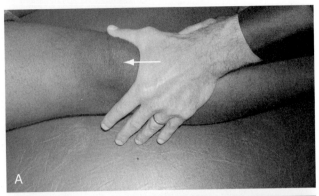

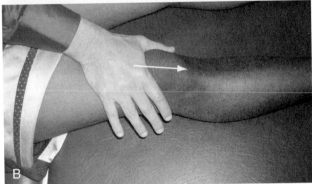

Figure 26-8 Superoinferior glide. Patient position: Supine. Contacts: Support the knee in slight flexion; contact the patella with the first web space at the base (superior) or the apex (inferior). Direction of movement: Glide **(A)** superiorly or **(B)** inferiorly.

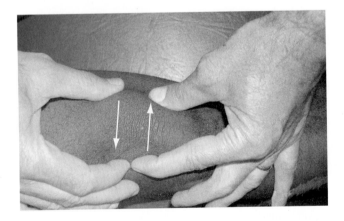

Figure 26-9 Medial or lateral glide. Patient position: Supine. Contacts: Use thumb tips and fingertips against the medial or lateral patellar borders. Direction of movement: Glide.

Tibiofemoral Joint

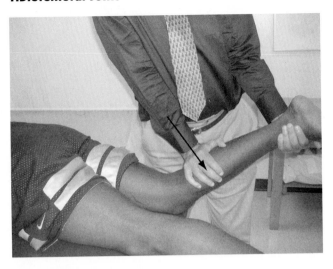

Figure 26-10 Anterior glide. Patient position: Prone, knee in approximately 45 degrees of flexion. Contacts: Stabilize with one distal lower leg proximal to ankle and contact with other hand the posterior aspect of the proximal lower leg. Direction of movement: Glide the tibia anteriorly.

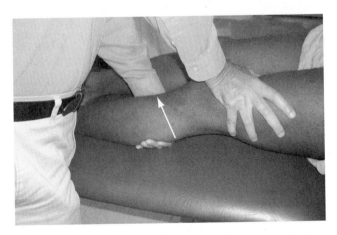

Figure 26-11 Anterior glide. Patient position: Supine, knee in slight flexion. Contacts: Stabilize the anterior aspect of the distal femur; grasp the posterior aspect of the proximal tibia. Direction of movement: Glide the tibia anteriorly on the femur.

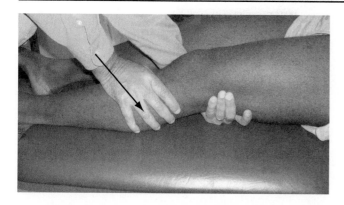

Figure 26-12 Posterior glide. Patient position: Supine, knee in slight flexion. Contacts: Stabilize the posterior aspect of the distal femur; grasp over the tibial tubercle. Direction of movement: Glide the tibia posteriorly.

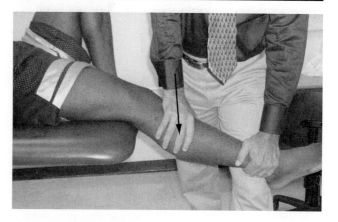

Figure 26-13 Posterior glide in flexion. Patient position: Supine, knee flexed to 45 degrees off the edge of the table. Contacts: Grasp the distal aspect of the tibia above the ankle and the other hand contacts the anterior surface and proximal aspect of the tibia. Direction of movement: Glide the tibia posteriorly.

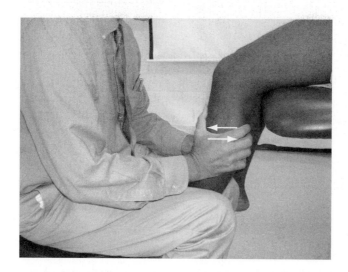

Figure 26-14 Anteroposterior glide. Patient position: Sitting, knee flexed to 90 degrees. Contacts: Grasp the proximal aspect of the tibia, thumbs anterior. Direction of movement: Glide the tibia anteriorly and posteriorly.

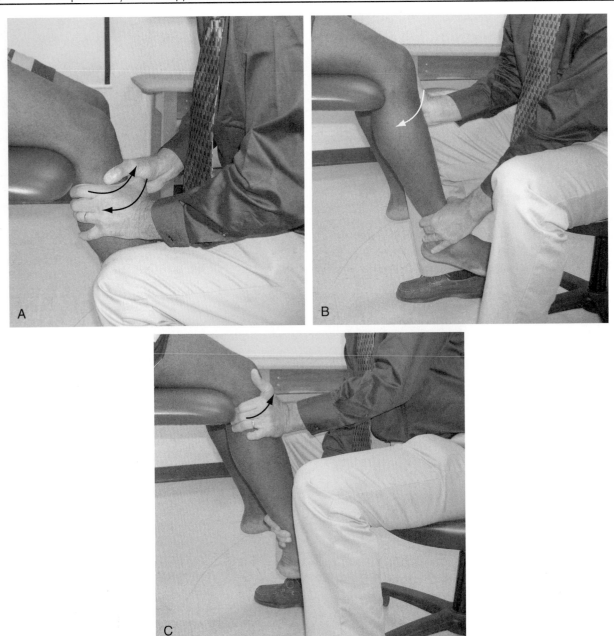

Figure 26-15 Mediolateral rotation. Patient position: Sitting, knee flexed to 90 degrees. Contacts: **A,** Grasp the proximal aspect of the tibia, thumbs anterior. Direction of movement: Medial and lateral rotation. **B,** Alternate contact with one hypothenar eminence of one hand on the lateral tibial tuberosity and the other hand grasping the distal tibia for lateral tibial rotation. **C,** Alternate contact with one hypothenar eminence of one hand on the medial tibial tuberosity and the other hand grasping the distal tibia for medial tibial rotation.

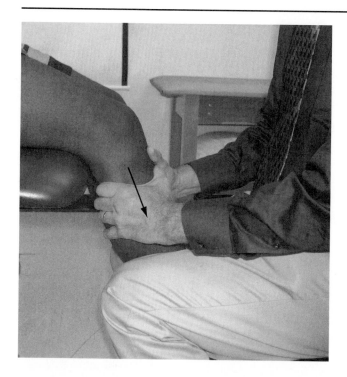

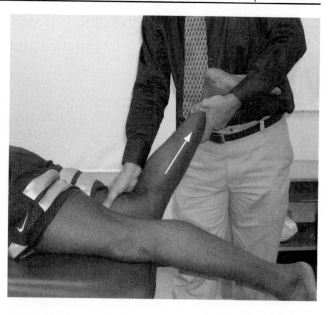

Figure 26-17 Distraction in flexion in prone. Patient position: Prone with knee flexed. Contacts: One hand stabilizes the distal femur, and the other hand grasps the distal tibia above the ankle. Direction of movement: Distract the lower leg along the long axis.

Figure 26-16 Distraction in flexion in sitting. Patient position: Sitting, knee flexed to 90 degrees. Contacts: Grasp the proximal aspect of the tibia, thumbs anterior. Direction of movement: Distract the lower leg downward; the therapist can assist distraction by holding the malleoli between the knees. Note: In this position, anteroposterior glides and rotations can also be applied while distracting.

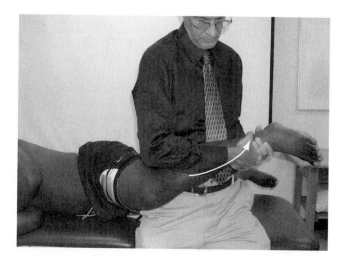

Figure 26-18 Distraction in flexion side lying. Patient position: Side lying with involved leg on superior. Contact. Patient wraps the knee around the examiner's body while the examiner grasps the lower leg with both hands above the ankle. Direction of movement: Examiner rotates the body away from the patient while holding contact, creating distraction in the tibiofemoral joint.

Superior Tibiofibular Joint

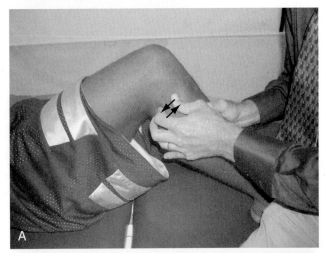

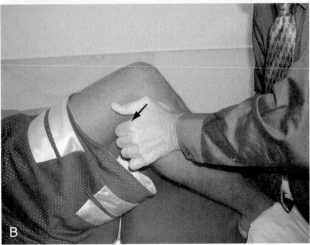

Figure 26-19 Anteroposterior glide. Patient position: Supine, knee flexed to 90 degrees. Contacts: Stabilize the medial aspect of the tibia; grasp the fibular head with the thumb and forefinger. Direction of movement: **A,** Glide the fibular head anteriorly and posteriorly. **B,** Same position as in **A,** except the hypothenar eminence is used to contact anteriorly and pads of fingers are used to contact posteriorly.

Foot and Ankle

Distal Tibiofibular Joint

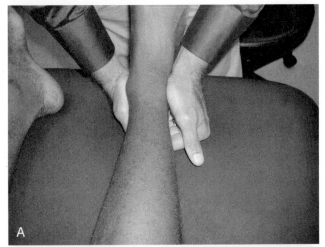

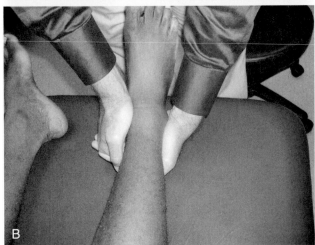

Figure 26-20 Fibular glides. Patient position: Supine. Contacts: Stabilize the medial malleolus against the carpal tunnel of the hand resting on the table; the carpal tunnel of the other hand contacts the anterior aspect of the lateral malleolus. Direction: **A,** Glide the fibula posteriorly on the tibia; **B,** reverse hand positions to glide the tibia posteriorly.

Talocrural (Mortise) Joint

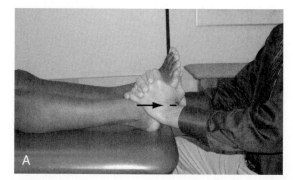

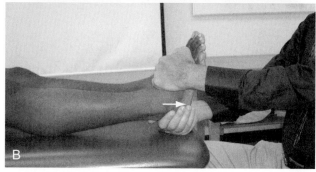

Figure 26-21 Distraction. Patient position: Supine. Contacts: **A,** Grasp the foot with the second, third, and fourth fingers of both hands interlocked over the dorsum, thumbs plantar, or **(B)** grasp with one hand dorsomedially while the other hand holds the calcaneus laterally. Direction of movement: Distract the talus from the mortise.

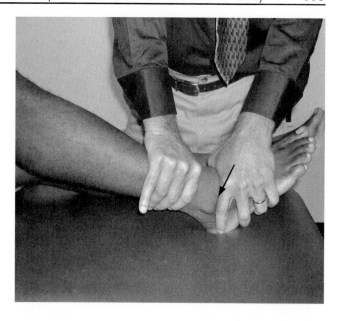

Figure 26-23 Posterior glide. Patient position: Supine, knee flexed, with the heel resting on the table. Contacts: Web contact along anterior surface of talus; the other hand grasps the anterior aspect of the lower leg above the malleoli. Direction of movement: Glide the talus posteriorly.

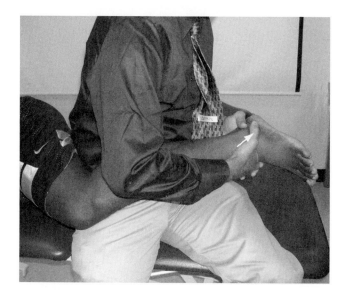

Figure 26-22 Distraction. Patient position: Side lying. Contacts: The posterior aspect of the femur is stabilized against the therapist's hip and iliac crest; the first web spaces grasp anterior and posterior to the talus. Direction of movement: Distract the talus from the mortise.

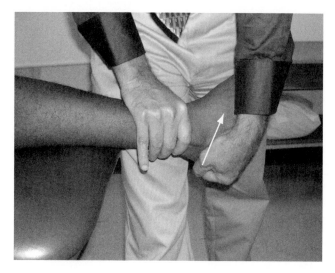

Figure 26-24 Anterior glide. Patient position: Supine, leg extended with the foot off the end of the table. Contacts: Stabilize the tibia and fibula by holding them against the table; the other hand cradles the calcaneus laterally. Direction of movement: Glide the calcaneus and talus upward (anteriorly).

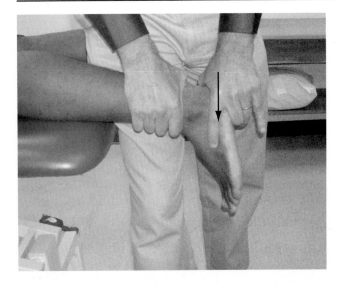

Figure 26-25 Anterior glide. Patient position: Prone, foot off the end of the table. Contacts: Stabilize the tibia and fibula by holding them against the table; the first web space of the other hand contacts the posterior aspect of the ankle. Direction of movement: Glide the calcaneus and talus downward (anteriorly) on the mortise.

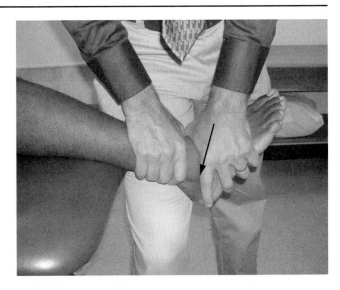

Figure 26-27 Posterior glide. Patient position: Supine, leg extended with the foot off the edge of the table. Contacts: Stabilize the tibia and fibula by holding them against the table; the other hand grasps the foot dorsolaterally, with the first web space against the anterior aspect of the talus.

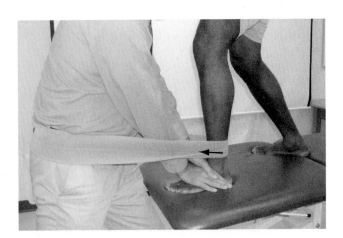

Figure 26-26 Mobilization with movement. Patient position: Standing with hip and knee flexed and involved foot resting on chair. Contacts: Stabilize anterior aspect of talus with both hands. Direction of movement: Place belt around posterior aspect of distal tibia and use trunk to provide a anterior glide of the tibia.

Subtalar joint

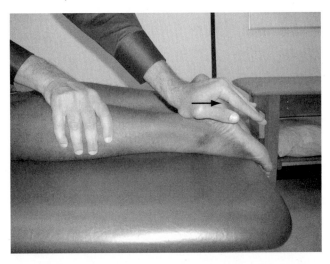

Figure 26-28 Distraction. Patient position: Prone, ankle plantar flexed, toes off the end of the table. Contacts: The therapist's carpal tunnel contacts the posterior aspect of the calcaneus near the insertion of the Achilles tendon. Direction of movement: Distract the calcaneus from the talus by pushing caudally.

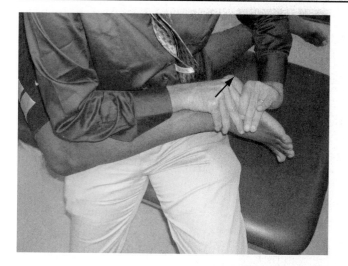

Figure 26-29 Distraction. Patient position: Side lying. Contacts: **A,** The posterior aspect of the femur is stabilized against the therapist's hip and iliac crest; **B,** first web spaces grasp the posterior and plantar aspects of the calcaneus. Direction of movement: Distract the calcaneus from the talus.

Talonavicular Joint (Medial Aspect of the Midtarsal Joint)

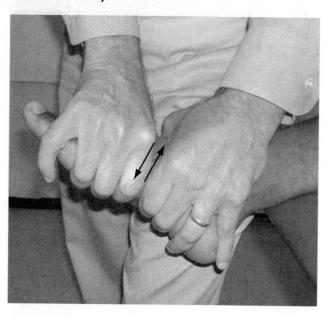

Figure 26-31 Talonavicular glide. Patient position: Supine. Contacts: With both hands on the medial aspect of the foot, stabilize the talus and grasp the navicular with the first web space. Direction of movement: Glide the navicular in dorsal and plantar directions.

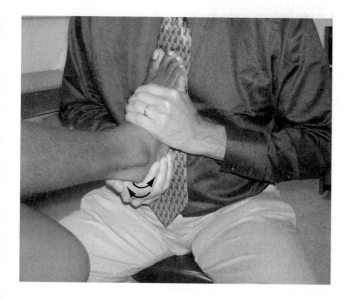

Figure 26-30 Distraction. Patient: Supine or sitting, foot off the end of the table. Contacts: Stabilize the foot by grasping it dorsomedially; the other hand grasps the calcaneus laterally. Direction of movement: Distract the calcaneus from the talus with inverting and everting (calcaneal rocking).

Calcaneocuboid Joint (Lateral Aspect of the Midtarsal Joint)

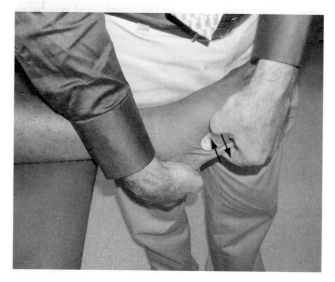

Figure 26-32 Calcaneocuboid glide. Patient position: Supine. Contacts: With both hands on the lateral aspect of the foot, stabilize under the calcaneus and contact cuboid with pad of thumb dorsally and fingers volarly. Direction of force: Dorsal and volar glides.

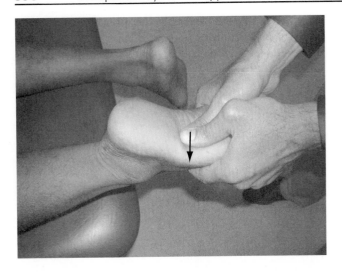

Figure 26-33 Cuboid whip.

First Metatarsophalangeal (MTP) joint

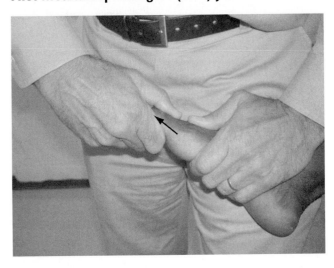

Figure 26-35 Distraction. Patient position: Supine. Contacts: Stabilize the first metatarsal head; the other hand grasps the proximal phalanx on its dorsal and plantar aspects. Direction of movement: Distract the phalanx from the metatarsal.

Intermetatarsal joints

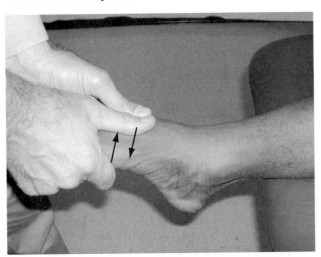

Figure 26-34 Intermetatarsal glides. Patient position: Supine. Contacts: With the thumbs and forefingers, grasp the first and second metatarsal heads; stabilize the second metatarsal head. Direction of movement: Glide the first metatarsal head in dorsal and plantar directions; repeat at the second, third, and fourth interspaces.

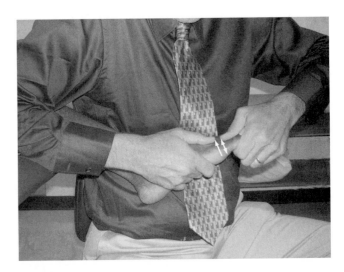

Figure 26-36 Dorsoplantar glides. Patient position: Supine. Contacts: Stabilize the first metatarsal head; the other hand grasps the dorsal and plantar aspects of the proximal phalanx. Direction of movement: Glide the phalanx in dorsal and plantar directions.

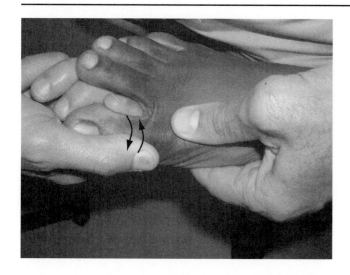

Figure 26-37 Rotation. Patient position: Supine. Contacts: Stabilize the first metatarsal head; the other hand grasps the medial and lateral aspects of the proximal phalanx. Direction of movement: Rotate the phalanx medially and laterally.

ACKNOWLEDGEMENTS

We thank Robert Metzger Jr., a Doctor of Physical Therapy student in the Division of Physical Therapy for serving as the model for this chapter.

SUGGESTED READINGS

Basmajian JV, MacConail C: Arthrology. In Warwick R, Williams P, editors: Gray's anatomy, ed 35, Philadelphia, 1973, WB Saunders.

Brooks-Scott J: Handbook of mobilization in the management of children with neurological disorders, London, 1998, Butterworth-Heinemann.

Butler D: Mobilization of the nervous system, Melbourne, 1991, Churchill Livingstone.

Corrigan B, Maitland GD: Practical orthopaedic medicine, London, 1985, Butterworths.

Cyriax J: Textbook of orthopaedic medicine, vol 1. Diagnosis of soft tissue lesions, London, 1978, Balliere Tindall.

Cyriax J, Cyriax P: Illustrated manual of orthopaedic medicine, London, 1983, Butterworths.

D'Ambrogio KJ, Roth GB: Positional release therapy: assessment and treatment of musculoskeletal dysfunction, St Louis, 1997, Mosby.

Donatelli RA, editor: Physical therapy of the shoulder, ed 3, Melbourne, 1986, Churchill Livingstone.

Glasgow EF, Twomey L, editors: Aspects of manipulative therapy, Melbourne, 1986, Churchill Livingstone.

Hoppenfeld S: Physical examination of the spine and extremities, East Norwalk, Conn, 1976, Appleton-Century-Crofts.

Konin JG, Wiksten DL, Isear JA: Special tests for orthopaedic examination, Thorofare, NJ, 1997, Slack Inc.

Loudon J, Bell S, Johnston J: The clinical orthopedic assessment guide, Champaign, Ill, 1998, Human Kinetics.

Magee DJ: Orthopedic physical assessment, Philadelphia, 1987, WB Saunders.

Maitland GD: Peripheral manipulation, London, 1978, Butterworths.

Mennell JM: Joint pain: diagnosis and treatment using manipulative techniques, Boston, 1964, Little, Brown.

CHAPTER

27

Gregory S. Johnson

Soft Tissue Mobilization

Manual treatment of the soft tissues has existed since the beginning of recorded history in the form of massage and manipulation.[1] The primary purpose of these approaches was apparently to treat symptomatic soft tissues. The functional orthopaedics approach to soft tissue mobilization (STM) has been developed not only to evaluate and treat soft tissue dysfunctions that precipitate myofascial pain but also to evaluate and treat those dysfunctions that alter structure and function and produce mechanical strains on symptomatic structures.[2] In addition, STM offers a functional approach for evaluating and improving the patient's capacity to achieve and maintain a balanced posture, which enhances the ability to learn and perform efficient body mechanics. This approach is integrated into a broader treatment strategy of joint mobilization and neuromuscular reeducation and is coupled with a specific training, conditioning, and flexibility program.

STM is intended to be used as a component of a complete manual therapy program that includes evaluation and treatment of articular, neurovascular, and neuromuscular dysfunctions. The approach encompasses evaluation of the soft tissue system and application of specifically directed manual therapy techniques to facilitate normalization of soft tissue dysfunctions.[2,3] This integrated treatment approach has been termed *functional mobilization*.[4]

This chapter defines STM and describes its contribution to the conservative care of musculoskeletal dysfunction. This is achieved by (1) defining the relevant soft tissue structures; (2) outlining a specific system of subjective, objective, and palpatory evaluations; (3) presenting basic treatment techniques; and (4) providing clinical correlations and case studies to develop an anatomic, biomechanical, and conceptual rationale for the use of STM.

SOFT TISSUE COMPONENTS

The four primary soft tissues of the body are epithelial, muscular, nervous, and connective.[5,6] All soft tissue structures have individual and unique functions, integrated into a dynamic biomechanical unit.[7,8] Grieve[7] emphasized this by stating that "the nerve, connective tissue, muscle, and articular complex produces multiple and varied arthrokinetic systems, which are functionally interdependent upon each other."

Many authorities have stated that dysfunctions of the soft tissue system play a primary role in the onset and perpetuation of musculoskeletal symptoms.[7,9-13] Grieve[7] stated the following: "An explanation of the incidence of vertebral joint syndromes, and of some unsatisfactory long-term therapeutic results, might be assisted by regarding joint problems in a wider context than that of the joint alone. Much abnormality presenting, apparently simply, as joint pain may be the expression of a comprehensive underlying imbalance of the whole musculoskeletal system, i.e., articulation, ligaments, muscles, fascial planes and intermuscular septa, tendons and aponeuroses ..."

The human system can develop to be efficient, strong, and flexible by responding appropriately to the various types of controlled physical, mental, and emotional stress.[14-16] When the system is unable to adapt appropriately, physical compensations occur (Figure 27-1).

The most common factor that precipitates soft tissue pain and functional impairment is trauma.[17,18] Trauma, whether from a significant external force or from repetitive internal or external microtraumas, can produce long-standing soft tissue changes (Box 27-1).[19,20] These soft tissue dysfunctions may be the primary source of symptoms or the secondary source through impeded structural and functional capacity.

All injuries, regardless of site, have a basic inflammation cascade. Inflammation has three distinct phases: (1) acute, (2) granulation, and (3) remodeling. The first phase, acute, occurs 0 to 4 days after injury. The ruptured cell releases debris and chemicals (prostaglandins) into the plasma, which attract leukocytes. The white blood cells clean out the bacteria and prevent infection. Prostaglandins are released from the injured cell, causing pain.[21]

The granulation phase is marked with the arrival of macrophages. Macrophages digest the cellular debris and secrete enzymes to aid the breakdown of ligament molecules. Macro-

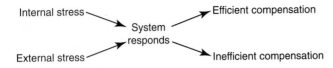

Figure 27-1 Internal and external stresses that affected the health of the system.

BOX 27-1 Macrotraumas and Microtraumas

External Macrotraumas	Internal or External Microtraumas
Blows	Faulty posture
Falls	Improper neuromuscular
Improper heavy lifting	mechanisms
Surgery	Poor body mechanics
Whiplash	Muscular imbalance
	Improper foot wear
	Repetitive stressful activities
	Poorly organized work surfaces
	Nonsupportive sitting and
	sleeping surfaces
	Chronic anxiety or depression
	Overweight

---

phages release growth factors, which stimulate the regeneration of blood vessels, intercellular matrix, and fibroblasts. Fibroblasts repair ligamentous cells. The combination new blood vessels and fibroblasts cause the fullness that can be felt at the injury site. Fibroblasts make massive amounts of collagen at the fibro-osseus junction—the site of ligament attachment to the bone.

During the third phase of healing, remodeling, the new collagen will be organized into a new ligament. The fibroblasts make single long molecules, which will begin to entwine to form a triple helix—a collagen fiber. The collagen fibers begin to contract, and the molecules become tighter and shorter. The collagen loses water with noted decreased laxity. The third phase lasts for weeks. Each phase is dependent on the previous phase for initiation of the next phases.[22] Occasionally, changes occur in the organization of collagen irregularities.[23]

Structurally, a balanced posture is no longer available because of the lack of flexibility of the soft tissue structures. This affects the efficient distribution of weight into the base of support and alters articular range of motion. These changes in soft tissue extensibility and mobility can cause abnormal forces and compressions to articular structures and can be a factor in precipitating and perpetuating pathologic and symptomatologic conditions.[7,9,11,24,25]

Soft tissue dysfunctions can be specifically identified through an organized and precise subjective, objective, and palpatory evaluation. The therapist should have a working knowledge of the body's normal functional anatomy, biomechanical function, and neuromuscular control to conduct and interpret this evaluation and to provide effective treatment. An understanding of soft tissue pathokinetic mechanisms is essential to correlate the objective findings with possible soft tissue dysfunction. STM primarily addresses the evaluation and treatment of four soft tissue structures: (1) irregular and regular connective tissues, (2) skin, (3) skeletal muscle, and (4) neurovascular components.[5,26-28] For an in-depth description of the connective-tissue structures, see Chapter 1.

CONNECTIVE-TISSUE STRUCTURES

The primary connective-tissue structures evaluated and treated by STM are the regular or dense tissues such as tendons and ligaments and the irregular or loose tissues such as fascia, intrinsic elements of muscle, articular capsules, and aponeuroses.

Fascia

All connective tissue is made up of fibers, proteoglycans, and glycoproteins. The fiber component, produced by fibroblasts, consists of collagen and elastin. Proteoglycans are core proteins with sulfated glycosaminoglycan (GAG) side chains. The GAG attachments absorb water to provide hydration of the extracellular matrix. Glycoproteins stabilize matrix of connective tissue and regulate cell functions and cell connection to the maxtrix.[29]

The delicate balance of each component within it determines the properties of connective tissue. Both collagen and elastin resist tensile loads. Proteoglycans and GAGs provide hydration within the matrix and resist compressive loads. Recent studies have shown that fibroblasts may also have the gene that can express contractile elements in fibers.[30] Imbalances of the connective-tissue matrix caused by disease and trauma can lead to regions of decreased mobility or restriction.

The fascial system is one of the primary soft tissues treated by STM. The fascial system ensheathes and permeates all tissues and structures; supplies the mechanical supportive framework that holds and integrates the body together and gives it form; provides passive support during lifting activities;[31] provides for the space and lubrication between all bodily structures; and creates pathways for nerves, blood, and lymphatic vessels.

Hollingshead[8] states the following: "If it were possible to dissolve out all the tissues of the body so as to leave only the fibrous (irregular) connective tissues, the essential organization of the body would still be represented and recognizable."

The fascial system is composed of laminated sheathes of connective tissues of varying thickness and density. These sheathes extend from the periosteum of bone to the basement membrane of the dermis. They are continuous throughout the body and are interconnected with the connective-tissue structures of muscle (intrinsic elements, tendons, and aponeuroses), the articular structures (ligaments and capsules), and the intrinsic elements of peripheral nerves (endoneurium, perineurium, and epineurium).[5,6,8,26] This ensheathing organization of fascia allows structures to have independent three-dimensional (3-D) mobility while connecting the system together into an integrated functional unit.[5,17]

Any system designed for function must have interfaces that allow motion. For the skeletal structures, these interfaces are termed *joints,* whereas in the soft tissue system these interfaces are termed *functional joints.*

Functional Joint Concept

Gratz[32] defined the normal spaces that are maintained between all structures by fascia as *functional joints.* He defined a functional joint as "a space built for motion." Each functional joint creates a mechanical interface that allows the adjoining structures to make 3-D movements in relation to each other.[2,13,17,32] In myofascial structures, the functional joints maintained by facial tissues include the spaces between individual muscle fibers on the micro level, as well as the spaces that exist between a muscle and the surrounding structures. All these spaces are maintained and lubricated by the amorphous ground substance. The amorphous ground substance is a viscous gel containing a high proportion of water (60% to 70%) and long chains of carbohydrate molecules called *mucopolysaccharides,* principally GAGs.[6,26,33]

In an optimal state, the 3-D mobility that exists at functional joints is termed *normal play.*[2,33,34] The degree of normal play varies according to the functional demands and requirements of the individual structures and their mechanical interface. When the normal extensibility, accessory mobility, and biomechanical function of the tissues and surrounding structures are restricted, this dysfunctional state is called *restricted* or *decreased play.* These dysfunctions are clinically identifiable through skilled palpation, range-of-motion testing, and observable alteration in function.[2,34]

Mennell[35] stated the following: "It is very remarkable how widespread may be the symptoms caused by unduly taut fascial planes. Though it is true that the fascial bands play a principal part in the mobility of the human body, they are often conducive to binding between two joint surfaces."

DYSFUNCTIONAL FACTORS

No exact scientific explanation exists for restricted play and decreased extensibility of tissues, and further research is needed to provide more in-depth physiologic understanding. However, some possible physiologic explanations include the following.

Scar Tissue Adhesions

After an injury, laceration, or surgery, fibroblastic activity forms new connective-tissue fibers to reunite the wound as part of the postinflammatory fibroplastic phase.[36,37] These fibers are formed through random fibroblastic activity. If the appropriate remodeling stimuli are not applied during the healing process, then the scar will become inextensible, with poor functional capacity.[10,14,38-41] Localized adhesions are generally produced as scar tissue forms.[10] In addition, often a restrictive matrix exists that has spiderweb-like tentacles attached to surrounding structures that can alter and limit their normal mobility.[42,43] For example, the restrictive matrix of the scar tissue that is

formed after abdominal surgery can often be palpated in other regions of the abdominal cavity.

Hollingshead[8] states that scar tissue "may be a major factor in altering the biomechanics of the whole kinematic chain, placing strain on all related structures." The abnormal strain caused by adherent and inextensible scar tissue may contribute to a chronic inflammatory process and further perpetuate symptoms.[10,42,44] The scar tissue matrix may also compromise neurovascular and lymphatic structures affecting the nerve conduction, the fluid balance, the exchange of metabolites, and the removal of waste products from the region.

Lymphatic Stasis and Interstitial Swelling

An increase in interstitial fluids alters the mechanical behavior of the adjacent structures and restricts normal mobility of the functional joints. This fluid imbalance may be related to immobility, poor lymphatic drainage, scar tissue blockage, or inflammation.[45,46]

Ground Substance Dehydration and Intermolecular Cross-Linking

Research has been conducted to determine the effects of forced immobilization on the periarticular tissues of various mammalian populations. This research has revealed that such immobilization contributes to soft tissue changes and development of restricted mobility of joints.[47-50] Researchers have identified biochemical and biomechanical compensations within the ligaments, tendons, capsule, and fascia of these restricted regions.[33,51] A primary component of these dysfunctions is ground substance dehydration.[33,47,48,52-54] Two results of this dehydration are (1) thixotropy and (2) loss of critical fiber distance.

Thixotropy is a state in which the ground substance becomes more viscous, resulting in increased tissue rigidity and stiffness. This increased viscosity of the ground substance requires more force to elongate and compress the tissues.[11,54]

With the loss of water from the ground substance, the critical distance that is required between fibers and structures is diminished. In this state a higher potential exists for and a significant increase in formation of restrictive intermolecular cross-link fibers (Figure 27-2).[40,47-49,54] These intermolecular cross-links restrict interfiber mobility and extensibility, and may be partially responsible for restricted soft tissue mobility and play. Furthermore, it has been shown that this reduced mobility affects the synthesis and orientation of new collagen fibrils, which further contributes to the pathogenesis of restricted fascial mobility.[54] (See Chapter 1 for a description of the effects of immobilization on connective tissue for biomechanical changes and intermolecular cross-linking.)

RESPONSE TO TREATMENT

It is reasonable to postulate a correlation between these research findings and the clinically identifiable decreased mobility and

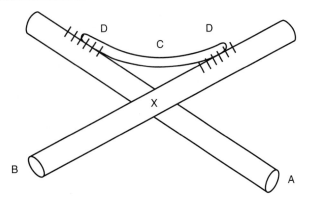

Figure 27-2 Idealized model of a collagen cross-link at the molecular level. **A-B,** Preexisting fibers; **C,** newly synthesized fibril; **D,** cross-link as the fibril joins the fiber; *(X)* nodal point where the fibers normally slide freely past one another. (From Akeson WH, Amiel D, Woo S: Immobility effects on synovial joint: the pathomechanics of joint contracture, Biorheology 17:95, 1980.)

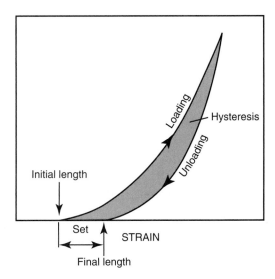

Figure 27-3 Hysteresis. When unloaded, a structure regains its shape at a rate different from that at which it deformed. Any difference between the initial and final shapes is the "set." (From Bogduk N, Twomey LT: Clinical anatomy of the lumbar spine, New York, 1987, Churchill Livingstone.)

play found in dysfunctional soft tissues. Clinically, through the application of STM, the mobility of these dysfunctional soft tissues can be improved. These results may be a result of one or more of the following factors: [55-58]

1. An alteration of the scar tissue matrix[42,50]
2. A redistribution of interstitial fluids[7]
3. The stimulation of GAG synthesis, restoring normal or improved lubrication and hydration
4. The breaking of restrictive intermolecular cross-links[43,54]
5. The mechanical and viscoelastic elongation of existing collagenous tissues through the phenomena of creep and hysteresis, as demonstrated by the stress-strain curve (Figure 27-3)[59-61]
6. A neuroreflexive response that may alter vascular, muscular, and biochemical factors related to immobility[62-66]

SKIN

The skin is composed of two layers: (1) an outer epidermis of ectodermal origin and (2) the deeper dermis of mesodermal origin.[67] The skin is continuous with the deep fascia and underlying structures through the attachment of the superficial fascia to the basement membrane of the dermis.[6] Because of the orientation and weave of the collagen and elastin fibers, the skin demonstrates considerable mechanical strength and a high degree of intrinsic flexibility and mobility. This intrinsic mobility allows the skin to have considerable extensibility and, because of its elastin content, the ability to recoil to its original configuration.[40,59] Because of the pliability of the superficial fascia, the skin also has extensive extrinsic mobility in all directions along the interface with deeper structures.[8,26] The skin in regions superficial to joints allows motion through its ability to fold and stretch in response to the underlying movements.[10,40]

The skin can lose normal mobility secondary to trauma, scar tissue formation, and immobility. With the loss of this mobil-

ity, the underlying structures can be impeded in their functional capacity, and the normal coordinated movement patterns of the kinetic chain can be altered.

Response to Treatment

Dysfunctions of the intrinsic and extrinsic mobility of the skin can be assessed and specific foci of restrictions identified. The mobility of these dysfunctions can be improved through the application of specific soft tissue techniques. These structural improvements are often clinically associated with dramatic reduction in pain and improved musculoskeletal function. These improvements may be related to the following possibilities:

1. More efficient biomechanical function because of release of fascial tension
2. Local and general changes in the vascular and lymphatic circulation[45,64]
3. A neuroreflexive inhibition of muscle tone and pain (This may be a response to the existing pathologic condition in deeper structures,[63,64] including that of underlying spinal dysfunctions.[7,68,69] These are passed through both afferent and autonomic pathways.[70])

SKELETAL MUSCLE

The two basic components of skeletal muscle are (1) the muscle fibers (the contractile components) and (2) the surrounding connective-tissue sheaths (the noncontractile components). The connective-tissue components are the endomysium, perimysium, and epimysium (Figure 27-4). They envelop each muscle fiber, fascicle, and muscle belly, respectively, and invest at the

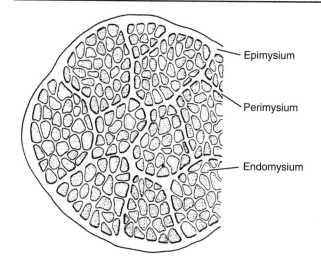

Figure 27-4 Connective-tissue components of muscle. (From Ham A, Cormack D: Histology, ed 8, Philadelphia, 1979, Lippincott Williams & Wilkins.)

muscle's terminus to form tendon, fascia, and aponeurosis.[6,26] These connective tissues provide for the following:

1. The mechanical and elastic characteristics of muscle for broadening during contraction and lengthening during passive elongation (functional excursion)[42,71] (They may be the major component affected by passive muscle stretching.[72])
2. The elastic property of muscle, possibly because of the parallel arrangement of these sheaths with the contractile components[73]
3. The tension regulation of the muscle, which influences contractile strength,[72] ability to withstand high-impact loads, and adaptive and recoil capability[74]
4. The support, cohesion, and protective restraint of the muscle[75]
5. The space and lubrication for normal extensibility and play of (a) the intrinsic contractile elements and (b) the muscle belly (through the epimysium) in relation to surrounding structures[8,10]
6. A soft tissue continuum (the myofascial unit) as they interconnect with each other, as well as the loose connective tissue and fascia surrounding the muscle through the superficial epimysium[13]
7. A conduit for blood vessels and nerve fibers (see Chapter 1)[6,26]

DYSFUNCTIONS OF THE MYOFASCIAL UNIT

Several authors believe that the myofascial unit is often the primary precipitator of pathologic conditions and symptoms.[9,12,76,77] The primary structural and functional dysfunctions of the myofascial unit include the following:
- Restrictive scar tissue[18]
- Restricted muscle play[78]
- Weakness or increased tone through impaired peripheral and central innervation

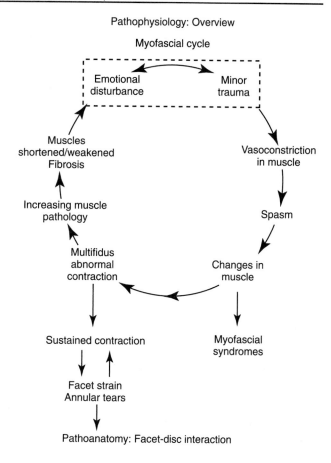

Figure 27-5 Myofascial cycle. (From Kirkaldy-Willis WH: Managing low lack pain, ed 3, New York, 1992, Churchill Livingstone.)

- Restricted extensibility and play of the connective-tissue elements (fibrosis)
- Adaptive muscle shortening, possibly through the loss of sarcomeres[10,13,46,79,80]
- Injury of the musculotendinous structures[72]
- Generalized hypertonus[1] and localized myofascial trigger points[12]
- Alteration in motor control and recruitment[9,81-83]

Myofascial Cycle

Dysfunctions of the myofascial cycle can be attributed to a variety of factors. Kirkaldy-Willis[9] has proposed a model for the evolution of spinal pathologic condition termed the *myofascial cycle*. This model presents possible courses of degeneration termed the *degenerative cascade,* which leads to spinal pathologic and symptomatologic conditions (Figure 27-5). This cycle begins with a minor trauma or emotional disturbance that facilitates a chronic neuromuscular response. This response facilitates chronic muscular changes such as fibrosis, weakness, limited extensibility, and altered recruitment patterns. Specifically, when the multifidi become dysfunctional, significant alteration of the arthrokinematic movements of the spinal segment occurs, leading to possible facet and disk deterioration.[84] Grieve,[7] in discussing tone, which Kirkaldy-Willis[9] refers to as the *chronic neuromuscular response,* states that tone in striated muscle is due to three sets of influences:

- The elastic tension of the connective-tissue elements
- The degree or extent of interdigitation overlap of the actin and myosin elements
- The number of active motor units

Myofascial Trigger Points

The number of active motor units can be influenced by multiple factors, such as trauma,[7,13] scarring from disease or injury,[13] supraspinal influences,[7] protective spasm, chronic reaction to situational stress, and repetitive habitual holding and movement patterns.[2,85] In a pathologic state, these foci of increased tone have been termed *myofascial trigger points* by Travell and Simons.[12]

Myofascial trigger points are defined as "hyperirritable spots, usually within a taut band of skeletal muscle or in the muscle's fascia, that are painful on compression and that can give rise to characteristic referred pain, tenderness, and autonomic phenomena."[12] Travell and Simons report that the palpable hardness identified with myofascial trigger points may be caused by increased fibrous connective tissue, edema, altered viscosity of muscle, ground substance infiltrate, contracture of muscle fibers, vascular engorgement, and fatty infiltration.[12] Within the STM system, myofascial trigger points are included in the category of specific or general muscle hypertonus.

A state of increased tone may be the primary source of symptoms[12] or a secondary one through a reflex response to underlying or related pathologic condition. In addition to local and referred pain, increased muscle tonus and myofascial trigger points may also precipitate altered movement patterns[86] and restricted range of motion.[9,12,42,81] Because of the individual variability of response to pain and the possibility that referred pain or protective spasm may be caused by the hypertonic state, the location of muscle tone or tenderness is often not a reliable indicator of the location of the source of pathologic condition.[7] Both muscular hypertonus and myofascial trigger points usually normalize in response to a treatment program of STM. However, if the hypertonus or trigger points are in protective or secondary spasm because of a primary dysfunction elsewhere, then the objective signs and symptoms often return, partially or completely, within a short period of time.[2]

NEUROMUSCULAR CONTROL

Another factor that must be taken into consideration when addressing the myofascial system is neuromuscular control. The movement control of the neuromuscular system must be precise and allow for few deviations to protect the articular and soft tissue structures.[17,76,87] Many authors report that dysfunctions of the myofascial unit are often preceded by faulty posture, poor neuromuscular control, and altered recruitment patterns.*

---

*References 17, 76, 82, 83, 88, 89.

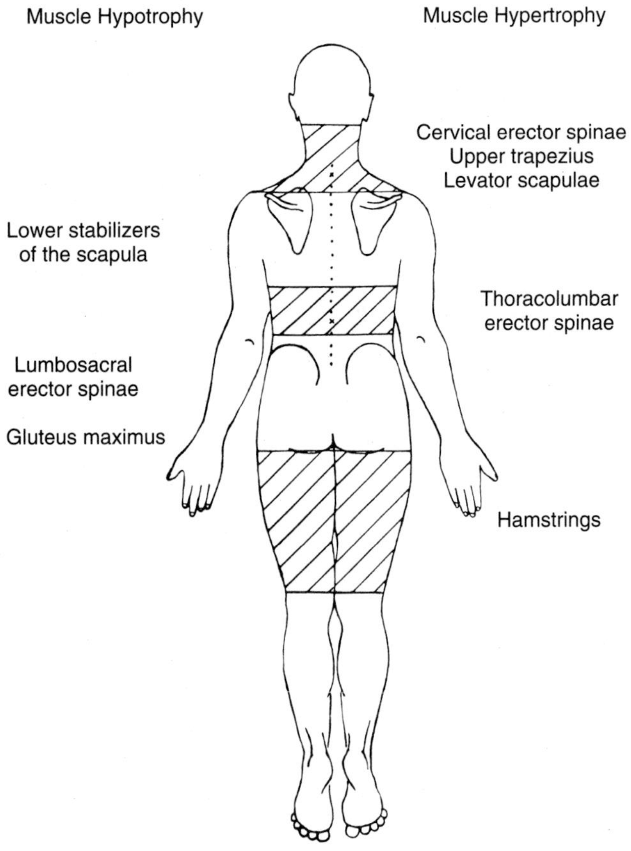

Figure 27-6 The layer syndrome. (From Jull G, Janda V: Muscles and motor control in low back pain: assessment and management. In Twomey LT, Taylor JR, editors: Physical therapy of the low back, New York, 1987, Churchill Livingstone, p 253.)

These conditions often lead to length-associated muscle imbalances between antagonistic muscle groups and affect the balanced force production, coordination, fine motor control, and distribution of forces necessary to protect the spinal segment during movement and static postures.[7,17,76]

For efficient neuromusculoskeletal function to occur, normal joint and soft tissue mechanics must be present. Normal voluntary and involuntary neuromuscular control is developed primarily through learned activities. Various factors may precipitate a state of altered recruitment patterns.[17,76] Janda[76] has observed that consistent neuromuscular patterns occur when altered recruitment exists. Muscles composed primarily of tonic (slow twitch) fibers become chronically facilitated and respond to stressful situations and pain by increased tone and tightness. Those that are primarily composed of phasic (fast twitch) fibers are inhibited, becoming weak, atrophied, and overstretched, thus creating length-associated muscle imbalances (Figures 27-6 and 27-7).[76,86]

Recent research[90,91] has confirmed the long-held proprioceptive neuromuscular facilitation (PNF) concept regarding the importance of the multifidus in stabilization of individual spinal segments and in controlling motion between those segments. In conjunction with the multifidus, researchers have

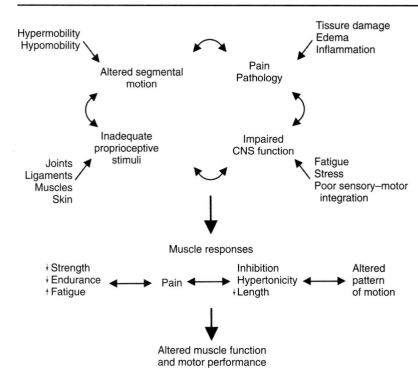

Figure 27-7 Sources of adverse stimuli and muscular responses. (From Jull G, Janda V: Muscles and motor control in low back pain: assessment and management. In Twomey LT, Taylor JR, editors: Physical therapy of the low back, New York, 1987, Churchill Livingstone.)

found that the transversus abdominis contracted before the other abdominal muscles and in conjunction with the multifidus to produce stability.[92-94] Other researchers have also found that the multifidus is inhibited in individuals with low-back pain.[95-98] Even in individuals with first-time acute episodes, the multifidi will frequently be inhibited and will not demonstrate the normal recruitment patterns. Research has found that the multifidus does not recover normal function after the episode has resolved. Therefore through the functional mobilization approach to rehabilitation, the following treatment strategy would be followed. Initially, manual therapy would be applied to normalize the condition of the myofascial and articular structures. Then specific training would be used to facilitate contractions of the deep stabilizing muscles (multifidus, transverse abdominis, deep fibers of the psoas and quadratus lumborum) through PNF trunk patterns and functional movement patterns (described later). Specific body mechanic training to use proper biomechanics and motor sequencing would follow this. An important aspect of the functional manual therapy approach is the facilitation of the core muscles' "tonic fibers." This is accomplished through the use of prolonged holds.

An example of an altered recruitment pattern is excessive activation and tightness of the trunk extensors during a poorly performed sit-up. In an individual who exhibits such an altered movement pattern, one can palpate the extensors while the sit-up is being performed and note substantial activation. This unnecessary activation of the extensors creates a state of neuromuscular imbalance that decreases the facilitation of the lower abdominals. This motor recruitment dysfunction is carried over to the performance of daily activities and alters the normal neuromuscular, postural, and mechanical dynamics of the lumbar spine. The treatment strategy for this condition would include STM and elongation of the shortened extensors,[2,11,76,86] strengthening of the weakened flexors,[11,79,98] neuromuscular reeducation to restore proper movement and recruitment patterns,[17,82,83,88,99] and body mechanics training to change stressful activities of daily living (ADL) patterns.[98]

Patients who are forced into inefficient postures because of soft tissue dysfunctions often have difficulty performing dynamic, coordinated, and balanced motions while simultaneously maintaining trunk stability and controlled mobility. STM directed toward improving posture often elicits an almost immediate improvement in neuromuscular control, recruitment patterns, and stabilization abilities.[2,98]

ABILITIES

Neurovascular Components

The connective-tissue components of the central nervous system (CNS) are the meninges and in the peripheral nervous system the mesoneurium, epineurium, perineurium and endoneurium. The vascular elements include the heart, arteries, and veins. It is important to understand that these neurovascular components have a mechanical interface with connective tissue, skin, and skeletal muscle. Often times these interfaces can have adherences that contribute to one having restricted range of motion, altered movement patterns, pain, adverse neural tension (discussed later), and impaired function. Through STM these adherences can be treated to restore the mobility of the neurovascular structures.[100]

Evaluation

A specific, organized evaluation system is an integral part of a rehabilitation and manual therapy program. The subjective and objective evaluation process is systematic and specific, providing baseline data from which to develop and perform a treatment program and to assess the effectiveness of treatment. The following components of evaluation can assist the therapist in identifying musculoskeletal dysfunction and determining the vigor of the treatment process:

- Patient's subjective report
- Structural analysis
- Motion analysis
- Palpation

Subjective Evaluation

Through a careful subjective evaluation, a therapist can identify many of the factors that cause and precipitate musculoskeletal symptoms. The subjective evaluation is the critical link between the patient's symptomatic and historical report and the objective findings. Cyriax and Cyriax[101] stated that most soft tissue dysfunctions have "distinctive histories."

The four primary goals of the initial subjective evaluation are as follows:

1. To develop rapport with the patient
2. To gather detailed historical information
3. To understand the specific symptoms and their irritability
4. To make the patient aware of his or her condition and of the need to take responsibility for his or her own care

Within the framework of a normal subjective evaluation, asking certain questions is important in determining soft tissue involvement. These questions[14,93,102] are designed to identify the following:

- Location and type of symptoms
- Course of symptoms and irritability
- Duration of symptoms
- Precipitating trauma or activity
- Previous traumas
- Previous surgeries
- Stressful employment, leisure, and recreational activities
- Postural and sleeping habits

Location and Type of Symptoms

The patient is guided in listing each symptom, beginning with the most bothersome and proceeding to the least bothersome. Each symptom is analyzed for its precise location, type, quality, and intensity.

Course of Symptoms and Irritability

Identifying the general or average course of symptoms assists in determining the degree of irritability and identifying the symptom-generating structures. The patient is asked to identify the postures and motions that exacerbate or ease the symptoms, and the therapist attempts to secure quantifiable measures of irritability.

Duration of Symptoms

The therapist should inquire primarily about those symptoms related to the chronic protective spasm and inactivity that could precipitate fibrotic changes within muscles and a remodeling of soft tissues.

Precipitating Trauma or Activity

It is important to carefully identify the direction of trauma and the movement pattern that occurred. This information is helpful in understanding the presenting symptoms, in analyzing the structural deviations, and in identifying which soft tissues should be evaluated. It is often important to know the patient's emotional state at the time of injury.[17]

Previous Traumas

One should look for earlier traumas that may have precipitated soft tissue changes, altered the biomechanics of the kinematic chain, or affected the performance of normal motor function. These alterations contribute to the presenting symptoms.

Previous Surgeries

It is important to inquire about previous surgeries, because scar tissue can dramatically affect efficient function in the whole kinematic chain. The authors have seen several cases in which restriction of scar tissue from abdominal surgery was a primary factor in the onset of shoulder symptoms. This was due to the restricted extensibility of the anterior region that altered the kinetics of throwing a ball and serving in tennis.

Stressful Employment, Leisure, and Recreational Activities

It is important to identify repeated patterns of postural dysfunction and aberrant movement patterns that may create dysfunctional soft tissue and muscular changes related to the presenting complaint.

Postural and Sleeping Habits

One should identify prolonged and habitual positions that may cause adaptive shortening of soft tissues and perpetuate symptoms.

OBJECTIVE EVALUATION

In clinical practice, therapists must make many choices every day in providing effective patient care. Some of these decisions are minor and obvious, whereas others are difficult and require careful analysis. Informed decision making is most effectively accomplished when all of the pertinent facts are gathered and analyzed. However, facts alone are not enough. Once the information is compiled, one must use discernment to sift through it. Discernment is drawn from previous experience; knowledge of anatomy, pathologic condition, and kinesiology; and a flexible scientific and intuitive decision-making process. This process requires a consistent and organized objective evaluation system.

A carefully performed objective evaluation provides a means to assess the physical and functional status of the whole patient. The objective evaluation assists in identifying abnormal postural and functional factors in both the symptomatic and the related asymptomatic regions. The organization and vigor of the objective evaluation are determined by data gained from the subjective evaluation (location, type, irritability, and nature of the symptoms). The components of an objective evaluation are observation (structural, movement, and functional analysis), palpation, neuromuscular control, and neurologic and special needs testing.

Data gathered through the objective evaluation will assist in developing a treatment plan, setting realistic goals, and objectifying the effectiveness of treatment.[86,103] Objective evaluation includes three components: (1) structural evaluation, (2) movement analysis, and (3) palpation assessment.

Structural Evaluation

Through careful observation, the postural and soft tissue components are analyzed for patterns of dysfunction that are directly or indirectly related to the patient's symptoms. They are observed through structural and postural analysis, as well as through soft tissue contours and proportions.

Structural and Postural Analysis

The structural and postural analysis is the building block of an objective evaluation and is based on the interrelationship that exists between structure and function. A system's inherent functional capacity is dependent on its structural integrity. Functionally, the body uses both static and dynamic postures. Static postures are primarily used for rest, whereas dynamic postures provide support for all functional activities.

Taking into account the natural asymmetrical state of each individual, efficient posture can be defined as the balanced 3-D alignment of the body's skeletal and soft tissue structures in an arrangement that provides for optimal weight attenuation, shock absorption, and functional capacity. This balanced posture is termed *neutral alignment.* This optimal skeletal arrangement provides for minimal energy expenditure and efficient neuromuscular control. In the neutral alignment, articulations are inherently protected in their midrange position, muscles are at an optimal length for function, and biomechanical potential is established for optimal coordinated function.

This should not imply that all functional activities occur in this neutral structural alignment. However, the capacity to assume this structural arrangement gives the neuromuscular system a flexible supportive structure and provides optimal function and protection for the articular and myofascial components.

Inefficient posture is often a major factor in the pathogenesis and perpetuation of symptoms.[17,104] Improper postural alignment places abnormal stress on sensitive structures and affects normal weight distribution, shock absorption, segmental biomechanics, and energy expenditure. These alterations can precipitate pathologic condition and symptoms in the articular and soft tissue structures. Poor skeletal alignment is especially significant clinically when symptom-producing postures are sustained and repeated for extended periods of time.

Inefficient alignment is usually a result of two closely interrelated factors: (1) structural and mechanical dysfunctions or (2) functional compensations.

Structural and Mechanical Dysfunctions

Structural and mechanical dysfunctions are defined as hyper- or hypomobility of articular and soft tissue structures that alter normal functional capacity.

Functional Compensations

Functional compensations are chronic or habitually held postures that alter the system's structural and functional capacity. Functional compensations develop because of either habitual use of stressful postures and motions or chronic unresolved emotional or mental physical responses.[86] The neuromuscular skeletal system compensates for these habitual or unresolved responses through unnecessary muscular effort, inefficient postural alignment, aberrant movement patterns, and reduced kinesthetic awareness. These functional compensations, when unidentified, may be primary factors in causing and perpetuating unresolved symptoms.

Observational evaluation begins with a global view of the patient that guides the therapist to regions in need of specific assessment. One should generally assess the overall body type,[14] as well as the contour, integrity, and balance of the patient's posture. The structural vertical and horizontal alignment should be evaluated for general patterns of imbalance and poor alignment, which may precipitate excessive stress on symptomatic structures.

Once regions and patterns of dysfunction are identified, a regional evaluation is conducted. A systematic regional structural evaluation begins with the analysis of the base of support and then progresses superiorly to scan each movement segment. (Figure 27-8 provides a block representation of the movement segments.) It is at the transitional zones between these general movement segments that many dysfunctions and symptoms occur. Each segment is assessed for position, relationship of the structural and soft tissue components, and relative structural proportions of each movement segment.[2,85,105-107] Special attention is given to the evaluation of the symptomatic region or regions, with a focus on the patient's capacity to assume a neutral posture.[2,86,104]

The regional assessment is followed by a specific evaluation to closely assess the dysfunctional regions for specific structural and movement dysfunctions. This evaluation is most effectively conducted in conjunction with exploratory palpation. Combining observation with palpation provides a valuable learning experience and an opportunity to correlate the observed structural changes and palpable findings. The specific evaluation can progress to the vertical compression test.[98,108]

The vertical compression test assesses the integrity and force attenuation capacity of the spine and extremities in weight-bearing positions. The test evaluates for the quality of weight distribution, the compliance of the structural components, and the symptoms produced by habitual postures.[78]

The vertical compression test is performed in weight-bearing postures such as standing, sitting, and on the hands and knees by applying a gentle vertical pressure to the head, shoulders, pelvis, or knees (Figure 27-9). During the application of vertical compression, the therapist evaluates the inherent stability of the weight-bearing structures.

When the test is applied in an optimal state, the structure will be stable, with the force felt and seen to be transmitted directly through each movement segment into the base of support. However, if a segment or a combination of segments is malpositioned, then vertical compression will produce noticeable buckling or pivoting at the transitional zones. These unstable transitional zones are often the regions of presenting symptoms, and they will be increased by the test if a postural component to the symptoms exists. These zones will often be used as primary fulcrums during functional activities. This excessive overuse of individual segments often alters neuromuscular patterns, precipitates degeneration, develops a low-grade inflammatory response, creates hypermobility, facilitates chronic muscular activity, and produces associated soft tissue adaptations.[109]

The therapist, while applying the vertical compression test, questions the patient about the status of the symptoms. Caution must be used with the force and number of retests applied, especially with highly irritable patients or those suspected of being load sensitive. The test can help patients recognize exist-

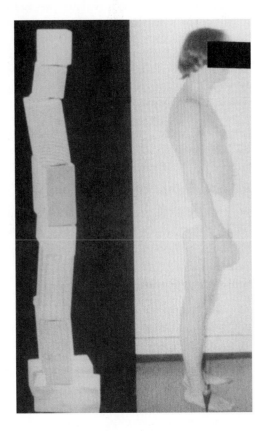

Figure 27-8 Positional relationships of movement segments.

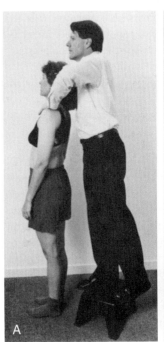 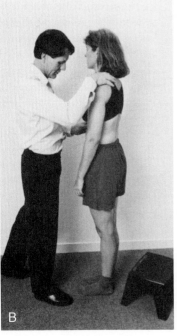 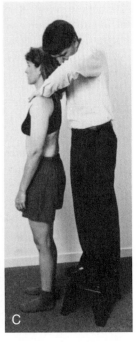

Figure 27-9 Vertical compression. **A,** Test. **B,** Correction. **C,** Retest.

ing postural deviations and their functional and symptomatic effects. The vertical compression test can be graded on a scale of 1 to 5, much like conventional manual muscle testing (MMT).

TREATMENT STRATEGY

Once the dysfunctional segments are identified and symptoms assessed, the next goal is to improve the patient's posture. Using both manual and verbal cues, the therapist guides each segment to a more balanced neutral position. When a more efficient alignment is achieved, vertical compression is again applied to reevaluate the vertical integrity and associated symptoms. Several postural corrections may be needed to achieve an optimal stable position. The retest also provides the patient with further kinesthetic feedback on the more stable and balanced alignment.

Those segments that cannot be repositioned because of structural limitations are identified for more in-depth soft tissue evaluation and treatment. For example, in the lumbar spine the most important and most frequently identified alignment problem is backward bending of the thoracic cage in relation to the pelvis.[2,101] The myofascial structures that are most often found to be dysfunctional are the deep fibers of the psoas, the lumbar extensors, and the anterior cervical muscles. When these and associated articular dysfunctions are normalized, the patient can assume a more balanced alignment with greater ease. Evaluation should progress to testing for the lumbar protective mechanism; balancing reactions and functional training should be emphasized.[98,108]

Except in cases in which a forced posture controls pain (e.g., maintaining a pelvic tilt to open the intervertebral foramens in cases of advanced foraminal stenosis), increased muscular effort should not be used to assume an improved posture against underlying soft tissue tension. The effort of forcing a fixed posture often causes secondary compensations, biomechanical stresses, and structural shortening.[2,83] Therefore restrictive soft tissues should be normalized through STM and stretching so that an improved alignment can be assumed with greater ease. This decreased effort enhances patient compliance and comfort.

With improved postural alignment, increased emphasis should be placed on body mechanics training and a conditioning exercise program to strengthen weak muscles, lengthen shortened structures, develop core muscle facilitation of the lumbar protective mechanism, reestablish proper movement patterns, and improve kinesthetic awareness and balancing reactions.

Soft Tissue Observation

A symbiotic relationship exists between the soft tissues and the underlying supportive bony structure. The following soft tissue components should be assessed for dysfunctional states:

- The surface condition for changes in texture, color, moisture, and scars

- The surface contours by assessing the body's outline for circumferential and segmental bands, regions of bulges or protrusions, and areas that appear flattened or tightened
- The soft tissue proportions by comparing the bulk of soft tissues between the front and back, right and left, and inferior and superior (Areas of imbalance can lead to the identification of regions of overdevelopment or a general deconditioned state or atrophy. Any proportional imbalances in soft tissue development require further evaluation and the initiation of an appropriate muscle-conditioning program.[2,85,106,107])
- The inherent patterns of dysfunction (The full structure is assessed using a global view to note any patterns in the organization of the soft tissue dysfunctions. These patterns often exist in observable and palpable zigzag and spiral patterns away from the central dysfunction. If a pattern is identified, then one should try to determine where the primary restrictions exist and if they are due primarily to underlying mechanical dysfunctions or to functional compensations (Figure 27-10). Frequently, normalization of these primary restrictions enhances the rehabilitation program by reducing the inherent stress placed on symptomatic structures.)
- The 3-D structural proportions (In the efficient state, each individual has an inherent proportional balance between the

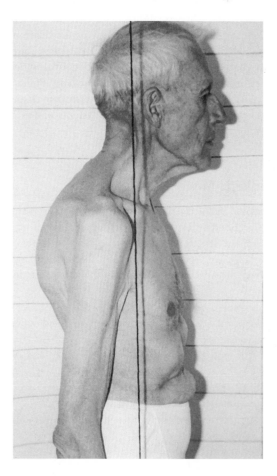

Figure 27-10 Evaluation of patterns of spiral and zigzag soft tissue compensations.

length, width, and depth of his or her structural components [skeletal and soft tissue systems]. Dysfunctions often diminish one dimension and restrict functional capacity and weight distribution.[85,106,107] The treatment strategy is to increase the diminished dimension through manual therapy and reeducation.)

Movement and Functional Analysis

Once postural abnormalities and soft tissue changes are identified, it is important to evaluate the mobility of these regions while the patient performs physiologic and functional movements. An important and often-overlooked assessment of the soft tissue system is the observation and palpation of these regions during the performance of guided motions and functional activities. Because the soft tissue system is continuous, movement that occurs in one region precipitates normal adjustments throughout the soft tissue and skeletal systems. However, dysfunctions in one region can affect the mobility and quality of movement in related regions, possibly altering the efficient function and overall adaptive potential of the entire kinematic chain.

Dysfunctional soft tissues impede efficient movement by limiting the ability of structures to elongate, fold, conform, and/or slide in relation to each other. Increased strain occurs as the motion transfers from regions of relative immobility to regions of relative hypermobility or vice versa, resulting in alterations in the function of the underlying articulations.

Through careful observation of the patient's ability to perform physiologic movement patterns, normal functional activities, functional movement patterns, and the adverse neural tension test, the therapist can identify soft tissue dysfunctions and grade the effects of those dysfunctions on movement performance.

Physiologic Movement Patterns

The conventional active range of motion (AROM) evaluation yields significant information about the mobility of articular and soft tissue structures. Movement evaluation is performed in weight-bearing postures such as standing, sitting, and quadruped. The evaluator should look and palpate for the following:

- Quality and sequencing of motion
- Range of movement (delineating structural and symptomatic limitations)
- Effect of movement on the intensity, location, and type of pain
- Mobility of individual segments
- Mobility of soft tissues in relation to each other
- Freedom of soft tissues to move in relation to underlying structures
- Ability of soft tissues to elongate and fold
- Proper use of the base of support

NOTE: Careful assessment and recording of specific limitations of physiologic motions provide the therapist with parameters for reevaluation and thus the ability to correlate the effects of soft tissue treatment.

Normal Functional Activities

Observation of an individual performing normal ADL, particularly those that produce symptoms, often reveals soft tissue dysfunctions associated with the presenting complaint and exacerbations. Many of the patients who have nontraumatic muscular skeletal symptoms have what is described as the *self-inflicted pain syndrome*. In any patient whose symptoms are perpetuated through stressful use, the aim of therapy is to assist the patient in becoming aware of the relationship between actions and pain, as well as educating the patient in the use of less stressful body mechanics.

A functional evaluation should include all functional activities frequently performed by the patient that may stress the symptomatic region, including the following:[85,98]

- Coming to sitting
- Sitting
- Rising to standing
- Walking
- Bending
- Reaching
- Pushing
- Pulling
- Lifting

Functional limitations such as a tight calf compartment, limitations in hip range of motion, and restrictions in shoulder girdle mobility are frequently identified through careful analysis.

Another critical component of a functional evaluation is the assessment of dynamic balance and balancing reactions. As anyone who has studied ballet, gymnastics, martial arts, or any athletic endeavor discovers, performance is often dependent on proper structural alignment, neuromuscular coordination, muscular strength, soft tissue compliance, and balancing capacity.

When a functional approach is used, the success of treatment can be gauged through documented improvements in the tested functional activities and abilities.[98]

Functional Movement Patterns

Functional movement patterns[3] were adapted primarily from the PNF diagonal movement patterns[88,99] and Awareness Through Movement lessons developed by Feldenkrais.[83] These movement patterns provide a means to quickly and effectively assess motor control; muscle recruitment patterns; soft tissue compliance; and articular mobility of specific body segments, regions, and/or the body as a whole. Functional movement patterns offer additional tools for evaluating specific limitations in dynamic range and sequencing of motion. For example, lower-quadrant movement patterns such as the pelvic clock, lower-trunk rotation, unilateral hip rotation, and pelvic diagonals can provide information about 3-D active compliance of the soft tissues, mobility of the underlying articulations, and quality of neuromuscular control. In addition, movement patterns such as side-lying shoulder girdle circles and arm circles reveal the mobility and compliance of the rib cage and upper-extremity soft tissues.

Treatment is applied through sustained pressure on the dysfunctional tissue or joint while the patient actively performs the functional movement pattern. The motion can vary from large excursions to very small ones. The purpose is to produce intermittent pressure and relaxation on the dysfunctions. After the resolution of these dysfunctions, the therapist performs neuromuscular reeducation by having the patient integrate the functional movement pattern into the new range in slow, controlled motions. Initial concern is evaluating the quality of contraction and strength of the core musculature in the region treated. This is accomplished through a prolonged hold. Motor control training immediately follows this, in which the therapist facilitates the patient to integrate the new range of motion in slow, coordinated combination of isotonic and isotonic reversals. The movement pattern can then be transferred to a home program for further training and strengthening.

Adverse Neural Tension Test

Adverse neural tension tests, as described by Maitland,[103] Elvey,[28] and Butler,[27] test the extensibility and mobility of the neural components from the dural tube through the peripheral aspects. Restricted motion and symptom production indicate a dysfunction through possible compression, adherence, or contractile and noncontractile restriction.[110]

Evaluations for both upper- and lower-limb neurovascular structures are performed by placing the individual nerves on selective tension through movement of the trunk and extremity. In the efficient state, when the neurovascular structures are placed at their lengthened range, a springy end feel is noted and the patient does not experience any discomfort. In a dysfunctional state, the range is restricted, palpable tension exists, and the patient reports reproduction of symptoms or discomfort. The most efficient procedure for evaluation of the peripheral nerve in all regions where it is accessible for palpation is to have the patient perform oscillatory motions of the distal component (using the wrist for the upper extremity and the ankle for the lower one). The therapist palpates the nerve along its course, assessing for free motion and efficient play. When restricted mobility is identified, sustained pressure is placed on the dysfunctional tissues while the oscillations continue to be performed at the distal and/or proximal components.[4]

Palpatory Evaluation

Palpatory evaluation is performed by placing selective tension on the tissues to be assessed. Through palpation, mechanical dysfunctions that restrict structures from their efficient functional excursion and independent play are identified.

Palpation evaluation is guided by the data gained through the subjective, postural, and movement evaluations and includes the specific assessment of the condition and the 3-D mobility of the individual layers of tissues. The soft tissues are initially evaluated in their resting positions; however, the associated functional deficits may be appreciated better by palpating the tissues during the performance of passive, active, or resisted motions.[3] The assessment is organized to evaluate the condition and the 3-D mobility of each layer, beginning superficially and progressing deeper. The individual layers are defined by the individual strata of muscles. This is important because skin, muscles, and neurovascular elements all exist in individual layers and compartments and are separated by loose connective tissue.[2,111]

Through proper layer palpation, most dysfunctional soft tissues can be identified. These dysfunctions exist within a specific layer or extend through several distinct layers. Such restricted regions have a single or several central epicenters of maximal restriction. Epicenters vary from the size of a pea to the size of a grain of sand. Most restrictions have spiral patterns of adherence that should be identified. A strong indicator of soft tissue dysfunction is tenderness to normal palpation. Therefore patients can assist in locating the epicenter of tenderness. It should be noted that some tissues without any identifiable dysfunction will be tender to normal palpation. These tissues may be in a state of low-grade inflammation, resulting in dysfunction of soft tissue structures.[2]

Referred pain is another clinical aspect of dysfunctional soft tissues. Referred pain patterns are elicited and assessed through normal palpation to epicenter restriction. By assessing these referred pain patterns, the therapist can discern whether the dysfunction is a primary or secondary source of symptoms or dysfunction.[63,101]

Although performing a palpatory evaluation, the therapist must remember that proper and sensitive palpation is a critical means of communication. One of the fastest ways to develop the patient's confidence is through a caring and competent touch. Often the difference between successful and unsuccessful manual treatment is the development of patient confidence, which influences the patient's ability to relax. It is recommended that the therapist strive to develop skills of touching and to assist this process by frequently asking patients for feedback and assistance.[112,113]

Soft tissue dysfunctions are identified through palpable changes in tissue extensibility, recoil, end feel, and independent play.[2]

Extensibility and Recoil

Tissue extensibility is the ability of tissues to elongate to an optimal range and still have a springy end feel. Tissue extensibility is evaluated through precise direct pressure on the tissues or through elongation of those tissues by joint motion. Recoil is evaluated by how the tissue returns to its normal resting length.

As soft tissues are deformed through their functional excursion, points of increased resistance may be palpated. These restrictions or changes in density may exist through all or part of the tissue excursion. The specific restrictive points, epicenters, and direction of greatest restriction must be identified because the treatment technique is applied to the adherent tissues at the point and direction of greatest restriction.

End Feel

Tissue end feel[42] is the quality of tension felt when a tissue is manually deformed to the limit of its physiologic or accessory range. In a healthy state, tissues have a springy end feel that can be compared with the quality of elasticity and recoil felt when a new rubber band is taken to end range. The excursion (range of deformation) of soft tissues varies throughout the body, but in a healthy state the end feel is consistently springy.

Dysfunctional tissues have varying degrees of hard end feel and motion loss. These limitations are defined by their specific 3-D limitation of precise depth, direction, and angle of maximal restriction. The goal of this evaluation process is to localize the dysfunction so that treatment can be more specific, more effective, and less invasive.[2]

Independent Play

All soft tissue structures in their efficient state have independent accessory mobility in relation to surrounding structures. The degree and extent of mobility vary from structure to structure. In a healthy state this is described as *normal play.* In a dysfunctional state, reduced play is noted between adjoining tissues. In myofascial tissue this is termed *restricted muscle play.* Dysfunctional tissues and structures can be evaluated most effectively by conducting palpation during passive and active movements that reveal associated functional limitations.

EVALUATION PROCEDURES FOR SOFT TISSUE STRUCTURES

The following are the individual structures specifically assessed through layer palpation: skin and superficial fascia, bony contours, and myofascial tissues (Figure 27-11).

Skin and Superficial Fascia Assessment

The skin is assessed for changes in tissue texture, temperature, and moisture by running the fingers or the back of the hand lightly over the surface of the skin. Changes in any of these parameters can guide the evaluation to underlying acute or chronic conditions.

The skin is evaluated for intrinsic and extrinsic mobility by fingertip palpation. The intrinsic mobility (within the skin) is assessed for extensibility, end feel, and recoil. The extrinsic mobility is assessed for independent play of the skin in relation to underlying structures.

Techniques for evaluation of the skin and superficial fascia include skin gliding, finger sliding, and skin rolling.

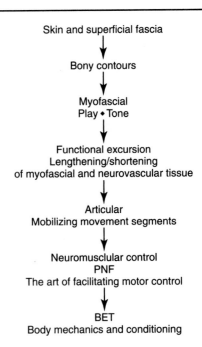

Figure 27-11 Selective and layer treatment progression. (Courtesy The Institute of Physical Art, Steamboat Springs, Colo.)

Skin Gliding

Skin gliding is performed by using either general (forearm, palm, elbow, knuckles) or specific (fingertips and thumbs) contacts. The skin's two-dimensional (2-D) mobility is evaluated for its ability to slide in relation to underlying structures (extrinsic mobility).

To evaluate, the manual contact point is fixed to the skin over the region to be assessed. The skin is pulled to the end range, evaluating the functional excursion, quality of extensibility, and end feel. The exact location of the adherence that is limiting its mobility is found through tracing and isolating along the direction of restriction. Restrictions are assessed using the clock face concept. Through this approach of evaluating the 360 degrees of 2-D motion around a single contact point, restrictions are localized.

Finger Sliding

Finger sliding evaluates the ease with which the fingertips slide across the skin (Figure 27-12). In normal tissue the finger slides with ease, creating a wave of skin in front. In restricted regions, the ability of the finger to slide across the skin is diminished. The goal is to isolate the specific location and direction of maximal restriction. Skin sliding is often used initially to trace and isolate regions of restriction, and finger sliding provides a means to localize the precise location and direction of restriction.

Skin Rolling

Skin rolling is performed by lifting the skin between the thumb and the index and middle fingers to evaluate its ability

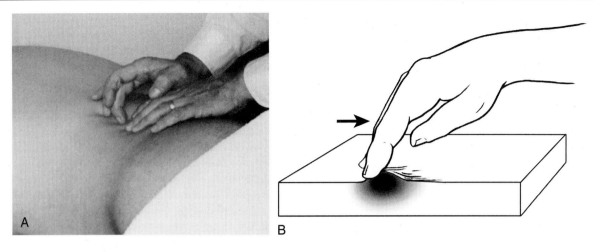

Figure 27-12 Skin and superficial fascia assessment: finger sliding.

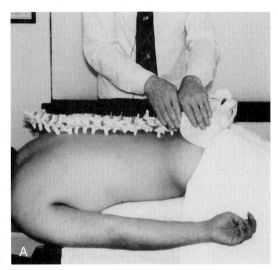

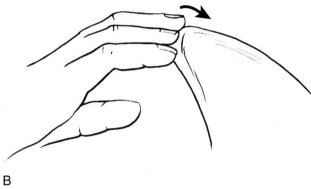

Figure 27-13 Assessment of bony contours.

to lift from underlying structures. Skin rolling is accomplished by keeping a wave of skin in front of the thumb while the finger feeds tissue toward the thumb. This procedure is especially effective over bony prominences.

Bony Contours Assessment

Scott-Charlton and Roebuck[114] state that "a great deal of spinal pain may well be pain felt where muscle, tendon, ligament and capsule are attached to sensitive periosteum of the spine." Therefore evaluation of the soft tissues along bony contours (i.e., iliac crest, vertebral bodies, scapula, tibia) may provide valuable information related to the overall condition of the multiple layers of soft tissues that attach to the bony contour. In addition, the bony contours are often the primary avenue for lymphatic drainage. If lymphatic drainage is impeded by restricted soft tissues, then further immobility may result.

A bony contour evaluation is performed by sliding the fingers parallel (longitudinally) at progressively deeper depths along the edges of the bone, noting any points of adherence and restricted mobility. The restrictions are defined by depth and direction, using the clock face concept (Figure 27-13). Corrective treatment often facilitates functional and symptomatic improvements, possibly because of enhancement of the normal dynamic soft tissue tension and mobility altering the stress on affected structures.

Myofascial Assessment

Evaluation of the myofascial structures should include assessment of the four conditions of (1) muscle tone, (2) muscle play, (3) muscle functional excursion, and (4) neuromuscular control.

Muscle Tone

Muscles in a state of increased tone feel harder, denser, and often tender to normal palpation.[32,115] When in a state of increased tone, myofascial tissue always has specific points or epicenters of maximal density. These points exist whether the entire muscle belly is involved or the dysfunction is localized to the individual foci of hypertonia. More specifically, the exact location, depth, and direction of the increased tone should be located and treated.

Muscle Play

Concepts of muscle play have been discussed previously in the section on the concepts of functional joints. The assessment of muscle play includes the following:

- The quality of accessory mobility of a muscle in relation to the surrounding structures, which allows full functional excursion and efficient biomechanical function during muscular contraction
- The ability of the muscle belly to expand during contraction, which allows full muscular shortening
- The ability of the muscle cell bundles to slide in relation to each other, which allows full passive and active functional excursion of that muscle

Muscle play is evaluated through perpendicular (transverse) deformation and parallel (longitudinal) separation of the muscle belly from surrounding structures. Each restriction is noted for its specific depth and direction. Because of the functional limitations caused by restricted muscle play, evaluation should also be conducted during passive and active motions.

Muscle Functional Excursion

Muscle functional excursion is defined as the muscle's capacity both to lengthen and narrow and to shorten and broaden. A muscle's ability to lengthen and narrow is evaluated by stretching the origin of the muscle from its insertion, identifying the specific direction of maximal restriction, and treating with STM in conjunction with contract or hold-relax techniques (Figure 27-14).[82,88,116] The patient can assist in the evaluation process by identifying where the stretch is felt when the muscle is positioned in a lengthened range.

The ability of a muscle to shorten and broaden can be evaluated through passive and active methods. Passive evaluation is performed through transverse fiber palpation to assess the play of the intrinsic fiber components. Active evaluation is similar, except that active or active-resisted movements may be performed during the evaluation, which offers additional information on the dynamic capacity of the muscle.

General Three-Dimensional Evaluation

A 3-D palpation involves evaluating the general ease or difficulty with which soft tissues surrounding a segment of the body move. An example is evaluation of the mobility of the circumferential soft tissues of the upper thigh, in which one hand is placed over the region of the quadriceps while the other hand is placed over the hamstrings (Figure 27-15). The therapist can evaluate the mobility of each layer circumferentially around the leg by moving the tissues in congruent motions of superior or inferior, internal or external circumferential rotation, or in a motion combining diagonal and spiral directions. Through this evaluation, one can identify those patterns in which the tissues are restricted and those in which they move freely. This distinction helps identify movement patterns that are frequently used to produce tissue mobility and those that are not used to create tissue immobility.[3,85]

Proprioceptive Neuromuscular Facilitation Patterns

Through the use of PNF patterns, one can identify inherent tissue tension patterns that limit the normal execution of the pattern. Because of the dynamic spiral nature of PNF patterns, many of the soft tissue restrictions that limit function can be identified (Figure 27-16). When those patterns of restriction are corrected, the PNF patterns that were previously restricted should be performed to reeducate movement within the new available range.[80,88,10]

Neuromuscular Control

Neuromuscular control is effectively evaluated and treated by using the principles and techniques of PNF (Figure 27-17).[88,99] Inefficient core muscle contraction coordination, recruitment,

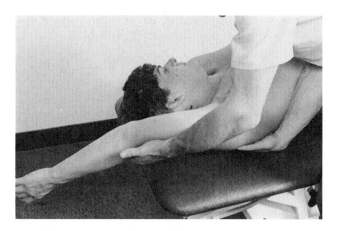

Figure 27-14 Evaluation of muscle functional excursion of the shoulder extensors.

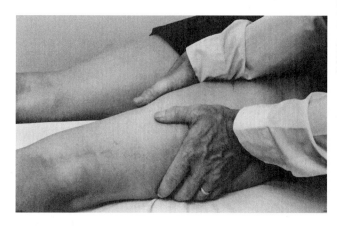

Figure 27-15 Three-dimensional (3-D) evaluation of the soft tissues of the thigh.

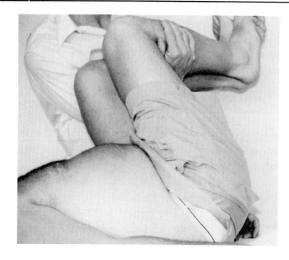

Figure 27-16 Proprioceptive neuromuscular facilitation (PNF) lower-trunk extension pattern with emphasis on the spinal intersegmental muscles and the quadratus lumborum.

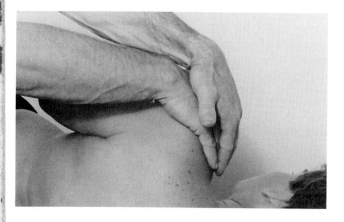

Figure 27-17 Performance of a proprioceptive neuromuscular facilitation (PNF) shoulder girdle anterior elevation pattern.

and sequencing of normal patterns of movement often lead to strain on the soft tissues. Improvement in neuromuscular control decreases the stress on articular structures and ensures long-term maintenance of improvement in posture, available movement, and symptoms.[84,98,103]

Associated Oscillations

Associated oscillations are rhythmic oscillatory motions that are manually applied to a body part. They are executed at a rate and excursion that will create wavelike motion in the soft tissues under evaluation. Associated oscillations are used to assess the patient's ability to relax, the mobility of the soft tissues, the play of muscles, and the ease of segmental motion.[2,3] Through the application of associated oscillations, the therapist can quickly identify general and specific sites of soft tissue restriction. These region are identified because of the fact that

dysfunctional tissues oscillate at a slower and impeded rate or are completely restricted and appear not to move. These restricted regions are termed *still points*.

Treatment Approach

Physical therapy is based on the ability to touch in a knowledgeable, conscious, therapeutic, and sensitive manner. The primary tools of the profession are based on the manual art of skilled palpation. This is an art that all therapists should develop. Initially, some students possess more enhanced natural palpation perception, but the ultimate mastery of the skill in all cases is achieved through experience and extensive directed practice. Because the ability to palpate is a foundational component of the profession, students should practice the art of palpation from the first day and continue throughout their undergraduate and postgraduate training.

Evaluation and treatment must be interrelated for the application of STM to be effective. Treatment is based on subjective and objective measures such as signs, symptoms, and the mechanical behavior of the symptomatic region.[103,117] The success of treatment is also dependent on the active involvement of the patient with the process through conscious relaxation and appropriate feedback.

Treatment Strategies

Two interrelated but distinct treatment strategies exist: (1) localized and (2) biomechanical.[3]

Localized Approach

The localized approach focuses primarily on evaluation of the painful or dysfunctional region, providing treatment of the localized symptomatic and dysfunctional structures. This treatment strategy is guided by changes in the presenting signs and symptoms.

Biomechanical Approach

The biomechanical approach is a systems analysis and treatment approach directed at optimizing the function of the kinematic chain. Through this approach, dysfunctions of posture, mobility, and neuromuscular control affecting the symptomatic region are identified and treated. These dysfunctions are often asymptomatic, but they precipitate perpetuation of symptoms and slowing of the healing processes through repeated irritation and reinjury. The primary evaluation tools used are analysis of the positional relationship of segments, vertical compression, 3-D proportions analysis, functional movement patterns, PNF, and functional activity evaluations.

The following example is provided to illustrate the use of the biomechanical approach. A load-sensitive right-lumbar problem that was not resolving with a localized treatment approach was assessed biomechanically.[118] It was noted that the patient's right shoulder girdle was positioned anterior and limited in its ability to be seated (like a yoke) and centered on the convexity of the rib cage. It appeared that the primary factor contributing to the patient's position was limited functional excursion of the right pectoralis minor. This dysfunctional position affected the shoulder girdle's normal arthrokinematics and force distribution capacity. Two primary biomechanical compensations were potentially affecting the lumbar spine.

Thoracic Spine

The shoulder girdle and arm were forced into an anterior position to the frontal plane, shifting the center of gravity of the upper body asymmetrically anterior of the vertical axis. The patient compensated for this imbalance by bending the thoracic cage backward from the midlumbar spine. This backward-bent position altered the vertical alignment, accentuated the lumbar lordosis, and increased the strain on the posterior elements of the symptomatic movement segments. Reproduction of symptoms and noticeable instability of the lumbar spine occurred during application of the vertical compression test.

Cervical Spine

When optimally positioned on the rib cage, the shoulder girdle distributes the weight and force of upper-extremity loading into the rib cage, the trunk, and the base of support. However, because of the protracted position of the patient's shoulder girdle, the primary mechanism of shoulder girdle support and force distribution was assumed by the shoulder girdle muscles attached to the cervical spine. This alteration in cervical muscular function placed abnormal strain on the cervical spine and precipitated myofascial adaptive shortening. The primary muscles affected were the longus coli, anterior scalenes, levator scapulae, upper trapezius, sternocleidomastoids, and suboccipitals. These myofascial restrictions precipitated a forward-head position with an accentuated cervical lordosis. This further altered the weight distribution and postural balance, increasing the strain on both the cervical and the lumbar spines.

As the patient's ability to position the shoulder girdle and assume a balanced alignment improved, she noted that she was able to be upright for longer periods of time without exacerbating her symptoms. This enhanced both her rehabilitative program and her functional capacity.

PRINCIPLES OF TECHNIQUE APPLICATION

Patient Preparation

Before providing any manual treatment, the therapist should describe to the patient the treatment that will be performed. The patient should also understand his or her responsibilities during the treatment process. Treatment is most effective when the patient is placed in a comfortable position that also allows for the greatest accessibility of the affected tissues. The patient is instructed to attempt to soften and relax the region being treated. Breathing is one of the most important adjuncts that can assist a patient in relaxation. In addition, the patient can be instructed to perform small, active oscillatory, physiologic, or functional movement patterns.

Soft Tissue Layer Concept

A foundational concept of this treatment method is to respect and treat according to the specific layer of tissue restriction or motion barrier. The superficial layers are evaluated and treated before attempting to correct the restrictions of deeper layers. By following this rule, the therapist will require the least amount of force to access the deeper restrictions. In addition, correction of superficial dysfunctions often improves the condition of restrictions of deeper layers. Dysfunctions are identified by specific depth, direction, and angle of restriction.

Technique Application

After assessing and localizing a soft tissue dysfunction, the therapist selects a specific STM technique and applies the appropriate amount of force in the direction of maximum density and/or restriction. The goal in applying soft tissue techniques is to achieve the desired results while using the least amount of force. It is important for the therapist to be patient and give the tissues time to respond and to allow both the mechanical and the viscoelastic effects to occur.

Degree of Force

Increased force is only used as a last resort when all other options for release have been attempted or when less mobile tissues such as scar adhesions and contractures are present. These tissues may require more force. The exact amount of force is dependent on the extent of restriction, the amount of discomfort, and the degree of irritability. The general rule is to place sufficient force on the restriction, in the precise depth, direction, and angle, to take and maintain the dysfunctional tissues to their end range. As the restriction begins to release, the therapist should continue to maintain pressure on the dysfunctional tissues and follow the path of the tissues that are releasing.

Progression of Technique

During application of a soft tissue technique, improvement in the dysfunction should be noted through a palpable normalization in tissue mobility or density. If a palpable improvement is seen in the restriction, then the subjective and objective signs should be reevaluated. If the restriction does not begin to improve within a short period of time (e.g., 10 seconds), then the therapist should alter or choose another technique. If after the application of two to three separate techniques no change is seen, then as a general rule the therapist should do the following:

- Reevaluate the region for underlying or more remote dysfunctions.

- Treat other dysfunctions and return to the unresponsive dysfunction later during the treatment session.
- Reassess and treat the dysfunction during subsequent treatment sessions.

NOTE: Dysfunctions related to scar tissue, decreased muscle play, or fascial tightness generally maintain the improvements gained during treatment. However, dysfunctions related to hypertonus or swelling and those of a neuroreflexive nature may return with time. Gains are more likely to be maintained if improved postures and range of motion are reinforced through application of resisted neuromuscular reeducation techniques, if the patient is trained in efficient body mechanics, and if a specific conditioning and rehabilitation program is designed to address the soft tissue dysfunction.

TREATMENT TECHNIQUES

Techniques are applied by using one hand to apply pressure on the restriction while the other hand assists to facilitate a release. The treatment hand can apply pressure through specific (fingers or thumb) or general (heel of the hand, elbow, forearm) contacts. The multiple options of manual contacts provide the therapist with a mosaic of treatment options. The selection of a general or specific contact surface depends on the type and size of dysfunctional tissue or tissues and the degree of irritability caused by the presenting symptoms.

Treatment pressure is applied in the direction of the restriction, and as it releases, the slack is taken up to keep a consistent pressure on the resolving restriction. The direction of the restriction often changes as the release occurs, and appropriate adjustments in the direction of force are needed to maintain the pattern of release. An inherent aspect of effective application of STM techniques is the therapist's use of proper body position and mechanics.

A natural progression of technique application exists. This progression generally begins with sustained pressure. If the restriction does not release, then the therapist should add or progress to additional techniques until the restriction begins to disappear (Figure 27-18).

Treatment Hand Techniques

Sustained Pressure

Pressure should be applied directly to the epicenter of the restricted tissue at the exact depth, direction, and angle of maximal restriction. The therapist should be positioned so that the technique can be applied either away from (pushing) or toward (pulling) his or her body. The pressure is sustained, and as the restriction resolves, the slack is taken up (Figure 27-19).

When applied to bony contours or myofascial tissues, sustained pressure is further defined according to the direction of motion in relation to the boundary of the structure.

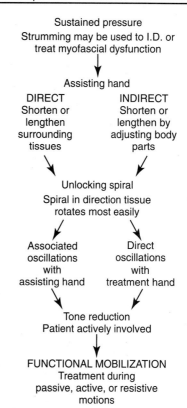

Figure 27-18 Cascade of techniques for progressive treatment of specific soft tissue restrictions. (Courtesy The Institute of Physical Art, Steamboat Springs, Colo.)

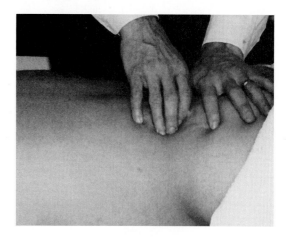

Figure 27-19 Sustained pressure with surrounding tissues placed on tension.

Unlocking Spiral

If a restriction does not resolve, the therapist can use an unlocking spiral to initiate a release. While maintaining a sustained pressure technique, the therapist assesses for the degree of tissue tension caused by clockwise and counterclockwise rotary motions. These motions are accomplished by moving the elbow away from or toward the body, spiraling the finger on the restriction as a screwdriver turns a screw. One motion creates greater tension in the tissues, while the other creates an easing of tension. When the direction of ease is identified, the therapist, while maintaining sustained pressure on the restriction, rotates in the direction of ease until the restriction begins to soften. At that point, the spiral motion is eased and the sustained pressure is continued following the pattern of release. On reassessment, the direction of tissue spiral that was of greater restriction (the opposite of the direction of ease) is evaluated for any remaining dysfunction and treated (Figure 27-20).

Direct Oscillations

The technique of direct oscillations involves an extension of the sustained pressure technique but with repeated, rhythmic, end-range deformation at the point of maxim dysfunction (grade III or IV of the Maitland system). These gentle oscillations places rhythmic pressure on and off a restriction (motion

barrier). As the restriction resolves, the tissue slack is taken up.[103]

Perpendicular Mobilization

Perpendicular mobilization involves sustained pressure applied at right angles or transverse to a bony contour or myofascial tissue to improve muscle and soft tissue play (Figure 27-21). Direct oscillation and unlocking spiral techniques can be used.

Parallel Mobilization

Parallel mobilization involves applying pressure longitudinally to restrictions along the edge of the muscle belly, to the seam between two muscles, or along bony contours. The purpose is to normalize the restriction and to improve muscle play and

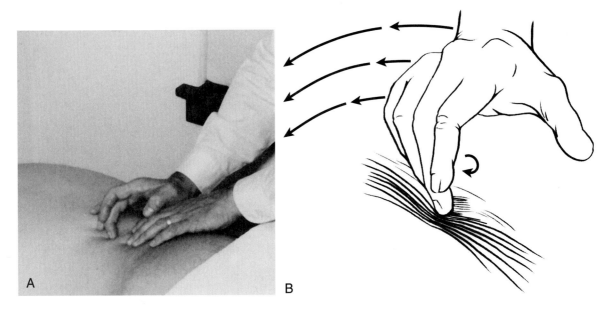

Figure 27-20 Unlocking spiral. The twisting action of the forearm and hand causes a spiral motion of fingers on restriction.

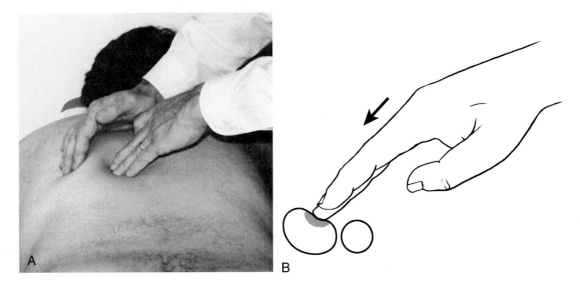

Figure 27-21 Perpendicular mobilization.

soft tissue mobility. Direct oscillations and unlocking spiral techniques can be used (Figure 27-22).

Perpendicular (Transverse) Strumming

Perpendicular strumming is used to evaluate for and treat increased tone and the loss of myofascial play. The technique is applied through repeated, rhythmic deformation of a muscle belly, as one would strum the string of a guitar. Perpendicular pressure is applied to the border of a muscle belly, deforming it until the end range is attained. The fingers are then allowed to slide over the top of the belly of the muscle as it springs back into position.

This technique produces rhythmic oscillations throughout the body. It allows the therapist to know if the patient is relax-ing, and it provides the relaxation qualities of oscillatory motions (mechanoreceptors) (Figure 27-23).

Friction Massage

Friction massage is a technique defined by Cyriax[42] involving repeated cross-grain manipulation of lesions of tendinous and ligamentous tissues.[44,101]

Assisting-Hand Techniques

The following procedures applied by the assisting hand can be used with any of the previously mentioned treatment hand procedures to hasten or facilitate resolution of tissues being treated.

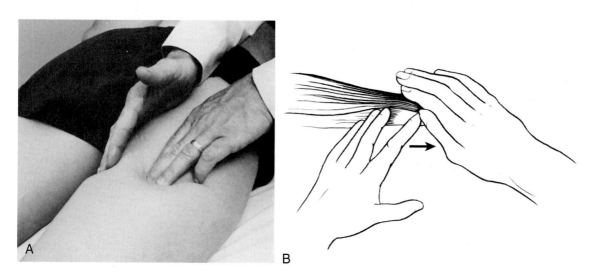

Figure 27-22 Parallel mobilization.

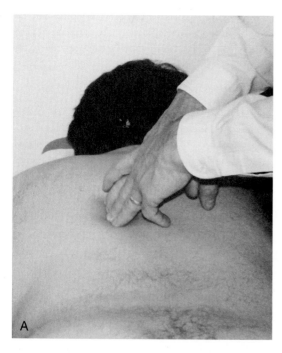

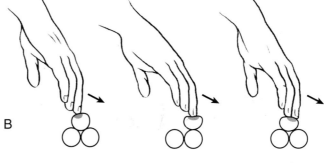

Figure 27-23 Perpendicular (transverse) strumming.

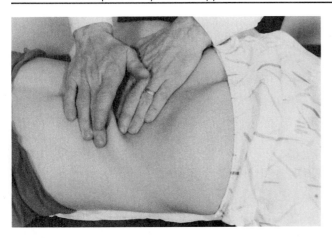

Figure 27-24 Placing tissues on slack with the assisting hand.

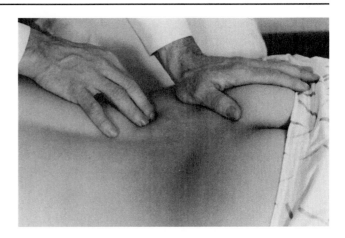

Figure 27-25 Placing tissues on tension with the assisting hand.

Placing Tissues on Slack

Placing tissues on slack involves adjusting the tissues surrounding the restriction in a shortened range to ease the tension on the restriction. This can occur from any direction in relation to the restriction (360 degrees). The tissues are shortened at the same tissue depth as the restriction.

Placing tissues on slack is generally the first assisting tool to be used, especially if the symptoms are acute or easily exacerbated. If a release does not begin within 10 seconds, then the therapist should choose another direction of shortening for the tissues or choose another assisting technique (Figure 27-24).

Placing Tissues on Tension

Placing tissues on tension involves adjusting the surrounding tissues in a lengthened range to place tension on the restriction. This technique is applied in the same manner as placing tissues on slack, with the exact depth and direction of tensing the surrounding tissues depending on the restriction. It is used more often in chronic conditions and as a means to place more demand on a restriction. All tissues should ultimately be checked in a lengthened position for the complete resolution of a restriction (Figure 27-25).

Using Both Hands

Conditions exist in which both hands are used together and no distinction is made between the treatment and assisting hands. For example, when performing a 3-D technique (which evolves from the 3-D evaluation covered in the previous section on palpatory evaluation), the two hands function together to improve the mobility of the tissues as an extension of the evaluation process.[3,85]

Passive Associated Oscillations

Trager first introduced the use of oscillations. This approach uses wavelike rhythmic oscillations to facilitate structural changes. Trager influenced the terms *associated oscillations, direct oscillations,* and *strumming.* Passive associated oscillations of a body part create a whole-body oscillation, but with focal oscillations on the restricted region. These oscillations are applied while sustained pressure is placed on the restriction. When used appropriately, these oscillations help the patient relax, decrease the discomfort of the pressure on the restriction, and promote normalization of the tissues. It is important to sense the degree to which the patient is able to relax and how well the oscillations translate through the body. The frequency of the oscillations varies according to the patient's body type and the type of dysfunction.[105,119]

Manual Resistance

While the treatment hand is maintaining pressure on restricted tissues, the assisting hand applies resistance to produce an isometric or isotonic contraction of the dysfunctional myofascial tissues. Many creative ways exist to use this assisting-hand tool. For example, in the side-lying position, treatment of dysfunctions of the soft tissues of the cervical spine can be enhanced by applying resistance to scapula patterns. These concepts are basic to the functional mobilization approach.[4,82]

Cascade of Techniques

The cascade of techniques flow chart can be used to better visualize and understand the options the therapist has for treating specific dysfunctions. This provides a mechanism for altering the treatment tools being used to meet the requirements of a specific restriction (Figure 27-26).

General Techniques

General techniques provide a larger contact surface to evaluate and treat larger regions of the body. They are often used when a general evaluation and treatment is desired, such as when a large region of restrictions is present and as an initial or completion stroke. General techniques are also useful to protect or reduce the use of fingertips and thumbs, which are stressed by the use of specific techniques (Figure 27-27).[120]

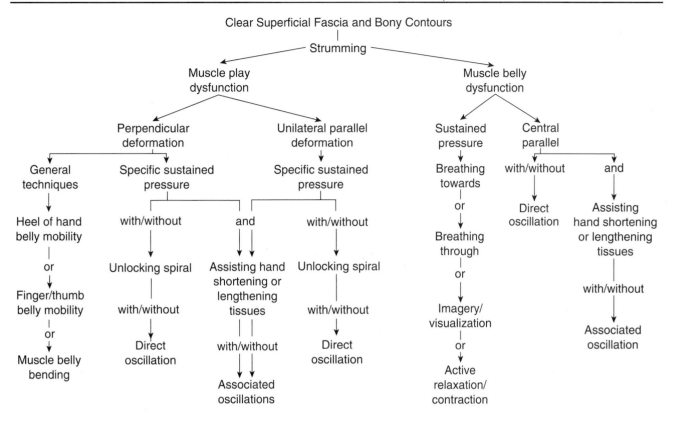

Figure 27-26 Myofascial cascade of techniques. (Courtesy The Institute of Physical Art, Steamboat Springs, Colo.)

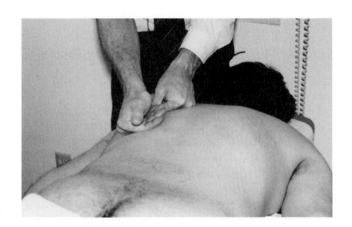

Figure 27-27 General techniques for the paraspinals.

Functional Mobilization

Functional mobilization is the integrated use of soft tissue and joint mobilization combined with the dynamic principles and procedures of PNF. This is a step-by-step evaluation and treatment approach, which combines mobilization or stabilization with neuromuscular reeducation. With the combined tools of PNF and STM, the therapist is able to combine the evaluation of the condition of the soft tissues, articulations, and neuromuscular control of multiple movement segments. (Figure 27-28).

PROGRESSION OF CARE

As noncontractile and contractile soft tissues regain their normal state of free and independent mobility, decreased tone, and normal physiologic length, the patient can assume a more efficient alignment and move with greater ease and coordination (see Figure 27-28). New postures and range of motion should be reinforced through application of resisted neuromuscular reeducation techniques,[88,99] and emphasis should be placed on a specific core muscle control, body mechanics training, and rehabilitation program.[98,117]

Precautions and Contraindications

As with any manual therapy approach, the application of any treatment technique needs to be done in a judicious manner, with recognition of the known pathologic conditions and irritabilities and with common sense. The following list of contraindications and precautions is provided as a guide. Therapists with extensive experience and training in manual therapy may judiciously treat a condition that less experienced therapists should avoid.

- Malignancy
- Inflammatory skin condition
- Fracture
- Sites of active hemorrhage
- Obstructive edema

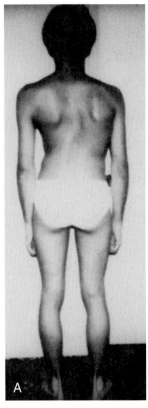
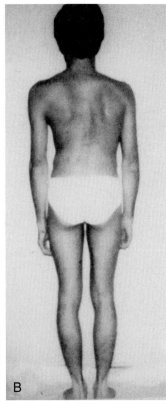
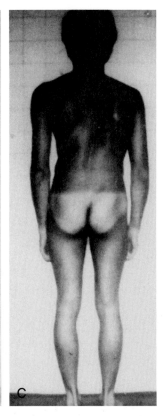

Figure 27-28 Postural changes after treatment. **A,** Initial. **B,** After 10 treatments. **C,** One year after discharge.

- Localized infections
- Aneurysm
- Acute rheumatoid arthritis
- Osteomyelitis
- Osteoporosis
- Advanced diabetes
- Fibromyalgia (while in an inflammatory state)
- Any symptoms that have previously been exacerbated by appropriately applied STM

CLINICAL CORRELATIONS

This overview of clinical correlations is intended to assist the reader in understanding the relevance of STM to the overall management of a patient and to illuminate the possible interaction of specific soft tissue restrictions with lumbar pathologic conditions. The lumbar spine has been chosen to illustrate the soft tissue dysfunctions associated with spinal dysfunction. Most of the functional changes reported are correlations made from observations after normalization of soft tissue dysfunctions.

SKIN AND SUPERFICIAL FASCIA

Improvements achieved through correction of skin restrictions are often dramatic in comparison with the subtleness of the restriction. The most frequently noted functional improvements (i.e., increased range of physiologic and functional motions, improvements in alignment and segmental spinal mobility, and reduced symptoms) are often noted after the treatment of abdominal or posterior surgical scars.[2,63]

Lumbar Muscles and Thoracolumbar Fascia

The lumbar muscles (Figure 27-29) can be divided into three groups and layers:[60] (1) the short intersegmental muscles (the interspinales and the intertransversarii), (2) the polysegmental muscles (the multifidus, the rotaries, and the lumbar components of the longissimus, spinalis, and iliocostalis), and (3) the long polysegmental muscles (represented by the thoracic components of the longissimus and iliocostalis lumborum that span the lumbar region from thoracic levels to the ilium and sacrum).

The deeper intersegmental and polysegmental muscles, particularly the multifidi, are primarily stabilizers controlling posture and assisting in fine adjustments and segmental movement.[8,9,26,121] The multifidus is also believed to protect against impingement of the facet capsule during joint movements because of its attachments to the joint capsules.[60] Kirkaldy-Willis[9] reports that uncontrolled contraction of the multifidus may be a primary factor in the production of torsional injury to the facet joints and disk. The more superficial and polysegmental muscles (erector spinae), the longissimus, spinalis, and iliocostalis, produce the grosser motions of thoracic and pelvic backward bending, side bending, and rotation that increase lumbar lordosis.[9,26,122] Some authors have reported that the erector spinae are active in maintaining upright posture.[122]

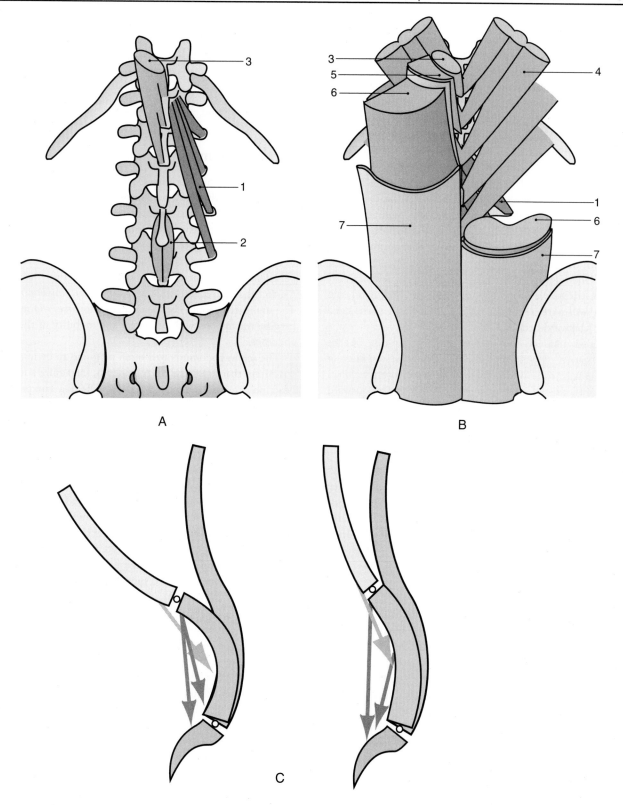

Figure 27-29 Lumbar musculature. *(1)* Transversospinalis, *(2)* interspinalis muscles, *(3)* spinalis muscle, *(4)* serratus posterior inferior, *(5)* longissimus, *(6)* iliocostalis, *(7)* aponeurosis of the latissimus dorsi. (From Kapandji: Physiology of the joints, vol 3. The Spinal column, pelvic girdle, and head, ed 6, Edinburgh, 2008, Churchill Livingstone.)

The extensive thoracolumbar fascia attaches to the transverse processes of the lumbar vertebrae, the iliac crest and iliolumbar ligament, the twelfth rib, the quadratus lumborum, the lateral portion of the psoas major, and the aponeurotic origin of the transversus abdominis.[26,123] Each layer of lumbar musculature is separated and compartmentalized by the thoracolumbar fascia and in an efficient state can be palpated for having independent mobility from surrounding structures. The lumbar musculature is most effectively assessed in the side-lying and prone positions. Its extensibility is most effectively appraised through evaluation of end ranges of PNF trunk patterns.

Restricted play of the erector spinae can limit range of motion of the lumbar spine because of the inability of the muscles to slide normally on each other. This is noted especially with the motions of side gliding (lateral shear), forward bending, and rotation. When muscles are in a state of increased tone or restricted play, they may have difficulty folding on each other and will restrict motions such as side bending to the same side and backward bending.

Increased tone of the deeper musculature can be the primary source of symptoms and can limit the mobility of individual segments. With unilateral soft tissue dysfunction, a deviation to the affected side often occurs during forward bending. In conjunction with the improvement of alignment, range of motion, and pain, improvement in the patient's ability to control active movement is often observed after treatment.

When the more lateral intertransversarii lateralis and quadratus lumborum have limited extensibility, the region often appears shortened and restricted in motions such as side bending and pelvic lateral shear (side gliding). The quadratus lumborum will often have restricted normal play in relation to the erector spinae and psoas, affecting most spinal motions.

Abdominal Scar

Scar tissue in the abdominal region often produces marked pathomechanics of the soft tissues and the articulations of the lumbopelvic girdle region. These scar tissue dysfunctions can alter efficient function from the superficial fascia to the deep abdominal region. Through careful palpation, spiderweb-like tentacles of restricted tissue can be traced, extending away from the central scar, possibly throughout the abdominal cavity, and to the posterior wall. If the palpation is performed with superimposed movement (e.g., a functional movement or PNF pattern), then the effects of these limitations and the altered biomechanics can be noted. This restricted matrix can affect proper alignment and functional movements such as forward bending (possibly because of the inability of the abdominal tissues to fold on themselves) and backward bending secondary to decreased extensibility of the anterior section.

In individuals with hypermobilities or spondylolisthesis, dramatic improvement in functional abilities has been observed through normalization of the abdominal scar. Improvement is often noted in static postures and in the performance of functional movement patterns such as the pelvic clock and lower-trunk rotation. Through appropriate STM the scar tissue may become more pliable, but the primary effect appears to be improved mobility of the surrounding structures and of the restricted spiderweb-like matrix. This probably facilitates a more neutral position of the lumbar spine and allows movement to be distributed through the spine into the pelvis more efficiently.

Rectus Abdominis

The rectus abdominis originates primarily from the costal cartilage of the fifth, sixth, and seventh ribs and inserts on the crest of the pubis. It is enclosed between the aponeuroses of the oblique and transversus, forming the rectus sheath, which separates it from the other abdominals.[26] If the rectus is adhered to the underlying structures, then motions such as rotation and pelvic lateral shearing are restricted because of the inability of the rectus abdominis to slide over the underlying abdominals. The umbilicus should also be evaluated for free 3-D mobility, because restrictions will also affect the mobility of the rectus abdominis.

The rectus abdominis will often be found to be in a shortened state that holds the rib cage down, increasing a forward-head posture and thoracic kyphosis. Often a compensatory backward bending of the thoracic cage occurs, increasing thoracolumbar or midlumbar lordosis. Clinicians often find shortened rectus abdominis muscles in individuals who do many sit-ups in a flexed position.

One of the myofascial complications of pregnancy is diastasis of the rectus abdominis. This is the separation of the two sections along the midline, the linea alba. Clinically, it has been observed that this separation occurs mostly in women who have restrictions of the lateral borders of the rectus abdominis, which prevent the muscle from stretching forward as a unit. This lack of mobility of the lateral aspect places excess stress on the central linea alba and produces separation.

Psoas and Iliacus Muscles

The psoas arises from the anterior surfaces and lower borders of the transverse processes of the twelfth thoracic vertebra and all of the lumbar vertebrae, creating a muscle with multiple distinct layers (Figure 27-30). At each segmental level it is attached to the margin of each vertebral body, the adjacent disk, and the fibrous arch that connects the upper and lower aspects of the lumbar vertebral body.[26,60] The iliacus originates primarily from the superior two thirds of the concavity of the iliac fossa and the upper surface of the lateral part of the sacrum, and most of the fibers converge into the lateral side of the psoas tendon.[26] The psoas and iliacus are covered with the iliac fascia, which attaches to the intervertebral disks, the margins of the vertebral bodies, and the upper part of the sacrum, and they are continuous with the inguinal ligament and the transversalis fascia. The iliopsoas flexes the femur on the pelvis or flexes the trunk and pelvis on the lower extremities. Some authors attribute a distinct postural component to the deeper spinal fibers of the psoas.[14,122]

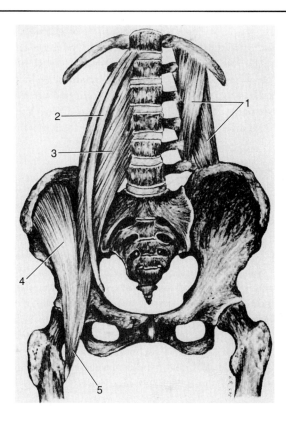

Figure 27-30 Muscles of the anterior spinal column. The intrinsic flexors of the lumbar spine: *(1)* two layers of the quadratus lumborum, *(2)* psoas minor, *(3)* psoas major, *(4)* iliacus, *(5)* conjoined attachment of the psoas and iliacus of and around the lesser femoral trochanter. (From Dupuis PR, Kirkaldy-Willis WH: The spine: integrated function and pathophysiology. In Cruess RL, Rennie WRJ, editors: Adult orthopaedics, New York, 1984, Churchill Livingstone.)

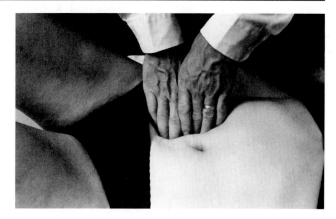

Figure 27-31 Evaluation and treatment of the psoas.

The iliopsoas muscles are often found to have limited extensibility, play, or increased tone at the level of spinal pathologic condition.[7,35,76,123] Because of the psoas' centralized biomechanical position, minor dysfunction of the psoas can have a dramatic effect on posture and the length of the lumbar region, and this can place excessive stress on the intervertebral disks and the performance of functional motions.[31,123] Restricted extensibility limits the posterior tilt of the pelvis, which increases lumbar lordosis. Such restrictions can decrease movement in all directions, especially limiting backward and forward bending. The function of the psoas is often altered by dysfunctions in the lower extremities, especially if the dysfunction is unilateral, thus altering the dynamics and the capacity for the two psoas muscles to act symmetrically during spinal function.

Through clinical experience it has been observed that, with improved length, play, and normalized tone of the psoas, an increase in forward bending of the lumbar spine often occurs. This improved mobility may be due to the ability of the psoas to fold on itself and the ability of the transverse processes, which are posterior to the central axis of motion, to separate from each other and allow the spine to bow convexly posteriorly. It has also been noticed that restricted play of a psoas at

a specific level can limit mobility of that segment, specifically affecting rotation and bending to the opposite side. Often pressure applied to the localized foci of tone will cause referred pain that duplicates the reported symptoms (Figure 27-31). In many cases, normalization of psoas mobility and improved neuromuscular control has facilitated dramatic improvements in symptoms and function.

Lower Extremities and Hip

Limited mobility of the myofascial structures of the lower extremities is a primary contributing factor that forces the individual to use the lumbar spine instead of the lower extremities as a primary axis of motion. Several authors have suggested a correlation between poor flexibility of the lower extremities and lumbar symptoms.[31,123] In addition, myofascial tightness of the lower extremities may cause a decrease in blood and lymph flow, which contributes to restricted mobility, fluid stasis, and greater muscular fatigability.

Of primary importance are dysfunctions that affect extensibility and normal play of the hip rotators, hamstrings, rectus femoris, iliotibial band, adductors, and gastrocsoleus (triceps surae).

Hip Rotators

Restricted play and decreased extensibility of these closely interrelated muscles limit hip mobility and affect pelvic motion and coordination for performance of forward-oriented tasks. The ability to rotate the body through the hips over a fixed base of support while maintaining a stable lumbar spine is affected when limited extensibility and play of the hip rotators is seen (Figure 27-32).

In addition, tightness of the hip capsule can be identified and treated in the prone position. In the efficient state, with the knee bent and the therapist palpating the posterior aspect of the greater trochanter, during passive internal and external rotation of the hip the femur remains in the same plane of motion. When it is restricted during external rotation, the femur migrates posteriorly; if it is restricted during internal rotation, the femur migrates anteriorly. Normalization of these

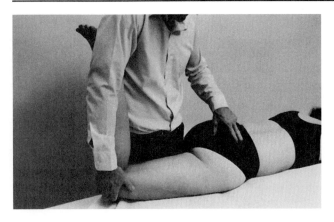

Figure 27-32 Function mobilization of the external rotators of the hip.

motions can be accomplished by impeding the dysfunctional motions and using contract-relax at the end ranges.

Hamstrings

Shortened hamstrings limit pelvic anterior tilt and therefore restrict a patient's ability to maintain a neutral spine while bending forward in standing and sitting. Restricted play between the three bellies can cause abnormal torsion on the ilium and affect the eccentric control of lower extremity and pelvic motions.

In the efficient state, the hamstrings fold around the femur during forward bending and rotational activities. This folding action provides additional range to the motions. However, the bellies of the hamstrings frequently become restricted together, preventing normal play. One of the most effective means to increase hamstrings range and function is to improve mobility at the interface between the hamstring bellies. The sciatic nerve between the bellies of the long head of the biceps femoris and the semitendinosus can be assessed. Restrictions of the hamstrings can be felt to restrict the mobility of the sciatic nerve.

Rectus Femoris

Decreased flexibility of the rectus femoris restricts the ability of the pelvis to tilt posteriorly on the head of the femur, often limiting the individual's ability to assume a neutral lumbar position in standing. Restricted mobility of the rectus femoris in relation to the sartorius, the tensor fascia lata, and the underlying quadriceps affects performance of each muscle's independent actions. Soft tissue restrictions within and around the rectus femoris can also limit hip extension during gait and result in compensatory backward bending of the lumbar spine.

Iliotibial Band

The iliotibial band is a lateral stabilizer and is important for maintaining posture during gait. Limited mobility and play of the iliotibial band is probably a major contributor to lumbar immobility and pain.[35] Tightness often reduces the individual's ability to shift weight over the base of support (because of lateral tightness) and to perform any lateral motion. In cases of sacroiliac hypermobility, limited extensibility of the iliotibial band is often seen on the side of hypermobility. Limited play, both at the lateral and medial borders and with the structures underneath, is the most common cause of limited iliotibial band extensibility. This limited play can be enhanced through directed STM, but mobilization also can occur through the use of small plungers or cupping devices.

Adductors

As with the iliotibial band, adductor tightness and limited play affect pelvic position, mobility, and the dynamics of lateral movements.

Gastrocsoleus

When the soleus is shortened, the heel lifts off the ground, decreasing the base of support and impairing balance during bending and lifting activities. This may further contribute to rearfoot deformities such as calcaneal valgus, which may cause aberrant lower-quadrant function. Restricted play between the bellies of the gastrocsoleus, and also between the soleus and the deeper toe flexors and posterior tibialis, can affect ankle coordination.

CASE STUDIES

Case Study 1
The following case study of a 38-year-old woman with right upper-quadrant symptoms illustrates the merging of STM in an integrated manual therapy program. This approach has been termed *functional mobilization.*[4]

Presenting Symptoms
The patient reported a 9-month duration of cervical and right upper-extremity pain with limited range secondary to involvement in a rear-end automobile accident. She denied experiencing any numbness, tingling, or weakness.

Mechanics of Injury
The patient was stopped at a traffic signal when another vehicle hit her from behind at approximately 40 miles per hour. At the time of impact her head was turned right, looking in the rearview mirror; her right hand was on the steering wheel, and her right foot was on the brake. This information is presented because the mechanical dysfunctions of the cervical spine, right shoulder, and pelvic girdle appear to have a bearing on the patient's posture and motion during the trauma.

CASE STUDY—cont'd

Symptom Onset and Progression
The patient reported an immediate onset of headache and cervical symptoms. Over the next 2 to 3 weeks, she developed right upper-extremity symptoms.

Test Results
Magnetic resonance imaging (MRI) revealed a minor disk bulging at the right C4-C5 level without thecal sac impingement.

Therapeutic Intervention and Symptomatic Progression
Initial therapeutic intervention consisted of antiinflammatory and muscle relaxant medications, which controlled the patient's symptoms so that she could return to her secretarial position within 1 week. One month after the trauma she continued to experience substantial symptoms, and her physician referred her for 6 weeks of physical therapy, three times per week, at another clinic. After 6 weeks of hot packs, ultrasound, cervical traction, and massage, the patient reported that she was experiencing increased symptoms, most notably in her right hand and wrist. On return to her physician, she was diagnosed as having carpal tunnel syndrome secondary to her frequent computer use and was given workman's compensation.

Six months later, she was referred to the clinic at the suggestion of a friend. She was still unable to return to work. Her presenting problems now included right shoulder limitation and pain. During the preceding 6-month period, she had received further physical therapy in addition to chiropractic care and acupuncture.

Diagnostic classification: Musculoskeletal 4B: Cervicalgia 723.1

Symptom Analysis
The following presenting symptoms are listed in the order of the patient's perceived intensity:
1. Right C7-T1 region: Pain at the approximate location of the first rib costovertebral articulation, described as a deep, boring aching pain.
2. Right C4-C5: Deep, sharp pain, especially with right rotation, side bending, and quadrant motions.
3. Right anterior and lateral shoulder pain. In addition to the range limitations, symptoms increased with flexion and abduction.
4. Right hand and wrist pain: Primarily the medial aspect of the hand, which increased with hand use.
5. Right medial scapula pain: Associated with forward oriented tasks.
6. Periodic right suboccipital and temporal headaches: Often precipitated with prolonged forward-oriented tasks or poor sleeping postures.

Significant Objective Findings
1. Cervical range of motion
   Right rotation: 50% with pain increasing at the right C4-C5

   Right extension quadrant: 30% with pain radiating into the right upper extremity to the hand
   Right side bending: 30% with pain radiating into the right-side neck and shoulder
2. Right first rib: Elevated with restricted caudal mobility, especially the posterior articulation
3. Right glenohumeral articulation range of motion
   Flexion: 140 degrees with the scapula stabilized
   Abduction: 80 degrees with pain in the subdeltoid region
   External rotation: 45 degrees
   Resisted test: Positive pain elicited with resisted abduction (supraspinatus) and external rotation (infraspinatus)
   Accessory mobility: Marked restriction of glenohumeral downward glide and acromioclavicular anterior mobility
4. Upper-limb nerve tension test: Tested according to the procedures of Butler[27] and Elvey[28]; positive with scapula depression, with radiation of symptoms into the hand; positive for the median nerve involvement
5. Right wrist: 70% extension
6. Pelvic girdle: Right innominate restricted in ability to extend and internally rotate (fixated in posterior torsion and outflare); region asymptomatic but functionally affecting the base of support, balance of the spine over the pelvis, and gait

Treatment Strategies
Treatment strategies for a patient with such complicated and system-wide problems require a multilevel and integrated approach. The following presentation emphasizes the progression and principles of treatment used for each dysfunctional region. Presented are the major components of the integrated treatment program:
1. Self-care was the initial emphasis of care. Training involved teaching the patient to use more efficient postures and body mechanics to reduce the self-perpetuated exacerbations. Education and training was the basic component of the treatment program and was addressed at each visit as symptoms and functional level improved.
2. During each visit a progressive and specific stretching, strengthening, and stabilization program was addressed. This program initially focused on the positive upper-limb tension sign, elevated first rib, limited cervical range of motion, self-resisted dorsal glide, and pivot prone for postural training.
3. In conjunction with education and training is the manual therapy treatment of the most obvious mechanical dysfunctions. This functional-mobilization approach includes STM, joint mobilization, and neuromuscular reeducation. The concept is to treat the soft tissue dys-

Continued

CASE STUDY—cont'd

functions before treatment of articular dysfunctions, combining each with neuromuscular reeducation.

The following is an overview of the treatment rendered to each dysfunctional region:

1. Thoracic girdle. The basic philosophy of functional mobilization is that dysfunctions of the base of support of a symptomatic segment should generally be normalized before treatment of the symptomatic structures. The thoracic girdle consists of the manubrium, the first ribs, and the first thoracic vertebra. The primary dysfunction of the thoracic girdle was the posterior aspect of the right first rib restricted in caudal glide.

Treatment strategy: The initial strategy was to normalize the superficial fascia, bony contours, and mobilization of the acromioclavicular articulation (Figure 27-33, *A*). In addition, STM was applied to the superior border of the scapula (Figure 27-33, *B*). There were significant restrictions of play and increased tone of the right anterior and medial scaleni muscles that, when reduced, improved the mobility of the first rib.

Mobilization of the first rib was performed in the supine position, with the soft tissues placed on slack through cervical right side bending. Sustained pressure was applied with the thumbs, the fingers, or the lateral first metacarpophalangeal to the most restricted portion and direction of the posterior first rib. Coupled with the sustained pressure was the use of directed breathing and contract relaxation (Figures 27-33, *C-D*).

Treatment progressed to sitting once the rib's mobility was returned to normal. The surrounding soft tissues were treated with the cervical spine in neutral and in left side bending to increase their functional excursion (Figure 27-34).

Home program: The patient was instructed to use a towel or strap to maintain the downward and posterior mobility of the first rib.

2. Cervical spine. Once the first rib was normalized, the amount of muscle spasm in the deep cervical musculature was reduced. Noted dysfunctions included the following:
   a. Marked superficial fascia tightness posterior along the spinous processes and in the right occipital and suboccipital region
   b. Adherence between the right semispinalis capitis and the splenius muscles, especially in the lower cervical spine (Figure 27-35, *A*)

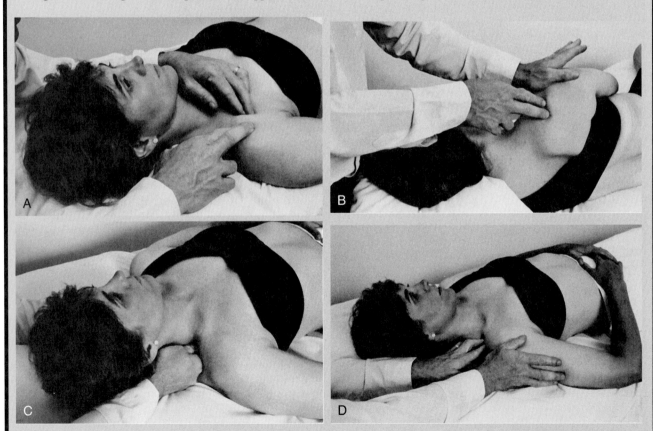

Figure 27-33 A, Mobilization of soft tissues of bony contours of the right clavicle and mobilization of the acromioclavicular joint. **B,** Mobilization of soft tissues of the superior right scapular border. **C,** Mobilization of the right first rib with soft tissues on slack. **D,** Mobilization of the right first rib with soft tissues on stretch.

CASE STUDY–cont'd

c. Dysfunctions of play and tone of the right longus coli, anterior and medial scaleni muscles, sternocleidomastoid, and upper trapezius (Figures 27-35, B-D)

d. Marked tenderness and swelling of the right C4-C5 articular facet

e. Limitation of C4 in left diagonal anterior glide and right rotation and side bending

f. General restriction of posterior longitudinal and interspinous ligaments, with most restriction at the C5-C6 level

Treatment strategy: The initial strategy was to treat the soft tissues to increase play and decrease tone. The tone of the muscles in the region of the right C4-C5 articular facet did not respond to tone-reducing techniques; therefore treatment progressed to improving mobility of that intervertebral segment. Using functional-mobilization techniques to localize the C4 restriction to the specific diagonal direction and using hold-relax procedures improved mobility and decreased the surrounding tone (Figure 27-36).

Additional treatment was used to reduce the tightness of the C5-C6 interspinous ligament by applying gentle fingertip traction to the C5 spinous process while the patient performed active axial extension. During the procedure the other hand performed STM to reduce anterior and posterior restrictions (Figure 27-37). To promote the ability of the cervical spine to balance on the rib cage, the O-1 and T1-T2 segments were mobilized (Figure 27-38).

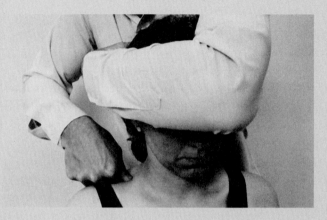

Figure 27-34 Mobilization of the right first rib in the sitting position coupled with cervical contraction and relaxation.

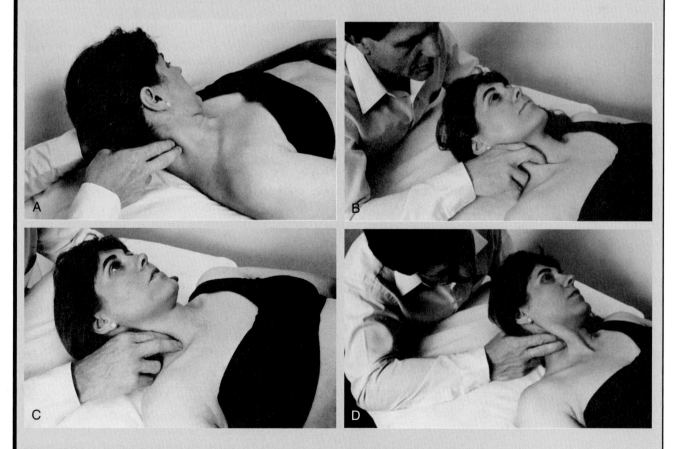

Figure 27-35 A, Parallel technique to improve play between the right semispinalis capitis and the splenius. **B,** Strumming of the right longus coli. **C,** Sustained pressure to the right anterior scalenus. **D,** Soft tissue mobilization (STM) of the right sternocleidomastoid.

Continued

CASE STUDY—cont'd

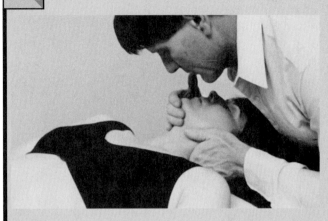

Figure 27-36 Functional mobilization to improve left anterior diagonal mobility of C4.

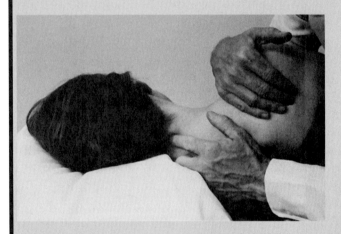

Figure 27-37 Mobilization of the interspinous ligament between C5 and C6 to increase extensibility.

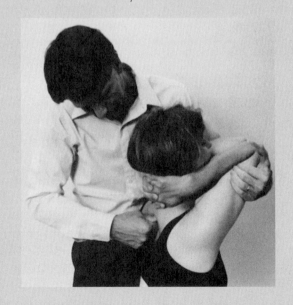

Figure 27-38 Mobilization of the upper-thoracic spine to increase backward bending of T1 and T2.

Home program: The home program consisted of resisted axial extension, short-neck and long-neck flexor strengthening, and resisted pivot prone to improve scapular stability.
3. Right shoulder. There were both subjective and objective gains in the shoulder after treatment of the first rib and cervical spine. Treatment was directed to the following primary dysfunctions:
   a. STM, primarily strumming of the bodies of the infra- and supraspinatus muscles (Figure 27-39, *A*)
   b. Friction massage to the supraspinatus and infraspinatus tendons (Figure 27-39, *B*)
   c. In the left side-lying position, selected PNF patterns to the right shoulder girdle in conjunction with STM (Figure 27-39, *C*)
   d. Mobilization of the scapular thoracic articulation by lifting the scapula from the rib cage (Figure 27-39, *D)*
   e. STM to the subscapularis and pectoralis minor muscles in the supine position (Figure 27-40, *A-B*)
   f. Distraction of the humeral head with STM and contract relaxation (Figure 27-41)
   g. Mobilization of the head of the humerus caudally, performed with the patient sitting and resting her right elbow on the table while the therapist placed downward pressure on the humerus (Figure 27-42)
   h. Neuromuscular reeducation of the rotator cuff through manual resistance applied in the same position, with emphasis on the humeral depressors
   i. Increasing range of motion of the right upper extremity by placing the arm at restricted ranges and performing STM and contract relaxation on the restricted tissues (Figure 27-43)
   j. Using upper-extremity PNF patterns to identify and treat weaknesses and motor recruitment problems (Figure 27-44, *A-B*)
Home program: This consists of rotator cuff and upper-extremity diagonal resistance using a sports cord, arm circles, and stretching to assist in maintaining and gaining range of motion (Figure 27-45).
4. Upper-limb nerve tension. After improvements in the mobility of the right first rib, C4-C5, and glenohumeral function, the upper-limb nerve tension test was negative with shoulder girdle depression.
   When the test was expanded to include a combination of shoulder girdle depression, 30 degrees of shoulder abduction, elbow extension, and wrist extension to 50%, the symptoms to the hand were elicited (Figure 27-46).[27,24]
   Treatment for these symptoms was addressed over several visits with three different protocols:
   a. Structures that may have been contributing to the adherent nerve (i.e., cervical spine, anterior and medial scaleni, clavicle, subclavius, first rib [also ribs two to four], clavicle, coracoid process, pectoralis minor, lateral boarder of

CASE STUDY—cont'd

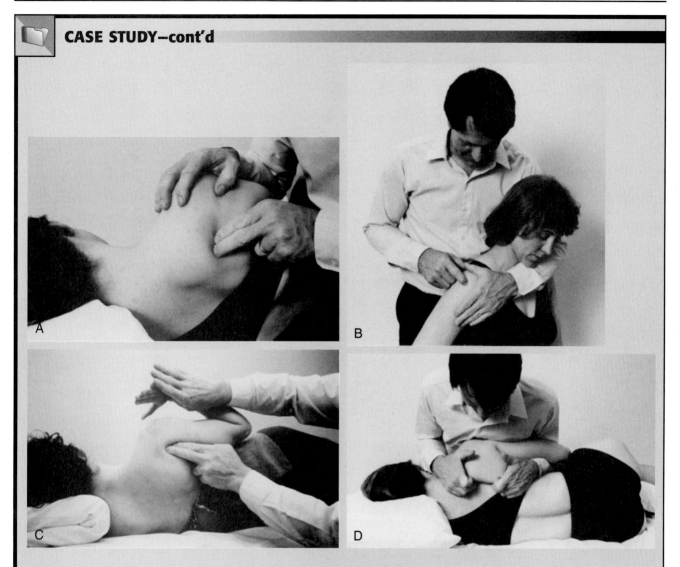

Figure 27-39 A, Strumming of the right infraspinatus. **B,** Friction massage of the right superspinatus tendon. **C,** Proprioceptive neuromuscular facilitation (PNF) for posterior depression, scapular pattern, with soft tissue mobilization (STM). **D,** Mobilization of the right scapulothoracic articulation.

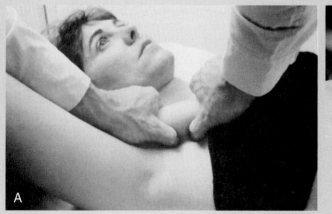

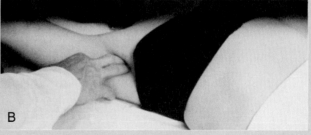

Figure 27-40 A, Soft tissue mobilization (STM) of the right pectoralis minor. **B,** Soft tissue mobilization (STM) of the right subscapularis.

Continued

CASE STUDY—cont'd

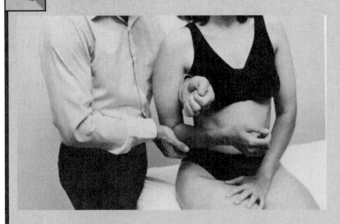

Figure 27-41 Distraction of the right glenohumeral articulation with contract relaxation.

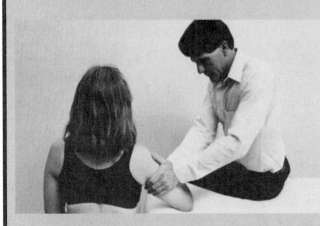

Figure 27-42 Caudal mobilization of the glenohumeral articulation with contract relaxation. Not shown is resistance to the depressors of the humeral head.

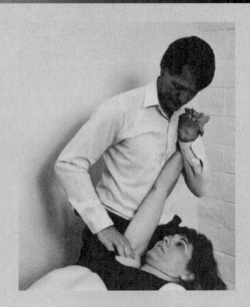

Figure 27-43 Proprioceptive neuromuscular facilitation (PNF) flexion abduction pattern with soft tissue mobilization (STM).

the scapula, soft tissues of the axilla arm and forearm region, and the nerves themselves) were evaluated and treated (Figure 27-47, *A*).

b. The upper-limb nerve tension test was performed, with the therapist moving the extremity until the patient or therapist first felt restriction. Through tracing and isolation, the therapist and patient identified restricted tissues and applied appropriate treatment techniques (Figure 27-47, *B*).

c. In the test position, the patient performed midrange wrist flexion and extension or cervical rotation and side bending while the therapist palpated the nerve to determine the locations of restrictions. This approach should not be used with irritable patients, because excessive motion will generally exacerbate symptoms.

Home program: The program was designed according to the protocol developed by Peter Edgelow.[124] This program includes diaphragmatic breathing, stretching of the upper thoracic spine and ribs over a fulcrum, and midrange oscil-

lations of the wrist in a position short of beginning resistance.

5. Right wrist. Treatment was performed to increase wrist extension and improve the mobility of the ligaments. The primary mechanical dysfunctions limiting wrist extension were a restriction of the ability of the distal ends of the radius and ulna to separate and volar mobility of the lunate. It is possible that these dysfunctions occurred at the time of the accident and were a factor in the onset of wrist and hand pain secondary to computer keyboard use.

The initial purpose of treatment was to mobilize the soft tissues and articulations of the wrist. As mobility improved, the extremity was placed at the end of the flexion abduction and extension abduction patterns to further treat the mechanical limitations of wrist extension and to initiate selective neuromuscular reeducation (Figure. 27-48, *A-B*). Treatment of the wrist in weight bearing was the final phase of functional mobilization (Figure 27-48, *C*). The patient was sitting on the table and bearing weight on her hand, which was placed at the side in varying degrees of rotation. Weight-bearing mobilization was applied while the patient actively moved over the fixed base of support.

Home program: This consisted of stretching in weight bearing and resisted PNF wrist pivots with a sports cord.

6. Pelvic girdle. During the patient's second visit, the pelvic girdle dysfunctions were normalized. The right innominate fixation in flexion and external rotation was probably precipitated during the accident secondary to the foot's position on the brake pedal. Pelvic girdle dysfunctions alter the normal weight distribution, base of

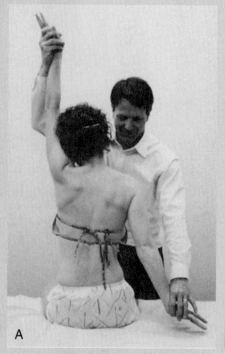
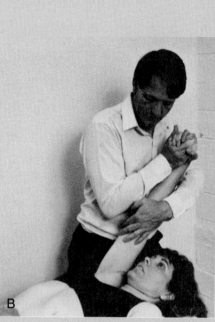

Figure 27-44 **A,** Extension adduction proprioceptive neuromuscular facilitation (PNF) pattern. **B,** Bilateral asymmetric reciprocal pattern for trunk and shoulder girdle stability while sitting.

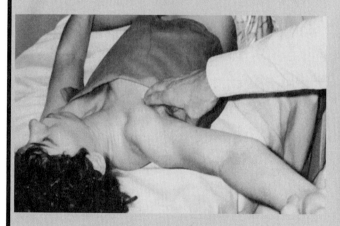

Figure 27-45 Functional movement pattern: arm circles with soft tissue mobilization (STM).

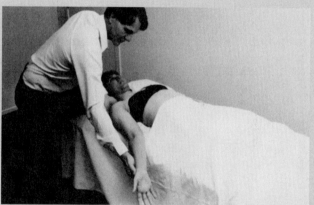

Figure 27-46 Position for the upper-limb nerve tension test.

support, and motor recruitment of the upper quadrant. It is the authors' belief that the pelvic girdle should be evaluated for dysfunctions whenever the present problem involves a weight-bearing structure.

The following soft tissue structures were evaluated and treated: the right psoas, iliacus, and piriformis (Figure 27-49, *A-C*). The following articulations were mobilized: the right sacral base with a fulcrum technique (Figure

27-50, *A-B*) and extension and internal rotation mobilization of the right innominate (Figure 27-51). Mobilization of the innominate was performed in a prone position, with the patient's left leg off the table to stabilize the lumbar spine. The right lower extremity was placed at the end range of the extension abduction pattern, and contract relaxation was performed toward flexion adduction. During performance of the contract relaxation technique, pressure was

Continued

CASE STUDY—cont'd

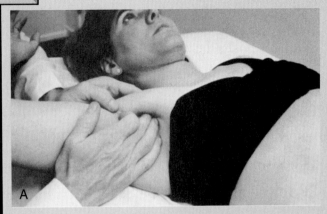
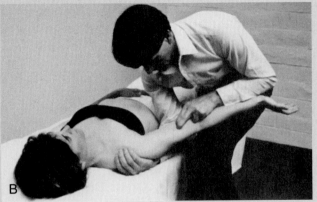

Figure 27-47 A, Mobilization of soft tissue around the axillary nerve track. **B,** Position for the upper-limb nerve tension test with tracing and isolating for soft tissue mobilization (STM).

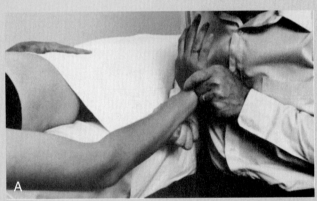
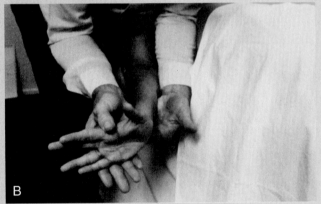
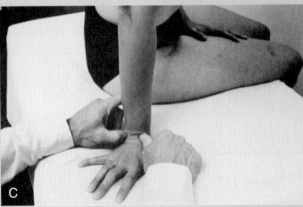

Figure 27-48 A, Wrist soft tissue and joint mobilization in the extension abduction pattern. **B,** Resisted reeducation of a tight wrist in extension abduction. **C,** Mobilization of the wrist in weight bearing.

applied on the upper lateral iliac crest to mobilize the superior innominate anterior and medially.

Treatment Progression and Results

The patient was seen initially for 7 visits over a 3-week period, with emphasis placed on education and training and manual therapy applied to the primary dysfunctions. After this period, the subjective and objective signs of the cervical spine and shoulder improved 70% to 80%. The upper-limb nerve tension improved 40% to 50% and became the primary emphasis of treatment. The patient was then seen once a week for the next 5 weeks for further training and treatment of the remaining dysfunctions. The emphasis of this component of treatment was on having the patient perform and progress in her exercise program and increase her level of daily activities.

At the end of this 5-week period, the patient returned to work. After 3 days of work she experienced increased cervical and peripheral symptoms, and treatment was initi-

CASE STUDY—cont'd

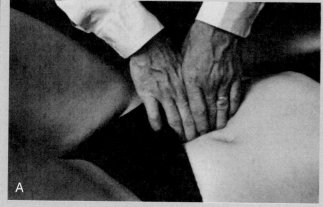

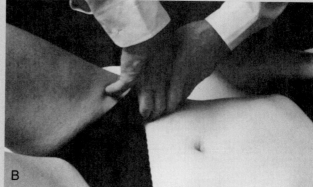

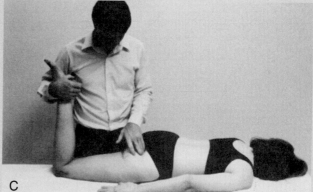

Figure 27-49 A, Strumming of the right psoas. **B,** Soft tissue mobilization (STM) of the right iliacus. **C,** Sustained pressure to the right piriformis with associated oscillations.

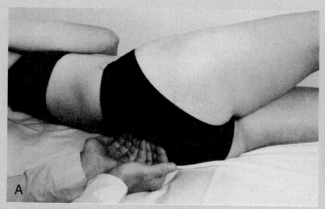

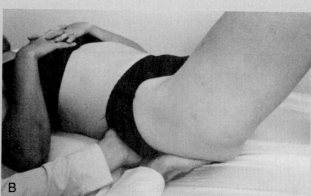

Figure 27-50 Fulcrum technique to mobilize the right sacral base. **A,** Finger position. **B,** Technique.

ated twice a week for the next 3 weeks to assist her transition to full-time employment. She was then seen for follow-up appointments every 3 to 4 weeks for 3 months.

At the end of 3 months she was discharged, with occasional peripheral symptoms secondary to excessive activity, but with the capacity to resolve and control these symptoms through self-management and a home program.

Case Study 2

The following case study illustrates the role that dysfunctional scar tissue can play in altering normal biomechanics and the results achieved with normalization.

The patient had right knee pain and dysfunction 1 year after anterior cruciate ligament (ACL) reconstructive surgery. She complained of lateral joint line and medial

Continued

CASE STUDY—cont'd

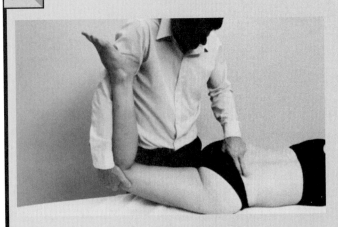

Figure 27-51 Functional mobilization of the right innominate into anterior torsion and inflare.

intrapatellar pain after extended use. She also stated that she was having difficulty developing strength and muscular bulk in the quadriceps, especially the vastus medialis obliquus. The functional evaluation revealed that she was tracking medially, with difficulty moving her knee over the lateral aspect of her foot. It was noted that the lateral scar tissue developed significant tightness during knee tracking, with restricted posterior mobility.

Diagnostic classification: Musculoskeletal 4I: ACL tear with internal derangement 717.8

Treatment of the scar was initially applied in nonweight bearing and progressed to weight bearing, with the patient attempting to track over the middle toe. The primary treatment technique used was unlocking spirals (Figure 27-52, A-B).

After normalization of the scar tissue, there was a natural tendency to track over the second toe. In addition, the patient was able to perform dynamic quadriceps setting exercises of the vastus medialis. This confirmed the limitations on lower-extremity function produced by the scar tissue.

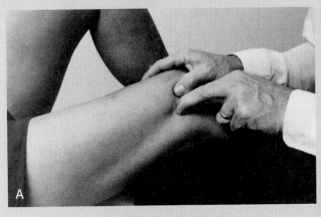
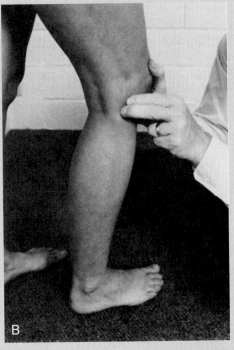

Figure 27-52 Scar tissue mobilization. **A,** Nonweight bearing. **B,** Weight bearing.

SUMMARY

The soft tissues of the body are often found to have inefficient mobility and tone, which precipitates and perpetuates many musculoskeletal symptoms. STM can play a valuable role in the treatment of these soft tissue dysfunctions. This treatment approach will achieve optimal results when used in conjunction with patient education, body mechanics training, a musculoskeletal conditioning program, and other manual therapy approaches (joint mobilization and neuromuscular education). A well-rounded and comprehensive conservative care program is required to return an individual to optimal function while avoiding nonconservative methods of management such as surgical intervention.

REFERENCES

1. Harris J: History and development of manipulation and mobilization. In Basmajian J, Nyberg R, editors: Rational manual therapies, Baltimore, 1993, Lippincott Williams & Wilkins.

2. Johnson GS, Saliba-Johnson VL: Functional orthopaedics I: course outline, San Anselmo, Calif, 2005, The Institute of Physical Art.

3. Johnson GS, Saliba-Johnson VL: Functional orthopaedics II: course outline, San Anselmo, Calif, 2008, The Institute of Physical Art.

4. Johnson GS, Saliba-Johnson VL: Functional mobilization UQ and LQ: course outlines, San Anselmo, Calif, 2008, The Institute of Physical Art.

5. Gray H: Anatomy of the human body, Philadelphia, 1966, Lea & Febiger.

6. Ham A, Cormack D: Histology, ed 8, Philadelphia, 1979, Lippincott Williams & Wilkins.

7. Grieve GP: Common vertebral joint problems, ed 2, London, 1988, Churchill Livingstone.

8. Hollingshead WH: Functional anatomy of the limbs and back: a text for students of the locomotor apparatus, Philadelphia, 1976, WB Saunders.

9. Kirkaldy-Willis WH: Managing low back pain, ed 2, New York, 1988, Churchill Livingstone.

10. Cummings GS, Crutchfield CA, Barnes MR: Orthopedic physical therapy, vol 1. Soft tissue changes in contractures, Atlanta, 1983, Strokesville.

11. Kendall HO, Kendall FP, Boynton DA: Posture and pain, Huntington, NY, 1977, Robert E Krieger.

12. Travell JG, Simons DG: Myofascial pain and dysfunction: the trigger point manual, vol I-II, Baltimore, 1992, Williams & Wilkins.

13. Woo S, Buckwalter JA: Injury and repair of the musculoskeletal soft tissues, Park Ridge, Ill, 1988, American Academy of Orthopedic Surgeons.

14. Porterfield J, DeRosa C: Mechanical low back pain, Philadelphia, 1991, WB Saunders.

15. Adams A: Effect of exercise upon ligament strength, Res Q 37:163, 1966.

16. Faulkner JA: New perspectives in training for maximum performance, JAMA 205:741, 1986.

17. Cailliet R: Soft tissue pain and disability, Philadelphia, 1977, FA Davis.

18. Woo S, Ritter MA, Amiel D, et al: The effects of exercise on the biomechanical and biochemical properties of swine digital flexor tendons, J Biomech Eng 103:51, 1981.

19. Ames DL: Overuse syndrome, J Fla Med Assoc 73:607,1986.

20. Sikorski JM: The orthopaedic basis for repetitive strain injury, Aust Fam Physician 17:81, 1988.

21. Tortora GJ, Grabowski SR: Principles of anatomy and physiology, ed 9, Hoboken, NJ, 2000, John Wiley & Sons Inc, p 152.

22. Clark RAF, Henson PM: The molecular and cellular biology of wound repair, ed 2, New York, 1996, Plenum Press.

23. Barbour TDA: Histology of the fascial-periosteal interface in lower limb chronic deep posterior compartment syndrome, Br J Sports Med 38(6):709-717, 2004.

24. Farfan HF: Mechanical factors in the genesis of low back pain. In Bonica JJ, editor: Advances in pain research and therapy, vol 3, New York, 1979, Raven Press.

25. Wadsworth CT: Manual examination and treatment of the spine and extremities, Baltimore, 1988, William & Wilkins.

26. Warwick R, Williams PL, editors: Gray's anatomy, ed 39, Edinburgh, 2005, Churchill Livingstone.

27. Butler D: The sensitive nervous system, Sidney, Australia, 2001, Norigroup Publications.

28. Elvey RL: Treatment of arm pain associated with abnormal brachial plexus tension, Aust J Physiother 32:224, 1986.

29. Culav EM, Clark CH, Merrilees MJ: Connective tissues: matrix composition and its relevance to physical therapy, Phys Ther 79(3):308-319, 1999.

30. Schleip R, Klingler W, Lehmann-Horn F: Active fascial contractility: fascial may be able to contract in a smooth muscle-like manner and thereby influence musculoskeletal dynamics, Medical Hypotheses 65:273-277, St Louis, 2005, Elsevier.

31. Farfan H, Gracovetsky S: The optimum spine, Spine 11:543, 1986.

32. Gratz CM: Air injection of the fascial spaces, Am J Roentgenol 35:750, 1936.

33. Donatelli R, Owens-Burkart H: Effects of immobilization on the extensibility of periarticular connective tissue, J Orthop Sports Phys Ther 3:67-72, 1981.

34. Mennell JM: Joint pain, Boston, 1964, Little, Brown.

35. Mennell JB: The science and art of joint manipulation, vol 2, London, 1952, Churchill Livingstone.

36. Forrest L: Current concepts in soft tissue wound healing, Br J Surg 70:133, 1983.

37. Woo S, Mathews JV, Akeson WH, et al: Connective tissue response to immobility: correlative study of biomechanical and biochemical measurements of normal and immobilized rabbit knees, Arthritis Rheum 18:257, 1975.

38. Nikolaou PK, MacDonald BL, Glisson RR, et al: Biomechanical and histological evaluation of muscle after controlled strain injury, Am J Sports Med 15:9, 1987.

39. Arem JA, Madden JW: Effects of stress on healing wounds. I. Intermittent noncyclical tension, J Surg Res 20:93, 1976.

40. Peacock E, VanWinkle W: Wound repair, ed 2, Philadelphia, 1976, WB Saunders.

41. Van der Muelen JCH: Present state of knowledge on processes of healing in collagen structures, Int J Sports Med 3:4, 1982.

42. Cyriax J: Textbook of orthopaedic medicine: diagnosis of soft tissue lesions, ed 8, Baltimore, 1984, Williams & Wilkins.

43. Noyes F: Functional properties of knee ligaments and alteration induced by immobilization: a correlative bio-

mechanical and histological study in primates, Clin Orthop 123:210, 1977.

44. Palastanga N: The use of transverse frictions for soft tissue lesions. In Grieve G, editor: Modern manual therapy of the vertebral column, London, 1986, Churchill Livingstone, p 819.

45. Ganong A: Textbook of medical physiology, ed 3, Philadelphia, 1968, WB Saunders.

46. Lowenthal M, Tobis JS: Contracture in chronic neurological disease, Arch Phys Med 38:640, 1957.

47. Amiel D, Frey C, Woo S, et al: Value of hyaluronic acid in the prevention of contracture formation, Clin Orthop 196:306, 1985.

48. Woo S, Gomez MA, Woo YK, et al: The relationship of immobilization and exercise on tissue remodeling, Biorheology 19:397, 1982.

49. Meyer K: Nature and function of mucopolysaccharides of connective tissue, Mol Biol 69, 1960.

50. Enneking W, Horowitz M: The intra-articular effects of immobilization on the human knee, J Bone Joint Surg 54A:973, 1972.

51. Amiel D, Akeson W, Woo S: Effects of nine weeks immobilization of the types of collagen synthesized in periarticular connective tissue from rabbit knees, TransOrthop Res Soc 5:162, 1980.

52. Akeson W: Wolff's law of connective tissue: the effects of stress deprivation on synovial joints, Arthritis Rheum 18(suppl 2):1, 1989.

53. Akeson W: Value of 17-/3-oestradial in prevention of contracture formation, Ann Rheum Dis 35:429, 1976.

54. Akeson WH, Amiel D, Woo S: Immobility effects on synovial joint: the pathomechanics of joint contracture, Biorheology 17:95, 1980.

55. Davidson C, Ganton L, Gehlsen G, et al: Rat tendon morphological and functional changes resulting from soft tissue mobilization, Med Sci Sports Exerc 29:313-319, 1997.

56. Gross M: Chronic tendonitis: pathomechanics of injury, factors affecting the healing response, and treatment, J Orthop Sports Phys Ther 16:248-261, 1992.

57. Leadbetter W: Cell-matrix response in tendon injury, Clin Sports Med 11:533-577, 1992.

58. Wong H, Wahl S: Tissue repair and fibrosis. In Zembala M, Asherman G, editors: Human monocytes, New York, 1989, Academic Press, pp 382-394.

59. Frankle VH, Nordin M: Basic biomechanics of the skeletal system, Philadelphia, 1980, Lea & Febiger.

60. Bogduk N, Twomey LT: Clinical anatomy of the lumbar spine, New York, 1987, Churchill Livingstone.

61. Frank C, Amiel D, Woo S, et al: Pain complaint-exercise performance relationship in chronic pain, Pain 10:311, 1981.

62. Cottingham JT, Porges SW, Richmond K: Shifts in pelvic inclination angle and parasympathetic tone produced by rolfing soft tissue manipulation, Phys Ther 68:1364, 1988.

63. Dicke E, Shliack H, Wolff A: A manual of reflexive therapy of the connective tissue (connective tissue massage) "bindegewebsmassage," Scarsdale, NY, 1978, Sidney S Simone.

64. Korr IM: The collected papers, Colorado Springs, Colo, 1979, American Academy of Osteopathy.

65. Levine P: Stress. In Coles MGH et al, editors: Psychophysiology: systems, processes, and applications, New York, 1986, Guilford Press, p 331.

66. Ward RC: The myofascial release concept. Course manual: tutorial on level 1 myofascial release technique, East Lansing, Mich, 1987, Michigan State University.

67. Basmajian JV: Grant's method of anatomy, ed 9, Baltimore, 1975, Williams & Wilkins.

68. Korr IM: The neurobiologic mechanisms in manipulative therapy, New York, 1978, Plenum Press.

69. Stoddard A: Manual of osteopathic practice, London, 1959, Hutchinson & Co.

70. Tappan F: Healing massage techniques: a study of eastern and western methods, Reston, Va, 1975, Prentice-Hall.

71. Sapega A, Quedenfeld T, Moyer R, et al: Biophysical factors in range-of-motion exercise, Phys Sportmed 9:57, 1981.

72. Malone TR: Muscle injury and rehabilitation, Baltimore, 1988, Williams & Wilkins.

73. Hill A: The mechanics of active muscle, Proc R Soc Lond B Biol Sci 141:104, 1953.

74. Komi PV: Training of muscle strength and power: interaction of neuromotoric, hypertrophic and mechanical factors, Int J Sports Med 7:10, 1986.

75. Locker LH, League NG: Histology of highly-stretched beef muscle: the fine structure of grossly stretched single fibers, J Ultrastruct Res 52:64, 1975.

76. Janda V: Muscle weakness and inhibition (pseudoparesis) in back pain syndromes. In Grieve G, editor: Modern manual therapy of the vertebral column, London, 1986, Churchill Livingstone, p 198.

77. Sahrmann SA: Course notes, 1988.

78. Saliba V, Johnson G: Lumbar protective mechanism. In White AH, Anderson R, editors: The conservative care of low back pain, Baltimore, 1991, Williams & Wilkins, p 112.

79. Grossmand MR, Sahrmann SA, Rose SJ: Review of length associated changes in muscle, Phys Ther 62:1799, 1982.

80. Tardieu C, Tarbary J, Tardieu G, et al: Adaptation of sarcomere numbers to the length imposed on muscle. In Gubba F, Marecahl G, Takacs O, editors: Mechanism of muscle adaptation to functional requirements, Elmsford, NY, 1981, Pergamon Press, p 103.

81. Dvorak J, Dvorak V: Manual medicine: diagnostics, Stuttgart, 1984, Georg Thieme Verlag.

82. Saliba V, Johnson G, Wardlaw C: Proprioceptive neuromuscular facilitation. In Basmajian J, Nyberg R, editors: Rational manual therapies, Baltimore, 1993, Williams & Wilkins, p 243.

83. Feldenkrais M: Awareness through movement, New York, 1977, Harper & Row.

84. Jowett RL, Fidler MW: Histochemical changes in the multifidus in the mechanical derangements of the spine, Orthop Clin North Am 6:145, 1975.

85. Aston J: Aston patterning, Incline Valley, Nev, 1989, Aston Training Center.

86. Jull GA: Examination of the lumbar spine. In Grieve G, editor: Modern manual therapy of the vertebral column, London, 1986, Churchill Livingstone, p 547.

87. Kirkaldy-Willis WH, Hill RJ: A more precise diagnosis for low back pain, Spine 4:102, 1979.

88. Knott M, Voss DE: Proprioceptive neuromuscular facilitation, ed 2, New York, 1968, Harper & Row.

89. Lewit K: The contribution of clinical observation to neurological mechanisms in manipulative therapy. In Korr I, editor: The neurobiologic mechanisms in manipulative therapy, New York, 1978, Plenum Press, p 3.

90. Hodges PW, Richardson CA: Contraction of the abdominal muscles associated with movement of the lower limb, Phys Ther 77:2, 1997.

91. Wilke HJ, Wolf S, Dlaes LE, et al: Stability of the lumbar spine with muscle groups—a biomechanical in vitro study, Spine 20:2, 1995.

92. Hodges PW, Richardson CA: Inefficient muscular stabilization of the lumbar spine associated with low back pain—a motor control evaluation of transversus abdominis, Spine 21:22, 1996.

93. Hodges PW, Richardson CA: Feed-forward contraction of transversus abdominis is not influenced by the direction of arm movement, Exp Brain Res 114:362, 1997.

94. Hides JA, Richardson CA, Jull GA: Multifidus muscle recovery is not automatic after resolution of acute, first-episode low back pain, Spine 21:23, 1996.

95. Hides JA, Stokes MJ, Saide M, et al: Evidence of lumbar multifidus muscle wasting ipsilateral to symptoms in patients with acute/subacute low back pain, Spine 19:2, 1994.

96. Hides JA, Richardson CA, Jull GA: Magnetic resonance imaging and ultrasonography of the lumbar multifidus muscle, Spine 20:1, 1995.

97. Kong WK, Goel VK, Gilbertson LG, et al: Effects of muscle dysfunction on lumbar spine mechanics, Spine 21:19, 1996.

98. Johnson GS, Saliba-Johnson VL: Back education and training: course outline, San Anselmo, Calif, 2005, Institute of Physical Art.

99. Johnson GS, Saliba-Johnson VL: PNFI: the functional approach to movement reeducation, San Anselmo, Calif, 2007, Institute of Physical Art.

100. Shacklock M: Clinical neurodynamics: a new system of musculoskeletal treatment, St Louis, 2005, Elsevier.

101. Cyriax J, Cyriax P: Illustrated manual of orthopaedic medicine, Bourough Green, England, 1983, Butterworths.

102. Paris S, Loubert P: Course notes, 1990.

103. Maitland GD: Vertebral manipulation, ed 7, London, 2005, Butterworths.

104. Jull G, Janda V: Muscles and motor control in low back pain: assessment and management. In Twomey LT, Taylor JR, editors: Physical therapy of the low back, New York, 1987, Churchill Livingstone, p 253.

105. Todd ME: The thinking body: a study of the balancing forces of dynamic man, Brooklyn, NY, 1937, Dance Horizons.

106. Klein-Vogelback S: Functional kinetics, London, 1990, Springer-Verlag.

107. Carriere B, Felix L: In consideration of proportions, Clin Management 4:93, 1993.

108. Johnson G, Saliba VA: Lumbar protective mechanism. In White A, Anderson R, editors: The conservative care of low back pain, Baltimore, 1991, Williams & Wilkins, p 113.

109. Paris S: Course notes, 1977.

110. Pacina M, Krmpotic-Nemanic J, Markiewitz A: Tunnel syndromes, ed 3, Boca Raton, Fla, 2001, CRC Press.

111. Greenman P: Principles of manual medicine, Baltimore, 1989, Williams & Wilkins.

112. Miller B: Learning the touch. In Physical therapy forum, vol 6, King of Prussia, Penn, 1987, Forum Publishing, p 3.

113. Montagu A: Touching: The human significance of skin, ed 2, New York, 1978, Harper & Row.

114. Scott-Charlton W, Roebuck DJ: The significance of posterior primary divisions of spinal nerves in pain syndromes, Med J Aust 2:945, 1972.

115. O'Brien J: Anterior spinal tenderness in low back pain syndromes, Spine 4:85, 1979.

116. Evjenth O, Hamberg J: Muscle stretching in manual therapy: a clinical manual, Alfta, Sweden, 1985, Alfta Rehab Forlag.

117. Morgan D: Concepts in functional training and postural stabilization for the low-back-injured, Top Acute Care Trauma Rehabil 2:8, 1988.

118. Vollowitz E: Furniture prescription for the conservative management of low back pain, Top Acute Care Trauma Rehabil 2:18, 1988.

119. Liskin J: Moving medicine: the life and work of Milton Trager, MD, Barrytowm NY, 1996, Barrytown/Station Hill Press.

120. Rolf R: Rolfing, Santa Monica, Calif, 1977, Dennis-Landman.

121. Wyke B: The neurology of joints, Ann R Coll Sur Engl 41:25, 1967.

122. Basmajian JV: Muscles alive: their functions revealed by electromyography, Baltimore, 1978, Williams & Wilkins.

123. Saal JS: Flexibility training, Phys Med Rehab 1:537, 1987.

124. Edgelow P: Adverse neural tension course notes, vol 26, Hayward, Calif, 1969, p. 716.

Somatosensory, Vestibular, and Visual Sensory Integration
Implications for Neuromuscular Control and Balance in Orthopaedic Practice

This chapter was written with several objectives in mind for the student. After studying this chapter the reader will be able to understand the need for consideration of sensory integration in orthopaedic practice, define neuromuscular control and its mechanisms, outline the neuroanatomy of neuromuscular control, define balance and dynamic joint stabilization as different expressions of neuromuscular control, describe evidence for measures of neuromuscular control and balance in orthopaedics, and design evidence-based, sensory-specific interventions for balance and cervical stabilization.

Clinicians tend to follow their interests into progressively specialized aspects of practice. At times, their focus becomes too narrow. This is reminiscent of the ancient Asian parable about the blind men and the elephant. The story tells of several blind men, each describing an elephant based on the individual part they are touching. The man touching the elephant's leg describes a tree, the one touching the elephant's trunk describes a snake and so forth.[1] This story parallels the author's experience while practicing simultaneously in the specialty areas of orthopaedic and vestibular physical therapy. At times, orthopaedic and vestibular perspectives on neuromuscular control appear very different. However, just as in the elephant fable, something (in this case a problem) is often described from a specialized but too often isolated focus. So it is in this light that the author hopes to enhance the orthopaedic rehabilitation specialist's practice by providing a view of neuromuscular control from perspectives traditionally reserved only for vestibular specialists.

THE RELEVANCE OF SENSORY INTEGRATION TO ORTHOPAEDIC PRACTICE

Several compelling reasons exist for an orthopaedic specialist to understand the role of sensory integration in neuromuscular

control (NMC). Most obvious is that many orthopaedic conditions display concomitant sensory impairment. For example, a large volume of research correlates lower-extremity injury with decreased somatosensory perception or proprioception[2-12] Similarly it is well established that neuromuscular training (NMT) programs emphasizing somatosensory perception significantly reduce the risk for anterior cruciate ligament (ACL) and other lower-extremity injury.[3-5,7,12-14] Evidence also links decreased NMC to shoulder instability.[14,15]

Many orthopaedic injuries such as ankle sprain, distal radius fracture, and hip fracture can be traced to poor balance resulting in falls.[16,17] In fact, it is estimated that by 2020 the national cost of falls related injuries will reach 43.8 billon dollars.[16] However, orthopaedic specialists often overlook the imbalance that caused the orthopaedic injury. Most geriatric fallers do so from multiple factors including decreased visual, somatosensory, and vestibular sensory perception.[17-25] Accurately assessing balance and risk for falls allows the orthopaedic professional to reduce the risk of reinjury or new injury and assists in difficult clinical decisions such as the recommended level of assistance.[16-26]

Orthopaedic specialists have treated and will continue to treat individuals with injury to the visual and vestibular system. For example, traumatic brain injury (TBI) has rapidly become the signature injury of the United States military forces sustaining casualties in Iraq and Afghanistan at the time of this writing.[27-30] This is due to the prevalence of improvised explosive devices (IEDs), which are in essence homemade bombs.[27-30] It is estimated that 20% of the soldiers injured in the Iraq war (some 4000 individuals to date) sustained TBI, often including damage to the peripheral or central aspects of the visual and vestibular systems.[27-30] As a result, Department of Defense and Veterans Affairs health care professionals are inundated with patients suffering from significant musculoskeletal and visual, vestibular sensory impairment.[31,32]

Less mortal but still morbid is the topic of mild traumatic brain injury (MTBI), commonly known as *concussion*.[32,33] MTBI is differentiated from TBI by the relative lesser degree of impairment and lack of pathologic findings on brain imaging. MTBI is most commonly associated with sports collisions but can occur with any head trauma. Current literature suggests that MTBI is commonplace in high school to professional level athletics but remains dramatically underreported.[32-36] It was previously assumed that patients suffering from MTBI would spontaneously recover if given adequate rest. However, some patients appear to suffer long-lasting postconcussive syndromes even when treated appropriately. Research in postconcussive syndromes suggests that for these individuals the difference between MTBI and TBI is very small indeed.[37,38] Furthermore, recent studies have identified an alarming inconsistency in the way MTBI is treated, which may delay or reduce recovery in both populations.[39] Orthopaedic rehabilitation specialists are often the first health care professionals to encounter individuals with MTBI. Recent studies suggest balance testing, measures of oculomotor coordination, and other forms of NMC assessment are more sensitive than history, symptom inventory, and neuropsychologic testing alone in detecting postconcussive problems.[40-48] Thus the orthopaedic specialist's skill in assessing NMC is at a premium.

The dramatic forces involved with motor vehicle accident (MVA) can result in a myriad of musculoskeletal injuries, especially whiplash-associated disorders (WAD). However, it is also well documented that post-MVA patients often report a wide variety of neurologic symptoms including dizziness, visual disturbance, and many others.[49-55] Numerous possible mechanisms such as MTBI, subclinical cervical instability, subclinical brainstem or cranial nerve injury, injury to the dura mater, depression, cervicogenic dizziness, and many others have been hypothesized. However, evidence for these hypotheses remains relatively low.[55-57] Perhaps this is due to previous narrow diagnostic criteria for the previously mentioned pathologic conditions or poor consistency in operational definitions in research on MVA. Regardless, the orthopaedic specialist who treats patients recovering from MVA can count on hearing these complaints. Further knowledge of sensory integration will improve the assessment and treatment of these patients.

Neck trauma, various systemic connective tissue disorders, and in some rare cases cervical manipulation are associated with clinical cervical spine instability (CCSI). CCSI can allow the atlas and dens of the axis to cause devastating injury to the vestibular, optic, abducens, oculomotor, trigeminal, and other vital brainstem nuclei and cranial nerves.[58-60] Likewise, the vertebral artery is subject to occlusion, functional insufficiency, vasospasm, or tearing. The tortuous pathway it takes through the upper cervical spine makes it susceptible to trauma in the form of whiplash mechanisms or in some rare instances cervical manipulation.[60,61] Significant vertebral artery insufficiency can result in transient abnormal function and in some cases damage to the same brainstem nuclei described previously.[60,61] Thus competent assessment of visual and vestibular sensory integra-

tion is key in identifying potentially catastrophic situations and helping patients access appropriate care.

Vestibular pathologic conditions can complicate differential diagnoses and interfere with orthopaedic manual therapies. Benign paroxysmal positional vertigo (BPPV) is regarded as the most common form of vestibular disorder diagnosed.[62-64] The prevalence of BPPV is estimated between 10 and 64 per 100,000 and possibly higher.[64] Vestibular neuronitis is the most common cause of unilateral peripheral vestibular hypofunction and has a prevalence of 1710 cases per million annually.[62,65] Meniere's disease is the most common form of unstable peripheral vestibular lesion and occurs at a rate of 500 cases per million per year.[62,65] Patients with these conditions often experience imbalance, vertigo, nausea, and/or visual disturbance, which are often provoked with common positioning for orthopaedic manual therapies and exercises.[62,65]

Vision is widely regarded as our primary sense but is typically taken for granted in musculoskeletal rehabilitation. Visual feedback affects head position, posture, ergonomics, accommodation to proprioceptive loss, and many other areas of orthopaedic practice.[66-70] This chapter explores the use of oculomotor NMC to improve visual sensory input and facilitate cervical stabilization.

Broadening awareness of sensory integration will also improve development of NMT programs. Research clearly shows sensory-specific drills provide for optimal NMT to improve balance, as well as joint stability of the extremities and spine. After completion of this chapter the reader will be able to optimize development of NMT programs by structuring them for correct sensory bias and the desired mechanism of NMC.

DEFINITION OF NEUROMUSCULAR CONTROL

Defining NMC is more difficult than it would appear. This is evidenced by a wide variety of operational definitions in the literature. Perhaps the most widely accepted is that offered by Williams et al. in 2001: "NMC ... involves the subconscious integration of sensory information that is processed by the central nervous system (CNS), resulting in controlled movement through coordinated muscle activity."[71] Put another way, NMC is how the body produces coordinated movement appropriate to the situational demands.

Perhaps variation of the definition of NMC has led to some misnomers about NMC in typical orthopaedic realms. For example, the terms *NMC* and *proprioception* are often used interchangeably. However, proprioception traditionally refers only to *joint position sense* and is derived by the processing of somatosensory information from specific touch, pressure, vibration, stretch, and tension receptors in connective tissues about the joint. NMC, on the other hand, is dependent on sensory integration of somatosensory, vestibular, and visual senses.[18,19,62,66,67] This illustrates another common misconception that the ability to balance is the same as proprioception. For example, many commonly used clinical tests of proprioception do not provide information about the effect of sensory deficit. Thus a patient with impaired somatosensory sensation common to orthopaedic injury could use his or her visual sense to compensate during single-leg stance with eyes open, producing a false-negative test of proprioception. To prevent this misunderstanding, it is necessary to have a rough understanding of how NMC is accomplished.

The computer-related terms *hardware* and *software* allow for a simplified explanation of the course of NMC. Sensory hardware in the form of end organs such as the somatosensory mechanoreceptors, vestibular apparatus, and eyes transduce sensory data from the environment into neural impulses, which are carried to the CNS by afferent peripheral nerves. Sensory integration refers to the accurate processing and weighting of the sensory data into meaningful information or an accurate perception of the environment.* Although many senses contribute to sensory integration, research shows somatosensory, vestibular, and vision are the primary senses involved in NMC. The CNS then compares this integrated perception to the desired goal and derives an error signal. Next it selects and grades the appropriate motor program to correct for the error signal and accomplish the given task.[19,20,62,72] This CNS processing, selection, and grading is likened to a computer running software. Finally motor hardware or motor neurons are recruited, resulting in the coordinated action of muscles to execute the correct motor response. Thus NMC is dependent on both sensory and motor hardware, as well as CNS software to provide accurate sensory integration and selection and grading of appropriate motor programs.

Feedback Versus Feed-Forward Neuromuscular Control

Depending on the situational need, the nervous system accomplishes NMC via two different but interrelated mechanisms. To achieve volitional movement requiring specific patterns and appropriate grading, the nervous system uses feedback NMC. As described previously, somatosensory, vestibular, and visual receptors transduce environmental stimuli into neural signals. These signals travel the ascending pathways to the CNS, where they are processed, resulting in the execution of specific and appropriate motor efferent signals to correct the body toward the desired goal.[19,20,62] However, specificity requires greater volumes of sensory data, which must be processed into meaningful information by the higher-order CNS hardware. Higher processing means neural signals must travel across a greater number of synapses and thus increase latency from stimulus to volitional movement; so production of specific motor response comes at the price of decreased speed. It appears the nervous system can produce a specific volitional motion in no faster than 120 ms, which is too slow for many situations such as recovery from tripping.[19,20,62]

Feed-forward NMC is the result of much lower-order nervous system processing. Because the neural impulses necessary for this lower-level processing cross fewer synapses, it is faster. Feed-forward NMC still very much relies on sensory afferent input, but the lower-level CNS processing results in selection of generalized and predictive motor programs.[19,62,66-68,70,71]

The most rapid form of feed-forward NMC is the monosynaptic arc or stretch reflex. Even in this case the afferent neural impulse must prorogate up the peripheral nerve, across one synapse in the spinal cord and back down the motor efferent, which takes 30 ms. Long loop reflexes to the brainstem travel a little farther and thus require 50 to 80 ms.[19,20,62] So for even the quickest of us, latency is involved in triggering human motion.

It is important to note that feedback and feed-forward NMC mechanisms work simultaneously to produce the symphony of human motion. For example, research suggests that normal walking is controlled by central pattern generators or software for the intricate muscle actions of bipedal gait.[19,62,72] These patterns are largely feed-forward in nature, but we use feedback NMC to modulate stride length, cadence, direction, and many other aspects of walking. Tripping on a curb still results in somatosensory, vestibular, and visual sensory input but in this case produces a feed-forward NMC response of stepping rapidly to increase the base of support in anticipation of the new position (and hopefully recovery of balance).

Triggered response is a hybrid of feedback and feed-forward NMC. It is believed that through practice the CNS can dramatically sensitize the response to sensory cues and select and execute the appropriate software within 80 to 120 ms.[19,62,73] Sports provide the most obvious example of triggered response. Hitting a ball traveling faster than 90 miles per hour requires hitters to swing where they anticipate the pitch will be when the ball is in range. Researchers hypothesize that NMT can increase the speed at which the CNS processes the sensory information to select the appropriate motor program whether for a baseball swing of postural sway.[3-12,18,19,62]

SENSORY NEUROANATOMY OF NEUROMUSCULAR CONTROL

This section will briefly review the specific neuroanatomy or hardware that provides the sensory afferent signal necessary for NMC. For ease of understanding, the sensory hardware is divided into somatosensory, vestibular, and visual sections. It is also important to note that sensory integration does not occur in one location of the CNS but rather is the result of the neural communication of all of the areas described.

Somatosensory

This broad category encompasses all forms of touch, pressure, vibration, and tension. As mentioned previously, the term *proprioception* refers to joint position sense and is the result of

---

*References 19, 20, 62, 66, 68, 70.

the integration of the information from all of these separate types of transducers. Research clearly shows degradation of somatosensory perception as we age.[73,74] This is thought to be a reflection of natural atrophy of the end organs.[73,74] Of the numerous discovered somatosensory receptors, the muscle spindles and Golgi tendon organs are thought to contribute the most pertinent sensory feedback used by the CNS to achieve NMC of joint stability.[2-12,71,75]

Muscle Spindles

Skeletal muscle is comprised of extrafusal fibers, which provide powerful muscle actions, and intrafusal fibers or muscle spindles, which house the sensory receptors. Spindle density (proportion of spindles or intrafusal fibers to extrafusal fibers) appears to be higher in the deeper, smaller muscles. This has prompted several researchers to hypothesize that smaller muscles may serve primarily as somatosensory receptors, as well as direct stabilizers.[76-78] Likewise, research suggests that the muscle spindles are primary sources of proprioceptive sensory information for all joints.[2-12,71,75]

As the name implies, *nuclear bag fibers* have circular or baglike nuclei clustered in the center of the intrafusal fiber. Quick stretches deform the bulbous center of the nuclear bag fiber first. This stimulates the annulospiral sensory endings, which wrap around the nuclear bag fibers and in turn depolarizes the primary afferent fiber of the spindle.[2-12,71,75]

Nuclear chain fibers have disclike nuclei stacked in series with the fiber. The proximal and distal aspects of the nuclear chain fibers are innervated by the flower spray endings. The nuclear chain fibers are thought to deform with slow prolonged stretches to the fiber because longer stretch times allow for more creep (because of the viscoelastic properties of muscle fiber). Thus slower prolonged stretches will stimulate the flower spray endings and in turn depolarize the secondary afferent fibers of the spindle.[2-12,71,75]

Both the primary and the secondary spindle afferents conduct neural impulses via the afferent aspect of the mixed peripheral nerve to the dorsal spinal nerve root and into the spinal cord. Once in the CNS, the afferent signal triggers a cascade of interneuron firing. The simplest of these is the monosynaptic reflex arc, which is formed by a single excitatory synapse between the dorsal root ganglion and the alpha motor neuron of the agonist muscle.[71,75] The result is that the stretched muscle exhibits greater motor unit recruitment for the most elementary form of feed-forward NMC. Ascending fibers carry the neural signal to the brainstem and cerebellum, providing for long loop reflexes, which is a slightly more complex form of feed-forward NMC. The sensory afferent fibers from the spindle also communicate with the antagonist muscle but via an inhibitory interneuron, resulting in decreased recruitment of the antagonist known as *reciprocal inhibition* (another form of feed-forward NMC).[75]

In addition, the dorsal root ganglion forms an excitatory synapse with the gamma motor neuron, which enervates the small contractile elements of the intrafusal fibers. This ensures that the intrafusal fiber will maintain a length proportional to

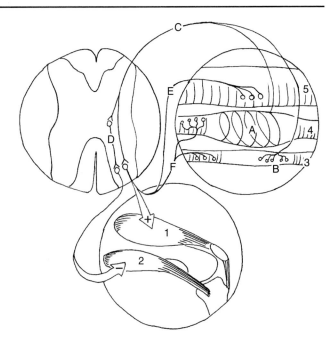

Figure 28-1 Muscle spindle diagram.

the extrafusal fiber. Thus the spindle can continue to transduce sensory information about muscle stretch regardless of muscle action (Figure 28-1). The dorsal root ganglion also initiates upward travel of the sensory signal via numerous interneuron connections to the cortex and other regions of the CNS for higher-level processing, allowing for slower but more precise and volitional feedback NMC.[75]

GOLGI TENDON ORGANS

Fibrous capsules in the tendon house weblike networks of collagen fibers (Figure 28-2). I beta afferent fibers perforate the capsules, allowing the free afferent endings to entangle with the collagen fibers. Tension causes deformation of the collagen fibers and in turn the free endings, thus stimulating the I beta afferent.[75] Tension sensory information in excess of the CNS set point (perceived point of danger to the tendon) stimulates the inverse myotatic reflex via an inhibitory interneuron to the alpha motor neuron of the agonist and an excitatory interneuron to the antagonist. The combined result is decreased tension and protection of the tendon.[75] This phenomenon is commonly observed as muscle tremors or outright failure during the eccentric muscle action of deconditioned individuals.

Vestibular Perception

The term *vestibular* arises from the inner chamber or vestibule of the ear. The delicate sensory end organs housed in the vestibule resemble a snail (Figure 28-3). The vestibular apparatus is housed in a thin bony shell, inside of which is the endolymphatic sac comprised of epithelial cells that secrete viscous endolymphatic fluid.[62]

The antennae of the snail make up the labyrinth named for the interconnected semicircular canals. The anterior and posterior canals are oriented at 45 degrees from the saggital plane but perpendicular to each other. They begin with the larger diameter ampulae of each respective canal just off the utricle (body of the snail) and then join together to form the common crus before reentering the utricle.[62,64] The horizontal canal is oriented at approximately 30 degrees superior to the transverse plane to match the slight downward head tilt typical of most

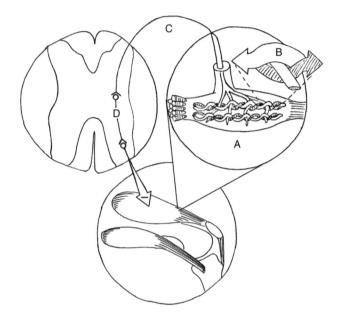

Figure 28-2 Golgi tendon organs.

upright movement.[62,64] The increased diameter of the ampluae houses the hair cell receptor. Each hair cell has a group of smaller stereocilia, which ramp in height as they connect to the larger kinocilium.[62] This arrangement ensures consistent movement of the hair cell in relation to relative motion between canal and endolymph. It also self-rights the hair cell after movement to ready it for new stimulation.[62,79,80]

With head rotation the viscous endolymph fluid remains relatively still thanks to inertia. As the hair cell is anchored to the moving labyrinth, it is dragged through the endolymph, causing it to bend. Bending the hair cell toward the larger kinocilium pulls on the receptor cell membrane, causing the ion channels to open, neurotransmitter release, and excitation of the respective branch of the vestibular nerve. Bending the hair cell away from the kinocilium closes the channels, thus inhibiting vestibular nerve firing.[62,79,80]

The utricle or body of the snail houses the otoliths, comprised of two sheets of gelatinous membranes. The macula is oriented to horizontal and the sacula to vertical. The otoliths are covered with a layer of otoconia, microscopic hexagonal-shaped calcium carbonate crystals. Otoconia enhance movement of the otoliths in response to linear acceleration, such as the pull of gravity when the head is tilted or changes in speed while riding in a car. Otoliths contain a variety of hair cells similar to kinocilium, so linear acceleration results in relative stimulation or inhibition of the branch of their respective branch of the vestibular nerve.[62,80,81]

Even with a perfectly still head, the vestibular nerves provide the CNS with a static firing rate of approximately 90 pulses per second.[62,79] The net result of the anatomy of the hair cells in the canals and otoliths described previously is that head rotation or tilt is excitatory to the vestibular nerve ipsilateral

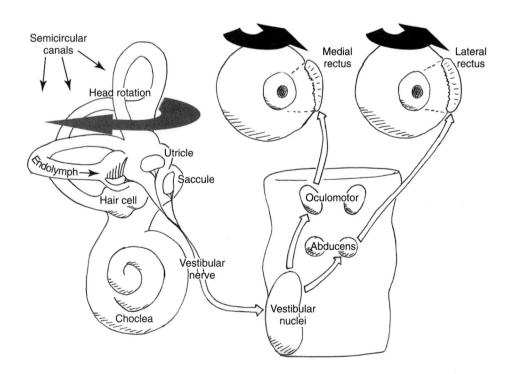

Figure 28-3 Vestibular apparatus.

to the direction of rotation or tilt while simultaneously inhibitory to the contralateral vestibular nerve. This is known as the *push and pull relationship* between vestibular sensory stimulation and modulation of peripheral vestibular nerve firing (see Figure 28-3).[62,80,81]

Peripheral vestibular sensory signals are initially processed in the vestibular nuclei of the brainstem; from there a cascade of interneurons fire to other brainstem nuclei, the cerebellum (particularly the vermis), and the cortex. Signals traveling upward to the higher cortical centers are used for more specific volitional movements or feedback NMC. Signals traveling along reflexive pathways in the brainstem or downward such as the vestibulospinal, vestibulocollic, and vestibuloocular reflexes will result in faster predictive feed-forward NMC.[62,79-81]

The "snail shell" is the cochlea, which transduces sound but is not discussed here. However, it is important to note that because of their close proximity in the vestibule, vertigo, equilibrium upset, and hearing loss often occur together.[62]

Visual Perception

Visual perception starts when light reflects off objects in the environment, travels through the eye, and excites the rods and cones of the retina. These visual sensory end organs transduce light photons into a neural signal, which travels along the optic nerve to the visual cortices allowing for visual perception.* However, not all parts of the human retina are created equally. The fovea of the retina contains the highest density of retinal receptors and thus provides high acuity but extremely narrow area of focal vision. As the name implies, *peripheral vision* comes from the edges of the retina. Although a vital part of visual perception, it is not useful for fine motor tasks or depth perception.†

Then how do humans perceive a very rich visual perception of the environment in most situations? It appears that ocular NMC allows for continuous targeting of foveal vision onto different areas of the environment. This detail-loaded visual memory of the foveal sensory perception is maintained until retargeting of foveal vision occurs and the CNS perception of vision is updated.[29,31,39] One way to think of this is to imagine a photographer continuously pointing and shooting huge amounts of quick snapshots and then placing them in a continually evolving mosaic. So we can state that ocular NMC allows for targeting of foveal vision or "pointing the camera" and is a prerequisite to allow for normal visual perception. The reader can gain personal awareness of this phenomenon of foveal visual perception by following the directions in Box 28-1.

Ocular NMC involves the complex interaction of three mechanisms. It was previously thought that smooth pursuit was initiated only with visual feedback, whereas saccades were more reflexive or feed-forward in nature. However, recent

---

BOX 28-1 Foveal Visual Perception Experience

- Focus your vision on this X.
- Next you will attempt to read a word from several lines below the X without moving your eyes. Have a friend give the signal to read the next word while he or she watches your eyes.
- The observer will note the eyes move whenever you attempt to read a few lines down.
- This illustrates the very narrow field of foveal or focal vision, as well as the need for ocular neuromuscular control (NMC) to target the foveal visual field.

---

research suggests smooth pursuit and saccades work in tandem to provide ideal ocular NMC.[83,84]

Smooth pursuits have reaction times or latencies in response to randomized direction targets of 80 to 100 degrees.[62,83] However, although relatively fast to initiate, the speed of tracking is relatively slow, less than 100 degrees per second.[62,83] Thus smooth pursuit is the ocular NMC mechanism used most when the goal is matching the velocity of a slow-moving target.* Saccadic latencies for randomized targets have been reported as 200 to 250 ms. However, although longer in reaction time, saccadic movement results in a much faster (up to 600 degrees per second) movement of the eye.[79,83] Thus saccades are used to change visual targeting rapidly or to reacquire a target that has drifted off of the fovea.[30,39,79,83]

Watching a tennis match is a classic example of the interaction of smooth pursuit and saccadic eye movement. As a slow-moving lob falls, the spectator uses smooth pursuit to track the ball. However, when the racquet strikes the ball, it moves rapidly. The speed of the ball outpaces the ability of smooth pursuit to track the ball, resulting in retinal slip of the image out of the fovea. This stimulus triggers a saccade to catch up or retarget the focal vision onto the ball's new location.

Recent studies have confirmed that smooth pursuit and saccades share CNS neuronal pathways but have segregated areas within each region. A very simplified explanation of the pathways is as follows. Optic flow is propagated along the optic nerves to the temporal, posterior parietal, and frontal aspects of the cortex. Complex interneuronal connections link the cortex to the pons and the cerebellum. The oculomotor vermis of the cerebellum sends neural impulses to the smooth pursuit and saccadic centers of the brainstem, which in turn stimulates the oculomotor and abducens nuclei to recruit appropriate muscle action in the extraocular muscles to move the eyes.[83]

Vergence refers to the ability of both eyes to point at the same target. This is often referred to as *teaming,* as with horse-drawn carriages that required a team of horses to go in the same direction. Humans share with most predatory mammals the anatomic placement of two slightly offset eyes in the front of the skull. This offset alignment allows the CNS slightly different

---

*References 18, 19, 26, 31, 39, 68.
†References 18, 19, 26, 39, 80, 82.

*References 30, 31, 39, 62, 79, 82, 84.

perspectives on the same target, which is crucial for accurate perception of depth or distance to a target.[39,82] This is similar to the principle of triangulation that is used in navigation and weapons targeting. The distances from two or more established positions (in this case the perspective from each eye) can be used to accurately calculate a third target position. Foveal retinal stimulation triggers the chain of events, causing each eye to move inwards (converge) or outwards (diverge) proportionate to the depth of the target.[82] Strabismus (commonly referred to as a *lazy eye*) or lack of one eye to coordinate movement with the other is a clinical disorder, which greatly affects depth perception. These clinical conditions are often overlooked as affecting orthopaedic conditions. In addition, recent research shows that many of those assumed to have normal vergence actually have subtle deficits affecting their visual depth perception and thus overall NMC.[30,31,39,66-69]

Orthopaedic professionals know that the cervical spine normally provides large amounts of head motion necessary for many daily activities. Other routine activities result in relatively low-amplitude head movements but with high-frequency oscillation of rotation or tilting. For example, driving or riding in an automobile typically results in head movement oscillations in excess of 5 Hz.[79] Running can result in head velocities up to 550 degrees per second and oscillation up to 20 Hz.[79] However, because the orbit is contained in the skull, head motion results in eye motion. The vestibular ocular reflex (VOR) acts to compensate for the effect of head motion on vision. The VOR consists of the sensory action of the vestibular apparatus (described previously) stimulating the vestibular nuclei in the brainstem. From there, excitatory tracts connect to the oculomotor nuclei, which in turn send efferent signals to the extraocular muscles. The neural hardware is arranged such that head rotation results in contralateral eye movement in the same plane.[79,82,85,86]

The theoretical optimal gain or ratio between head movement and resulting eye movement to provide stable gaze would be 1.0 (or a 1:1 ratio). However, study of VOR in healthy subjects found the actual VOR gain to be 0.75 or less, suggesting multiple mechanisms of gaze stabilization.[87] In subjects with vestibular injury the gain can decrease to 0.35, resulting in the phenomenon of oscillopsia often described as jumpy or even double vision by patients.[87,86] Research also suggests that injured and older subjects compensate for reductions in VOR performance with the cervical ocular reflex (COR), corrective saccades, and various other mechanisms. The COR is similar to the VOR in that it produces eye movement contralateral to head motion but it is stimulated by cervical somatosensation as opposed to the vestibular apparatus. In addition, it does not appear to function well at speeds over 1.0 Hz, which is insufficient for many sports and daily activities.[54,79,85,87]

It is important to note that all of the previously mentioned mechanisms of ocular NMC operate simultaneously with nearly all visual activities.* Any visual targeting involves the same

---

*References 30, 31, 39, 68, 79, 82, 85.

extra ocular muscles and nervous hardware. The difference is the CNS software or programming involved. A driver uses smooth pursuit to track other cars but also performs numerous saccades to check the rearview mirror, sideview mirror, blind spots, and other potential road hazards. Likewise his or her eyes are continuously diverging and converging as they look at targets with differing depths inside the vehicle, such as the dashboard displays, audio-visual devices, cell phones, passengers, and eventually back to the road. Because driving results in oscillatory head movement in excess of 5.0 Hz, the driver simultaneously uses the VOR to sustain accurate targeting despite the head movement. Understanding the individual mechanisms of ocular NMC allows the rehabilitation professional to more accurately assess impairments affecting visual sensory perception and thus design specific programs to improve his or her NMT programs. Later in this chapter the author discusses how the same knowledge base will allow for cervical stabilization.

ALTERED SENSORY INTEGRATION IN ORTHOPAEDICS

The intricate sensory organs described previously provide for some of the nervous system's elegant redundancy. If one sense is impaired or processed inappropriately, then the CNS can call on other senses to determine body position in relation to the desired target and still arrive at effective NMC. However, this assumes effective sensory integration occurs. Multiple streams of sensory information are only useful if they agree. Many cases in orthopaedic practice show this does not occur as automatically as people would wish. For example, research demonstrates that most musculoskeletal injuries result in decreased somatosensory perception, more commonly labeled *proprioception* in orthopaedic literature. This is hypothesized to be from direct loss of somatosensory receptors with tissue disruption or from habituation of pressure receptors secondary to increased fluid pressure with edema. However, almost immediately the CNS reweights its sensory perception to favor visual input. This compensation is effective in regaining NMC of volitional movement but can leave these individuals somewhat dependent on vision. They will likely display inaccurate NMC in any situation that distorts visual sensory input such as walking to the bathroom in a dark house. Visual compensation will not carry over to the situational demand of joint stabilization in response to perturbation; research shows this situation requires feed-forward NMC based on somatosensory input.[2-12,71] Understanding altered sensory integration allows the rehabilitation professional to better detect the underlying impairments, which set up poor NMC.

Vertigo

In extreme cases, incorrect sensory integration can result in dramatically altered perceptions of reality such as vertigo, an abnormal sense of motion. One way to explain the phenomenon of vertigo is to relate it to a common shared experience. For example, a driver at a stop light has a bus next to him or her pull forward. For a brief period the driver is uncertain as to whether the bus was moving forward or the driver's car is rolling backward. This abnormal sense of motion or vertigo occurs because the bus takes up the majority of the visual field; when the bus moves, it provides the same visual stimulus the driver would see if his or her car was rolling backwards. Thus the CNS misinterprets the information, resulting in inaccurate sensory integration (i.e., the false sense of rolling backwards). This misperception of backward motion produces an incorrect response to slam on the brakes.

However, for most people the abnormal sense of rolling backwards quickly dissipates. This is because correct sensory integration occurs as the CNS rapidly processes alternate streams of information to regain accurate perception of the environment. For example, when the driver looks forward, the distance to an object ahead has not increased. The otoliths do not detect a change in linear acceleration, which would happen with rolling backwards. No change in pressure receptors occurs on the back of the body (somatosensory), which would occur with rolling backwards because of the inertia of the body.

This example has great clinical use in explaining the phenomenon of vertigo (an abnormal sense of motion). Unfortunately, this condition is common in patients with injury to the peripheral vestibular sensory organs or the CNS structures that process vestibular data. When exposed to this kind of visual or other stimuli, they cannot rely on accurate vestibular input to reference for sensory integration and thus have difficulty regaining a normal perception of being stationary. However, through programmatic sensory exposure or deprivation these patients can often learn to reweigh their perception of somatosensory and visual senses (sensitization) and recalibrate their perception of the skewed vestibular sense (habituation).[62,80,81]

Definition of Dynamic Joint Stabilization

Dynamic joint stabilization is the maintenance of optimal joint alignment via restraint of potentially destructive forces.

Although the term *dynamic joint stabilization* is often considered synonymous with NMC, it is actually the result of appropriate NMC. To move the human body, larger muscles must produce significant amounts of torque to propel it. However, this produces intrinsic and ground reaction forces that must be counteracted to maintain the joint center near the instantaneous axis of rotation. This ensures optimal muscle length-tension relationships, allows efficient movement, and prevents tissues from reaching the point of injury. No doubt exists that these potentially destructive forces are restrained by noncontractile tissues such as ligaments and fibrocartilage. However, research clearly shows that conditions with recurrent instability and pain correlate with impaired NMC even when ligamentous integrity has been restored.[3-15,88] Likewise, evidence clearly validates NMT as the preferred intervention to restore dynamic joint stability.[3-14,88] Box 28-2 outlines a simple clinical analogy for the role of NMC in dynamic joint stabilization.

BOX 28-2 Clinical Analogy for Neuromuscular Control and Dynamic Joint Stabilization

- Shake hands and note the wrist naturally assumes an efficient position. Move the patient's wrist into flexion or extension and it loses efficiency as the tissues are stretched or compressed respectively (and could eventually result in injury).
- Instruct the patient that you will attempt to move his or her wrist slowly out of position while he or she maintains the desired position. This is an analogy for feedback neuromuscular control (NMC), because the patient has advanced warning of what will happen and can plan a specific volitional response based on all of the different sensory inputs.
- Perform the same activity but this time without warning as to when you will move the wrist and with the patient's eyes closed. This is the analogy for feed-forward NMC, because the patient has to react predictively. This will also lead into an explanation of the need for perturbation with a somatosensory-biased condition to train dynamic joint stabilization of any joint.
- Note: Some patients will react to either of these situations by preemptively gripping firmly. Although effective, it is inefficient because one cannot grip all the time. This is a fair analogy for maladaptive muscle spasm common with instabilities.

Definition of Balance

"Balance is maintenance of the center of gravity over the base of support."[18]

Another common misconception is that balance and NMC are synonymous. But just as with dynamic joint stabilization, balance is really one expression of NMC. For example, a martial artist who falls is by this definition out of balance. However, he or she can still use NMC to alter his or her body position while falling and disperse the effect over multiple body parts. Because balance is well-defined, it can be measured. This section will provide an overview of commonly used measures of balance and the evidence of their clinical use. In addition, because balance and dynamic joint stabilization are both expressions of NMC, it is very common to see some of the same balance measures used as indirect measures of dynamic joint stabilization for the lower extremities.

EVIDENCE-BASED ASSESSMENT OF NEUROMUSCULAR CONTROL AND BALANCE FOR ORTHOPAEDICS

In possibly more than any other realm of practice, advancing technologies allow for reliable, valid, and sensitive clinical measurement of postural NMC and balance. Computerized posturography systems use force plate technology to provide a highly accurate measurement of the center of pressure (from which the center of mass can be inferred) in relation to the base of support or specific targets. The Modified Clinical Test of Sensory Integration and Balance (MCTSIB) measures performance of the motor task of static balance under the sensory-biased conditions of firm and compliant surfaces with eyes open and closed. When performed on computerized posturography platforms, data on postural sway can be quantified and with some systems analyzed in comparisons to normative models.[86,89-92] The Sensory Organization Test (SOT), available on the Smart Balance Master, uses the same sensory-biasing principles with the addition of perturbation to allow for true quantitative analysis of feed-forward NMC referred to as *computerized dynamic posturography* (Figure 28-4).[86,89-93] The Shuttle Balance by Shuttle Systems holds great promise as a lower-technology assessment (and training) tool for feed-forward NMC. These tests can provide the clinician with vital information about somatosensory, vestibular, and visual sensory integration. NeuroCom International Inc., makers of the Balance Master line have long been the industry leader in the manufacture of computerized posturography and dynamic posturography (CDP) (Figure 28-5). More recently, several new manufacturers such as Vestibular Technologies have introduced systems for computerized posturography with their CAPS line.

Although these systems have exceptional clinical use, one criticism voiced by some in orthopaedics is their expense. The continued efforts of these manufacturers are making computerized posturography a reality for more orthopaedic practitioners. In the meantime, some reliable and valid, but less sensitive, clinical tests exist for even the smallest budget.

The MCTSIB was originally designed as a stand-alone clinical test without the aid of computerized posturography (Figure 28-6). The subject attempts to stand as still as possible in a comfortable stance on a firm surface with eyes open and then closed for 20 seconds per each trial. The therapist makes qualitative observations about postural sway, balance motor strategies, and patient report of symptoms. Falls are also noted and at what time they occur in the trial. This is repeated while the patient stands on a piece of medium-density foam (60 kg/m³, load deflection 80 to 90 kg). Patients with difficulty balancing on the firm surface with the eyes closed are thought to have difficulty integrating somatosensory information. However, patients who cannot perform well on the compliant foam surface with eyes closed have difficulty integrating vestibular information. When testing is performed in this way, the clinician can obtain a rough idea of the patient's sensory integration.[86,89,92]

The Balance Error Scoring System (BESS) uses similar sensory conditions but omits the eyes open (visual biased) conditions because these are less sensitive in detecting abnormal NMC (Figure 28-7). The subject is asked to maintain balance with hands on hips and eyes closed in three postures: (1) feet together, (2) on one foot, and (3) tandem stance on a firm floor. Then the same postures are performed on a piece of 10 cm–thick medium-density foam. Errors are noted during the 20-second trials over each of the six sensory conditions. A higher number of errors indicate poor NMC. Control subjects committed an average of nine errors over the six trials. Higher

Table 28-1	Sample Data Sheet for Balance Error Scoring System (BESS)

Subject attempts to balance for 20 seconds with hands on iliac crest and eyes closed for all conditions following:

Balance errors following = 1 point per error

Average in controls = 9 errors

Low score = good neuromuscular control (NMC)

Hands off iliac crest

Open eyes

Step, stumble, or fall

Hip more than 30 degrees flexion or abduction

Lift forefoot or heel

Out of the test position >5 seconds

Firm Surface:

Double-leg stance

Single-leg stance

Tandem stance

Foam surface:

Double-leg stance

Single-leg stance

Tandem stance

Total Errors

number of errors with eyes-closed, firm-surface conditions suggests difficulty with somatosensory integration. A higher number of errors with eyes closed on foam suggest difficulty integrating vestibular sensory input. A sample data sheet for the BESS can be found in Table 28-1.

The BESS has been shown to have good test-retest reliability and to correlate well with computerized balance tests examining sensory integration but requires only a level floor and piece of foam.[94-96] Some research has shown a mild learning effect with the BESS, which indicates it may best serve as a screening tool for suspected postconcussive patients or as a sensory-specific measure of balance in any patient but perhaps administered less frequently as a postintervention test.[95] Similarly, research showed that fatigue increased the number of errors on the BESS, suggesting it is best administered when the athlete has at least 20 minutes of rest after exercise.[96]

The Berg Balance Scale (BBS) is highly reliable between raters and correlates well with other efficacious measures of standing balance (a sample data sheet for the BBS can be found in Table 28-2). In previous retrospective studies, subjects who scored below a cutoff point of 45/56 on the BBS were found more likely to fall than those scoring higher than 45.[20-22,97,98] Unfortunately, misunderstanding of the original findings led to inappropriate analysis of the BBS using a dichotomous scale (greater than 45/56 indicating not at risk for falling, 45 or less indicating at risk for falls).[98,99] However, in a recent prospective clinical trial, Muir et al.[99] demonstrated use of the BBS with a dichotomized scale (45/56 cutoff point) actually had poor specificity and sensitivity in predicting falls.[99] Instead, analysis of the BBS using likelihood ratios scored over divisions of the range of test scores allowed for accurate grading of risk for multiple falls. They found that patients with BBS scores of 40

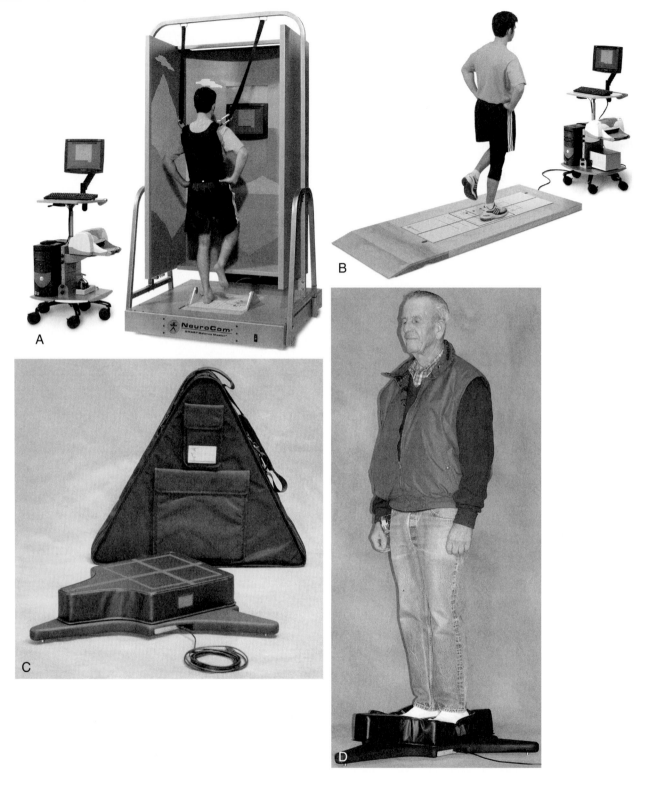

Figure 28-4 A-D, Neurocom and vestibular technologies stock photos. (**A-B** courtesy NeuroCom International, Clackamas, Oregon; **C-D** courtesy Vestibular Technologies, Cheyenne, Wyoming.)

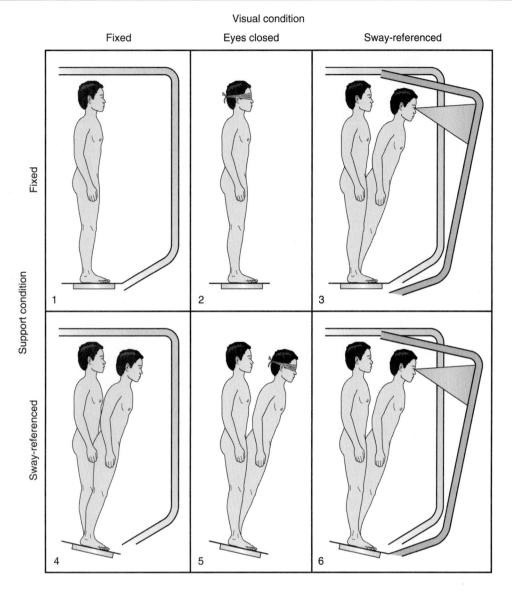

Figure 28-5 Support and visual conditions for the Sensory Organization Test (SOT). (From Cameron MC, Monroe LH: Physical rehabilitation: evidence-based examination, evaluation, and intervention. St Louis, 2007, Saunders.)

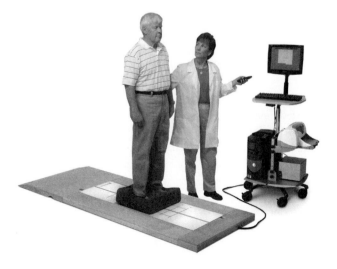

Figure 28-6 Modified Clinical Test of Sensory Integration and Balance (MCTSIB) stand alone. (Courtesy NeuroCom International, Clackamas, Oregon.)

to 44/56 were 2.07 times more likely to have multiple falls; patients with BBS scores less than 40 were 5.19 times more likely to have multiple falls.[99] Other research suggests that a change of 1 point on the BBS can be considered a clinically significant change in balance.[20] A 6-point change in the BBS can be considered clinically significant in patients suffering from cerebral vascular accident.[100] This test offers the clinician an efficacious test of standing balance that does not require any equipment except a step stool, chair, and tape measure.

Further studies showed a short-form BBS with a condensed 3-point scoring scale (7-Item BBS-3P) (Table 28-3) was reliable, offered as good concurrent validity and psychometric properties as the original BBS, but took less time in clinic to administer.[22] Although this form of the test is very efficient, many clinicians may prefer the original format because it allows for direct observation of functional goals such as reaching and transfers.

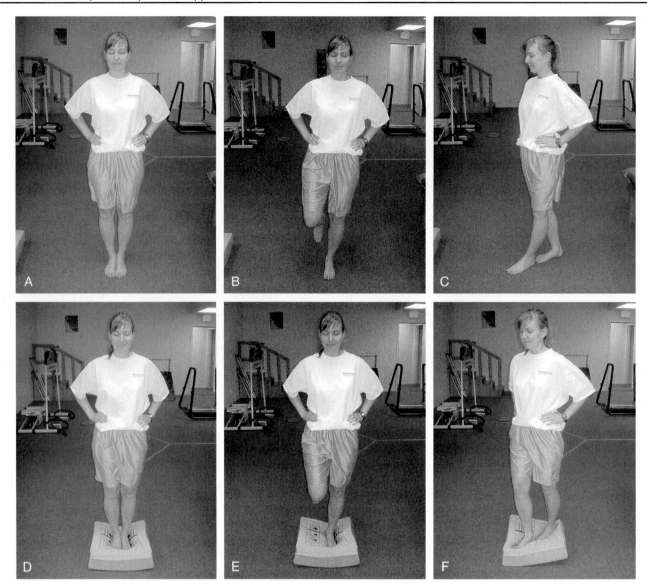

Figure 28-7 A-F, BESS.

The Dynamic Gait Index (DGI) is another low-technology clinical test that provides efficient assessment of balance and aspects of sensory integration (Table 28-4). It has been shown to have excellent intrarater and interrater reliability in numerous patient populations, including those living in the community, in assistive facilities, and those with vestibular pathologic conditions.[23,101] A score of less than 19/24 indicates the patient is at risk for falling.[23] This makes the DGI a widely accepted clinical outcomes measure for any patient with imbalance or conditions affecting gait. The DGI consists of eight physical tasks performed while walking, which are scored on a 4-point scale (0 is severely impaired, whereas 3 is normal ability). Evidence indicates that the eight subcomponents of the DGI have varying degrees of difficulty related to the type and number of sensory demands.[102] Thus some clinicians administer the test in progressive order of difficulty to put patients at ease. Low scores with horizontal and vertical head turns, as well as pivot turn, may be suggestive of vestibular loss.[101]

Similar to the BBS a Four-Item DGI (Table 28-5) has been developed that is reliable, holds good concurrent validity with, and has similar psychometric properties to the original DGI. More research is required to determine if the Four-Item DGI will hold the same predictive value of fallers.[103]

Rehabilitation professionals are often asked to determine the need for assistive devices by patients, their families, or other health professionals. Because the BBS and DGI are both predictive of falls, they can help the clinician decide if an assistive device is required to improve patient safety. Deciding what level of assistive device is always a compromise between safety and energy efficiency.

Table 28-2	Sample Data Sheet for Berg Balance Scale (BBS)

Circle the Score for Each Component   Total Score = _____ /56

40-44 = 2.07 Times More Likely to Have Multiple Falls
<40 = 5.19 Times More Likely to Have Multiple Falls

Sit Unsupported

4 = Sits safely × 2 minutes
3 = Sits × 2 minutes with supervision
2 = Sits × 30 seconds
1 = Sits × 10 seconds
0 = Unable to sit without support × 10 seconds

Sit to Stand

4 = Stands, stabilize independent no hands
3 = Stands independently using hands
2 = Stands using hands, more than one attempt
1 = Minimal assist to stand or stabilize
0 = Moderate to maximal assist to stand

Stand Unsupported

4 = Stand safely × 10 seconds
3 = Stand × 10 seconds with supervision
2 = Stand × 3 seconds
1 = Able to stand <3 seconds
0 = Cannot perform

Stand Eyes Closed

4 = Stand safely × 10 seconds
3 = Stand × 10 seconds with supervision
2 = Stand × 3 seconds
1 = Stand <3 seconds
0 = Cannot perform

Stand with Feet Together

4 = Places feet together, stands × 1 minute
3 = As previously mentioned but requires supervision
2 = Places feet together, stand × 30 seconds
1 = Help to position, stand × 15 seconds
0 = Cannot perform

Forward Reach

4 = Reach forward confidently >10 inches
3 = Reach forward safely >5 inches
2 = Reach forward safely >2 inches
1 = Reach forward with supervision
0 = Needs help to prevent fall

Retrieve Object From Floor

4 = Able to pick up object and stand safely
3 = Picks up object but requires supervision
2 = Unable to retrieve, within 2 inches safely
1 = Unable to retrieve, supervision while trying
0 = Cannot perform

Turn to Look Behind

4 = Looks behind both sides, good weight shift
3 = Looks behind one side only
2 = Turns sideways only, maintains balance
1 = Needs supervision while turning
0 = Needs assistance to prevent fall

Turn 360 degrees

4 = Turns safely in <4 seconds, left, right
3 = Turns safely in <4 seconds, one direction
2 = Turns safely in >4 seconds
1 = Needs close supervision or verbal cues
0 = Cannot perform

Alternating Stool Touch

4 = Safely completes eight steps in 20 seconds
3 = Safely completes eight steps in >20 seconds
2 = Safely completes four steps
1 = Completes two steps with supervision
0 = Cannot perform

Tandem Stance

4 = Places feet independent, hold × 30 seconds
3 = Places foot in front of other in 30 seconds
2 = Small step independent, hold × 30 seconds
1 = Assist to place feet, holds × 15 seconds
0 = Cannot perform

Stand on One Foot

4 = Able to lift one leg & hold >10 seconds
3 = Able to lift one leg & hold 5-10 seconds
2 = Able to lift one leg & hold 3-4 seconds
1 = Lifts one leg & holds <3 seconds
0 = Cannot perform

Stand to Sit

4 = Sit safely minimal use of hands
3 = Controls descent with use of hands
2 = Controls descent with back of legs on chair
1 = Sits independent but uncontrolled descent
0 = Requires assist to sit

Transfers

4 = Transfers safely, minor use of hands
3 = Transfers safely, must use hands
2 = Transfers safely, verbal cues or supervision
1 = One-person assist
0 = Two-person assist

From Berg K, Wood-Dauphinee S, Williams JI, et al: Measuring balance in the elderly: validation of an instrument, Can J Public Health 2(suppl):S7-S11, 1992; Berg K, Wood-Dauphinee S, Williams JI, et al: Measuring balance in the elderly: preliminary development of an instrument, Physiother Can 41:304-311, 1989.

Table 28-3	**Sample Data Sheet for 7-Item Berg Balance Scale, 3-Level Scale**

Circle the Score for Each Component   Total Score =_____/56

Under 45 Indicates Increased Risk for Falls
Score Change of 6 Points Clinically Significant

Forward Reach

4 = Reach forward confidently >10 inches
2 = Reach forward safely >5 inches
2 = Reach forward safely >2 inches
2 = Reach forward with supervision
0 = Needs help to prevent fall

Stand Eyes Closed

4 = Stand safely × 10 seconds
2 = Stand × 10 seconds with supervision or
2 = Stand × 3 seconds or
2 = Stand <3 seconds
0 = Cannot perform

Tandem Stance

4 = Places feet independent, hold × 30 seconds
2 = Places foot in front of other in 30 seconds
2 = Small step independent, hold × 30 seconds
2 = Assist to place feet, hold × 15 seconds
0 = Cannot perform

Turn to Look Behind

4 = Looks behind both sides, good weight shift
2 = Looks behind one side only or
2 = Turns sideways only, maintain balance or
2 = Needs supervision while turning
0 = Needs assistance to prevent fall

Retrieve Object From Floor

4 = Able to pick up object and stand safely
2 = Picks up object but requires supervision or
2 = Unable to retrieve, within 2 inches safely
2 = Unable to retrieve, supervision while trying
0 = Cannot perform

Stand on One Foot

4 = Able to lift one leg and hold >10 seconds
2 = Able to lift one leg and hold 5-10 seconds or
2 = Able to lift one leg and hold 3-4 seconds or
2 = Lifts one leg and hold <3 seconds
0 = Cannot perform

Sit to Stand

4 = Stands, stabilize independent no hands
2 = Stands independently using hands or
2 = Stands using hands, more than one attempt
2 = Minimal assist to stand or stabilize
0 = Moderate to maximal assist to stand

> ### Clinical Tip
>
> Rehabilitation professionals are often asked to determine the need for assistive devices by patients, their families, or other health professionals. Because the BBS and DGI are both predictive of falls, they can help the clinician decide if an assistive device is required to improve patient safety. Deciding what level of assistive device is always a compromise between safety and energy efficiency.

The Functional Gait Assessment (FGA) is an extension of the DGI that provides a higher degree of difficulty in testing, which may be useful in assessing athletes or any patients that may experience a ceiling effect with the DGI (Table 28-6). It consists of the original DGI, minus the stepping around obstacles component but with the addition of three more challenging components: (1) gait with narrow base of support, (2) gait with eyes closed, and (3) ambulating backwards.[102] The scoring scale remains the same as the DGI but with a maximum possible score of 30 reflecting the new test components. It appears to have good reliability and validity.[102]

The Star Excursion Balance Test (SEBT) is a simple, cost-effective, reliable clinical test of lower-extremity NMC and balance, which provides robust predictive value of ankle injury (Figure 28-8) (Table 28-7).[104-108] Its current form represents the culmination of extensive prior research to refine the test from earlier versions to improve reliability and validity in predicting injury. Because of its validity in predicting injury or reinjury, the SEBT is particularly useful as a functional outcome measure and in return-to-sport decisions.[104-108]

To perform the test, it is helpful to tape three intersecting lines on the floor at 120 degrees from each other (a goniometer helps with this). The patient stands with the stance foot placed so that the toes are just inside the intersection of the lines. The patient reaches with the contralateral leg as far as possible along the three lines. After six practice trials the tester measures the maximum reach in each distance obtained over three trials. The subject must maintain the stance with one foot flat on the floor while the other foot reaches and returns to the start position without touching the floor.[108] To obtain normalized reach distance (NRD), the reach distance is divided by the subject's leg length as measured from the anterior superior iliac spine of the pelvis to the lateral malleolus. A composite NRD of 94% or lower was associated with significant increased risk of injury for all athletes (especially female athletes). Similarly, a difference between the left and right anterior reach distance of more than 4 cm was associated with increased risk of injury.[108]

Table 28-4	**Sample Data Sheet for Dynamic Gait Index (DGI)**

Circle the Score for Each Component   Total Score =_____/24

Under 19 Indicates at Risk for Falls

Around Obstacles

3 = Walks around two cones, no change in speed or balance

2 = Slows down and adjusts steps

1 = Must stop first or requires cueing

0 = Cannot perform without assistance

Speed Change: 5 Feet at Average, Slow, and Fast

3 = Significant change in speed, good balance

2 = Mild gait deviations or not a significant change in speed or uses a device

1 = Only minor change in speed or changes speed with significant deviation or changes speed with loss of balance

0 = Cannot change speeds or loss of balance, requires outside support

Stairs—Ascend and Descend

3 = Alternating feet, no rail

2 = Alternating feet, must use rail

1 = Two feet to a step, must use rail

0 = Cannot perform safely

Pivot Turn

3 = 3-Second turn, no loss of balance

2 = >3-Second turn, no loss of balance

1 = Slow with imbalance

0 = Cannot turn safely, requires assist

Over Obstacles

3 = No change in speed or imbalance

2 = Slows down or has to adjust steps to clear

1 = Must stop before stepping over the box

0 = Cannot perform without assistance

Vertical Head Turn

3 = Turns head smoothly, no change in gait

2 = Turns head smoothly with minor change in gait or uses devices

1 = Turns head with signs of imbalance

0 = Severe disruption to gait, loss of balance, or staggers and reaches for wall

Level Walking

3 = No devices, normal speed and pattern, steady

2 = Uses devices, slow, mild deviations

1 = Imbalance, slow, abnormal pattern

0 = Cannot walk 20 feet, severe deviation, imbalance

Horizontal Head Turn

3 = Turns head smoothly, no change in gait

2 = Turns head smoothly with minor change in gait or uses devices

1 = Turns head with signs of imbalance

0 = Severe disruption to gait, loss of balance or staggers and reaches for wall

From Herdman SJ: Vestibular rehabilitation, ed 2, Philadelphia, 2000, FA Davis; Shumway-Cook A, Woollacott M: Motor control theory and applications, Baltimore, 1995, Williams & Wilkins, pp 323-324.

Table 28-5	**Sample Data Sheet for Four-Item Dynamic Gait Index (DIG) (Four-Item DGI)**

Circle the Score for Each Component   Total Score =_____/12

Level Walking

3 = No devices, normal speed and pattern, steady

2 = Uses devices, slow, mild deviations

1 = Imbalance, slow, abnormal pattern

0 = Cannot walk 20 feet, severe deviation, imbalance

Vertical Head Turn

3 = Turns head smoothly, no change in gait

2 = Turns head smoothly with minor change in gait or uses devices

1 = Turns head with signs of imbalance

0 = Severe disruption to gait, loss of balance, or staggers and reaches for wall

Speed Change: 5 Feet at Average, Slow, Fast

3 = Significant change in speed, good balance

2 = Mild gait deviations or not a significant change in speed or uses a device

1 = Only minor change in speed or changes speed with significant deviation or changes speed with loss of balance

0 = Cannot change speeds or loss of balance, requires outside support

Horizontal Head Turn

3 = Turns head smoothly, no change in gait

2 = Turns head smoothly with minor change in gait or uses devices

1 = Turns head with signs of imbalance

0 = Severe disruption to gait, loss of balance, or staggers and reaches for wall

MEASURES OF OCULAR NEUROMUSCULAR CONTROL

As with balance testing, computerized testing suites allow for highly reliable, sensitive, and specific testing of oculomotor function.[109-114] Micromedical has long been an industry standard, but recently NeuroCom International Inc. and Vestibular Technologies have entered this field. Unassisted clinical examination can still help the orthopaedic clinician in identifying sensory deficits common with diagnosis of TBI, MTBI, CCSI, and vestibular pathologic conditions.

The Northeastern State University College of Optometry (NSUCO) Oculomotor Test (also referred to as the *Maples test*) is an excellent clinical measure of smooth pursuit and saccadic

Table 28-6   Sample Data Sheet for Functional Gait Assessment (FGA)

Circle the Score for Each Component   Total Score = _____/30

Stairs—Ascend and Descend

3 = Alternating feet, no rail
2 = Alternating feet, must use rail
1 = Two feet to a step, must use rail
0 = Cannot perform safely

Over Obstacles

3 = No change in speed or imbalance
2 = Slows down or has to adjust steps to clear
1 = Must stop before stepping over the box
0 = Cannot perform without assistance

Level Walking

3 = No devices, normal speed and pattern, steady
2 = Uses devices, slow, mild deviations
1 = Imbalance, slow, abnormal pattern
0 = Cannot walk 20 feet, severe deviation, imbalance

Speed Change: 5 Feet at Average, Slow, Fast

3 = Significant change in speed, good balance
2 = Mild gait deviations or not a significant change in speed,
    or uses a device
1 = Only minor change in speed, or changes speed with
    significant deviation, or changes speed with loss of balance
0 = Cannot change speeds or, loss of balance, requires outside
    support

Pivot Turn

3 = 3-Second turn, no loss of balance
2 = >3-Second turn, no loss of balance
1 = Slow with imbalance
0 = Cannot turn safely, requires assistance

Vertical Head Turn

3 = Turns head smoothly, no change in gait
2 = Turns head smoothly with minor change in gait or uses devices
1 = Turns head with signs of imbalance
0 = Severe disruption of gait, loss of balance, or staggers and reaches for wall

Horizontal Head Turn

3 = Turns head smoothly, no change in gait
2 = Turns head smoothly with minor change in gait or uses devices
1 = Turns head with signs of imbalance
0 = Severe disruption to gait, loss of balance, or staggers and reaches for wall

Gait with Narrow Base of Support

3 = Normal—10 steps heel to toe in 12 feet
2 = 7-9 Steps heel to toe
1 = 4-7 Steps heel to toe
0 = <4 Steps heel to toe or cannot perform

Gait with Eyes Closed

3 = 20 Feet no assistive devices, good speed, no imbalance, normal pattern,
    deviates no more than 6 inches outside 12-inch path
2 = 20 Feet, uses assistive device, slower speed, mild gait deviations, deviates
    more than 6-10 inches outside of 12-inch path
1 = 20 Feet, slow speed, abnormal pattern, imbalance, deviates 10-15 inches
    outside of 12-inch path, requires more than 9 seconds to walk 20 feet
0 = Cannot perform without assist

From Shumway-Cook A, Woollacott MH: Motor control: theory and practical applications, Baltimore, 1995, Lippincott Williams & Wilkins.

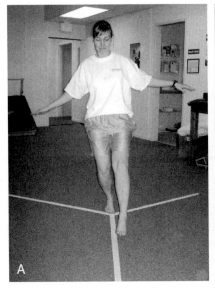
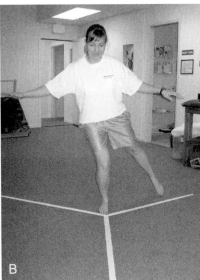
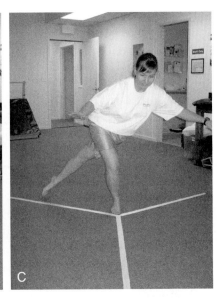

Figure 28-8 A-C, Star Excursion Balance Test (SEBT).

Table 28-7	Sample Data Sheet Star Excursion Balance Test (SEBT)				
	Left Reach (right stability)	Right Reach (left stability)	Male Norms	Female Norms	Combined Norms
Leg-length (cm) (anterior superior iliac spine [ASIS] to medial malleolus)					
Anterior reach (cm)			82.3	73.1	78.2
Posteromedial reach (cm)			113.6	98.9	107
Posterolateral reach (cm)			106.4	93	100.4
Normalized reach distance = distance as percent of leg length					
Anterior normalized reach distance (NRD)			84.1	81.4	83.9
Posteromedial NRD			116.1	110.1	113.4
Posterolateral NRD			108.7	103.6	106.4
Composite NRD = sum of all reaches/3 × leg length			103	98.4	100.9

Note: Scores recorded by reach leg; however, this reflects stability of stance leg. Direction of reach is named in reference to stance leg.
Male or female subject with anterior reach distance difference greater than 4 cm are 2.5 times more likely to injure ankle.
Female subjects with composite NRD of 94% or less are 6.5 times more likely to injure ankle.

performance (Figure 28-9). It has been shown to have good between-rater reliability for all subcomponents of test, with the exception of fair between-rater reliability with saccades accuracy and head movement with smooth pursuits. Test-retest reliability was excellent for all test components.[115-118] The subject stands in front of the clinician with the feet shoulder-width apart. No specific instructions are given to the subject regarding head movement. To test for saccadic movement, the tester holds two targets 10 cm to each side while the subject looks from target to target as quickly as possible for five cycles. Saccades may also be tested in vertical and diagonal planes. The tester records over- or undershoots, ability to complete the task, and compensatory head or body movements.[115-118] To test smooth pursuit, the patient stands while the tester holds a target approximately 40 cm from the patient. The tester then moves the target in a 20 cm circle twice in each direction while the subject follows the target with the eyes only. The tester records the subject's ability to complete the circles and maintain gaze on the target, as well as any compensatory movements of the head or body.[115-118]

The NSUCO has been shown to be a valid measure of oculomotor control and predictor of academic performance in optometric research (Table 28-8).[115-118] Table 28-9 outlines the minimum acceptable scores by age and gender, which represents the bottom 31% of performance in normals. Scoring below minimum acceptable is the benchmark for intervention in the field of behavioral optometry with regard to prevention or remediation of learning disabilities. The author feels it is reasonable to use the same guidelines to classify saccadic and smooth pursuit performance as impaired for the orthopaedic rehabilitation setting and thus serve as a guideline for intervention and/or appropriate outside referral.

The Brock string test is a time-honored but qualitative clinical test of vergence that requires only three or more beads strung on a 6- to 10-foot string (Figure 28-10). The subject holds one end of the string just under the nose while the other end is held or tied taut just below eye level. The beads are spaced approximately equidistant from each other. The subject is instructed to look precisely at only one bead. This should produce a single focused image of the bead with a slightly blurry image of two crossed strings. The cross is formed by the artifact of each eye's separate perspective of the string. Ideally this cross should occur directly through the target bead, indicating both eyes are correctly verging on the target. If the cross occurs *in front* of the target bead, then it means the subject is verging closer than the actual target, whereas *behind* means verging farther than the actual target. Either result indicates poor vergence, which can affect depth perception for balance, hand-eye coordination, and cervical NMC.

The head thrust test (HTT) is a valid clinical test of VOR function, which requires nothing more than the clinician's hands (Figure 28-11). The clinician places the subject's head in 30 degrees of downward tilt to align the horizontal semicircular canal to true horizontal and thus maximize horizontal angular acceleration. The subject is asked to focus on a stationary target such as the clinician's nose bridge. The clinician then gently moves the head in a 5 to 10 degrees lateral rotation arc, followed by an unpredictable highly rapid thrust to one side. A subject with normal functioning VOR will maintain gaze on target regardless of the thrust. Vestibular sensory loss will result in decreased gain (ratio of eye-to-head movement) in the VOR, allowing the eyes to move with the head and thus off target. A positive test occurs when the clinician observes a corrective saccade to bring the subject's gaze back on target. When performed in this manner, the HTT was 71% sensitive for unilateral peripheral vestibular hypofunction and 84% sensitive for bilateral with a specificity of 82%, which is actually superior to the previous gold standard of caloric electronystagmography. This test has great clinical use in identifying patients with peripheral vestibular loss and who will require training to compensate for decreased gain in the VOR.[119]

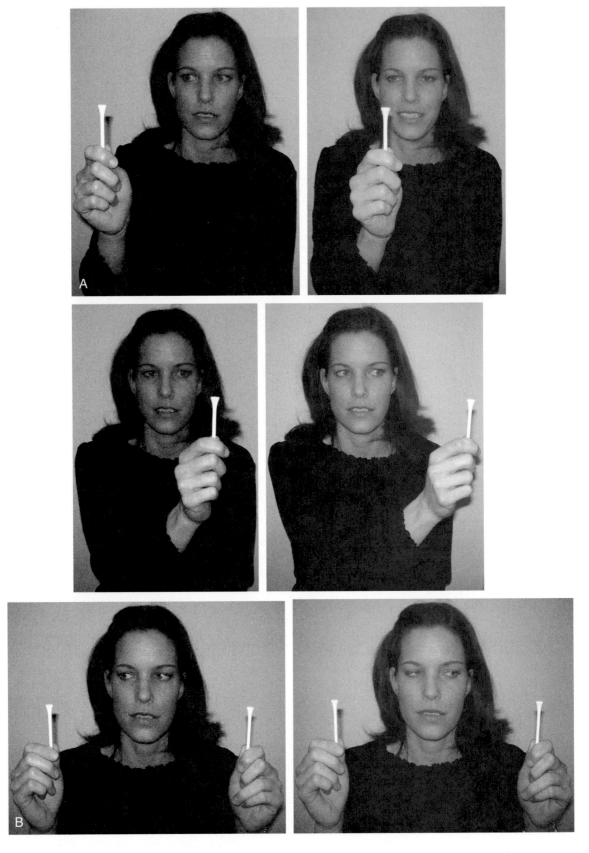

Figure 28-9 Northeastern State University College of Optometry (NSUCO) Oculomotor Test (also referred to as the *Maples Test*). These tests are depicted here with the patient holding the targets, but when performed in testing, the therapist should be holding the targets. **A,** Smooth pursuit; **B,** Saccadic performance.

Table 28-8	Sample Data Sheet for Northeastern State University College of Optometry (NSUCO) Oculomotor Test

The Patient Performs the Test Standing with Feet Shoulder-Width Apart, Directly in Front of the Examiner. No Instructions are Given Regarding Head Movement During Testing.

Saccades–Circle Appropriate Performance For Each Area.

Ability	1	Completes less than two roundtrips (one target to the other and back)
	2	Completes two roundtrips
	3	Completes three roundtrips
	4	Completes four roundtrips
	5	Completes five roundtrips
Accuracy	1	Large over/undershoots noted one or more times
	2	Moderate over/undershoots noted one or more times
	3	Constant slight over/undershoots noted more than 50% of the time
	4	Intermittent slight over/undershoots noted less than 50% of the time
	5	No over/undershoots noted
Head movements	1	Large movement of head at any time
	2	Moderate movement of head at any time
	3	Slight movement of head more than 50% of time
	4	Slight movement of head less than 50% of time
	5	No movement of head
Body movements	1	Large movement of body at any time
	2	Moderate movement of body at any time
	3	Slight movement of head more than 50% of time
	4	Slight movement of head less than 50% of time
	5	No movement of body

Smooth Pursuit–Circle Appropriate Performance for Each Area.

Ability	1	Cannot complete ½ rotation in either direction
	2	Completes ½ rotation in either direction
	3	Completes one rotation in either direction but not two rotations
	4	Completes two rotations in one but less than two in other direction
	5	Completes two rotations in each direction
Accuracy	1	No attempt to follow the target or requires greater than 10 refixations
	2	Refixations 5-10 times
	3	Refixations 3-4 times
	4	Refixations 1-2 times
	5	No refixations
Head movements	1	Large movement of head at any time
	2	Moderate movement of head at any time
	3	Slight movement of head more than 50% of time
	4	Slight movement of head less than 50% of time
	5	No movement of head
Body movements	1	Large movement of body at any time
	2	Moderate movement of body at any time
	3	Slight movement of head more than 50% of time
	4	Slight movement of head less than 50% of time
	5	No movement of body

From Maples WC: NSUCO Oculomotor Test, Chicago, 1995, Optometric Extension Program.

EVIDENCED-BASED SENSORY-SPECIFIC INTERVENTIONS FOR BALANCE AND CERVICAL STABILIZATION

Neuromuscular Training for Balance

Evidence exists for improving balance with protocols to improve lower-extremity strength, range of motion, and flexibility.[120-127] Likewise, protocols emphasizing balance drills on a variety of unstable surfaces regardless of their sensory bias have also been shown to improve balance.[120-127] However, the best evidence for NMT improving balance comes from programmatic vestibular rehabilitation, which applies the principles of sensory integration.[128-135] Understanding the client's sensory strengths and weaknesses allows for prescription of exercises to train true recovery of a specific sensory perception or compensation with other senses.

Table 28-9	Minimal Acceptable Scores for Northeastern State University College of Optometry (NSUCO) Oculomotor Test (Indicating Bottom 31% of Normal Performance)

	Age																			
	5		6		7		8		9		10		11		12		13		≥14	
Saccades	M	F	M	F	M	F	M	F	M	F	M	F	M	F	M	F	M	F	M	F
Ability	5	5	5	5	5	5	5	5	5	5	5	5	5	5	5	5	5	5	5	5
Accuracy	3	3	3	3	3	3	3	3	3	3	3	3	3	3	3	3	3	3	4	3
Head movements	2	2	2	3	3	3	3	3	3	3	3	4	3	4	3	4	3	4	3	4
Body movements	2	2	2	3	3	3	3	3	3	3	3	4	3	4	3	4	3	4	3	4

	Age																			
	5		6		7		8		9		10		11		12		13		≥14	
Smooth pursuit	M	F	M	F	M	F	M	F	M	F	M	F	M	F	M	F	M	F	M	F
Ability	4	5	4	5	5	5	5	5	5	5	5	5	5	5	5	5	5	5	5	5
Accuracy	2	3	2	3	3	3	3	4	3	4	4	4	4	4	4	4	5	4	5	4
Head movements	2	3	2	3	3	3	3	3	3	3	4	4	4	4	4	4	4	4	4	4
Body movements	3	4	3	4	3	4	4	4	4	4	4	5	4	5	5	5	5	5	5	5

From Maples WC: NSUCO Oculomotor Test, Chicago, 1995, Optometric Extension Program.

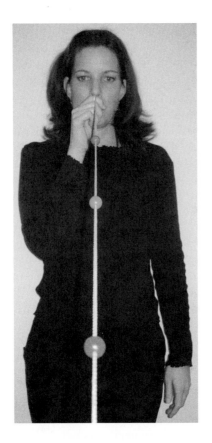

Figure 28-10 Brock string test.

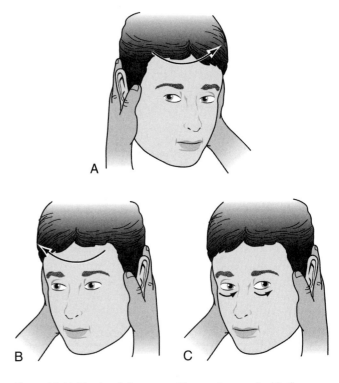

Figure 28-11 The head thrust test. The test is started with the eyes fixated on a target, and the head in 30 degrees of cervical flexion to improve test sensitivity. **A,** Normal response to rapid head thrust to the left: the eyes smoothly move to the right, maintaining fixation on the target. **B,** Abnormal response to rapid head thrust to the right. The eyes initially lose the target and move with the head then **(C)** make small saccades to the left to regain fixation on the target. (From Cameron MC, Monroe LH: Physical rehabilitation: evidence-based examination, evaluation, and intervention. St Louis, 2007, Saunders.)

Whenever possible, true recovery of any impairment is preferable, but in many cases compensatory gains are highly effective.[80,130,131] As with strengthening or other common orthopaedic exercises, most patients naturally gravitate toward compensatory solutions rather than address the impairments directly. By the same token, patients will prefer compensatory drills biased toward their unaffected senses because they have relative success. However, clients typically do not like balance training biased toward their specific sensory deficit because they have great difficulty. As mentioned before, patients with vestibular loss can often suffer from vertigo, which will often be provoked with vestibular sensory-biased balance training. Although compliance with a balance program that includes both approaches can be a bit of a tough sell, the author has experienced great success with educating patients as to the benefits of gaining as much reintegration of each sense as possible.

For example, a clinician wishing to train recovery of somatosensory loss (common with nearly all orthopaedic injuries) should prescribe balance activities on firm surfaces with deprivation (eyes closed) or degradation (blinking or low light) of vision. Conversely a client with long-standing peripheral neuropathy may never regain somatosensory sensation and will benefit from compensatory balance training on compliant surfaces and degraded vision to emphasize vestibular compensation. A client with vestibular loss will benefit from balance training in somatosensory conditions (firm surface, vision degraded or deprived) to allow for compensation. As they progress, patients will benefit from balance drills in vestibular-biased conditions (compliant surface, vision degraded or deprived).[19,80,129] The human nervous system preference for visual input is so strong that essentially any balance activity with the eyes open will bias toward visual sensory integration. This is still useful as a compensatory strategy for the initial phase of a balance-training program, especially when partnered with oculomotor exercises described following. Balancing with eyes open can also help acutely within a training session to familiarize a patient with a chosen surface before closing the eyes.

Regardless of the sensory biasing prescribed by the clinician, progression of exercise parameters is essential to provide continued error signal and force CNS adaptations, which lead to improved balance.[80] Width of stance, degree of perturbation (moving the surface), dynamic versus static balance tasks (weight shifting or stepping), concurrent motor tasks (catch, throw, kick), and concurrent cognitive tasks (math problems or conversing) are all parameters that can be manipulated to increase the difficulty of maintaining balance.[62,80,128-135] Computerized platforms (e.g., the CAPS Pro by Vestibular Technologies Inc.) can provide for easy tracking of progression of exercise and appropriate sensory biasing. The Smart Balance Master by Neurocom provides these features and computerized perturbation via automated tilting and translation of the platform. The Shuttle Balance by Shuttle Systems provides for nonautomated perturbation by adjusting of the chains suspending the platform and/or manual translation of the platform by the therapist.

Strong evidence exists for gains in balance and reduction of falls with the practice of several forms of tai chi (an ancient Chinese martial art form focusing on slow rhythmic weight shifting through various forms or positions).[136-138] Again, results with tai chi practice may be further enhanced by applying sensory-specific biasing via surface and visual deprivation based on the patient's unique impairments.[62,80,129,131]

Oculomotor Neuromuscular Training

Some clients with a history of cerebral vascular accident, TBI, or MTBI will have marked impairment of oculomotor control and may benefit from oculomotor drills to recover visual sensation.[27-31,39,139] However, more commonly in orthopaedics, clinicians will encounter clients with normal or minimally affected oculomotor control. For these patients, oculomotor exercises can enhance the speed and accuracy of foveal visual targeting and thus provide visual compensation for the loss of somatosensory or vestibular sensation.[62,67,79,140]

Orthopaedic rehabilitation specialists commonly use open kinetic chain exercises to isolate weak links before prescribing multiple muscle closed kinetic chain drills. Similarly it is usually easier to train each mechanism of oculomotor control separately before combining them to allow for more carryover to functional tasks. Any clinician who is able to assess these mechanisms should be able to train them with a little creativity. To review, following a slow-moving target without moving the head will train smooth pursuit. Rapid movements with the head still train saccadic eye movement.[62,141-144] Rapidly changing focus between near and far targets will address vergence. Focusing on an initially still target with the head moving will produce improved gain in the VOR (Figure 28-12).[62,79,140,131]

Clinical Note for Vertigo

Most patients with vestibular impairment will experience vertigo, imbalance, and nausea secondary to head movement as with the VOR drills. This is the direct result of asymmetrical vestibular stimulation into the CNS, as well as the indirect result of visual-vestibular conflict (poor sensory integration between visual and vestibular senses). Over time the CNS will adapt or habituate, resulting in less provocation of vertigo in response to the stimulus of head rotation. VOR exercises also produce sensitization to head rotation, increasing gain in the VOR and COR to provide gaze stabilization with head movement and thus relatively less visual-vestibular conflict. In the short term it can help clients to perform a compensation exercise by pressing into the pelvis (maximizing somatosensory input via the receptor-rich skin of the hands and pelvis) while looking at a stationary object (visual compensation).

Visual targets can be fingers, pens, or objects in the gym or patient's home. Objects with distinct text or pictures are often helpful to confirm the patient is actually targeting with focal vision. Laser pointers are useful tools for the clinician and patients who have difficulty moving or holding a target still in the hand. All of the previously mentioned exercises should

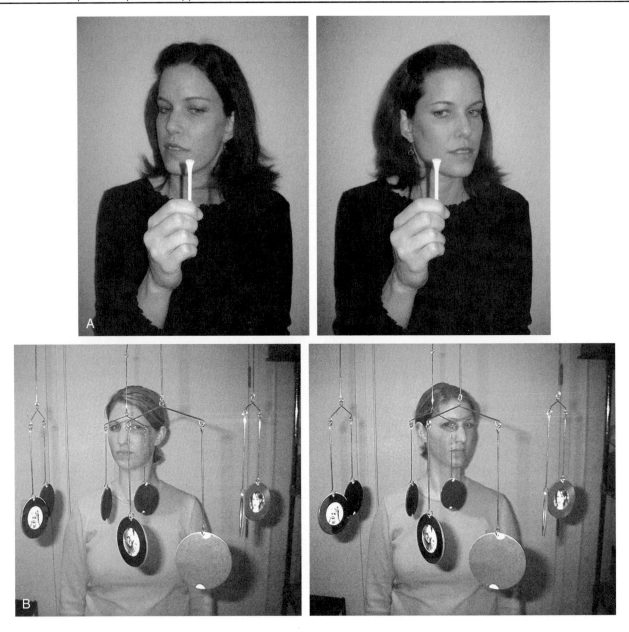

Figure 28-12 Ocular neuromuscular control (NMC) exercises. **A,** Vestibular ocular reflex (VOR) times 1; **B,** Integrated ocular NMC: mobiles.

be performed with targets moving in horizontal, vertical, diagonal, and then random directions.

Progression of all oculomotor drills is accomplished by manipulating the following variables. Increasing the speed with smooth pursuit, saccades, vergence, and VOR drills will add challenge. However, clinicians must keep in mind that a ceiling speed exists for smooth pursuit at which point all clients will naturally transition to a saccade.[141-144] All of the oculomotor drills mentioned previously can also be performed in conjunction with the balance progressions described earlier. Similarly, adding progressively more complex and/or moving backgrounds makes it harder for patients to locate their visual target and thus increases challenge.[63,80,85,132,133]

Clinical Note on Motion Sensitivity or Sickness

Motion sensitivity or sickness refers to nausea, vertigo, and even imbalance created by a visual-vestibular sensory conflict (a form of abnormal sensory integration). The visual-vestibular conflict is common in clients with vestibular loss because they cannot rely on normal vestibular input. Motion sensitivity or sickness can also be provoked with complex or moving backgrounds or during oculomotor NMT. This is because tracking a moving target in front of a stationary background produces the visual equivalent of a moving background. Use of a laser pointer or other far visual targets will decrease motion sensitiv-

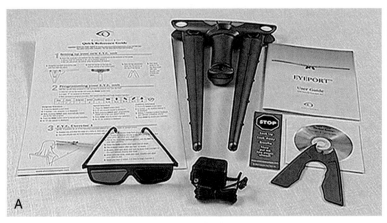
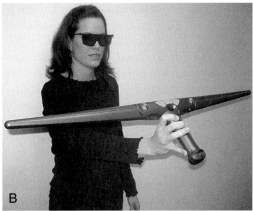

Figure 28-13 A-B, EYEPORT. (**A** courtesy Exercise your eyes, Wailuka, Hawaii.)

ity with oculomotor training by decreasing the relative perception of moving background. This is a similar phenomenon to sitting in the back of a movie theater versus the front row. In addition, the same compensations of hands on pelvis and looking at a stationary target away from the moving background can help the patient acutely control symptoms and better comply with oculomotor NMT.

As with balance training, new technologies are available to train oculomotor performance. The EYEPORT was developed by leading researchers in the field of behavioral optometry. It uses light-emitting diodes to provide moving visual targets for training of smooth pursuits, saccades, and vergence (Figure 28-13). The targets can be adjusted to move in a predictable or random manner and at varying speeds. The EYEPORT also allows for unique training paradigms only possible by exploiting the phenomenon of chromatic aberration. The red- and blue-colored targets emit slightly different wavelengths of light, which will penetrate different depths on the retina (similar to how different wavelengths of ultrasound waves penetrate more superficial or deep in to tissues). This drives CNS adaptation for control of smooth muscle action on the lens of the eye for more rapid and precise focus of the image on the retina. In addition, the patient wears training glasses with one red and one blue lens. Thus depending on the color of the illuminated target, only one eye will receive visual sensory input. This unique feature also prevents monocular vision compensations by forcing individual reception of visual information through each eye and thus CNS adaptation for more precise vergence.[145] Laukkanen and Rabin[145] showed that despite less than optimal subject compliance, the EYEPORT has the potential to improve visual performance and reading ability in normal subjects, and it is gaining widespread use in the treatment of vision-related learning disabilities. Use of the EYEPORT in home exercise programs has been shown to improve performance in baseball and law enforcement–based pistol marksmanship.[146,147]

NEUROMUSCULAR CONTROL APPROACH TO CERVICAL STABILIZATION

A great deal of research using fine wire electromyography and real-time ultrasound (RTUS) identified the transversus abdominis, deep fascicles of the lumbar multifidus, and the pelvic floor as local stabilizers in the lumbopelvic spine, which fire in anticipation of motion or in response to perturbation of the extremities. This is thought to be a feed-forward mechanism of NMC whereby these muscles stiffen the spine to dampen the reaction forces produced with gross movement. The latency of the local stabilizers is increased as much as 200 ms in subjects with chronic episodic low-back pain.[76-78,148-153] Similar research identified the longus coli and longus capitis, or deep cervical flexors (DCFs), as the primary local stabilizer of the cervical spine and indicated that abnormal recruitment patterns correlated with tension headaches, abnormal posture, neck pain, and disability.[154-156]

In these studies the more superficial, larger, nonsegmentally innervated muscles were referred to as *global stabilizers*. Other authors have referred to these larger muscles as *mobilizers* to describe their role in moving joint segments.[75,148-156] Although many authors do not agree with the local versus global stabilization classification schema, parallels exist for this abnormal pattern of NMC in other areas of the body. For example, delayed activation of the peroneals and rotator cuff are observed with unstable ankles and shoulders respectively.[13-15,88]

Regardless, the debate may be rendered moot because previous mechanical models of spinal stability have been revised to describe spinal stability as a function of NMC. In short, it is believed that clinical injury begins with subclinical injury to passive stabilizing structures such as the intervertebral discs, ligaments, and facet capsules. This results in decreased function of the somatosensory receptors set in these tissues, which leads to degraded sensory reception and, in turn, abnormal motor response.[76-78] Under a NMC model for spinal stability, CNS software allows for feed-forward anticipatory firing of smaller local stabilizers slightly before the larger global stabilizers or mobilizers.

Initial research into local cervical stabilization protocols emphasizing the use of pressure feedback tools to retrain volitional movement of the DCFs produced similar results to global protocols examining generalized neck strength and/or endurance training.[157-161] Falla et al.[157] demonstrated that although both local and global stabilization protocols improved neck pain and disability, only local DCF protocols improved neck posture with seated tasks.

Based on the plethora of research using RTUS and its commercial availability, the author sees increasing use of RTUS. It appears RTUS provides good intra- and interrater reliability of the cross-sectional area in select lumbar and cervical spinal muscles when viewing the same image but has yet shown to be reliable when rating images from different days. Research has shown RTUS to be an effective means of visual feedback NMT of the lumbar multifidus in healthy normals and subjects with low-back pain.[162-178] Similar research shows pressure feedback devices can provide feedback NMT to retrain volitional recruitment of the DCFs.[154] However, commentary on these studies pointed out the lack of experimental groups performing the same local stabilization exercises without the feedback. Further research into the therapeutic effects of multiple modes of feedback on spinal stabilization is ongoing.

Both RTUS and pressure-based protocols are feedback forms of NMT. The author finds it interesting that one of the key findings of the initial basic research into local spinal stabilization is that the local stablizers are driven by feed-forward NMC. If this is the case, then why do clinicians predominantly use feedback techniques of NMT when attempting to retrain spinal stabilization? A wealth of research demonstrates the efficacy of feed-forward NMT programs in producing dynamic joint stability in the extremities.[3-15,88] These researchers hypothesize that the mechanism for feed-forward NMT improving stability of the extremities is sensitization of the CNS to specific sensory input, allowing for faster triggering of reflexive, predictive pathways of NMC. Similar reflexes assist in the NMC task of maintaining head and neck position. Several recent studies have acknowledged the role of feed-forward NMT for stabilization of the neck.

The cervicocollic reflex consists of somatosensory afferent signals resulting in cervical muscle actions to right the head on the body. Thus just as clinicians address an unstable ankle with balance drills on firm, perturbing surfaces, apparently they can stimulate cervical somatosensory receptors with perturbation using head weighting or trunk movement to produce stabilization of the neck.[169-174] One study reported significant acute changes in posture after just 5 minutes with light anterior weighting of the head and perturbation via a free-moving multiaxis chair.[170] Blouin et al.[174] showed that seated subjects exposed to repeated linear translation of the trunk anterior on the spine resulted in effective NMT because the CNS learned to decrease scalene activity to modulate cervical muscle stress.

The cervicospinal reflex is actually a collection of short and long loop reflexes, which result in extension of the shoulder on the side of head rotation with simultaneous flexion of the contralateral shoulder. It is thought that the cervicospinal reflex helps compensate for vestibulospinal reflex to maintain balance and head attitude when vestibular loss is present. It now appears that the reflexive connection may work both ways.[175,176] Falla et al.[175] demonstrated feed-forward NMC of the deep cervical flexors, anterior scalene, and sternocleidomastoid as they fired less than 50 ms after upper-extremity volitional movement. Conversely, the authors found significant delays in firing of the same muscles in subjects with a history of chronic neck pain. Further research into the therapeutic effect of the cervicospinal reflex on cervical stabilization is clearly warranted.

Although its exact neural pathways have yet to be described, the vestibulocollic reflex acts to counter head movements sensed by the vestibular apparatus and assist in maintaining head orientation in relation to the earth. Borel et al.[178] examined head position in subjects with vestibular deficit and found significant impairment in head orientation. They also found that recovery of the ability to stabilize the head in relation to space occurred primarily through the use of visual sensation (and next via increased COR activity if vision was unavailable). These studies have shown that subjects with vestibular deficit may have altered cervical posture and will benefit from oculomotor NMT, as well as upper-extremity and cervical perturbation to stimulate the COR, cervicospinal reflexes, and cervicocollic reflexes, respectively.[178-182] In addition, many orthopaedic patients experience abnormal cervical postures but without clinical vestibular loss. These patients may benefit from the same type of exercises to stimulate a return to normal posture via the same reflexive pathways. Likewise, they may also benefit from bouncing on a Gymnic ball and head rotation in a short, pain-free arc because their intact vestibular pathways allow for cervical stabilization via the vestibulocollic reflex (Figure 28-14).

Oculomotor Neuromuscular Training for Cervical Stabilization

As mentioned previously the COR is a loop between cervical somatosensation and ocular movement counter to head motion. It is shown to help compensate for decreased gain in the VOR seen with vestibular injury.[53-55,79,140,178] To understand the additional clinical implications of the COR, it is helpful to think of the function of the neck. It is true that the neck functions as part of the axial skeleton to hold up the cranium and as a flexible and protective conduit for the spinal cord. However, much as the shoulder serves to preposition the hand, the cervical spine functions like a multiplanar swivel to preposition the head to receive visual sensory information. As mentioned previously, humans, like most other predatory mammals, have two eyes located on the front of the head that allow for binocular vision essential for judging distance to a target.[52-54,79,140] Although the ocular NMC described earlier provides a high degree of visual scanning, the addition of cervical motion multiplies the range of visual scanning. Therefore it is not totally

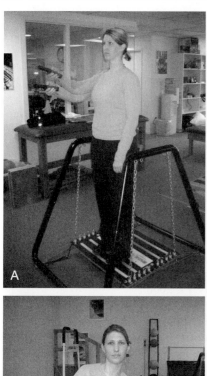

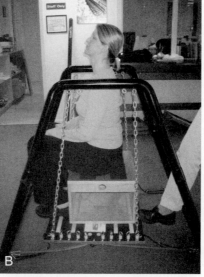

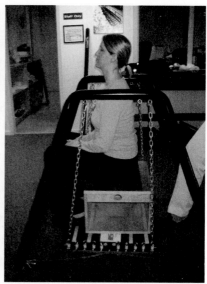

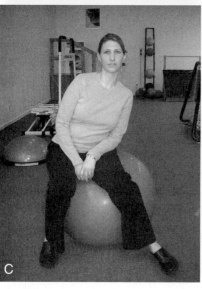

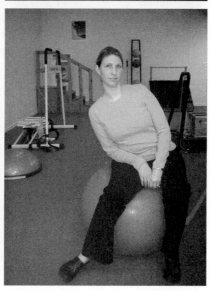

Figure 28-14 A, Upper-extremity perturbations; **B,** direct cervical perturbation; **C,** otolith stimulation.

surprising that recent studies have linked cervical muscle activity to extraocular muscle activity.

Research demonstrates the COR may work both ways (i.e., cervical to ocular and ocular to cervical). Andre-Deshays et al.[183] demonstrated increased neural impulse to the splenius cervicis in the same direction as horizontal gaze while the head was stationary. A follow-up study found splenius cervicis phasic changes in muscle activity that correlated with oculomotor saccades, suggesting coupling of eye and head motion with both visual fixation and during the saccadic movement.[183] In a more recent study, Bexander et al.[184] examined the effect of gaze on eye-neck coupling while the neck was rotating. They demonstrated that visual gaze to the same direction as head rotation increased activation of the sternocleidomastoid multifidus. The splenius capitis showed a nonsignificant trend toward increased activity with eye movement. Obliquus capitis inferior did not change with gaze.[184] Another study found a multimodal rehabilitation protocol that included visual fixation drills produced superior outcomes to education-only and

home exercise protocols, as measured by self-reported benefit.[185] These studies suggest that many of the oculomotor exercises described earlier may be incorporated into cervical stabilization programs to preferentially retrain the sternocleidomastoid and cervical multifidus. Smooth pursuit and saccades drills with the head still may be more useful in recruiting the splenius capitis. However, the cervical and upper-extremity perturbation discussed earlier may be preferential in neuromuscular reeducation of the longus coli, scalenes, and obliquus capitis.

Several studies have documented oculomotor abnormalities in patients suffering cervical trauma with WAD. Kelders et al.[185] demonstrated the COR is increased in post-MVA patients suffering WAD. Treleaven et al.[51] studied the smooth pursuit neck torsion test between 50 patients with WAD who reported dizziness and 50 patients with WAD who did not report it; they found significant impairment as compared with 50 control subjects. Montfort et al.[53] found increases in COR gain without change in VOR gain in patients with WAD. They hypothesized that this increased gain was due to changes in cervical somatosensation. Although Kongstead et al.[186] did not find oculomotor changes in subjects with WAD, their study design examined only smooth pursuit, which may not have been a broad enough measure to identify changes. Thus evidence exists linking cervical conditions addressed commonly by the orthopaedic rehabilitation professional to impaired oculomotor function. Furthermore, Storaci et al.[52] found abnormal posturography in 40 subjects with WAD and was able to obtain good outcomes as measured by pain, disability, and reduction of dizziness if oculomotor NMT was initiated promptly after injury. However, these outcomes were significantly reduced in patients who used cervical collars for longer than 3 weeks. This clearly demonstrates the need to assess and treat oculomotor NMC in WAD clients to allow for optimal functional outcomes.

SUMMARY

In conclusion, it is clear that the orthopaedic rehabilitation specialist will routinely encounter clients with altered sensory integration regardless of the pathologic condition. Altered sensory integration can significantly affect NMC and thus balance and dynamic joint stabilization. Use of clinical assessment tools previously limited to the realm of vestibular rehabilitation and new orthopaedic-based measures of NMC will assist clinicians in their assessment. This leads to the design of sensory-specific feedback and feed-forward NMT protocols, which produce superior outcomes for clients with imbalance and instability. More recent studies illustrate the use of applying the same approaches, including the prescription of oculomotor NMT, to clients with neck pain and WAD.

REFERENCES

1. James R: The poems of John Godfrey Saxe, Boston, 1873, Osgood & Company, p 77.
2. Hewett TE, Myer GD, Ford KR, et al: Biomechanical measures of neuromuscular control and valgus loading of the knee predict anterior cruciate ligament injury risk in female athletes, Am J Sports Med 33(4):492-592, 2005.
3. Cerulli G, Benoit DL, Carffa A, et al: Proprioceptive training and prevention of anterior cruciate ligament injuries in soccer, J Orthop Sports Phys Ther 31(11):655-660, 2001.
4. Meyers GD, Patterno MV, Ford KR, et al: Rehabilitation after anterior cruciate ligament reconstruction: criteria-based progression through return to sport, J Orthop Sports Phys Ther 36(6):385-402, 2006.
5. Chmielewski TL, Hurd WJ, Randolph KS, et al: Perturbation training improves knee kinematics and reduces muscle co-contraction after complete unilateral anterior cruciate ligament rupture, Phys Ther 85:740-754, 2005.
6. Cowley HR, Ford KR, Myer GD, et al: Difference in neuromuscular strategies between landing and cutting tasks in female basketball and soccer athletes, J Athl Train 41(1):57-73, 2006.
7. Grindstaff TL, Hammill RR, Tuzon AE, et al: Neuromuscular control training programs and noncontact anterior cruciate ligament injury rates in female athletes: a

8. numbers-needed-to-treat analysis, J Athl Train 41(4):450-456, 2006.
8. Swanik CB, Lephart SM, Swanik KA, et al: Neuromuscular dynamic restraint in women with anterior cruciate ligament injuries, Clin Orthop Relat Res 425:189-199, 2004.
9. Ross SE, Guskiewicz KM: Examination of static and dynamic postural stability in individuals with functionally stable and unstable ankles, Clin J Sport Med 14:332-338, 2004.
10. Houck JR, DeHaven KE, Maloney M: Influence of anticipation on movement in subjects with ACL injury classified as non-copers, J Orthop Sports Phys Ther 37(2):56-64, 2007.
11. Plisky PJ, Rauh MJ, Kaminski TW, et al: Star Excursion Balance Test as a predictor of lower extremity injury in high school basketball players, J Orthop Sports Phys Ther 36(12):911-919, 2006.
12. Risberg MA, Holm I, Myklebust G, et al: Neuromuscular training versus strength training during the first 6 months after anterior cruciate ligament reconstruction: a randomized clinical trial, Phys Ther 87:737-750, 2007.
13. Hale SA, Hertel J, Olmsted-Kramer LC: The effect of a 4-week comprehensive rehabilitation program on postural control and lower extremity function in individuals with chronic ankle instability, J Orthop Sports Phys Ther 37(6):303-311, 2007.
14. Forwell LA, Carnahan H: Proprioception during manual aiming in individuals with shoulder instability and controls, J Orthop Sports Phys Ther 23(2):111-120, 1996.
15. Brindle TJ, Nitz AJ, Uhl TL, et al: Measures of accuracy for active shoulder movement at 3 different speeds with kinesthetic and visual feedback, J Orthop Sports Phys Ther 34:468-478, 2004.
16. Day S, Munski J: Role of the orthopaedist in fracture prevention, Tech Orthop 19(3):115-120, 2004.
17. Anacker SL, DiFabio RP: Influence of sensory inputs on standing balance in community-dwelling elders with a recent history of falling, Phys Ther 72:575-584, 1992.
18. Shumway-Cook A, Woolacoot M: Motor control theory and practical applications, Baltimore, Md, 1995, Williams & Wilkins.
19. Shumway-Cook A, Horak FB: Assessing the influence of sensory integration on balance; suggestions from the field, Phys Ther 66:1548-1559, 1986.
20. Shumway-Cook A, Baldwin M, Polissar NL, et al: Predicting the probability for falls in community-dwelling older adults, Phys Ther 77:812-819, 1997.
21. Bogle-Thorbahn LD, Newton RA: Use of Berg balance test to predict falls in elderly persons, Phys Ther 76:576-585, 1996.
22. Chou CY, Chien CW, Hsuch IP, et al: Developing a short form of the Berg Balance Scale for people with stroke, Phys Ther 86:195-204, 2006.
23. Hall CD, Schubert MC, Herdman SJ: Prediction of fall risk reduction as measured by Dynamic Gait Index in

individuals with unilateral vestibular hypofunction, Otol Neurotol 25:746-751, 2004.

24. Day L, Flides B, Gordan I, et al: Randomized factorial trial of falls prevention among older people living in their own homes, BMJ 325:128-135, 2002.

25. Chang JT, Morton SC, Rubenstein LZ, et al: Interventions for the prevention of falls in older adults: systematic review and meta-analysis of randomized clinical trials, BMJ 328:680-688, 2004.

26. DiFabiio RP, Emasithi A: Aging and the mechanisms underlying head and postural control during voluntary motion, Phys Ther 77:458-475, 1997.

27. Ciuffreda KJ, Kapoor N: Traumatic brain injury and the nation, J Behavior Optometry 18(3):58, 2007.

28. VanRoekel C: Military optometry in the care of traumatic brain injury patients, J Behavior Optometry 18(3):60-61, 2007.

29. Townsend JC: Traumatic brain injury: a new challenge for optometry, neuro-optometric rehabilitation, and our nation, J Behavior Optometry 18(3):63-66, 2007.

30. Ciuffreda KJ, Kapoor N, Rutner D, et al: Occurrence of oculomotor dysfunctions in acquired brain injury: a retrospective analysis, Optometry 78:155-161, 2007.

31. Stelmack J: Measuring outcomes of neuro-optometric care in traumatic brain injury, J Behavior Optometry 18(3):67-71, 2007.

32. Barnes BC, Cooper L, Kirkendall DT, et al: Concussion history in elite male and female soccer players, AJSM 26(3):433-438, 1998.

33. Ferrara MS, McCrea M, Peterson CL et al: A survey of practice patterns in concussion assessment and management, J Athl Train 36(2):145-149, 2001.

34. Guskiewicz KM, Bruce SL, Cantu RC, et al: National Athletic Trainers' Association position statement: management of sport-related concussion, J Athl Train 39(3):280-297, 2004.

35. Guskiewicz KM, Bruce SL, Cantu RC, et al: Research based recommendations of management of sport related concussion: summary of the National Athletic Trainers' position statement, Br J Sports Med 40:6-10, 2006.

36. Tommasone BA, Valovich McLeod TC: Contact sport concussion incidence, J Athl Train 41(4):470-472, 2006.

37. McCrea M, Guskiewicz KM, Marshall SW, et al: Acute effects and recovery time following concussion in collegiate football players, The NCAA concussion study, JAMA 290(19):2556-2563, 2003.

38. McCrory P: When to retire after concussion, Br J Sports Med 35:380-382, 2001.

39. Ciuffreda KJ, Kapoor N: Oculomotor dysfunctions, their remediation, and reading-related problems in mild traumatic brain injury, J Behavior Optometry 18(3):72-77, 2007.

40. Mendez CV, Hurley RA, Lassonde M, et al: Mild traumatic brain injury: neuroimaging of sports-related concussion, J Neuropsychiatry Clin Neurosci 17(3):297-304, 2005.

41. Barr WB: Methodological issues in neuropsychological testing, J Athl Train 36(3):297-302, 2001.

42. Valovich McLeod TC, Barr WB, McCrea M, et al: Psychometric and measurement properties of concussion assessment tools in youth sports, J Athl Train 41(4):399-408, 2006.

43. Basford JR, Chour LS, Kaufman KR, et al: An assessment of gait and balance deficits after traumatic brain injury, Arch Phys Med Rehabil 84:343-349, 2003.

44. Catena RD, van Donkelaar P, Chou LS: Cognitive task effects on gait stability following concussion, Exp Brain Res 176(1):23-31, 2006.

45. Catena RD, van Donkelaar P, Chou LS: Altered balance control following concussion is better detected with an attention test during gait, Gait Posture 25(3):406-411, 2006.

46. Parker TM, Osternigh LR, Van Donkelaar P, et al: Gait stability following concussion, Med Sci Sports Exerc 38(6):1032-1040, 2006.

47. Parker TM, Osternigh LR, Van Donkelaar P, et al: The effect of divided attention on gait stability following concussion, Clin Biomech (Bristol, Avon) 20:389-395, 2005.

48. Pearson BC, Armitage KR, Horner CWM, et al: Saccadometry: the possible application of latency distribution measurement for monitoring concussion, Br J Sport Med 41:610-612, 2007.

49. Bunketorp L, Nordholm L, Carlsson J: A descriptive analysis of disorders in patients 17 years following motor vehicle accidents, Eur Spine J 11:227-234, 2002.

50. Mallinson AI, Longridge NS: Dizziness from whiplash and head injury, differences between whiplash and head injury, Am J Otol 19:814-818, 1998.

51. Treleaven J, Jull G, LowChoy N: Smooth pursuit neck torsion test in whiplash-associated disorders: relationship to self-reports of neck pain and disability, dizziness and anxiety, J Rehabil Med 37:219-223, 2005.

52. Storaci R, Manelli A, Schiavone N, et al: Whiplash injury and oculomotor dysfunctions: clinical-posturographic correlations, Eur Spine J 15:1811-1816, 2006.

53. Montfort I, Kelders WP, Van Der Geest JN, et al: Interaction between ocular stabilization reflexes in patients with whiplash injury, Invest Opthalmol Vis Sci 47:2881-2884, 2006.

54. Kelders WPA, Kleinrensink GJ, Vand Der Geest JN, et al: The cervico-ocular reflex is increased in whiplash injury patients, J Neurotrauma 22(1):133-137, 2005.

55. Brandt T, Bronstein AM: Nosological entities? Cervical vertigo, J Neurol Neurosurg Psychiatry 71:8-12, 2001.

56. Reid SA, Rivett DA: Manual therapy treatment of cervicogenic dizziness: a systematic review, Man Ther 10:4-13, 2005.

57. Endo K, Ichimaru K, Komagata M et al: Cervical vertigo and dizziness after whiplash injury, Eur Spine J 15:886-890, 2006.

58. Labler L, Eid K, Platz A, et al: Atlanto-occipital dislocation: four case reports of survival in adults and review of literature, Eur Spine J 13:172-180, 2004.

59. Cook C, Brismee JM, Fleming R, et al: Identifiers suggestive of clinical cervical spine instability: a Delphi study of physical therapists, Phys Ther 85:895-906, 2005.

60. DiFabio RP: Manipulation of the cervical spine: risks and benefits, Phys Ther 79:50-65, 1999.

61. Manipulation Education Committee of the APTA Manipulation Task Force: Manipulation education manual for Physical Therapist Professional Degree Programs, Alexandria, Va, 2004, American Physical Therapy Association.

62. Herdman SJ: Vestibular rehabilitation, ed 2, Philadelphia, 2000, FA Davis.

63. Woodworth BA, Gillespie MB, Lambert PR: The Canalith repositioning procedure for benign positional vertigo: a meta-analysis, Laryngoscope 114:1143-1146, 2004.

64. Froehling DA, Silverstein MD, Mohr DN, et al: Benign positional vertigo: incidence and prognosis in a population-based study in Olmsted county, Minnesota, Mayo Clin Proc 66(6):596-601, 1991.

65. Gill-Body KM, Beninato M, Krebs DE: Relationship among balance impairments, functional performance, and distability in people with peripheral vestibular hypofunction, Phys Ther 80:748-758, 2000.

66. Guitton D, Kearney RE, Wereley N et al: Visual, vestibular, and voluntary contributions to human head stabilization, Exp Brain Res 64(1):56-69, 1986.

67. Wade MG, Jones G: The role of vision and spatial orientation in maintenance of posture, Phys Ther 77:619-628, 1997.

68. Subramanian A, Dickinson C: Spatial localization in visual impairment, Invest Ophthalmol Vis Sci 47:78-85, 2006.

69. Keefe JE, Jin CF, Weih LM, et al: Vision impairment and older drivers: who's driving? Br J Opthalmol 86(10):1118-1124, 2002.

70. Kershner EA, Kenyon RV, Langston J: Postural responses exhibit multisensory dependencies with discordant visual and support surface motion, J Vestibular Res 14:307-319, 2004.

71. Williams GN, Chmielewski T, Rudolph KS, et al: Dynamic knee stability: current theory and implications for clinicians and scientists, J Orthop Sports Phys Ther 31(10):546-566, 2001.

72. MacKayy-Lyons M: Central pattern generation of locomotion: a review of the evidence, Phys Ther 82:69-83, 2002.

73. Woollacott MH, Shumway-Cook A: Changes in posture control across the life span—a systems approach, Phys Ther 70:799-807, 1990.

74. Shaffer SW, Harrison AL: Aging of the somatosensory system: a translational perspective, Phys Ther 87:193-207, 2007.

75. Donatelli R: Sports-specific rehabilitation, St Louis, 2007, Elsevier.

76. Panjabi MM: A hypothesis of chronic back pain: ligament subfailure injuries lead to muscle control dysfunction, Eur Spine J 15:668-676, 2006.

77. Hodges P, Holm AK, Hansson T, et al: Rapid atrophy of the lumbar multifidus follows experimental disc or nerve root injury, Spine 31:2926-2933, 2006.

78. Hides JA, Stokes MJ, Saide M, et al: Evidence of lumbar multifidus muscles wasting in ipsilateral to symptoms in patients with acute/subacute low back pain, Spine 19(2):165-177, 1994.

79. Schubert MC, Minor LB: Vestibulo-ocular physiology underlying vestibular hypofunction, Phys Ther 84:373-385, 2004.

80. Black FO, Pesznecker SC: Vestibular adaptation and rehabilitation, Curr Opin Otolaryngol Head Neck Surg 11:355-360, 2003.

81. Black FO, Gianna-Poulin C, Pesznecker SC: Recovery from vestibular ototoxicity, Otol Neurotol 22:662-671, 2001.

82. Lewis RF, Clendaniel RA, Zee, DS: Vergence-dependent adaptation of the vestibulo-ocular reflex, Exp Brain Res 152:335-340, 2003.

83. Burke MR, Burns GR: Quantitative differences in smooth pursuit and saccadic eye movements, Exp Brain Res 175:596-603, 2006.

84. Mandellos D, Anastasopoulos D, Becker W: Smooth pursuit rather than visual signals mediate short-term adaptation of the cervico-ocular reflex in humans, Exp Brain Res 169:153-161, 2006.

85. Riijkaart DC, van der Geest JN, Kelders WP, et al: Short-term adaptation of the cervico ocular reflex, Exp Brain Res 156:124-128, 2004.

86. Horak FB: Clinical measurement of postural control in adults, Phys Ther 67:1881-1885, 1987.

87. Han YH, Kumar AN, Reschke MF, et al: Vestibular and non-vestibular contributions to eye movements that compensate for head rotations during viewing of near targets, Exp Brain Res 165:292-304, 2005.

88. Ross SE, Guskiewicz KM: Examination of static and dynamic stability in individuals with functionally stable and unstable ankles, Clin J Sport Med 14:332-338, 2004.

89. Cohen H, Blatchly CA, Gombash LL: A study of the clinical test of sensory integration and balance, Phys Ther 73:346-351, 1993.

90. DiFabio RP: Sensitivity and specificity of platform posturography for identifying patients with vestibular dysfunction, Phys Ther 75:290-305, 1995.

91. Black FO: Clinical status of computerized dynamic posturography in neurotology, Curr Opin Otolaryngol Head Neck Surg 9:314-318, 2001.

92. Huxham FE, Goldie PA, Patla AE: Theoretical considerations in balance assessment, Aust J Physiother 47:89-100, 2001.

93. Chaundry H, Findley T, Quigely KS, et al: Measures of postural stability, J Rehabil Res Dev 41(5):713-720, 2004.

94. Riemann BL, Guskiewicz KM: Effects of mild head injury on postural stability as measured through clinical balance testing, J Athl Train 35(1):19-25, 2000.

95. Valovich TC, Perrin DH, Gansneder BM: Repeat administration elicits a practice effect with the balance error score system but not with the standard assessment of concussion in high school athletes, J Athl Train 38(1):51-56, 2003.

96. Wilkins JC, Valovich McCleod TC, Perrin DH, et al: Performance on the balance error scoring system decreases after fatigue, J Athl Train 39(2):156-161, 2004.

97. Boulgarides LK, McGinty SM, Willett JA, et al: Use of clinical and impairment-based tests to predict falls by community-dwelling older adults, Phys Ther 83:328-339, 2003.

98. Berg KO, Wood-Dauphinee SL, Williams JI, et al: Measuring balance in the elderly: validation of an instrument, Can J Public Health S2:S7-S11, 1992.

99. Muir SW, Berg K, Chesworth B, et al: Use of the Berg Balance Scale for predicting multiple falls in community-dwelling elderly people: a prospective study, Phys Ther 88:449-459, 2008.

100. Stevenson TJ: Detecting change in patients with stroke using the Berg Balance Scale, Aust J Physiother 47:29-38, 2001.

101. Chiu YP, Fritz SL, Light KE, et al: Use of item response analysis to investigate measurement properties and clinical validity of data for the dynamic gait index, Phys Ther 86:778-787, 2006.

102. Wrisley DM, Marchetti GF, Kuharsky DK, et al: Reliability, internal consistency, and validity of data obtained with the functional gait assessment, Phys Ther 84:906-918, 2004.

103. Marchetti GF, Whitney SL: Construction and validation of the 4-item dynamic gait index, Phys Ther 86:1651-1660, 2006.

104. Kinzey SJ, Armstrong CW: The reliability of the Star-Excursion Test in assessing dynamic balance, J Orthop Sports Phys Ther 27(5):356-361, 1998.

105. Olmstead LC, Carcia CR, Hertel J, et al: Efficacy of the Star Excursion Balance Tests in detecting reach deficits in subjects with chronic ankle instability, J Athl Train 37(4):501-506, 2002.

106. Lanning CL, Uhl T, Ingram C, et al: Baseline values of trunk endurance and hip strength in collegiate athletes, J Athl Train 41(4):427-434, 2006.

107. Hertel J, Braham RA, Hale SA, et al: Simplifying the Star Excursion Balance Test: analysis of subjects with and without chronic ankle instability, J Orthop Sports Phys Ther 36:131-137, 2006.

108. Plisky PJ, Rauh MJ, Kaminski TW, et al: Star Excursion Balance Test as a predictor of lower extremity injury in high school basketball players, J Orthop Sports Phys Ther 36(12):911-919, 2006.

109. Banks PM, Moor LA, Liu C, et al: Dynamic visual acuity: a review, S Afr Optom 63(2):58-64, 2004.

110. Herdman SJ, Tusa RJ, Blatt P, et al: Computerized dynamic visual acuity test in the assessment of vestibular deficits, Am J Otol 19:790-796, 1998.

111. Schubert MC, Herdman SJ, Tusa RJ: Vertical dynamic visual acuity in normal subjects and patients with vestibular hypofunction, Otol Neurotol 23:372-377, 2002.

112. Bronstein AM: Vestibular reflexes and positional maneuvers, J Neurol Neurosurg Psychiatry 74:289-293, 2003.

113. Tian J, Shubayev I, Demer JL: Dynamic visual acuity during passive and self generated transient head rotation in normal and unilaterally vestibulopathic humans, Exp Brain Res 142:486-495, 2002.

114. Gottshall K, Drake A, Gray N, et al: Objective vestibular tests as outcome measures in head injury patients, Laryngoscope 113:1746-1750, 2003.

115. Maples WC, Ficklin TW: Interrater and test-retest reliability of smooth pursuits and saccades, J Am Optom Assoc 59(7):549-552, 1988.

116. Maples WC, Atchley J, Ficklin TW: Northeastern State University College of Optometry's oculomotor norms, J Behav Optom 3:143-150, 1992.

117. Maples WC, Ficklin TW: Comparison of eye movement skills between above average and below average readers, J Behav Optom 1:87-91, 1991.

118. Maples WC: NSUCO Oculomotor Test, Santa Ana, Calif, 1995, Optometric Extension Program.

119. Schubert MC, Tusa RJ, Grime LE, et al: Optimizing the sensitivity of head thrust for identifying vestibular hypofunction, Phys Ther 84:151-158, 2004.

120. Chang JT, Morton SC, Rubenstein LZ, et al: Interventions for the prevention of falls in older adults: systematic review of meta-analysis of randomized clinical trials, BMJ 328:680-689, 2004.

121. Feder G, Cryer C, Donovan S, et al: Guideline for the prevention of falls in people over 65, BMJ 321:1007-1011, 2000.

122. Khan KM, Liu-Ambrose T, Donaldson MG, et al: Physical activity to prevent falls in older people: time to intervene in high risk groups using falls as an outcome, Br J Sports Med 35:144-145, 2001.

123. Wolf B, Feys H, DeWeerdt W, et al: Effect of physical therapeutic intervention for balance problems in the elderly: a single-blind, randomized, controlled multicentre trial, Clin Rehab 15:624-636, 2001.

124. Perrin PP, Gauchard GC, Perrot C, et al: Effects of physical and sporting activities on balance control in elderly people, Br J Sports Med 33:121-126, 1999.

125. Carter ND, Khan KM, McKay HA, et al: Community-based exercise program reduces risk factors for falls in 65- to 75-year-old women with osteoporosis: randomized controlled trial, CMAJ 167(9):997-1004, 2002.

126. Day L, Flides B, Gordan I, et al: Randomized factorial trial of falls prevention among older people living in their own homes, BMJ 325:128-135, 2002.

127. Chang JT, Morton SC, Rubenstein LZ, et al: Interventions for the prevention of falls in older adults: systematic review and meta-analysis of randomized clinical trials, BMJ 328:680-688, 2004.

128. Nitz JC, Choy NL: The efficacy of a specific balance-strategy training program for preventing falls among older people: a pilot randomized controlled trial, Aging 33:52-58, 2004.

129. Westlake KP, Wu Y, Culham EG: Sensory-specific balance training in older adults: effect on position movement, and velocity sense at the ankle, Phys Ther 87:560-568, 2007.

130. Black OF, Angel CR, Pesznecker SC, et al: Outcome analysis of individualized vestibular rehabilitation protocols, Am J Otol 21:543-551, 2000.

131. Herdman SJ, Blatt PJ, Schubert MC: Vestibular rehabilitation of patients with vestibular hypofunction or with benign paroxysmal positional vertigo, Curr Opin Neruol 13:39-43, 2000.

132. Brown KE, Whitney SL, Wrisley DM, et al: Physical therapy outcomes for persons with bilateral vestibular loss, Laryngoscope 111:1812-1817, 2001.

133. Nisbino LK, DeFreitas Gananca C, Manso A, et al: Personalized vestibular rehabilitation: medical chart survey with patients seen at the ambulatory clinic of otoneurology of I.S.C.M.S.P., Rev Bras Otorrinolaringol 71(4):440-447, 2005.

134. Whitney SL, Wrisley DM, Marchetti GF, et al: The effect of age on vestibular rehabilitation outcomes, Laryngoscope 112:1785-1790, 2002.

135. Pellecchia GL: Dual-task training reduces impact of cognitive task on postural sway, J Mot Behav 37(3):239-246, 2005.

136. Xu D, Hong Y, Chan K: Effect of tai chi exercise on proprioception of ankle and knee joints in old people, Br J Sports Med 38:50-54, 2004.

137. Tsang WWN, Hui-Chan CWY: Effect of 4-and 8-wk intensive tai chi training on balance control in the elderly, Med Sci Sports Exerc 36(4):648-658, 2004.

138. Tsang WWN, Hui-Chan CWY: Effects of exercise on joint sense and balance in elderly men: tai chi versus golf, Med Sci Sports Exerc 36(4):658-667, 2004.

139. Schieman W, Michell L, Cotter S, et al: A randomized clinical trial of treatments in convergence insufficiency in children, Arch Ophthalmol 123:14-24, 2005.

140. Cromwell R, Newon RA, Carlton LG: Horizontal plane head stabilization during locomotor tasks, J Mot Behav 33(1):49-58, 2001.

141. Ciuffreda KJ: The scientific basis for efficacy of optometric vision therapy in nonstrabismic accommodative and vergence disorders, Optometry 73:735-762, 2002.

142. Rawstron JA, Burley CD, Elder MJ: A systematic review of the applicability and efficacy of eye exercises, J Pediatr Opthalmol Strabismus 42:82-88, 2005.

143. Scheiman M, Mitchell L, Cotter S, et al: A randomized clinical trial of treatments for convergence insufficiency in children, Arch Opthalmol 123:14-24, 2005.

144. Clarke MP, Wright CM, Hrisos S, et al: Randomized controlled trial of treatment of unilateral visual impairment detected at preschool vision screening, BMJ 327:1251-1257, 2003.

145. Laukkanen H, Rabin J: A prospective study of the EYEPORT Vision Training System, Optometry 77:508-514, 2006.

146. Bowen T, Horth L: Use of the EYEPORT™ vision training system to enhance the visual performance of little league baseball players, J Behav Optom 16(6):143-148, 2005.

147. Liberman J, Horth L: Use of the EYEPORT™ vision training system to enhance the visual performance of police recruits: a pilot study, J Behav Optom 17(4):87-92, 2006.

148. Richardson CA, Jull GA, Richardson BA: A dysfunction of the deep abdominal muscles exists in low back pain patients. In Proceedings World Confederation of Physical Therapists, Washington, DC, 1995, p 932.

149. Hides J, Richardson C, Jull G: Multifidus muscle recovery is not automatic following resolution of acute first episode low back pain, Spine 21:2763-2769, 1996.

150. Hodges PW, Richardson CA: Inefficient muscular stabilization of the lumbar spine associated with low back pain. A motor control evaluation of transversus abdominis, Spine 21(22):2640-2650, 1996.

151. Hodges PW, Richardson CA, Jull GA: Evaluation of the relationship between the findings of a laboratory and clinical test of transversus abdominis function, Physiother Res Int 1:28-40, 1996.

152. Richardson CA, Jull G, Hodges P, et al: Therapeutic exercise for spinal segmental stabilization in low back pain; scientific basis and clinical approach, Philadelphia, 1999, Churchill Livingston.

153. Richardson CA, Snijders CJ, Hides JA, et al: The relationship between the transversus abdominis muscles, sacroiliac joint mechanics, and low back pain, Spine 27(4):399-405, 2002.

154. Falla D, Jull G, Dall'Alba P, et al: An electromyographical analysis of deep cervical flexor muscles in performance of cranicervical flexion, Phys Ther 83:899-906, 2003.

155. O'Leary SP, Vicenzino BT, Jull GA: A new method of isometric dynamometry for the craniocervical flexor muscles, Phys Ther 85:556-564, 2005.

156. Harris KD, Heer DM, Roy TC, et al: Reliability of a measurement of neck flexor muscle endurance, Phys Ther 85:1349-1355, 2005.

157. Falla D, Jull G, Russell T, et al: Effect of neck exercise on sitting posture in patients with chronic neck pain, Phys Ther 87(4):408-417, 2007.

158. Mansell J, Tierney RT, Sitler MR, et al: Resistance training and head-neck segment dynamic stabilization in male and female collegiate soccer players, J Athl Train 40(4):310-319, 2005.

159. Alriscsson M, Harms Ringdahl K, Larsson B, et al: Neck muscle strength and endurance in fighter pilots: effects

of a supervised training program, Aviat Space Environ Med 75:23-28, 2004.

160. Seng KY, Lam PM, Lee VS: Acceleration effects on neck muscle strength in pilots vs. non-pilots, Aviat Space Environ Med 74:164-168, 2003.

161. Ang B, Linder J, Harms-Ringdahl K: Neck strength and myoelectric fatigue in fighter and helicopter pilots with a history of neck pain, Aviat Space Environ Med 76:375-380, 2005.

162. Hodges PW, Pengel LHM, Herbert RD, et al: Measurement of muscle contraction with ultrasound imaging, Muscle Nerve 27:682-692, 2003.

163. Wallwork TL, Hide JA, Stanton WR: Intrarater and interrater reliability of assessment of lumbar multifidus muscle thickness using rehabilitative ultrasound imaging, J Orthop Sports Phys Ther 37:608-612, 2007.

164. Hides JA, Miokovic T, Belavy DL, et al: Ultrasound imaging assessment of abdominal muscle function during drawing-in of the abdominal wall: an intrarater reliability study, J Orthop Sports Phys Ther 37(8):480-486, 2007.

165. Stokes M, Hides J, Elliot J, et al: Rehabilitative ultrasound imaging of the posterior paraspinal muscles, J Orthop Sports Phys Ther 37(10)581-595, 2007.

166. Van K, Hides JA, Richardson CA: The use of real-time ultrasound imaging for biofeedback of lumbar multifidus muscle contraction in healthy subjects, J Orthop Sports Phys Ther 36(12):920-925, 2006.

167. Hides JA, Richardson CA, Jull G: Use of real-time ultrasound imaging for feedback in rehabilitation, Man Ther 3:125-131, 1998.

168. Hides JA, Jull GA, Richardson CA: Long-term effects of specific stabilizing exercises for first-episode low back pain, Spine 26:E243-248, 2001.

169. Morningstar MW, Pettibon BR, Schlappi H, et al: Reflex control of the spine and posture: a review of the literature from a chiropractic perspective, Chiropr Osteopat 13:16-24, 2005.

170. Saunders ES, Woggon D, Cohen C, et al: Improvement of cervical lordosis and reduction of forward head posture with anterior head weighting and proprioceptive balancing protocols, JVSR April:1-5, 2003.

171. Thuresson M, Linder AB, Harms Ringdahl K: Neck muscle activity in helicopter pilots: effect of position and helmet-mounted equipment, Aviat Space Environ Med 74:527-532, 2003.

172. Knight JF, Baber C: Neck muscle activity and perceived pain and discomfort due to variations of head load and posture, Aviat Space Environ Med 75:123-131, 2004.

173. De Nunzio AM, Nardone A, Schieppati M: Head stabilization on a continuously oscillating platform: the effect of a proprioceptive disturbance on balance strategy, Exp Brain Res 165: 261-272, 2005.

174. Blouin JS, Descarreaux M, Belanger-Gravel A, et al: Attenuation of human neck muscle activity following repeated imposed trunk-forward linear acceleration, Exp Brain Res 150:458-464, 2003.

175. Falla D, Jull G, Hodges PW: Feedforward activity of the cervical flexor muscles during voluntary arm movements is delayed in chronic neck pain, Exp Brain Res 157:43-48, 2004.

176. Cordero AF, Levin O, Li Y, et al: Posture control and complex arm coordination: analysis of multijoint coordinative movements and stability of stance, J Mot Behav 39(3):215-226, 2007.

177. Knox JJ, Coppieter MW, Hodges PW: Do you know where your arm is if you think your head has moved, Exp Brain Res 173:95-101, 2006.

178. Borel L, Harlar F, Magnan J, et al: Deficits and recovery of head and orientation and stabilization after unilateral vestibular loss, Brain 125:880-894, 2002.

179. Kershner EA: Head-trunk coordination during linear anterior-posterior translations, J Neurophysiol 89:1891-1911, 2003.

180. Kershner EA, Hain TC, Chen KJ: Predicting control mechanisms for human head stabilization by altering passive mechanics, J Vestib Res 9:423-434, 1999.

181. Keshner EA: Modulating active stiffness affects head stabilizing strategies in young and elderly adults during trunk rotations in vertical plane, Gait Posture 11:1-11, 2000.

182. Cavanaugh JT, Goldvaser D, McGibbon A, et al: Comparison of head- and body-velocity trajectories during locomotion among healthy and vestibulopathic subjects, J Rehabil Res Devel 42(2):191-198, 2005.

183. Andre-Deshays C, Berthoz A, Revel M: Eye-head coupling in humans I. Simultaneous recording of isolated motor units in dorsal neck muscles and horizontal eye movements, Exp Brain Res 69:399-406, 1988.

184. Bexander CSM, Mellor R, Hodges PW: Effect of gaze direction on neck muscle activity during cervical rotation, Exp Brain Res 167:422-432, 2005.

185. Kelders WPA, Klenrensink GJ, vand der Geest JN et al: Compensatory increase of the cervico-ocular reflex with age in healthy humans, J Physiol 553(1):311-317, 2003.

186. Kongsted A, Jorgensen LV, Bendix T, et al: Are smooth pursuit eye movements altered in chronic whiplash-associated disorders? A cross-sectional study, Clin Rehabil 21:1038-1049, 2007.

Exercises for the Trunk, Shoulder, Hip, and Knee
Electromyographic Evidence

The purpose of this chapter is to provide guidelines for exercises that may be effective for the rehabilitation of the trunk, shoulder, hip, and knee based on evidence gathered by electromyography (EMG). Evidence indicates that a strong relationship exists between the EMG signal amplitude and the amount of force produced by a muscle.[1-3]

When EMG data for a muscle during an exercise are normalized, the result is the percentage of muscle activity produced during the exercise compared with the activity the muscle can produce during a maximum contraction. The contraction is usually a maximum voluntary isometric contraction (MVIC). For the purpose of clinical practice, the percent of MVIC determined by electromyography should relate quite well to a corresponding percent of one repetition maximum (the amount of weight an individual can lift during an exercise one time, and one time only).

In untrained individuals, loads of 45% to 50% of one repetition maximum have been shown to increase strength.[4,5] Therefore those exercises that produce EMG signal amplitude in a muscle of greater than 45% MVIC may provide sufficient stimulus for strength gains in some patients, especially after injury. Individuals that are better conditioned or more advanced in their rehabilitation program will need higher levels of stimulus to obtain a strengthening response. Those exercises that produce levels of EMG signal amplitude in a muscle of less than 45% MVIC should be considered exercises best suited for endurance or motor control training.

EXERCISE FOR STRENGTH AND ENDURANCE TRAINING OF THE LOW BACK

Literature reviews have been performed regarding the effectiveness of exercise for patients with chronic low-back pain (LBP).[6-12] The authors of these reviews have concluded that exercise is beneficial for the treatment of patients with chronic LBP, but none of the reviews demonstrated that one exercise is better than another. Faas[10] concluded that intensive exercise may be more effective than mild exercising. The literature seems to provide very little evidence to indicate that exercise is any more beneficial for patients with acute LBP when compared with advice to a patient to resume normal daily activities as soon as possible, even when experiencing some pain.

Even though a lack of good evidence exists for exercise for patients with acute LBP, one could conclude that all patients with either acute or chronic LBP could benefit from appropriate exercise programs. Wilke et al.[13] demonstrated in a biomechanical study that the lumbar multifidus muscle provides more than two thirds of the stiffness increase at the L4-5 lumbar segment, and therefore is a very important muscle for lumbar segmental stability. Atrophy and weakness of the lumbar multifidus may then lead to instability. The lumbar multifidus muscle has been shown to atrophy at the dysfunctional segment in patients with acute LBP.[14,15] In patients with chronic LBP, the whole muscle will tend to atrophy from disuse and may become infiltrated with fatty tissue.[16-20]

In addition, evidence exists of motor control dysfunction in the transversus abdominis (TrA) and lumbar multifidus muscles in patients with LBP.[13,21-26] In normal subjects, these two muscles have been shown to be recruited before extremity movements, and their activation does not appear to be directional but will contract with movements of the limbs in any direction.[23,14,25] In patients with LBP, these muscles tend to have a delay in activation contracting after the initiation of limb movements, rather than before. This delay in activation may result in a lack of protective stabilization for the spine before movement of the body. Ferreira et al.[27] also demonstrated with ultrasound imaging that the TrA muscle contracts with less thickness in patients with LBP. Moseley et al.[28] found an independent activation pattern of the deep versus superficial parts of the lumbar multifidus muscles. The deep fibers seem to have nondirectional activation causing compression and stability for the segment, whereas the superficial fibers tend to function more as movers of the spine. Moseley et al.[29] also found an increase of deep multifidus fiber activity in anticipation of trunk loading that is not observed in the more superficial fibers. It is felt that the deep part of the lumbar multifidus and the TrA muscles work in synergy for optimal segmental stabilization of the spine.[30,31]

Hides et al.[14] demonstrated less lumbar multifidus muscle segmental atrophy in patients who had acute LBP after a 10-week stabilization exercise program compared with patients who did not exercise. Reduced recurrence rates of LBP has also been demonstrated for patients that performed this exercise program.[32] O'Sullivan et al.[33] used a similar exercise approach in patients with chronic LBP having spondylolysis and spondylolisthesis and demonstrated significant reduction in disability after the exercise program. Goldby et al.[34] also demonstrated positive results with the exercise program in other patients with chronic LBP. The exercise program used in these studies emphasized the facilitation of an active, isometric contraction of the lumbar multifidus muscle with cocontraction of the deep abdominal muscles during specific exercises and activities. This exercise program was performed at very low–intensity levels with a goal of improving motor control of the TrA, internal oblique abdominis (IO), and lumbar multifidus muscles. However, Koumantakis et al.[35] compared a lumbar stabilization exercise approach to a more general strengthening program in patients with subacute and chronic nonspecific LBP and did not find any significant difference in outcomes when comparing the two groups. Risch et al.[36] and Manniche et al.[37] have demonstrated benefits of an intensive strengthening program for patients with chronic LBP.

More exercise studies need to be performed involving patients with LBP classified into homogeneous groups with similar signs and symptoms before clinicians can make definitive conclusions about what types of exercises are most effective. In patients with acute LBP, exercise programs may be most effective for reducing recurrence rates.

Lumbar Extension Exercises

Active lumbar extension exercises from the prone-lying position will maximally activate the lumbar multifidus and erector spinae muscles. These exercises are performed at an intensity level that should produce a strengthening response in the muscles. However, because these exercises activate the muscles to their highest level, greater compression occurs on the lumbar spine, which some patients may not tolerate.[38]

When subjects extended the lumbar spine by raising both upper and lower extremities off the table into a "Superman position" (Figure 29-1, A), researchers have recorded activity in the lumbar multifidus and erector spinae muscles ranging from 48% to 66% MVIC.[38-40] When subjects extended the lumbar spine by just raising the upper body off the table with the feet stabilized (Figure 29-1, B), other researchers have found EMG signal amplitude levels ranging from 80% to 84% MVIC in the multifidus and erector spinae muscles respectively.[41,42] Drake et al.[43] recorded lower levels of 43% to 69% MVIC in the multifidus and erector spinae respectively during prone trunk extension with the arms abducted to 90 degrees.

Researchers have recorded muscle activity in the lumbar multifidus and erector spinae ranging from 45% to 81% MVIC when subjects extended the spine to neutral when positioned with the trunk over the end of a table.[40,44] Arokoski et al.[45]

found that women had higher levels of muscle activity at 56% MVIC as compared with men at 36% MVIC during the same exercise.

Shirado et al.[46] found an increase in erector spinae muscle activity during active trunk extension if the pelvis is first stabilized with muscle contractions of the abdominal and gluteus maximus muscles with the neck maximally flexed. Mayer et al.[47] studied the effect of hip position on the lumbar paraspinal muscle activity during lumbar extension exercise with the feet stabilized. They recorded 18% greater paraspinal activity when the hips were internally rotated as compared with externally rotated hips.

When comparing men and women during lower-extremity lifts in the prone position with the trunk stabilized, Arokoski et al.[48] recorded EMG signal amplitudes ranging from 34% to 50% MVIC in the lumbar multifidus muscles. A prone bilateral lower-extremity lift to maximum range over the edge of a table produced muscle activity in the multifidus that ranged from 61% to 77%.[48] Ng and Richardson[44] found similar levels of muscle activity during the same exercise that ranged from 61% to 73% MVIC.

Also of interest is that the activity of the gluteus maximus muscle increases at a greater extent than that of the paraspinal muscles as increased resistance is applied during the prone lumbar extension exercise.[49] The gluteus maximus muscle seems to be responsible for accommodating additional external loads. Leinonen et al.[50] had previously studied the activity of the lumbar paraspinals and gluteus maximus muscle in patients with LBP during standing active flexion and the return to the upright position. The activity of the gluteus maximus muscle during the flexion-extension cycle was reduced in patients with LBP. Therefore the gluteus maximus function and strength should be considered during the rehabilitation of patients with LBP.

LUMBAR STABILIZATION EXERCISES IN NEUTRAL SPINE POSITION

Lumbar stabilization exercises are often performed in the supine position. The lumbar spine is held in a neutral position with abdominal muscle contraction (many use the abdominal hollowing maneuver by drawing the umbilicus in and up toward the spine) while the subject performs various movements with either the upper or lower extremities (Figure 29-2).[30] Some authors stress that patients should learn isolated, active contraction of the lumbar multifidus muscle before advancing to more difficult stabilization exercises so that cocontraction occurs with the abdominal muscles.[30,31] EMG signal amplitudes ranging from 6% to 7% MVIC in the rectus abdominis (RA), 15% to 19% MVIC in the external oblique abdominis (EO), and 4% to 7% MVIC in the multifidus and erector spinae muscles have been recorded during the abdominal hollowing exercise in patients with and without LBP.[51,52]

The stabilization exercises can then be made more difficult with movements of either the upper or lower extremities while

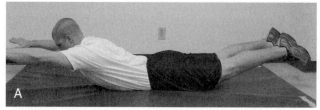

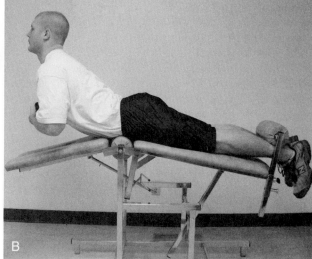

Figure 29-1 A, Lumbar extension with the upper and lower extremities raised. **B,** Active lumbar extension.

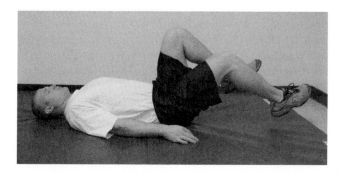

Figure 29-2 Lumbar stabilization exercise with deep abdominal muscle contraction.

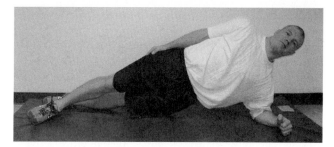

Figure 29-3 Side-support exercise with the spine in neutral position.

the lumbar spine is maintained in a neutral spine position. The ability to maintain the lumbar spine in neutral is often monitored by a pressure transducer placed under the lumbar spine. Davidson and Hubley-Kozey[53] performed an exercise progression with movements of the lower extremities, with the most difficult exercise being bilateral lower-extremity extension with the heels slightly off the table while maintaining a neutral spine position.[53] During the exercise progression, the activity in the RA and EO muscles ranged from 15% MVIC up to 39% MVIC. There was very low muscle activity in the erector spinae and lumbar multifidus ranging from 3% to 7% MVIC during the exercise progression. Souza et al.[54] studied the dying bug exercise using both upper-extremity flexion and lower-extremity extension motions simultaneously while maintaining the lumbar spine in a neutral position. The muscle activity in the erector spinae remained quite low at about 6% MVIC or less, even during the most difficult part of the exercise. The highest level of muscle activity in the RA and EO was about 40% MVIC.

Side-Support Exercise

This exercise is performed with the patient on the side and supported on the elbow and feet with the spine aligned in the

neutral position (Figure 29-3). Ekstrom et al.[55] recorded EMG amplitudes of 40% and 42% MVIC respectively in the longissimus thoracis and lumbar multifidis muscles and 69% MVIC in the EO muscle on the side of the supporting elbow and feet. McGill[38] and McGill et al.[56] had previously recorded EMG signal amplitude levels of 43% MVIC in the EO, 36% MVIC in the IO, 39% MVIC in the TrA, 54% MVIC in the quadratus lumborum, and 24% MVIC in the erector spinae. Kavcic et al.[57] demonstrated similar results for the erector spinae and lumbar multifidus muscles. This is considered a good back exercise, because of the cocontraction of the abdominal, paraspinal, and the quadratus lumborum muscles.

Bridge Exercise

The bridge exercise is performed from the crook-lying position (Figure 29-4). The hips are raised only to a point where the hips and low back are aligned and the spine is maintained in a neutral position. Ekstrom et al.[55] recorded muscle activity of 39% MVIC in both the lumbar multifidus and the longissimus thoracis muscles during a bilateral bridge, and 44% and 40% MVIC respectively in these muscles on the side of the lower-extremity support during a unilateral bridge. Kavcic et al.[57] recorded lower EMG signal amplitudes ranging from 15% to

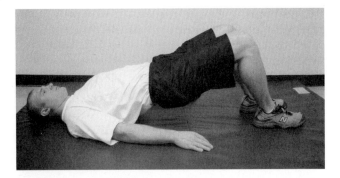

Figure 29-4 Bridging exercise.

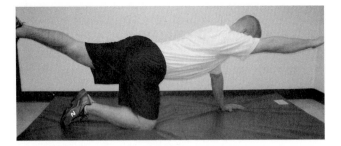

Figure 29-5 Quadruped arm and leg lift exercise.

20% MVIC in these muscles during these same two exercises. Arokoski et al.[48] found that men and women varied considerably in the muscle activity of the low back during these exercises. In the lumbar multifidus muscle, they recorded activity of 33% MVIC for men and 53% MVIC for women during the bilateral bridge and 34% MVIC for men and 65% MVIC for women during the unilateral bridge. This exercise seems to be most appropriate for endurance training of the spinal muscles, but in some women a strengthening effect may occur as well.

Quadruped Lower- and Upper-Extremity Lift

The patient performs this exercise by raising one lower extremity and the opposite upper extremity up to the point that the patient can still maintain a neutral spine position in the quadruped position (Figure 29-5). EMG signal amplitude levels of 36% and 46% MVIC have been recorded in the longissimus thoracis and lumbar multifidus muscles respectively on the side of the lower-extremity lift during this exercise.[55] Others have recorded values ranging from about 20% to 50% MVIC for the erector spinae and 27% to 56% MVIC for the lumbar multifidus muscle.* From the level of muscle activity produced, one could conclude that this exercise is best for endurance training of the lumbar spinal musculature (Box 29-1).

ABDOMINAL EXERCISES

Abdominal exercises are usually performed to help individuals improve fitness level or athletic performance by improving core

---

*References 38, 40, 41, 43, 45, 48, 57, 58.

strength and control. They also are commonly prescribed for patients with low-back problems with the goal to improve control and endurance of the muscles and to teach the patient how to stabilize the pelvis and spine during functional activities. The abdominal muscles are the RA, TrA, EO, and IO.

Many of the abdominal exercises commonly performed do not stress the muscles to levels that will significantly improve strength but are better suited for improving endurance. Because the abdominal muscles are both postural and prime movers of the trunk, the stress on endurance training would seem to be appropriate.

Abdominal Hollowing Exercise (Abdominal Drawing-In Maneuver)

The patient performs this abdominal exercise by hollowing the abdomen by drawing the navel up and in toward the spine. The goal of the exercise is to attempt to cocontract the TrA and the deep fascicles of the lumbar multifidus muscles at a very low level with minimal contraction of other abdominal muscles and erector spinae in the back as the spine is maintained in a neutral position.[30] This exercise approach has become very popular with clinicians during the initial stages of teaching stabilization exercises. When the patient has learned to perform cocontraction of the TrA and lumbar multifidus muscle, they are progressed to more advanced stabilization exercises. This exercise routine has been demonstrated to be effective in restoring lumbar multifidus muscle size in patients with acute LBP[15] and in reducing pain and disability in patients with documented lumbar instability.[33] However, it is unknown whether this is the most effective method for retraining motor control of the deep trunk muscles.

During a gentle abdominal hollowing maneuver, the TrA muscle is activated minimally at about 1% to 2% MVIC, and it may contract independently of the other abdominal muscles.[30] However, most subjects are unable to isolate abdominal activity only to the TrA muscle. As the demand for stabilization of the spine increases, the EO and IO muscles become more active and the TrA muscle can no longer contract in isolation.[51,53,59]

Other researchers have recorded EMG signal amplitudes ranging from 5% to 6% MVIC in the lower RA, 6% to 12% MVIC in the upper RA, 15% to 19% MVIC in the EO, and 4% to 5% MVIC in the lumbar multifidus muscle during the hollowing exercise.[51,52,60]

Maximum contraction of the pelvic floor muscles during the hollowing exercise will increase the EMG signal amplitude levels in all the abdominal muscles (but to a greater amount in the TrA muscle, especially at lower levels of effort).[61] Critchley[62] demonstrated greater activation of the TrA as compared with the EO and IO muscles with the pelvic floor contracted during abdominal hollowing when performed in the quadruped position.

During the abdominal hollowing exercise, additional stress can be placed on the abdominal muscles by adding movements of the upper or lower extremities as the spine is maintained in a neutral position. Many of these exercises have been developed.[30,53,54] During the most difficult exercises, the abdominal muscles tend to be equally recruited with EMG signal amplitudes ranging from 37% to 40% MVIC in both the RA and the EO muscles.[53,54]

Although the abdominal hollowing exercise seems to be effective for retraining cocontraction of the abdominal, pelvic floor, and segmental back muscles, it is not the best maneuver for establishing spinal stability during functional activities. It has been demonstrated that abdominal bracing is more effective in creating trunk stability than the hollowing maneuver when perturbations are applied to the trunk.[63,64]

Abdominal Bracing Exercise

The abdominal bracing exercise is performed with emphasis on the coactivation of all the abdominal and back muscles to a level that increases torso stiffness with the spine maintained in a neutral position. When this is performed, the EO and IO muscles contract very strongly so that the abdominal wall contracts and expands laterally. Richardson et al.[65] recorded EMG signal amplitude levels of 12% MVIC during the abdominal hollowing maneuver and 32% MVIC during the bracing maneuver in the EO muscle.

Abdominal bracing is similar to an abdominal contraction that occurs during the Valsalva maneuver. The patient should learn to perform the contraction with a normal breathing pattern. Abdominal bracing should be practiced and taught to patients during lifting and other heavy functional activities to prevent undue stress on the spine.[65]

Posterior Pelvic Tilt Exercise

During the posterior pelvic tilt exercise, the abdominal muscles are contracted and the lordosis of the lumbar spine is reduced or flattened. This exercise can be used for general range of motion of the lumbar spine or for training a patient to maintain the spine in reduced lordosis if they have an increased lordotic curve causing LBP. This exercise has been shown to produce EMG signal amplitudes of 13% MVIC in the lower RA, 12% to 16% MVIC in the upper RA, and 26% to 32% in the EO

when performed in a supine position.[51,52] Filho et al.[66] had subjects perform a maximum-effort posterior pelvic tilt and recorded bilateral EMG signal amplitude levels of 25% to 29% MVIC in the RA, 26% to 29% MVIC in the EO, and 35% to 49% MVIC in the IO. It therefore appears that this exercise, when performed at low levels, will recruit the EO to higher levels than the RA, but with greater effort the muscle activity between those two muscles is very similar. The IO seems to be recruited to the greatest level when comparing the three muscles during maximum efforts.

Some clinicians may teach patients to perform a posterior pelvic tilt for stabilization during lifting and other functional activities. However, McGill[38] warns against using the posterior pelvic tilt before loading, because the posterior pelvic tilt may flex and flatten the lumbar spine too much and preload the disc. He suggested it is better to perform stabilization with the spine in a neutral position during functional activities.

Sit-Up Exercises

The sit-up exercise has been used extensively for strengthening the abdominal muscles. During a full sit-up, the iliopsoas muscles must work to flex the hips as the abdominal muscles flex the trunk. Kendall et al.[67] have stressed that a subject needs good abdominal control during the full sit-up to counteract the pull of the iliopsoas muscles, otherwise the lumbar spine may be pulled into hyperlordosis and place strain on the lumbar spine. If one does not have good abdominal control, then the full sit-up exercise should not be performed. In addition, the contraction of the iliopsoas will place higher compressive forces on the lumbar spine as compared with a curl exercise, so some patients with LBP may not tolerate the exercise.[38,68]

No significant difference of muscle activity is seen for any of the hip flexor or abdominal muscles when comparing the straight-leg sit-up and the bent-knee sit-up.[59] During either sit-up, the RA and EO muscles were activated to levels ranging from 43% to 55% MVIC. The TrA and IO muscles were activated to fairly low levels during the two exercises with EMG signal amplitudes ranging from 10% to 16% MVIC. Escamilla et al.[69] recorded EMG signal amplitude level of 49% MVIC in the IO, which is significantly higher, but their recordings for the RA and EO were not significantly different from those of Juker et al.[59]

Psoas muscle activity ranged from 24% to 28% MVIC during the two exercises.[38,59] Clinicians have advocated a "press-heels" sit-up, which activates the hip extensors during the sit-up. The theory has been that this will cause reciprocal inhibition of the psoas muscle, and therefore reduce compressive forces on the spine. This, however, has been proven to be false. This maneuver increased the activity of the psoas muscle to 34% MVIC.[38,59]

The muscle activity during the bent-knee sit-up has been compared with the muscle activity produced when using abdominal exercise devices, and it has been shown to be just as effective. An exception is the slide-out devices that significantly increase the RA activity.[69,70] A slide-out exercise is per-

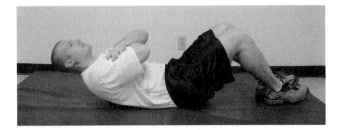

Figure 29-6 Curl-up exercise.

formed in the quadruped position with a track or wheel, which allows the upper extremities to go into flexion as far as possible as one attempts to keep the spine in a neutral position.

Curl-Up Exercises

Curl-up exercises are usually performed in the supine position with the hips flexed to 45 degrees and the knees flexed to 90 degrees with the feet on the floor or else with the hips and knees both flexed to 90 degrees (Figure 29-6). The head and shoulders are raised until the scapulae just clear the floor or table. To attempt to stress the obliques to a greater extent, a twist of the trunk to the left or right is often incorporated.

It has been demonstrated that the RA is the most active muscle during the curl-up exercises.[38,59] The activity in the RA was found to be 62% MVIC with all of the other abdominal muscles having activity of less than 19% MVIC and the psoas muscle activity of about 10% MVIC. In a more recent study, Lehman and McGill[71] recorded less muscle activity in the RA (38% MVIC) during a curl-up with the hands placed behind the lumbar spine, but the EO activity was similar at 20% MVIC. During the active curl-up, Willett et al.[72] and Escamilla et al.[69] recorded similar activity of the RA but higher levels of activity in the EO and IO muscles ranging from 27% to 42% MVIC. Willett et al.[72] and Juker et al.[59] did not find that the EO muscle activity increased during a curl-up with a twist to the opposite side, but Escamilla et al.[70] demonstrated a tendency toward increased EO activity.

Karst and Willett[73] reported on strategies to emphasize either the RA or oblique muscles during a curl-up exercise. For the RA they instructed subjects to push the belly button out by tightening the stomach muscles and then curl up, shortening the distance between the xiphoid and the pubic symphysis, drawing the rib cage down and inward. To emphasize oblique activity, they instructed the subject to suck in the stomach, flatten the lower back to the table, and then curl up while focusing on flaring out the rib cage. The instructions for the RA changed muscle activity very little as compared with a curl-up with no instructions; however, the RA activity was greater than EO activity in both cases. The instructions for emphasis on oblique activity increased IO and EO muscle activity by about 20% and at the same time reduced RA activity. The EO and IO muscle activity was now greater than the RA activity.

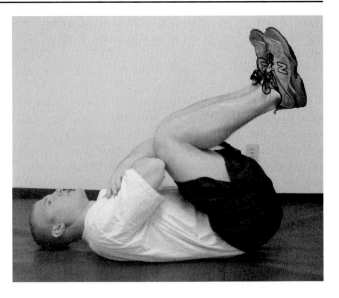

Figure 29-7 Reverse curl-up exercise.

The muscle activity in all the abdominal and psoas muscles can be significantly increased during a curl-up with isometric resistance by pushing the hand against the opposite knee with the hip flexed to about 90 degrees.[59] This increased RA muscle activity up to 74% MVIC and EO activity to 68% MVIC. IO activity increased to 48% MVIC, TrA activity to 44% MVIC, and the psoas muscle activity to 58% MVIC.

Another way to increase abdominal muscle activity is to perform curl-ups on an unsteady surface. Vera-Garcia et al.[74] demonstrated significant increases in the RA and EO muscles when performing the curl-up when lying with the back on a gymnastic ball or on a wobble board.

Reverse Curl

The reverse curl is performed by actively bringing the knees to the chest as far as possible, curling the spine inferiorly to superiorly (Figure 29-7). The upper-extremity position may change the difficulty of the exercise. Willett et al.[72] had subjects cross their arms over the chest and Escamilla et al.[69] had the subjects place their arms along their sides. With the arms at the side a tendency may exist for a subject to push down with the upper extremities and therefore assist the abdominal muscles. Willett et al.[72] recorded EMG signal amplitude levels of up to about 90% MVIC in the lower RA and 66% MVIC in the EO muscle, whereas Escamilla et al.[69] recorded muscle activity levels of 41% MVIC in the RA, 39% MVIC in the EO, and 52% in the IO.

Escamilla et al.[69] also studied this exercise with the subjects placed on a 30-degree incline and found that the EMG activity significantly increased, especially in the RA and IO muscles. The IO activity increased to a level of 86% MVIC. During this exercise the subject grabbed onto a bar overhead for stabilization. It would appear that the reverse curl exercise is at a difficulty level that could qualify it as both a strengthening and an endurance exercise for the abdominal muscles.

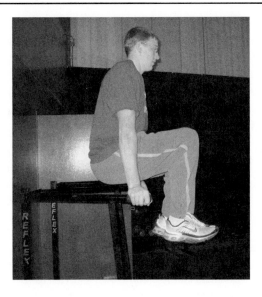

Figure 29-8 Hanging abdominal exercise with hip flexion.

Hanging Hip Flexion Exercises

This exercise is similar to a reverse curl, but is performed against gravity. The exercise can be performed while hanging from a chin-up bar or with the hands supported on parallel bars (Figure 29-8). The hips are then flexed as far as possible, either with the knees flexed or extended. With the knees and hips actively flexed as far as possible, Escamilla et al.[69] reported high levels of muscle activity in all the abdominal muscles, with 77% MVIC in the upper RA, 53% MVIC in the lower RA, 79% MVIC in the EO, and 85% MVIC in the IO when hanging from a bar. Axler and McGill[68] reported even higher levels of EMG amplitudes in the RA and EO when the subjects were hanging from a chin-up bar. Hip flexion with the knees extended increased the muscle activity by about 10% to 15%, as compared with performing the exercise with the knees flexed.

Bilateral Straight-Leg Raises

Filho et al.[66] studied the bilateral leg-lowering exercise. They recorded the greatest activity in the EO muscle as compared with the RA and IO muscles. The activity level of all the abdominal muscles stayed fairly constant from 70 to 30 degrees of hip flexion, and then all muscle activity gradually decreased, especially at 10 degrees. The RA muscle reached a maximum activity level of 43% MVIC, as compared with 55% MVIC for the EO, and 28% MVIC for the IO. They used a pressure cuff under the low back to monitor a subject's ability to keep the back flat against the table. A gradual decrease occurred in the pressure cuff in all subjects as the lower extremities were lowered. This exercise also required psoas muscle activity of about 35% MVIC.[59] In another study, EMG signal amplitude levels were recorded at 47% MVIC in the RA and 38% MVIC in the EO with the lower extremities raised 25 cm off the table.[71] There does not appear to be any advantage in using this exercise over other abdominal exercises that elicit high levels

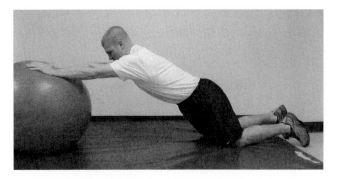

Figure 29-9 Roll-out abdominal exercise.

of muscular activity. In many subjects it may place a strain on the low back because of the psoas muscle activity.[59]

Isometric Side-Support Exercise

To perform the isometric side-support exercise, a subject is positioned on the side and resting on the elbow. The subject then raises the hips off the table until the spine is in neutral alignment. This exercise activates the abdominal, paraspinal, hip abductor, and quadratus lumborum muscles on the side of support. It is thought to be a very good trunk stabilization exercise, because of the cocontraction of the abdominal and back muscles.

EMG signal amplitudes ranging from 39% to 43% MVIC were recorded in the EO, IO, and TrA, but the RA was activated to a lesser degree at 22% MVIC on the side of support.[38,59] When performed dynamically a slightly higher recording was noted, but the increase was not significant. Axler and McGill[68] and Ekstrom et al.[55] recorded higher EMG signal amplitudes ranging from 50% to 69% MVIC in the EO and 34% to 50% MVIC in the RA muscle during an isometric hold. The muscle activity in the quadratus lumborum has been recorded at 54% MVIC, the lumbar multifidus at 42% MVIC, and in the longissimus thoracic at 40% MVIC.[55]

The exercise may also be performed with support on the elbow and knees, which reduces the difficulty of the exercise for patients that may have back pain. It should be considered as a core exercise in a back rehabilitation program.

Slide-Out or Rollout Exercise

The slide-out or roll-out exercise is performed with devices such as the Power Wheel, Torso Track, or Ab Slide.[69,70] Starting in the quadruped position with the hands on one of these devices, the shoulders are gradually flexed with the knees remaining on the floor (Figure 29-9). The shoulders are flexed to a point where it takes maximum effort to maintain the spine in a neutral position and then the shoulders are extended so that the body is brought back to the starting quadruped position. This exercise using the three devices has produced EMG signal levels ranging from 61% to 81% MVIC in the RA muscle. The Ab Slide and Torso Track devices did not appear to be any better than a bent-knee sit-up or a curl-up exercise for producing activity in the EO and IO muscles.[70] However,

BOX 29-2**Exercises Generating the Greatest to the Least Amount of EMG Signal Amplitude for the Rectus Abdominis Muscle**

Strengthening Exercises

- Upper-extremity slide-out or roll-out from the quadruped position
- 30-Degree incline reverse curl
- Reverse curl
- Hanging hip flexion with the knees flexed or extended
- Curl-up with isometric resistance with the hand against the opposite knee
- Curl-up

Endurance Exercises

- Sit-up
- Supine stabilization exercises with transversus abdominis (TrA) contraction
- Posterior pelvic tilt
- Abdominal hollowing

BOX 29-3 **Exercises Generating the Greatest to the Least Amount of EMG Signal Amplitude for the External Oblique Abdominis Muscle**

Strengthening Exercises

- Hanging hip flexion with the knees flexed or extended
- Curl-up with isometric resistance with the hand against the opposite knee
- 30-Degree incline reverse curl
- Reverse curl

Endurance Exercises

- Sit-up
- Upper-extremity slide-out or roll-out from the quadruped position
- Bilateral lower-extremity lifts
- Supine stabilization exercises with transversus abdominis (TrA) contraction
- Posterior pelvic tilt
- Abdominal hollowing

---

the exercise with the Power Roller did show a tendency for greater activity (Box 29-2, Box 29-3).[69]

UPPER- AND LOWER-EXTREMITY MUSCLE ACTIVATION

Pain-free muscle activation during any exercise is felt to be important for recovery from a variety of musculoskeletal conditions, including those of the shoulder, hip, and knee joints. Many studies have assessed muscle activation in single sessions, which is helpful to determine the level of muscle activation with a particular activity or exercise. However, few studies have conducted strengthening programs for 6 weeks or longer, as suggested by the American College of Sports Medicine[75] with pre- and posttesting to determine if the muscle activation identified in the single test session does in fact create a strength-

ening effect. In addition, many of the studies involving specific exercises have been performed on normal subjects, with a limited number of studies incorporating randomization when performed on subjects with specific conditions.

Open Kinetic Chain Exercise versus Closed Kinetic Chain Exercise

It would be difficult to discuss exercises involving the extremities without discussing open and closed kinetic chain exercise. Considerable interest has been focused on the use of both open kinetic chain and closed kinetic chain exercise during rehabilitation programs for patients with various knee conditions, but most frequently for patients with unstable knees because of ligamentous injury. For a review of the history, scientific rationale, and clinical application of the concepts important to both open kinetic chain exercise and closed kinetic chain exercise, the reader is referred to the work by Davies et al.[76] Open kinetic chain exercises are commonly thought of as those exercises in which the distal segment is not fixed, not in contact with another surface, and only one joint moves during the motion. Typically, open kinetic chain exercises tend to isolate a particular muscle during a specific joint movement. One example would be seated leg extension (quadriceps muscle activation) in which the tibia is moving on the femur. A second example would be an exercise involving arm flexion and curl (biceps brachii and brachialis muscle activation) in which movement is occurring at the elbow joint (ulna and radius moving on humerus), but the shoulder joint is not involved in the activity. A third example would be a straight-leg raise (SLR) in which the movement is occurring at the hip joint (femur moving on the acetabulum), but the knee and ankle joints are not involved in the movement. Closed kinetic chain exercises are described as those movements or exercises in which the distal extremity is fixed and multiple joints are moving simultaneously during the activity. An example of this would be a leg press in which an individual is lying on a platform with the feet in contact with a footplate that moves separately from the platform. When the individual pushes on the footplate, either the footplate or the platform moves, and the hip, knee, or ankle joints (tibia moving on talus) are all moving simultaneously. Closed kinetic chain exercise provides simultaneous activation of multiple muscles (both single- and multiple-joint muscles) because of concurrent multiple-joint movements. The following exercises typically fit one of these two kinetic movement patterns.

Shoulder Girdle and Glenohumeral Joint Exercises

A rehabilitation program for the shoulder should include exercises not only for muscles controlling the glenohumeral joint but also for exercises for strengthening the scapular muscles. Scapular control is important as a foundation on which the glenohumeral joint can function in a normal manner.

Normal scapulohumeral rhythm must be maintained during elevation of the upper extremity. That is, during full elevation of the shoulder through about 180 degrees, the scapula should upwardly rotate about 60 degrees while the humerus flexes or abducts about 120 degrees. This requires good coordinated function of the rotator cuff and deltoid muscles at the glenohumeral joint, as well as scapular control by the serratus anterior and trapezius muscles. The following information provides evidence for exercises that may be used for strengthening the various muscles of the shoulder girdle and glenohumeral joint. Of special interest to many is how to best activate the muscles of the rotator cuff.

Military Press

Several authors have performed EMG studies to evaluate the muscle activation levels during the military press exercise.[77-80] The anterior and middle deltoid, supraspinatus, upper trapezius, and serratus anterior muscles have been shown to be highly activated with EMG signal amplitudes of 62% MVIC or greater.[77-79] Townsend et al.[78] demonstrated high levels of supraspinatus muscle activity of 80% MVIC even during exercise of moderate intensity.

Horizontal Bench Press, Incline Press, and Decline Press

Barnett et al.[77] compared pectoralis major, anterior deltoid, and triceps brachii muscle activity during all three exercises. They found maximum activity in the sternocostal head of the pectoralis major during the horizontal bench press and maximum activity in the clavicular head of the pectoralis major during an incline press, especially with a narrower handgrip. Hand spacing did not affect the muscle activity of the sternocostal head of the pectoralis major.

Glass and Armstrong[81] compared just the incline (30 degrees) and decline (−15 degrees) bench press positions and found greater activity in the sternocostal part of the pectoralis major during the decline position but no significant difference in the clavicular head during the two exercises.

The anterior deltoid activity increased in activity during the incline press. Welsch et al.[82] recorded peak levels of muscle activity in the pectoralis major and anterior deltoid of 56% MVIC during a horizontal barbell bench press exercise performed at six-repetition maximum. The triceps brachii muscle activity was greatest during the horizontal bench press. Narrow hand spacing increased its activity as compared with a wider handgrip.[77]

Because great difference is not found in muscle activity in the decline, incline, or horizontal bench press, any position could be used during rehabilitation. Progressing from a horizontal bench press to increasing levels of an incline press is a good method of gradually progressing to overhead activities.

Scapular Protraction Exercises

Shoulder protraction at the end phase of a bench press exercise is often used for strengthening the serratus anterior muscle. However, Ekstrom et al.[83-85] demonstrated that this exercise is not optimal for producing activity in the serratus anterior muscle. During a maximally resisted muscle test in this position, the EMG amplitude reached only levels of 54% ± 27% MVIC in the serratus anterior and an exercise performed at 5 repetition maximum (RM) intensity produced EMG amplitude levels of 62% ± 19% MVIC. The serratus anterior muscle reaches maximum EMG amplitude levels only when upward rotation of the scapula is resisted.

Other scapular protraction exercises for serratus anterior strengthening such as the forward punch, serratus anterior punch, and dynamic hug exercises have been studied.[86,87] Hintermeister et al.[86] found that the forward punch exercise performed with moderate resistance produced EMG amplitudes of 49% MVIC in the serratus anterior muscle. Decker et al.[87] recorded peak EMG amplitude levels ranging from 94% to 109% MVIC in the serratus anterior during the serratus punch and dynamic hug exercises. One must take into consideration the MVIC performed for normalization of these data. The authors of these two studies performed a baseline muscle test for the serratus anterior using scapular protraction as the MVIC. As found by Ekstrom et al.,[85] this muscle test produced only about 54% MVIC. A maximum muscle test for the serratus anterior must include an upward-rotation component of the scapula such as in the muscle test proposed by Kendall et al.[67] Taking this into consideration, these exercises are not optimal for strengthening the serratus anterior, but they may be used as low-level exercises early in a rehabilitation program.

The push-up plus exercise performed with full scapular protraction has been shown to produce high levels of muscle activity in the serratus anterior muscle.[83] Ekstrom et al.[83] found that this exercise produced EMG amplitude of 78% ± 24% MVIC. Lear and Gross[88] found that increased resistance can be added to the serratus anterior during this exercise if the feet are elevated onto a stool or chair. The reason that this exercise produces greater muscle activity in the serratus anterior than straight protraction exercises is that the thoracic spine goes into kyphosis (ribs pulled posteriorly), which produces upward rotation of the scapula in relationship to the rib cage (Figure 29-10).

Decker et al.[87] recorded near maximum muscle activity in the upper subscapularis, supraspinatus, and infraspinatus during the push-up plus exercise. They also demonstrated peak amplitudes in the subscapularis muscle of 49.8% MVIC during the forward punch exercise and 94.1% MVIC during the dynamic hug exercise. Therefore these exercises may be of value in strengthening and retraining the rotator cuff.

Abduction in the Scapular Plane and Other Humeral Elevation Exercises

The scapular plane is generally about 30- to 45-degrees anterior from the frontal plane in individuals and is considered the best functional position of the humerus when performing abduction exercises. The muscles most active are the glenohumeral joint elevators and the scapular upward rotators. The primary glenohumeral joint elevators are considered to be the deltoid and supraspinatus muscles, and the scapular upward

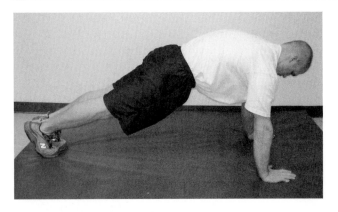

Figure 29-10 Push-up plus exercise with scapular protraction.

rotators are the serratus anterior and trapezius muscles. The rotator cuff muscles must keep the humeral head centered in the glenoid fossa during this exercise. All of the previously mentioned muscles maintain normal scapulohumeral rhythm.

It is recommended that abduction in the plane of the scapula be performed with moderate lateral rotation (thumb-up position) of the shoulder to minimize the possibility of impingement. Kelly et al.[89] compared the muscle activity of the supraspinatus during exercises in the plane of the scapula with external rotation (thumb up) and internal rotation (thumb down) and found no significant difference between the two exercises. During low-intensity scaption exercises with external rotation, Townsend et al.[78] recorded muscle activity levels in the supraspinatus and infraspinatus ranging from 62% to 64% MVIC and 71% to 72% MVIC in the anterior and middle deltoid muscles. Alpert et al.[90] recorded very comparable activity in the supraspinatus and infraspinatus but significantly lower levels of muscle activity in the teres minor during this exercise. They recorded high levels of muscle activity in the anterior and middle deltoid but relatively low levels of activity in the posterior deltoid.

Authors have demonstrated increasing activity of both the trapezius and the serratus anterior muscles from the beginning range to the end range of shoulder abduction.[79,84,91,92] Ekstrom et al.[84] found that abduction in the plane of the scapula above 120 degrees performed at 5 RM intensity produced 96% ± 24% MVIC in the serratus anterior muscle.

This finding agreed with that of Moseley et al.,[79] who found maximum activation of the serratus anterior between 120 and 150 degrees of elevation. This finding is not surprising because about two thirds of the serratus anterior muscle has its insertion into the inferior angle of the scapula, acting as an upward rotator of the scapula. Some patients with shoulder problems may tolerate this exercise if midrange abduction is avoided to help minimize impingement and a painful arc of movement at the glenohumeral joint.

Hardwick et al.[92] studied the wall slide exercise above 90 degrees of flexion and found it to produce comparable EMG amplitude in the serratus anterior muscle as compared with shoulder abduction in the plane of the scapula. Pushing the ulnar border against the wall as the hand slides upward can increase resistance. For some patients this shoulder elevation exercise may be easier to perform because of the support on the wall, which allows for assistance in control of the exercise.

Shoulder External Rotation Exercises

External rotation of the shoulder will activate the posterior deltoid, infraspinatus, teres minor, and the scapular retractor and depressor muscles. Shoulder external rotation exercises can be performed with a patient in a variety of positions including side lying with 0 degrees of shoulder abduction, prone with the shoulder abducted to 90 degrees, or in varying degrees of abduction in either the plane of the scapula or frontal plane with the subject in either a sitting or standing position. Reinold et al.[93] recently demonstrated a trend toward greater activation of the infraspinatus and teres minor muscles with external rotation at 0 degrees of abduction with subjects positioned in the side-lying position as compared with external rotation with the shoulder at 90-degrees abduction with the subject prone. However, they did not find a statistical difference in the activity of these muscles when external rotation was performed in five different positions at a 10 RM intensity. Myers et al.[94] also did not find a significant difference in the activation of these muscles when exercised with external rotation at 0 degrees or 90 degrees of shoulder abduction. The supraspinatus is activated to about the same levels as the infraspinatus and teres minor during external rotation exercises. The posterior deltoid was more active during external rotation at 90-degrees abduction in both prone and standing positions when compared with 0-degrees abduction when side lying.[93]

During isokinetic testing, Greenfield et al.[95] determined that subjects could produce significantly more torque in external rotation with the shoulder abducted to 45 degrees in the plane of the scapula as compared with the frontal plane. It has also been demonstrated that prone external rotation with the shoulder abducted to 90 degrees is a good exercise for activating the lower trapezius muscle.[84,96] During external rotation performed at 5 RM intensity, the activity in the lower trapezius muscle was 79% MVIC.[84] This exercise causes maximum depression of the scapula and tends to isolate lower trapezius activity from the middle and upper trapezius.[84]

Shoulder Internal Rotation Exercises

The internal rotation muscles of the shoulder are the subscapularis, pectoralis major, latissimus dorsi, teres major, and the anterior deltoid. Shoulder internal rotation can be performed in a variety of positions including 0 degrees of abduction, 90 degrees of abduction, and at any angle in between those two positions. It can also be performed in the frontal plane, plane of the scapula, or with varying degrees of shoulder flexion.

Kronberg et al.[80] found the greatest amount of muscle activity in the subscapularis, pectoralis major, and latissimus dorsi when the shoulder was internally rotated at 0 degrees of abduction. However, as the shoulder was abducted to 90 degrees, the subscapularis muscle activity remained quite high with a decrease of pectoralis major muscle activity. Suenaga et al.[97] performed maximum isometric contractions of the internal rotator muscles during several positions of the shoulder. They demonstrated slightly greater EMG signal amplitude (96% MVIC) of the subscapularis when abducted to 90 degrees as compared with the 0-degree abducted position. They also found that the pectoralis muscle activity greatly decreased at 90 degrees of abduction, but the latissimus dorsi activity decreased only slightly. Anterior deltoid activity was relatively low during all the internal rotation exercises. Decker et al.[98] performed tubing exercises at 10-repetition maximum intensity and found a trend toward higher EMG peak signal amplitude levels in the upper subscapularis muscle at 90-degrees abduction (91% MVIC) as compared with abduction at 45-degree (87% MVIC) and 0-degree shoulder abduction (84% MVIC), but the values were not significantly different. Myers et al.[94] also did not find a significant difference in the subscapularis activity in the two positions when performing tubing resistance exercises. Therefore there seems to be a tendency for greater levels of subscapularis muscle activity during internal rotation with the shoulder abducted to 90 degrees.

Greis et al.[99] studied the Gerber lift-off test. During this test, the hand is placed behind the back in the midlumbar area and the subject is asked to lift the hand away from the back. They concluded the subscapularis is primarily responsible for performing this motion because this test requires internal rotation at end range. They recorded peak EMG signal amplitudes in the subscapularis of 78% MVIC during the active test and 100% MVIC during a resisted test. During the active and resisted tests, the muscle activity in the pectoralis major ranged from 3% to 3.8% MVIC, compared with 15% and 33% MVIC for the teres major and 12% and 38% MVIC for the latissimus dorsi. Tokish et al.[100] found similar results during the active lift-off test. Suenaga et al.[97] reported results that followed a similar pattern. However, during the active lift-off test, they only recorded EMG signal amplitude of 45% MVIC in the subscapularis and 21% MVIC in the latissimus dorsi, with minimal activity in the pectoralis major and anterior deltoid. During the resisted lift-off test, Suenaga et al.[97] recorded high levels of muscle activity in both the subscapularis (91% MVIC) and the latissimus dorsi (73% MVIC). They also recorded fairly high activity of the posterior deltoid (50% MVIC), which may indicate they applied resistance not only to internal rotation but also to shoulder extension. The authors of this chapter suggest that the lift-off motion with internal rotation at end range may be another way to strengthen the subscapularis if an individual has the available range of motion to perform the exercise.

Tokish et al.[100] also studied the belly-press test for subscapularis muscle activity. This test is performed by pressing the hand against the belly while keeping the elbow in the frontal plane, which creates resisted internal rotation of the shoulder. This test produced greater activity in the upper subscapularis than the active lift-off test (86% MVIC versus 57% MVIC) but less activity in the lower subscapularis (59% MVIC versus 80% MVIC). The test produced activity of less than 23% MVIC in all the other internal rotators. Therefore this would be an excellent isometric exercise for the subscapularis muscle.

Prone Shoulder Horizontal Abduction Exercise at 90, 100, and 135 Degrees of Abduction

Shoulder horizontal abduction exercises in the prone position are often performed for strengthening the trapezius, rhomboids, posterior deltoid, and infraspinatus muscles. Very high levels of EMG activity ranging from 66% to 108% MVIC have been recorded in the three parts of the trapezius during these exercises.[79,84] Slightly higher activity of the middle trapezius is seen than in the upper or lower trapezius when performed at 90 degrees of abduction.[84] When performed at 135 degrees of abduction with the thumb-up position, maximum activity occurs in both the middle and the lower trapezius.[84]

Townsend et al.[78] and Reinold et al.[93] recorded very high levels of activity in the posterior and middle deltoid when the shoulder is horizontally abducted with either internal or external rotation. Townsend et al.[78] performed the exercise at 90 degrees of abduction and Reinold et al.[93] performed the exercise at 100 degrees of abduction.

Townsend et al.[78] also recorded peak EMG signal amplitudes of 88% MVIC in the infraspinatus muscle when the shoulder was horizontally abducted with external rotation, but Reinold et al.[93] only recorded values of 39% and 44% MVIC in the infraspinatus and teres minor muscles respectively. However, they recorded very high levels of muscle activity in the supraspinatus (82% MVIC) during horizontal abduction. Some discrepancy exists between the findings of these two studies, and it may be because of the 10-degree difference of abduction at which the exercise was performed. The Blackburn prone position for muscle testing the supraspinatus is also performed with the shoulder abducted to 100 degrees and has been shown to activate the supraspinatus to levels that are not significantly different when compared with a muscle test at 90 degrees of abduction in the plane of the scapula when sitting. Therefore horizontal abduction exercises appear to be good exercises for strengthening and training of the rotator cuff.

Researchers have demonstrated less activity in the trapezius when horizontal abduction is performed with the shoulder internally rotated as compared with the externally rotated position.[85] When the shoulder is internally rotated, the scapula elevates, so one can speculate that increased activity occurs in the rhomboid and levator scapula muscles.

Dumbbell Fly Exercise

The dumbbell fly exercise is performed by horizontally adducting the shoulders with dumbbells in the hands while lying in the supine position. Welsch et al.[82] compared the muscle activity of the pectoralis major and anterior deltoid muscles during the dumbbell fly exercise and barbell bench press performed at 6 RM. They did not find any significant difference in the peak EMG signal amplitudes of the muscles when comparing the two exercises; however, the time of activation during the dumbbell fly exercise was slightly less when compared with the barbell bench press.

Ferreira et al.[101] found increased muscle activity in both the clavicular head of the pectoralis major and the anterior deltoid during the dumbbell fly exercise in an inclined position rather than horizontal or declined position. This may be because these muscles are not only working as horizontal adductors but also as elevators of the humerus to resist gravity.

Rowing Exercises

Rowing exercises are usually performed to help improve the strength of the scapular adductors and shoulder extensor muscles. Bilateral or unilateral rowing can be performed in sitting or standing using a pulley system or elastic tubing for resistance, or it can be performed unilaterally in the prone position, with the upper extremity hanging over the side of a treatment table with a dumbbell weight in the hand.

Several studies have evaluated unilateral rowing in the prone position.[78,79,84] The humerus is usually moderately abducted about 30 degrees during this exercise. Moseley et al.[79] performed this exercise with low intensity and recorded peak muscle activity in the upper trapezius of 112% MVIC, middle trapezius of 59% MVIC, lower trapezius of 67% MVIC, and rhomboids of 56% MVIC. Ekstrom et al.[84] performed the prone unilateral row at 5 RM intensity and recorded 63% MVIC in the upper trapezius, 79% in the middle trapezius, and 45% MVIC in the lower trapezius. Myers et al.[94] evaluated the unilateral row while standing with moderate resistance from elastic tubing and recorded peak values of 51% MVIC in the lower trapezius and 59% MVIC in the rhomboids.

When performed with the shoulder in minimal abduction, the scapula will downwardly rotate as the shoulder is extended during the rowing motion. One can then speculate that the rhomboids would be more active in this position and less active if the shoulder is abducted to 90 degrees during the rowing motion. On the other hand, the trapezius would be expected to be more active as the shoulder is abducted because of the upward rotation of the scapula. This may be the case because it has been demonstrated that the trapezius is more active during horizontal abduction of the shoulder than with rowing.[84]

The shoulder muscles that are active during rowing exercises are the posterior deltoid, latissimus dorsi, teres major, and teres minor. Townsend et al.[78] recorded very high levels of muscle activity in the posterior deltoid (88% MVIC), and Myers et al.[94] recorded muscle activity of 40% MVIC in the latissimus dorsi and very high activity in the teres minor of 109% MVIC.

Shoulder Shrug

The shoulder shrug exercise is performed to strengthen the scapular elevators, which are the levator scapulae and upper trapezius muscles. Both of these muscles have been shown to be highly activated during this exercise.[79,86] With some patients

it may be desirable to try to isolate upper trapezius activation from the levator scapulae muscle. Because the upper trapezius is an upward rotator of the scapula and the levator scapulae is a downward rotator, one may be able to better isolate upper trapezius muscle activity if shoulder shrugging is performed with the scapula upwardly rotated. The military press or the wall slide exercise with the arms overhead as described by Sahrmann[102] would be appropriate for strengthening the upper trapezius muscle. During the wall slide exercise, the subject strongly elevates the scapula as the hands slide up the wall. Dumbbell weights can be held in the hands to increase the resistance.

When the shoulder shrug is performed against resistance with the shoulder adducted, all the rotator cuff muscles are activated to a moderate degree to help prevent inferior subluxation of the humerus.[86] Therefore the shrug could be considered a low-level exercise for the rotator cuff musculature.

Press-Up Exercise

The press-up exercise is performed in the sitting position by pressing down with the upper extremities to lift the buttock off a bench or table. A high level of muscle activity has been demonstrated in the pectoralis major (84% MVIC) and minor (89% MVIC) muscles during the press-up exercise, with lesser muscle activity in the latissimus dorsi (55% MVIC).[78,79] This exercise will also activate the scapular stabilizing muscles to a lesser degree.

Push-Up Exercise

The muscles thought to be highly activated during the push-up exercise are the pectoralis major, anterior deltoid, and the triceps brachii. Cogley et al.[103] studied the muscle activity of the pectoralis major and triceps brachii during a push-up exercise with the hand positions at shoulder width, wider than shoulder width, and closer than shoulder width apart. For the triceps brachii, the mean EMG signal amplitudes ranged form 99% to 109% MVIC, with the narrow base hand position producing significantly greater EMG signal amplitudes in the triceps brachii when compared with the wide base. The results for the pectoralis major were similar, with the EMG signal amplitudes ranging from 83% to 101% MVIC. Therefore to increase muscle activity in both these muscle groups, one would want to narrow the hand spacing.

Pull-Down Exercise

The muscles thought to be exercised with the pull-down exercise are the latissimus dorsi, teres major, pectoralis major, and posterior deltoid muscles, which are the primary adductors or extensors of the shoulder. The pull-down exercise can be performed with either shoulder adduction, extension, or a combination of both, depending on the handgrip and position of the arms during the exercise.

Signorile et al.[104] performed an EMG analysis of the muscles already mentioned, plus the long head of the triceps brachii during pull-down exercises with the hands in four different positions. The hand positions included hands close together in neutral pronation and supination, grip with the hands supinated and shoulder-width apart, and a wide grip with the hands pronated. The bar was brought down in front of the head during these three exercises. A fourth exercise was performed with a wide grip, with the hands pronated with the bar pulled down behind the head. A narrow handgrip would promote extension of the shoulder during the pull-down, and a wide grip promotes more shoulder adduction during the pull-down. All the exercises were performed at 10 RM intensity.

They found that the pull-down anterior to the head with a wide grip produced significantly greater activity in the latissimus dorsi when compared with the other three exercises. The pull-down close grip exercise tended to produce greater muscle activity in the pectoralis major and posterior deltoid than the other grip positions, but the difference was not significant. No significant difference was noted for the teres major with any of the grips. It appears that there would not be a reason to perform pull-downs behind the head for any of these muscles; however, this exercise could be beneficial for other muscles that were not analyzed, such as the scapular retractor muscles.

Diagonal Shoulder Exercise With Extension-Adduction-Internal Rotation

Decker et al.[105] performed the extension-adduction-internal rotation diagonal exercise at 10 RM using elastic tubing for resistance. This exercise produced peak EMG signal amplitudes of 104% MVIC for the pectoralis major, 98% MVIC for the upper subscapularis, 76% MVIC for the supraspinatus, and 49% MVIC for the latissimus dorsi muscles. Because the exercise direction is in line with the sternocostal head of the pectoralis major, it is an excellent exercise for its development, as well as for general activation of the rotator cuff.

Diagonal Exercise With Flexion-Adduction-Lateral Rotation

The flexion-adduction-lateral rotation diagonal exercise pattern highly activates the anterior and middle parts of the deltoid, as well as the pectoralis major (clavicular head) muscle.[106] In addition, maximal activation of the serratus anterior muscle occurs at 100% MVIC.[84] This exercise requires maximal protraction and upward rotation of the scapula. When the scapula is fully protracted, the trapezius activity tends to decrease during shoulder elevation, transferring more of the load for upward rotation to the serratus anterior muscle.

Upper-Extremity Weight-Bearing Exercises

Uhl et al.[107] studied muscle activity of the infraspinatus, supraspinatus, anterior deltoid, posterior deltoid, and pectoralis major muscles during progressive weight bearing through the upper extremity. The progressive weight-bearing exercises were as follows: kneeling with weight on hands, quadruped position, quadruped with one arm lift, quadruped with arm

and lower-extremity lift, push-up, push-up with feet elevated, and push-up position with weight on only one upper extremity with the elbow straight (Figure 29-11). Muscle activity during the easiest to most difficult exercise ranged from 2% to 29% MVIC in the supraspinatus, 4% to 86% MVIC in the infraspinatus, 2% to 46% MVIC in the anterior deltoid, 4% to 74% MVIC in the posterior deltoid, and 7% to 44% MVIC in the pectoralis major. The one-arm support in the push-up position substantially increased the EMG activity as compared with other exercises, especially in the infraspinatus and posterior deltoid (Boxes 29-4 and 29-5).

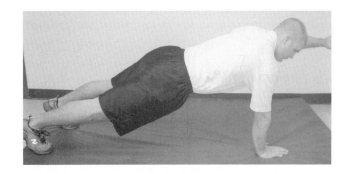

Figure 29-11 Upper-extremity unilateral weight-bearing exercise.

BOX 29-4   Exercises for the Serratus Anterior

The serratus anterior requires upward rotation during the exercise for full activation. Protraction exercises do not provide adequate stimulus for strengthening of the serratus anterior muscle.

The following exercises provide adequate stimulus for strengthening the serratus anterior muscle:

- Shoulder abduction in the plane of the scapula above 120 degrees
- Wall slides with the ulnar border of the hand against the wall during shoulder flexion
- Push-up plus exercise

BOX 29-5   Exercises for Rotator Cuff Training

- Abduction in the plane of the scapula with some external rotation (thumb up) to avoid impingement
- External rotation in any degree of abduction up to 90 degrees
- Internal rotation in any degree of abduction up to 90 degrees
- For better isolation of subscapularis muscle activity, two exercises may be beneficial: (1) lifting the hand off the small of the back with internal rotation or (2) the isometric hand belly press as the elbow is kept in the frontal plane
- Push-pull exercises
- Upper-extremity closed chain exercises

Hip Exercises

Exercises involving the hip musculature are not as widely studied compared with exercises for the spine, shoulder, and knee. The exercises studied in the past have been based on traditional and common exercises. However, recent interest has been shown in studying the hip musculature as it relates to the acetabular labrum, its role in pathologic conditions of the hip,[108-110] and the role of the hip in anterior cruciate ligament (ACL) injuries, particularly in women.[111-114] Recent work has addressed the multisegmental activity of the hip musculature in a weight-bearing position—particularly the gluteus medius.[115,116] The hip and pelvis are intimately linked to the lumbar spine and knee, and exercises at the hip can influence lumbar spine function, as well as function at the knee and ankle.

Hip Extension Exercise

Common positions used to perform resisted hip extension are standing resisted hip extension, prone hip extension, and supine hip extension performing a "bridging exercise" (described previously). Sakamoto et al.[117] studied the normal firing pattern of the hip and spine muscles during prone hip extension with the knee extended, with the knee flexed, and with the thigh laterally rotated and the knee either extended or flexed. They found that the muscle activation pattern for prone hip extension was similar for the knee extended, knee flexed, and thigh laterally rotated with knee extended positions such that the semitendinosus, contralateral erector spinae, ipsilateral erector spinae, and gluteus maximus contracted in sequence. For prone hip extension with the thigh laterally rotated with knee flexed position, the ipsilateral and contralateral erector spinae contracted almost simultaneously, with the gluteus maximus again being the last muscle activated before movement occurring. Oh et al.[118] studied the effect on hip extensor and medial hamstring muscles while performing hip extension in combination with an abdominal drawing-in maneuver. They found that when the abdominal drawing-in maneuver was performed simultaneously with hip extension, the hip extensor muscle activity was increased and the erector spinae muscle activity was decreased. In addition, less movement of the pelvis in the direction of an anterior tilt was noted. Furlani et al.[119] investigated the various actions at the hip joint that involve the gluteus maximus and found it to be active during extension of the thigh, abduction of the thigh, abduction of the thigh with the thigh flexed to 90 degrees, abduction with the trunk flexed, and when straightening up from touching the toes.

Ekstrom et al.[55] studied a variety of exercises using surface EMG. Three of the exercises studied were traditional rehabilitation exercises involving the motion of hip extension in which the gluteus maximus, as well as the gluteus medius, received moderate levels of activation. The three hip extension exercises were quadruped alternate arm flexion and leg extension and supine double-leg and single-leg bridging. They found that the level of activation for the gluteus maximus was 56% of MVIC

for the quadruped arm and lower-extremity lift, 40% MVIC for the supine unilateral bridge, and 25% MVIC for the supine bridge when both lower extremities were used. Gluteus medius activation was 42% of MVIC for the quadruped arm and lower-extremity lift, 47% of MVIC for the supine unilateral bridge, and 28% of MVIC for the supine bilateral bridge. Of all the exercises studied by these authors, the quadruped arm and lower-extremity lift created the greatest activation for the gluteus maximus.

Wall Slide and Wall Squat Exercise (Hip Muscle Activation)

Ayotte et al.[120] studied a variety of lower-extremity muscles during five unilateral weight-bearing activities, including single-leg wall slide. For the wall slide, subjects were instructed to maintain contact with the back on the supporting surface (wall) to ensure they kept the pelvis level and the head upright. The heel of the support limb was positioned 30 cm from the wall. Subjects were instructed to keep the contralateral leg off the floor by keeping the knee straight and the hip flexed enough so that the foot did not touch the floor. The individual's body weight was used during this activity—no additional weight was added. These authors found that the single-leg wall slide provided the best activation among the positions tested for gluteus maximus, gluteus medius, and biceps femoris. The authors felt that gluteus maximus activation at 86% MVIC and gluteus medius activation at 52% MVIC was high enough to have a strengthening effect. Biceps femoris activation was 15% MVIC, and therefore felt to have insufficient activation to create a change in strength. Blanpied[121] also examined hip muscle activity during a single-leg wall slide using only the individual's body weight and two different foot positions (foot in line with hip and foot 50 cm forward of hip), as well as two support locations for the trunk (one at the level of the scapula and the other at the level of the hip). The author found that the forward foot position required greater activation of the gluteus maximus muscle for either position of trunk support. As reported by Blanpied,[121] the normalized EMG activation for the gluteus maximus muscle during the wall slide was 27% MVIC for the foot-forward position, with wall contact at the level of the hip, and 18% MVIC for the foot position in vertical alignment with the hip, with the wall contact at the level of the hip. These values are less than reported by Ayotte et al.[120] The difference may be the result of differences in the depth of the squat performed (60 degrees by Blanpied[121] but no specific angle documented by Ayotte et al.) or differences in the method of normalization. Blanpied[121] performed the normalization contraction in prone with the hip in extension and neutral rotation with the knee flexed to 90 degrees. Ayotte et al.[120] performed their normalization contraction in supine, with the hip flexed to 30 degrees and the distal pad of the isokinetic device just proximal to the popliteal fossa.

It would appear that a wall slide exercise performed with the heel between 30 and 50 cm from the wall and a squat depth to 60-degrees knee flexion may provide sufficient activation of the gluteus maximus and gluteus medius to create a strengthening effect.

Hip Abduction Exercise

Maintenance of a level pelvis or stabilizing the pelvis during gait is felt to be an important functional activity of the hip abductor muscles.[115,116,122-124] Hip abductor muscle rehabilitation performed in the frontal plane is the traditional method for strengthening the gluteus medius. The gluteus medius has a proximal attachment on the lateral wall of the ilium from the iliac crest down to the middle (anterior) gluteal line, with a distal attachment at the anterior surface of the greater trochanter. Bolgla and Uhl[122] examined three nonweight-bearing and three weight-bearing hip exercises and documented gluteus medius muscle activation. The exercises consisted of nonweight-bearing hip abduction (side-lying abduction), nonweight-bearing standing hip abduction (hip in extension), nonweight-bearing standing flexed hip abduction (hip and knee flexed 20 degrees), pelvic drop exercise (see the following for a description and discussion), weight-bearing hip abduction, and weight-bearing with flexion (hip and knee flexed 20 degrees) hip abduction. For the nonweight-bearing exercises, the researchers placed an ankle cuff weight equivalent to 3% of the subject's mass on the extremity performing the abduction motion. The weight-bearing hip abduction exercises involved having the subject stand on one leg (the leg with EMG electrodes attached), while performing abduction and adduction of the nonstance leg 25 degrees in each direction while maintaining a level pelvis. The authors found that the activation of the gluteus medius ranged from 28% MVIC for nonweight-bearing (standing) flexed hip abduction, 33% MVIC for nonweight-bearing hip abduction in standing, 42% MVIC for the side-lying hip abduction exercise and weight-bearing hip abduction exercise, 46% MVIC for the weight-bearing with flexion hip abduction exercise to the pelvic drop maneuver having the greatest activation of the gluteus medius at 57% MVIC. Because there appeared to be a gradation from least to highest activation, the authors recommend the lowest-level activation exercises (flexed hip abduction and the nonweight-bearing hip abduction in standing) for patients requiring muscle activation at lower levels or who may be postoperative and just beginning a rehabilitation program.

Ekstrom et al.[55] studied side-lying active hip abduction in the frontal plane and side-lying side bridge—also in the frontal plane. The side-lying active hip abduction exercise consisted of having the subject lying on the side with the lateral trunk and lateral thigh in contact with the support surface. The hip on the nonweight-bearing extremity was abducted in the frontal plane to an angle of approximately 30 degrees with the hip in neutral rotation. In the side bridge exercise, the subject was positioned as described previously in the low-back exercise section. During the side bridge exercise, the individual was instructed to lift the hip to neutral spine alignment. The side-lying active hip abduction exercise activated the gluteus

medius to 39% of MVIC, which is very similar to the 42% MVIC reported by Bolgla and Uhl[122] as noted previously. The side bridge exercise performed during the study by Ekstrom et al.[55] activated the gluteus medius to 74% MVIC.

Pelvic Drop Exercise

The pelvic drop exercise has been found to provide high-level activation of the gluteus medius muscle.[122] To perform a pelvic drop exercise, an individual stands on an elevated platform such as a step and lowers one leg to the surface below the step (Figure 29-12). This is different from performing a step-down maneuver in that during the pelvic drop exercise the individual maintains both knees in an extended position. Therefore during the lowering phase of the movement, the pelvis on the stance leg is adducting toward the femur, creating an eccentric contraction of the gluteus medius on the stance leg side. On the return to the starting position, the gluteus medius on the stance leg is performing a concentric contraction as the pelvis is returned to a level position.

Bolgla and Uhl[122] studied muscle action during the pelvic drop. They found that the pelvic drop exercise activated the

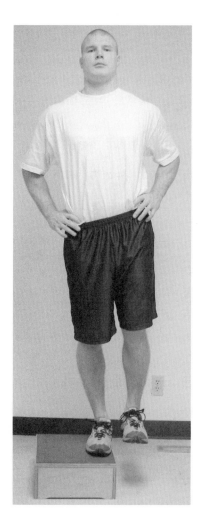

Figure 29-12 Pelvic-drop exercise for hip abductor strengthening.

gluteus medius to 57% MVIC, which was significantly more than weight-bearing hip abduction with the knees and trunk straight, as well as exercises performed in nonweight-bearing positions. They stated, "The pelvic drop exercise would be more appropriate for patients needing a more challenging exercise."[122]

Unilateral Minisquat (Hip Musculature Activation)

The minisquat exercise is commonly performed to activate the thigh muscles such as the quadriceps after trauma or pathologic condition involving the knee joint. Because of the frequency that this exercise is used in clinical practice, the authors felt it may be helpful for clinicians to be aware of hip muscle activation that is present during the unilateral minisquat. Ayotte et al.[120] studied the gluteus maximus and gluteus medius muscles during a unilateral minisquat exercise. In their study, the subjects were instructed to perform a minisquat to a depth of 15 cm while keeping the trunk and head in an upright position and the pelvis level (Figure 29-13). They found the minisquat activated the gluteus maximus to 57% MVIC and the gluteus medius to 36% MVIC. It would appear that the minisquat provides adequate activation of the gluteus maximus for a possible strengthening effect, whereas the gluteus medius muscle activation appears below the recommended level for a strengthening effect.

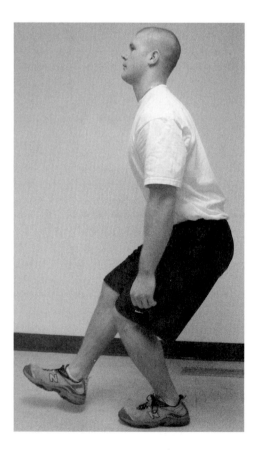

Figure 29-13 Single-leg minisquat.

Lunge Exercise (Hip Musculature Activation)

The lunge exercise is commonly used for rehabilitation for a variety of patient problems affecting the knee and hip joints. Ekstrom et al.[55] studied the forward lunge exercise in which the forward leg was flexed at both the hip and the knee to a 90-degree angle. The gluteus maximus muscle was activated to 36% MVIC, and the gluteus medius muscle was activated to 29% MVIC. Both of these muscles appear to be activated at a level below what is necessary for a strengthening effect in this study.

Step-Up Exercise (Hip Musculature Activation)

Forward, side, and backward stepping onto various height steps is commonly used for rehabilitation of clients with a variety of lower-extremity conditions. Typically, the target muscle group is the quadriceps. However, the hip musculature certainly contributes to the movement. All three stepping directions have been investigated with EMG and are reviewed following.

Forward (Front) Step-Up

This activity involves the typical movements associated with climbing a flight of stairs or stepping up a curb. Ayotte et al.[120] studied the front step-up movement using a 15 cm step height. They found the gluteus maximus muscle was activated to 74% MVIC and the gluteus medius muscle was activated to 44% MVIC.

Lateral Step-Up

This activity involves the movement of hip abduction of both the stance (abducting in a closed kinetic chain manner) and the nonstance limb (open chain abduction) to place the foot on the step followed by closed chain adduction of the pelvis toward the limb on the step to complete the motion. Ayotte et al.[120] and Ekstrom et al.[55] found that the gluteus maximus is activated to 56% MVIC and 29% MVIC, respectively. The gluteus medius was found to be activated to 38% MVIC by Ayotte et al.[120] and 43% by Ekstrom et al.[55] Some of the difference between the results for the gluteus maximus MVIC may be accounted for by the difference in the movement, as well as the normalization method. Ayotte et al.[120] performed MVIC in supine using an isometric contraction against an isokinetic device, whereas Ekstrom et al.[55] performed manual resistance to standardized muscle test positions. In addition, step heights of 15 cm and 20 cm were used by Ayotte et al.[120] and Ekstrom et al.[55] respectively. Ekstrom et al.[55] used a 5-second hold at the point of maximal knee flexion, with a 30-second rest between repetitions for the lateral step-up.

Retro (Rear) Step-Up

This activity involves the movement of going up a step backward. Ayotte et al.[120] found that the gluteus maximus is activated to 59% MVIC and the gluteus medius is activated to 37% MVIC when performed on a step of 15 cm in height.

It would appear that forward step-up onto a 15 cm step creates the best activation of the gluteus maximus, whereas gluteus medius activation is relatively constant for step-ups in each of the three directions studied (44% MVIC for forward step-up, 38% to 43% for lateral step-up, and 37% for retro step-up).

Closed Chain Hip Rotation

There has been recent interest in identifying exercises that activate the anterior portion of the gluteus medius because of its involvement in medial (internal) rotation of the femur and the posterior portion of gluteus medius for its influence on femoral lateral (external) rotation. In a closed chain action in which the femur is relatively fixed, contraction of the anterior portion of the gluteus medius muscle creates closed chain medial (internal) rotation at the hip joint (acetabulum on femur). Conversely, if the posterior fibers of the gluteus medius muscle contract in a weight-bearing state, then lateral (external) rotation at the hip joint (acetabulum on femur) occurs. Schmitz et al.[116] studied the activity of the gluteus medius in response to isometric and submaximal external rotation forces with the hip in neutral, as well as in a flexed position during weight bearing (standing). They used three different trunk positions (upright with the hip and knee in extension, forward bent 20 degrees at the hip and the knee in extension, and forward bent 20 degrees at the hip and 20- to 30-degrees flexion at the knee), as well as three different levels of rotational load for each stance condition. The load (8.9 to 26.7 N) was applied to the nonstance side of the pelvis such that the pelvis was being rotated in a lateral rotation direction with reference to the stance limb (i.e., the force was directed from anterior to posterior on the nonstance side of the pelvis). The exact direction of the force application (horizontal versus oblique) was not clearly described. The authors merely stated that the force was "posteriorly directed," implying that the force was in a horizontal plane. The authors found that the gluteus medius muscle activity increased with increasing load applied in a rotary direction at the pelvis in their weight-bearing study. They also determined that the gluteus medius muscle activity decreases with forward bending of the trunk when compared with the upright position.

Earl[115] also conducted a study of gluteus medius response to various loading conditions in a standing weight-bearing position. The stated purpose of this study was to determine which combination of hip abduction and rotation loading created the greatest activation of gluteus medius. Three isometric loading conditions occurred in which a cable column was used to create the static loading. The pulley for the cable column was in the lowest position (near the floor), with the end of the cable attached to a belt worn by the subjects. Surface EMG recordings measured anterior and middle gluteus medius muscle activity. Two loading conditions were performed: one using 2.26 kg and the other using 4.53 kg. The results indicated significantly more muscle activity for the anterior gluteus

medius versus middle gluteus medius with the 4.53 kg load, as well as during the abduction and internal rotation position (force was applied at a 45-degree angle to the vertical for the abduction component, and the rotator force was applied from anterior to posterior, both with the subject facing away from the pulley system). Therefore both Schmitz et al.[116] and Earl[115] felt that the gluteus medius was important for maintaining transverse plane stability for the hip joint, and this approach to activating the anterior gluteus medius may be of benefit in patients having difficulty with pelvic stability during gait.

Hip Flexion Exercise

Hip flexion is a movement that is common in everyday life for such activities as walking on level surfaces, as well as stepping up curbs and stairs. In addition, sporting activities that involve running and sprinting require additional muscle activation and speed of contraction for normal function. The muscles that are primarily responsible for this action are the iliacus, psoas major, sartorius, and the rectus femoris (RF) muscles. The iliacus muscle and the psoas major muscle are single-joint muscles (even though the psoas major muscle attaches to the transverse processes of the lumbar vertebrae and could technically be described as *multijoint* in function), whereas the sartoris muscle and RF muscle are two-joint muscles with action at both the hip joint (flexion) and the knee joint (flexion for sartorius and extension for RF). Investigation of hip flexion exercises typically involves RF and sartorius because of ease of access with surface electrodes. Very little evidence exists to verify the activity of the iliacus and the psoas major muscles, possibly because of their location in the anterior hip region. They are in very close proximity (as a common tendon called the *iliopsoas*) to the femoral artery and the femoral nerve, making any needle sampling of the muscles somewhat treacherous. In addition, the muscle bellies for both of these muscles lie within the pelvic cavity, necessitating insertion of a needle within the pelvic cavity to study the muscle action. Surface EMG may be possible, but the abdominal oblique muscles and the TrA muscles overlie this area and would create considerable "cross-talk," limiting the value of the information gained through surface EMG.

Andersson et al.[125] performed an EMG study of various activities and exercises involving the trunk and hip musculature. They used surface electrodes to study RF and sartorius muscles, as well as indwelling fine wire electrodes in the distal iliacus muscle below the inguinal ligament (verified with diagnostic ultrasonography). They found that the hip flexor muscles were activated to a low level in all types of trunk flexion ("curl-up" exercise) in which the hips remained in an extended position. However, when hip flexion was performed (sit-up exercise [i.e., trunk flexing on the hip, acetabulum moving on the femur]), the hip flexor muscles were activated to 50% to 75% MVIC. When a nonresisted leg lift (SLR [i.e., femur moving on acetabulum]) was performed, the iliacus and sartorius muscle activation tended to increase from 32% to 88% MVIC when the hip joint was flexed between 10 and 60 degrees

BOX 29-6	Exercises for Gluteus Maximus Strengthening

- Single-leg wall squat
- Forward step-up onto 15 cm step
- Retro step-up onto 15 cm step

BOX 29-7	Exercises for Gluteus Medius Strengthening

- Side-lying bridge
- Pelvic drop

irrespective of double-leg lift or single-leg lift. However, the RF was activated to 42% MVIC with hip flexion at 10 degrees but decreased to approximately 31% MVIC as the hip flexion increased to 60 degrees, irrespective of double-leg lift or single-leg lift (Boxes 29-6 and 29-7).

Lower-Extremity Exercise: The Knee Joint

Muscle action and joint movement at the knee has received considerable interest over the past 15 to 20 years because of various pathologic knee conditions such as patellofemoral arthralgia, as well as knee injuries involving meniscal tears and ligament injuries such as the ACL. As a result, considerable interest has been expressed in identifying exercises or positions that create activation of the quadriceps and hamstring musculature during rehabilitation for patients with a variety of conditions such as anterior knee pain, knee instability, patella-femoral arthralgia, degenerative joint disease, and many other conditions affecting the knee (meniscal tear, chondral surface injury). The quadriceps muscle group has been recognized as important for a variety of functional tasks such as climbing stairs, rising from and sitting down in a chair, kicking a ball, and walking backward to name a few. Many exercises have been identified that create muscle activation of the quadriceps musculature (some of which are outlined following.)

The hamstring muscles are two-joint muscles that have a proximal attachment at the ischial tuberosity of the pelvis and a distal attachment at the fibular head (biceps femoris), posterior superior tibia (semimembranosus), and pes anserinus (semitendinosus). Because of their attachment sites, the hamstring muscles can influence both the hip and the knee joints directly, with indirect influence on the lumbar spine through the pelvis and the ankle through the tibia. The hamstrings act to flex the knee and extend the hip. The hamstring muscles are also felt to provide a stabilizing force (cocontraction with the quadriceps) at the knee during various activities.[126-128] Several authors have studied the action of the hamstrings during a squat maneuver.[126-132]

Isometric Exercise

Isometric exercise is commonly used with patients who are beginning a rehabilitation program after knee injury or surgery.

Even though no joint movement is occurring, activation of a specific muscle group is often the aim of the isometric exercise. With respect to the quadriceps muscle, the degree of knee flexion used during isometric quadriceps contraction will vary depending on the intent and purpose of the exercise and any precautions in place at the time the exercise program is performed. Soderberg and Cook[133] chose to use a position of 40 degrees of knee flexion in their study on isometric knee extension based on their pilot data. They found that the vastus medialis (VM) was significantly more active in isometric knee extension (103% MVIC) than in a resisted SLR (63% MVIC), whereas the RF was significantly more active in the resisted SLR (93% MVIC) versus isometric knee extension (52% MVIC). Brownstein et al.[134] chose to assess isometric quadriceps muscle activity in 10-degree increments from 10 degrees from terminal knee extension to 90 degrees of knee flexion. They found that "the VMO is least active in the extended position," with greatest torque at 50 degrees of knee flexion and VMO EMG activity highest at 80 degrees of knee flexion.[134] They did not represent their EMG data as a percentage of MVIC, so comparisons cannot be made.

Bandy and Hanten[135] investigated changes in quadriceps muscle torque and EMG activity after an isometric training program that lasted 8 weeks. Subjects performed isometric knee extension contractions at different degrees of knee flexion. One group exercised with the knee flexed to 30 degrees, another group exercised with the knee flexed to 60 degrees, and a third group exercised with the knee flexed to 90 degrees. Each subject performed 20 contractions at the selected knee angle. Each maximal contraction was held for 6 seconds. Pre- and posttesting involved examining torque generation at 15-degree increments from 15 degrees to 105 degrees of knee flexion. They found that performance of isometric strengthening at any of the three angles significantly increased torque generation when compared with the control group. The group that exercised at the 90-degree angle demonstrated the greatest change in torque generation over the widest range of angles (from 15 to 90 degrees). The group that exercised at the 90-degree angle also demonstrated greater EMG activity compared with the control group for angles from 30 to 105 degrees. The authors presented their EMG data in millivolts (mV), not as a percentage of MVIC, so comparisons are not possible.

Nonweight-Bearing Exercise Performed Through an Arc of Motion

Nonweight-bearing exercises performed through an arc of motion are commonly used during rehabilitation of a variety of knee conditions. These exercises may focus on terminal knee extension (the last 30 degrees), full arc range of motion (typically 100 to 0 degrees), or any other arc of motion based on patellofemoral contact area and compressive force or specific concerns relative to the patient's condition. The arc of motion being used during an exercise program may have significance for certain patient conditions. For example, a patient with an anterior cruciate–deficient knee is discouraged from performing short-arc quadriceps (SAQ) exercises during the last 45 degrees of knee extension (45 degrees of knee flexion to 0 degrees [in which 0 degrees represents a fully straight knee]) because of the increased amount of anterior shear that occurs between the tibia and the femur as a result of the quadriceps force applied to the tibia at the tibial tubercle.[136-141] However, the performance of hamstring strengthening through an arc of motion from 0 to 90 degrees is encouraged because of the stabilization effect provided by hamstring muscle contraction (i.e., the hamstrings are an anterior cruciate protagonist), as suggested by More et al.[142] Additionally, patients who have a tendency toward patellar instability are discouraged from performing terminal knee extension exercises because of the tendency for muscle imbalances to occur in the terminal range of knee extension (most commonly excessive lateral patellar glide toward terminal knee extension). In contrast, patients with patellofemoral arthralgia may be helped by performing quadriceps-strengthening exercises with the knee in greater angles of knee flexion if the area of articular damage is on the more distal portions of the patellar articular surface.

Straight-Leg Raising

Many postoperative and postinjury rehabilitation programs for knee patients incorporate SLR. Some therapists and physicians feel that this exercise provides good activation of the quadriceps musculature with minimal trauma to the knee joint. Soderberg and Cook[133] studied SLR and isometric quadriceps muscle setting in an attempt to quantify the muscle activity occurring during performance of these activities. They found that the RF was significantly more active (93% MVIC) than the VM (63% MVIC) during a resisted SLR activity. Gryzlo et al.[143] also studied the quadriceps muscle electrical activity for the SLR maneuver during a variety of arcs of motion from 0 to 75 degrees. In their study they found that the vastus medialis oblique (VMO), vastus lateralis (VL), and RF were not statistically different in their EMG activity for any of the arcs of motion studied. They did find that the RF did have a higher degree of muscle activation than the VMO and VL, but it was not statistically significant (at 0 to 15-degrees arc of motion, VMO was 26% MVIC, VL was 29% MVIC, RF was 42% MVIC; at 60 to 75-degrees arc of motion, VMO was 24% MVIC, VL was 27% MVIC, RF was 34% MVIC). This agrees with the work by Andersson et al.[125] for the RF muscle (as noted in "Hip Flexion Exercise" earlier in the chapter). The studies by Soderberg and Cook[133] and Gryslo et al.[143] appear to contradict one another. However, in the study by Soderberg and Cook,[133] manual resistance (not quantified) was applied at the ankle during the SLR, whereas Gryzlo et al.[143] studied the SLR without any resistance applied. Because most clinical applications typically involve a gradation from no resistance to increasing resistance for a SLR, the therapist must recognize that as the resistance to SLR increases, the activity of the RF increases, as does the VMO and VL muscle activity.

In the studies by Gryzlo et al.[143] and Andersson et al.,[125] the normalized EMG values were below the accepted muscle activation level to create a strengthening effect, whereas in the Soderberg and Cook study,[133] the normalized values for both the VM and the RF were within the range to increase strength. Therefore the performance of a SLR without resistance will provide activation of the VM, as well as the RF, and may be appropriate for more acute patients, whereas the addition of resistance may be more appropriate for patients who are less acute and able to tolerate the increased muscle demands of a resisted SLR without pain or risk of injury.

Seated Knee Extension

Seated knee extension is a commonly used form of nonweight-bearing strengthening for the quadriceps musculature after injury to the knee joint. This exercise can be performed in a variety of knee joint angles, from 120-degree knee flexion to 0-degree flexion (knee fully straight). The most common arc of motion is 90 to 100 degrees of knee flexion to 0 degrees. Seated knee extension exercise has received some scrutiny in the past 20 years because of the potential for anterior shear of the tibia on the femur that occurs when the movement takes place from 90 degrees of flexion to 0 degrees of extension.[144-146] Recent work has indicated that if anterior tibial shear is a concern, then use of an arc of motion from 90-degree knee flexion to 50-degree knee flexion is felt to be safer (less shear occurs in this arc of motion).[138,147] Matheson et al.[148] conducted a study to investigate various seated knee extension exercises used to activate the quadriceps musculature. They found that isokinetic resistance at 60 degrees per second angular velocity provided the best activation of the quadriceps musculature (peak EMG amplitude of 91.3% RF, 87.2% VL, and 90.6% VM) during the concentric phase of the movement. Free-weight and elastic-tubing resistance did not provide the same level of activation as the isokinetic resistance at 60 degrees per second. Free-weight exercise performed at 60 degrees per second with 7.9 Kg resistance, provided muscle activation in the 29.9% to 40.5% of MVIC range. Elastic-tubing resistance provided a load of 47 to 168 N. When knee extension was performed at 60 degrees per second in the same arc of motion, muscle activation was in the 27 to 31% MVIC range.[148] Anderson et al.[149] found that the isolated knee extension exercise using heavy resistance (10 repetition maximum) created the best activation of the quadriceps musculature (arc of motion from 100-degrees flexion to 0-degrees extension). They compared the muscle activation of the quadriceps muscles during isolated knee extension (10 RM), squat (10 RM), leg press (10 RM), static quadriceps contraction, supine hip extension, and static quadriceps contraction with lateralization of the patella. They found that the quadriceps muscles were activated to 68% to 74% of MVIC during isolated knee extension, which would indicate the potential for increased strength when performed in a strengthening program. Wilk et al.[150] found that the maximum quadriceps muscle activation occurred during the arc from 35 to 11 degrees during nonweight-bearing isotonic knee extension (started and ended at 100-degrees flexion), with experienced lifters performing four repetitions of their 12-repetition maximum. This agrees with the work by Gryzlo et al.[143] but does not agree with the work by Brownstein et al.[134] for isometric quadriceps muscle contractions. In their study, Gryzlo et al.[143] noted that "the muscle activity of the RF, VMO, and VL increased as the knee approached full extension." They noted that the VMO had 56% MVIC and the VL had 58% MVIC during the last 15 degrees of extension (15 to 0 degrees), which was significantly greater than the previous arcs of motion in their study. Wilk et al.[150] noted, however, that the maximum torque produced during open chain knee extension occurred "during the concentric (ascending) phase of motion when the knee was flexed between 56 to 70 degrees," which would agree with the findings by Brownstein et al.[134] for isometric contraction.

Evetovich et al.[151] performed a quadriceps-strengthening program using seated resisted leg extension exercises on an isokinetic device at 90 degrees per second for 12 weeks. They demonstrated a 15.5% increase in peak quadriceps muscle torque for the extremity performing the strengthening program, but they also noted a 5.5% increase in the peak torque of the untrained limb. The authors also performed pre- and postassessment of quadriceps muscle electrical activity, but were unable to demonstrate any difference in the EMG amplitude despite the changes in peak torque generation. Shin et al.[152] also conducted a 12-week strengthening program and studied changes in EMG signal and muscle strength. They found a significant increase in quadriceps muscle strength when compared with a control group, as well as an average of 2.06 cm increase in thigh girth for the group who performed the 12-week strengthening program. In addition, they found a linear pattern for the changes in electrical activity during the 12-week training program for their subjects. Cresswell and Ovendal[153] studied isokinetic knee extension when performed bilaterally versus unilaterally to determine if any difference occurred in muscle activation between the two conditions. They found better activation of the quadriceps musculature when exercises are performed unilaterally. This certainly has implications for patients who are attempting to recover muscle function in an involved limb.

With respect to open kinetic chain strengthening, it appears that the highest muscle activation of the quadriceps occurs in the last 35 degrees of knee extension during the ascending (concentric) portion of the movement, with maximum torque production occurring between 56 and 70 degrees of knee flexion. Unfortunately, the arc of motion from 35 to 0 degrees is also a portion of the knee range of motion, with the greatest pressure per unit area on the patella, as well as the portion of the knee range of motion in which the greatest anterior shear of the tibia is felt to occur in open chain exercise. Therefore this exercise may not be appropriate or safe for all patients.

Isolated Hamstring Curl

Isolated hamstring strengthening is also a common exercise program performed with individuals who have sustained a knee injury. The exercise can be performed in a variety of ways, including seated hamstring curls, prone hamstring curls, and standing hamstring curls. Andersen et al.[149] investigated isolated hamstring curls, as well as static quadriceps muscle setting, rhythmic stabilization, pelvic bridging, free-weight squat, horizontal seated leg press, and isolated knee extension. They found that "hamstring muscle activity was highest during isolated hamstring muscle curl, with normalized EMG amplitude values of 67% to 70% MVIC."[149]

Open Kinetic Chain Exercise versus Closed Kinetic Chain Exercise

This section reviews several articles in which the authors compared open kinetic chain exercises with closed kinetic chain exercises. Alkner et al.[1] compared the EMG/force relationship of individual quadriceps femoris muscles in the single-joint knee extension exercise and the multijoint leg press at various loads equivalent to 20%, 40%, 60%, and 80% MVIC in normal subjects. They found that "the EMG/force relationship of all quadriceps muscles studied appears to be similar in isometric multijoint leg press and single-joint knee extension actions at a knee angle of 90 degrees." Stensdotter et al.[154] also compared quadriceps muscle activation in both closed and open kinetic chain exercises. However, they studied isometric muscle contractions of the lower-extremity muscles with the hip in 90 degrees of flexion and the knee within 30 degrees of full extension. They found that "exercise in the isometric closed chain promotes more balanced initial quadriceps activation than does exercise in open kinetic chain."[154] Unfortunately, Stensdotter et al.[154] did not represent the muscle activity in percentage of MVIC, so comparisons cannot be made concerning differences in muscle activation between open kinetic chain exercises and closed kinetic chain exercises.

Wilk et al.[150] investigated the electrical activity of the quadriceps and hamstring muscles during the standing squat, leg press, and leg extension activities, with 10 normal (noninjured) athletes. The exercises were performed through an arc of knee flexion motion ranging from 12 to 104 degrees for the squat, 18 to 101 degrees for the leg press, and 12 to 101 degrees for open kinetic chain knee extension. The participants performed four repetitions of their 12-repetition maximum for each exercise. They found that the maximum EMG signal amplitude of the quadriceps was 59% MVIC during the squat from 88 to 102 degrees of flexion during the ascending phase, 51% MVIC during the leg press from 88 to 102 degrees during the extending phase, and 52% MVIC during the extending phase of open kinetic chain knee extension from 35 to 11 degrees. Based on this information, it appears that the best muscle activation for the quadriceps when performing a squat or leg press occurs in 90 to 100 degrees of knee flexion. The percentage of MVIC for the leg press and squat in the study by Wilk et al.[150] appears to be on the lower end of that necessary for strength change with inexperienced or deconditioned individuals, as noted in the literature (although the subjects in the Wilk et al.[150] study were experienced weight lifters performing four repetitions with their 12-repetition maximum weights).

Therefore if the emphasis is on increased strength, then an increase in the amount of weight may be necessary so that the individual is performing at 6- to 8-repetition maximum; however, this may not be possible or safe in clinical rehabilitation until near the end of the rehabilitation.

The ability for a closed kinetic chain exercise to increase the strength of the quadriceps is often used as a rationale for rehabilitation. The evidence to support this philosophy, however, is somewhat mixed. Wawrzyniak et al.[155] conducted a 6-week leg press strengthening program using 30 college-aged females and demonstrated improvement in isokinetic peak torque values for the quadriceps when the leg press was performed through an arc of 0 to 90 degrees. The individuals in this study performed single-leg press strengthening three times per week, with resistance loads adjusted at each training session with the intention of providing maximal overload. Reynolds et al.[156] and Worrell et al.[157] each conducted a lateral step-up exercise protocol in which pre- and posttest assessments for changes in quadriceps muscle torque generation were conducted. Neither study demonstrated any change in quadriceps muscle isokinetic strength at the conclusion of the study. Reynolds et al.[156] used gradually increasing step height from 4 inches (10.2 cm) to 12 inches (35 cm) during their study, whereas Worrell et al.[157] used an 8-inch (20.3 cm) step height throughout the study but varied the amount of resistance by having the subjects hold onto a weight while performing the step-ups. Koenig et al.[158] also conducted a 10-week bench step program in which they measured pre- and postisokinetic quadriceps strength. They found a decrease in quadriceps muscle strength, with no change in quadriceps muscle power or endurance based on isokinetic testing. Step heights of 10.2 and 15.2 cm were randomly assigned to the subjects in their study.

It would appear that high-resistance closed kinetic chain exercise may be able to stimulate changes in quadriceps muscle strength, but step-ups are unable to demonstrate similar changes.

Several authors have stated that closed kinetic chain exercises are more functional than open kinetic chain exercises. One must remember, however, that all movements contain components of both activities; therefore components of both open kinetic chain exercises and closed kinetic chain exercises would ideally be included in most exercise programs, as recommended by Davies et al.[76] and Mikkelsen et al.[159] In the next section a variety of both open and closed chain exercises is described.

Weight-Bearing Exercises

Weight-bearing exercises that activate the quadriceps and hamstring musculature are numerous. They include step-up exercise, either forward or lateral; wall slides in which a subject is supported by a wall and performs a squat maneuver; and standard squats, either with both legs or a single leg. Resistance may be applied with body weight only or with weight added to the subject's body weight during leg press, minisquats, lunges, and ambulation activities such as backward walking. Elastic tubing can also be used to provide resistance during squats or standing terminal knee extension exercise. This list is by no means complete, but it forms the basis for this review of literature on weight-bearing exercise, because many of these exercises are used during various rehabilitation programs.

Forward Step-Ups

Beutler et al.[131] studied a forward step-up with the step height being adjusted to correspond with tibial plateau height for each subject. They found the maximum quadriceps muscle activation to be 207% MVIC at 83 degrees of knee flexion.

Lateral Step-Up

Brask et al.[160] studied quadriceps muscle activity during a lateral step-up, with step heights of 4 and 8 inches in normal subjects. They found that the VM activity during the concentric phase of the lateral step-up was 60% MVIC for the 8-inch step height and 43% MVIC for the 4-inch step height. All other muscles (RF, biceps femoris, semimembranosus, semitendinosus) were below 23% MVIC, and therefore would not be expected to increase in strength. Cook et al.[161] also found the lateral step-up onto an 8-inch step provided better quadriceps muscle activation than a stepping machine. The VM was activated to 47% MVIC for the extension (concentric) phase of the lateral step-up and 42% for the flexion (eccentric) phase as compared with 37% and 10% for the stepping machine, respectively. Ekstrom et al.[55] also studied the lateral step-up using an 8-inch step height with a 5-second hold at the maximum angle of knee flexion. They found that the VMO was activated to 85% MVIC, and the hamstrings were activated to 10% MVIC.

Wall Slides

Blanpied[121] conducted a study to look at a variety of muscles and their activation patterns during wall slides and the use of a squat machine. He found that "the quadriceps was better facilitated by using hip support and placing the foot forward. The wall slide was better than the squat-machine exercise for activating the quadriceps in this experiment, using body weight only."[121] This agrees with the work of Ayotte et al.[120] with respect to the performance of a unilateral limb wall squat with the foot of the stance limb placed in front of the hip. Ninos et al.[129] investigated the change in quadriceps and hamstring muscle activation that would occur as a result of changes to lower-limb position (30-degree medial or lateral rotation) during the performance of the squat exercise. They did not find any change in muscle activation based on lower limb and foot position, but they did find that the VM and VL were significantly more active during the 50- to 60-degree arc of motion for both the descending (eccentric) and ascending (concentric) phases of the squat.

Squat

Several authors have investigated the muscle activation for various hip and thigh muscles during the squat.[126,130,131,150,162] Beutler et al.[131] compared the single-leg standing squat with forward step-ups onto varying height steps in normal subjects. They found that the greatest concentric and eccentric quadriceps muscle activation (as represented by MVIC) for both the single-leg squat and the forward step-up occurred at knee angles between 70 and 105 degrees of knee flexion, with the greater knee angle producing higher EMG values. This agrees with the findings of Wilk et al.,[150] who found that the greatest quadriceps muscle activation occurred between 88 and 102 degrees during the concentric (ascending) phase of the double-leg squat. Isear et al.[162] also found that the VMO and VL had their greatest activity (68% and 63% MVIC, respectively) during the 60- to 90-degree arc of motion (ascending phase) for a double-leg squat using body weight only. Ebben and Jensen[163] investigated the addition of a metal chain or elastic bands to the performance of a traditional squat to determine if there was any advantage to their addition to a traditional squat exercise. They found that the concentric phase of the squat provided greater muscle activation than the eccentric phase, as noted previously. They did not find any significant difference with the addition of either chains or elastic-band resistance to the traditional squat.

Isear et al.[162] and Wilk et al.[150] noted that the quadricep muscles (VM and VL) were activated at their highest levels during the double-leg squat on the initiation of ascending (concentric contraction) from the deepest portion of the squat movement (68% MVIC and 59% MVIC, respectively). The subjects in the study by Isear et al.[162] performed a double-leg squat without resistance, whereas the subjects in the Wilk et al.[150] study performed a squat with resistance equivalent to their 12 RM. The squat depth at which maximal quadriceps activation occurred was an average of 94 degrees in the study by Isear et al.[162] and ranged between 88 and 102 degrees in the study by Wilk et al.[150] These studies do not agree with the results of a study by Caterisano et al.[130] in which they also studied resisted double-leg squats (100% to 125% of body weight) at varying depths. They found that the quadriceps muscles did not vary in their recruitment for either the eccentric (lowering) phase of the squat or the concentric (upward) phase of the squat. The activation of the quadriceps was between 18% MVIC and 29% MVIC in their study. Beutler et al.[131] studied a single-leg squat (no resistance) in which the individuals squatted to a depth of 96 to 120 degrees and documented quadriceps muscle activation of 197% to 205% MVIC.

Hamstring muscle activation during a double-leg squat maneuver was also studied by Caterisano et al.,[130] Isear et al.,[162] Vakos et al.,[164] and Wilk et al.[150] Caterisano et al.[130] and Wilk et al.[150] found the hamstrings to be activated to 19% to 28% MVIC and 33% to 36% MVIC respectively, whereas Isear et al.[162] found hamstring muscle activation to be no higher than 17% MVIC. Vakos et al.[164] found hamstring muscle (biceps femoris and semitendinosus) activation in the 5% to 10% MVIC range, with no significant variation based on lumbar spine posture (kyphotic versus lordotic posture). Beutler et al.[131] found that maximum hamstring muscle activation of 81% MVIC occurred at 86-degrees flexion in the single-leg squat.

Quadriceps muscle activation appears to be adequate during a squat exercise for a strengthening effect based on the work of Beutler et al.,[131] Isear et al.,[162] and Wilk et al.[150] Irrespective

of whether the squat was resisted or not, hamstring muscle activation does not appear adequate for a strengthening effect.[130,150,162,164] In addition, Isear et al.[162] felt that the hamstrings did not provide sufficient cocontraction force to stabilize the knee during an unloaded squat maneuver. The single-leg study by Beutler et al.[131] demonstrated that hamstring activation appeared to be adequate for a strengthening effect.

Studies assessing changes to lower-extremity rotation (neutral versus 30-degree lower-extremity turnout) positions and foot position (supination versus pronation) with the use of orthotic devices have not demonstrated any changes in muscle activation patterns for the squat.[129,165]

Leg Press

The leg press is a common exercise incorporated during rehabilitation for a variety of lower-extremity conditions. Stensdotter et al.[154] compared the muscle activation of the quadriceps muscles during an isometric leg extension and an isometric leg press. They determined that the quadriceps muscles were activated simultaneously during the isometric leg press. Andersen et al.[149] determined that the seated horizontal leg press provided better activation of the quadriceps muscles than the free-weight squat. The leg press performed in their study provided approximately 65% MVIC activation of the quadriceps compared with approximately 40% MVIC activation for the free-weight squat. Seated leg extension activated the quadriceps to approximately 68% to 74% MVIC in their study. Wilk et al.[150] found that RF muscle activation was 39% MVIC, VM muscle activation was 52% MVIC, VL activation was 48% MVIC, lateral hamstring muscle activation was 12% MVIC, and medial hamstring muscle activation was 14% MVIC during the leg press. Each of these maximal muscle activation events occurred between 88 and 102 degrees of knee flexion on the ascent (concentric muscle contraction) portion of the exercise cycle, except the lateral hamstring, which occurred at 60 to 74 degrees of knee flexion on the ascent portion of the cycle. Alkner et al.[1] studied the EMG/force relationship for knee extension and leg press. They determined that the estimated force for the knee flexors was 7% to 8% of knee extensor force, irrespective of the level of force performed. The purpose of their study was to compare the EMG/force relationship, so they did not report quadriceps muscle MVIC data.

One-Quarter (Mini) Squat and Elastic-Tubing Exercises in Weight Bearing

Hopkins et al.[127] conducted an investigation of four closed chain exercises consisting of the unilateral one-quarter squat, the lateral step-up, the FlexCord front pull, and the FlexCord back pull. The unilateral one-quarter squat involved having the subject perform a single-leg squat to 30 degrees of knee flexion and return to the extended position in one complete motion. The lateral step-up involved standing on a 10 cm step with one leg and bending the stance knee until the opposite foot touched the floor while keeping the trunk and head upright (knee flexed to approximately 30 degrees with this maneuver). The FlexCord front pull involved placing elastic tubing around one foot at a specified distance from the other attachment point of the elastic tubing. While standing on the other leg (facing away from the elastic-tubing attachment site), the individual moved the leg with the elastic tubing attached (nonstance limb) from a starting position of hip extension through a hip flexion motion in the sagittal plane (EMG electrodes attached to the stance leg). The FlexCord back pull was the opposite of the front pull (subject facing the attachment site of the elastic tubing), and the subject went from a starting position of hip flexion to an ending position of hip extension (EMG electrodes attached to the stance leg). They found "the flex cord front pull produced higher levels of VM activity than the unilateral one-quarter squat, lateral step-up, and Flex-Cord back pull during knee extension."[127] Unfortunately, they did not express the muscle activation in percentage of MVIC but presented activation in millivolts. Therefore it is not possible to compare their work with that of others.

Schulthies et al.[166] investigated the use of the elastic-tubing exercises with subjects who were postoperative after ACL reconstruction. They studied the front pull and back pull exercises as described previously. They also studied a crossover exercise and a reverse crossover exercise. The crossover exercise consisted of having elastic tubing connected to the subject's ankle (noninjured side) and anchored to a wall at the level of the ankle on the same side as the ankle it was attached to (i.e., if the tubing was attached to the left ankle, the tubing was attached to the wall on the subjects left side). The subject stood perpendicular to the attachment site. The subject then performed adduction of the hip on the extremity with the tubing attached until the leg crossed the midline, and the lower extremity was then returned to the starting position. The reverse crossover involved having the anchor point for the elastic tubing on the side opposite the extremity performing the motion. The subject began with the lower extremity adducted and performed abduction of the hip against the resistance of the elastic tubing. These authors found that the front pull exercise created greater hamstring muscle (biceps femoris and semitendinosus) activation (on the stance leg) than quadriceps muscle activation (57% MVIC for semitendinosus and 49% MVIC for biceps femoris versus 42% MVIC for VMO and 35% MVIC for VL). The back pull exercise created similar activation of the biceps femoris (39% MVIC) and quadriceps muscle activation (37% MVIC for VMO and 38% MVIC for VL). The semitendinosus activation was 13% MVIC for the back pull. The crossover exercise demonstrated 31% MVIC for the VMO, 27% MVIC for the VL, 40% MVIC for the semitendinosus, and 27% MVIC for the biceps femoris. The reverse crossover demonstrated 32% MVIC for the VMO, 35% MVIC for the VL, 16% MVIC for the semitendinosus, and 25% MVIC for the biceps femoris.

It appears that the front pull exercise creates adequate hamstring muscle activation for a potential strengthening effect and provides cocontraction stabilization for the knee joint in this closed kinetic chain exercise.

Weight-Bearing Terminal Knee Extension

Willett et al.[167] investigated a terminal knee extension exercise performed in standing with resistance to terminal knee extension provided by elastic tubing placed against the posterior knee at the popliteal fossa area. The length of the elastic tubing was adjusted to ensure consistent tension for the performance of the exercise. There were 16 healthy volunteers who completed this study. They studied muscle activation without resistance for terminal knee extension from 30 degrees of knee flexion to 0 degrees of knee extension. In addition, they studied muscle activation for the same 30-degree movement with green elastic-tubing resistance for each of three foot positions (neutral, 30-degree internal rotation, 30-degree external rotation). The authors noted that "significantly higher VMO and VL EMG activity occurred during all conditions in which elastic resistance was used, regardless of foot position, as compared with the no elastic resistance condition with the foot in neutral."[167] Muscle activation for VMO and VL was reported to be 45% MVIC or higher for the resisted movements, whereas the muscle activation without resistance appears to be 28% to 30% MVIC. In addition, the authors did not detect any preferential activation of either the VMO or the VL for any of the exercise conditions studied.

Backward Walking

Backward walking is currently used as an exercise program for patients undergoing rehabilitation for a variety of knee conditions such as patellofemoral arthralgia and postoperative ACL rehabilitation, as well as other nonoperative and postoperative knee conditions. Cipriani et al.[168] examined quadriceps muscle activation during backward walking on a treadmill at three different elevations. They studied four muscles on each of three different treadmill elevations (0%, 5%, and 10%). They compared treadmill backward-walking electrical activity to forward walking at 0% elevation (i.e., no MVIC was performed). They found that significant changes occurred for all muscles (gastrocnemius, RF, hamstrings, tibialis anterior) during all three treadmill elevations. Increased RF muscle activity occurred during loading response and heel-off phases of the gait cycle. Of interest, the hamstring muscle activity decreased as the treadmill elevation increased.

Lunges

Lunges are commonly used exercises intended to provide activation of the quadriceps musculature, with coactivation of the hamstring musculature to assist with knee stabilization. Ekstrom et al.[55] found that VM activation was 76% MVIC and hamstring muscle activation was 11% MVIC during the forward lunge maneuver. This indicates good activation of the quadriceps muscles with a very low level of hamstring muscle activity during the forward lunge, thus bringing the concept of functional hamstring muscle coactivation into question. However, the specific level of hamstring muscle activation necessary to stabilize the knee during functional activities is presently unknown.

Selective and Isolated VMO/VL Quadriceps Muscle Activation

Clinicians have found selective activation of the VMO to be important when managing patients with patellofemoral arthralgia (in an attempt to "normalize" patellar position). Brownstein et al. stated that "it may be possible to selectively strengthen the VMO because of the attachment of the VMO to the adductor magnus" [134] (as suggested by Zakaria et al[169]). However, they were not able to identify any preferential activation of the VMO in their study of normal female subjects in a nonweight-bearing position. This is in agreement with the work of Hertel et al.[170] for combined hip adduction in a single-leg weight-bearing position while squeezing an object between the knees. However, combining the activation of hip adductors with weight-bearing exercises for the quadriceps muscles appears to have a positive effect on increased muscle activation of the VM and VL in healthy subjects according to the work of Earl et al.[171] Coqueiro et al. used healthy subjects and subjects with patellofemoral arthralgia and found that the addition of adduction during a double-leg semisquat exercise "produced a more overall quadriceps activity and could be indicated for clinical rehabilitation or muscle strengthening programs."[172] They also noted that the muscle activation of the VM and VL was significantly increased with the addition of adduction during the double-leg semisquat exercise when compared with the muscle activation without the adduction component. Neither of the studies demonstrated a preferential activation of the VMO, however. Earl et al.[171] performed a wall squat in which the heels and buttocks remained in contact with the wall during a squat to a depth of 30-degrees flexion at the knee joint. Coqueiro et al.[172] had their subjects perform a double-leg squat in a standing position with a knee angle to 45 degrees while performing isometric hip adduction against an object between their knees.

Bevilaqua-Grossi et al.[173] studied the effect of hip abduction on VL muscle activation in normal subjects in a nonweight-bearing position. They found "no selective EMG activation was observed when comparison was made between the VMO, vastus lateralis longus and vastus lateralis obliquus muscles while performing maximum knee extension at 90 degrees of flexion and maximum hip abduction at 0 and 30 degrees of abduction for both male and female subjects."[173] This finding is in agreement with Hertel et al.[170] for a standing activity involving hip abduction combined with isometric quadriceps contraction in a position of 60 degrees of knee flexion.

Walking, Walking Up and Down a Ramp, Ascending and Descending Stairs

Ciccotti et al.[174] studied lower-limb muscle electrical activity for a variety of activities such as walking on level surfaces, walking up and down a ramp (up to 10% grade), ascending and descending stairs, as well as running and cutting. They

---

BOX 29-8	Quadriceps Muscle-Strengthening Exercises

- Forward step-up (tibial plateau height)
- Single-leg squat
- Isometric knee extension performed in 40-degree knee flexion
- Resisted SLR (RF)
- Isokinetic knee extension at 60 degrees per second (RF, VMO, VL)
- Forward lunge
- Seated leg extension
- Squat (VMO, VL)—ascending phase
- Resisted SLR
- Lateral step-up (8-inch step height)

SLR, Straight-leg raising; *RF,* rectus femoris; *VMO,* vastus medialis oblique; *VL,* vastus lateralis.

BOX 29-9	Hamstring-Strengthening Exercises

- Single-leg squat
- Isolated hamstring curl
- Front pull elastic-tubing exercise—semitendinosus

---

found that level walking, going up or down a ramp, and ascending and descending stairs were very similar activities. In addition, they found that running and cutting were very different when compared with each other or when compared with walking or climbing stairs or ramps. Colby et al.[175] studied the muscle activity and kinematics of cutting maneuvers. They found that "there is high level quadriceps muscle activation beginning just before foot strike and peaking in mid-eccentric motion" (Boxes 29-8 and 29-9). [175]

REFERENCES

1. Alkner B, Tesch P, Berg H: Quadriceps EMG/force relationship in knee extension and leg press, Med Sci Sports Exerc 32(2):459-463, 2000.
2. Marras WS, Davis KG: A non-MVC EMG normalization technique for the trunk musculature. I. Method development, J Electromyogr Kinesiol 11(1):1-9, 2001.
3. DeLuca C: The use of electromyography in biomechanics, J Appl Biomech 13:135, 1997.
4. Sale DG, Jacobs I, MacDougall JD, et al: Comparison of two regimens of concurrent strength and endurance training, Med Sci Sports Exerc 22(3):348-356, 1990.
5. Stone WJ, Coulter SP: Strength/endurance effects from three resistance training protocols with women, J Strength Cond Res 8(4):231-234, 1994.
6. Hayden JA, van Tulder MW, Malmivaara AV, et al: Meta-analysis: exercise therapy for nonspecific low back pain, Ann Intern Med 142(9):765, 2005.
7. Abenhaim L, Rossignol M, Valat J, et al: The role of activity in the therapeutic management of back pain: report of the International Paris Task Force on Back Pain, Spine 25(suppl 4):1S-S33, 2000.

8. Liddle SD, Baxter GD, Gracey JH: Exercise and chronic low back pain: what works? Pain 107(1-2):176-190, 2004.

9. Maher C, Latimer J, Refshauge K: Prescription of activity for low back pain: what works? Aust J Physiother 45(2):121-132, 1999.

10. Faas A: Exercises: which ones are worth trying, for which patients, and when? With commentary by Battie MC and Malmivaara A, Spine 21(24):2874-2879, 1996.

11. van Tulder M, Malmivaara A, Esmail R, et al: Exercise therapy for low back pain: a systematic review within the framework of the Cochrane Collaboration Back Review Group, Spine 25(21):2784-2796, 2000.

12. Rainville J, Hartigan C, Martinez E, et al: Exercise as a treatment for chronic low back pain, Spine J 4(1):106-115, 2004.

13. Wilke HJ, Wolf S, Claes LE, et al: Stability increase of the lumbar spine with different muscle groups: a biomechanical in vitro study, Spine 20(2):192-198, 1995.

14. Hides JA, Stokes MJ, Saide M, et al: Evidence of lumbar multifidus muscle wasting ipsilateral to symptoms in patients with acute/subacute low back pain, Spine 19(2):165-172, 1994.

15. Hides JA, Richardson CA, Jull GA: Multifidus muscle recovery is not automatic after resolution of acute, first-episode low back pain, Spine 21(23):2763-2769, 1996.

16. Hodges P, Holm AK, Hansson T, et al: Rapid atrophy of the lumbar multifidus follows experimental disc or nerve root injury, Spine 31(25):2926-2933, 2006.

17. Barker KL, Shamley DR, Jackson D: Changes in the cross-sectional area of multifidus and psoas in patients with unilateral back pain: the relationship to pain and disability, Spine 29(22):E515-E519, 2004.

18. Cooper RG, St Clair Forbes W, Jayson MI: Radiographic demonstration of paraspinal muscle wasting in patients with chronic low back pain, Br J Rheumatol 31(6):389-394, 1992.

19. Danneels LA, Vanderstraeten GG, Cambier DC, et al: CT imaging of trunk muscles in chronic low back pain patients and healthy control subjects, Eur Spine J 9(4):266-272, 2000.

20. Keller A, Brox JI, Gunderson R, et al: Trunk muscle strength, cross-sectional area, and density in patients with chronic low back pain randomized to lumbar fusion or cognitive intervention and exercises, Spine 29(1):3-8, 2004.

21. Cresswell AG, Oddsson L, Thorstensson A: The influence of sudden perturbations on trunk muscle activity and intra-abdominal pressure while standing, Exp Brain Res 98(2):336-341, 1994.

22. Hodges PW, Richardson CA: Feed-forward contraction of transversus abdominis is not influenced by the direction of arm movement, Exp Brain Res 114(2):362-370, 1997.

23. Hodges PW, Richardson CA: Inefficient muscular stabilization of the lumbar spine associated with low back pain: a motor control evaluation of transversus abdominis, Spine 21(22):2640-2650, 1996.

24. Hodges PW, Richardson CA: Contraction of the abdominal muscles associated with movement of the lower limb, Phys Ther 77(2):132, 1997.

25. Hodges PW, Richardson CA: Delayed postural contraction of transversus abdominis in low back pain associated with movement of the lower limb, J Spinal Disord 11(1):46-56, 1998.

26. MacDonald DA, Hodges PW, Moseley L: The function of the lumbar multifidus in unilateral low back pain. Paper presented at the fifth Interdisciplinary World Congress on Low Back and Pelvic Pain, Melbourne, 2004.

27. Ferreira PH, Ferreira ML, Hodges PW: Changes in recruitment of the abdominal muscles in people with low back pain: ultrasound measurement of muscle activity, Spine 29(22):2560-2566, 2004.

28. Moseley GL, Hodges PW, Gandevia SC: Deep and superficial fibers of the lumbar multifidus muscle are differentially active during voluntary arm movements, Spine 27(2):E29-E36, 2002.

29. Moseley GL, Hodges PW, Gandevia SC: External perturbation of the trunk in standing humans differentially activates components of the medial back muscles, J Physiol 547:581-587, 2003.

30. Richardson C, Jull G, Hodges P, et al: Therapeutic exercise for spinal segmental stabilization in low back pain: scientific basis and clinical approach, Edinburgh, 1999, Churchill Livingstone.

31. MacDonald DA Jr: Physiotherapeutic management of lumbar spine pathology, Halifax, 2005, Novont Health Publishing Limited.

32. Hides JA, Jull GA, Richardson CA: Long-term effects of specific stabilizing exercises for first-episode low back pain, Spine 26(11):E243-E248, 2001.

33. O'Sullivan PB, Phyty GD, Twomey LT, et al: Evaluation of specific stabilizing exercise in the treatment of chronic low back pain with radiologic diagnosis of spondylolysis or spondylolisthesis, Spine 22(24):2959-2967, 1997.

34. Goldby LJ, Moore AP, Doust J, et al: A randomized controlled trial investigating the efficiency of musculoskeletal physiotherapy on chronic low back disorder, Spine 31(10):1083-1093, 2006.

35. Koumantakis GA, Watson PJ, Oldham JA: Trunk muscle stabilization training plus general exercise versus general exercise only: randomized controlled trial of patients with recurrent low back pain, Phys Ther 85(3):209-225, 2005.

36. Risch SV, Norvell NK, Pollock ML, et al: Lumbar strengthening in chronic low back pain patients: physiologic and psychological benefits, Spine 18(2):232-238, 1993.

37. Manniche C, Lundberg E, Christensen I, et al: Intensive dynamic back exercises for chronic low back pain: a clinical trial, Pain 47(1):53-63, 1991.

38. McGill SM: Low back exercises: evidence for improving exercise regimens, Phys Ther 78(7):754-765, 1998.

39. Plamondon A, Serresse O, Boyd K, et al: Estimated moments at L5/S1 level and muscular activation of back extensors for six prone back extension exercises in healthy individuals, Scand J Med Sci Sports 12(2):81-89, 2002.

40. Callaghan JP, Gunning JL, McGill SM: The relationship between lumbar spine load and muscle activity during extensor exercises, Phys Ther 78(1):8-18, 1998.

41. Danneels LA, Coorevits PL, Cools AM, et al: Differences in electromyographic activity in the multifidus muscle and the iliocostalis lumborum between healthy subjects and patients with sub-acute and chronic low back pain, Eur Spine J 11(1):13-19, 2002.

42. Andersson EA, Oddsson L, Nilsson J, et al: The flexion-relaxation phenomenon revisited and interactions between quadratus lumborum and erector spinae for back stability. In Hakkinen K et al, editors: XVth Congress of the International Society of Biomechanics, July 2-6, 1995, Jyvaskyla: book of abstracts, Jyvaskyla, Finland, 1995, University of Jyvaskyla, pp 56-57.

43. Drake JDM, Fischer SL, Brown SHM, et al: Do exercise balls provide a training advantage for trunk extensor exercises? A biomechanical evaluation, J Manipulative Physiol Ther 29(5):354-362, 2006.

44. Ng J, Richardson C: EMG study of erector spinae and multifidus in two isometric back extension exercises, Aust J Physiother 40(2):115-121, 1994.

45. Arokoski JP, Kankaanpaa M, Valta T, et al: Back and hip extensor muscle function during therapeutic exercises, Arch Phys Med Rehabil 80(7):842-850, 1999.

46. Shirado O, Ito T, Kaneda K, et al: Electromyographic analysis of four techniques for isometric trunk muscle exercises, Arch Phys Med Rehabil 76(3):225-229, 1995.

47. Mayer JM, Verna JL, Manini TM, et al: Electromyographic activity of the trunk extensor muscles: effect of varying hip position and lumbar posture during Roman chair exercise, Arch Phys Med Rehabil 83(11):1543-1546, 2002.

48. Arokoski JP, Valta T, Airaksinen O, et al: Back and abdominal muscle function during stabilization exercises, Arch Phys Med Rehabil 82(8):1089-1098, 2001.

49. Clark BC, Manini TM, Mayer JM, et al: Electromyographic activity of the lumbar and hip extensors during dynamic trunk extension exercise, Arch Phys Med Rehabil 83(11):1547-1552, 2002.

50. Leinonen V, Kankaanpaoao M, Airaksinen O, et al: Back and hip extensor activities during trunk flexion/extension: effects of low back pain and rehabilitation, Arch Phys Med Rehabil 81(1):32-37, 2000.

51. Vezina MJ, Hubley-Kozey CL: Muscle activation in therapeutic exercises to improve trunk stability, Arch Phys Med Rehabil 81(10):1370-1379, 2000.

52. Hubley-Kozey CL, Vezina MJ: Muscle activation during exercises to improve trunk stability in men with low back pain, Arch Phys Med Rehabil 83(8):1100-1108, 2002.

53. Davidson KLC, Hubley-Kozey CL: Trunk muscle responses to demands of an exercise progression to improve dynamic spinal stability, Arch Phys Med Rehabil 86(2):216-223, 2005.

54. Souza GM, Baker LL, Powers CM: Electromyographic activity of selected trunk muscles during dynamic spine stabilization exercises, Arch Phys Med Rehabil 82(11):1551-1557, 2001.

55. Ekstrom RA, Donatelli RA, Carp KC: Electromyographic analysis of core trunk, hip, and thigh muscles during 9 rehabilitation exercises, J Orthop Sports Phys Ther 37(12):755-768, 2007.

56. McGill S, Juker D, Kropf P: Appropriately placed surface EMG electrodes reflect deep muscle activity (psoas, quadratus lumborum, abdominal wall) in the lumbar spine, J Biomech 29(11):1503-1507, 1996.

57. Kavcic N, Grenier S, McGill SM: Quantifying tissue loads and spine stability while performing commonly prescribed low back stabilization exercises, Spine 29(20):2319-2329, 2004.

58. Stevens VK, Vleeming A, Bouche KG, et al: Electromyographic activity of trunk and hip muscles during stabilization exercises in four-point kneeling in healthy volunteers, Eur Spine J 16(5):711-718, 2007.

59. Juker D, McGill S, Kropf P, et al: Quantitative intramuscular myoelectric activity of lumbar portions of psoas and the abdominal wall during a wide variety of tasks, Med Sci Sports Exerc 30(2):301-310, 1998.

60. Allison GT, Godfrey P, Robinson G: EMG signal amplitude assessment during abdominal bracing and hollowing, J Electromyogr Kinesiol 8(1):51-57, 1998.

61. Sapsford RR, Hodges PW, Richardson CA, et al: Co-activation of the abdominal and pelvic floor muscles during voluntary exercises, Neurourol Urodyn 20(1):31-42, 2001.

62. Critchley D: Instructing pelvic floor contraction facilitates transversus abdominis thickness increase during low-abdominal hollowing, Physiother Res Int 7(2):65-75, 2002.

63. Grenier SG, McGill SM: Quantification of lumbar stability by using 2 different abdominal activation strategies, Arch Phys Med Rehabil 88(1):54-62, 2007.

64. Vera-Garcia FJ, Elvira JLL, Brown SHM, et al: Effects of abdominal stabilization maneuvers on the control of spine motion and stability against sudden trunk perturbations, J Electromyogr Kinesiol 17(5):556-567, 2007.

65. Richardson CA, Snijders CJ, Hides JA, et al: The relationship between the transversus abdominis muscles, sacroiliac joint mechanics, and low back pain, Spine 27:399-405, 2002.

66. Filho Rde F, de Brito Silva P, Ito MA, et al: Stabilization of lumbo-pelvic region and electromyography of the abdominal muscles, Electromyogr Clin Neurophysiol 46(1):51-57, 2006.

67. Kendall FP, McCreary EK, Provance PG, et al: Muscles: testing and function with posture and pain, vol 5, Baltimore, 2005, Lippincott Williams & Wilkins.

68. Axler CT, McGill SM: Low back loads over a variety of abdominal exercises: searching for the safest abdominal challenge, Med Sci Sports Exerc 29(6):804-811, 1997.

69. Escamilla RF, Babb E, DeWitt R, et al: Electromyographic analysis of traditional and nontraditional abdominal exercises: implications for rehabilitation and training, Phys Ther 86(5):656-671, 2006.

70. Escamilla RF, McTaggart MSC, Fricklas EJ, et al: An electromyographic analysis of commercial and common abdominal exercises: implications for rehabilitation and training, J Orthop Sports Phys Ther 36(2):45-57, 2006.

71. Lehman GJ, McGill SM: Quantification of the differences in electromyographic activity magnitude between the upper and lower portions of the rectus abdominis muscle during selected trunk exercises, Phys Ther 81(5):1096-1101, 2001.

72. Willett GM, Hyde JE, Uhrlaub MB, et al: Relative activity of abdominal muscles during commonly prescribed strengthening exercises, J Strength Cond Res 15(4):480-485, 2001.

73. Karst GM, Willett GM: Effects of specific exercise instructions on abdominal muscle activity during trunk curl exercises, J Orthop Sports Phys Ther 34(1):4-12, 2004.

74. Vera-Garcia FJ, Grenier SG, McGill SM: Abdominal muscle response during curl-ups on both stable and labile surfaces, Phys Ther 80(6):564-569, 2000.

75. Kraemer WJ, Adams K, Cafarelli E, et al: American College of Sports Medicine position stand. Progression models in resistance training for healthy adults, Med Sci Sports Exerc 34(2):364-380, 2002.

76. Davies GJ, Heiderscheit BC, Manske R, et al: The scientific and clinical rationale for the integrated approach to open and closed kinetic chain rehabilitation, Orthop Phys Ther Clin N Am 9(2):247-267, 2000.

77. Barnett C, Kippers V, Turner P: Effects of variations of the bench press exercise on the EMG activity of five shoulder muscles, J Strength Cond Res 9(4):222-227, 1995.

78. Townsend H, Jobe FW, Pink M, et al: Electromyographic analysis of the glenohumeral muscles during a baseball rehabilitation program, Am J Sports Med 19(3):264-272, 1991.

79. Moseley JB Jr, Jobe FW, Pink M, et al: EMG analysis of the scapular muscles during a shoulder rehabilitation program, Am J Sports Med 20(2):128-134, 1992.

80. Kronberg M, Nemeth G, Brostrom LA: Muscle activity and coordination in the normal shoulder. An electromyographic study, Clin Orthop Relat Res (257):76-85, 1990.

81. Glass SC, Armstrong T: Electromyographical activity of the pectoralis muscle during incline and decline bench presses, J Strength Cond Res 11(3):163-167, 1997.

82. Welsch EA, Bird M, Mayhew JL: Electromyographic activity of the pectoralis major and anterior deltoid muscles during three upper-body lifts, J Strength Cond Res 19(2):449-452, 2005.

83. Ekstrom RA, Bifulco KM, Lopau CJ: Comparing the function of the upper and lower parts of the serratus anterior muscle using surface electromyography, J Orthop Sports Phys Ther 34(5):235-243, 2004.

84. Ekstrom RA, Donatelli RA, Soderberg GL: Surface electromyographic analysis of exercises for the trapezius and serratus anterior muscles, J Orthop Sports Phys Ther 33(5):247-258, 2003.

85. Ekstrom RA, Soderberg GL, Donatelli RA: Normalization procedures using maximum voluntary isometric contractions for the serratus anterior and trapezius muscles during surface EMG analysis, J Electromyogr Kinesiol 15(4):418-428, 2005.

86. Hintermeister RA, Lange GW, Schultheis JM, et al: Electromyographic activity and applied load during shoulder rehabilitation exercises using elastic resistance, Am J Sports Med 26(2):210-220, 1998.

87. Decker MJ, Hintermeister RA, Faber KJ, et al: Serratus anterior muscle activity during selected rehabilitation exercises, Am J Sports Med 27(6):784-791, 1999.

88. Lear LJ, Gross MT: An electromyographical analysis of the scapular stabilizing synergists during a push-up progression, J Orthop Sports Phys Ther 28(3):146-157, 1998.

89. Kelly B, Kadrmas W, Speer K: The manual muscle examination for rotator cuff strength. An electromyographic investigation, Am J Sports Med 24(5):581-588, 1996.

90. Alpert SW, Pink MM, Jobe FW, et al: Electromyographic analysis of deltoid and rotator cuff function under varying loads and speeds, J Shoulder Elbow Surg 9(1):47-58, 2000.

91. Guazzelli Filho J, de Freitas V, Furlani J: Electromyographic study of the trapezius muscle in free movements of the shoulder, Electromyogr Clin Neurophysiol 34(5):279-283, 1994.

92. Hardwick DH, Beebe JA, McDonnell MK, et al: A comparison of serratus anterior muscle activation during a wall slide exercise and other traditional exercises, J Orthop Sports Phys Ther 36(12):903-910, 2006.

93. Reinold MM, Wilk KE, Fleisig GS, et al: Electromyographic analysis of the rotator cuff and deltoid musculature during common shoulder external rotation exercises, J Orthop Sports Phys Ther 34(7):385-394, 2004.

94. Myers JB, Pasquale MR, Laudner KG, et al: On-the-field resistance-tubing exercises for throwers: an electromyographic analysis, J Athl Train 40(1):15-22, 2005.

95. Greenfield BH, Donatelli R, Wooden MJ, et al: Isokinetic evaluation of shoulder rotational strength between the plane of scapula and the frontal plane, Am J Sports Med 18(2):124-128, 1990.

96. Ballantyne B, O'Hare S, Paschall J, et al: Electromyographic activity of selected shoulder muscles in commonly used therapeutic exercises, Phys Ther 73(10):668-677; discussion 677-682, 1993.

97. Suenaga N, Minami A, Fujisawa H: Electromyographic analysis of internal rotational motion of the shoulder in

various arm positions, J Shoulder Elbow Surg 12(5):501-505, 2003.

98. Decker MJ, Tokish JM, Ellis HB, et al: Subscapularis muscle activity during selected rehabilitation exercises, Am J Sports Med 31(1):126-134, 2003.

99. Greis PE, Kuhn JE, Schultheis J, et al: Validation of the lift-off test and analysis of subscapularis activity during maximal internal rotation. Presented at the 21st annual meeting of the AOSSM, Toronto, Ontario, Canada, July 1995, Am J Sports Med 24(5):589-593, 1996.

100. Tokish JM, Decker MJ, Ellis HB, et al: The belly-press test for the physical examination of the subscapularis muscle: electromyographic validation and comparison to the lift-off test, J Shoulder Elbow Surg 12(5):427-430, 2003.

101. Ferreira MI, Ball ML, Vitti M: Electromyographic validation of basic exercises for physical conditioning programmes. IV. Analysis of the deltoid muscle (anterior portion) and pectoralis major muscle (clavicular portion) in frontal-lateral cross, dumbbells exercises, Electromyogr Clin Neurophysiol 43(2):67-74, 2003.

102. Sahrmann S: Diagnosis and treatment of movement impairment syndromes, St Louis, 2002, Mosby.

103. Cogley RM, Archambault TA, Fibeger JF, et al: Comparison of muscle activation using various hand positions during the push-up exercise, J Strength Cond Res 19(3):628-633, 2005.

104. Signorile JF, Zink AJ, Szwed SP: A comparative electromyographical investigation of muscle utilization patterns using various hand positions during the lat pull-down, J Strength Cond Res 16(4):539-546, 2002.

105. Decker M, Tokish J, Ellis H, et al: Subscapularis muscle activity during selected rehabilitation exercises, Am J Sports Med 31(1):126-134, 2003.

106. Ekholm J, Arborelius UP, Hillered L, et al: Shoulder muscle EMG and resisting moment during diagonal exercise movements resisted by weight-and-pulley-circuit, Scand J Rehabil Med 10(4):179-185, 1978.

107. Uhl T, Carver T, Mattacola C, et al: Shoulder musculature activation during upper extremity weight-bearing exercise, J Orthop Sports Phys Ther 33(3):109-117, 2003.

108. Binningsley D: Tear of the acetabular labrum in an elite athlete, Br J Sports Med 37(1):84-88, 2003.

109. McCarthy JC, Noble PC, Schuck MR, et al: The Otto E. Aufranc Award: the role of labral lesions to development of early degenerative hip disease, Clin Orthop Relat Res (393):25-37, 2001.

110. McCarthy JC: The diagnosis and treatment of labral and chondral injuries, Instr Course Lect 53:573-577, 2004.

111. Anderson AF, Dome DC, Gautam S, et al: Correlation of anthropometric measurements, strength, anterior cruciate ligament size, and intercondylar notch characteristics to sex differences in anterior cruciate ligament tear rates, Am J Sports Med 29(1):58-66, 2001.

112. Chandrashekar N, Slauterbeck J, Hashemi J: Sex-based differences in the anthropometric characteristics of the anterior cruciate ligament and its relation to intercondylar notch geometry: a cadaveric study, Am J Sports Med 33(10):1492-1498, 2005.

113. Garrison JC, Hart JM, Palmieri RM, et al: Lower extremity EMG in male and female college soccer players during single-leg landing, J Sport Rehabil 14(1):48-57, 2005.

114. Russell KA, Palmieri RM, Zinder SM, et al: Sex differences in valgus knee angle during a single-leg drop jump, J Athl Train 41(2):166-171, 2006.

115. Earl JE: Gluteus medius activity during 3 variations of isometric single-leg stance, J Sport Rehabil 14(1):1-11, 2004.

116. Schmitz RJ, Riemann BL, Thompson T: Gluteus medius activity during isometric closed-chain hip rotation, J Sport Rehabil 11(3):179-188, 2002.

117. Sakamoto ACL, Teixeira-Salmela LF, de Paula-Goulart FR, et al: Muscular activation patterns during active prone hip extension exercises, J Electromyogr Kinesiol, 2009 (in press).

118. Oh J, Cynn H, Won J, et al: Effects of performing an abdominal drawing-in maneuver during prone hip extension exercises on hip and back extensor muscle activity and amount of anterior pelvic tilt, J Orthop Sports Phys Ther 37(6):320-324, 2007.

119. Furlani J, Berzin F, Vitti M: Electromyographic study of the gluteus maximus muscle, Electromyogr Clin Neurophysiol 14(4):379-388, 1974.

120. Ayotte N, Stetts D, Keenan G, et al: Electromyographical analysis of selected lower extremity muscles during 5 unilateral weight-bearing exercises, J Orthop Sports Phys Ther 37(2):48-55, 2007.

121. Blanpied PR: Changes in muscle activation during wall slides and squat-machine exercise, J Sport Rehabil 8:123-134, 1999.

122. Bolgla LA, Uhl TL: Electromyographic analysis of hip rehabilitation exercises in a group of healthy subjects, J Orthop Sports Phys Ther 35(8):487-494, 2005.

123. Murray MP, Sepic SB: Maximum isometric torque of hip abductor and adductor muscles, Phys Ther 48(12):1327-1335, 1968.

124. Neumann DA, Soderberg GL, Cook TM: Comparison of maximal isometric hip abductor muscle torques between hip sides, Phys Ther 68(4):496-502, 1988.

125. Andersson EA, Nilsson J, Ma Z, et al: Abdominal and hip flexor muscle activation during various training exercises, Eur J Appl Physiol Occup Physiol 75(2):115-123, 1997.

126. Shields RK, Madhavan S, Gregg E, et al: Neuromuscular control of the knee during a resisted single-limb squat exercise, Am J Sports Med 33(10):1520-1526, 2005.

127. Hopkins JT, Ingersoll CD, Sandrey MA, et al: An electromyographic comparison of 4 closed chain exercises, J Athl Train 34(4):353-357, 1999.

128. Isear JA Jr, Erickson JC, Worrell TW: EMG analysis of lower extremity muscle recruitment patterns during an unloaded squat, Med Sci Sports Exerc 29(4):532-539, 1997.

129. Ninos JC, Irrgang JJ, Burdett R, et al: Electromyographic analysis of the squat performed in self-selected

lower extremity neutral rotation and 30 degrees of lower extremity turn-out from the self-selected neutral position, J Orthop Sports Phys Ther 25(5):307-315, 1997.

130. Caterisano A, Moss R, Pellinger T, et al: The effect of back squat depth on the EMG activity of 4 superficial hip and thigh muscles, J Strength Cond Res 16(3):428-432, 2002.

131. Beutler A, Cooper L, Kirkendall D, et al: Electromyographic analysis of single-leg, closed chain exercises: implications for rehabilitation after anterior cruciate ligament reconstruction, J Athl Train 37(1):13-18, 2002.

132. Stuart MJ, Meglan DA, Lutz GE, et al: Comparison of intersegmental tibiofemoral joint forces and muscle activity during various closed kinetic chain exercises, Am J Sports Med 24(6):792-799, 1996.

133. Soderberg GL, Cook TM: An electromyographic analysis of quadriceps femoris muscle setting and straight leg raising, Phys Ther 63(9):1434-1438, 1983.

134. Brownstein BA, Lamb RL, Mangine RE: Quadriceps torque and integrated electromyography, J Orthop Sports Phys Ther 6(6):309-314, 1985.

135. Bandy WD, Hanten WP: Changes in torque and electromyographic activity of the quadriceps femoris muscles following isometric training, Phys Ther 73(7):455-465; discussion 465-457, 1993.

136. Kvist J, Gillquist J: Sagittal plane knee translation and electromyographic activity during closed and open kinetic chain exercises in anterior cruciate ligament-deficient patients and control subjects, Am J Sports Med 29(1):72-82, 2001.

137. Barber-Westin S, Noyes F, Heckmann T, et al: The effect of exercise and rehabilitation on anterior-posterior knee displacements after anterior cruciate ligament autograft reconstruction, Am J Sports Med 27(1):84-93, 1999.

138. Beynnon B, Fleming B, Johnson R, et al: Anterior cruciate ligament strain behavior during rehabilitation exercises in vivo, Am J Sports Med 23(1):24-34, 1995.

139. Fleming B, Oksendahl H, Beynnon B: Open- or closed-kinetic chain exercises after anterior cruciate ligament reconstruction? Exerc Sport Sci Rev 33(3):134-140, 2005.

140. Heijne A, Werner S: Early versus late start of open kinetic chain quadriceps exercises after ACL reconstruction with patellar tendon or hamstring grafts: a prospective randomized outcome study, Knee Surg Sports Traumatol Arthrosc 15(4):402-414, 2007.

141. Risberg MA, Lewek M, Snyder-Mackler L: A systematic review of evidence for anterior cruciate ligament rehabilitation: how much and what type? Phys Ther Sport 5(3):125-145, 2004.

142. More RC, Karras BT, Neiman R, et al: Hamstrings—an anterior cruciate ligament protagonist: an in vitro study, Am J Sports Med 21(2):231-237, 1993.

143. Gryzlo SM, Patek RM, Pink M, et al: Electromyographic analysis of knee rehabilitation exercises, J Orthop Sports Phys Ther 20(1):36-43, 1994.

144. Yak H, Collins C, Whieldon T: Comparison of closed and open kinetic chain exercise in the anterior cruciate ligament-deficient knee, Am J Sports Med 21(1):49-54, 1993.

145. Henning CE, Lynch MA, Glick KR Jr: An in vivo strain gage study of elongation of the anterior cruciate ligament, Am J Sports Med 13(1):22-26, 1985.

146. Markolf KL, Gorek JF, Kabo JM, et al: Direct measurement of resultant forces in the anterior cruciate ligament: an in vitro study performed with a new experimental technique, J Bone Joint Surg Am 72(4):557-567, 1990.

147. Beynnon BD, Fleming BC: Anterior cruciate ligament strain in-vivo: a review of previous work, J Biomech 31(6):519-525, 1998.

148. Matheson JW, Kernozek TW, Fater DC, et al: Electromyographic activity and applied load during seated quadriceps exercises, Med Sci Sports Exerc 33(10):1713-1725, 2001.

149. Andersen LL, Magnusson SP, Nielsen M, et al: Neuromuscular activation in conventional therapeutic exercises and heavy resistance exercises: implications for rehabilitation, Phys Ther 86(5):683-697, 2006.

150. Wilk K, Escamilla R, Fleisig G, et al: A comparison of tibiofemoral joint forces and electromyographic activity during open and closed kinetic chain exercises, Am J Sports Med 24(4):518-527, 1996.

151. Evetovich TK, Housh TJ, Housh DJ, et al: The effect of concentric isokinetic strength training of the quadriceps femoris on electromyography and muscle strength in the trained and untrained limb, J Strength Cond Res 15(4):439-445, 2001.

152. Shin H, Cho S, Lee Y, et al: Quantitative EMG changes during 12-week DeLorme's axiom strength training, Yonsei Med J 47(1):93-104, 2006.

153. Cresswell AG, Ovendal AH: Muscle activation and torque development during maximal unilateral and bilateral isokinetic knee extensions, J Sports Med Phys Fitness 42(1):19-25, 2002.

154. Stensdotter A, Hodges P, Mellor R, et al: Quadriceps activation in closed and in open kinetic chain exercise, Med Sci Sports Exerc 35(12):2043-2047, 2003.

155. Wawrzyniak J, Tracy J, Catizone P, et al: Effect of closed chain exercise on quadriceps femoris peak torque and functional performance, J Athl Train 31(4):335-340, 1996.

156. Reynolds NL, Worrel TW, Perrin DH: Effect of a lateral step-up exercise protocol on quadriceps isokinetic peak torque values and thigh girth, J Orthop Sports Phys Ther 15(3):151-155, 1992.

157. Worrell T, Borchert B, Erner K, et al: Effect of a lateral step-up exercise protocol on quadriceps and lower extremity performance, J Orthop Sports Phys Ther 18(6):646-653, 1993.

158. Koenig JM, Jahn DM, Dohmeier TE, et al: The effect of bench step aerobics on muscular strength, power and endurance, J Strength Cond Res 9(1):43-46, 1995.

159. Mikkelsen C, Werner S, Eriksson E: Closed kinetic chain alone compared to combined open and closed kinetic chain exercises for quadriceps strengthening after anterior cruciate ligament reconstruction with respect to return to sports: a prospective matched follow-up study, Knee Surg Sports Traumatol Arthrosc 8(6):337-342, 2000.

160. Brask B, Lueke RH, Soderberg GL:. Electromyographic analysis of selected muscles during the lateral step-up exercise, Phys Ther 64(3):324-329, 1984.

161. Cook TM, Zimmermann CL, Lux KM, et al: EMG comparison of lateral step-up and stepping machine exercise, J Orthop Sports Phys Ther 16(3):108-113, 1992.

162. Isear JA Jr, Erickson JC, Worrell TW: EMG analysis of lower extremity muscle recruitment patterns during an unloaded squat, Med Sci Sports Exerc 29(4):532-539, 1997.

163. Ebben WP, Jensen RL: Electromyographic and kinetic analysis of traditional, chain, and elastic band squats, J Strength Cond Res 16(4):547-550, 2002.

164. Vakos JP, Nitz AJ, Threlkeld AJ, et al: Electromyographic activity of selected trunk and hip muscles during a squat lift: effect of varying the lumbar posture, Spine 19(6):687-695, 1994.

165. Hung Y, Gross MT: Effect of foot position on electromyographic activity of the vastus medialis oblique and vastus lateralis during lower-extremity weight-bearing activities, including commentary by Soderberg GL with author response, J Orthop Sports Phys Ther 29(2):93-105, 1999.

166. Schulthies S, Ricard M, Alexander K, et al: An electromyographic investigation of 4 elastic-tubing closed kinetic chain exercises after anterior cruciate ligament reconstruction, J Athl Train 33(4):328-335, 1998.

167. Willett GM, Paladino JB, Barr KM, et al: Medial and lateral quadriceps muscle activity during weight-bearing knee extension exercise, J Sport Rehabil 7(4):248-257, 1998.

168. Cipriani DJ, Armstrong CW, Gaul S: Backward walking at three levels of treadmill inclination: an electromyographic and kinematic analysis, J Orthop Sports Phys Ther 22(3):95-102, 1995.

169. Zakaria D, Harburn KL, Kramer JF: Preferential activation of the vastus medialis oblique, vastus lateralis, and hip adductor muscles during isometric exercises in females, J Orthop Sports Phys Ther 26(1):23-28, 1997.

170. Hertel J, Earl JE, Tsang KKW, et al: Combining isometric knee extension exercises with hip adduction or abduction does not increase quadriceps EMG activity, Br J Sports Med 38(2):210-213, 2004.

171. Earl J, Schmitz R, Arnold B: Activation of the VMO and VL during dynamic mini-squat exercises with and without isometric hip adduction, J Electromyogr Kinesiol 11(6):381-386, 2001.

172. Coqueiro K, Bevilaqua-Grossi D, Bérzin F, et al: Analysis on the activation of the VMO and VLL muscles during semisquat exercises with and without hip adduction in individuals with patellofemoral pain syndrome, J Electromyogr Kinesiol 15(6):596-603, 2005.

173. Bevilaqua-Grossi D, Monteiro-Pedro V, de Vasconcelos RA, et al: The effect of hip abduction on the EMG activity of vastus medialis obliquus, vastus lateralis longus and vastus lateralis obliquus in healthy subjects, J Neuroeng Rehabil 3:13, 2006.

174. Ciccotti MG, Kerlan RK, Perry J, et al: An electromyographic analysis of the knee during functional activities. I. The normal profile, Am J Sports Med 22(5):645-650, 1994.

175. Colby S, Francisco A, Yu B, et al: Electromyographic and kinematic analysis of cutting maneuvers. Implications for anterior cruciate ligament injury, Am J Sports Med 28(2):234-240, 2000.

Evaluation and Treatment of Neural Tissue Pain Disorders

Advances in the pain sciences in recent years have opened the eyes of many physiotherapists, who now have a better understanding of how pain develops and how the nervous system reacts to trauma and inflammation. Dysfunction of the nervous system is increasingly recognized as an important contributing factor to a variety of chronic musculoskeletal pain disorders, even those disorders thought previously to be isolated to musculotendinous structures. Similarly, more and more we see the importance of central nervous system (CNS) sensitization, its effects on chronic pain, and its influence on physiotherapy examination and intervention. This information is driving change in patient management.

When diagnosing injury to the peripheral nervous system, musculoskeletal medicine generally only considers injury to have occurred when clinical evidence indicates axonal conduction loss.[1] Conduction loss occurs with readily diagnosable forms of peripheral neuropathy such as nerve root compression, peripheral nerve entrapments, transections, and stretch injuries, but these are relatively uncommon in comparison with the array of disorders to which physiotherapists regularly manage.[2,3]

Pain in the upper or lower quarter in the absence of any clinical evidence of neurologic deficit—and in the absence of relevant information from diagnostic tests such as radiologic imagery—is a common clinical presentation. In recent years considerable interest has developed in the role that neural tissue may play in this type of pain disorder. Of particular interest is the possible involvement of peripheral nerve sensitization causing heightened responses to mechanical stress applied to the peripheral nerve trunk along its length.[1]

A number of studies have found evidence of peripheral nerve sensitization in disorders as diverse as nonspecific arm pain, whiplash, carpal tunnel syndrome (CTS), and lateral epicondylalgia.[4-8] However, little research reports on the proportion of sufferers of specific disorders that have peripheral nerve sensitization as the primary cause of pain. Hall et al.[9] investigated subjects with chronic shoulder pain and found, through clinical examination, that approximately one third had peripheral nerve sensitization as the dominant cause of their pain. Further studies are required to investigate this, but sufficient evidence necessitates examination of the nervous system in the

management of the patient with upper- or lower-quarter pain. Identification of the source of pain is essential before administration of physical treatment or the prescription of exercise programs.

The concept of physical examination and manual treatment techniques of the nervous system is not new.[10,11] What has changed in recent years is the contemporary understanding of pain-related physiologic conditions and how this might relate to neural tissue involvement in pain disorders, as well as the management of those disorders.[12-14] This knowledge requires careful consideration regarding the indication for manual therapy. Some disorders, particularly those involving significant signs of CNS sensitization may not be suitable to manual therapy, and an alternative approach should be used.

This chapter presents a brief overview of neuropathic pain, distinguishing various subclassifications based on pathomechanisms, including central sensitization, denervation, and peripheral nerve sensitization.[15] Following this is a scheme for the clinical examination necessary to evaluate the involvement of neural tissue in a musculoskeletal disorder. In addition, a treatment approach is outlined for each subclassification.

NEUROPATHIC PAIN

In the evaluation of pain and the various types of pain patterns that may accompany disorders of the upper and lower quarters, it is essential for the clinician to keep an open mind with respect to the tissue pertaining to the origin of pain. Although symptoms such as tingling, burning, paresthesia, and numbness are generally thought to indicate pathologic condition affecting the nerve root or peripheral nerve trunk, this may not always be the case, and pain unaccompanied by paresthesia may be very difficult to analyze in terms of tissue of origin.

Pain has been traditionally divided into two types: (1) inflammatory and (2) neuropathic (some pain may also be a combination of both).[15] Inflammatory pain arises from chemically induced impulses from damage to nonneural tissues, whereas neuropathic pain arises from damage to the nervous system itself. However, with the recent advances in pain sciences, and the knowledge of peripheral and central pain mechanisms, the distinction between neuropathic and inflammatory pain has become less clear.[16] One recent viewpoint suggests that all pain is inflammatory,[17] whereas another posits that neuropathic pain may be impossible to isolate[16] (because inflammation can cause nerve damage, and nerve damage can cause inflammation).

It is undoubtedly true that neuropathic pain arises from damage to neural structures.[18] However, the degree of damage required to cause a neuropathic disorder is currently of contention.[12] It is becoming increasingly apparent that minor nerve damage, clinically difficult to detect on standard neurologic assessment, is capable of causing pain.[5,19,20] The nervi nervorum is the sensory supply of the peripheral neural system, innervating the connective tissue layers protecting the nerve trunks.[21-23] Hence damage of a peripheral nerve trunk, CTS for example, is likely to involve inflammation and therefore sensitization of nervi nervorum afferents.

Pain arising from noxious stimulation of the nervi nervorum does not appear to have been classified as either *nociceptive* or *neuropathic*. Although physiologically it is inflammatory, pain must be considered as arising from stimulation of the nervi nervorum to be included in the neuropathic category. Hence clinically, in the presence of nerve trunk damage, any combination of inflammatory and neuropathic pain may exist, either local or referred. A good example of this would be a lumbar radiculopathy, with radicular pain, secondary to a disc prolapse. It is likely that a significant proportion of the symptoms may be composed of referred pain arising from inflammatory sensitization of afferents within the damaged annular layers. Similarly, a large proportion may also arise from damage to, and inflammation of, the adjacent compromised nerve root. Pain disorders rarely fit into one category. It cannot be assumed that all leg pain is a neuropathic disorder of the sciatic nerve, because the disc and zygapophyseal joints have been shown to be capable of causing referred symptoms,[24] even as far as the foot.[25] O'Neill et al.[26] performed an experiment on patients with low-back pain, noxiously stimulating (with variable intensity) the symptomatic lumbar disc. Their study showed that the distal extent of referred leg pain depends on the intensity of stimulation and that disc stimulation may reproduce pain that extends below the knee.

The term *peripheral neuropathic pain* has been suggested to embrace the combination of positive and negative symptoms and signs in patients in whom pain is due to pathologic changes or dysfunction in neural tissues distal to the dorsal horn.[27] These structures include peripheral nerve trunks, plexuses, dorsal and ventral rami, nerve roots, and dorsal root ganglion. Positive features occur in response to increased excitability of the nervous system, whereas negative features are associated with reduced axonal conductivity. Table 30-1 shows a composite of positive and negative, motor and sensory features typically found in peripheral neuropathic pain.

Two types of pain after peripheral nerve injury have been recognized: (1) dysesthetic pain and (2) nerve trunk pain.[28] Dysesthetic pain results from volleys of impulses arising in damaged or regenerating nociceptive afferent fibers. Character-

Table 30-1	Positive and Negative Features (Signs and Symptoms) of Peripheral Neuropathic Disorders	
	Motor	Sensory
Positive	Spasm	Pain
	Dystonia	Paresthesia
	Cramp	Hyperesthesia
		Allodynia (thermal and mechanical)
		Hyperalgesia
		Hyperpathia
		Dysaesthesia
Negative	Weakness	Anesthesia
	Wasting	Hypoesthesia
	Hyporeflexia	

istically, dysesthetic pain is felt in the peripheral sensory distribution of a sensory or mixed nerve. This pain has features that are not found in deep pain arising from either somatic or visceral tissues. These features include abnormal or unfamiliar sensations (frequently having a burning or electrical quality), pain felt in the region of the sensory deficit, pain with a paroxysmal brief shooting or stabbing component, and the presence of allodynia.[27,29]

In contrast, nerve trunk pain has been attributed to increased activity in chemically sensitized nociceptors within the nerve sheaths or axons themselves.[21] This kind of pain is said to follow the course of the nerve trunk. It is commonly described as deep and aching, familiar like a toothache, and worsened with movement, nerve stretch, or palpation.

Peripheral nerve trunks, nerve roots, and dorsal root ganglia are known to be mechanosensitive because their connective tissues possess afferents, the nervi nervorum, which are capable of mechanoreception.[22,30] Many of the nervi nervorum are unmyelinated—forming a sporadic plexus in all the connective tissues of a peripheral nerve—and have predominantly free endings.[22]

Electrophysiologic studies have demonstrated that at least some nervi nervorum have a nociceptive function because they respond to noxious mechanical, chemical, and thermal stimuli.[31] Most nervi nervorum studied by Bove and Light[21] were sensitive to excess longitudinal stretch of the entire nerve they innervated, as well as to local stretch in any direction and to focal pressure. They did not respond to stretch within normal ranges of motion. Clinical studies support this evidence by showing that, under normal circumstances, nerve trunks and nerve roots are insensitive to nonnoxious mechanical stimuli.[32,33]

The nervi nervorum contain neuropeptides including substance P and calcitonin gene-related peptide, indicating a role in neurogenic vasodilation.[21,23] It has been suggested that local nerve inflammation is mediated by the nervi nervorum, especially in cases with no intrafascicular axonal damage. In keeping with this suggestion, it has been postulated that the spread of mechanosensitivity along the length of the nerve trunk distant from the local area of pathologic condition seen in nerve trunk pain is mediated through neurogenic inflammation via the nervi nervorum.[34] The entire nerve trunk then behaves as a sensitized nociceptor, generating impulses in response to minor mechanical stimuli.[35]

The mechanism of neurogenic inflammation may help to explain mechanical allodynia of structurally normal nerve trunks in which the pathologic condition is more proximal in the nerve root. An alternative explanation is that nonnociceptive input from the presumed nerve trunk mechanoreceptors is being processed abnormally within the CNS.[32] This is probably the result of a sustained afferent nociceptive barrage from the site of the nerve,[30] a pathologic process termed *central sensitization.*[36]

More recently it has been suggested that the nervi nervorum may not be the only cause of mechanosensitization of inflamed nerve trunks.[37] Bove et al.[19] demonstrated in a rat model that some intact nerve fibers become sensitive to pressure at the site of inflammation and that that axons themselves develop properties of pressure mechanosensitivity.[19,20,37] Furthermore Dilley et al.[20] showed evidence of stretch sensitivity in a small proportion of structurally normal, but inflamed, A and C nerve fibers. Most responsive fibers fired to only 3% stretch, which is within the range of nerve stretch seen during normal limb movements.[20] The mechanisms underlying mechanosensitivity of axons are complex. Disruption of axoplasmic flow and axonal transport because of pressure changes around the inflamed site leads to the accumulation of ion channels at the lesion site.[19,20,38] Ion channel expression is also altered, resulting in a change in type and density of ion channels produced by the cell body.[39,40] The result is that axons become capable of generating impulses to mechanical stimuli when they would normally not do so.

The studies by Bove et al.[19] and Dilley et al.[20] provide very good explanations for the frequent clinical finding of peripheral nerve trunk mechanosensitivity in a range of musculoskeletal disorders[41] in which normal neurologic function is found on electrodiagnostic tests and no apparent structural abnormality is seen on radiologic imaging. This mounting evidence, supporting the concept of mechanosensitivity of structurally normal nerves, should put a stop to the criticism of such a notion.[42]

The most commonly cited form of spinal neuropathic disorder is nerve root compression or radiculopathy. In the lumbar spine this most commonly results from intervertebral disc herniation. However, it can also be caused by age-related changes, including slow-growing osteophytes from lumbar vertebral bodies at the disc margins and from zygapophyseal joints, which can compress the nerve root in the intervertebral foramen, lateral recess, or spinal canal.[43] Although pain is not always a feature of nerve root compression and spinal stenosis,[44-47] true radiculopathic pain in the absence of inflammation of the nerve root is presumably the result of chronic compression, causing hypoxia, vascular compromise, and subsequent damage of axons within the nerve root. Under these circumstances, there may be minimal peripheral nerve sensitization and little evidence of neural tissue mechanosensitivity with neural tissue provocation tests such as straight-leg raise (SLR).[46,48]

Patients with a denervation disorder typically report pain associated with movement or postures that compress the neural structures. The classic example is spinal canal or foraminal stenosis. Spine extension is typically provocative, because it further reduces the space available for the nerve root. However, for extension to compromise the neural structures, a reduction must occur in the volume of the canal or foramen to begin with, usually by some degenerative process as mentioned previously. Characteristically, sustained standing and walking both promote extension and provoke leg symptoms.[49] Clinical evaluation of deep tendon reflexes, muscle power, skin sensation tests, and vibration perception reveal neurologic dysfunction. In addition to these typical clinical findings, radiologic and electrodiagnostic evidence of compressive neurologic compromise must exist.

Alternatively, radicular pain, even when severe, may occur in the absence of frank axonal damage,[50,51] but the nerve trunk is highly sensitized mechanically. In this case, clinical neurologic and electrodiagnostic test findings may be normal. What appears to be the significant factor is inflammation[52-54] that causes mechanosensitization of the peripheral nerve trunks.

As a result of damage to, or inflammation of, innervated tissues, noxious input will bombard the CNS, leading to profound changes that are collectively termed *central sensitization.* Central sensitization represents a state of heightened sensitivity of dorsal horn neurons such that their threshold of activation is reduced and their responsiveness to synaptic inputs is augmented.[55] Central sensitization is a normal, short-term event that takes place after any kind of tissue injury, because it contributes to the normal repair processes. Damaged tissues are rendered sensitive to mechanical stimuli, thus forcing the protection and repair of the damaged part. However, central sensitization also plays a major role in the ongoing pain in neuropathic disorders (e.g., some unfortunate individuals with reflex sympathetic dystrophy experience permanent pain). A number of different mechanisms have been described that are responsible for the enhanced pain processing associated with central sensitization; these include sensitization of nociceptive-specific dorsal horn neurons (especially wide dynamic range [WDR] neurons), disinhibition, deafferentation, phenotypic switch and sprouting of AΔ fibers, as well as changes in cortical and subcortical brain regions.[13]

After peripheral nerve injury, as a result of change to the structure of the nerve, C-fiber input may arise spontaneously and drive central sensitization.[55] Stimulus independent, spontaneous pain is a common feature of neuropathic disorders. In addition, A fibers, that normally signal innocuous events such as light touch, change their function through a process of altered gene transcription, behaving more like C fibers, which enable them now to drive central sensitization.[56] Pain is provoked by either light touch (allodynia) or to pin prick (hyperalgesia) stimuli. Now the normally innocuous stimuli of light touch, joint movement, or muscle contraction produce or maintain central sensitization.[39]

The upshot of this brief overview is that it is possible to subclassify neuropathic pain into three groups based on underlying mechanisms.[13] These are (1) central sensitization with a dominance of the positive features of allodynia and hyperalgesia, (2) denervation with evidence of significant axonal compromise, and (3) peripheral nerve sensitization with significant nerve trunk mechanosensitization. This classification is important because it drives treatment priorities (discussed later). The following section details the clinical examination that enables the clinician to correctly classify the disorder.

CLINICAL EXAMINATION

The purpose of the clinical examination is to determine the source of the patient's symptoms, to make a diagnosis, and to prescribe appropriate management. To effectively evaluate a particular disorder from a manual therapy perspective, the clinician must first conduct a thorough subjective examination. An intimate knowledge of the subjective complaint will allow the clinician to plan the scope and range of physical examination tests necessary to elicit a sufficient number of consistent signs to make an appropriate diagnosis. It is also particularly important that the nature of those signs on physical examination is consistent with the severity, degree of trauma, and history of the patient's symptoms. For example, minor signs of increased upper-quarter neural tissue mechanosensitivity in a clinical presentation of severe neck, scapula, and arm pain would not be consistent with a classification of peripheral nerve sensitization. An alternative diagnosis would be appropriate and the dominant dysfunctional structures identified.

In a patient with nerve injury (e.g., lumbar radiculopathy after disc prolapse), inflammatory and neuropathic pain are both likely to be present.[46] For this reason, it may be difficult to distinguish between referred pain arising from damaged musculoskeletal structures such as the disc and referred pain arising from neural tissues.[16,57,58]

The pain and paresthesia that occur in cervical and lumbar radiculopathy may not be well localized anatomically because different nerve roots have similar dermatomal distributions. In a series of 841 patients with cervical radiculopathy, only 55% had pain after a typical discrete dermatomal pattern.[59] The remainder had diffuse nondermatomally distributed pain. Rankine et al.[58] found that the location of pain and paresthesia was not a good predictor of the presence of lumbar nerve root compression.

A number of screening tools have been developed to help the clinician determine the predominance of neuropathic pain in a patients presenting complaint. These include the Neuropathic Pain Questionnaire (NPQ),[60] the French Douleur Neuropathique 4 (DN4),[61] the Leeds Assessment of Neuropathic Symptoms and Signs (LANSS),[62] painDETECT,[63] and ID-pain.[64] Each tool attempts to identify the presence of neuropathic pain in a different way. For example the ID-pain is purely subjective,[64] whereas the LANSS and DN4 consist of questionnaires regarding pain description, together with items relating to the bedside clinical examination. Table 30-2 lists the relative strengths of each screening tool, identified by studies reporting sensitivity and specificity.

Table 30-2 Best Evidence for Use of Neuropathic Screening Tools

Tool	Evidence
NPQ[65]	Sensitivity = 66%
	Specificity = 74%
DN4[61]	Sensitivity = 83%
	Specificity = 90%
LANSS[66-68]	Sensitivity =>82%
	Specificity =>80%
painDETECT[63]	Sensitivity = 85%
	Specificity = 80%
	Diagnostic accuracy = 83%

DN4, Douleur Neuropathique 4; *LANSS,* Leeds Assessment of Neuropathic Symptoms and Signs; *NPQ,* Neuropathic Pain Questionnaire.

Some authors have postulated that a given pain disorder may be more or less neuropathic. Although this concept is relatively untested, it seems to have construct validity[15,69,70] and fits well with basic science opinion regarding chronic pain mechanisms.[70] As is always the case, information from the subjective examination should be interpreted with caution and within the context of the complete clinical evaluation.

The subjective examination provides the majority of the evidence for a patient to be classified into a neuropathic disorder with predominant central sensitization. Patients with this classification report primarily positive symptoms such as paresthesias, dysaesthesias, hyperalgesia, dynamic mechanical allodynia, and stimulus-independent pain.[13] The LANSS scale[62] forms a useful tool to identify these patients, with those scoring greater than 12 classified as *positive* in this group.

Physical evaluation of neural tissue follows the same principles used in examination of any other structure in the body. For example, a clinical presentation of hamstring pain after an injury such as a "pulled muscle" requires a number of physical examination tests (with findings that correlate with each other) before a diagnosis of muscle strain can be supported. Such tests would include static isometric muscle contraction, hamstring muscle stretch, and palpation of the muscle. These physical tests provide mechanical stimuli to the injured muscle tissue and so are provocative tests seeking a subjective pain response. It is therefore apparent that no test in isolation is sufficient to provide a consistently accurate diagnosis.

To determine the degree to which peripheral nerve sensitization is present in a given patient's presentation, a similar but more sophisticated process of clinical reasoning must be used. A number of specific correlating signs must be present. For instance, it is not possible to say that a SLR test is positive or negative in the diagnosis of a lumbosacral nerve root pathologic condition. The mechanical stress of SLR is not isolated to the neural structures,[71] because the SLR test induces posterior pelvic rotation within a few degrees of lifting the leg from the horizontal[72] (with concomitant effects on the structures in the posterior thigh, pelvis, and lumbar spine). The findings of the SLR test must be interpreted within the clinical context of a number of other procedures before a diagnosis of nerve root pathologic condition can be made.

The following details the scope of physical assessment to determine the degree to which peripheral nerve sensitization contributes to a presenting pain complaint (based on Elvey and Hall)[73]:

1. Posture
2. Active movement dysfunction
3. Passive movement dysfunction, which correlates with the degree of active movement dysfunction
4. Adverse responses to neural tissue provocation tests, which must relate specifically and anatomically to tests two and three
5. Mechanical allodynia in response to palpation of specific nerve trunks, which relates specifically and anatomically to tests two and four
6. A musculoskeletal-related cause of peripheral nerve sensitization, relating to neural structures found positive in tests four and five

In addition to being a conductive system, the peripheral nervous system is well adapted to movement. Under normal circumstances, peripheral nerve trunks slide and glide with movement, relative to the associated movement of surrounding structures, adapting to positional changes of the trunk and limbs.[11,74-76] In addition, the spinal cord, nerve roots, and spinal meninges can readily adapt to movements of the spinal column with changes in length and tension.[77,78] With a sound knowledge of applied anatomy and biomechanics of the nervous system, the clinician can selectively stress nerve trunks and nerve roots as part of a comprehensive physical examination.

When neural tissue is sensitized or inflamed, limb movement and positional change cause a provocative mechanical stimulus, resulting in pain and noncompliance. This lack of compliance is demonstrated by painful limitation of movement caused by antagonistic muscles trying to prevent further pain. Muscle contraction, as measured by electromyography (EMG), in response to provocation of neural tissue has been demonstrated in both animal and in vivo human experiments.[32,79-84] In patients with heightened neural tissue mechanosensitivity, muscle activity occurs at the onset of pain provocation, whereas in normal subjects, muscle activity occurs according to the level of the subject's pain tolerance.[80] It appears that muscles are recruited via CNS processes to prevent pain associated with the provocation of neural tissue.[32,85]

Posture

An antalgic posture may be the first clinical indicator of pain associated with a neural tissue disorder, with adaptation being dependent on the type and severity of neural tissue problem. For example, in the presence of moderate to severe pain arising from peripheral nerve sensitization, the patient usually adopts a posture that shortens the anatomic distance over which the sensitized peripheral nerve trunk courses. In contrast, in the presence of neuropathic pain with denervation arising from a compressed, stenotic nerve root, the patient will subconsciously adopt a posture that increases the available space surrounding

the nerve root. Two examples of antalgic posture assumed in response to sensitization of upper- and lower-quarter neural tissue are presented in Figures 30-1A and B.

The first example (see Figure 30-1A) is a patient with neck, shoulder, and arm pain associated with a brachial plexopathy. The posture adopted to relieve provocation of the sensitized neural tissue is a combination of shoulder girdle elevation, cervical spine ipsilateral lateral flexion, and elbow flexion. In the second example (see Figure 30-1B) of a patient with buttock and leg pain, the posture adopted to relieve provocation of the sensitized S1 nerve root is a combination of knee flexion, ankle plantar flexion, and lumbar spine ipsilateral lateral flexion.

When sensitization of a lumbar nerve root is associated with an acute, painful intervertebral disc prolapse, the added problem of minimizing the stress on the disc exists. The bulge will compromise the nerve root more on extension or ipsilateral flexion.[86] The conflict between minimizing the disc bulge and reducing the provocation of neural tissue is resolved in a variety of postures, one of which, seen commonly, is a list toward the painful side together with a flattened lumbar lordosis.

Guarded postures to avoid movement of the sensitized nerve site have been demonstrated in an animal model.[87] In animal experiments, Hu et al.[82,83] showed that the application of a small fiber irritant to cervical neuromeningeal tissues resulted in increased electromyographic activity in the upper trapezius and jaw muscles. It appears that the most likely mechanism for altered posture is protective muscle contraction or spasm.

Active Movement

In the majority of less painful disorders, active movement dysfunction may be the first aspect of the physical examination that provides evidence of involvement of the neural system. As with active movement at any joint complex, the clinician should inquire about symptom reproduction, as well as observe the quantity and quality of movement.

In the presence of neuropathic pain with denervation arising from a compressed nerve root, active movement limitation will be consistent with the severity of the disorder. In this case the patient is likely to suffer from limb symptoms. Those active movements that provoke the peripheral symptoms are sought. Typically, movements that reduce the space for the surrounding nerve root are provocative. For example, in the cervical spine, extension and ipsilateral rotation have been shown to reduce the volume of the intervertebral foramen, whereas flexion increases it.[88,89] Furthermore, combinations of these movements are likely to be more symptomatic. A modification of the Spurling maneuver, using extension, ipsilateral rotation, lateral flexion, and compression, has been shown to have good sensitivity (77%) and specificity (92%), as well as good positive and negative predictive value (respectively, 80% and 91%).[90]

Figure 30-2 demonstrates active shoulder abduction. In this example, the patient has compensated for the lack of compliance of neural tissue in the upper quarter by adopting ipsilat-

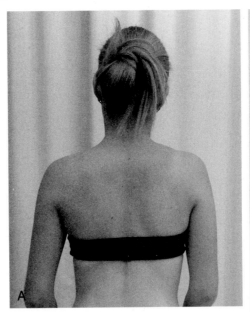

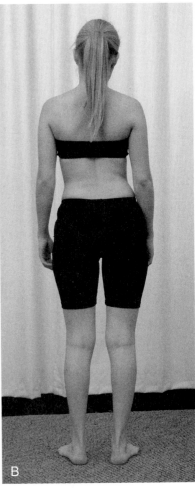

Figure 30-1 A, Antalgic posture associated with severe right upper-quarter neural tissue sensitization. **B,** Antalgic posture associated with severe left lower-quarter neural tissue sensitization.

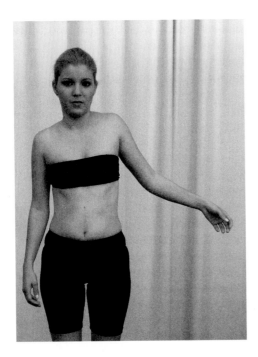

Figure 30-2 Active shoulder abduction with compensatory mechanisms.

eral cervical spine lateral flexion, shoulder girdle elevation, and elbow flexion. This pattern of movement dysfunction can be observed in many disorders involving the shoulder girdle, and a hypothesis of peripheral nerve sensitization must be supported by a series of other specific examination procedures.

With an understanding of applied anatomy, the clinician can examine active movements in various ways to support the clinical hypotheses of a peripheral nerve sensitization disorder. In the upper quarter, various active movements will be affected, depending on the particular nerve tract involved. Shoulder abduction and contralateral lateral flexion of the cervical spine will increase the mechanical stress on the brachial plexus and associated tracts of neural tissue.[11,91-94] Therefore these are the movements most likely to be affected by increased mechanosensitivity of the neural tissues forming the brachial plexus.

If active shoulder abduction or cervical spine contralateral lateral flexion is painful or limited in range, the clinician can differentiate between a local pathologic condition and a neural tissue pathologic condition by repeating the movement with neural-sensitizing maneuvers such as wrist extension. Wrist extension will place greater provocation on the neural tissue of the upper quarter via the median nerve trunk.[91,95,96] Likewise,

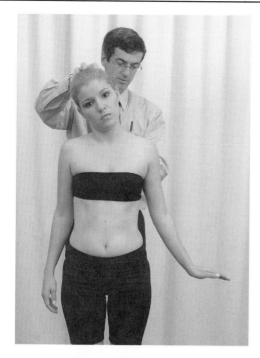

Figure 30-3 Active shoulder abduction with cervical spine contralateral lateral flexion and the shoulder girdle lightly stabilized.

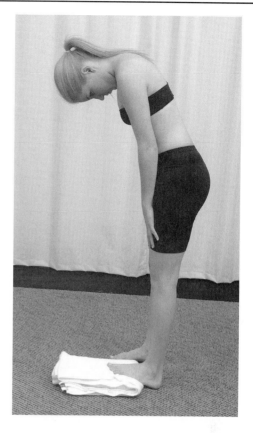

Figure 30-4 Lumbar active flexion with the ankle in end-range dorsiflexion.

medial rotation of the shoulder with wrist and finger flexion will increase the stress along the course of the radial nerve.[97]

Figure 30-3 demonstrates shoulder abduction with the cervical spine positioned in contralateral lateral flexion and the wrist extended. Great care must be taken to avoid changing the position of the shoulder girdle complex. A typical response to cervical spine contralateral lateral flexion when upper-quarter neural tissue is peripherally sensitized is for the patient to elevate the shoulder girdle in an attempt to compensate for the additional mechanical stress of side flexion. The clinician can maintain a consistent shoulder girdle position through the range of abduction with light fixation over the acromion. Using this hand position, the clinician is able to detect compensatory involuntary upper-trapezius muscle activity, which can be associated with upper-limb neural tissue provocative maneuvers.[98] Without this careful handling, the clinician may misinterpret the outcome of this examination procedure.

> ### Clinical Tip
> Figures 30-3 and 30-4 are useful screening tools for rapidly identifying the likelihood of peripheral nerve sensitization. If these tests are positive, then further examination of the nervous system is warranted to confirm or refute the presence of peripheral nerve sensitization.

In the lower-quarter lumbar flexion with hip flexion, knee extension and ankle dorsiflexion are provocative to the sciatic nerve, its terminal branches, and the L4 and S3 nerve roots.[75,99-101] If pain is provoked or range of movement is limited on active lumbar flexion in standing, then the clinician

may consider using a process to differentiate between pathologic condition in the lumbar musculoskeletal structures and neural tissues. The ankle is positioned in dorsiflexion or the cervical spine in flexion, and the movement is repeated (Figure 30-4). If the neural tissue associated with the sciatic nerve is sensitized anywhere along its course, then the response to active lumbar flexion is more painful and the range of movement is more limited. Again, the clinician must take great care to prevent compensatory involuntary movement of knee flexion, which is presumably a protective hamstring muscle response.

In contrast to the sciatic nerve, the femoral nerve arises from the L2 to L4 nerve roots and lies anterior to the coronal axis for sagittal plane movements of the hip and knee. As a consequence, the femoral nerve and L2 to L4 nerve roots are mechanically stressed by a combination of lumbar contralateral lateral flexion, hip extension, and knee flexion.[74,102,103]

Differentiation of musculoskeletal structures and neural structures as the source of pain can be considered by using a combination of remote movements sensitizing the neural structures, as previously outlined. Figure 30-5 demonstrates assessment of active lumbar lateral flexion with the knee positioned in flexion. It is essential that the position of the femur and the lumbopelvic posture not be changed between trials; otherwise, the test is invalidated. If significant sensitization of the femoral nerve and the L2 to L4 nerve roots exists, then range of lumbar lateral flexion will be diminished or more painful with the knee in flexion compared with extension.

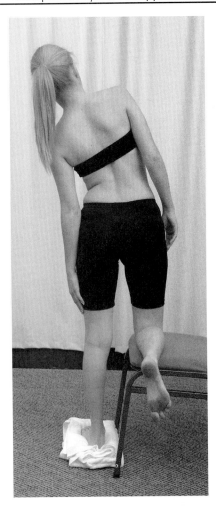

Figure 30-5 Active lumbar lateral flexion with the knee flexed provoking the femoral nerve.

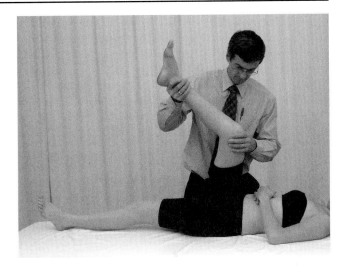

Figure 30-6 Hip flexion adduction maneuver with neural tissue provocation.

This is a basic approach to analysis of active movement in the physical evaluation of neural tissue. With some thought to applied anatomy, the clinician can examine active movements in different directions and in various ways to support a clinical hypothesis formed at this early stage of evaluation. For example, a disorder of the C5-6 motion segment may involve the C5 nerve root or the spinal nerve, which may cause an observable dysfunction of shoulder abduction and movement of the hand behind the back (because of the mechanically induced stimulus produced by these movements on the suprascapular and axillary nerve trunks). Contralateral flexion of the head and neck would increase the dysfunction of shoulder abduction in this example.[1]

PASSIVE MOVEMENT DYSFUNCTION

Both active and passive movement have similar effects in terms of mechanical stress applied through lengthening of neural tissues. Therefore in the presence of peripheral nerve sensitization disorders, consistent pain provocation and limitation of movement should occur during both passive and active movement. However, in addition to assessment of range and pain provocation, the clinician must evaluate any change in the feel of the movement, which is perceived as a change in the nature and quality of resistance.[104]

The flexion and adduction maneuver of the hip and the quadrant position of the shoulder[105] are two important passive movement tests of those joints. These movements stress not only the hip joint and shoulder complex but also certain peripheral nerve trunks.[73,99]

For example, the sciatic nerve lies posterior and lateral to the axis of motion of hip flexion adduction, so this movement will be provocative to the sciatic nerve and hence to the L4 to S2 nerve roots. Possible neural tissue involvement in which flexion adduction of the hip is painful and limited in range can be determined by performing the same movement with the knee more extended (Figure 30-6). A significant decrease in range of movement should be seen if neural tissue is involved in the condition.

In the quadrant position of the shoulder,[105] the humeral head has an upward fulcrum effect on the overlying neurovascular bundle in the region of the axilla.[11] Therefore it is possible to use this test not only for the shoulder but also for the compliance of the neurovascular tissues to the quadrant position. In the context of this chapter, this test specifically includes the neural tissues of the brachial plexus and its proximal and distal extensions. To differentiate between pain evoked from musculoskeletal structures and pain from neural tissue, the test can be performed with the shoulder girdle in elevation and depression and with the head and neck in ipsilateral and contralateral lateral flexion.[73] If the source of pain is musculoskeletal structures, then little change in response should occur between these positions. By contrast, a predictable change in pain response should be noted if pain is arising from peripheral nerve sensitization.

ADVERSE RESPONSES TO NEURAL TISSUE PROVOCATION TESTS

Neural Tissue Provocation Tests (NTPTs) are passive tests applied to selectively stress neural tissues to assess their sensitivity to mechanical provocation. A variety of tests have been suggested to mechanically provoke various components of the neural system. The most common of these is the SLR test.[75] Other tests include the slump test,[77] the femoral nerve stress test,[103] the passive neck flexion test,[106] the median nerve stress test,[95] and the brachial plexus tension test.[107] In the upper limb these tests have also been called *Upper-Limb Tension Tests* (ULTT), with variants described ULTT1, ULTT2a, ULTT2b, and ULTT3.[108] In the authors' opinion, this kind of nomenclature it is not descriptive of the test and is therefore not helpful in communication with other health professionals.

In the past, criticism has been expressed regarding the concept of neural mobilization (especially NTPT), with questions raised as to whether these tests can selectively stress nerve trunks without affecting neighboring musculoskeletal structures.[42] Since Elvey[11] and Butler[10] put forward the concept of the assessment and treatment of the nervous system, a great deal of research has investigated the validity of NTPT.[4,20,100,109-114] For example, an experimental pain model was used to determine the specificity of a median nerve NTPT in the differential diagnosis of hand symptoms.[109] Sensory responses to this test were unchanged by the presence of experimentally induced muscle pain in the hand, illustrating high specificity for this test. Other studies have similarly demonstrated high sensitivity for this test to identify patients with CTS.[115] Similarly, this test was found to be the single clinical test item with the highest reliability and sensitivity in making a diagnosis of cervical radiculopathy.[115] The lower-limb and experimental pain model (involving the tibialis anterior muscle) was used to examine the validity of the SLR and slump tests.[111] Sensory responses during these tests were unchanged by the presence of induced muscle pain in the leg, illustrating high specificity for the SLR and slump tests. Furthermore, a cadaver study showed that strain in nerves around the ankle and foot could be selectively increased by a NTPT without affecting adjacent musculoskeletal structures such as the plantar fascia.[100] Many additional biomechanical and anatomic studies illustrate the validity of NTPTs.

Range and sensory responses to NTPTs are governed by the severity of the disorder being evaluated. For instance, in severe cervicobrachial pain conditions, only limited range of shoulder abduction and lateral rotation can be achieved. Therefore it is unrealistic to use a standardized provocation test such as ULTT1. The clinician is required to formulate a test according to each patient's signs and symptoms.

A methodological approach to neural tissue provocation tests for the upper quarter has been documented.[1,116] This approach offers guidelines for examination that allow the test technique to be tailored to the severity of the particular pain disorder. The suggested approach incorporates provocative maneuvers directed to the median, radial, and ulnar nerve trunks, with stress applied from a proximal to a distal direction and vice versa.

Figure 30-7 illustrate the test technique from distal to proximal. For confirmation, to verify the responses to the tests just described, it is important to apply provocative maneuvers from proximal to distal. Figure 30-8 illustrate these maneuvers. It is not always necessary to apply both sets of maneuvers. For example, in the presence of severe pain arising from peripheral nerve sensitization, the tests from distal to proximal may be too provocative to perform and only tests from proximal to distal are required.

It has been suggested that the sequence in which the various component movements are applied during NTPT is of importance because it provides information to the site of neural tissue pathologic condition.[117,118] This conjecture is unsupported in the literature, and it may be that responses to neurodynamic sequencing may simply be the result of the attention placed on the first of a combination of movements.[119] Again, the informed clinician will combine information from the whole examination, rather than that from one test in isolation.

A similar flexible approach is recommended for the lower quarter, although it is not feasible to undertake passive tests from proximal to distal. For a disorder involving the lumbar spine, provocative maneuvers directed to the sciatic, femoral, and obturator nerve trunks are required. The use of sensitizing maneuvers is a necessary part of each test. For the SLR test (Figure 30-9) these include, among others, ankle dorsiflexion, medial hip rotation, and hip adduction, which have all been shown to increase mechanical provocation on the sciatic nerve tract.[75,100] Although cervical spine flexion has also been shown to move (and tension) lumbar nerve roots in an animal cadaver model,[101] the clinical use of cervical spine flexion as a sensitizing maneuver for SLR has been shown to be questionable.[80]

Neural tissue provocative maneuvers directed to the femoral nerve trunk are shown in Figure 30-10. Lumbar spine lateral flexion can be used as a sensitizing maneuver for this test. The slump test[117] is an important procedure when determining the involvement of neural tissue mechanosensitivity in lower-quarter pain disorders. This test may be performed as described by Maitland,[117] with the patient sitting on the edge of the examination table (Figures 30-11A and B) or in the side-lying position.[120] Hall et al.[120] demonstrated that, in the side-lying position, changing the lumbosacral L5-S1 junction from end-range flexion to end-range extension has a significant sensitizing effect on sciatic nerve extensibility. Lumbosacral extension increases provocation on the L4 and L5 roots because of the change in their anatomic course over the alar of the sacrum. In contrast, the S1 root has a less tortuous path[120] and is thus not provoked by extension. This information may be useful in the differential diagnosis of lumbosacral nerve root disorders.

Neural tissue provocation tests are passive movement tests. The examiner must appreciate changes in muscle tone or activity in addition to a subjective pain response. Increased muscle

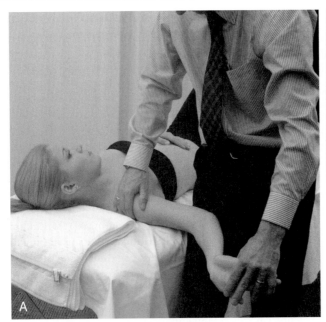

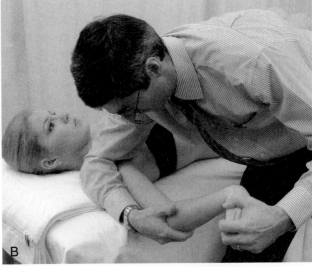

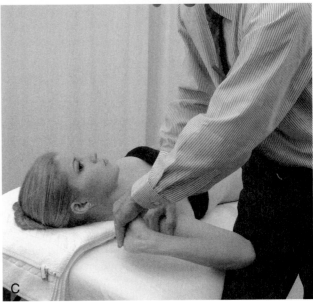

Figure 30-7 A, Neural tissue provocation test biased to the median nerve trunk (distal to proximal). **B,** Neural tissue provocation test biased to the radial nerve trunk (distal to proximal). **C,** Neural tissue provocation test biased to the ulnar nerve trunk (distal to proximal).

activity is a reflection of increased mechanosensitivity of the neural tissue being tested and is indicated by an increase in resistance to movement.[84] This increase in resistance, because of the onset of protective muscle activity, should coincide with the patient's report of onset of pain[80] and reproduction of the pain complaint. Symptom reproduction is the second important response. *Moments* is a more appropriate biomechanical term to describe angular forces during limb movement. Figure 30-12 is typical of the subjects in this study and represents the moment of stretched tissue, measured objectively by a load cell, during SLR (in the clinical context, moment of stretched tissue is perceived by the examiner as resistance).[81] In this example, the subject tested had significant evidence of sciatic nerve sensitization. A change in moment (increased resistance) occurs only at the onset of muscle activity. The change in resistance, associated with the onset of muscle activity, is readily appreciable to the clinician during all passive neural tissue provocation procedures.

MECHANICAL ALLODYNIA IN RESPONSE TO PALPATION OF SPECIFIC NERVE TRUNKS

An important step in the classification of peripheral nerve sensitization is palpation of the nerve trunks. If pain is provoked through lengthening of the nerve, then focal pressure directly over the nerve trunk should also be painful.

It is widely known that under normal circumstances, peripheral nerve trunks and nerve roots do not evoke pain in response to nonnoxious mechanical stimuli.[32,33,121,122] By contrast, inflamed nerve roots are exquisitely sensitive to even mild mechanical provocation.[33,122] Similarly, Dyck[123] reported that the entire extent of the sciatic nerve trunk is invariably tender when a lumbosacral nerve root is traumatized. Comparable findings have been reported in cervical radiculopathy.[32]

The spread of mechanosensitivity along the length of the nerve trunk after proximal nerve trauma has been reported

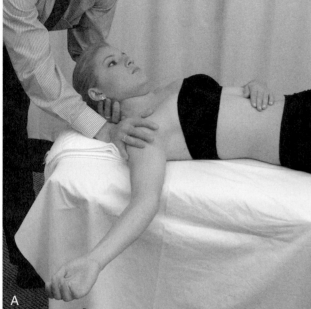

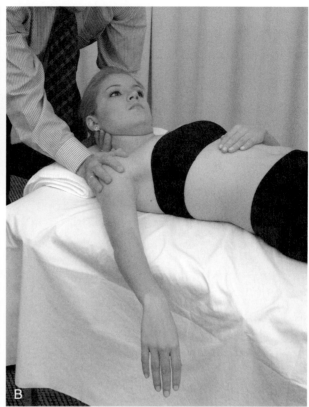

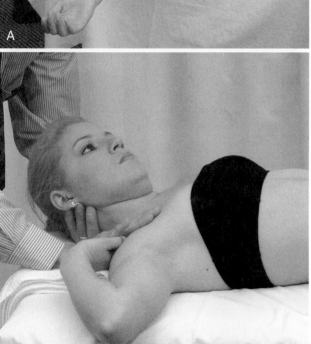

Figure 30-8 A, Neural tissue provocation test biased to the median nerve trunk (proximal to distal). **B,** Neural tissue provocation test biased to the radial nerve trunk (proximal to distal). **C,** Neural tissue provocation test biased to the ulnar nerve trunk (proximal to distal).

elsewhere,[124] and it has been interpreted as reflecting mechanosensitivity of regenerating axon sprouts, either freely growing or arrested in disseminated microneuromas. An alternative interpretation suggests that abnormal responses to mechanical provocation of neural tissue in radiculopathy arise from the nervi nervorum.[21] The spread of sensitization of the nervi nervorum has been attributed to neurogenic inflammation.[34] Activation of the nervi nervorum in response to nerve insult is likely to result in neuropeptide release leading to intraneural edema. This edema, particularly within the epineurium, is likely to spread longitudinally, because peripheral nerves and spinal nerve roots at the level of the intervertebral foramen have very poor lymphatic drainage.[125] The endoneurium and epineurium act as closed compartments[126] that become distorted by fluid pressure[127] and therefore cause further sensitization of the

nervi nervorum. The spread of inflammatory mediators within the edema along the course of the nerve may also sensitize the nervi nervorum.

Palpation of neural tissue must be undertaken with care. When sensitized, peripheral nerve trunks can be exquisitely tender to even very gentle palpation. In addition to assessing for pain, the clinician should be watching and palpating for associated reflex muscle responses or withdrawal reactions.[128]

Mild nonnoxious pressure, enough to blanch the nail bed of the palpating finger, should be applied to the nerve trunks on the uninvolved side first to allow the patient to make a comparison. In some instances, palpation can be made directly over the nerve trunk, which can be identified as a distinct structure. In other locations, nerve trunks must be palpated through muscle or they are so closely associated with vascular tissues

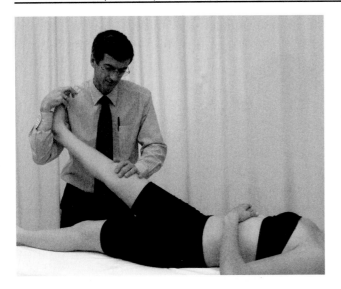

Figure 30-9 Straight-leg raise (SLR) with ankle dorsiflexion.

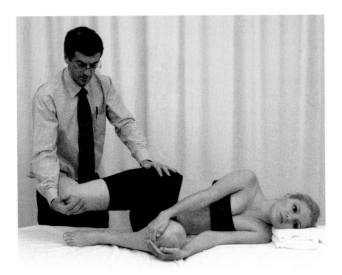

Figure 30-10 Femoral nerve provocation test in the side lying position.

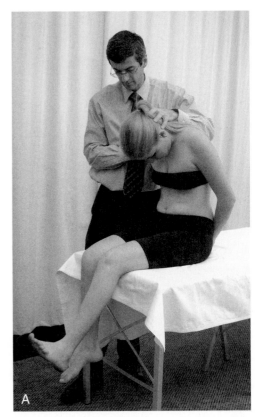

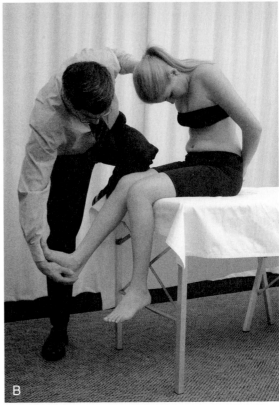

Figure 30-11 A, Slump test performed actively. **B,** Slump test performed passively.

that it is difficult to distinguish the nerve as a structure. When this is the case, broad-based pressure is applied in the area of the nerve trunk and the response is compared with that on the uninvolved side. Care must be taken when palpating nerve trunks directly overlying bone, because a distinct possibility exists of an iatrogenic compression neuropathy with overzealous pressure.

Although nerve palpation has not been investigated to a great degree, studies have shown that manual palpation is reliable in the upper limb[128] and lower limb.[129] Using an algometer to measure pressure pain threshold may increase the precision to which nerve mechanosensitivity can be determined and has been shown to demonstrate high reliability in the upper limb[130] and lower limb.[131]

Many nerves can be readily palpated, but in the clinical context of upper- and lower-quarter pain syndromes, the

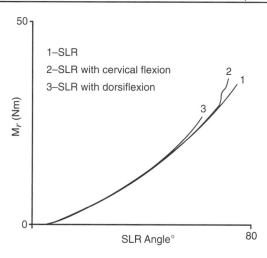

Figure 30-12 Moment of stretched tissue plotted against the straight-leg raise (SLR) angle during SLR, SLR with dorsiflexion, and SLR with cervical spine flexion. (From Hall T, Zusman M, Elvey R: Adverse mechanical tension in the nervous system? Analysis of straight leg raise, Man Ther 3(3):140-146, 1998.)

most relevant and commonly palpated nerves include the following:

• Ventral and dorsal rami as they exit from the gutters of the transverse processes of C4 to C6
• Upper and middle trunks of the brachial plexus
• Neurovascular bundle of the cords of the brachial plexus and axillary nerve underlying the tendon of the pectoralis minor
• Neurovascular bundle in the axilla incorporating the axillary artery and vein together with the median, radial, and ulnar nerves
• Median, radial, ulnar, axillary, suprascapular, and dorsal scapular nerves

Figure 30-13A demonstrates palpation of the upper and middle trunks of the brachial plexus, which lie posterior to the sternocleidomastoid and between the belly of the scalenus anterior and scalenus medius. Figures 30-13B and C demonstrates palpation of the median nerve in the upper arm and the neurovascular bundle in the axilla.

In the lower quarter, the following neural structures can be examined:

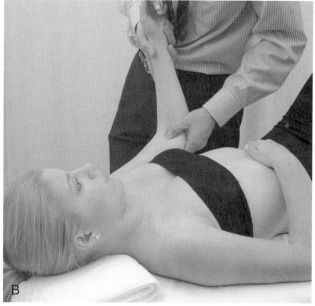

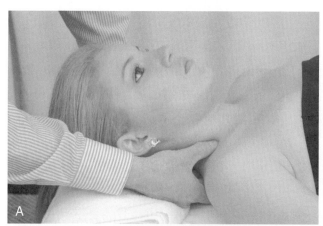

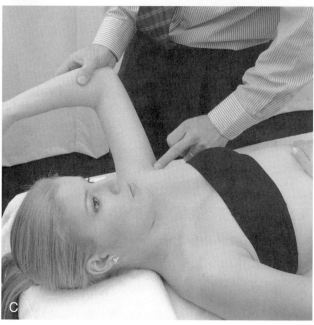

Figure 30-13 A, Palpation of the upper and middle trunk of the brachial plexus. **B,** Palpation of the median nerve in the upper arm. **C,** Palpation of the neurovascular bundle in the axilla.

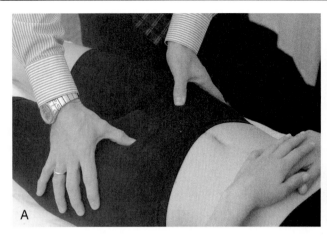

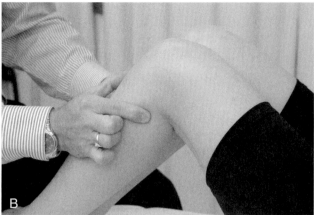

Figure 30-14 A, Palpation of the femoral nerve in the inguinal region. **B,** Palpation of the common fibular nerve at the neck of the fibula.

- Sciatic nerve in the gluteal region and posterior thigh
- Tibial, common fibular, and femoral nerves

Figure 30-14 demonstrate palpation of the femoral and common fibular nerves. To verify that a particular nerve trunk is sensitized, the clinician is advised to examine a number of different sites along the course of the nerve trunk. For example, the median nerve can be palpated within the neurovascular bundle in the axilla, as well as the upper arm (see Figures 30-13 *B* and *C*), medial to the biceps tendon in the cubital fossa, and immediately proximal to the carpal tunnel. If the median nerve trunk is sensitized, then a consistent pain response should exist throughout it, with greater pain provocation when the nerve is palpated closer to the site of pathologic condition. For example, if the median nerve were inflamed and subsequently sensitized in the carpal tunnel, then a stronger pain response would be expected when palpating the median nerve close to the wrist than when palpating the neurovascular bundle in the axilla.

EVIDENCE OF A LOCAL-AREA PATHOLOGIC CONDITION

The examination procedures presented so far have focused on identification of the presence or absence of peripheral nerve sensitization and denervation. Once this has been established, it is important to identify a local cause for the neuropathic state. On physical examination, many peripheral neuropathic pain disorders display all the features discussed. This does not mean that they are amenable to manual therapy treatment. It is quite possible for conditions, such as diabetic neuropathy or a neuropathy caused by tumor infiltration, to cause all of the features discussed so far, including limitation of active and passive movement.[73] Therefore the clinician must determine a cause for the neuropathic pain disorder. In other words, he or she must identify the underlying pathologic condition or the musculoskeletal site at which the nerve is being affected.

For example, in the upper quarter, an intervertebral disc pathologic condition will often result in radicular arm pain and can be traced to a specific cervical spine motion segment, which

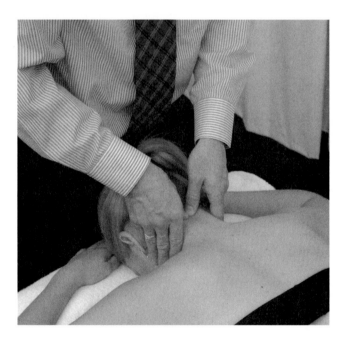

Figure 30-15 Manual examination to identify painful spinal segment.

is dysfunctional. Manual examination consists of pain provocation tests and passive segmental mobility tests to identify the dysfunctional motion segment. Abnormal findings are aberrant segmental mobility associated with pain (Figure 30-15). For example a patient with a C7 radiculopathy, would have many of the features previously discussed, together with a C6–7 motion segment dysfunction. This would suggest a spinal cause of the arm pain. Without the manual diagnostic findings, it may not be possible to determine such a cause, and further medical investigation would be necessary to exclude disorders such as Pancoast's tumor in the lung masquerading as a radiculopathy.

Neurologic Examination

An important aspect of the evaluation of neural tissue disorders is the assessment of neurologic function. In the clinical setting,

Table 30-3	Best Evidence for Use of Lumbar Dermatomal Maps

Level	Dermatome
L4	88% probability of L4 denervation if sensory hypoaesthesia in this region
L5	82% probability of L5 denervation if sensory hypoaesthesia in this region
S1	83% probability of S1 denervation if sensory hypoaesthesia in this region

the neurologic examination is the only means of determining the presence of axonal conduction loss. The neurologic examination incorporates both subjective inquiry and physical tests of nerve function.

The subjective examination must delineate the specific type and area of symptoms, including paresthesias and sensory loss. These areas can then be compared with typical dermatomal, sclerotomal, and myotomal maps. The clinician should not rely purely on dermatomal charts when determining the segmental origin of pain because they are not the ideal diagnostic reference[132] (because of significant overlap of innervation from adjacent nerve roots, in addition to there being much variability between individuals[133,134]). In this respect, myotomal and sclerotomal charts[135] are more helpful.[132]

In the lumbar spine, Nitta et al.[136] studied areas of sensory loss associated with lumbar radicular pain and was able to improve on the diagnostic accuracy for the three most commonly involved lumbosacral nerve root disorders, L4, L5, and S1 (see Table 30-3 for more details).

Physical neurologic examination procedures include tests for sensation, tendon reflexes, and muscle strength. Although a number of studies have investigated the reliability and diagnostic validity of the neurologic examination, its value is still not well established.[137-140] Interobserver reliability and agreement are best achieved by incorporating the subjective history together with the physical examination findings.[138,141] Reliability was shown to be good for muscle strength[141-144] and sensory loss[141] but controversial for reflex changes.[141,145,146] Wainner et al.[139] investigated the diagnostic accuracy of a range of cervical physical tests (e.g., range of motion, Spurling maneuver, muscle strength and reflexes) to identify cervical radiculopathy and reported that a cluster of physical examination tests were more useful for identifying cervical radiculopathy than any single test item.

Other tests of nerve function include electrodiagnostic tests such as EMG. These are invasive procedures that are more specific in the evaluation of motor or sensory conduction loss,[147] but they are not helpful if the problem is related to increased mechanosensitivity of the nerve trunk. Additionally, it is well established that only a modest correlation exists between strength deficits on physical examination and EMG results in radiculopathies, with weakness detected in some individuals with normal EMG findings and abnormal EMG results in cases with normal strength examinations.[144] Other diagnostic tests

such as magnetic resonance imaging (MRI), radiographic tests, and other radiologic investigations have, in the past, been largely unhelpful in visualizing pathologic peripheral neural tissue. In addition, these tests have been particularly unhelpful when the disorder is one of peripheral nerve sensitization rather than mechanical compression and conduction loss. Advances in MRI and ultrasound neurography have enabled the visualization of peripheral neural tissues, including nerve roots and peripheral nerve trunks.[148,149] These tests show promise for the future, but further studies are required to investigate the correlation between abnormal neurography and the findings from the clinical examination.

The examination protocol outlined enables the clinician to broadly classify patients with pain into one of four categories:[13]

1. Central sensitization—comprising major features of CNS sensitization (based on the LANSS scale[62])
2. Denervation—arising from significant axonal compromise, without evidence of CNS changes (based on the neurologic assessment)
3. Peripheral nerve sensitization—arising from nerve trunk inflammation without clinical evidence of significant denervation (based on NTPT and nerve palpation)
4. Musculoskeletal pain—referred from nonneural structures

Classification is based on dominant findings following an order of priority, with central sensitization first, denervation second, peripheral nerve sensitization third, and musculoskeletal pain last. This classification system has been shown to have good reliability,[150] as well as validity,[151] and it is predictive of response to treatment.[151]

Treatment

In this chapter a distinction is made between three types of peripheral neuropathic pain disorder: (1) central sensitization, (2) denervation, and (3) peripheral nerve sensitization. This distinction is important in regard to manual therapy treatment options, which are different for each classification. Central sensitization, as previously discussed, is a disorder categorized by abnormal processing of sensory information because of various CNS pathomechanisms. Patients classified with this disorder are unlikely to respond to manual therapy techniques such as neural mobilization. Rather, cognitive behavioral retraining (CBT) programs would be more appropriate management. The basis of CBT it to provide basic understanding of pain mechanisms in chronic, acute, and neuropathic pain; to relieve anxiety and fear; to teach appropriate pacing strategies; and to provide graded activity exposure.

For patients fulfilling the denervation classification, neural tissue mobilization techniques, particularly those that attempt to lengthen or stretch the nerve such as "tensioners,"[152] would be contraindicated at that time. This is particularly important in the acute or subacute stage of the disorder in which the nerve trunk is physiologically vulnerable to lengthening.

Normally, peripheral nerve trunks are protected from the effects of stretch and compression.[81] As the fasciculi are stretched, their cross-sectional area is reduced, the intrafascicular pressure is increased, nerve fibers are compressed, and the intrafascicular microcirculation is compromised.[153] Even slight pressure on the nerve can lead to external hyperemia, edema, and demyelination of some axons lasting for up to 28 days.[21] Elsewhere it has been observed that 8% elongation of a defined nerve segment may result in impaired venous flow. At elongation of approximately 10% to 15%, an upper stretch limit is reached in which complete arrest of all blood flow in the nerve exists.[154,155] Furthermore, severe conduction loss may occur at strains as low as 6%.[156]

In a neuropathic pain disorder, it is likely that nerve microcirculation is compromised and minimal nerve stretch may lead to further hypoxia and concomitant nerve damage. For these reasons, it is unwise to treat a damaged, compressed, or edematous nerve trunk with stretching or lengthening techniques. However, this does not prevent the clinician using other forms of manual therapy to treat patients classified as *denervation.* For example an acute cervical radiculopathy, with evidence of conduction loss, may be conservatively treated with a manual therapy regime that aims to increase the space surrounding the nerve in an attempt to "unload" it, to optimize the recovery over time.

The treatment of nerve trunk pain can involve the use of passive movement techniques, but the authors of this chapter believe that nerve "lengthening" or stretching techniques are contraindicated. Instead, the use of gentle, controlled oscillatory passive movements of the anatomic structures surrounding the affected neural tissues (close to or at the site of involvement) is advocated. At no time should pain be evoked. Treatment can be progressed by using passive movement techniques in a similar manner but involving movement of the surrounding anatomic tissues or structures and the affected neural tissues together in an oscillatory movement.[157]

Cervical Lateral Glide

A cervical lateral glide technique described by Elvey[157] is an example of a treatment approach that is not only clinically useful but also one of the few neural tissue mobilization techniques supported by evidence for its efficacy.[9,112,113,158,159] For a patient with C6 nerve root involvement, the arm on the affected side should be positioned in approximately 30 degrees of abduction, with the elbow flexed and the hand resting on the abdomen. The technique involves a gentle transverse glide of the C5-6 motion segment to the contralateral side in a slow, oscillating manner. The glide should be carried out for approximately 60 seconds and repeated five times, again depending on the sensitivity, the irritability, and nature of the disorder.

During the technique, the treating clinician will be aware of the onset of protective muscle activity that represents the limit in range of lateral glide, termed the *treatment barrier.*[73] The treatment barrier will be dependent on the sensitivity of the disorder. If the barrier is not reached, then the patient's arm is positioned in greater range of abduction or elbow extension (Figure 30-16). If the technique is too aggressive, then this usually results in an immediate or latent exacerbation of symptoms.

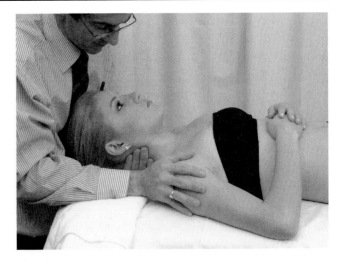

Figure 30-16 Cervical lateral glide technique.

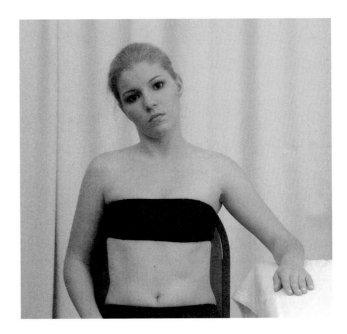

Figure 30-17 Home exercise upper quarter.

Progression of the technique on subsequent days is made by performing the technique with the shoulder in gradually increasing range of abduction. The purpose of the technique is to desensitize the overly sensitive peripheral neural system. At an early point in the management of the disorder, a home exercise program should be provided to compliment the neural mobilization technique. Home exercise should be introduced only when significant signs of improvement to the hands-on manual techniques exist. An example is shown in Figure 30-17. It is important that no pain occurs during this movement; the exercise should not stretch the neural tissues. Generally the patient is asked to carry out three sets of 10 repetitions of the home treatment exercise.

Evidence of the efficacy of this approach has been demonstrated in subjects with lateral elbow pain and cervicobrachial pain (see Table 30-4 for more details).

Table 30-4	Best Evidence for the Use of the Efficacy of the Lateral Cervical Glide for Elbow and Cervicobrachial Pain
Investigators	**Summary**
Allison et al.[158]	A single-blind randomized controlled trial investigating the efficacy of two different manual therapy interventions for chronic cervicobrachial pain (Neural mobilization, including the cervical lateral glide, was more effective than joint mobilization. Both regimes were better than a control in improving pain intensity, pain quality scores, and functional disability levels immediately after treatment and at 8 weeks follow-up.)
Coppieters et al.[112]	A randomized controlled trial investigating the immediate effects of the cervical lateral glide versus ultrasound for subacute cervicobrachial pain (For the neural mobilization group, significant improvements were noted in pain measures and range of motion but no change for the ultrasound intervention.)
Coppieters et al.[113]	A randomized controlled trial investigating the immediate effects of the cervical lateral glide on pain and protective responses during Neural Tissue Provocation Test (NTPT) in subjects with chronic cervicobrachial pain (Significant improvement was noted in the active intervention only.)
Cowell et al.[160]	A single case study with ABC design, investigating the cervical lateral glide for a patient with chronic cervicobrachial pain (Significant improvement in pain, functional capacity and range of motion was maintained at 1-month follow-up.)
Hall et al.[9]	A case control study investigating chronic cervicobrachial pain (Significant improvements were found in pain, functional capacity, and mobility after a 4-week treatment period. Improvement was maintained at 3-month follow-up.)
Saranga et al.[161]	A single-blind placebo-controlled trial investigating the effect of cervical lateral glide on range of motion during a median nerve NTPT in asymptomatic subjects (Significant immediate improvements were noted in range of motion in the active intervention group compared with the placebo and control group.)
Vicenzino et al.[159]	A randomized, double-blind, placebo-controlled trial investigating the immediate effects of the cervical lateral glide for lateral epicondylalgia (Significant improvement was noted in pressure-pain threshold, pain-free grip strength, and NTPT range of motion and pain.)

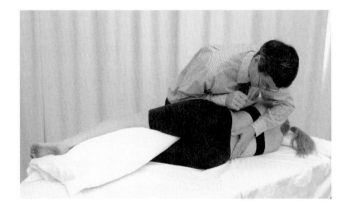

Figure 30-18 Right lateral flexion at L5-S1 for left leg pain.

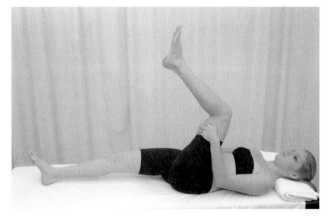

Figure 30-19 Home exercise: Lower quarter.

In the lower quarter, a similar approach can be used. A lateral glide is not possible; instead, a modified lateral flexion maneuver has been found to be clinically effective (Figure 30-18). The example seen in Figure 30-18 is for the treatment of a left L5 nerve root involvement. The symptomatic leg is positioned in approximately 50 degrees of hip flexion, with the knee flexed to at least 30 degrees of flexion. The leg is supported to prevent adduction, medial rotation, and further provocation of the neural tissue. The range of hip and knee flexion is dependent on the severity and irritability of the disorder. The motion segment to be mobilized is positioned in flexion. The clinician localizes the movement to the L5–S1 segment by transverse pressure to the right via the L5 spinous

process, with an attempt to restrict movement above this level. The clinician applies gentle force through the pelvis to create lumbar spine contralateral lateral flexion in a slow, oscillating manner.

As with the cervical lateral glide, the treating clinician will be aware of the onset of protective muscle activity that represents the treatment barrier while using this technique. If this barrier is not reached, then the patient's uppermost leg is positioned in a greater range of hip flexion and thereby greater neural tissue provocation.

The treatment is progressed on subsequent days by performing the technique with progressively greater range hip flexion. An additional, slider technique[152] involving movement of the entire course of the nerve in relation to its interface (but without increasing tension) can also be used. In the side-lying position, hip flexion is performed through range with concomitant knee flexion, starting from a position just short of provocation of back or limb symptoms. At no time should the patient's symptoms or any paresthesias be evoked.

The patient can perform a similar slider technique as a home exercise (Figure 30-19). The knee is flexed while the hip is flexed and vice versa, to prevent stretching of the neural elements. Again, the patient must understand that the exercise should not cause pain or paresthesias.

Sliding techniques are a logical, safe form of mobilization of the nervous system because they do not stress the nerve by increasing tension and reducing nerve vascularity.[4,110] However, to date only minimal evidence supports their use.[162]

CASE STUDIES

CASE STUDY 1

History

A 36-year-old female subject had pain as per the body chart (Figure 30-20). The problem evolved 18 months previously after a particularly vigorous 3-hour dinghy sailing session. No specific incident occurred, but midthoracic, shoulder, and arm pain developed gradually during the evening after sailing and worsened over subsequent days. The patient sought advice from her medical practitioner, who prescribed nonsteroidal antiinflammatory drugs (NSAIDs), rest, and a shoulder radiograph, which was normal. Feeling no improvement over the next 2 weeks, she sought treatment from an osteopath, who manipulated her neck and back, which relieved the thoracic pain. Subsequent treatment gave no relief from the shoulder or arm pain. Since this time, the patient has "learned to live with it." The disorder did not progress, but it worsened temporarily if she tried to perform any physical activity such as sailing. Subsequent investigations by the medical practitioner revealed no abnormality on cervical spine radiograph or ultrasound imaging of the shoulder. No evidence suggested dominance of positive features; therefore the patient's condition could not be classified as *neuropathic pain with central sensitization*.

Physical Evaluation

At the initial evaluation, active right shoulder function was recorded as 70 degrees of abduction, 30 degrees of external rotation, and 120 degrees of flexion. A poor pattern of scapulohumeral rhythm was noted for both flexion and abduction, with excessive scapula movement. Active cervical mobility was restricted in left lateral flexion compared with lateral flexion to the right. Of further interest was the fact that active shoulder mobility was more painful and more restricted in range when the head and neck were positioned in left lateral flexion and when the right wrist was extended.

Neural tissue provocation tests were carried out from central to peripheral and vice versa for the median, radial, and ulnar nerve trunks. With the arm positioned in 60 degrees of abduction and the cervical spine in contralateral lateral flexion, wrist and finger extension reproduced the arm pain. Cervical left lateral flexion with the arm positioned in 60 degrees of abduction and shoulder girdle depression reproduced the arm and shoulder pain. Provocative maneuvers of the ulnar nerve were not symptomatic. Mild pressure over the median, radial, axillary, and suprascapular nerve trunks of the right upper quarter, as well as over the upper trunk of the brachial plexus and the neurovascular bundle in the axilla, produced painful responses that were not present on the left side.

Manual diagnosis revealed dysfunction at C5 and C6, and no evidence was seen of a neurologic deficit.

The physical findings correlated accurately with the subjective complaint and supported a diagnosis of cervicobrachial pain syndrome, in which there was strong evidence to classify the disorder as *peripheral nerve sensitization*. Although there were signs of glenohumeral joint dysfunction, these were minor in relation to the neural problem originating at the C6 nerve root.

Diagnostic classification: Neuromuscular 5F: Cervical Nerve Root Disorder (353.0)

Treatment

As there were no signs of denervation and central sensitization was not overriding, treatment commenced with a gentle, controlled oscillation of left lateral glide of C5 on C6. The right arm was positioned in 20 degrees of abduction, with the elbow flexed to 90 degrees and the hand resting on the abdomen. Treatment was initially carried out three times per week. The patient was asked to refrain from any activity involving shoulder abduction or shoulder girdle depression. In the authors' experience, a significant part of treatment is the advice that is given to the patient about initially avoiding activities that provoke symptoms.

Subjective improvement occurred within the first few treatments; concomitant improvement occurred in active and passive shoulder mobility. After 2 weeks of treatment, active shoulder abduction was 120 degrees and flexion was 160 degrees. Cervical lateral glide was continued with the arm in a progressively greater range of abduction but with the elbow maintained at 90 degrees of flexion. A home exercise program was also introduced that involved sitting sideways at a table with the right arm supported on a pillow

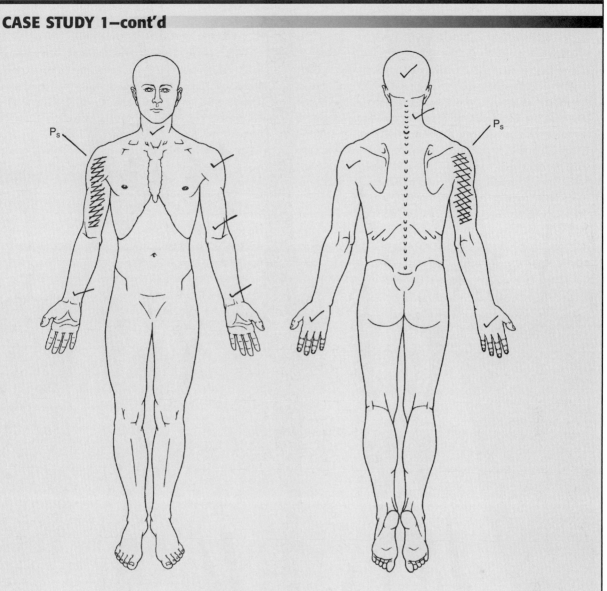

Figure 30-20 Body chart Case Study 1.

to achieve 30 degrees of abduction. Active cervical left lateral flexion was performed without pain. Progression of this exercise was made by positioning the shoulder in greater range of abduction.

After 4 weeks of treatment, manual therapy techniques directed at restoring normal mobility of the glenohumeral joint were added to the previous treatment. At the completion of the management program, the patient had regained 90% of her shoulder mobility and was able to undertake daily tasks without discomfort.

This case is an example of the situation in which treatment is initially directed at the sensitized neural tissue as the primary source of symptoms, but it was also necessary to address the dysfunctional glenohumeral joint as a secondary contributing factor. In the authors' experience, if the treatment approach had been reversed and the glenohumeral joint treated first, then the outcome would have been poor.

CASE STUDY 2

History

A 43-year-old male subject had pain as per the body chart (Figure 30-21). The problem developed 3 months before assessment as a result of unloading a pallet stacked with boxes of photocopy paper. The patient was aware of pain in the low back that gradually worsened overnight and spread to his left leg. The patient saw the company doctor, who sent him home with muscle relaxants, painkillers, and NSAIDs. The doctor subsequently ordered a lumbar radiograph and a computed tomography (CT) scan. According to the radiologist's report, the CT scans revealed evidence of an L4-5 broad based posterior disc bulge, which did not impinge on the thecal sac; no evidence of nerve root compromise was seen. The patient had a history of previous low-back pain associated with lifting injuries at work; however, no history of leg pain was reported. The previous low-back episode occurred 3 years previously, at which time a CT scan revealed the same findings. No change in the radiologic findings was seen between the two scans, and no other abnormality was detected apart from a mild scoliosis. The patient had attempted to return to work with light duties, working in the company office, but this had been unsuccessful.

As a result of the work trial, the patient was referred to a pain specialist, who requested physiotherapy management.

Physical Evaluation

At the initial examination, the patient had an antalgic posture, the left hip and knee were flexed, and the left iliac crest was elevated with respect to the right. The lumbar spine was laterally flexed to the left. Correction of the deformity increased the leg pain.

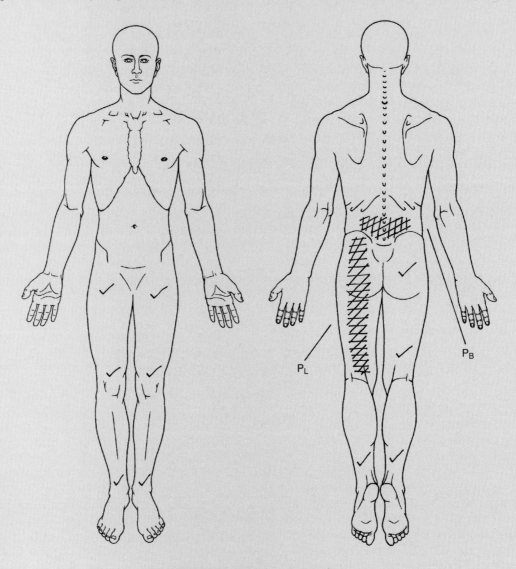

Figure 30-21 Body chart Case Study 2.

CASE STUDY 2–cont'd

Active lumbar mobility was recorded as flexion—fingertips to the knee joint line limited by left leg pain; side flexion to the right fingertips 6 cm above the knee joint line limited by back pain; side flexion to the left and extension both symptom free. Of further interest was the fact that active lumbar flexion and right lateral flexion were more painful and more restricted in range when the left ankle was positioned in dorsiflexion and the cervical spine flexed.

Neural tissue provocation tests were carried out for the sciatic and femoral nerve trunks. SLR was limited to 40 degrees and reproduced the leg pain, which was made worse when the ankle was dorsiflexed. SLR was limited to 80 degrees, without pain on the right side. Provocative maneuvers to the femoral nerve trunks did not produce symptoms. Left knee extension with the left hip in 90 degrees of flexion, tested in the right side-lying position, was more painful and restricted in range when the L5-S1 segment was positioned in extension compared with flexion.

Mild pressure over the sciatic and common peroneal (fibular) nerve trunks of the lower quarter produced painful responses that were not present on the right side. No responses to pressure were seen over the femoral nerve trunk or the tibial nerve on either side.

Manual diagnosis revealed dysfunction at the L4-5 and L5-S1 levels. Sacroiliac joint stress tests produced no symptoms, and no evidence of a neurologic deficit was seen.

Diagnostic classification: Neuromuscular 5F: Lumbar Nerve Root Disorder (353.1)

Treatment

Treatment commenced with a gentle oscillation of right lateral flexion at L4-5 with the left leg positioned in 50 degrees of hip and knee flexion. Treatment was initially carried out three times per week. The patient was advised to avoid provocative movements to the lower-limb neural tissues.

Subjective improvement occurred gradually over 3 weeks. Significant improvement occurred in active and passive lumbar and hip mobility. After 3 weeks of treatment, active lumbar flexion was to midshin and SLR was 70 degrees. Localized L4-5 lateral flexion was continued with the leg positioned in a progressively greater range of hip flexion and with the knee flexed to 30 degrees.

A home exercise program was also introduced, which involved sitting sideways at a low table with the left leg supported on the table and with the left knee flexed to 30 degrees. Active lumbar right lateral flexion was performed without pain. A further addition to treatment was a slider technique involving passive left hip flexion combined with left knee flexion. The endpoint of hip flexion was always short of symptom reproduction.

After 4 weeks the patient returned to light duties in an office environment. After 6 weeks he was introduced to a gradual work hardening program based in a gym. After a period of reconditioning, the patient returned to his original duties.

SUMMARY

In this chapter a distinction is made between three categories of neuropathic pain disorders based on underlying mechanisms: (1) central sensitization, (2) denervation, and (3) peripheral nerve sensitization. Although it is not possible as yet to diagnose pain mechanisms by clinical evaluation, a comprehensive examination protocol consisting of screening for central sensitization, a neurologic examination, and assessment of nerve tissue mechanosensitization enables the clinician to appropriately classify the neuropathic disorder. Examples of appropriate treatment options for each classification are outlined here.

REFERENCES

1. Hall TM, Elvey RL: Management of mechanosensitivity of the nervous system in spinal pain syndromes. In Boyling G, Jull G, editors: Grieve's modern manual therapy, Edinburgh, 2004, Churchill Livingstone, pp 413-431.
2. Bogduk N, Twomey LT: Clinical anatomy of the lumbar spine, ed 2, Melbourne, 1991, Churchill Livingstone, pp 197.
3. Drye C, Zachazewski J, editors: Peripheral nerve injuries. In Zachazewski J, Magee D, Quillen W, editors: Athletic injuries and rehabilitation, Philadelphia, 1996, WB Saunders.
4. Coppieters MW, Alshami AM: Longitudinal excursion and strain in the median nerve during novel nerve gliding exercises for carpal tunnel syndrome, J Orthop Res 25(7):972-980, 2007.
5. Greening J, Dilley A, Lynn B: In vivo study of nerve movement and mechanosensitivity of the median nerve in whiplash and non-specific arm pain patients, Pain 115(3):248-253, 2005.
6. Sterling M, Jull G, Vicenzino B, et al: Sensory hypersensitivity occurs soon after whiplash injury and is associated with poor recovery, Pain 104(3):509-517, 2003.
7. Sterling M, Treleaven J, Jull G: Responses to a clinical test of mechanical provocation of nerve tissue in whiplash-associated disorder, Man Ther 7(2):89-94, 2002.
8. Yaxley G, Jull G: A modified upper limb tension test: an investigation of responses in normal subjects, Aust J Physiother 37:143-152, 1991.
9. Hall T, Elvey R, Davies N, et al: Efficacy of manipulative physiotherapy for the treatment of cervicobrachial pain. In Proceedings of the Tenth Biennial Conference of the Manipulative Physiotherapists Association of Australia, Melbourne, 1997.

10. Butler DS: Adverse mechanical tension in the nervous system: a model for assessment and treatment, Aust J Physiother 35(4):227-238, 1989.

11. Elvey R: Brachial plexus tension tests and the pathoanatomical origin of arm pain. In Idczak R, editor: Aspects of manipulative therapy, Melbourne, 1979, Lincoln Institute of Health Sciences, pp 105-110.

12. Greening J, Lynn B: Minor peripheral nerve injuries: an underestimated source of pain, Man Ther 3(4):187-194, 1998.

13. Schafer A, Hall TM, Briffa K: Classification of low back related leg pain—a proposed pathomechanism based approach, Man Ther 14(2):222-230, 2008.

14. Zusman M: Forebrain-mediated sensitization of central pain pathways: 'non-specific' pain and a new image for MT, Man Ther 7(2):80-88, 2002.

15. Backonja MM: Defining neuropathic pain, Anesth Analg 97(3):785-790, 2003.

16. Bennett GJ: Can we distinguish between inflammatory and neuropathic pain? Pain Res Manag 11(suppl A):11A-15A, 2006.

17. Omoigui S: The biochemical origin of pain: the origin of all pain is inflammation and the inflammatory response. II. Inflammatory profile of pain syndromes, Med Hypotheses 69(6):1169-1178, 2007.

18. Elliott KJ: Taxonomy and mechanisms of neuropathic pain, Semin Neurol 14(3):195-205, 1994.

19. Bove GM, Ransil BJ, Lin HC, et al: Inflammation induces ectopic mechanical sensitivity in axons of nociceptors innervating deep tissues, J Neurophysiol 90(3):1949-1955, 2003.

20. Dilley A, Lynn B, Pang SJ: Pressure and stretch mechanosensitivity of peripheral nerve fibbers following local inflammation of the nerve trunk, Pain 117(3):462-472, 2005.

21. Bove G, Light A: The nervi nervorum: missing link for neuropathic pain? *Pain* forum 6(3):181-190, 1997.

22. Hromada J: On the nerve supply of the connective tissue of some peripheral nervous system components, Acta Anat (Basel) 55:343-351, 1963.

23. Zochodne D: Epineural peptides: a role in neuropathic pain, Can J Neurol Sci 20:69-72, 1993.

24. Fukui S, Ohseto K, Shiotani M, et al: Distribution of referred pain from the lumbar zygapophyseal joints and dorsal rami, Clin J Pain 13(4):303-307, 1997.

25. Mooney V, Robertson J: The facet syndrome, Clin Orthop Relat Res 115:149-156, 1976.

26. O'Neill CW, Kurgansky ME, Derby R, et al: Disc stimulation and patterns of referred pain, Spine 27(24):2776-2781, 2002.

27. Devor M: Neuropathic pain and injured nerve: peripheral mechanisms, Br Med Bull 47(3):619-630, 1991.

28. Asbury AK, Fields HL: Pain due to peripheral nerve damage: an hypothesis, Neurology 34:1587-1590, 1984.

29. Fields HL: Pain, New York, 1987, McGraw Hill, pp 133-169.

30. Thomas PK, Berthold C-H, Ochoa J: Microscopic anatomy of the peripheral nervous system. In Dyck PJ, Thomas PK, editors: Peripheral neuropathy, Philadelphia, 1993, WB Saunders, pp 28-91.

31. Bove G, Light A: Unmyelinated nociceptors of rat paraspinal tissues, J Neurophysiol 73:1752-1762, 1995.

32. Hall T, Quintner J: Responses to mechanical stimulation of the upper limb in painful cervical radiculopathy, Aust J Physiother 42(4):277-285, 1996.

33. Kuslich SD, Ulstrom CL, Cami JM: The tissue origin of low back pain and sciatica: a report of pain responses to tissue stimulation during operations on the lumbar spine using local anesthesia, Orthop Clin North Am 22(2):181-187, 1991.

34. Quintner J: Peripheral neuropathic pain: a rediscovered clinical entity. In Proceedings of the Annual General Meeting of the Australian Pain Society, Hobart, Australia, 1998.

35. Devor M: The pathophysiology of damaged peripheral nerves. In Wall P, Melzack R, editors: Textbook of pain, Edinburgh, 1989, Churchill Livingstone, pp 63-81.

36. Woolf CJ: Generation of acute pain: central mechanisms, Br Med Bull 47:523-533, 1991.

37. Eliav E, Herzberg U, Ruda MA, et al: Neuropathic pain from an experimental neuritis of the rat sciatic nerve, Pain 83(2):169-182, 1999.

38. Devor M, Seltzer Z: Pathophysiology of damaged peripheral nerves in relation to chronic pain. In Wall P, Melzack R, editors: Textbook of pain, Edinburgh, 1989, Churchill Livingstone, pp 129-164.

39. Campbell JN, Meyer RA: Mechanisms of neuropathic pain, Neuron 52(1):77-92, 2006.

40. Costigan M, Woolf CJ: Pain: molecular mechanisms, J Pain 1(suppl 3):35-44, 2000.

41. Nee R, Butler DS: Management of peripheral neuropathic pain: integrating neurobiology, neurodynamics, and clinical evidence, Phys Ther Sport 7:36-49, 2006.

42. Di Fabio R: Neural mobilization: the impossible, J Orthop Sports Phys Ther 31(5):224-225, 2001.

43. Epstein JA, Epstein BS, Levine LS, et al: Lumbar nerve root compression at the intervertebral foramina caused by arthritis of the posterior facet, J Neurosurg 39:362-369, 1973.

44. Kjaer P, Leboeuf-Yde C, Korsholm L, et al: Magnetic resonance imaging and low back pain in adults: a diagnostic imaging study of 40-year-old men and women, Spine 30(10):1173-1180, 2005.

45. Macnab I: The mechanism of spondylogenic pain. In Hirsch C, Zotterman Y, editors: Cervical pain, New York, 1972, Pergamon Press, pp 89-95.

46. Rydevik B, Garfin SR: Spinal nerve root compression. In Szabo RM, editor: Nerve compression syndromes: diagnosis and treatment, New York, 1989, Slack.

47. Wiesel SW, Tsourmas N, Feffer HL, et al: A study of computer-assisted tomography. I. The incidence of positive CAT scans in an asymptomatic group of patients, Spine 9:549-551, 1984.

48. Amundsen T, Weber H, Lilleas F, et al: Lumbar spinal stenosis: clinical and radiologic features, Spine 20(10):1178-1186, 1995.

49. Takahashi K, Kagechika K, Takino T, et al: Changes in epidural pressure during walking in patients with lumbar spinal stenosis, Spine 20(24):2746-2749, 1995.

50. Boos N, Weissbach S, Rohrbach H, et al: Classification of age-related changes in lumbar intervertebral discs: 2002 Volvo Award in basic science, Spine 27(23):2631-2644, 2002.

51. Ohnmeiss DD, Vanharanta H, Ekholm J: Degree of disc disruption and lower extremity pain, Spine 22(14):1600-1605, 1997.

52. Brisby H: Nerve root injuries in patients with chronic low back pain, Orthop Clin North Am 34(2):221-230, 2003.

53. Olmarker K, Brisby H, Yabuki S, et al: The effects of normal, frozen, and hyaluronidase-digested nucleus pulposus on nerve root structure and function, Spine 22(5):471-476; discussion 476, 1997.

54. Olmarker K, Rydevik B: Pathophysiology of sciatica, Orthop Clin North Am 22(2):223-234, 1991.

55. Woolf CJ: Dissecting out mechanisms responsible for peripheral neuropathic pain: implications for diagnosis and therapy, Life Sci 74(21):2605-2610, 2004.

56. Decosterd I, Allchorne A, Woolf CJ: Progressive tactile hypersensitivity after a peripheral nerve crush: non-noxious mechanical stimulus-induced neuropathic pain, Pain 100(1-2):155-162, 2002.

57. Dalton PA, Jull GA: The distribution and characteristics of neck-arm pain in patients with and without a neurological deficit, Aust J Physiother 35:3-8, 1989.

58. Rankine J, Fortune D, Hutchinson C et al: Pain drawings in the assessment of nerve root compression: a comparative study with lumbar spine magnetic resonance imaging, Spine 23(15):1668-1676, 1998.

59. Henderson CM, Hennessy R, Shuey H: Posterior lateral foraminotomy for an exclusive operative technique for cervical radiculopathy: a review of 846 consecutively operated cases, J Neurosurg 13:504-512, 1983.

60. Galer BS, Jensen MP: Development and preliminary validation of a pain measure specific to neuropathic pain: the Neuropathic Pain Scale, Neurology 48(2):332-338, 1997.

61. Bouhassira D, Attal N, Alchaar H, et al: Comparison of pain syndromes associated with nervous or somatic lesions and development of a new neuropathic pain diagnostic questionnaire (DN4), Pain 114(1-2):29-36, 2005.

62. Bennett M: The LANSS Pain Scale: the Leeds Assessment of Neuropathic Symptoms and Signs, Pain 92(1-2):147-157, 2001.

63. Freynhagen R, Baron R, Gockel U, et al: painDETECT: a new screening questionnaire to identify neuropathic components in patients with back pain, Curr Med Res Opin 22(10):1911-1920, 2006.

64. Portenoy R: Development and testing of a neuropathic pain screening questionnaire: ID Pain, Curr Med Res Opin 22(8):1555-1565, 2006.

65. Krause SJ, Backonja MM: Development of a Neuropathic Pain Questionnaire, Clin J Pain 19(5):306-314, 2003.

66. Kaki AM, El-Yaski AZ, Youseif E: Identifying neuropathic pain among patients with chronic low-back pain: use of the Leeds Assessment of Neuropathic Symptoms and Signs pain scale, Reg Anesth Pain Med 30(5):422-428, 2005.

67. Potter J, Higginson IJ, Scadding JW, et al: Identifying neuropathic pain in patients with head and neck cancer: use of the Leeds Assessment of Neuropathic Symptoms and Signs Scale, J R Soc Med 96(8):379-383, 2003.

68. Yucel A, Senocak M, Kocasoy Orhan E, et al: Results of the Leeds Assessment of Neuropathic Symptoms and Signs pain scale in Turkey: a validation study, J Pain 5(8):427-432, 2004.

69. Attal N, Bouhassira D: Can pain be more or less neuropathic? Pain 110(3):510-511, 2004.

70. Bennett MI, Smith BH, Torrance N, et al: Can pain can be more or less neuropathic? Comparison of symptom assessment tools with ratings of certainty by clinicians, Pain 122(3):289-294, 2006.

71. Kleynhans AM, Terrett AGJ: The prevention of complications from spinal manipulative therapy. In Glasgow EF, Twomey LT, editors: Aspects of manipulative therapy, Melbourne, 1986, Churchill Livingstone, pp 171-174.

72. Fahlgren Grampo J, Reynolds HM, Vorro J, et al: 3-D motion of the pelvis during passive leg lifting. In Anderson PA, Hobart DJ, Danoff JV, editors: Electromyographical kinesiology, St Louis, 1991, Elsevier Science Publishers, pp 119-122.

73. Elvey R, Hall T: Neural tissue evaluation and treatment. In Donatelli R, editor: Physical therapy of the shoulder, New York, 1997, Churchill Livingstone, pp 131-152.

74. Breig A: Adverse mechanical tension in the central nervous system: relief by functional neurosurgery, Stockholm, 1978, Almquist & Wiksell.

75. Goddard MD, Reid JD: Movements induced by straight leg raising in the lumbo-sacral roots, nerves and plexus and in the intrapelvic section of the sciatic nerve, J Neurol Neurosurg Psychiatry 28:12-18, 1965.

76. McLellan D, Swash M: Longitudinal sliding of the median nerve during movements of the upper limb, J Neurol Neurosurg Psychiatry 39:566-570, 1976.

77. Louis R: Vertebroradicular and vertebromedullar dynamics, Anat Clin 3:1-11, 1981.

78. Troup JDG: Straight-leg-raising (SLR) and the qualifying tests for increased root tension: their predictive value after back and sciatic pain, Spine 6(5):526-527, 1981.

79. Balster S, Jull G: Upper trapezius muscle activity during the brachial plexus tension test in asymptomatic subjects, Man Ther 2(3):144-149, 1997.

80. Hall T, Zusman M, Elvey R: Manually detected impediments during the straight leg raise test. In Proceedings

of the Manipulative Physiotherapists Association of Australia, Ninth Biennial Conference, Queensland, Australia, 1995.

81. Hall T, Zusman M, Elvey R: Adverse mechanical tension in the nervous system? Analysis of straight leg raise, Man Ther 3(3):140-146, 1998.

82. Hu JW, Vernon H, Tatourian I: Changes in neck electromyography associated with meningeal noxious stimulation, J Manipulative Physiol Ther 18(9):577-581, 1995.

83. Hu JW, Yu XM, Vernon H, et al: Excitatory effects on neck and jaw muscle activity of inflammatory irritant applied to cervical paraspinal tissues, Pain 55(2):243-250, 1993.

84. Jaberzadeh S, Scutter S, Nazeran H: Mechanosensitivity of the median nerve and mechanically produced motor responses during upper limb neurodynamic test 1, Physiotherapy 91:94-100, 2005.

85. Elvey RL: Nerve tension signs. In Proceedings of the Fifth International Conference of the International Federation of Manipulative Therapists, Vail, Colo, 1992.

86. Troup JDG: Biomechanics of the lumbar spinal canal, Clin Biomech (Bristol, Avon) 1:31, 1986.

87. Laird JMA, Bennett GJ: An electrophysiological study of dorsal horn neurons in the spinal cord of rats with an experimental peripheral neuropathy, J Neurophysiol 69(6):2072-2085, 1993.

88. Muhle C, Resnick D, Ahn JM, et al: In vivo changes in the neuroforaminal size at flexion-extension and axial rotation of the cervical spine in healthy persons examined using kinematic magnetic resonance imaging, Spine 26(13):E287-E293, 2001.

89. Yoo JU, Zou D, Edwards WT, et al: Effect of cervical spine motion on the neuroforaminal dimensions of human cervical spine, Spine 17(10):1131-1136, 1992.

90. Sandmark H, Nisell R: Validity of five common manual neck pain provoking tests, Scand J Rehabil Med 27(3):131-136, 1995.

91. Coppieters MW, Stappaerts KH, Everaert DG, et al: Addition of test components during neurodynamic testing: effect on range of motion and sensory responses, J Orthop Sports Phys Ther 31(5):226-235; discussion 236-227, 2001.

92. Ginn K: An investigation of tension development in upper limb soft tissues during the upper limb tension test. In Proceedings of the International Federation of Orthopaedic Manipulative Therapists Conference, Cambridge, UK, 1988.

93. Wilgis EF, Murphy R: The significance of longitudinal excursion in peripheral nerves, Hand Clin 2(4):761-766, 1986.

94. Wright TW, Glowczewskie F, Wheeler D, et al: Excursion and strain of the median nerve, J Bone Joint Surg Am 78(12):1897-1903, 1996.

95. Kleinrensink GJ, Stoeckart R, Vleeming A, et al: Mechanical tension in the median nerve. The effects of joint positions, Clin Biomech (Bristol, Avon) 10(5):240-244, 1995.

96. Lewis J, Ramot R, Green A: Changes in mechanical tension in the median nerve: possible implications for the upper limb tension test, Physiotherapy 84(6):254-261, 1998.

97. Kleinrensink GJ, Stoeckart R, Mulder PG, et al: Upper limb tension tests as tools in the diagnosis of nerve and plexus lesions: anatomical and biomechanical aspects, Clin Biomech (Bristol, Avon) 15(1):9-14, 2000.

98. van der Heide B, Allison GT, Zusman M: Pain and muscular responses to a neural tissue provocation test in the upper limb, Man Ther 6(3):154-162, 2001.

99. Breig A, Troup JDG: Biomechanical considerations of the straight-leg-raising test, Spine 4(3):242-250, 1979.

100. Coppieters MW, Alshami AM, Babri AS et al: Strain and excursion of the sciatic, tibial, and plantar nerves during a modified straight leg-raising test, J Orthop Res 24(9):1883-1889, 2006.

101. Lew PC, Morrow CJ, Lew AM: The effect of neck and leg flexion and their sequence on the lumbar spinal cord: implications in low back pain and sciatica, Spine 19(21):2421-2425, 1994.

102. O'Connell JEA: Protrusions of the lumbar intervertebral disc, J Bone Joint Surg 33B(1):8-17, 1951.

103. Sugiura K, Yoshida T, Katoh S et al: A study on tension signs in lumbar disc hernia, Int Orthop 3:225-228, 1979.

104. Jull GA, Bullock M: A motion profile of the lumbar spine in an ageing population assessed by manual examination, Physiother Theory Pract 3:70-81, 1987.

105. Maitland GD: Peripheral manipulation, ed 3, London, 1991, Butterworth-Heinemann.

106. Yuan Q, Dougherty L, Margulies S: In vivo human cervical spinal cord deformation and displacement in flexion, Spine 23(15):1677-1683, 1998.

107. Elvey RL: Brachial plexus tension tests and the pathoanatomical origin of arm pain. In Glasgow EF et al, editors: Aspects of manipulative therapy, Melbourne, 1985, Churchill Livingstone, pp 116-122.

108. Butler DS: Mobilization of the nervous system, Melbourne, 1991, Churchill Livingstone, pp 161-181.

109. Coppieters MW, Alshami AM, Hodges PW: An experimental pain model to investigate the specificity of the neurodynamic test for the median nerve in the differential diagnosis of hand symptoms, Arch Phys Med Rehabil 87(10):1412-1417, 2006.

110. Coppieters MW, Butler DS: Do 'sliders' slide and 'tensioners' tension? An analysis of neurodynamic techniques and considerations regarding their application, Man Ther 2008, 13(3):213-221.

111. Coppieters MW, Kurz K, Mortensen TE, et al: The impact of neurodynamic testing on the perception of experimentally induced muscle pain, Man Ther 10(1):52-60, 2005.

112. Coppieters MW, Stappaerts KH, Wouters LL, et al: The immediate effects of a cervical lateral glide treatment technique in patients with neurogenic cervicobrachial pain, J Orthop Sports Phys Ther 33(7):369-378, 2003.

113. Coppieters MW, Stappaerts KH, Wouters LL, et al: Aberrant protective force generation during neural provocation testing and the effect of treatment in patients with neurogenic cervicobrachial pain, J Manipulative Physiol Ther 26(2):99-106, 2003.

114. Dilley A, Odeyinde S, Greening J, et al: Longitudinal sliding of the median nerve in patients with non-specific arm pain, Man Ther 13(6):543-546, 2008.

115. Wainner RS, Fritz JM, Irrgang JJ, et al: Development of a clinical prediction rule for the diagnosis of carpal tunnel syndrome, Arch Phys Med Rehabil 86(4):609-618, 2005.

116. Hall TM, Elvey RL: Nerve trunk pain: physical diagnosis and treatment, Man Ther 4(2):63-73, 1999.

117. Maitland G: The slump test: examination and treatment, Aust J Physiother 31(6):215-219, 1985.

118. Shacklock M: Clinical neurodynamics, Edinburgh, 2005, Elsevier.

119. Butler DS, Coppieters MW: Neurodynamics in a broader perspective, Man Ther 12(1):e7-e8, 2007.

120. Hall TM, Hepburn M, Elvey RL: The effect of lumbosacral postures on the modified SLR test, Physiotherapy 79(8):566-570, 1993.

121. Howe JF, Loeser JD, Calvin WH: Mechanosensitivity of dorsal root ganglia and chronically injured axons: a physiological basis for the radicular pain of nerve root compression, Pain 3:25-41, 1977.

122. Smyth MJ, Wright V: Sciatica and the intervertebral disc: an experimental study, J Bone Joint Surg 40A:1401-1418, 1958.

123. Dyck P, editor: Sciatic pain. In Watkins R, Collis J, editors: Lumbar discectomy and laminectomy, Rockville, 1987, Aspen, Colo, pp 5-14.

124. Devor M, Rappaport HZ: Pain and pathophysiology of damaged nerve. In Fields HL, editor: Pain syndromes in neurology, Oxford, 1990, Butterworth Heinemann, pp 47-83.

125. Sunderland S: Nerve injuries and their repair. A critical appraisal, Edinburgh, 1991, Churchill Livingstone, pp 333-350.

126. Rydevik B, Brown MD, Lundborg G: Pathoanatomy and pathophysiology of nerve root compression, Spine 9(1):7-14, 1984.

127. Lundborg G, Myers R, Powell H: Nerve compression injury and increased endoneurial fluid pressure: a miniature compartment syndrome, J Neurol Neurosurg Psychiatry 46:1119-1124, 1983.

128. Jepsen JR, Thomsen G: A cross-sectional study of the relation between symptoms and physical findings in computer operators, BMC Neurol 6:40, 2006.

129. Walsh J, Hall T: Reliability and validity of nerve trunk palpation in subjects with low back related leg pain. In: Proceedings of the 9th International Federation of Manipulative Therapy Conference, Rotterdam, Holland, 2008.

130. Sterling M, Jull G, Carlsson Y et al: Are cervical physical outcome measures influenced by the presence of symptomatology? Physiother Res Int 7(3):113-121, 2002.

131. Walsh J, Hall T: Reliability, validity and diagnostic accuracy of palpation of the sciatic, tibial and common peroneal nerves in the examination of low back related leg pain. Man Ther doi:10.1016/j.math.2008.12.007, 2009.

132. Bove GM, Zaheen A, Bajwa ZH: Subjective nature of lower limb radicular pain, J Manipulative Physiol Ther 28(1):12-14, 2005.

133. Slipman CW, Plastaras CT, Palmitier RA, et al: Symptom provocation of fluoroscopically guided cervical nerve root stimulation. Are dynatomal maps identical to dermatomal maps? Spine 23(20):2235-2242, 1998.

134. Wolff AP, Groen GJ, Crul BJ: Diagnostic lumbosacral segmental nerve blocks with local anesthetics: a prospective double-blind study on the variability and interpretation of segmental effects, Reg Anesth Pain Med 26(2):147-155, 2001.

135. Inman VT, Saunders JBdM: Referred pain from skeletal structures, J Nerv Ment Dis 99:660-667, 1944.

136. Nitta H, Tajima T, Sugiyama H et al: Study on dermatomes by means of selective lumbar spinal nerve block, Spine 18(13):1782-1786, 1993.

137. Viikari-Juntura E: Interexaminer reliability of observations in physical examinations of the neck, Phys Ther 67(10):1526-1532, 1987.

138. Viikari-Juntura E, Porras M, Laasonen EM: Validity of clinical tests in the diagnosis of root compression in cervical disc disease, Spine 14(3):253-257, 1989.

139. Wainner RS, Fritz JM, Irrgang JJ, et al: Reliability and diagnostic accuracy of the clinical examination and patient self-report measures for cervical radiculopathy, Spine 28(1):52-62, 2003.

140. Wainner RS, Gill H: Diagnosis and nonoperative management of cervical radiculopathy, J Orthop Sports Phys Ther 30(12):728-744, 2000.

141. Vroomen PC, de Krom MC, Knottnerus JA: Consistency of history taking and physical examination in patients with suspected lumbar nerve root involvement, Spine 25(1):91-96; discussion 97, 2000.

142. Jepsen J, Laursen L, Hagert C, et al: Diagnostic accuracy of the neurological upper limb examination 1: interrater reproducibility of selected findings and patterns, BMC Neurol 6(8):1-11, 2006.

143. Jepsen J, Laursen L, Larsen A, et al: Manual strength testing in 14 upper limb muscles: a study of inter-rater reliability, Acta Orthop Scand 75(4):442-448, 2004.

144. Rainville J, Noto DJ, Jouve C, et al: Assessment of forearm pronation strength in C6 and C7 radiculopathies, Spine 32(1):72-75, 2007.

145. Litvan I, Mangone CA, Werden W, et al: Reliability of the NINDS Myotatic Reflex Scale, Neurology 47(4):969-972, 1996.

146. Stam J, van Crevel H: Reliability of the clinical and electromyographic examination of tendon reflexes, J Neurol 237(7):427-431, 1990.

147. Haldeman S: The electrodiagnostic evaluation of nerve root function, Spine 9(1):42-48, 1983.

148. Kim S, Choi JY, Huh YM, et al: Role of magnetic resonance imaging in entrapment and compressive neuropathy—what, where, and how to see the peripheral nerves on the musculoskeletal magnetic resonance image. I. Overview and lower extremity, Eur Radiol 17(1):139-149, 2007.

149. Lew HL, Chen CP, Wang TG, et al: Introduction to musculoskeletal diagnostic ultrasound: examination of the upper limb, Am J Phys Med Rehabil 86(4):310-321, 2007.

150. Schafer A, Hall T, Ludtke K, Mallwitz J, Briffa N, et al: Interrater Reliability of a new classification system for patients with neural low back-related leg pain. Journal of Manual & Manipulative Therapy 2009. (available on-line at http://jmmtonline.com/epub/#schafer#ixzz0D O2OeKRm&B).

151. Schafer A, Hall TM, Briffa K, et al: Classification of low back related leg pain: difference in treatment responses between diagnostic groups, Man Ther 2007 (in press).

152. Shacklock M: The normal response when the SLR is added to plantarflexion/inversion and the effect of passive neck flexion as support of a neural cause of symptoms. In Proceedings of the Manipulative Physiotherapists Association of Australia, Seventh Biennial Conference, New South Wales, Australia, 1991.

153. Sunderland S: The anatomy and physiology of nerve injury, Muscle Nerve 13:771-784, 1990.

154. Lundborg G, Rydevik B: Effects of stretching the tibial nerve of the rabbit: a preliminary study of the intraneural circulation and the barrier function of the perineurium, J Bone Joint Surg 55B(2):390-401, 1973.

155. Ogato K, Naito M: Blood flow of peripheral nerves: effects of dissection, stretching and compression, J Hand Surg [Am] 11:10, 1986.

156. Kwan MK, Wall EJ, Massie J, et al: Strain, stress and stretch of peripheral nerve: rabbit experiments in vitro and in vivo, Acta Orthop Scand 63(3):267-272, 1992.

157. Elvey R: Treatment of arm pain associated with abnormal brachial plexus tension, Aust J Physiother 32:225-230, 1986.

158. Allison GT, Nagy BM, Hall T: A randomized clinical trial of manual therapy for cervico-brachial pain syndrome—a pilot study, Man Ther 7(2):95-102, 2002.

159. Vicenzino B, Collins D, Wright A: Cervical mobilization: immediate effects on neural tissue mobility, mechanical hyperalgesia and pain free grip strength in lateral epicondylitis, Gold Coast, Australia, 1995, Manipulative Physiotherapists Association of Australia.

160. Cowell IM, Phillips DR: Effectiveness of manipulative physiotherapy for the treatment of a neurogenic cervico-brachial pain syndrome: a single case study—experimental design, Man Ther 7(1):31-38, 2002.

161. Saranga J, Green A, Lewis J, et al: Effects of a cervical lateral glide on the upper limb neurodynamic test 1: a blinded placebo-controlled investigation, Physiotherapy 89(11):678-684, 2003.

162. Coppieters MW, Bartholomeeusen KE, Stappaerts KH: Incorporating nerve-gliding techniques in the conservative treatment of cubital tunnel syndrome, J Manipulative Physiol Ther 27(9):560-568, 2004.

Manual Therapy Techniques for the Thoracolumbar Spine

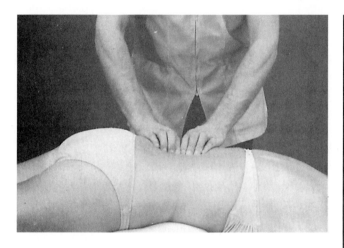

Figure A1-1 The patient is prone, with the lumbar spine in a neutral position. The therapist, with fingertips in a row lateral to the spinous process, uses a pulling motion to stretch the erector spinae muscle mass at right angles to the spine.

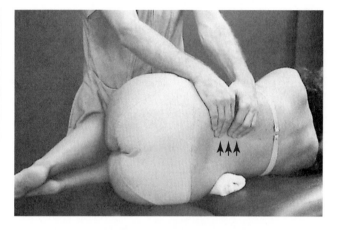

Figure A1-3 The therapist flexes the patient's knees and, with the thighs, pushes against the patient's knees, causing the lumbar spine to flex. With the erector spinae in some degree of stretch, the therapist pulls the erector spinae mass in a transverse direction. Altering pressure on the knees varies the tension on the erector spinae muscle.

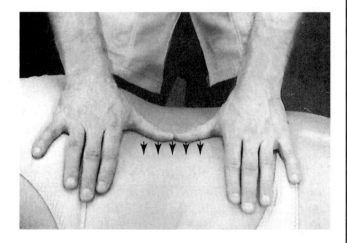

Figure A1-2 This technique uses the same principles as in Figure App 1-1. The therapist's thumbs push the opposite erector spinae laterally, at right angles to the spinous processes. A scooping motion of the thumb assists the lateral movement of the muscle.

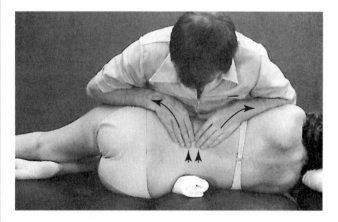

Figure A1-4 The therapist applies outward pressure with both forearms, causing the lumbar spine to arch and stretching the quadratus lumborum and erector spinae muscles. Arching is assisted by placing a roll under the patient's lumbar spine and flexing the patient's bottom hip, as well as by the therapist pulling up with the fingers on the erector spinae mass.

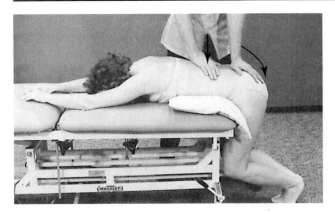

Figure A1-5 While increasing the flexion of the lumbar spine in the prone position, the therapist stabilizes the T12 and Ll segment and presses against the patient's sacrum. Further stretch may be achieved by the therapist pushing downward along the patient's thighs.

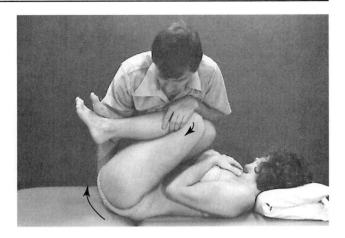

Figure A1-6 The therapist stretches the lumbar extensors by pressing on the patient's knees while simultaneously lifting the patient's sacrum. Further stretch may be achieved by pushing downward along the patient's thighs.

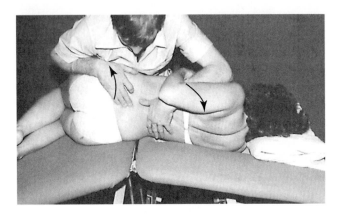

Figure A1-7 Technique to increase extension, left rotation, and right side bending. A cushion under the waist may be used to produce right side bending if the bed does not elevate in the middle. As the patient exhales, the therapist pushes the left shoulder and thorax posteriorly and cranially while pulling the left ilium forward and caudally.

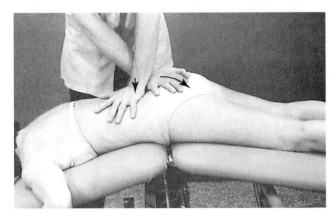

Figure A1-8 Technique to increase the flexion of L5 on S1. The middle of the couch is elevated. A roll may be placed under the abdomen. As the patient exhales, the therapist pushes the sacrum caudally and ventrally. This technique may be used for all the lumbar segments. The therapist's hypothenar eminence stabilizes the proximal lumbar segment.

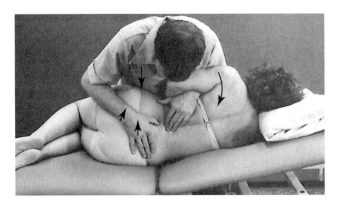

Figure A1-9 Technique to increase flexion and left rotation and side bending at the L2-L3 level. The pelvis may be stabilized with a belt. As the patient exhales, the therapist pushes the patient's left shoulder and thorax backward. The head of the bed is progressively elevated to side bend the lumbar spine to the left. Rotation may be enhanced by pulling the right arm and shoulder forward. The pelvis is stabilized between the therapist's chest and forearm, as well as by the therapist placing a hand over the sacrum. The patient's upper leg may be extended, and a roll may be put under the lower lumbar spine.

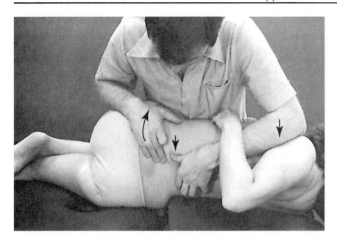

Figure A1-10 Technique to increase flexion and left rotation and side bending of L5 on S1. The upper lumbar spine is flexed and right side bent, causing right rotation, thus locking the upper-lumbar segments. If the midsection of the bed will not lift, use a roll. As the patient exhales, the therapist pulls the pelvis forward and cranially.

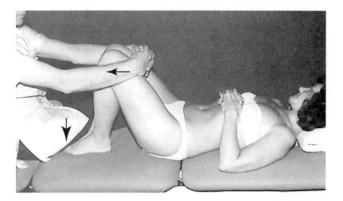

Figure A1-11 Surprisingly effective manual traction may be applied in crook lying through the patient's hips when the therapist leans back. The therapist's thighs fix the patient's feet. The angle of pull may be guided by the patient's response.

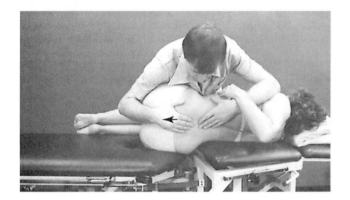

Figure A1-12 Specific distraction in lumbar flexion is facilitated by the use of a mobilization bed to side bend and by the use of accessories to assist with distraction. The patient's pelvis is stabilized by the therapist's shoulder, chest, forearm, and hand.

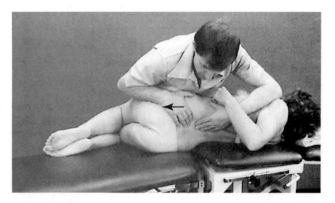

Figure A1-13 Specific distraction in lumbar extension. The patient's pelvis may also be stabilized with a belt. Side bending of the lumbar spine may be prevented by a pillow if the bed does not lift.

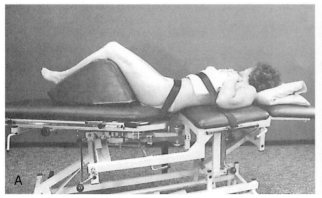

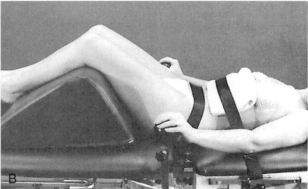

Figure A1-14 A-B, Different degrees of rotation and side bending may be incorporated to reduce discomfort. Traction may be applied by the therapist or the patient with the use of appropriate accessories.

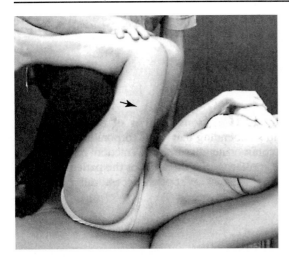

Figure A1-15 Treatment for a forward bending dysfunction of L1. Flexion of the thoracolumbar junction is assisted by lifting the end of the bed. Further flexion is produced by the therapist's knees against the back of the patient's thigh, with slight rotation of the patient's knee toward the side of tenderness. The position is one of marked flexion, rotation away, and side bending toward the restriction. The position is held and the tender spot monitored for 90 seconds.

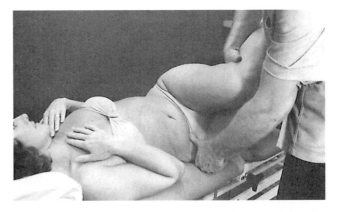

Figure A1-16 Treatment for abdominal L2 dysfunction. The hips are flexed, the pelvis is rotated to the right, and the patient's feet are lifted to the left to side bend the lumbar spine. Adductor strain can be reduced by slightly lifting behind the upper knee.

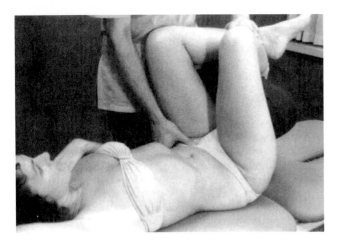

Figure A1-17 Treatment for iliacus dysfunction. A tender point is located in the iliac fossa. The hips are flexed, the ankles crossed, and the thighs externally rotated.

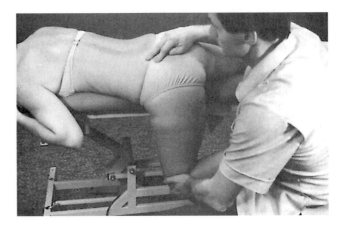

Figure A1-18 Treatment for L5 dysfunction. Approximately 20 degrees of pelvic rotation plus adduction of the thigh reduces the tender spot under the index finger. The third finger marks the posterior superior iliac spine.

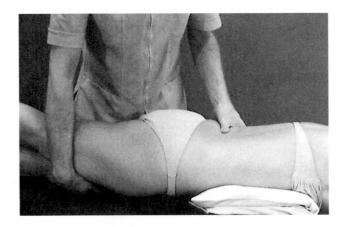

Figure A1-19 Treatment for L3, L4, and L5 dysfunctions. Adduction of the thigh is necessary at all levels. More rotation is needed for L3, whereas L5 requires more extension.

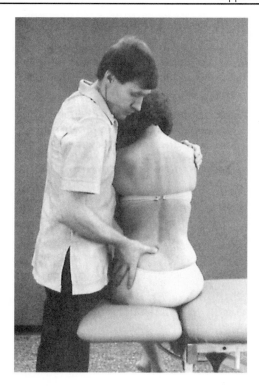

Figure A1-20 Starting position for a functional technique for lumbar dysfunction. The therapist palpates changes in tissue tension with the right thumb.

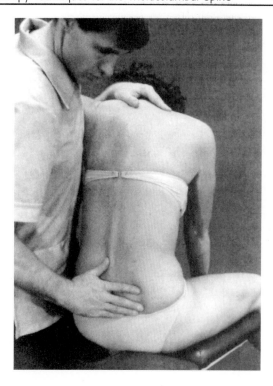

Figure A1-21 End position of a functional treatment technique. The point of greatest tissue relaxation determines the movement and position of the patient.

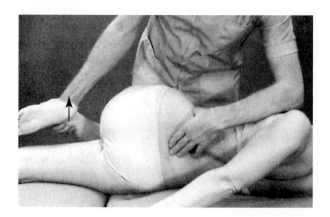

Figure A1-22 Technique for correcting an L5 that is flexed, rotated right, and side bent right (FRSR). The aim of treatment is to extend, rotate, and side bend left (ERSL). The patient resists lifting up of the left ankle. The patient may look over the left shoulder to reduce stress on the upper thoracic spine.

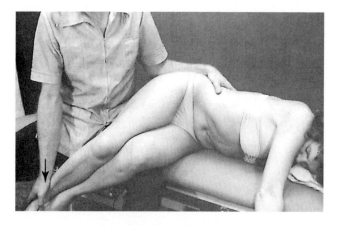

Figure A1-23 Technique for correcting an L5 that is extended, rotated right, and side bent right (ERSR). The aim of treatment is to flex, rotate, and side bend left (FRSL). The patient resists pushing down of both feet. The therapist protects the patient's left thigh from the edge of the bed by supporting it with his or her own left thigh.

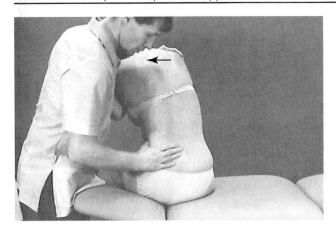

Figure A1-24 Technique for correcting an L4 that is extended, rotated right, and side bent right (ERSR) in a sitting position. The therapist flexes and rotates the patient to the segment involved; the patient resists side bending further to the left. The aim of treatment is to flex, rotate, and side bend left (FRSL) L4.

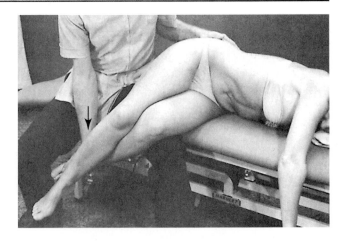

Figure A1-25 Technique for correcting a forward left sacral torsion (L/L). This is an often forgotten technique to restore full function of the L5-S1 segment. The aim of treatment is to restore symmetry and motion to the sacrum by reciprocally inhibiting the right piriformis by contracting the left. The patient resists pushing down with the left leg but allows the right leg to fall in the relaxation phase or to be gently stretched.

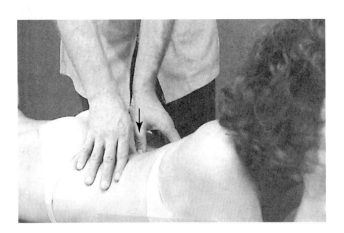

Figure A1-26 Specific posteroanterior central pressure to increase extension.

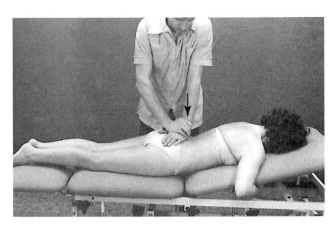

Figure A1-27 Specific extension mobilization with the pisiform. As mobility increases, the end of the bed may be elevated farther.

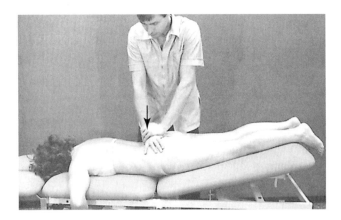

Figure A1-28 Specific extension mobilization with the pisiform as a contact. The caudal end of the bed is elevated as much as mobility allows.

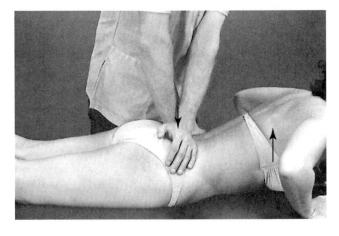

Figure A1-29 Specific stabilization over the transverse processes as the patient attempts extension.

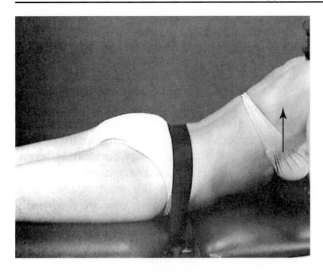

Figure A1-30 Specific stabilization using a belt as the patient attempts extension.

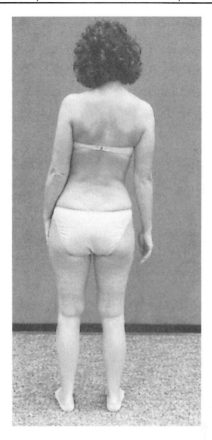

Figure A1-31 Typical presentation in which the lumbar spine is shifted slightly to the right.

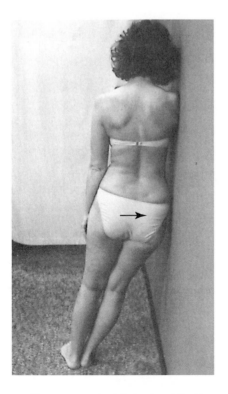

Figure A1-32 Self-correction of a right lumbar shift. Alternatively, the patient may stand in a doorway and let the pelvis sag to the right.

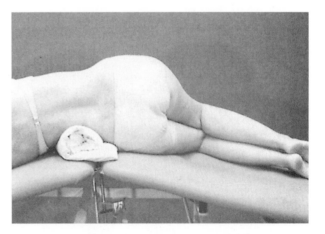

Figure A1-33 Positional traction in the side-lying position to correct a right lumbar shift to the left.

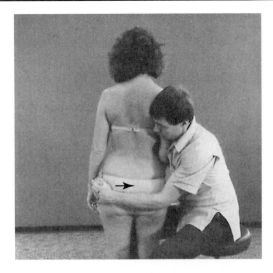

Figure A1-34 The therapist assists in correcting a right deviated spine. The therapist stabilizes with the shoulder while pulling on the patient's pelvis. A slow, constant pull is most beneficial. A slight overcorrection may be needed.

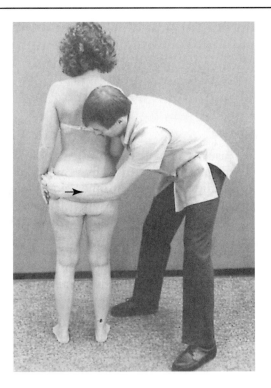

Figure A1-35 The therapist assists in correcting a right deviated lumbar spine. This technique is not recommended because it involves poor body mechanics by the therapist, and frequently the stabilization provided by the therapist's shoulder is too high.

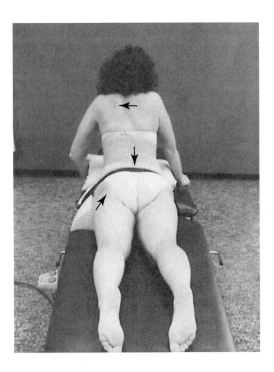

Figure A1-36 Correction of a right deviated lumbar spine in the prone position. The technique is assisted by belt stabilization, a foam wedge under the hip opposite the deviation, and extending to the left when pressing up. If a three-dimensional (3-D) mobilization bed is used instead, it may be adjusted accordingly.

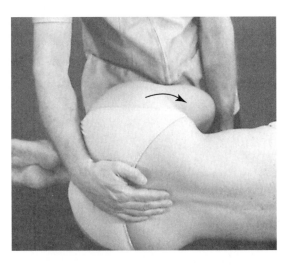

Figure A1-37 One of the basic positions for applying lumbar flexion. The patient's knees rest on the therapist's abdomen, and the therapist's left hand guides the knees into flexion as the therapist side bends or sways at the hips. The fingers of the therapist's right hand palpate the interspaces for movement.

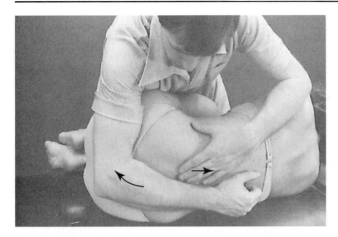

Figure A1-38 Very strong flexion is applied by a combination of full hip flexion and a strong pull with the therapist's right forearm against a firm pull by the therapist's left hand on a spinous process. Strain on the therapist's back is reduced by leaning on the patient's left hip, which assists in stabilization. The therapist must adopt a wide stance.

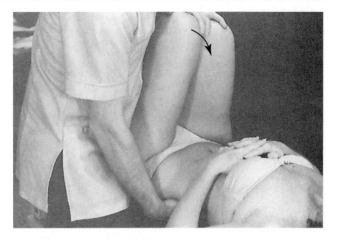

Figure A1-39 Suitable techniques for thin subjects. The therapist flexes the patient's hips with the left hand. The therapist's right hand may palpate the intraspinous process or stabilize the spinous process.

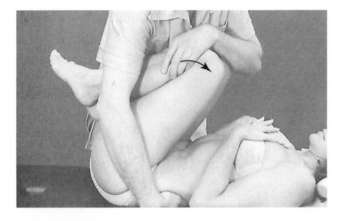

Figure A1-40 Fairly forceful flexion may be applied by the therapist leaning on the patient's knees. The therapist guides with the left hand and palpates or stabilizes with the right hand.

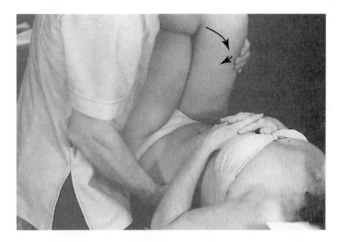

Figure A1-41 Crossing the patient's knees induces slight side bending; the therapist's left hand adds flexion. The right hand palpates or stabilizes the spinous process.

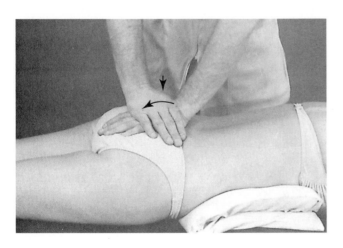

Figure A1-42 The therapist applies firm ventral pressure over the sacrum and then applies a rocking motion caudally to flex the lumbosacral joint. A pillow under the patient's abdomen is recommended.

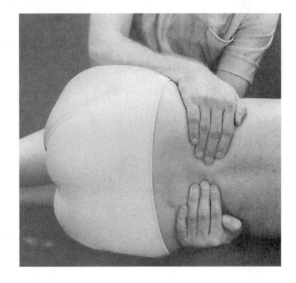

Figure A1-43 The patient's knees are pushed toward the pelvis as the therapist pulls ventrally on the lumbar segment, causing extension.

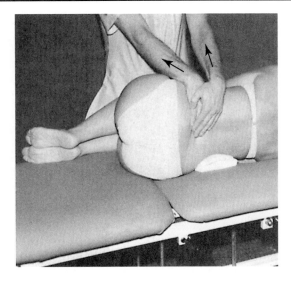

Figure A1-44 An alternative method for extending the lumbar spine.

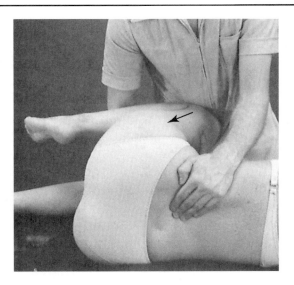

Figure A1-45 The therapist flexes the patient's left hip to approximately a right angle and supports the patient's knee with the abdomen and right forearm. The therapist pushes along the patient's thigh, pushing the left side of the pelvis back and causing extension and left rotation of the lumbar vertebrae. Stabilization can be provided by placing the thumb against the side of the spinous process, or the fingers may palpate for mobility.

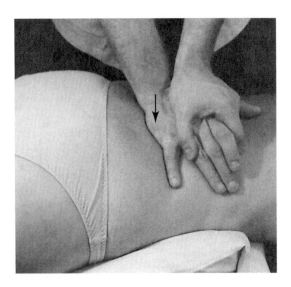

Figure A1-46 Specific extension over the spinous process with the pisiform bone of one hand, reinforced by the other hand. The therapist's arms are straight. Note the quality and quantity of movement of each lumbar segment.

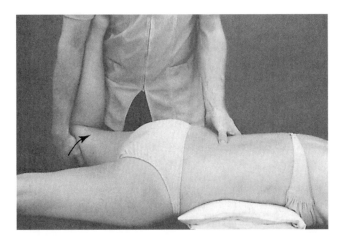

Figure A1-47 Specific technique to assess or increase left side bending of the lumbar segment with the patient prone. The therapist's thumb palpates the lateral aspect of the interspinous space. Lumbar spine extension may be increased without the use of a pillow. The therapist steadies the patient's leg and knee with a firm grip while abducting the patient's hip beyond its physiologic barrier.

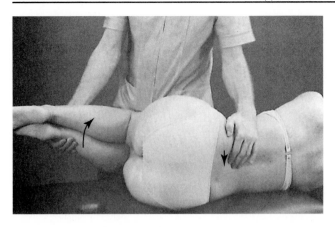

Figure A1-48 Specific technique to assess or increase left side bending in the side-lying position. The patient's knees are supported by the therapist's abdomen or groin. The therapist palpates the lateral aspect of the interspinous space while lifting up on the patient's leg above the ankle.

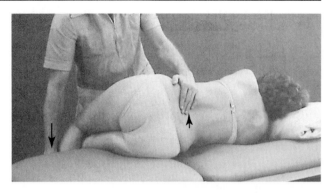

Figure A1-49 Specific technique to assess or increase right side bending. While pushing down on the patient's legs, the therapist palpates for interspinous movement or stabilizes the lateral aspect of the spinous process. The reader should note the degree of side bending that can be produced by increased downward movement of the patient's legs. The edge of the bed on the patient's lower thigh may be uncomfortable.

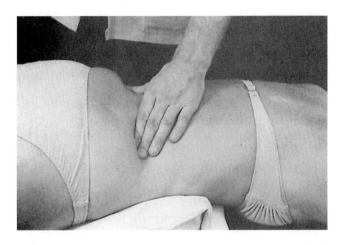

Figure A1-50 Basic hand position used to apply side-to-side rocking of a lumbar segment. The thumb and index finger are over the transverse process of the vertebrae.

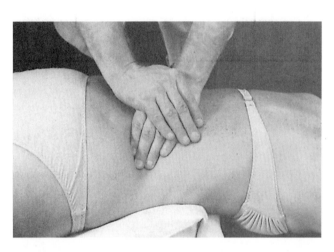

Figure A1-51 With support from the other hand, the therapist rocks the lumbar segment from side to side. Pressure is applied to attempt a lateral shift motion rather than side bending.

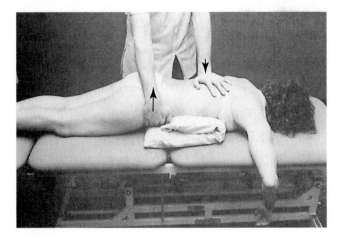

Figure A1-52 Nonspecific technique to increase left rotation of the lumbar spine. A pillow may be used to reduce lumbar extension. The therapist fixes the thoracolumbar junction and lifts with a comfortable but firm grip of the ilium over the anterior superior iliac spine.

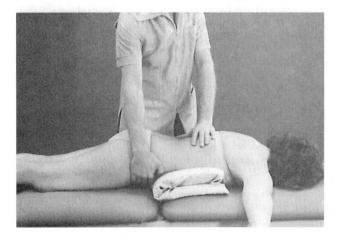

Figure A1-53 Specific technique to increase or assess left rotation of a lumbar segment. The therapist stabilizes the cranial vertebrae by applying pressure against the lateral aspect of the spinous process and lifts with a comfortable grip over the anterior superior iliac spine.

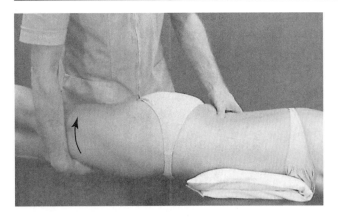

Figure A1-54 Minimal effort is required to lift the patient's crossed right thigh with the right forearm, causing rotation of the pelvis to the right. The therapist's right hand grasps the patient's anterior left thigh. The patient's thighs are stabilized at the edge of the bed by the therapist's right thigh.

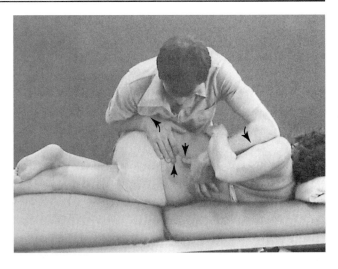

Figure A1-55 Probably the most common basic position for treating a rotation restriction of the lumbar spine. The patient's left knee is flexed until movement is palpated at a specific lumbar level. The patient's right shoulder is then pulled forward, and the left shoulder is rotated backward to lock the thoracolumbar spine at the desired level. This is further assisted by pressure of the left thumb on the lateral aspect of the cranial spinous process. Gapping of the left apophyseal joint is accomplished by (1) simultaneous opposing thrusts of the therapist's left and right forearms, (2) the therapist pulling forward with the right hand, and (3) the therapist lifting up with the index or middle finger of the right hand on the underside of the caudal spinous process.

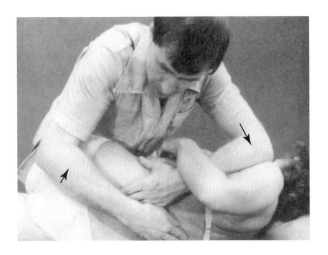

Figure A1-56 A variation of a nonspecific basic position in which the therapist uses the inner aspect of the forearm against the posterior ilium, allowing for more extension. The therapist palpates with the fingers of the left hand and stabilizes the patient's left shoulder with the left forearm.

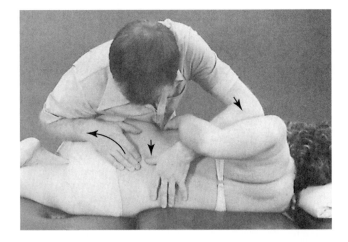

Figure A1-57 A variation of a specific position in which the patient's left shoulder and cranial lumbar segment are stabilized by the therapist's left thumb. The fingers of the therapist's right hand pull up on the underside of the spinous process. The patient's left knee lies over the edge of the table, with the left foot hooked comfortably behind the right knee. If the edge of the midsection of the bed does not lift up, a cushion may be placed under the patient's side. Additional distraction may be applied by the therapist's right hand and forearm.

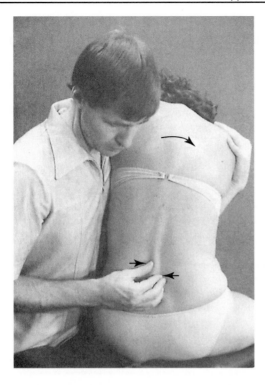

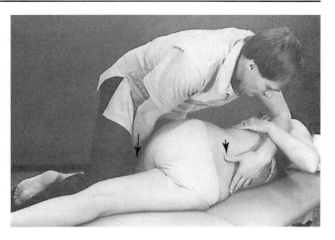

Figure A1-58 The therapist's left arm is placed under the patient's folded arms, and the therapist reaches across the patient's chest while firmly holding the right shoulder. The patient leans forward as the therapist rotates the patient to the left. The therapist assists the rotation with the right thumb pushing on the lateral aspect of the spinous process while stabilizing the caudal spinous process with the second finger, reinforced by the third. Alternatively, the therapist may resist rotation of the caudal spinous process by stabilizing with the thumb instead of the fingers.

Figure A1-59 Specific technique to gap the left lumbosacral facet joint. With the patient lying close to the edge of the bed, the left knee is flexed and allowed to hang over the edge of the bed. If the patient cannot comfortably keep the left foot behind the right knee, the therapist can place his or her own flexed right knee on the bed, allowing the patient's left ankle to rest on the posterior aspect of the therapist's right leg. The therapist places the thumb and index finger on either side of the patient's left knee, with the popliteal space covered by the web of the hand. The therapist's right forearm is along the posterior aspect of the patient's left thigh. Leaning well forward, the therapist thrusts through the popliteal space. Stabilization of L5 is provided by the therapist's left forearm and thumb, which are on the lateral aspect of the spinous process of L5. Because a wide range of angles exist for the lumbosacral facets, the degree of left hip flexion will vary to accommodate the sagittal or more coronal joint plane.

Table A1-1 Relative Contraindications to Manipulation

Condition	References	Condition	References
Articular Derangements		Paget's disease	Sandoz & Lorenz[3]
Ankylosing spondylitis after the acute stage	Bollier[1]		Nwuga[14]
	Rinsky et al.[2]		Lindner[15]
	Sandoz and Lorenz[3]	Scheuermann's disease	Beyeler[16]
	Stoddard[4]		Hauberg[17]
Articular deformity	Cyriax[5]		Janse[8]
Basilar impression	Kaiser[6]		Maigne[9]
Congenital anomalies	Grillo[7]		Nwuga[14]
	Janse[8]	Spondylolisthesis, spondylolysis	Hauberg[17]
	Maigne[9]		Sandoz and Lorenz[3]
	Sandoz[10]		
	Valentini[11]	**Disc Lesion**	
	Yochum[12]	Posterolateral and posteromedial disc protrusions	
Hypertrophic spondyloarthritis		Degenerative disease	Jaquet[18]
Osteoarthritis	Sandoz and Lorenz[3]		Odom[19]
Osteochondrosis with defective "holding apparatus"	Stoddard[4]		Stoddard[4]
		Neurologic Dysfunction	
Bone Weakening and Modifying Disease		Myelopathy	Cyriax[5]
Hemangioma	Siehl[13]		Stoddard[4]

Continued

Table A1-1   Relative Contraindications to Manipulation—cont'd

Condition	References	Condition	References
Dysfunction of nonvertebral origin	Nwuga[14] Stoddard[4]	Pregnancy	Cyriax[5] Nwuga[14] Sandoz and Lorenz[3]
Pyramidal tract involvement	Cyriax[5]		
Radicular pain from disc lesion	Gutmann[20] Stoddard[4]	Scoliosis	Stoddard[4]
Viscerosomatic reflex pain	Gutmann[20] Nwuga[14] Stoddard[4]	**Lumbar Spine**	
		Accessory sacroiliac joints	
Unclassified		Baastrup's disease	Maigne[9] Grillo[7]
Abdominal hernia	Sandoz and Lorenz[3]	Cleft vertebra in the sagittal plane	Grillo[7]
Asthma	Beyeler[16] Sandoz[21]	Facet tropism	Grillo[7] Janse[8]
Basilar ischemia	Bourdillon[22] Cyriax[5] Nwuga[14]	Knife clasp syndrome	
		Nuclear impression	Grillo[7]
		Pseudosacralization	Grillo[7] Janse[8]
Dysmenorrhea	Sandoz[21]	Sacralization, lumbarization	Grillo[7] Janse[8]
Epicondylitis	Droz[23]		
Postspinal operations	Nwuga[14]	Spina bifida occulta	Janse[8]
Peptic ulcer	Janse[8]	Spondylolisthesis	Janse[8]

Modified from Haldeman S: Modern developments in the principles and practice of chiropractic, East Norwalk, Conn, 1980, Appleton Century Crofts.

Table A1-2   Contraindications for Manipulation

Condition	References	Condition	References
Articular Derangements		Hypermobility	Gutmann[20] Kaltenborn[27] Maitland[24] Stoddard[4] Grieve[26] Haldeman[25]
Arthritides			
Acute arthritis of any type	Hauberg[17] Janse[8] Maigne[9] Maitland[24] Stoddard[4] Yochum[12] Haldeman[25] Grieve[26]		
		Bone Weakening and Destructive Disease	
		Calvé's disease	Lindner[15]
Rheumatoid arthritis	Bourdillon[22] Janse[8] Maigne[9] Stoddard[4] Yochum[12] Grieve[26] Haldeman[25]	Fracture	Gutmann[20] Heilig[28] Maigne[9] Nwuga[14] Rinsky et al.[2] Siehl[13] Stoddard[4] Haldeman[25]
Acute ankylosing spondylitis	Bollier[1] Droz[23] Hauberg[17] Janse[8] Nwuga[14] Stoddard[4] Haldeman[25] Grieve[26]	Malignancy (primary or secondary)	Bourdillon[22] Gutmann[20] Maigne[9] Maitland[24] Nwuga[14] Timbrell-Fisher[29] Stoddard[4] Grieve[26] Haldeman[25]

Table A1-2 **Contraindications for Manipulation—cont'd**

Condition	References	Condition	References
Osteomalacia	Lindner[15]	**Disk Lesions**	
Osteoporosis	Bollier[1]	Prolapse with serious neurologic changes (including cauda equina syndrome)	Bourdillon[22]
	Bourdillon[22]		Cyriax[5]
	Maigne[9]		Hooper[30]
	Nwuga[14]		Jaquet[18]
	Siehl[13]		Jennett[31]
	Stoddard[4]		Nwuga[14]
	Grieve[26]		Odom[19]
	Haldeman[25]		Stoddard[4]
Osteomyelitis	Hauberg[17]		Haldeman[25]
	Nwuga[14]		Grieve[26]
	Sandoz and Lorenz[3]		
	Stoddard[4]	**Neurologic Dysfunction**	
Tuberculosis (Pott's disease)	Bourdillon[22]	Micturition with sacral root involvement	Cyriax[5]
	Hauberg[17]		Stoddard[4]
	Maigne[9]		Haldeman[25]
	Siehl[13]		Grieve[26]
	Stoddard[4]	Painful movement in all directions	Maigne[9]
	Timbrell-Fisher[29]	**Unclassified**	
		Infectious disease	Maigne[9]
			Nwuga[14]
		Patient intolerance	Maigne[9]
			Lescure[32]

Modified from Haldeman S, editor: Modern developments in the principles and practice of chiropractic, East Norwalk, Conn, 1980, Appleton Century Crofts.

REFERENCES

1. Bollier W: Inflammatory infections and neoplastic disease of the lumbar spine, Ann Swiss Chiropract Assoc 1960.

2. Rinsky LA, Reynolds GG, Jameson RM, et al: Cervical spine cord injury after chiropractic adjustment, Paraplegia 13:233, 1976.

3. Sandoz R, Lorenz E: Presentation of an original lumbar technique, Ann Swiss Chiropract Assoc 1:43, 1960.

4. Stoddard A: Manual of osteopathic practice, London, 1969, Hutchinson of London.

5. Cyriax J: Textbook of orthopaedic medicine, ed 8, vol 2, London, 1971, Bailliere Tindall.

6. Kaiser G: Orthopaedics and traumatology (translated from the German), Beitr Orthop 20:581, 1973.

7. Grillo G: Anomalies of the lumbar spine, Ann Swiss Chiropract Assoc 1:56, 1960.

8. Janse J: Principles and practice of chiropractic: an anthology. In Hildebrandt R, editor: National College of Chiropractic, Lombard, Ill, 1976.

9. Maigne R: Orthopaedic medicine: a new approach to vertebral manipulations (translated by WT Liberson), Springfield, Ill, 1972, Charles C Thomas.

10. Sandoz R: Newer trends in the pathogenesis of spinal disorders, Ann Swiss Chiropract Assoc 5, 1971.

11. Valentini E: The occipito cervical region, Ann Swiss Chiropract Assoc 4:225, 1969.

12. Yochum TR: Radiology of the Arthritides (lecture notes), Melbourne, 1978, Int Coll Chiro.

13. Siehl D: Manipulation of the spine under anaesthesia. In 1967 Yearbook, Academy of Applied Osteopathy, Carmel, Calif, 1967.

14. Nwuga V: Manipulation of the spine, Baltimore, 1976, Lippincott, Williams & Wilkins.

15. Lindner H: A synopsis of the dystrophies of the lumbar spine, Ann Swiss Chiropract Assoc 1:143, 1960.

16. Beyeler W: Scheuermann's disease and its chiropractic management, Ann Swiss Chiropract Assoc 1:170, 1960.

17. Hauberg GV: Contraindications of the manual therapy of the spine (translated from the German), Hippokrates, Stuttgart, 1967.

18. Jaquet P: Clinical chiropractic: a study of cases, Geneva, 1978, Chrounauer.

19. Odom GL: Neck ache and back ache. In Proceedings of the NINCDS Conference on Neck Ache and Back Ache, Charles C Thomas, Springfield, Ill, 1970.

20. Gutmann G: Chirotherapie, Grundlagen, Indikationen, Genenindikationen and objektivier, Barkeit Med Welf Bd 1978.

21. Sandoz R: About some problems pertaining to the choice of indications for chiropractic therapy, Ann Swiss Chiropract Assoc 3:201, 1965.

22. Bourdillon JF: Spinal manipulation, London, 1973, W Heinemann.

23. Droz JM: Indications and contraindications of vertebral manipulations, Ann Swiss Chiropract Assoc 5:81, 1971.

24. Maitland GD: Vertebral manipulation, ed 4, London, 1977, Butterworth-Heinemann.

25. Haldeman S: Spinal manipulative therapy in the management of low back pain. In Finneson BE, editor: Low back pain, ed 2, Philadelphia, 1981, JB Lippincott.

26. Grieve GP: Mobilization of the spine, ed 3, Edinburgh, 1979, Churchill Livingstone.

27. Kaltenborn FM: Mobilization of the extremity joints, Oslo, 1980, Olaf Norlis Bokhandel.

28. Heilig D: Whiplash mechanics of injury: management of cervical and dorsal involvement. In 1965 Yearbook, Academy of Applied Osteopathy, Carmel, Calif, 1965.

29. Timbrell Fisher AG: Treatment by manipulation, London, 1948, HK Lewis,

30. Hooper J: Low back pain and manipulation paraparesis after treatment of low back pain by physical methods, Med J Aust 1:549, 1973.

31. Jennett WB: A study of 25 cases of compression of the cauda equina by prolapsed IVD, J Neurol Neurosurg Psychiatry 8:19, 1956.

32. Lescure R: Incidents, accidents, contreindications des manipulations de la colonne vertebrae, (translated from the French), Med Hyg 12:456, 1954.

Index

Page numbers followed by f indicate figures; t, tables; b, boxes.